Practical Cardiac Electrophysiology

Practical Cardiac Electrophysiology

Editors

Kartikeya Bhargava
MD DNB FACC FISHNE FHRS
Senior Consultant Cardiology
Division of Cardiac Electrophysiology and Pacing
Medanta Heart Institute
Medanta-The Medicity
Gurgaon, Delhi-NCR, Haryana, India

Samuel J Asirvatham
MD FACC FHRS
Consultant, Division of Cardiovascular Diseases and Internal Medicine
Division of Pediatric Cardiology and
Department of Physiology and Biomedical Engineering
Professor of Medicine and Pediatrics
Mayo Clinic College of Medicine
Program Director, EP Fellowship Program
Mayo Clinic, Rochester, MN, USA

Forewords

George Klein
Eric N Prystowsky

JAYPEE The Health Sciences Publisher

New Delhi | London | Philadelphia | Panama

Jaypee Brothers Medical Publishers (P) Ltd.

Headquarters

Jaypee Brothers Medical Publishers (P) Ltd.
4838/24, Ansari Road, Daryaganj
New Delhi 110 002, India
Phone: +91-11-43574357
Fax: +91-11-43574314
E-mail: jaypee@jaypeebrothers.com

Overseas Offices

J.P. Medical Ltd.
83, Victoria Street, London
SW1H 0HW (UK)
Phone: +44-20 3170 8910
Fax: +44(0) 20 3008 6180
E-mail: info@jpmedpub.com

Jaypee-Highlights Medical Publishers Inc.
City of Knowledge, Building 235, 2nd floor
Clayton, Panama City, Panama
Phone: +1 507-301-0496
Fax: +1 507-301-0499
E-mail: cservice@jphmedical.com

Jaypee Medical Inc.
325, Chestnut Street
Suite 412, Philadelphia, PA 19106
USA
Phone: +1 267-519-9789
E-mail: support@jpmedus.com

Jaypee Brothers Medical Publishers (P) Ltd.
17/1-B, Babar Road, Block-B
Shaymali, Mohammadpur
Dhaka-1207, Bangladesh
Mobile: +08801912003485
E-mail: jaypeedhaka@gmail.com

Jaypee Brothers Medical Publishers (P) Ltd.
Bhotahity, Kathmandu, Nepal
Phone: +977-9741283608
E-mail: kathmandu@jaypeebrothers.com

Website: www.jaypeebrothers.com
Website: www.jaypeedigital.com

Inquiries for bulk sales may be solicited at: jaypee@jaypeebrothers.com

Practical Cardiac Electrophysiology

First Edition: **2017**

ISBN: 978-93-86056-79-5

Printed at: Ajanta Offset & Packagings Ltd., Faridabad, Haryana

Dedicated to

My mother, Dr Satya Bhargava, a classical singer and an author in the field of music, a true example of dedication and determination, for being a constant source of inspiration; my wife, Rekha Bhargava, for her patience and unconditional support and my lovely daughters, Devpriya and Shivpriya, for allowing me to devote time that should have been rightfully theirs.

—Kartikeya Bhargava

My mother-in-law, Kamala Aravamudan (née Ramanujam), a wonderful person whose nature is to be kind and pleasant yet has the strength and persistence to say and do what may be difficult but needed for the betterment of those around her.

—Samuel J Asirvatham

Contributors

SP Abhilash MD DNB DM
Assistant Professor
Department of Cardiology
Sree Chitra Tirunal Institute for Medical Sciences and Technology
Thiruvananthapuram, Kerala, India

Arnon Adler MD
Department of Cardiology
Tel Aviv Sourasky Medical Center and Sackler School of Medicine
Tel Aviv University
Tel Aviv, Israel

Masood Akhtar
MD FACC FACP FAHA MACP FHRS
Clinical Adjunct Professor of Medicine
University of Wisconsin School of Medicine and Public Health
Director, Electrophysiology Research and Cardiovascular Continuing Medical Education Program
Aurora Cardiovascular Services
Aurora Sinai/Aurora St. Luke's Medical Centers
Milwaukee, WI, USA

Noora Al-Jefairi MD
IHU LIRYC, Electrophysiology and Heart Modeling Institute
Foundation Bordeaux Université
Bordeaux University Hospital (CHU)
Cardiac Electrophysiology and Cardiac Stimulation Team
Pessac, France

Sana Amraoui MD
IHU LIRYC, Electrophysiology and Heart Modeling Institute
Foundation Bordeaux Université
Bordeaux University Hospital (CHU)
Cardiac Electrophysiology and Cardiac Stimulation Team
Pessac, France

Charles Antzelevitch
PhD FACC FHRS FAHA
Professor and Executive Director
Cardiovascular Research Program
Lankenau Institute for Medical Research
Wynnewood, PA, USA

Rishi Arora MD
Associate Professor
Department of Medicine
Director, Experimental Cardiac Electrophysiology
Northwestern University Feinberg School of Medicine
Chicago, IL, USA

Samuel J Asirvatham MD FACC FHRS
Consultant, Division of Cardiovascular Diseases and Internal Medicine
Division of Pediatric Cardiology and Department of Physiology and Biomedical Engineering
Professor of Medicine and Pediatrics
Mayo Clinic College of Medicine
Program Director, EP Fellowship Program
Mayo Clinic
Rochester, MN, USA

Moustapha Atoui MD
Department of Cardiology
University of Kansas Medical Center
Kansas City, KS, USA

Nitish Badhwar MD
Professor, Department of Medicine
Section of Cardiac Electrophysiology
Division of Cardiology
University of California
San Francisco, CA, USA

Benjamin Berte MD
IHU LIRYC, Electrophysiology and Heart Modeling Institute
Foundation Bordeaux Université
Bordeaux University Hospital (CHU)
Cardiac Electrophysiology and Cardiac Stimulation Team
Pessac, France

Kartikeya Bhargava
MD DNB FACC FISHNE FHRS
Senior Consultant Cardiology
Division of Cardiac Electrophysiology and Pacing
Medanta Heart Institute
Medanta-The Medicity
Gurgaon, Delhi-NCR, Haryana, India

Zalmen Blanck MD FHRS
Staff Electrophysiologist
South Texas Medical Center
Cardiology Clinic of San Antonio
San Antonio, TX, USA

Shomu Bohora MD DM
Associate Professor, Cardiology
UN Mehta Institute of Cardiology and Research Center
Ahmedabad, Gujarat
Consultant Electrophysiologist and Device Specialist
Vadodara, Gujarat, India

Noel G Boyle MD PhD
Professor of Medicine
UCLA Cardiac Arrhythmia Center
UCLA Health System
University of California
Los Angeles, CA, USA

José Angel Cabrera MD PhD
Professor of Cardiology and Chairman
Department of Cardiology
Hospital Quirón-Madrid
European University of Madrid
Madrid, Spain

Ivan Cakulev MD
Assistant Professor
Department of Medicine
Case Western Reserve University
University Hospitals Case Medical Center
Cleveland, OH, USA

Hugh Calkins MD
Nicholas J Fortuin MD Professor of Cardiology
Director, Cardiac Arrhythmia Services
Electrophysiology Laboratory and John Hopkins ARVD/C Program
Division of Cardiology
John Hopkins University
Baltimore, MD, USA

David Callans MD
Professor
Department of Medicine
University of Pennsylvania
Philadelphia, PA, USA

Bryan Cannon MD
Associate Professor
Department of Pediatrics
Mayo Clinic
Rochester, MN, USA

Riccardo Cappato MD FHRS
Chief
Arrhythmia and Electrophysiology Research Center
Humanitas Clinical and Research Center
Rozzano (Milan), Italy

Sergio Castrejón MD
Department of Cardiology
Hospital Quirón-Madrid
European University of Madrid
Madrid, Spain

Peter Cheung MD FACC FHRS
Assistant Professor of Medicine
Texas A & M University Health Science Center
Section of Cardiac Electrophysiology and Pacing
Division of Cardiology
Baylor Scott and White Health
Temple, TX, USA

Tahmeed Contractor MD
Assistant Professor of Medicine
Clinical Cardiac Electrophysiology
Division of Cardiology
Loma Linda University Medical Center
Loma Linda, CA, USA

Ralph J Damiano Jr MD
Evarts A Graham Professor of Surgery
Chief, Division of Cardiothoracic Surgery
Co-Chairman, Heart and Vascular Center
Washington University School of Medicine
St. Louis, MO, USA

Mithilesh K Das MD MRCP FACP
Professor of Medicine
Krannert Institute of Cardiology
Indiana University School of Medicine
Indiana University Health
Indianapolis, IN, USA

Freddy Del-Carpio Munoz MD MSc FACC FHRS
Consultant
Division of Cardiovascular Diseases
Assistant Professor of Medicine
Mayo Clinic College of Medicine
Mayo Clinic, Rochester, MN, USA

Arnaud Denis MD
IHU LIRYC, Electrophysiology and Heart Modeling Institute
Foundation Bordeaux Université
Bordeaux University Hospital (CHU)
Cardiac Electrophysiology and Cardiac Stimulation Team
Pessac, France

Nicolas Derval MD
IHU LIRYC, Electrophysiology and Heart Modeling Institute
Foundation Bordeaux Université
Bordeaux University Hospital (CHU)
Cardiac Electrophysiology and Cardiac Stimulation Team
Pessac, France

Abhishek Deshmukh MD
Division of Cardiology
Mayo Clinic
Rochester, MN, USA

Anwer Dhala MD FACC FHRS
Clinical Adjunct Associate Professor of Medicine
Cardiovascular Disease Section
Department of Medicine
University of Wisconsin School of Medicine and Public Health
Aurora Cardiovascular Services
Aurora Sinai/Aurora St. Luke's Medical Centers
Milwaukee, WI, USA

Sanjay Dixit MD
Associate Professor of Medicine
University of Pennsylvania School of Medicine
Director, Cardiac Electrophysiology
Philadelphia VA Medical Center
Philadelphia, PA, USA

Katherine Duello MD
Division of Cardiovascular Diseases
Mayo Clinic
Jacksonville, FL, USA

Paul Friedman MD FHRS
Professor of Medicine
Vice-Chair, Cardiovascular Medicine
Vice-Chair for Academic Affairs and Faculty Development
Medical Director, Remote Monitoring
Division of Cardiology
Mayo Clinic
Rochester, MN, USA

Antonio Frontera MD
IHU LIRYC, Electrophysiology and Heart Modeling Institute
Foundation Bordeaux Université
Bordeaux University Hospital (CHU)
Cardiac Electrophysiology and Cardiac Stimulation Team
Pessac, France

Edward P Gerstenfeld MD
Chief, Section of Cardiac Electrophysiology
Melvin Scheinman Professor of Medicine
University of California
San Francisco, CA, USA

Sampath Gunda MD MHA
Assistant Professor of Medicine
Cardiology Hospitalist
Virginia Commonwealth University
Richmond, VA, USA

Michel Haissaguerre MD
Chief, Department of Cardiac Electrophysiology
IHU LIRYC, Electrophysiology and Heart Modeling Institute
Foundation Bordeaux Université
Univ. Bordeaux, Centre de recherche Cardio-Thoracique de Bordeaux
Bordeaux University Hospital (CHU)
Cardiac Electrophysiology and Cardiac Stimulation Team
Pessac, France

Haris M Haqqani MBBS(Hons) PhD
Senior Lecturer and Electrophysiologist
School of Medicine
University of Queensland
Department of Cardiology
The Prince Charles Hospital
Brisbane, Queensland, Australia

Matthew C Henn MD MS
Division of Cardiothoracic Surgery
Washington University School of Medicine
St. Louis, MO, USA

Mélèze Hocini MD PhD
Professor
LIRYC institute, Hopital du Haut-Lévèque et University de Bordeaux, Pessac, France

Darren Hooks MD MBChB FRACP
IHU LIRYC, Electrophysiology and Heart Modeling Institute
Foundation Bordeaux Université
Bordeaux University Hospital (CHU)
Cardiac Electrophysiology and Cardiac Stimulation Team
Pessac, France

Shoei K Stephen Huang
MD FACC FAHA FHRS
Chair Professor of Medicine
Tzu Chi University School of Medicine
Hualien, Taiwan
Former Professor of Medicine with Tenure
Texas A&M University School of Medicine
Temple, TX, USA

Rahul Jain MD MPH FHRS
Assistant Professor
Indiana University School of Medicine
Department of Medicine
Krannert Institute of Cardiology
Indianapolis, IN, USA

Pierre Jais MD
CHU Bordeaux
Université de Bordeaux
LIRYC, Bordeaux, France

Aravdeep S Jhand MD
Sparrow Thoracic and Cardiovascular
Institute, Michigan State University
Lansing, MI, USA

Mark E Josephson MD
Chief, Division of Cardiovascular Medicine
Beth Israel Deaconess Medical Center
Herman Dana Professor of Medicine
Harvard Medical School
Director, Harvard-Thorndike
Electrophysiology Institute and
Arrhythmia Service
Boston, MA, USA

Jonathan M Kalman MBBS PhD
Department of Cardiology and Medicine
The Royal Melbourne Hospital
University of Melbourne
Parkville, Victoria, Australia

Vikas Kalra MBBS
Indiana University School of Medicine
Krannert Institute of Cardiology
Indianapolis, IN, USA

Demosthenes G Katritsis
MD PhD FRCP
Director, Department of Cardiology
Athens Euroclinic
Athens, Greece
Lecturer, Department of Medicine
Division of Cardiology
Beth Israel Deaconess Medical Center
Harvard Medical School
Boston, MA, USA

Bradley P Knight MD FACC FHRS
Director, Cardiac Electrophysiology
Bluhm Cardiovascular Institute of
Northwestern University, Chicago
Professor, Department of Medicine
Feinberg School of Medicine
Northwestern University
Chicago, IL, USA

Karl-Heinz Kuck PhD MD
Professor and Head
Department of Cardiology
Asklepios Klinik St. Georg
Hamburg, Germany

Dhanunjaya Lakkireddy
MD FACC FHRS
Professor of Medicine
Director, Center for Excellence in AF and
Complex Arrhythmias
University of Kansas Medical Center
Kansas City, KS, USA

Dennis H Lau MBBS PhD
Robert J Craig Lecturer
Centre for Heart Rhythm Disorders (CHRD)
South Australian Health and
Medical Research Institute (SAHMRI)
University of Adelaide and
Royal Adelaide Hospital
Adelaide, Australia

Adam Lee MBBS BSc(Hons) Mmed
Department of Cardiology
The Prince Charles Hospital
Brisbane, Queensland, Australia

Jianqing Li MD
Division of Cardiology
Winthrop University Hospital
Mineola, NY, USA

Jackson J Liang DO
University of Pennsylvania
Philadelphia, PA, USA

Watchara Lohawijarn MD
Sparrow Thoracic and
Cardiovascular Institute
Michigan State University
Lansing, MI, USA

Gerard Loughlin MD
Department of Cardiology
Hospital General Universitario
Gregorio Marañon
Madrid, Spain

Rajiv Mahajan MD PhD
NHMRC Early Career Fellow and
Leo J Mahar Lecturer
Center for Heart Rhythm Disorders (CHRD)
South Australian Health and
Medical Research Institute (SAHMRI)
University of Adelaide and
Royal Adelaide Hospital
Adelaide, Australia

Tilman Maurer MD
Department of Cardiology
Asklepios Klinik St. Georg
Hamburg, Germany

John M Miller MD
Professor of Medicine
Director, Clinical Cardiac Electrophysiology
Indiana University School of Medicine
Department of Medicine
Krannert Institute of Cardiology
Indianapolis, IN, USA

Jeffrey Munro DO
Mayo Clinic
Phoenix, AZ, USA

Chrishan J Nalliah BSc MBBS
Department of Cardiology and Medicine
The Royal Melbourne Hospital
University of Melbourne
Parkville, Victoria, Australia

Narayanan Namboodiri
MD DM DNB PDF(SCT) FIC(RAH)
Additional Professor
Department of Cardiology
Sree Chitra Institute for Medical Sciences
and Technology
Thiruvananthapuram, Kerala, India

Calambur Narasimhan MD DM
Director, Arrhythmia and
Electrophysiology Services
CARE Hospital
Hyderabad, Telangana, India

Venkata A Narla MD MAS
Section of Cardiac Electrophysiology
Division of Cardiology
Department of Medicine
University of California
San Francisco, CA, USA

Akihiko Nogami MD PhD
Professor of Cardiology
Faculty of Medicine
University of Tsukuba
Tsukuba, Japan

Peter A Noseworthy MD
Assistant Professor of Medicine
Mayo Clinic
Rochester, MN, USA

Karen Ordovas MD MAS
Associate Professor of Radiology
Director of Cardiac Imaging
Department of Medicine and Radiology
University of California
San Francisco, CA, USA

Benzy J Padanilam MD
Director, Electrophysiology Labs
St. Vincent Medical Group
St. Vincent Hospital
Indianapolis, IN, USA

Thomas Pambrun MD
Hôpital Cardiologique du Haut-Lévêque
and the Université de Bordeaux
Bordeaux, France

Bence Patocskai MD
Clinician/Postdoc Research Fellow
University Medical Center Mannheim
University of Heidelberg
Mannheim, Germany

Daniel Pelchovitz MD FACC
Attending Electrophysiologist
The Christ Hospital
Cincinnati, OH, USA

B Hygriv Rao MD DM FACC FISE
Senior Consultant Cardiologist
Director, Division of Pacing and
Electrophysiology
Krishna Institute of Medical Sciences
(KIMS) Hospitals
Hyderabad, Telangana, India

Raphael Rosso MD
Department of Cardiology
Tel Aviv Sourasky Medical Center and
Sackler School of Medicine
Tel Aviv University
Tel Aviv, Israel

Chawannuch Ruaengsri MD
Visiting Researcher
Division of Cardiothoracic Surgery
Washington University School of Medicine
St. Louis, MO, USA

Frédéric Sacher MD PhD
IHU Liryc, Electrophysiology and
Heart Modeling Institute
Bordeaux University
Bordeaux University Hospital (CHU)
Pessac, France

Daljeet Kaur Saggu MD DM
Consultant Cardiologist and
Electrophysiologist
CARE Hospital
Hyderabad, Telangana, India

Negar Salehi MD
Sparrow Thoracic and Cardiovascular
Institute
Michigan State University
Lansing, MI, USA

Damián Sánchez-Quintana MD PhD
Professor of Human Anatomy
Department of Anatomy and Cell Biology
Faculty of Medicine
University of Extremadura
Badajoz, Spain

Prashanthan Sanders MBBS PhD
Knapman Professor of Cardiology
Research
Center for Heart Rhythm Disorders (CHRD)
South Australian Health and
Medical Research Institute (SAHMRI)
University of Adelaide and
Royal Adelaide Hospital
Adelaide, Australia

Melvin Scheinman MD
Professor
Department of Medicine
University of California
San Francisco, CA, USA

Matthew R Schill MD
Resident Physician
Department of Surgery
Washington University School of Medicine
St. Louis, MO, USA

John William Schleifer MD
Division of Cardiovascular Diseases
Mayo Clinic
Rochester, MN, USA

Richard B Schuessler PhD
Professor of Surgery
Division of Cardiothoracic Surgery
Washington University School of Medicine
St. Louis, MO, USA

Raja J Selvaraj MD DNB
Associate Professor
Jawaharlal Institute of Postgraduate
Medical Education and Research (JIPMER)
Puducherry, India

Ashok Shah
MBBS MD DM CCDS
Consultant Cardiac Electrophysiology
Peel Health Campus
Mandurah, WA, Australia

George Shaw MD
University of Pennsylvania
Philadelphia, PA, USA

Win-Kuang Shen MD
Professor of Medicine
Mayo Clinic College of Medicine
Chair, Department of Cardiovascular
Diseases
Mayo Clinic
Phoenix, AZ, USA

Kalyanam Shivkumar MD PhD
Professor of Medicine and Radiology
Director, UCLA Cardiac Arrhythmia
Center and EP Programs
UCLA Health System
University of California
Los Angeles, CA, USA

Vini Singh MD
Sparrow Thoracic and Cardiovascular
Institute
Michigan State University
Lansing, MI, USA

Dan Sorajja MD
Assistant Professor of Medicine
Department of Cardiovascular Diseases
Mayo Clinic
Phoenix, AZ, USA

Antonio Sorgente MD PhD
Staff Physician
Cleveland Clinic
Abu Dhabi, United Arab Emirates

Komandoor Srivathsan MD
Director, Cardiac Electrophysiology
Mayo Clinic
Phoenix, AZ, USA

Leonard A Steinberg MD
Pediatric Electrophysiologist
Peyton Manning Children's Hospital
St. Vincent Hospital
Indianapolis, IN, USA

Taresh Taneja MD FACC FHRS
Cardiac Electrophysiology
The Permanente Medical Group
Sacramento, CA, USA

Ajit Thachil MD DM CCDS
Cardiac Electrophysiologist
Lisie Hospital
Kochi, Kerala, India

Ranjan K Thakur
MD MPH MBA FRCP FACC FHRS
Cardiac Electrophysiology Laboratory
Sparrow Thoracic and Cardiovascular Institute
Michigan State University
Lansing, MI, USA

Roderick Tung MD
Associate Professor of Medicine
Director of Cardiac Electrophysiology
University of Chicago
Chicago, IL, USA

Darragh Twomey MBBS
Research Associate
Center for Heart Rhythm Disorders (CHRD)
South Australian Health and
Medical Research Institute (SAHMRI)
University of Adelaide and
Royal Adelaide Hospital
Adelaide, Australia

Amar Upadhyay MD
Senior Resident
Jawaharlal Institute of Postgraduate
Medical Education and Research (JIPMER)
Puducherry, India

KL Venkatachalam MD
Assistant Professor of Medicine
Consultant, Cardiovascular Diseases
Division of Cardiovascular Diseases
Mayo Clinic
Jacksonville, FL, USA

Nishant Verma MD MPH
Assistant Professor of Medicine
Northwestern University
Feinberg School of Medicine
Chicago, IL, USA

Sami Viskin MD
Department of Cardiology
Tel Aviv Sourasky Medical Center and
Sackler School of Medicine
Tel Aviv University
Tel Aviv, Israel

Philip Wackel MD
Assistant Professor of Pediatrics
Division of Pediatric Cardiology
Mayo Clinic
Rochester, MN, USA

Albert L Waldo MD PhD(Hon)
Professor of Medicine
Case Western Reserve University
University Hospitals Case Medical Center
Cleveland, OH, USA

Edward P Walsh MD
Chief, Cardiac Electrophysiology Division
Department of Cardiology
Boston Children's Hospital
Professor of Pediatrics
Harvard Medical School
Boston, MA, USA

Erik Wissner MD FACC FHRS
Senior Consultant Cardiology/
Electrophysiology
Director Stereotaxis Laboratory
Asklepios Klinik St. Georg
Hamburg, Germany

Takumi Yamada MD
Associate Professor of Medicine
Division of Cardiovascular Disease
University of Alabama at Birmingham
Birmingham, AL, USA

Seigo Yamashita MD
IHU Liryc, Electrophysiology and
Heart Modeling Institute
Foundation Bordeaux Université
Bordeaux University Hospital (CHU)
Cardiac Electrophysiology and Cardiac
Stimulation Team, Pessac, France

Yanfei Yang MD
Associate Director
Medical Affairs and Medical Safety
Boston Scientific
San Francisco, CA, USA

Foreword

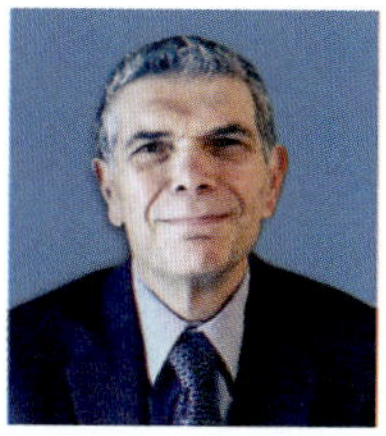

Drs Kartikeya Bhargava and Samuel J Asirvatham have carefully selected a well-known group of international experts to contribute to this multi-authored, comprehensive and up-to-date textbook of cardiac electrophysiology. *Practical Cardiac Electrophysiology* is largely clinically oriented and constitutes 47 chapters covering the spectrum of clinical diagnosis and management of arrhythmias, in and out of the electrophysiology laboratory. There is extensive coverage of all our "tools" including mapping equipment, ablation catheters and lab setup. There is an excellent chapter on practical cardiac anatomy, a must read for the serious student of the electrophysiology.

The book not only covers the most current fashionable entities and procedural skills, but also covers the less glamorous but necessary areas such as sinus node function testing.

This is not a "quick read" but individual chapters can be used as an excellent starting point for studying an area of interest for the electrophysiologist be they novice or more experienced. It would also serve well as a basis for study for board review as there is virtually no area of clinical electrophysiology not covered.

Overall, a useful addition to the shelf of any serious student of electrophysiology.

George Klein
Professor of Medicine
University of Western Ontario
London, Ontario
Canada

Foreword

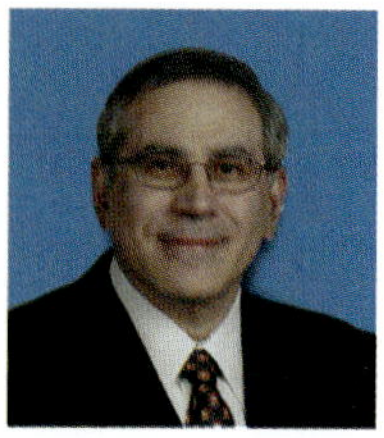

I was asked to write a Foreword for *Practical Cardiac Electrophysiology* edited by Drs Kartikeya Bhargava and Samuel J Asirvatham. This book contains 47 chapters authored by experts from around the world and includes topics as basic as how to do an electrophysiology study to complex imaging techniques and approaches to ablation of supraventricular and ventricular arrhythmias. While I admit, I had an opportunity to do a cursory journey through the various chapters in this textbook, my role is not one of a reviewer. Rather, I will address a more fundamental question, why bother to do such a project.

I grew up in an era of medical education where we "cherished" our textbooks. The chapters were read, key sections underlined, often reread, and kept on a shelf for ready reference. It was important to read journals to keep abreast of new observations (actually, not so new by the time the journal arrived). However, during teaching rounds, quotes from Friedberg's or Hurst's Textbook of Cardiology reigned supreme. The years moved on and a few specialty textbooks in electrophysiology became available, including one from my co-author Dr George Klein and me. Scores of journals entered the cardiovascular space, several specializing in cardiac arrhythmias. But in the distance, a looming shadow appeared that produced a sea change in how we access information: The Internet.

What a marvelous educational tool the Internet is, constantly available at your fingertips and nearly always willing to answer your queries. A search of a topic can not only provide the latest literature on it but also an abundance of non-vetted information of questionable worth – good luck on sorting through it! There are more blogs and commentary sites than "Carter has Little Liver Pills" (you youngsters will need to search the Internet for that reference). Still, it is an incredible fountain of knowledge, the modern-day Pierian Spring.

So, I ask again, why bother assembling more than 2 score chapters from even more authors yielding hundreds of pages of information, even if it can be put into an electronic format? The reason is that reference books such as this are needed and provide a cohesive source of information for a novice or expert in clinical electrophysiology. The chapters and authors have been "vetted" by two accomplished electrophysiologists, Dr Asirvatham, who is one of the world's leading educators and a past recipient of the Distinguished Teacher award from Heart Rhythm Society (HRS), and Dr Kartikeya Bhargava. Thus, the reader has a single reference source to answer most questions about cardiac arrhythmias. Any such textbook will be somewhat out of date by the nature of how fast our field is moving, but in my experience this accounts, mostly for changes in therapy or sometimes an ablation technique, but not in the core principles of our field. I previously stated that my responsibility is not to review the content of this thorough textbook, but I must admit that I did do more than a "peek" in some of the chapters. I was delighted to see that the authors used "AV node-dependent arrhythmias" in one of their overall sections, a term that we initially used in our textbook in 1994, and I have found this is a useful way to teach concepts of supraventricular arrhythmias.

In summary, my congratulations to the editors for compiling such a complete and excellent resource for clinical electrophysiologists. It is worth having on your electronic bookshelf.

Eric N Prystowsky MD
Director, Cardiac Arrhythmia Service
St. Vincent Hospital, Indianapolis, IN, USA
Consulting Professor of Medicine
Duke University Medical Center
Durham, NC, USA

Preface

"Education is not the learning of facts, but the training of the mind to think."

—Albert Einstein

The complexity of cardiac electrophysiology is simultaneously a source of never-ending challenge and ever-fulfilling satisfaction for practitioners of this art. To attempt good invasive electrophysiology practice without learning the facts and being conversant in the fundamental principles is futile. Yet, the cornerstones themselves are insufficient in guiding a practitioner through the impasse between success and complication. This textbook begins with a recognition that the basics of anatomy, physiology, biophysics, and electrocardiography require mastery before progress can be made. In addition, the focus on practical understanding and training the electrophysiologist's mind to be able to apply these principles in real-time when confronted by challenging arrhythmias permeates the book.

There already exist outstanding textbooks of electrophysiology which are often comprehensive treatises or collected case studies. The present work, we hope, benefits all practitioners; those in the developing world may stand to benefit the most. The large number of patients, sometimes suboptimal resources, and in certain cases the lack of access to the standard books and journals have been kept in mind by keeping this book practical and easy to use.

We acknowledge the time and effort of an international panel of master electrophysiologists, who have authored the works that reflect their specific areas of expertise.

Extensive illustrations, case-based discussions, and brief summaries provided at the end of most chapters will provide a perspective on the topic covered in the chapter and guide the readers in applying this information in their daily work.

Kartikeya Bhargava
Samuel J Asirvatham

Acknowledgments

We acknowledge with gratitude the untiring meticulous work from Jennifer A Mears, BA and Susan E Bisco, MA, without their assistance and organizational skills, this textbook would not have made it out to be of value for our present generation!

We thank Ms Shivangi Pramanik for all her help in getting this project completed.

We are grateful to Shri Jitendar P Vij (Group Chairman), Mr Ankit Vij (Group President), Mr Tarun Duneja (Director-Publishing), Mr Mohit Bhargava (Production Coordinator), Ms Swati Thapar (Development Editor), and the entire team of M/s Jaypee Brothers Medical Publishers (P) Ltd., New Delhi, India, for their help in bringing out the book.

List of Abbreviations

18-F-FDG	Flourine-18 Fluorodeoxyglucose
3D	Three Dimensional
AAD	Anti-arrhythmic Drug
AAV	Adeno-associated Virus
ACE	Angiotensin Converting Enzyme
ACLS	Advanced Cardiac Life Support
ACTN-2	Alpha Actinin-2
AEF	Atrioesophageal Fistula
AEGM	Atrial Electrogram
AF	Atrial Fibrillation
AFl	Atrial Flutter
AFP	Atriofascicular Pathway
AHA	American Heart Association
AIV	Anterior Interventricular Vein
ALARA	As Low As Reasonably Achievable
AMC	Aortomitral Continuity
AMP	Adenosine Mono Phosphate
ANS	Autonomic Nervous System
AP	Accessory Pathway
APL	Action Potential
APC	Atrial Premature Contraction
APD	Atrial Premature Depolarization
ARI	Activation Recovery Intervals
ARP	Absolute Refractory Period
ART	Antidromic Reciprocating Tachycardia
ARVC	Arrhythmogenic Right Ventricular Cardiomyopathy
ARVD/C	Arrhythmogenic Right Ventricular Dysplasia/ Cardiomyopathy
ASC	Aortic Sinus Cusps
AT	Atrial Tachycardia
ATP	Antitachycardia Pacing
ATT	Antitubercular Treatment
AV	Atrioventricular
AVN	Atrioventricular Node
AVNERP	Atrioventricular Nodal Effective Refractory Period
AVNRT	Atrioventricular Nodal Reentrant Tachycardia
AVRT	Atrioventricular Reciprocating or Reentrant Tachycardia
AWP	Alternating Wenckebach Periods
BB	Bundle Branch
BBB	Bundle Branch Block
BBR	Bundle Branch Reentry
BBRVT	Bundle Branch Reentrant Ventricular Tachycardia
BLS	Basic Life Support
BrS	Brugada Syndrome
BT	Bypass Tract
CA	Cardiac Arrest
CICR	Calcium induced Calcium Release
CAD	Coronary Artery Disease
cAMP	Cyclic Adenosine Monophosphate
CASPER	Cardiac Arrest Survivors with Preserved Ejection Fraction Registry
CCAVB	Congenital Complete Atrioventricular Block
CCB	Calcium Channel Blocker
CCW	Counter-clockwise
CF	Contact Force
CFAE	Complex Fractionated Atrial Electrograms
CFB	Central Fibrous Body
CHD	Congenital Heart Disease
CHF	Congestive Heart Failure
CL	Cycle Length
CMIV	Cox-Maze IV Procedure
CMP	Cardiomyopathy
CMP	Cox-Maze Procedure
CMR	Cardiac Magnetic Resonance Imaging
CMRR	Common-Mode Rejection Ratio
CPVT	Catecholaminergic Polymorphic Ventricular Tachycardia
CRD	Cournard
CRT	Cardiac Resynchronization Therapy
CS	Coronary Sinus
CT	Crista Terminalis
CTB	Cardiac Tuberculosis
CTCA	Computed Tomography Coronary Angiogram
CTI	Cavo-Tricuspid Isthmus
CW	Clockwise
DAD	Delayed Afterdepolarization
DC	Direct Current
DCM	Dilated Cardiomyopathy
DE	Delayed Enhancement
DPP-6	Dipeptidyl aminopeptidase-like protein-6
DS	Desmosomal
DSC	Desmocollin
DSG	Desmoglein
DSP	Desmoplakin
DSP	Digital Signal Processing
DWR	Double Wave Reentry
EAD	Early Afterdepolarization
EAM	Electro-anatomical Map/mapping
EAT	Ectopic Atrial Tachycardia
ECG	Electrocardiogram

ECGI	Electrocardiographic Imaging
ECMO	Extra Corporeal Membrane Oxygenation
EGM	Electrogram
E-IDC	Electrograms with Isolated Delayed Components
EMB	Endomyocardial Biopsy
EP	Electrophysiology
EPS	Electrophysiology Study
ER	Early Repolarization
ERP	Early Repolarization Pattern
ERP	Effective Refractory Period
ERS	Early Repolarization Syndrome
ES	Electrical Storm
EUS	Electrically Unexcitable Scar
FDG	Fluorodeoxyglucose
FO	Fossa Ovalis
FP	Fast Pathway
fQRS	Fragmented QRS
FRP	Functional Refractory Period
GA	General Anesthesia
GCV	Great Cardiac Vein
Gd	Gadolinium
GM	Granulomatous Myocarditis
GP	Ganglionated Plexus/Plexi
GWAS	Genome Wide Association Studies
HA	His Bundle-Atrial
HB	His Bundle
HCM	Hypertrophic Cardiomyopathy
HIFU	High Intensity Focused Ultrasound
HOP	His Overdrive Pacing
HP	His-Purkinje
HPE	Histopathological Examination
HPF	High Pass Filter
HPS	His-Purkinje System
HRA	High Right Atrium
IABP	Intra-aortic Balloon Pump
IART	Intra-atrial Reentrant Tachycardia
IAS	Interatrial Septum
ICD	Implantable Cardioverter-Defibrillator
ICE	Intracardiac Echocardiography
IF-VT	Interfascicular Ventricular Tachycardia
IHR	Intrinsic Heart Rate
IIR	Intra-isthmus Reentry
IP	Isolated Potential
iPSC-CM	Induced Pluripotent Stem Cell-derived Cardiac Myocytes
IST	Inappropriate sinus tachycardia
IVC	Inferior vena cava
IVCD	Intraventricular Conduction Defect
JET	Junctional Ectopic Tachycardia
JPB	Junctional Premature Beat
JSN	Josephson
JT	Junctional Tachycardia
JUP	Plakoglobin
LA	Left Atrium/Atrial
LAA	Left Atrial Appendage
LAD	Left Anterior Descending
LAFB	Left Anterior Fascicular Block
LAO	left Anterior Oblique
LASER	Light Amplification by Stimulated Emission of Radiation
LAVA	Local Abnormal Ventricular Activity
LB	Left Bundle
LBB	Left Bundle Branch
LBBB	Left Bundle Branch Block
LCC	Left Coronary Cusp
LCx	Left Circumflex
LF	Left Fascicle
LGE	Late Gadolinium Enhancement
LICU	Low Intensity Collimated Ultrasound
LLR	Lower Loop Reentry
LMCA	Left Main Coronary Artery
LMWH	Low Molecular Weight Heparin
LN	Lymph Node
LOM	Ligament of Marshall
LP	Late Potential
LPF	Low Pass Filter
LPFB	Left Posterior Fascicular Block
LQTS	Long QT Syndrome
LSPV	Left Superior Pulmonary Vein
LSVC	Left Superior Vena Cava
LV	Left Ventricle
LVEF	Left Ventricular Ejection Fraction
LVOT	Left Ventricular Outflow Tract
MA	Mitral Annulus
MAP	Monophasic Action Potential
MAT	Multifocal Atrial Tachycardia
MB	Moderator Band
MDCT	Multidetector Computerized Tomography
MET	Metabolic Equivalent
MI	Myocardial Infarction
MM	Monomorphic
MR	Magnetic Resonance
MRI	Magnetic Resonance Imaging
MTB	Mycobacterium *tuberculosis*
MW	Microwave energy
NCC	Non-coronary cusp
NCX	Sodium-Calcium ion Exchanger
NOAC	Novel Oral Anticoagulant
NSIVCD	Non-specific Intraventricular Conduction Defect
NSVT	Non-Sustained Ventricular Tachycardia
ORT	Orthodromic Reciprocating Tachycardia
OTVT	Outflow Tract Ventricular Tachycardia
OVM	Oblique Vein of Marshall
P2R	Phase 2 Reentry
PA	Pulmonary Artery
PAC	Premature Atrial Complex /Contraction
PAF	Paroxysmal Atrial Fibrillation
PAM	Papillary Muscles
PCL	Paced/Pacing cycle length
PCR	Polymerase Chain Reaction

PDE Phosphodiesterase
PES Programmed Electrical Stimulation
PET Position Emission Tomography
PET-CT Positron Emission Tomography – Computed Tomography
PI Preexcitation Index
PJRT Permanent Junctional Reciprocating Tachycardia
PKP Plakophilin
PLN Phospholamban
PLVT Pleomorphic Ventricular Tachycardia
PMVT Polymorphic Ventricular Tachycardia
PNP Phrenic Nerve Palsy
POTS Postural Orthostatic Tachycardia Syndrome
PPI Postpacing Interval
PSVT Paroxysmal Supraventricular Tachycardia
PTSD Post-traumatic Stress Disorder
PV Pulmonary Vein
PVAC Pulmonary Vein Ablation Catheter
PVC Premature Ventricular Complex/Contraction
PVI Pulmonary Vein Isolation
QTc Corrected QT interval
RA Right Atrium
RAA Right Atrial Appendage
RAO Right Anterior Oblique
RB Right Bundle
RBB Right Bundle Branch
RBBB Right Bundle Branch Block
RCA Right Coronary Artery
RCC Right Coronary Cusp
RCT Randomized Clinical Trials
RF Radiofrequency
RFA Radiofrequency Ablation
RIPV Right Inferior Pulmonary Vein
RMS Room Mean Squared
RRP Relative Refractory Period
RSPV Right Superior Pulmonary Vein
RV Right Ventricle
RVOT Right Ventricular Outflow Tract
RYR Ryanodine Receptor
SA Sinoatrial
SA Stimulus to Atrial
SAECG Signal Averaged Electrocardiogram
SAN Sinoatrial Node
SCD Sudden Cardiac Death
SEMA3A Semaphorin 3A
SERCA Sarcoplasmic Reticulum Calcium Adenosine Triphosphatase
SF Safety Factor
SHD Structural Heart Disease
SIDS Sudden Infant Death Syndrome
SMT Septomarginal Trabeculation
SMVT Sustained Monomorphic Ventricular Tachycardia
SN Sinus Node
SND Sinus Node Dysfunction
SNRT Sinus Node Recovery Time
SOO Site of Origin
SP Slow Pathway
SQTS Short QT Syndrome
SR Sarcoplasmic Reticulum
SR Sinus Rhythm
SSFP Steady State Free Precession
SVC Superior Vena Cava
SVT Supraventricular Tachycardia
TA Tricuspid Annulus
TB Tuberculosis
TCL Tachycardia Cycle Length
TEE Transesophageal Echocardiography
TFC Task Force Criteria
TGFβ Transforming Growth Factor Beta
TMEM43 Transmembrane Protein 43
TRPM4 Transient Receptor Potential Melastatin Protein 4
TTE Transthoracic Echocardiogram
TTN Titin
TWI T-wave inversion
TZI Transition Zone Index
ULR Upper Loop Reentry
VA Ventriculoatrial
VA or VArr Ventricular Arrhythmia
VEGM Ventricular Electrogram
VES Ventricular Extrastimulus
VES Ventricular Extrasystole
VF Ventricular Fibrillation
VGLA Visually Guided Laser Ablation
VPC Ventricular Premature Complex/Contraction
VSD Ventricular Septal Defect
VT Ventricular Tachycardia
WACA Wide Area Circumferential Ablation
WCT Wilson Central Terminal
WPW Wolff-Parkinson-White

Contents

SECTION C SUPRAVENTRICULAR TACHYARRHYTHMIAS: AV NODE-DEPENDENT TACHYCARDIAS

SECTION D SUPRAVENTRICULAR TACHYARRHYTHMIAS: ATRIAL TACHYCARDIA, FLUTTER AND FIBRILLATION

SECTION F MISCELLANEOUS

SECTION A

Introduction and Basics of Cardiac Electrophysiology

CHAPTER 1

Ajit Thachil

Electrophysiology Study: Indications, Hardware and Set-up, Catheter Placement

LIST OF ABBREVIATIONS

AV	Atrioventricular	JSN	Josephson
CRD	Cournard		

INTRODUCTION

A cardiac electrophysiology study is a procedure that entails evaluation of the cardiac conduction system and induction and analysis of various arrhythmias so as to identify targets for ablation as a means of treatment. The study entails introduction of various catheters into the heart through which signals can be recorded and electrical stimulation performed in order to induce and study arrhythmias.

INDICATIONS FOR ELECTROPHYSIOLOGY STUDIES

The indications for an electrophysiology study can be broadly categorized as:

- To evaluate the nature of a documented tachycardia.
- To evaluate whether undocumented palpitation is due to an inducible arrhythmia.
- To evaluate the presence of a potentially causative bradyarrhythmia or tachyarrhythmia in a patient with undiagnosed syncope.
- To evaluate the potential for future sustained tachyarrhythmia in asymptomatic patients deemed to be at higher than normal risk for such arrhythmia.
- To evaluate the potential for future bradycardia due to atrioventricular conduction block in asymptomatic patients deemed to be at higher than normal risk for such bradycardia.
- To evaluate the outcome of a pharmacological or non-pharmacological therapy (e.g. radiofrequency ablation) administered for a tachyarrhythmia.

These indications have been characterized in detail in guidelines for electrophysiology studies published by various societies.[1]

HARDWARE AND SET-UP FOR ELECTROPHYSIOLOGY STUDY AND RADIOFREQUENCY ABLATION

The hardware required for electrophysiology study includes catheters used for intracardiac recording and ablation, cables used to connect these catheters to the electrophysiology unit, the electrophysiology and radiofrequency ablation unit per se, and low resistance grounding patches connecting the radiofrequency current generator to the patient to complete the circuit. **Figures 1.1A to D** depict the schematic of a typical electrophysiology and radiofrequency ablation set-up.

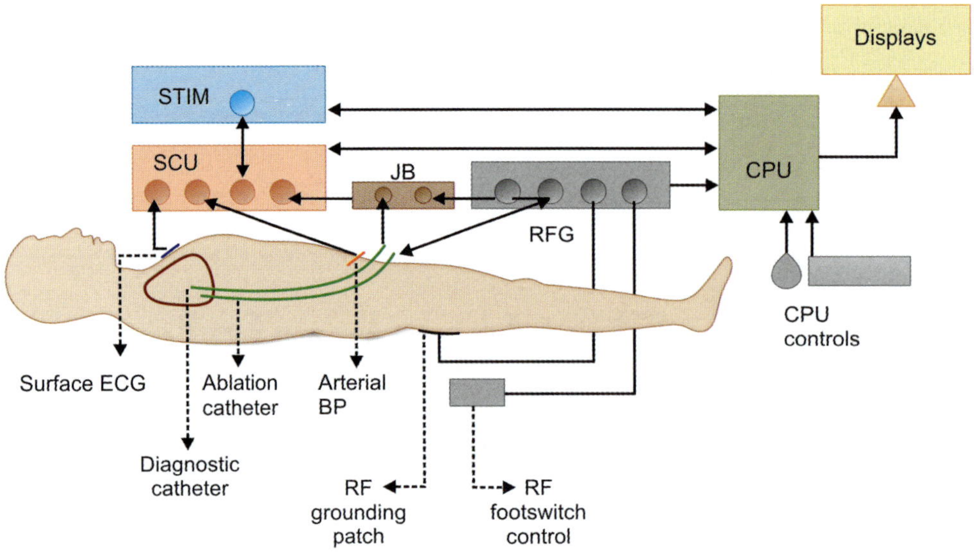

Figure 1.1A: Typical set-up for electrophysiology study and radiofrequency ablation

Abbreviations: STIM, stimulator unit; SCU, signal conditioning unit; JB, junction box; RFG, radiofrequency current generator; CPU, central processing unit ("Computer"); RF, radiofrequency

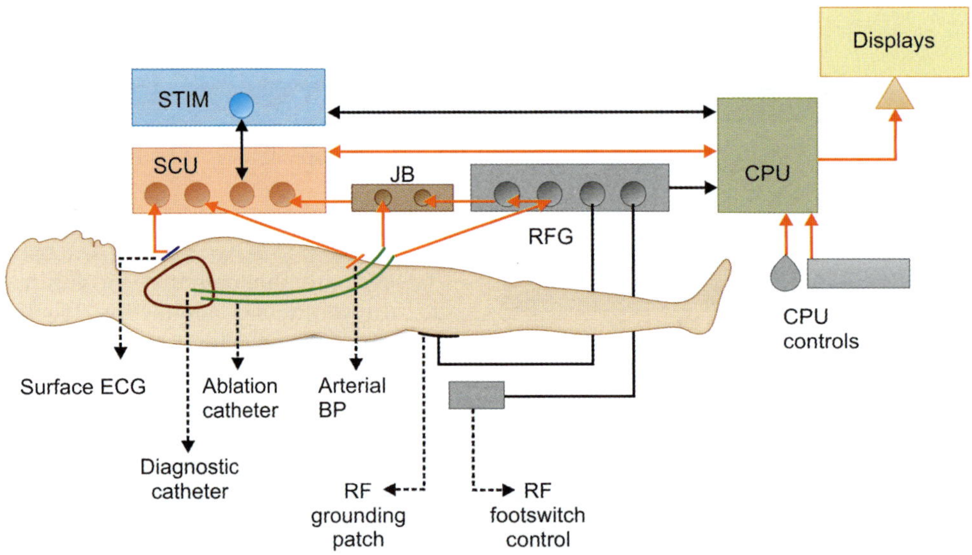

Figure 1.1B: The sensing circuit. Red lines depict the active components. Three sets of signals (surface ECG, arterial blood pressure, intracardiac signals from the various diagnostic catheters and the ablation catheter) are received by the SCU which processes (filtering, amplification, etc.) them as per the instructions conveyed by the CPU, converts them to binary digital signals, and relays the processed digital signals to the CPU. The CPU processes this digital information into a format in which they are displayed graphically on the monitor(s)

Abbreviations: STIM, stimulator unit; SCU, signal conditioning unit; JB, junction box; RFG, radiofrequency current generator; CPU, central processing unit ("Computer"); RF, radiofrequency

The typical set-up used for electrophysiology study and radiofrequency ablation combines three different circuits—a sensing circuit, which is always operational, a pacing circuit and a unipolar ablation circuit. The pacing and ablation circuits may be turned on separately or together along with the sensing circuit. **Figures 1.1A to D** illustrate how these components of the circuit work.

ELECTRODE CATHETERS

The catheters used for electrophysiology study and radiofrequency ablation are composed of multiple insulated wires in a flexible insulated casing, usually made of polyurethane. Some of the catheters are also made of wires encased in woven Dacron. The electrode catheters are typically

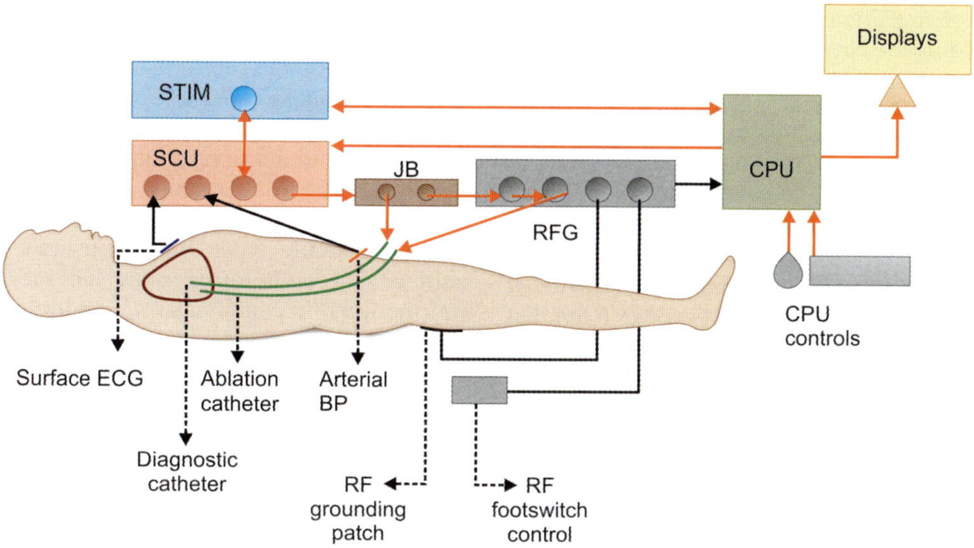

Figure 1.1C: The pacing circuit. Red lines depict the active components. The CPU instructs the stimulator to deliver the specified type of pacing impulse through the specified channel(s); pacing can be simultaneously or sequentially delivered through one to four channels. Each pacing channel is a route that extends from CPU–> STIM–> SCU–>JB–>diagnostic catheter –> patient, or CPU–> STIM–> SCU –> JB –> RFG –> ablation catheter –> patient. The CPU instructs the SCU regarding which port in the junction box to route each pacing channel through, and regarding the timing of the stimuli. The stimulator communicates back to the CPU when the pacing impulse is being delivered, so that this timing is noted in the recording. The SCU filters out the delivered stimulus from the sensing circuit
Abbreviations: STIM, stimulator unit; SCU, signal conditioning unit; JB, junction box; RFG, radiofrequency current generator; CPU, central processing unit ("Computer"); RF, radiofrequency

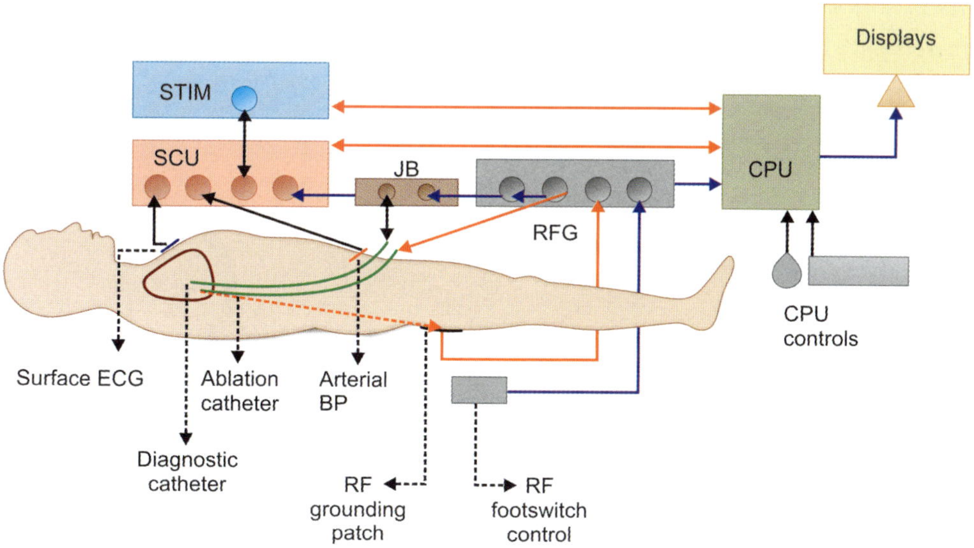

Figure 1.1D: The ablation circuit. Components of the circuit that are utilized to deliver energy during unipolar radiofrequency ablation (the most commonly used from of radiofrequency ablation) are highlighted in red. Other parts of the circuit that are activated are highlighted in blue. Upon command, usually delivered via a footswitch, radiofrequency energy passes from the RFG to the tissue in contact with the tip of the ablation catheter, from where it travels through the path of least resistance in the patient's body to the grounding patch and then back to the RFG to complete the loop. The RFG continuously monitors and relays details pertaining to radiofrequency energy delivery to the CPU. Upon signal from the RFG, the SCU filters out radiofrequency energy frequencies from the sensing circuit
Abbreviations: STIM, stimulator unit; SCU, signal conditioning unit; JB, junction box; RFG, radiofrequency current generator; CPU, central processing unit ("Computer"); RF, radiofrequency

available in 4 French to 8 French diameters and are typically 120 cm long. They may be classified as diagnostic catheters and radiofrequency ablation catheters. The diagnostic catheters record electrical signals and can deliver pacing stimuli through their electrodes. The electrical signals may be recorded in a unipolar configuration from any of the electrodes in reference to a designated ground electrode, or in a bipolar configuration between any pair of electrodes. The ablation catheters, in addition to serving as diagnostic catheters, can also deliver unipolar radiofrequency energy between their tip electrode and the grounding patch applied to the patient's body.

The distal tip of diagnostic catheters is composed of a 1 or 2 mm long electrode. The tip electrode of ablation catheters is either 4 mm or 8 mm long. The ablation catheters have a total of four electrodes whereas diagnostic catheters have 2 to 20 electrodes. The electrodes are separated by specific interelectrode distances, and are numbered starting from the tip. The tip electrode is numbered as electrode 1, and the more proximally located electrodes are serially numbered from 2 to 20 as required **(Figures 1.2A to C)**.

Electrode catheters can have a fixed or deflectable tip (also called a steerable tip). The steerable catheters allow deflection of the tip of the catheter in one or two directions in a single plane. Deflection is controlled by a manual mechanism located at the proximal end of the catheter. The catheters that can be deflected in two directions (in the same plane) are called bidirectional steerable tip catheters; some of them have asymmetrical bidirectional deflectable curves. **Figures 1.3A to E** show various types of deflectable tip catheters.

Some of the catheters have a straight shape up to the tip, whereas some others have preshaped tips designed to reach specific locations in the heart. **Figure 1.4** shows some such catheters designed for access to specific areas of the heart. Some multielectrode catheters like the basket catheter **(Figure 1.5A)** and the pentaray catheter **(Figure 1.5B)** can be used for simultaneous recordings from multiple areas in a chamber.

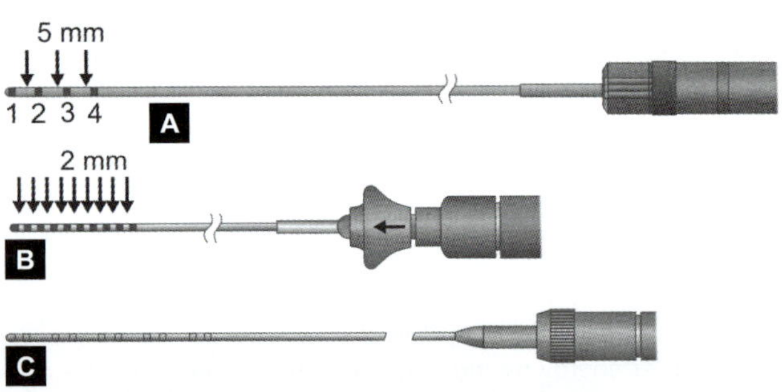

Figures 1.2A to C: Numbering of catheter electrodes. (A) Catheter with four electrodes numbered 1–4 starting from the distal electrode. The electrodes are 2 mm each in diameter, and separated by uniform interelectrode distances of 5 mm. This catheter is described as a 5-5-5 spaced quadripolar catheter; (B) Decapolar catheter with 2-2-2 spacing; (C) Decapolar catheter with 2-5-2-5-2-5-2-5-2 spacing. The electrode diameter remains at 2 mm in A to C

Ablation Catheters

Whereas diagnostic catheters only record electrical signals, ablation catheters can also deliver radiofrequency energy. Ablation catheters have one or more specialized sensors near their tip to aid precise manipulation and safe titration of energy delivery. All ablation catheters have a temperature sensor near their tip, which may be of a thermistor type or thermocouple type. These sensors allow the ablation catheter to continuously relay catheter tip temperature information to the ablator unit. In addition, certain ablation catheters are equipped with additional tip sensors that allow navigation in a magnetic field, and monitoring of the contact force generated by the catheter on the tissue **(Figure 1.6)**. Irrigated tip ablation catheters that allow creation of deeper radiofrequency lesions are also available. Such catheters allow continuous saline irrigation of the catheter tip to cool the catheter tip and catheter-tissue interface, thereby enabling greater amount of energy delivery. Unlike previously available closed loop irrigation technology, current catheters have open loop irrigation that involves catheter tip cooling by saline sprayed out through the holes near the tip **(Figure 1.6)**.

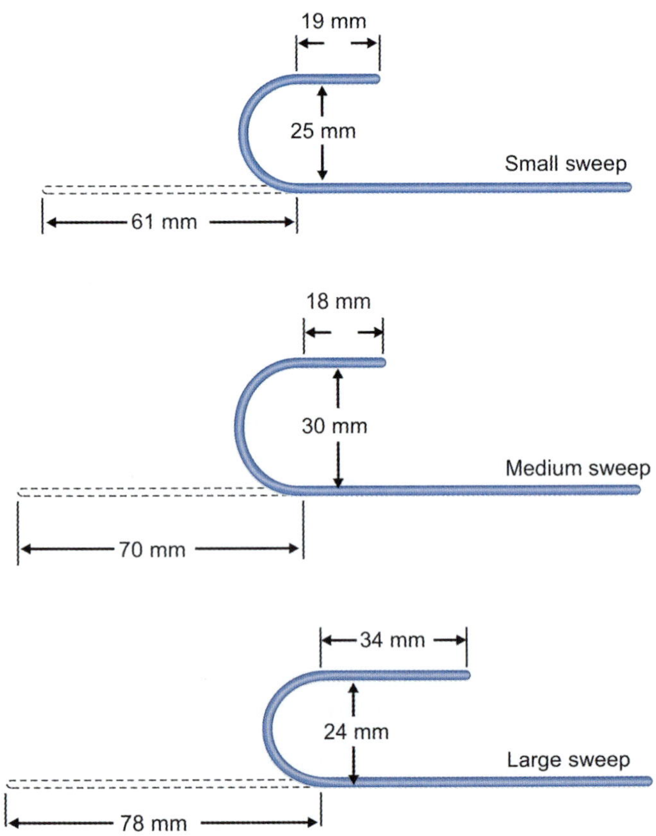

Figure 1.3A: Unidirectionally deflectable diagnostic and ablation catheters of various sweeps. The large sweep catheter also has an extended reach

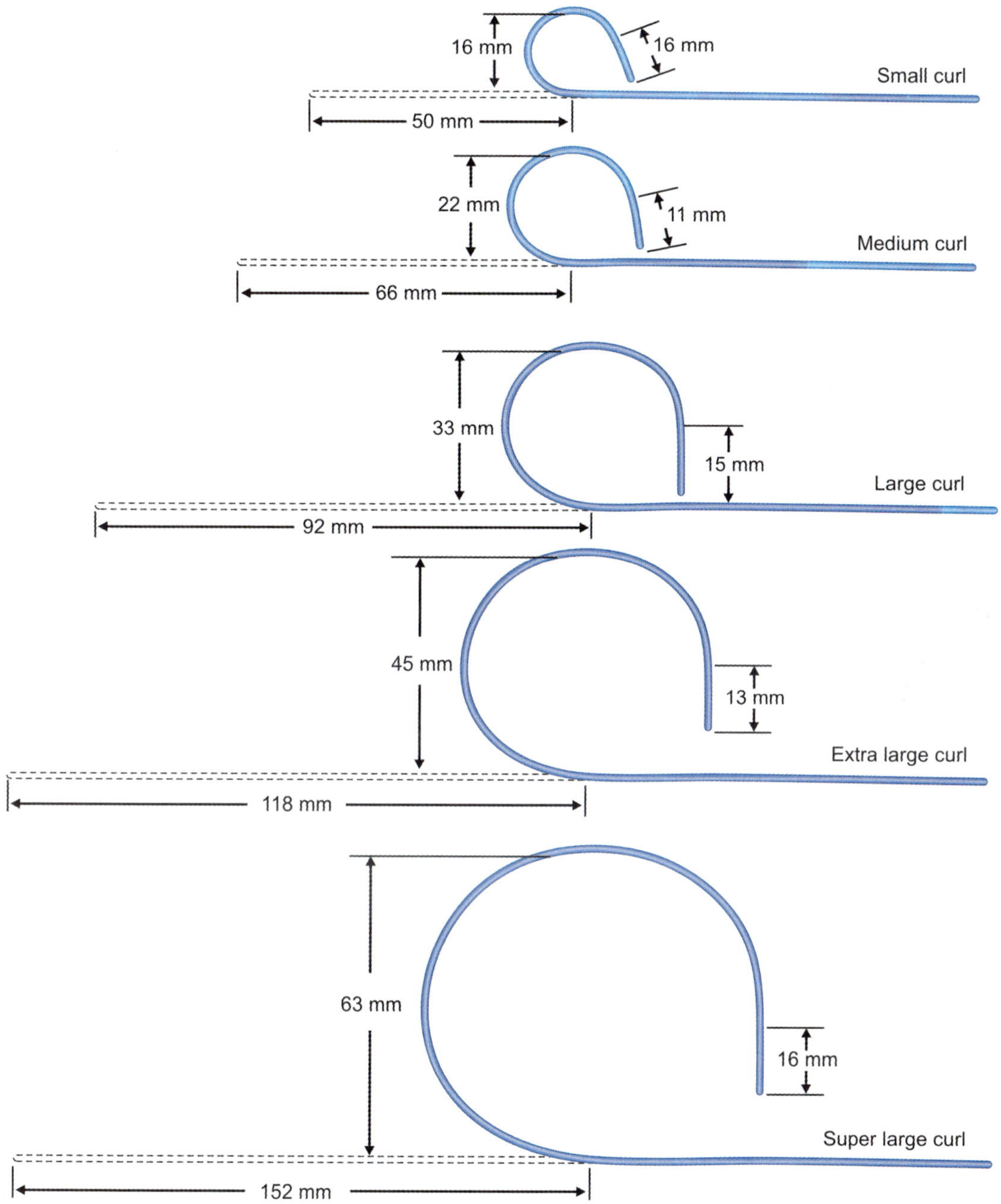

Figure 1.3B: Unidirectionally deflectable diagnostic catheters of various curls. These catheters can be deflected 360° to form circular loops

Connecting Cables

Specific cables are used to connect each catheter to the electrophysiology/radiofrequency ablation unit. The connector pin that connects the cable to the catheter is specific to the configuration of that catheter. The pins at the other end of the cable (the pins that insert into the junction box/ radiofrequency current generator) are standardized only for diagnostic catheters; therefore any diagnostic catheter may be plugged into the junction box of any electrophysiology system using the same cable **(Figure 1.7A)**. The connector pins of the cables that connect to the radiofrequency current generator are specific to the manufacturer. Specific cables are therefore, required to connect a St. Jude Medical ablation catheter to a St. Jude Medical radiofrequency current generator, a St. Jude Medical ablation catheter to

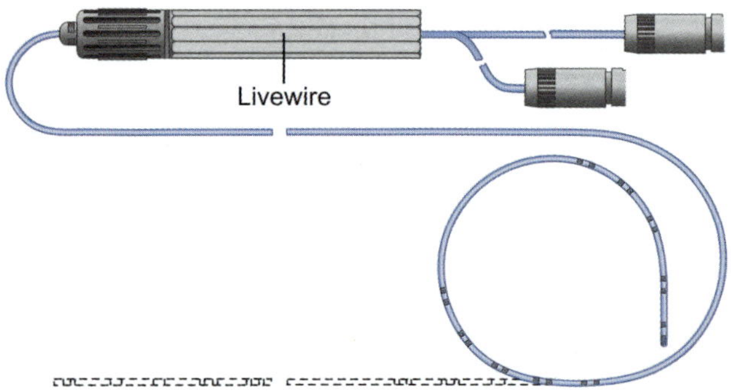

Figure 1.3C: Unidirectionally deflectable super large curl duodecapolar diagnostic catheter with 2-5-2-5-2-5-2-5-2-60-2-5-2-5-2-5-2-5-2 spacing, intended for simultaneous recording from the coronary sinus and free wall of the right atrium, when introduced via the jugular approach

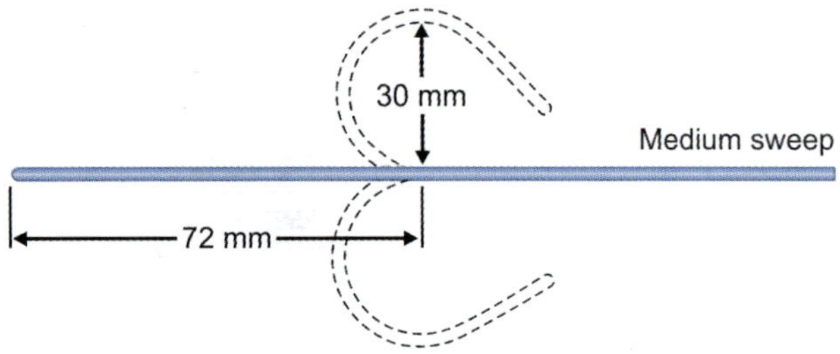

Figure 1.3D: Bidirectionally deflectable symmetrical medium sweep catheter. Both the deflections are in the same plane

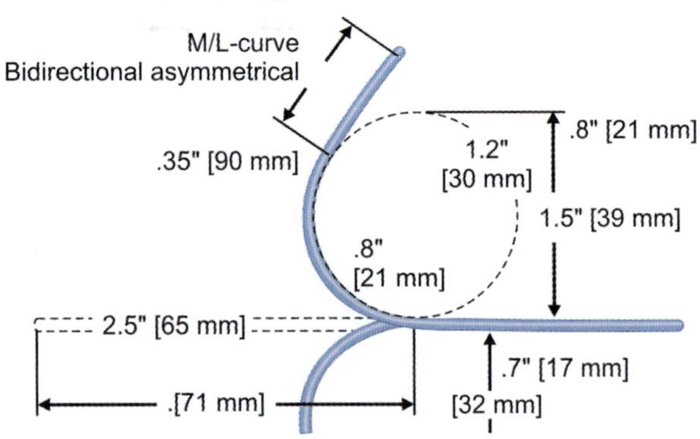

Figure 1.3E: Bidirectionally deflectable asymmetrical medium/large sweep catheter. Both the deflections are in the same plane

a Stockert EP Shuttle radiofrequency current generator, a Biosense Webster thermocouple type ablation catheter to a Stockert EP Shuttle radiofrequency current generator, a Biosense Webster thermistor type ablation catheter to a Stockert EP Shuttle radiofrequency current generator and so on **(Figure 1.7B)**.

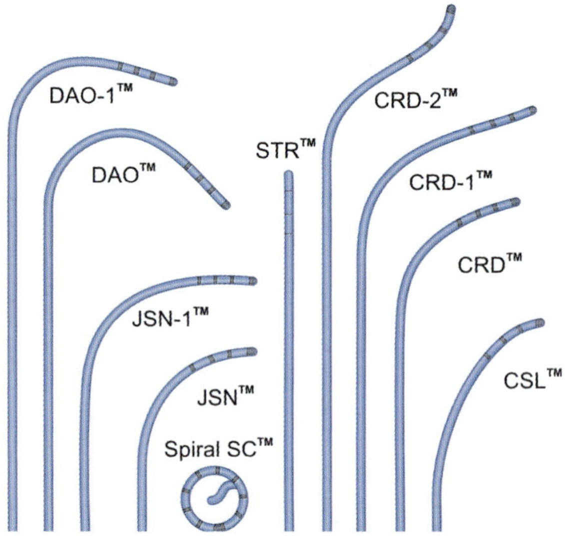

Figure 1.4: Catheters with precurved tips designed to access specific areas in the heart. The DAO and JSN curves are designed for access to the right ventricular apex. The CRD-2 curve designed to rest on the septum in the area of the His bundle. The CSL curve is designed for access to the coronary sinus, and is specifically useful to negotiate a valve at the ostium of the coronary sinus when introduced from the jugular approach. The Spiral catheter can be curled into a tight or a loose curve (variable curve spiral), has a deflectable shaft, and fits into pulmonary veins and other such vessels to record electrical activity from the circumference of the vessel; this catheter is often called the "lasso" catheter

Abbreviations: DAO, damato; JSN, josephson; CRD, cournard; STR, straight

CATHETER PLACEMENT FOR ELECTROPHYSIOLOGY STUDIES

Access Sites

Transluminal percutaneous access for electrophysiology study is typically obtained via one or both femoral veins and arteries, and via the right internal jugular vein. Other access sites, usually used when these sites are unavailable or unsuitable include the brachial and subclavian or axillary veins, the left internal jugular vein, and the subclavian or axillary artery. These sites provide direct access to the endocardium, as well as indirect access (by recording through the arterial and/or venous lumen) to areas of the epicardium that lie in proximity to the coronary vascular system. In addition, direct access to a large area of the epicardium can be obtained via a subxiphoid approach. Subxiphoid epicardial access is usually obtained via fluoroscopically directed needle puncture, and occasionally through a surgically created window. In occasional cases, direct access to the epicardium may have to be obtained through a thoracotomy.

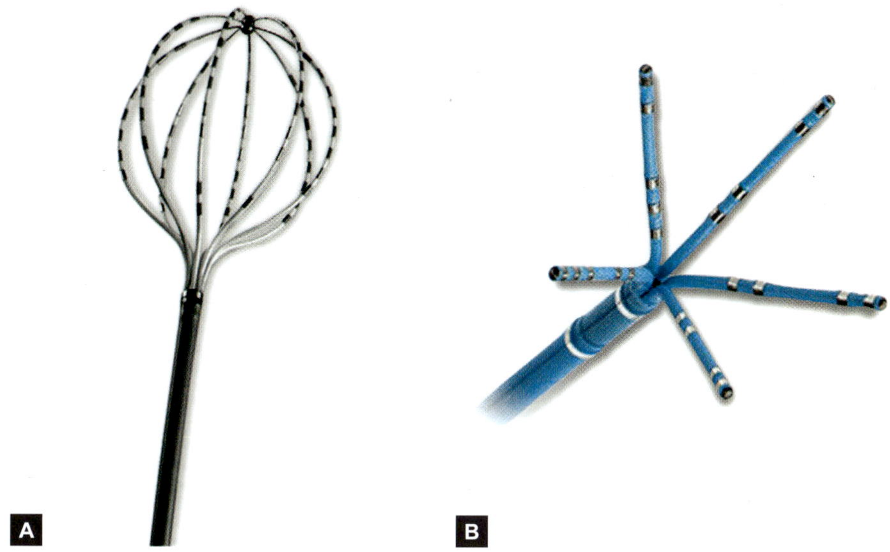

Figures 1.5A and B: The basket (A) and pentaray (B) catheters are used for simultaneous recording from multiple areas in the same chamber

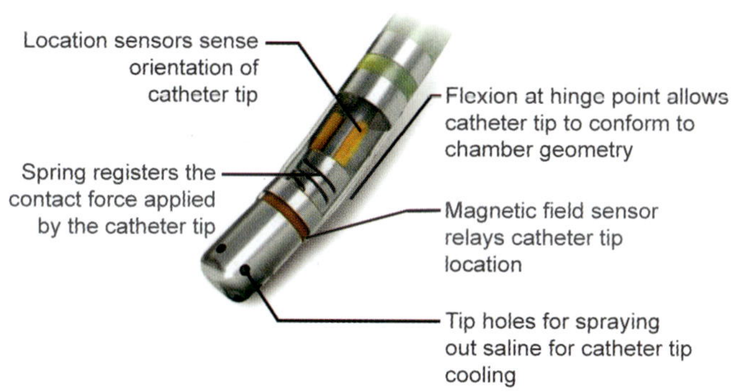

Figure 1.6: The Thermocool Smart Touch™ catheter. In addition to the catheter tip temperature sensor, it has the additional functions illustrated above

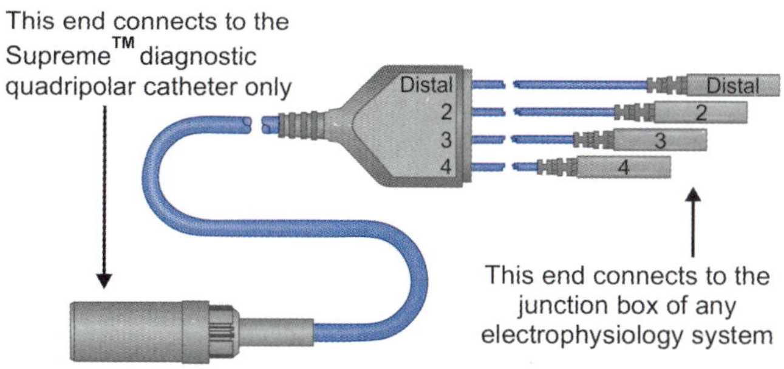

Figure 1.7A: Cable to connect a Supreme™ model diagnostic quadripolar catheter to the junction box of any electrophysiology system

Sheaths for Vascular Access

One or more sheaths, ranging from 4 French to 12 French in diameter, are typically introduced into the selected vessel(s) via the modified Seldinger technique under local anesthesia. Depending on the requirement, up to three or rarely four separate sheaths are typically introduced per vein; alternatively, a single 12 French triport sheath that can accommodate three catheters can also be used. Sheaths with a "locking facility" may help to stabilize catheters in case of excessive to-and-fro catheter movement. Alternatively, the catheter and sheath may sometimes be sutured onto the skin to prevent excessive catheter movement. This may be specifically applicable to the coronary sinus catheter, especially when used as an anatomical/electrical reference during a procedure using a 3-dimensional electroanatomical mapping system.

Sheaths for Intracardiac Access to Specific Sites

Long sheaths (typically, 63 cm long sheaths introduced over 67 cm long dilators), usually introduced through the femoral veins, are often used to gain access to and attain stability at specific sites within the heart. Such sheaths are available in two categories: precurved sheaths designed to access specific areas of the heart, and deflectable sheaths that may be variably curved by the operator using handle-mounted controls. Several of the precurved sheaths are curved in more than one plane, allowing access to only specific areas of the heart. Deflectable sheaths of shorter length are often

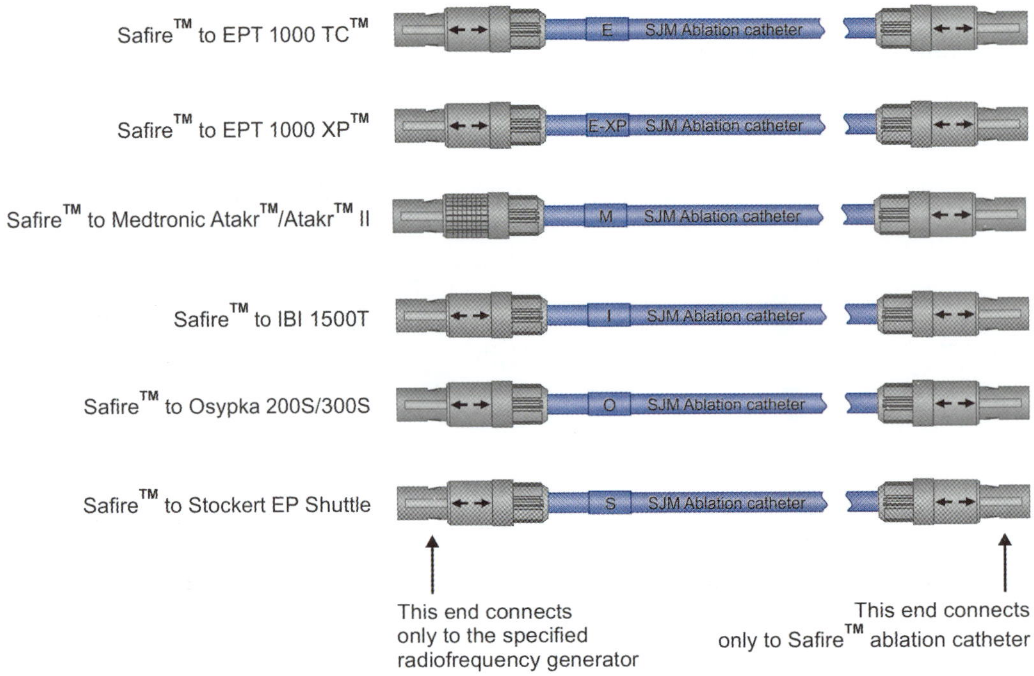

Figure 1.7B: Specific cables to connect a Safire™ model ablation catheter to specific radiofrequency current generators

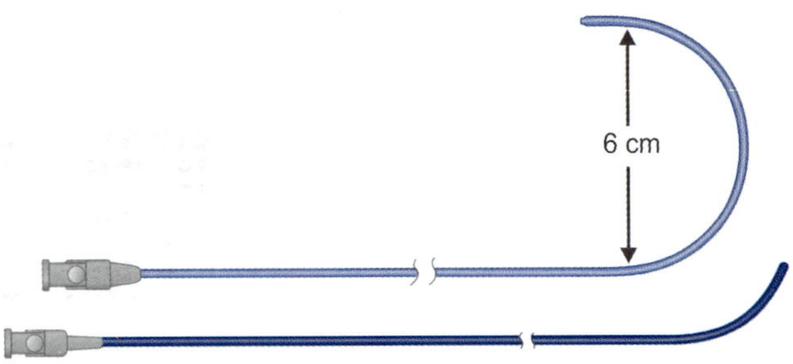

Figure 1.8A: The Mullin's type sheath, used for trans-septal access to the mitral annulus or left ventricle. The sheath has a fixed curve in a single plane. A similar sheath with a smaller curve may be used for stabilization of the ablation catheter on the inferior interatrial septum during ablation in the Koch's triangle for AV nodal re-entry

used during subxiphoid epicardial access. **Figures 1.8A to C** depict some of the commonly used long sheaths, and lists some of the areas typically accessed using them. These long sheaths also have valved side ports which allow contrast injection for visualization of intracardiac anatomy.

Catheter Placements in Specific Locations

As a general principle, intracardiac anatomy is best appreciated in the 20 to 30° right anterior oblique **(Figure 1.9)** and 40 to 60° left anterior oblique projections. Though a left anterior oblique projection with cranial angulation profiles the interventricular and interatrial septa better than the plain left anterior oblique projection, cranial and caudal angulations are rarely used in the electrophysiology laboratory.

Right Atrium and Right Ventricle

Right atrial and right ventricular recording and stimulation may be accomplished using deflectable or fixed curve catheters. Quadripolar catheters are conventionally used for this purpose. The right atrial catheter is often placed in the high right atrium just below the anterior part of the junction of the superior vena cava and the right atrium. Alternately, it may be positioned in the right atrial appendage, the base of which is located in the anterior part of the right atrium above the anterosuperior aspect of the tricuspid annulus. These areas are most readily located in the right anterior oblique projection. The superior vena cava-right atrium junction location records the area of earliest electrical activation in the right atrium during sinus rhythm, and corresponds to the sinus node. Catheter stability at this location may be less than in the right atrial appendage. Besides, inferoposterior displacement of a catheter located at the superior vena cava-right atrium junction may sometimes cause stimulation of the phrenic nerve which is often located on the epicardial aspect at this area, especially when higher outputs are used for pacing. The right ventricular catheter is conventionally placed at the right ventricular apex due to stability, reproducibility, ease of positioning, and good electrical parameters. Recording and stimulation from areas other than the right ventricular apex may be required in specific situations.

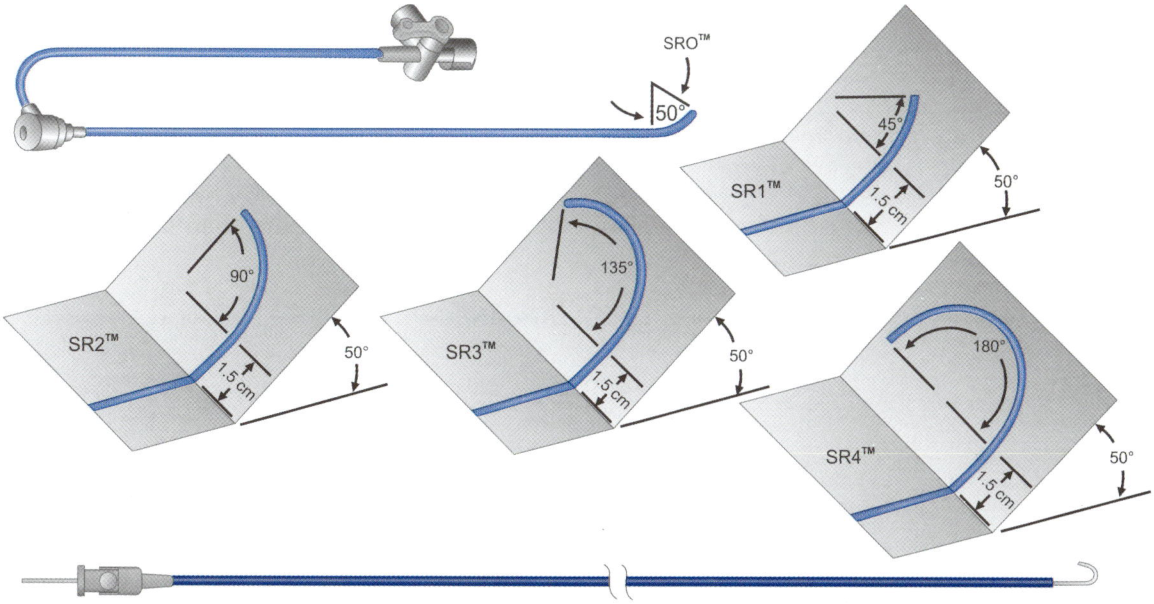

Figure 1.8B: The Swartz Right (SR) sided series of sheaths for catheter stabilization onto various areas of the tricuspid annulus, depicted along with a straight dilator. The SR 0 curve is useful for catheter stabilization onto the Koch's triangle. The SR 1,2,3 and 4 curves direct to the anterosuperior, anterolateral, lateral to posterolateral and posterolateral to posterior areas of the tricuspid annulus respectively. These sheaths have tips with fixed curves in more than one plane. A similar series of left sided sheaths that curve in the opposite direction is also available

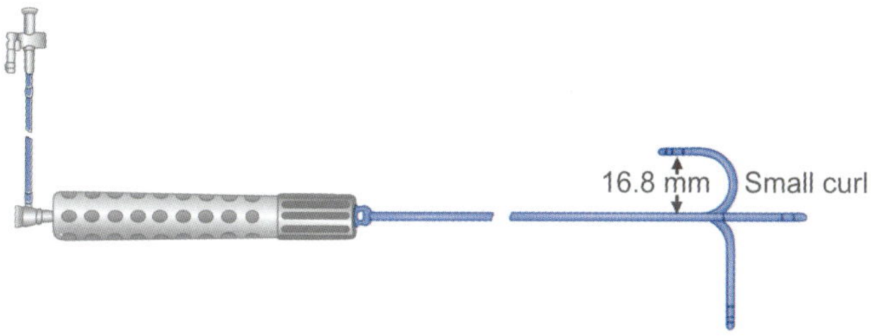

Figure 1.8C: The Agilis NxT bidirectionally deflectable steerable sheath. The tip deflection is controlled by the handle mechanism

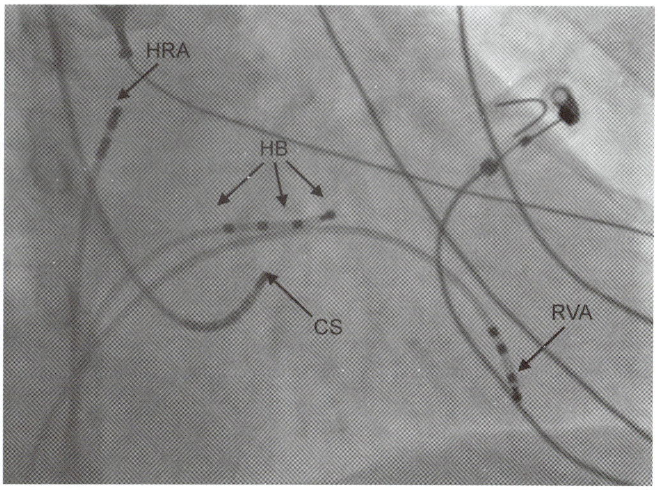

Figure 1.9: Right anterior oblique projection showing usual catheter locations used to record electrical activity from the right atrium, His bundle, right ventricle and coronary sinus

Abbreviations: HRA, high right atrium; HB, His bundle; RVA, right ventricular apex; CS, coronary sinus

Coronary Sinus

The coronary sinus may be accessed from the superior vena caval or either femoral venous access. The former is often easier, especially when a prominent Eustachian valve is present at the ostium of the coronary sinus. A fixed curve or a deflectable-tip catheter may be used to cannulate the coronary sinus from the superior vena caval approach, whereas the inferior vena caval approach usually requires a deflectable-tip catheter. Fixed curve catheters of the CSL type curve (*See* **Figure 1.4**) are specifically designed for coronary sinus access via the right superior vena caval route, and are especially helpful in the presence of a very prominent valve at the coronary sinus ostium. The coronary sinus catheter is usually the first catheter to be introduced in the right side of the heart as presence of other catheters may hamper the manipulation required to position the coronary sinus catheter.

To engage the coronary sinus from the superior vena caval access, the catheter is first directed to the region of the coronary sinus ostium in the right anterior oblique or posteroanterior projection, before manipulating it into the coronary sinus in the left anterior oblique projection.

The coronary sinus ostium lies close to the inferior and posterior-most part of the tricuspid annulus at an area often marked by a fat-pad translucency in the right anterior oblique fluoroscopic projection. With experience, this area may also be located in the postero-anterior fluoroscopic projection. The catheter tip is directed towards this area with a slight curve at its tip **(Figure 1.10A)**. Once the ostium is located, the catheter shaft is rotated to make the distal part of the catheter face towards the spine in the left anterior oblique projection **(Figure 1.10B)**. With the catheter in this orientation, the ostium of the coronary sinus is probed with gentle forward pressure on the catheter. It may be required to move the catheter slightly up and down the interatrial septum to identify the exact location of the ostium, especially when guarded by a prominent valve. Once the ostium is crossed, the catheter usually "jumps" into the coronary sinus with

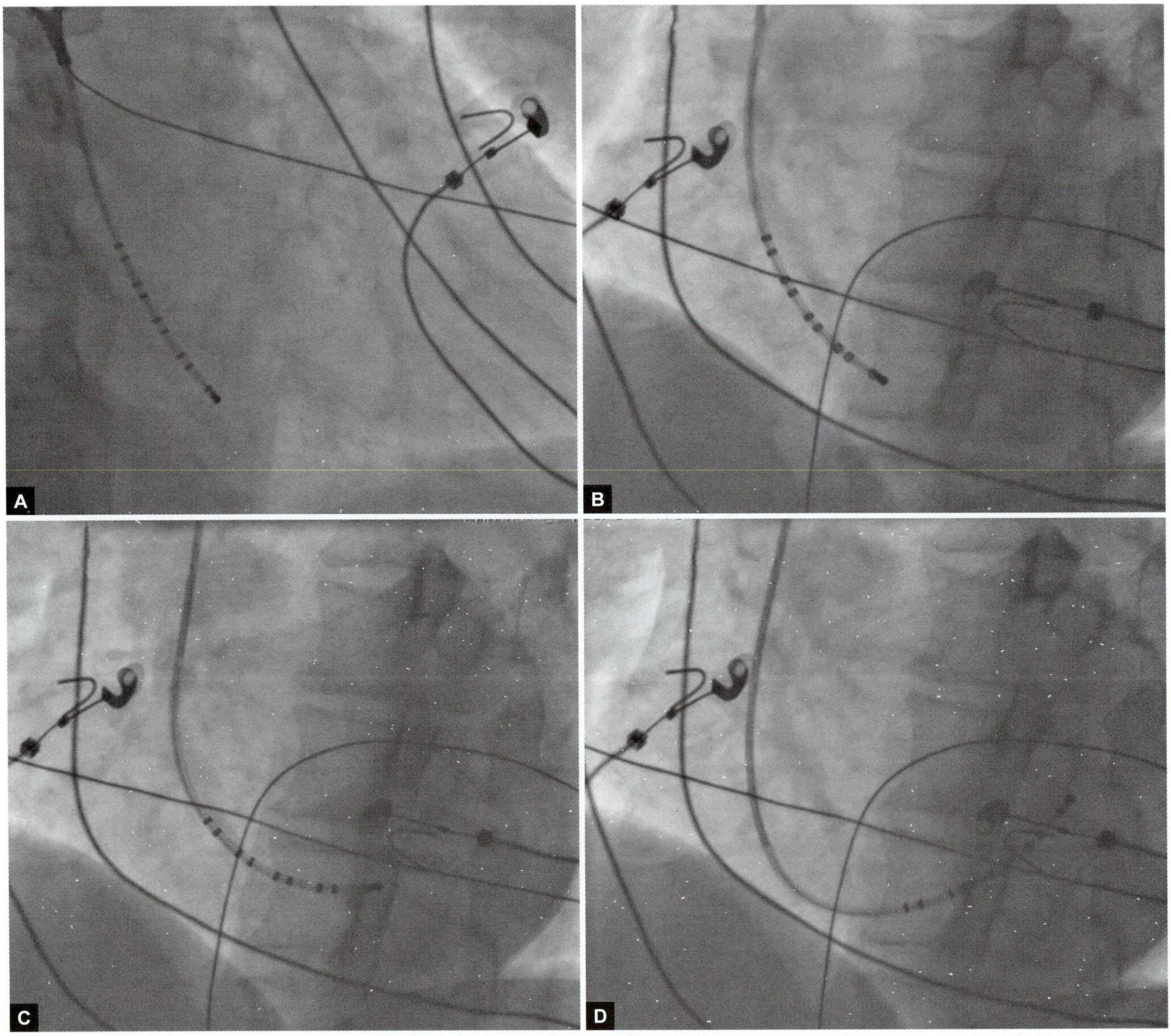

Figures 1.10A to D: Steps in positioning a catheter in the coronary sinus from the superior approach. The catheter is first directed in the right anterior oblique projection to just superior to the translucent fat pad adjoining the inferior end of the tricuspid annulus (A). The projection is then switched to left anterior oblique with the catheter in the same orientation (B). The catheter is now gently deflected up in the left anterior oblique projection and the ostium of the coronary sinus is probed; a slight clockwise turn may be required at this point (C). Once the ostium is located, the catheter usually "jumps" into the coronary sinus with minimal forward pressure; it is now advanced gently through the coronary sinus (D). With experience, the entire maneuver may be performed in the left anterior oblique or anteroposterior projection

minimal forward pressure, except in situations with very prominent Eustachian valves **(Figures 1.10C and D)**. When deflectable-tip catheters are used, maintaining a slight deflection of the catheter tip assists this movement.

The trajectory of the coronary sinus from the ostium onwards usually describes a smooth upward arc in the left anterior oblique projection. When the subsequent course of the catheter after engaging the coronary sinus ostium is more or less straight towards the outer border of the heart rather than in an upward arc, one must take care to ensure that the catheter is entering the coronary sinus itself, rather than a posterior or lateral tributary of the coronary sinus (*See* **Figure 1.24**). The electrogram recorded often gives a clue in this situation. The coronary sinus electrogram has atrial and ventricular components, with the atrial component usually being larger in amplitude than the ventricular component. As the tributaries of the coronary sinus overlie the left ventricle, electrograms recorded from them often show a ventricular electrogram that is larger in amplitude than the atrial electrogram. In case of doubt, recording the levophase of the left coronary angiogram in the left anterior oblique projection with the coronary sinus catheter in place will readily delineate its location. Another source of confusion while cannulating the coronary sinus is movement of the catheter into the right ventricular outflow tract. A catheter in the right ventricular outflow tract will record only ventricular electrograms, in contrast to the dual atrial and ventricular electrograms recorded from the coronary sinus. Catheter movement into the right ventricle/right ventricular outflow tract often triggers ventricular ectopy, whereas catheter movement into the coronary sinus usually does not cause any ectopy or sometimes causes atrial ectopy. On pushing further, a catheter located in the right ventricular outflow tract will move superiorly rather than towards the left heart border. Progressively greater degrees of left anterior oblique projection (up to ~ 60°) will make a catheter in the coronary sinus appear progressively more towards the outer border of the left ventricle. Greater degrees of left anterior oblique projection (up to ~ 60°) will make a catheter located in the right ventricular outflow tract appear progressively more towards the center of the heart.

To engage the coronary sinus from the femoral venous approach **(Figures 1.11A to E)**, the catheter is deflected down from the mid right atrial location to the area of the coronary sinus ostium in the right anterior oblique projection using the fluoroscopic landmark previously described. Subsequently, a manipulation combining slight de-deflection, clockwise torque and slight forward pressure, performed in the left anterior oblique projection usually makes the catheter enter the coronary sinus. Once the catheter enters the coronary sinus, the downward deflection and clockwise torque must be completely released to let it slide up the coronary sinus.

An alternate method of coronary sinus cannulation via transfemoral access is sometimes used when the previously described approach fails. This method involves turning the downwardly deflected catheter towards the inferior part of the right atrial free wall in the left anterior oblique projection and then gently pushing it into the coronary sinus after it moves from the lateral to the medial part of the inferior tricuspid annulus. If a coronary angiogram is performed along with the electrophysiology study, it is useful to record a levophase angiogram of the left coronary artery to visualize the coronary sinus prior to cannulation.

His Bundle

Electrical activity of the His bundle may be recorded via catheters placed on the membranous atrioventricular/proximal interventricular septum on the right side of the heart, the base of the noncoronary cusp of the aorta, or on the atrioventricular/proximal interventricular septum on the left side of the heart. The various catheters and accesses used for this purpose are detailed in this section.

His bundle recordings are typically obtained using quadripolar catheters with fixed or deflectable curves at the tip. Fixed curve catheters readily allow recording of His bundle activity when introduced via the femoral venous route. Fixed curve quadripolar catheters with the Josephson (JSN) or Cournard (CRD) type curves provide His bundle recordings, and can be moved to obtain recordings from other areas of the heart. Fixed curve catheters with the Cournard-2 (CRD-2) type curve are specifically designed to rest on the His bundle area when introduced via the femoral vein **(Figure 1.9)**. When recording the His bundle activity using these catheters, the catheter is passed across the cranial aspect of the tricuspid annulus in the right anterior oblique view until it is clearly in the right ventricle. It is then withdrawn across the tricuspid orifice while maintaining a slight clockwise torque until the desired potential is recorded. At the more apical locations, a large ventricular electrogram is the only electrogram observed. As the catheter is withdrawn, the right bundle branch potential (recognized as a high frequency spike recorded less than 30 milliseconds before the ventricular electrogram) is additionally observed. As the catheter is withdrawn further, a third electrogram—a small atrial electrogram—also appears proximal to the high frequency signal; this is the location of the distal His bundle. With further withdrawal of the catheter, the atrial electrogram progressively increases in amplitude. The catheter is withdrawn up to the proximal—most location where the three deflections are still visible; this is the location of the proximal His bundle, and is the site from which the HV interval should be measured **(Figures 1.12A and B)**. Once the His bundle is located, the recording catheter usually rests at the desired location on its own. Occasionally it may be required to manually maintain the clockwise torque to retain the catheter at the His bundle location. In this situation, forming a small clockwise loop on the connecting cable helps to maintain the position of the His bundle catheter, thereby freeing the operator's hand. It is often possible to record the

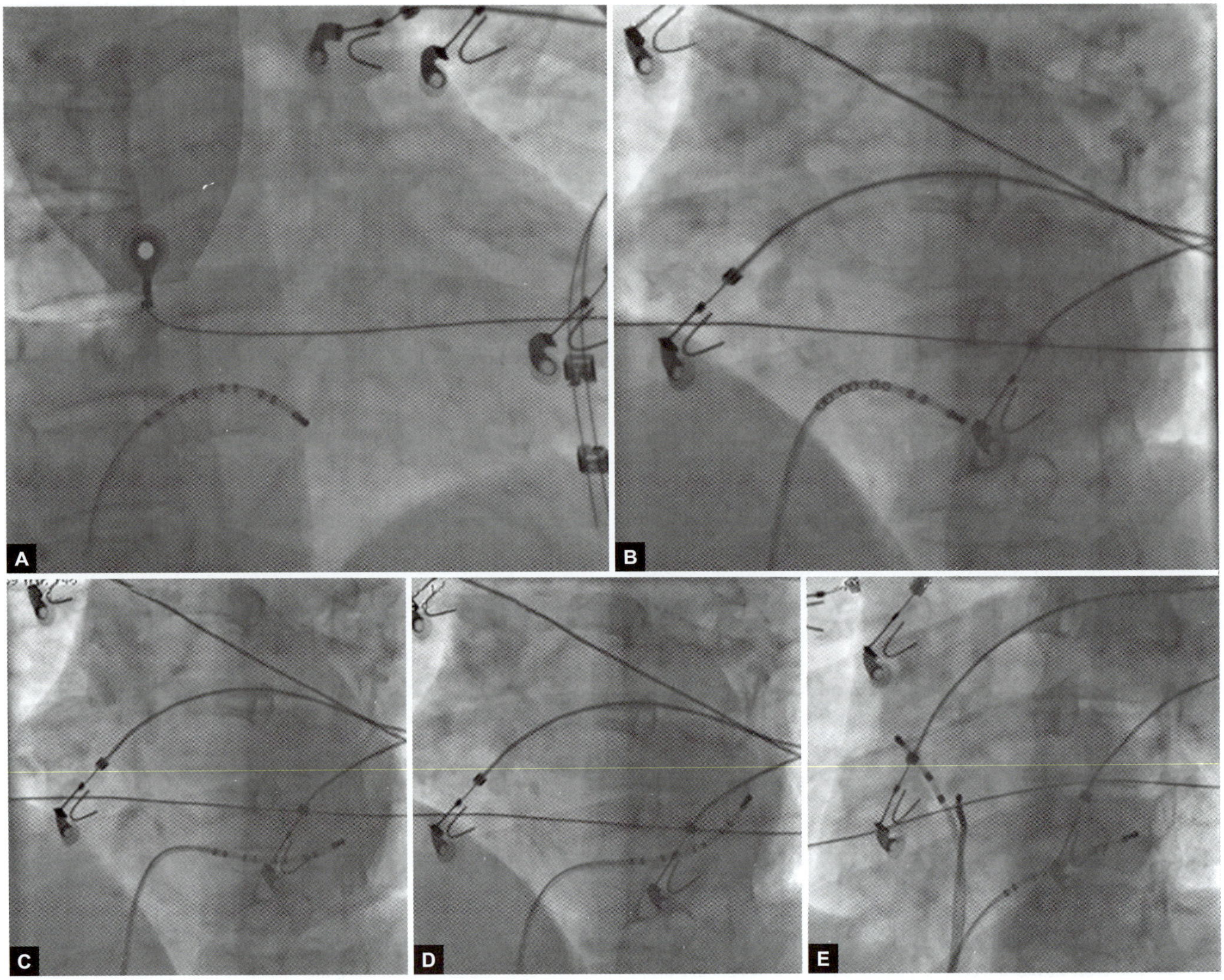

Figures 1.11A to E: Steps in positioning a catheter in the coronary sinus from the inferior approach. The catheter is first directed in the right anterior oblique projection to just superior to the translucent fat pad adjoining the inferior end of the tricuspid annulus (A). The projection is then switched to left anterior oblique with the catheter in the same orientation (B). The catheter is now subjected to a maneuver comprising of dedeflection, clockwise torquing, and forward pressure to probe the ostium of the coronary sinus (C). Once the ostium is located, the catheter is advanced gently through the coronary sinus (D). In some cases, especially when the valve at the coronary sinus ostium is not prominent, the coronary sinus catheter describes a straighter course when introduced via the inferior vena cava (E)

His bundle activity while entering the right ventricle itself, rather than having to enter distally and then pull back as just described. This second, simpler technique is more likely to work if entry into the right ventricle can be accomplished via the cranial-most aspect of the tricuspid annulus, and especially so if a Cournard-2 (CRD-2) type curve catheter is used.

Deflectable tip catheters are preferred when recording the His bundle activity through accesses other than the femoral vein, and may be useful when the anatomy of the His bundle region is altered. To record the His bundle activity from the noncoronary cusp, the deflectable catheter is moved retrogradely up the descending aorta via the femoral arterial approach on either side. It is often helpful to use the right anterior oblique projection to negotiate the arch of the aorta. In the right anterior oblique projection, the tip of the catheter is deflected anteriorly to negotiate the aortic arch. Once the catheter enters the ascending aorta, it may be de-deflected and gently pushed downwards. The operator must be careful to not point the catheter anteriorly in the proximal ascending aorta, as the coronary artery ostia are normally located anteriorly. The catheter is gently pushed down the ascending aorta in the right anterior oblique projection while maintaining a posterior deflection to reach the base of the noncoronary cusp to record the His bundle deflection. The noncoronary cusp location of the catheter tip can be confirmed by its central location in the left anterior oblique projection **(Figures 1.12A and B)**.

The above two are the most commonly used approaches to record the His bundle activity. His bundle recordings may also be obtained from the left ventricle by deflecting a catheter onto the membranous atrioventricular/proximal interventricular septum on the left side of the heart via the antegrade, trans-septal or the retrograde, aortic approach **(Figures 1.13A and B)**.

His bundle activity may also be recorded by a catheter introduced via the superior vena cava and deflected onto the His bundle area via the cranial-most aspect of the tricuspid annulus in the right anterior oblique projection. It is comparatively more difficult to record His bundle activity from the superior vena caval approach. The use of closely spaced (2 mm or 1 mm interelectrode distance) Hexapolar catheters allow more precise recording of His bundle conduction. This may be required when elucidation of intra-Hisian conduction delays or direction of His bundle activation (proximal to distal versus distal to proximal) are crucial to the study.

Manipulation in the His bundle/right bundle area can sometimes cause catheter trauma-induced right bundle branch block. This is usually transient and resolves within few seconds to minutes. Catheter trauma-induced right bundle branch block can uncommonly persist for hours, and rarely be permanent. Gentle manipulation to avoid this is crucial when presence of intact right bundle conduction is required for the electrophysiology study. Manipulation in the His bundle/right bundle area should be performed with great care in the presence of left bundle branch block, as catheter trauma to the right bundle can sometimes cause transient complete atrioventricular (AV) block in this scenario. In the presence of left bundle branch block, it may be preferable to try to obtain the His bundle deflection while advancing the catheter gently forward through the His bundle area, rather than while withdrawing from the right ventricle across the right bundle to avoid this complication. Another useful precaution in this scenario is to first keep back-up right ventricular apical pacing ready through a catheter introduced through the caudal aspect of the tricuspid annulus. In presence of left bundle branch block, in case the His bundle deflection cannot be obtained via the transtricuspid route after significant manipulation, it may be prudent to switch to the aortic route of obtaining the His bundle deflection to avoid this complication.

The Fascicular System

Recording of activity from the right and left fascicular systems is important in mapping and ablation of certain arrhythmias like tachyarrhythmias involving atriofascicular bypass tracts, fascicular ventricular tachycardia, bundle branch re-entry, and other Purkinje-fiber mediated tachyarrhythmias. Besides, knowledge of the distribution of the normal fascicular system is useful in differentiating fascicular potentials from myocardial activity. Recording of right bundle activity can be accomplished by simply pushing the

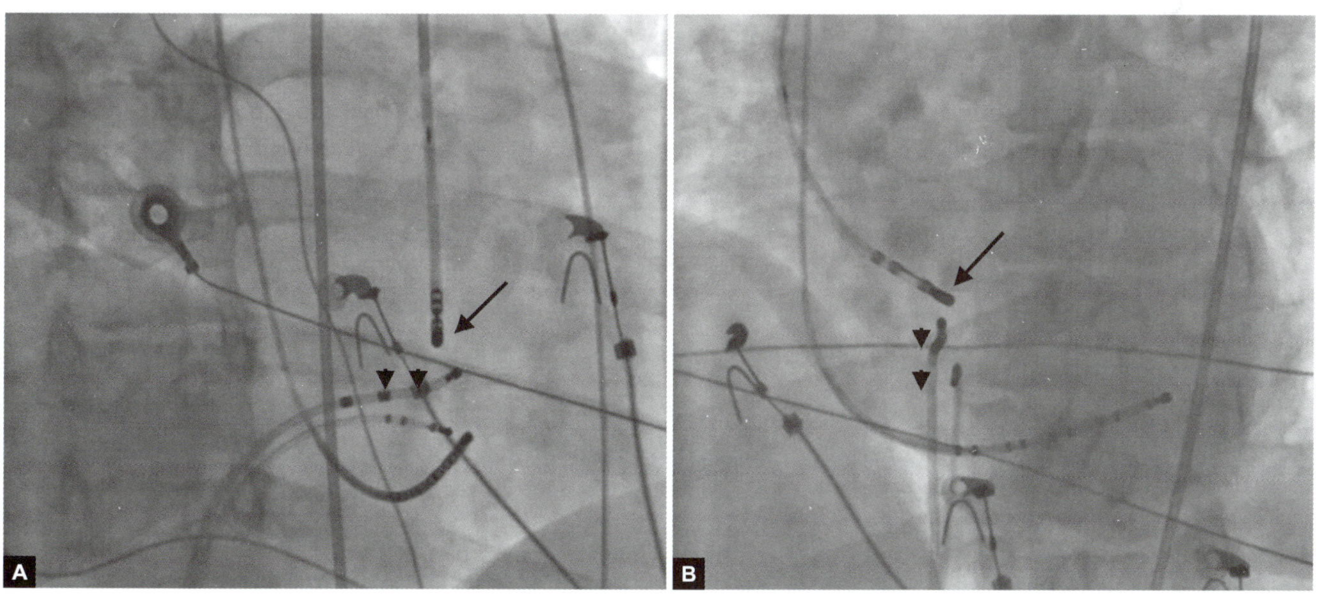

Figures 1.12A and B: Catheter positions used to record His bundle activity. The ablation catheter (single arrow) is positioned to record the His bundle electrogram through the noncoronary cusp, and the Cournard-2 diagnostic quadripolar catheter (multiple arrowheads) is positioned to record His bundle activity via the femoral venous route. Catheter positions are shown in right anterior oblique (A) and left anterior oblique (B) projections

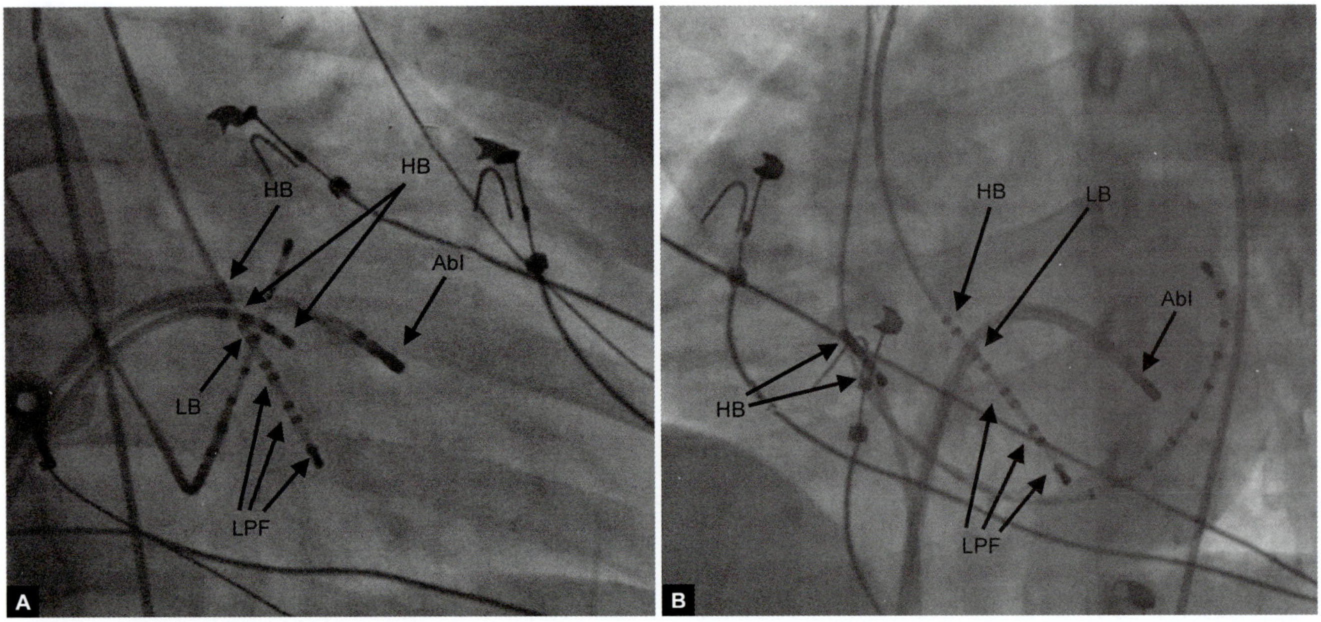

Figures 1.13A and B: (A) (Right anterior oblique projection) and (B) (Left anterior oblique projection). Catheter positions to record left bundle branch activity. The decapolar catheter introduced into the left ventricle through the retrograde approach records the His bundle deflection in bipole 9–10, the left bundle deflection in bipole 7–8, and the proximal part of the left posteroseptal fascicle in electrodes 1–6. The quadripolar catheter introduced via the femoral vein records the His bundle deflection from the right side of the septum
Abbreviations: HB, His bundle; LB, left bundle; LPF, left posteroseptal fascicle. The ablation catheter (Abl) is in the left ventricle through the trans-septal approach

catheter into the right ventricle along the septum from the point of distal His bundle recording. This may be done in the right anterior oblique projection, where the interventricular septum is located along the middle third of ventricular silhouette or in the left anterior oblique projection, where the septum lies parallel to the spine. A 2-5-2 spaced deflectable decapolar catheter may be positioned with its proximal bipole at the level of the proximal His bundle to provide simultaneous recording of the entire His bundle-right bundle system **(Figures 1.14A and B)**. Right bundle activation can be recorded from the distal bipoles using this technique. This technique is useful when elucidation of the sequence of His bundle-right bundle activation is critical to the study, as in mapping of right sided atriofascicular accessory pathways.

The left bundle branch and the posteroinferior part of the left fascicular system can be mapped with either a decapolar catheter placed along the left side of the interventricular septum in the left anterior oblique projection via the retrograde route, or by moving a quadripolar catheter along the septum via the same approach **(Figures 1.15A and B)**. The retrograde approach to the left ventricle provides better access to the posteroinferior part of the left fascicular system as compared to the antegrade, trans-septal approach. The anterolateral left ventricular fascicular system can be mapped by deflecting a catheter onto the basal and mid anterolateral wall of the left ventricle. Catheter placement in this location is guided by both right anterior oblique and left anterior oblique projections as depicted.

Trans-septal Access

The trans-septal approach allows access to the left atrium, pulmonary veins, mitral annulus and the left ventricle. This access should be obtained through the fossa ovalis, preferably at its thinnest part. Puncture of the area between the superior border of the fossa ovalis and the superior vena cava should be avoided as this area, although referred to as the "septum secundum", is an infolding of the atrial wall filled with adipose tissue. A needle puncturing this area is likely to exit the cardiac cavity and track along the roof of the left atrium. Occasionally, a needle might puncture both folds of the atrium in this location to gain access to the left atrium. In such cases, bleeding with/without tamponade might result immediately or subsequently.[2]

The equipment for trans-septal access consists of one of several long sheaths (standard adult sheath length 63 cm, inner dilator length 67 cm), 0.035" or 0.032" J-tipped wire for tracking the sheath into the superior vena cava, the septal puncture needle (standard adult needle length 71 cm), and an 0.028" or 0.032" wire of 140 cm length for tracking the sheath into the left atrium. The 175 cm, 0.025" stainless steel Torayguide™ wire is our preferred wire for tracking

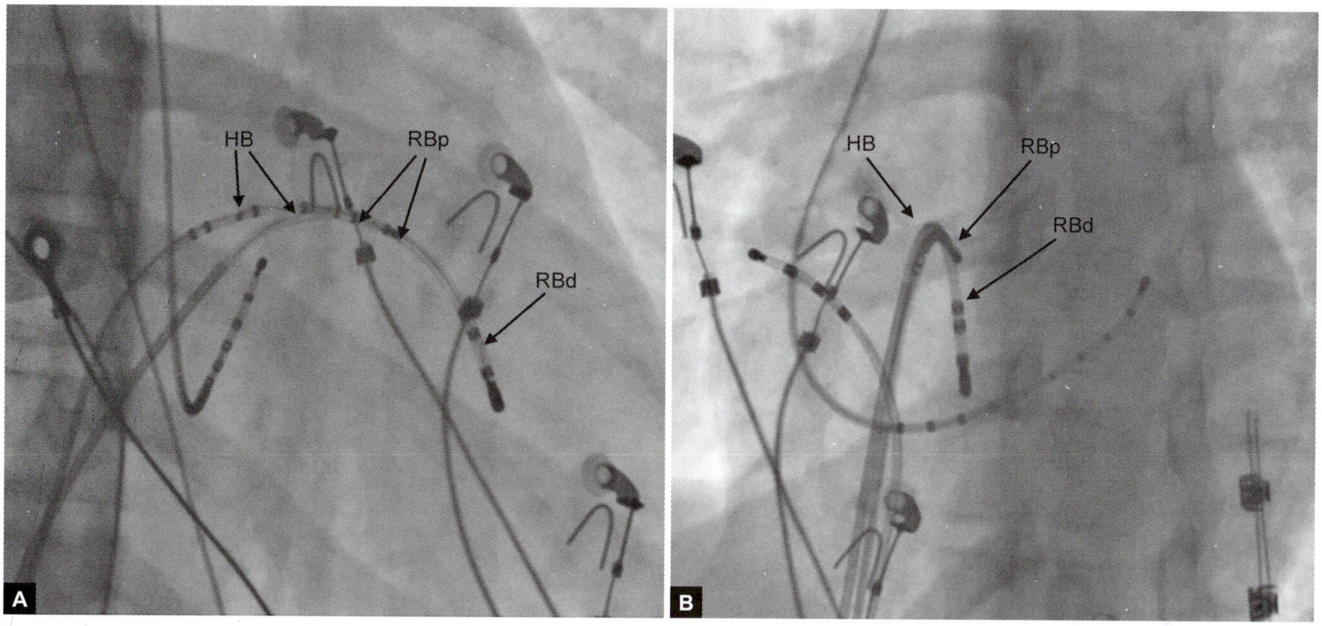

Figures 1.14A and B: Catheter position to record activity from the His bundle and right bundle, seen in right anterior oblique (A) and left anterior oblique (B) projections
Abbreviations: HB, His bundle; RBp, proximal right bundle; RBd, distal right bundle

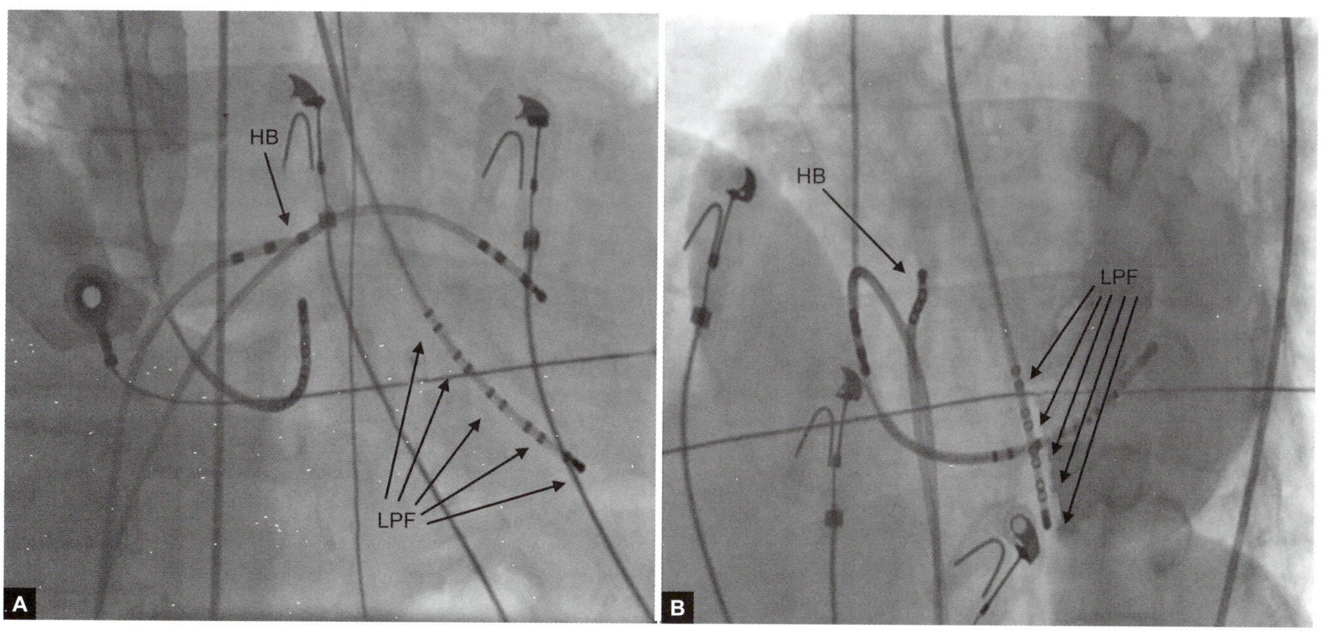

Figures 1.15A and B: Position of a decapolar catheter to record activity from the posteroseptal area of the left posteroseptal fascicular system, in right anterior oblique (A) and left anterior oblique (B) projections
Abbreviations: HB, His bundle; LPF, left posterior fascicle

the sheath into the left atrium. This wire has a coiled tip which ensures that the wire curls downward within the left atrium upon entry, ensuring that no structure is damaged by the wire tip after entry into the left atrium. This wire also provides adequate support to track a sheath or dilator across a tough septum, and makes the sheath curve down towards the mitral annulus.

The sheath may be of fixed curve type, like the Mullin's or one of the Swartz left sided sheaths, or deflectable tip type, like the Agilis sheath. Sheaths for trans-septal access should have valves at the proximal end to prevent entry of air, and should preferably have side ports that allow periodical flushing/irrigation/injection of contrast. The commonly used needle is the Brockenbrough needle, with an angulation at its tip. The Brockenbrough-1 type needle has a greater degree of angulation at its tip, and may be useful when an unusually vertically oriented interatrial septum cannot be engaged with the standard curve Brockenbrough needle **(Figure 1.16)**. Septal puncture using the standard Brockenbrough needle is by mechanical pressure. A blunt-tipped Brockenbrough curve needle which uses radiofrequency energy for septal puncture (NRG® RF Transseptal Needle, Baylis Medical, Montreal, Canada) is also available, and may be particularly useful for puncture of thick or aneurysmal septae, and in presence of significantly altered septal anatomy.[3]

Septal puncture may be guided by fluoroscopic landmarks, transesophageal echocardiography, or by intracardiac echocardiography. The use of transesophageal echocardiography for septal puncture is cumbersome and uncomfortable for the unanesthetized patient, and has largely been abandoned in presence of normal anatomy; this technique should be kept in mind as an option in presence of altered anatomy. Fluoroscopic landmarks suffice to guide puncture of the fossa ovalis in the majority of cases. Intracardiac echocardiography helps to tailor the site of puncture within the fossa to the site that requires to be accessed for mapping/ablation; for example, puncture of a more posterior part of the septum is desirable for pulmonary vein isolation whereas puncture of the mid part of the fossa provides easier access to the anterior part of the mitral annulus. Intracardiac echocardiography is also helpful in situations altering septal anatomy, as in a dilated aortic root distorting the orientation of the septum, or in guiding puncture of an unusually thick septum.

Though septal puncture may be accomplished via either femoral vein, it is easier through the right femoral venous approach. The procedure is done under continuous invasive arterial pressure monitoring. Some centers prefer to perform septal puncture before administration of heparin, whereas

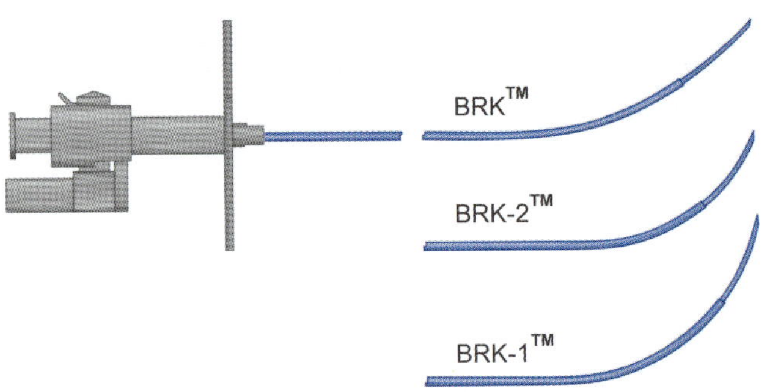

Figure 1.16: Brockenbrough ("BRK") type needles of varying tip angulations designed for interatrial septal puncture with manual pressure. These needles are available in pediatric (56 cm) and various adult (71, 89 and 98 cm) lengths. Needles of greater curve are used for septae that are less convex towards the right atrium

some others administer up to 2500 units of intravenous heparin at the time of vascular access prior to septal puncture. The coronary sinus and/or the His bundle catheters may be introduced before septal puncture, and mark the locations of the posterior wall of the left atrium and the base of the noncoronary cusp of the aorta respectively. A coronary sinus catheter introduced via the superior vena cava may hamper manipulation of the septal puncture hardware at the point at which the catheter curves into the coronary sinus ostium. If so, it may have to be withdrawn into the high right atrium to prevent this. The Brockebrough needle is flushed with heparinized saline before septal puncture. It is then connected via a short extension tubing to a manifold with two three-way stop cocks to allow flushing and injection of contrast through one port, and recording of pressure through another port. The J-tipped 0.035" or 0.032" wire is now introduced into the superior vena cava. It is easier if the wire is manipulated a few centimeters into the innominate vein. The long sheath and its dilator are now tracked together atop this wire into the superior vena cava or preferably the innominate vein, with its curve facing medially. The wire is now removed, and the sheath-dilator assembly is flushed with heparinized saline. The needle with the attached manifold is now introduced through the dilator with its curve directed in the same orientation as that of the sheath and dilator. The tip of the needle is maintained just inside the dilator until the puncture is made. There is an arrowhead like marker near the needle hub to guide its orientation. When viewed from the foot end, this arrowhead usually faces towards approximately the 3 O'clock position at this point in the procedure. For fluoroscopically-guided puncture, the base of the noncoronary cusp is now located, usually guided by the position of the His bundle catheter, or using the location of a pigtail catheter placed in the noncoronary cusp. The entire septal puncture assembly consisting of the sheath, dilator and needle are withdrawn into the right atrium in either the right anterior oblique or the posteroanterior projection, while applying a slight posterior and clockwise torque. The relative positions of the sheath, dilator and needle are maintained by stabilizing the sheath with the operator's left hand, and the needle with the right hand. The septal puncture assembly should face towards the aortic root during this movement **(Figures 1.17A to E)**. During gentle downward withdrawal, three abrupt "dips" are usually felt, each corresponding to an abrupt slightly more posterior and leftward movement of the assembly. The first of these occurs as the assembly enters the right atrium from the superior vena cava. The second occurs as the lower border of the aortic root is crossed. The first two dips may be very gentle, and may not be perceived at all. The third dip occurs as the needle crosses the superior limbus of the fossa ovalis. This third and final dip occurs just below the lower border of the noncoronary cusp, is usually the most prominent of the three, and is often associated with a slight spontaneous clockwise turn of the needle-sheath assembly. The downward withdrawal is stopped once this dip is felt.

If this dip does not occur spontaneously, applying more clockwise torque on the assembly by rotating the needle hub at the location of the expected dip can be helpful; the arrowhead marker on the needle hub faces between 3 and 6 O'clock at the end of this movement. The position of the marker on the needle hub is only an indicator of needle tip position. The marker position that corresponds to a needle tip position at the center of the fossa ovalis may vary depending on alterations in septal anatomy. In case the foramen ovale is patent, the tip of the dilator would now enter the left atrium through it, and this access to the left atrium usually suffices. In the majority of cases, it is necessary to proceed with puncture of the fossa ovalis as described below. The tip of the dilator should now be located approximately one-half to one vertebral space below the lower border of the noncoronary cusp, and should face towards the noncoronary cusp in the right anterior oblique projection; minor adjustments may be made to attain this orientation **(Figures 1.17A to E)**. The position of the dilator tip is now inspected in the left anterior oblique or lateral projection. It should face towards the posterior wall of the left atrium, and should be located approximately midway between posterior part of the aortic root and the posterior wall of the left atrium **(Figures 1.17A to E)**. If it is not, the assembly is rotated to attain such an orientation. The tip of the dilator should snugly abut the interatrial septum such that the pulsations of the left atrium can be felt by the operator through the assembly. Slight forward pressure may be exerted on the sheath dilator assembly using the left hand (while maintaining steady needle position with the right hand) to make the assembly abut the septum snugly. The pressure recording from the needle should now reveal a damped tracing in the form of a flat line. Septal location of the sheath tip may be confirmed by contrast injection through the needle in the left anterior oblique or lateral projection. The contrast stain of the septum often provides an idea about the septal thickness at the point at which the sheath-dilator assembly has engaged it. The slight forward pressure exerted on the assembly "tents" the septum; this tenting may be visible in the contrast stain **(Figures 1.17A to E)**. The sheath and dilator are now stabilized with the left hand and the septum is punctured with an abrupt forward movement of the needle using the right hand. At the point of septal puncture, an abrupt give-way of resistance is felt. The tented septum falls back onto the needle at the moment of puncture; this too, may be visible on the contrast stain **(Figures 1.17A to E)**. It is important to arrest forward movement of the needle at this precise point. Entry into the left atrium is confirmed by appearance of left atrial pressure waveforms. A small puff of contrast injected through the needle at this point, in the left anterior oblique/lateral/anteroposterior/right anterior oblique projection helps to confirm entry into the left atrium as well as to assess the distance from the point of puncture to the roof and the posterior wall of the left atrium **(Figures 1.17A to E)**. It is imperative to confirm that the needle has entered the left atrium before the next step. If it has not, the assembly can be withdrawn and another puncture may be attempted if the hemodynamics remain stable. Introduction of the dilator-sheath assembly into a structure other than the left atrium (like the aortic root, or the pericardial reflection of the septum secundum area), or its passage through the roof or posterior wall of the left atrium due to excessive forward/posterior/superior movement of the needle after septal puncture can be catastrophic, whereas isolated needle puncture of these areas usually seals off without such consequences. Once septal puncture is accomplished, the dilator and sheath are pushed over the needle to just beyond the needle tip, the needle is removed, the sheath is aspirated and flushed with heparinized saline, and the 0.025"/0.028"/0.032" wire is introduced into the left atrium though the sheath. The puncture needle is removed with the right hand while maintaining the dilator-sheath assembly steady with the left hand. Until the operator is sufficiently experienced, it is recommended to fluoroscopically visualize the tip of the sheath-dilator system during this step, as removal of the needle can sometimes cause partial rotation of the sheath-dilator assembly and its exit back into the right atrium. A bolus of 2500 to 4000 units of heparin (depending on the amount administered prior to septal puncture) is administered soon after the wire accesses the left atrium. The sheath is now tracked into the left atrium over the wire while the dilator is simultaneously removed. The wire is then removed, and the desired catheter is introduced into the sheath. Subsequent heparinization is guided by the activated clotting time value checked 10 minutes after the heparin bolus. It is important to realize that puncture of the interatrial septum is a painless procedure.

The septal puncture needle might occasionally slide up the septum without puncturing it. If this happens, one should confirm in the right anterior oblique/anteroposterior projection that it does not slide above the limbus of the fossa ovalis at the point of puncture. Engaging the sheath-needle assembly at a slightly more leftward part of the septum in the left anterior oblique projection can sometimes help to prevent this sliding movement. Upward sliding of the Brockenbrough needle during attempted puncture sometimes occurs because the septum is more vertical than usual. In such cases, using the more curved Brockenbrough-1 needle helps to overcome the problem. In all situations where the septal puncture assembly is manipulated in the left anterior oblique/lateral projection to adjust its orientation, the final orientation should be confirmed as facing towards the aortic root in the right anterior oblique projection prior to puncture. In some situations, usually in the presence of a very dilated/unfolded aortic root (as may happen in elderly, hypertensives, and in the presence of significant aortic stenosis/regurgitation), the interatrial septum is pushed to a more horizontal orientation than usual. Comparing the orientation of the interatrial septum in **Figures 1.17A to E** (usual orientation) and **Figures 1.18A to C** (horizontal

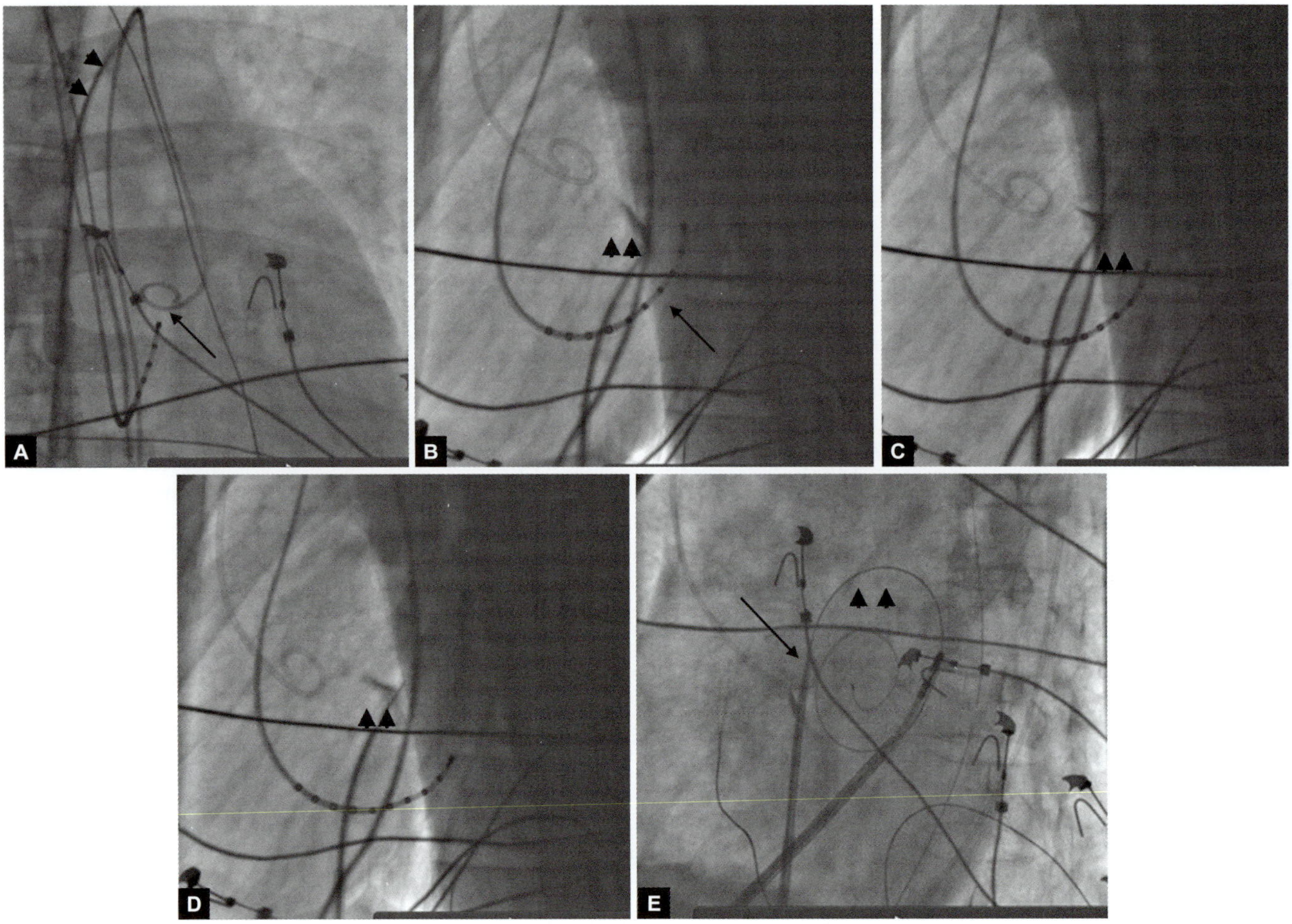

Figures 1.17A to E: Steps in fluoroscopically-guided septal puncture in presence of a normally-oriented interatrial septum. (A) is in right anterior oblique projection; (B to D) are in lateral projection; (E) is in the left anterior oblique projection. Prior to the puncture, the location of the septal puncture assembly is confirmed in right anterior oblique and left anterior oblique/lateral views; the puncturing movement per se may be performed in the right anterior oblique/left anterior oblique/lateral projection as per operator preference. First, the location of the noncoronary cusp of the aorta is ascertained using a pigtail catheter positioned in the posterior-most aortic cusp in the right anterior oblique projection (A, single arrow); alternatively, the location of a catheter recording the compact His bundle deflection may be used as surrogate. (A) also shows the initial position of the septal puncture assembly. At this point, the tip of the needle is just within the dilator, the tip of the dilator is within the left innominate vein (dual arrowheads), and the marker on the needle hub points to approximately 3 O'clock. (B) Shows the position of the septal puncture assembly just before puncture. The needle tip is still within the dilator. The coronary sinus catheter (single arrow) may be used to mark the posterior border of the left atrium as shown. The tip of the dilator firmly abuts the septum, which has been stained by a puff of contrast (dual arrowheads). At this point, the marker on the needle hub usually points to between 5 and 6 O'clock. (C) Shows the position just prior to the moment of puncture. The septum has been stretched ("tented") towards the left atrium (dual arrowheads) by the needle tip which has been protruded out of the dilator by a sharp forward movement of the operator's right hand. Note that the assembly has slid up a few mm compared to its location in (B). This amount of sliding may happen, and is acceptable. If it is felt that the assembly has slid up beyond the superior border of the fossa ovalis, further movement should be arrested immediately, and needle tip position should be confirmed to be below the inferior-most margin of the noncoronary cusp in the right anterior oblique projection. Some operators prefer to deliberately pull the assembly down by a few mm before the puncturing motion in anticipation of this slight upward sliding. (D) Shows the needle tip across the septum. The tented septum has now fallen back onto the needle (dual arrowheads); needle movement is immediately arrested. A small puff of contrast injected through the needle at this point confirms entry into the left atrium. This injection, usually performed in the right anterior oblique/left anterior oblique/anteroposterior view, also helps to assess the distance from the point of septal puncture to the posterosuperior left atrial roof; this gives an idea of how far the dilator-sheath assembly can be safely pushed forward over the needle. (E) Shows the coil shaped Inoue wire (dual arrowheads) introduced into the left atrium through the dilator to allow tracking of the sheath into the left atrium over the wire. The extent to which the dilator-sheath assembly has been pushed into the left atrium beyond the point of puncture (arrow) can also be appreciated in this panel

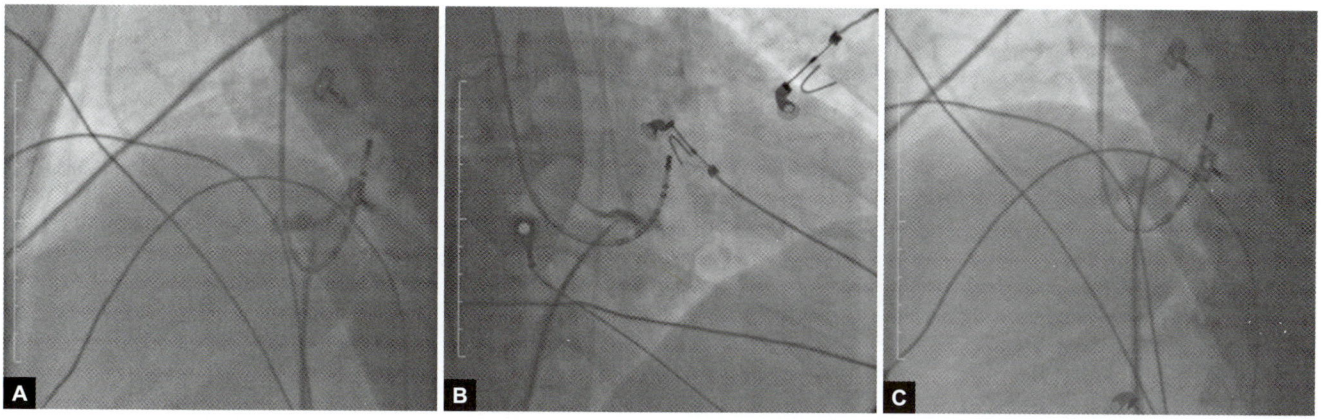

Figures 1.18A to C: (A) Lateral projection; (B) Right anterior oblique projection; and (C) (Lateral projection) depict steps in septal contrast stain-guided fluoroscopic puncture of an interatrial septum that is oriented more horizontally than usual due to an unfolded aortic root

orientation) provides an idea of some of the alterations that occur in interatrial septal anatomy. Fluoroscopically-guided puncture with standard equipment is still possible in altered septal anatomies, after injecting contrast to stain the septum prior to puncture. Use of intracardiac echocardiography to guide puncture is preferable in such situations as it may not be possible to engage the relatively thinner area of the septum under fluoroscopic guidance in presence of altered septal anatomy.

For intracardiac echocardiography-guided septal puncture, the intracardiac echocardiography catheter is usually introduced into the right atrium through the left femoral vein. The His bundle/aortic root catheter is not required during intracardiac echocardiography-guided septal puncture. The intracardiac echocardiography catheter is initially positioned in the mid right atrium with the controls in neutral position to view the tricuspid valve and the right ventricle. This view is called the "home view" **(Figure 1.19)**.

Gradual clockwise rotation from this view allows sequential visualization of anterior to posterior structures starting with the aortic root and the pulmonary artery, followed by the mitral valve and the left atrial appendage along with the anterior aspect of the fossa ovalis, and finally the pulmonary venous ostia along with the posterior aspect of the fossa ovalis. Slight posterior and/or leftward deflection of the transducer tip may be required for adequate visualization of the fossa ovalis. Septal puncture must be accomplished in a plane posterior to the plane of the aortic root, at an area where there is adequate space from the interatrial septum to the posterior wall of the left atrium. The site of puncture should also be a relatively thin area of the interatrial septum. With the needle tip just inside the dilator, the appropriate site in the septum is engaged by the septal puncture assembly under intracardiac echocardiography guidance. Tenting of the septum at this area is visualized on snugly engaging the septum **(Figure 1.20)**. Subsequently, the septum is punctured with the needle, at which point sudden loss of resistance is felt on the needle, and the tented part of the septum abruptly collapses back onto the needle.

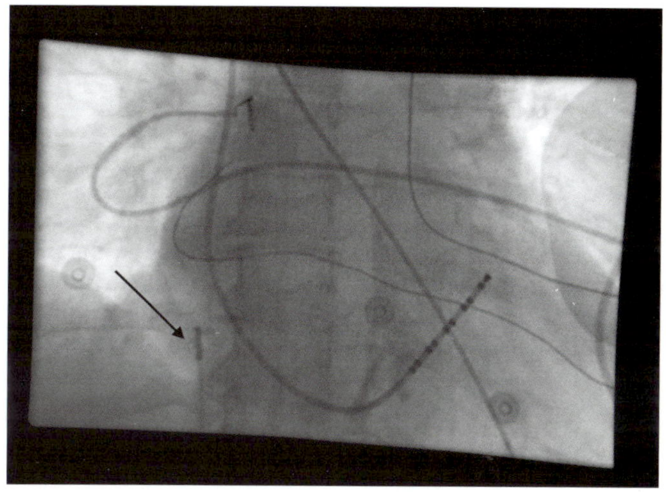

Figure 1.19: Fluoroscopic orientation of the intracardiac echocardiography catheter (arrow) (shown in anteroposterior projection) to obtain the "home view". A slight tilt/rotation (as shown in the figure) may sometimes be required to obtain an adequate home view

Advancement of the needle is promptly arrested, and the rest of the assembly is introduced into the left atrium as described previously. Radiofrequency energy for septal puncture is preferred in situations where an unusually thick septum precludes puncture by manual pressure exerted through the Brockenbrough needle. In cases where two transseptal accesses are required, two separate septal punctures may be made adjacent to each other, or two accesses may be obtained via a single septal puncture. To obtain two accesses via a single puncture, the sheath and dilator are introduced into the left atrium through the initial puncture, so that the site of puncture is dilated. The left atrial access wire is retained in the left atrium, and the sheath and dilator are withdrawn into the right atrium. The second sheath-dilator

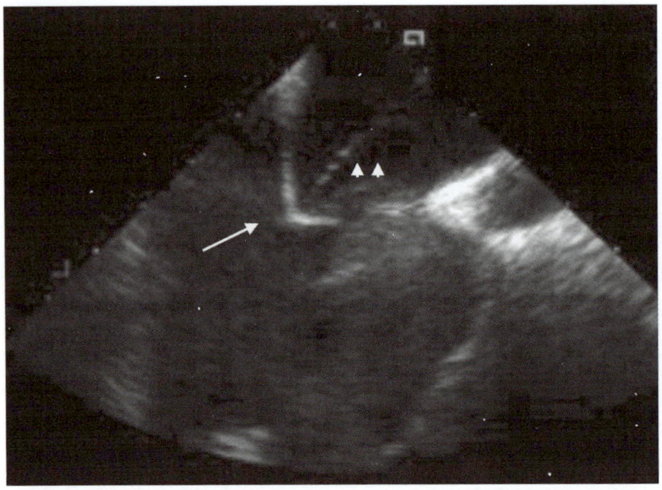

Figure 1.20: Tenting of the interatrial septum (arrow) by the septal puncture needle (dual arrowheads) visualized on intracardiac echocardiography just prior to septal puncture

assembly is now tracked into the right atrium over a 0.032" or 0.035" wire, and the dilator is removed. A deflectable catheter is introduced through this second sheath into the right atrium, and the septal orifice made by the first puncture is located by probing the septum adjacent to the retained left atrial wire from the first puncture. Once the deflectable catheter enters the left atrium, the sheath-dilator assembly from the first puncture, and the sheath for the second trans-septal access are tracked into the left atrium over the left atrial wire and the deflectable catheter respectively. Alternatively, a straight 0.032" or 0.035" wire may be introduced into the left atrium beside the initial left atrial access wire, and a sheath-dilator assembly may be tracked into the left atrium over each of these wires.

Retrograde or Transaortic Access

This approach, usually obtained via the right femoral artery, is used to access the left ventricle and the mitral annulus. In comparison to antegrade approach to the left ventricle across the interatrial septum, this approach is particularly good for accessing areas of the left ventricular outflow tract just below the coronary cusps. In general, if certain areas of the left ventricle or mitral annulus cannot be accessed adequately by either the antegrade or the retrograde approach after reasonable amount of catheter manipulation, it is prudent to switch to the other approach.

For retrograde access, a deflectable catheter whose tip is curled into a tight J curve in the descending aorta is passed up to the aortic root while maintaining this curve. In the right anterior oblique projection, the base of the J curve is made to rest on the aortic leaflets. The curled catheter is now allowed to prolapse gently across the aortic valve **(Figures 1.21A to D)**. It is important to not let the J curve open anteriorly while in the aortic root, as it may engage the ostia of the coronary arteries, which are located anteriorly in the aortic root. The straight catheter tip must never be used to cross the aortic valve as this can damage the aortic leaflets, and provides less control over catheter tip movement at the point of entry into the left ventricle as compared to a curled catheter entering the left ventricle. Occasionally, the 'J' curl at the catheter tip may not be small enough to allow passage across the aortic arch, especially if large curve catheters are required for mapping the left ventricle. In such situations, the straight catheter is passed through the descending aorta up to the aortic arch. Once the area of the aortic arch is reached, the catheter is gently deflected anteriorly in the right anterior oblique projection, just enough to negotiate across the aortic arch and down into the ascending aorta. The J curl is now made in the aortic root, and the aortic valve is crossed as previously described. Continuous heparinization similar to trans-septal access is maintained during retrograde access as well.

The Outflow Tracts and Coronary Cusps

The right ventricular outflow tract is usually accessed via the transfemoral route. Bidirectionally deflectable catheters are particularly helpful in accessing the right ventricular outflow tract. When rotation within the right ventricular outflow tract is difficult, it is easier to rotate the catheter to the appropriate septal or free wall location in the pulmonary artery and to then pull the catheter down in the desired plane. Certain areas of the right ventricular outflow tract septum may be better accessed via the internal jugular route than the femoral route.[4] The coronary cusps and left ventricular outflow tract are accessed via the transfemoral, retrograde approach as described above.

Mitral and Tricuspid Annuli

The entire mitral annulus can be accessed via the antegrade trans-septal approach, by using a deflectable tip catheter of the medium to large size curves **(Figures 1.22A to D)**. Parts of the mitral annulus, especially the areas between 2 and 7 O'clock in the left anterior oblique projection, may also be accessed via the retrograde transaortic approach **(Figures 1.22A to D)**. This is best accomplished using medium and small sized catheter curves. For this approach, the catheter is made to face posteriorly towards the coronary sinus catheter in the right anterior oblique projection after left ventricular entry, and then deflected up towards the mitral annulus. Subsequently, rotation and deflection/de-deflection of the catheter provides access to various parts of the annulus. As a general principle, until the operator is sufficiently experienced, it is preferable to do all pushing movements towards either ventricle in the right anterior oblique projection. This visualization will confirm the

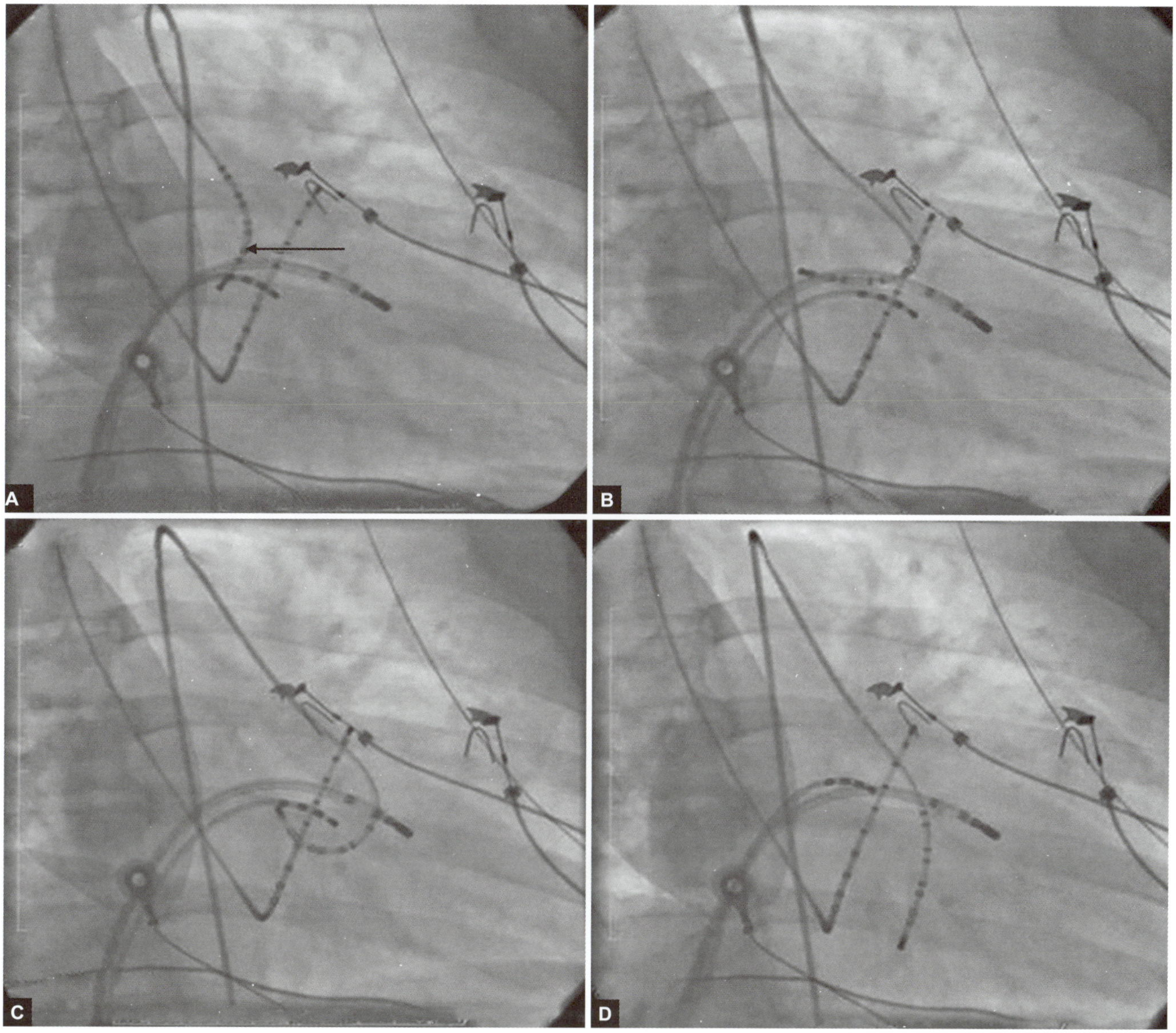

Figures 1.21A to D: Retrograde access to the left ventricle, obtained in the right anterior oblique projection. The deflectable catheter for left ventricular access is introduced into the noncoronary cusp of the aorta, facing posteriorly and with its tip curved slightly (A). The tip is now curved more (alternatively, this curve may be made in the descending aorta also) (B). Upon gentle forward pressure, the loop begins to prolapse into the left ventricle during aortic valve opening (C). A slight forward push of the catheter at this point makes the loop prolapse fully into the left ventricle; the loop opens out as it prolapses in the left ventricle (D)

catheter as entering the ventricle rather than pushing against the free wall. Once the plane of the annulus is located in the right anterior oblique projection (by inspecting the electrograms from the distal bipole), the circumference of the annulus may be navigated in the left anterior oblique projection.

To navigate the tricuspid annulus, entry to the right ventricle is secured via the inferior vena caval approach in the right anterior oblique projection using a deflectable catheter of medium or large sized curves. The catheter is then pulled back gradually while maintaining the downward deflection. Appearance of atrial and ventricular electrograms in the recording indicates annular location of the catheter. Once the annulus is thus located, navigation along the annulus is performed in the left anterior oblique projection **(Figures 1.23A to F)**. Starting from approximately 5 O'clock on the tricuspid annulus, counterclockwise rotation while maintaining the downward deflection allows navigation

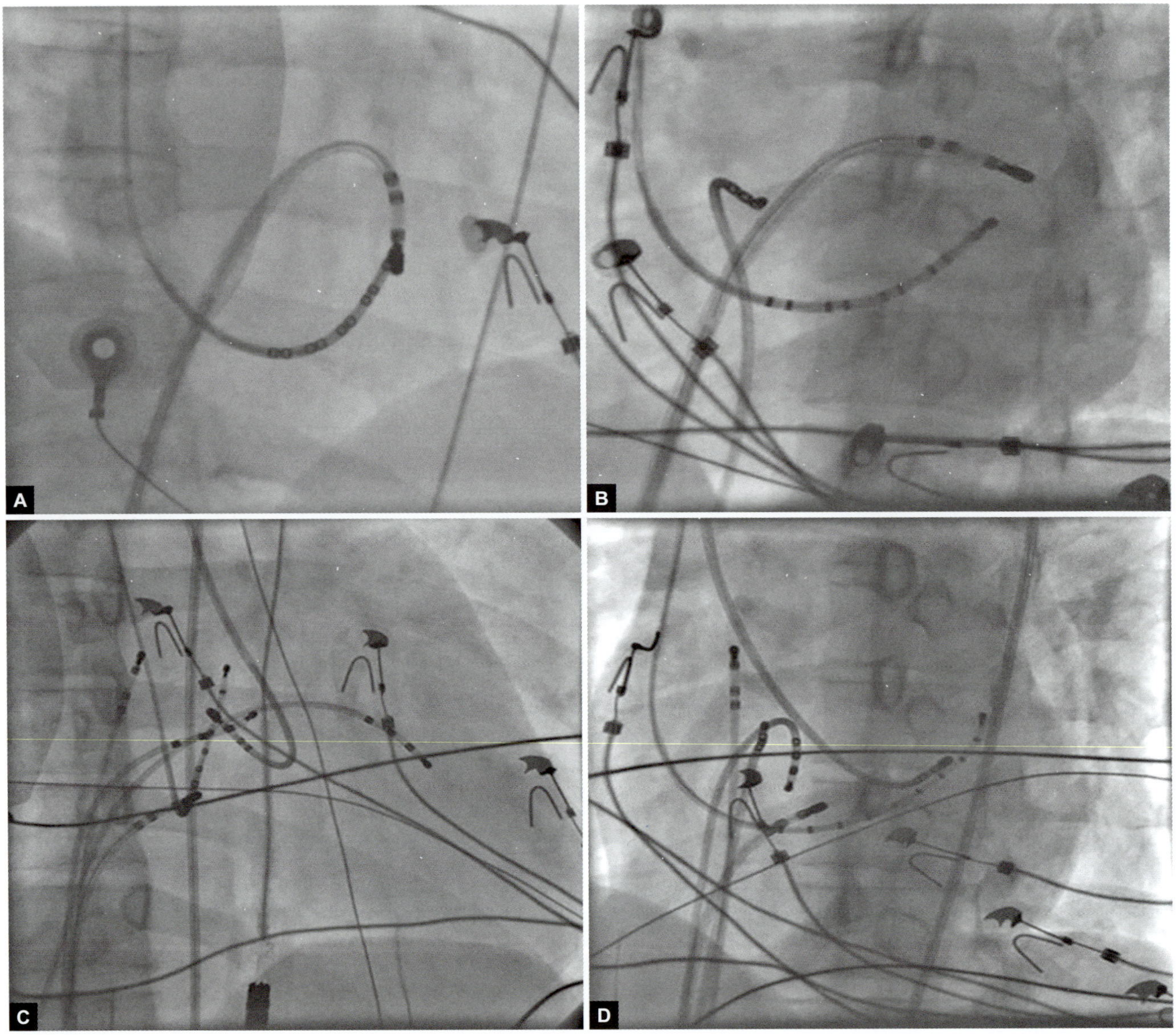

Figures 1.22A to D: Access to the mitral annulus through antegrade, trans-septal (A and B) and retrograde (C and D) approaches. (A) and (C) are in right anterior oblique projection; (B) and (D) are in left anterior oblique projection. Note that the plane of the coronary sinus catheter approximates, but does not always depict the plane of the endocardial mitral annulus

from approximately 5 O'clock to 8 O'clock locations on the annulus. De-deflection from the 8 O'clock location allows access up to the 12 O'clock location, whereas de-deflection from the 5 O'clock location allows access to the mid and anteroseptal locations. Counterclockwise rotation of the de-deflected catheter from the anteroseptal location allows access to the anterior tricuspid annulus. The anteroseptal, anterior and posterior parts of the tricuspid annulus may also be accessed via the transjugular approach using deflectable catheters of medium or small sized curves. This approach gives good catheter tip stability, albeit with less maneuverability. For this approach, the catheter is first introduced into the right ventricle and then deflected up to curve around the tricuspid leaflet to wedge into the ventricular aspect of the annulus. A similar method may occasionally be adopted via the inferior vena caval route to access the right ventricular aspect of the posteroinferior tricuspid annulus, especially in patients with dilated right ventricles. This approach usually requires the use of a precurved long sheath like a Mullin's sheath to enter the right ventricle at approximately 5 O'clock location on the tricuspid annulus followed by backward deflection of the catheter to the desired area.

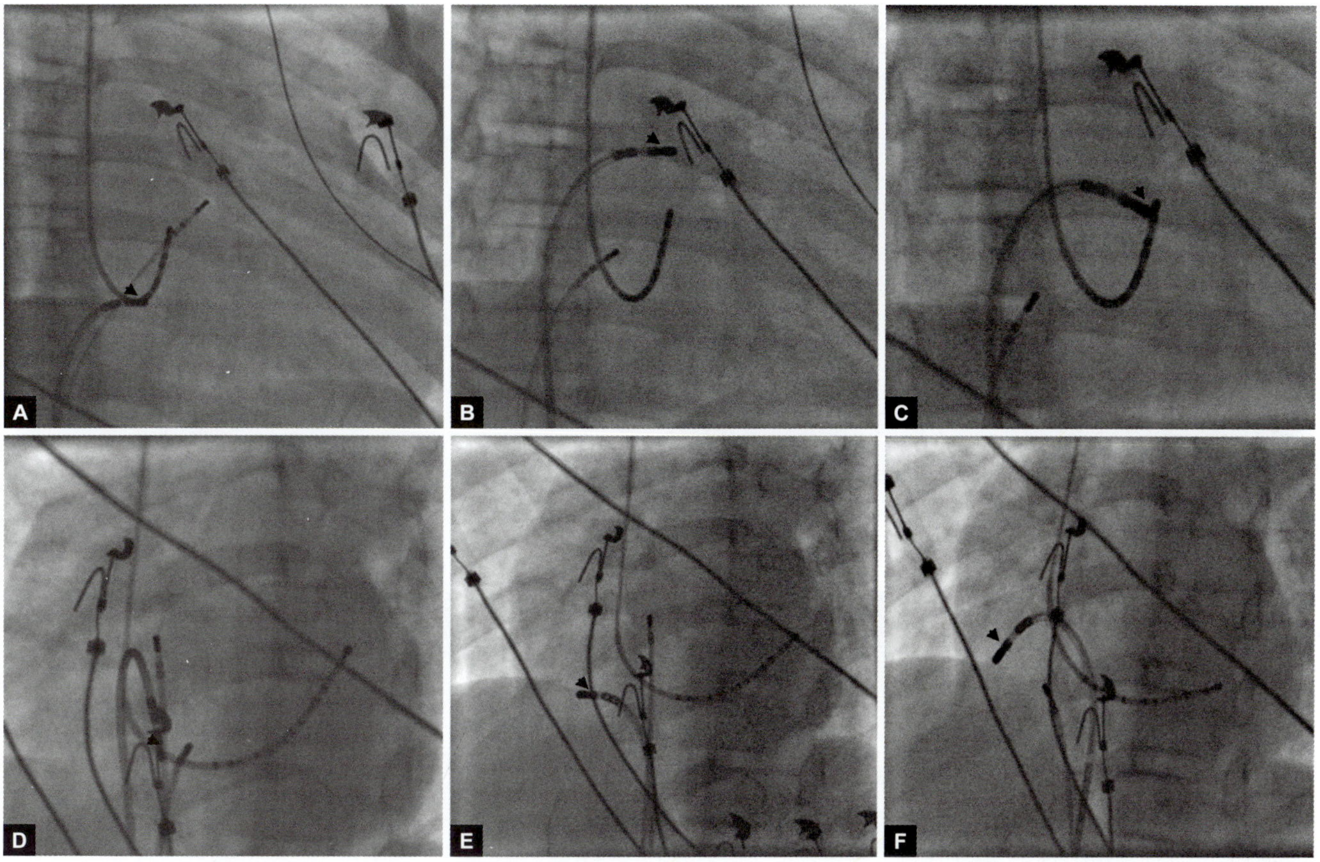

Figures 1.23A to F: Catheter locations along the tricuspid annulus (arrowheads). (A to C) Show 5, 12 and 8 O'clock locations respectively along the tricuspid annulus in the right anterior oblique projection; (D to F) Show 5, 7 and 8 O'clock locations respectively along the tricuspid annulus in the left anterior oblique projection

Energy delivery to the tissue around the anteroseptal tricuspid annulus may also be achieved via the noncoronary cusp of the aorta. To accomplish this, a catheter positioned in the noncoronary cusp is deflected posteroinferiorly towards the His bundle area in the right anterior oblique projection.

Accessory pathways may sometimes be located in relation to diverticula of the coronary sinus. These diverticula usually occur in relation to the proximal coronary sinus, and are best visualized by contrast injection into the proximal coronary sinus in the left anterior oblique projection through a catheter like the AL1 (Amplatz Curve Left-1) coronary diagnostic catheter **(Figure 1.24)**. The usual site of successful ablation of accessory pathways related to coronary sinus diverticula is near the neck of the diverticulum.

The Koch's Triangle

The slow input area into the AV node ("slow pathway") is the usual site of ablation for AV nodal reentrant tachycardia. This area is usually located in the posteroinferior part of the Koch's triangle, on the inferior interatrial septum between the ostium of the coronary sinus and the tricuspid annulus. In the most common technique used for ablation of AV nodal reentrant tachycardia, care is taken to not injure the fast input area into the AV node ("fast pathway). The fast pathway area is usually located in the part of the Koch's triangle that is anterosuperior to the slow pathway area. **Figures 1.25A to F** depict catheter positioning in various areas of the Koch's triangle. **Figures 1.26 and 1.27** depict the usual locations in the Koch's triangle where the slow pathway may be selectively ablated. It is important to remember that in an individual patient, the fast pathway area may be more posteroinferior and the slow pathway area may be more anterosuperior compared to what is depicted in the illustration.

Epicardial Access

Limited, transluminal recording of epicardial electrical activity may be obtained by catheters introduced into the coronary venous system. A limited, unipolar mapping via the more extensive coronary arterial system can be obtained

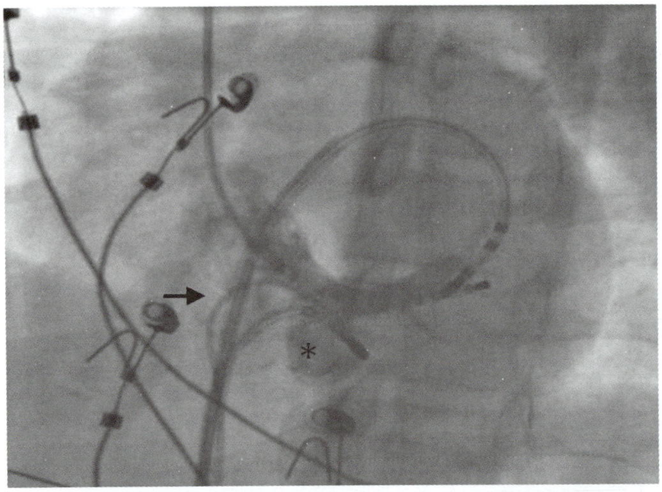

Figure 1.24: Contrast injection via an AL-1 diagnostic catheter (arrow) in left anterior oblique projection to facilitate catheter positioning in a diverticulum (*) associated with the coronary sinus. Coronary sinus diverticula are usually narrow-necked (as shown in the Figure). Accessory pathways are usually ablated at the level of the neck of the diverticulum, rather than within the diverticulum as shown in this figure. The figure also shows an ablation catheter positioned on the mitral annulus via the trans-septal approach, as well as a decapolar catheter in the coronary sinus, the tip of which is in a posterolateral tributary rather than in the coronary sinus per se

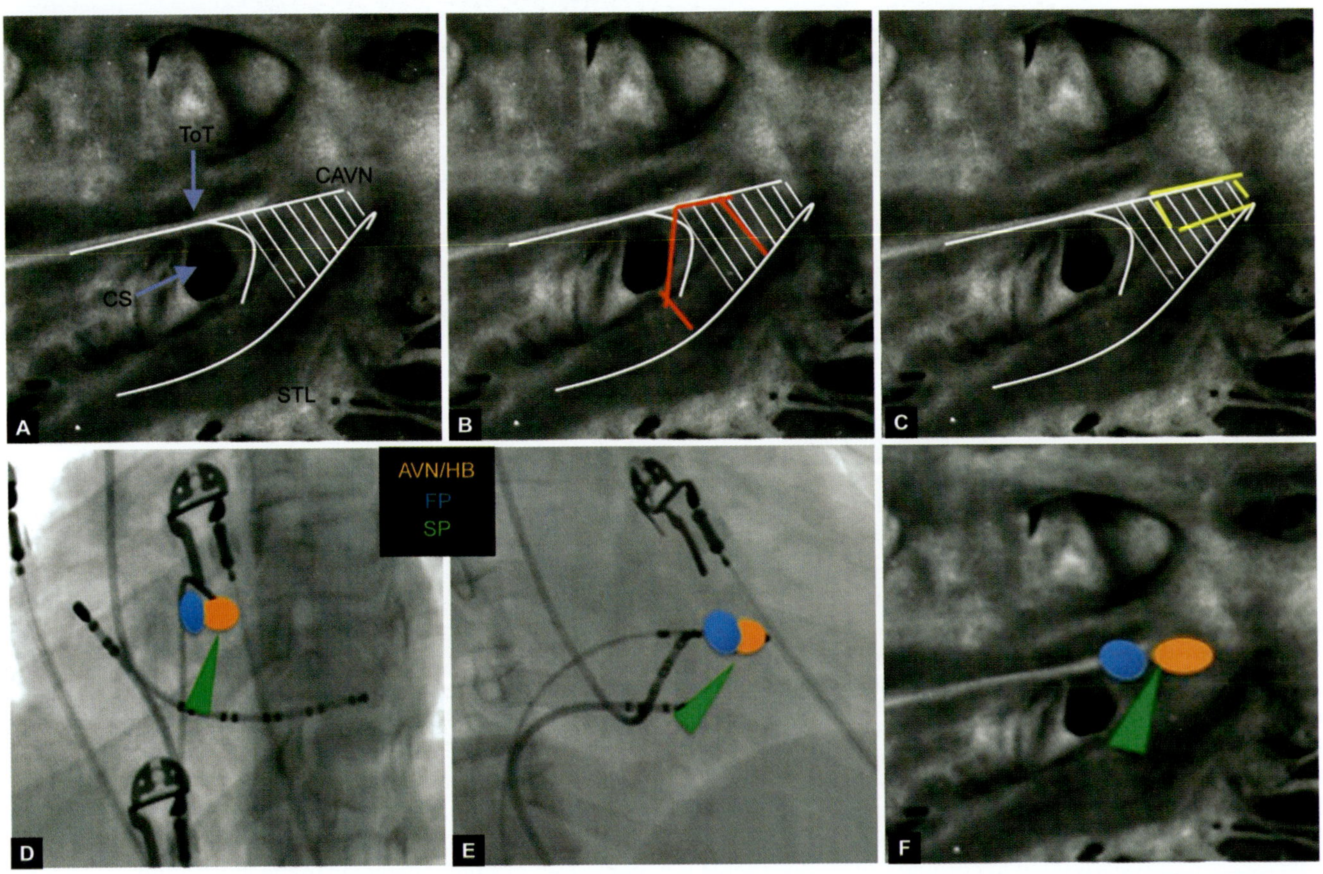

Figures 1.25A to F: The Koch's triangle and catheter positioning within it. In this dissection of the heart, the parallel white lines in (A to C) show the Koch's triangle, bounded by the ostium of the coronary sinus (CS), the Tendon of Todaro (ToT), and the septal tricuspid valve leaflet (STL). The compact AV node (CAVN) lies at the apex of the Koch's triangle, and approximately corresponds to the location of the recording of the His bundle deflection. The area bounded by the red lines in (B) depicts the usual location of the slow pathway input into the AV node. The area bounded by the yellow lines in (C) depicts the usual location of the fast pathway input into the AV node; (D) (Left anterior oblique projection); and (E) (Right anterior oblique projection) show the fluoroscopic locations corresponding to the usual slow pathway and fast pathway locations; and (F) Shows a dissection correlate of (D and E)

Abbreviations: AVN, compact AV node; HB, His bundle; FP, fast pathway; SP, slow pathway

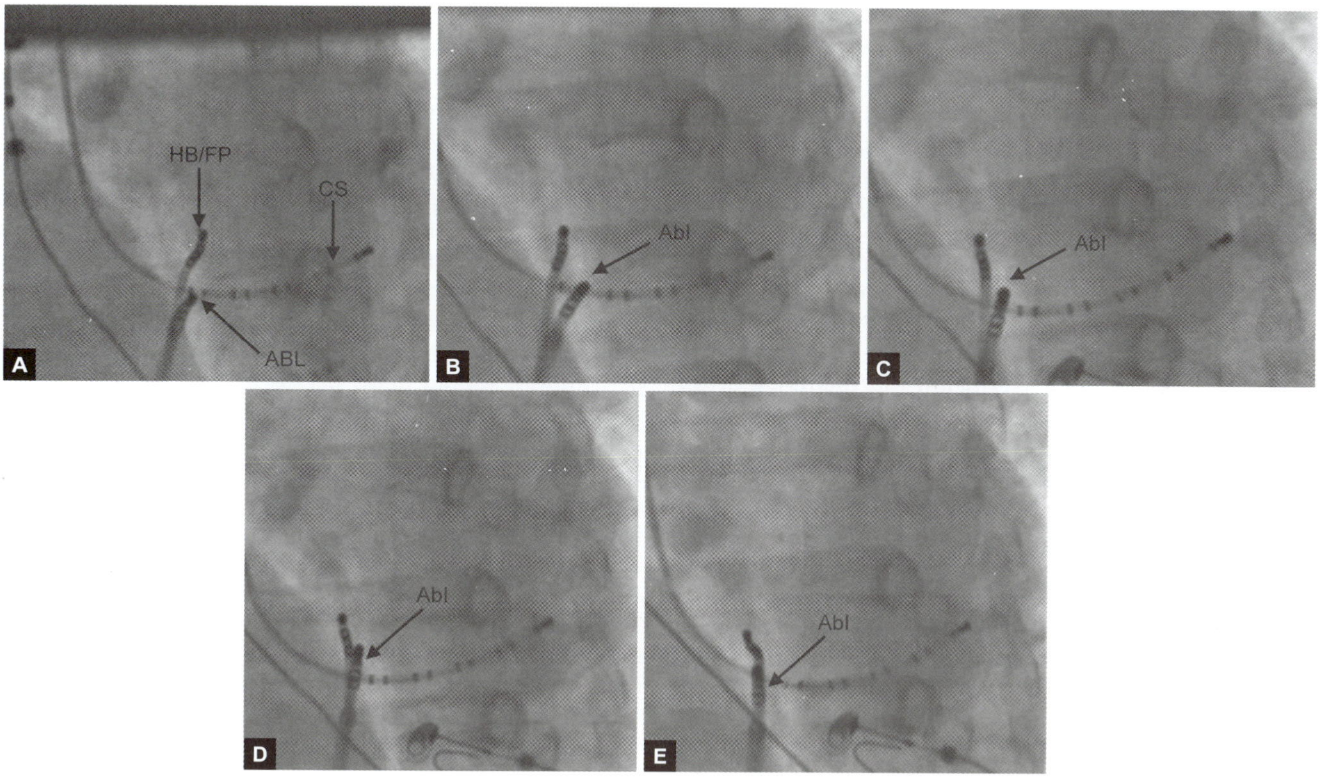

Figures 1.26A to E: Left anterior oblique projection showing ablation catheter locations used to ablate the slow pathway within the Koch's triangle, in presence of a relatively vertical interatrial septum. Contrast the images with those in Figure 1.27, where the ablation catheter is positioned in various locations in the Koch's triangle to ablate the slow pathway in the presence of a septum that is more convex towards the right atrium

Abbreviations: HB, His bundle; FP, fast pathway; CS, coronary sinus; Abl, Ablation catheter

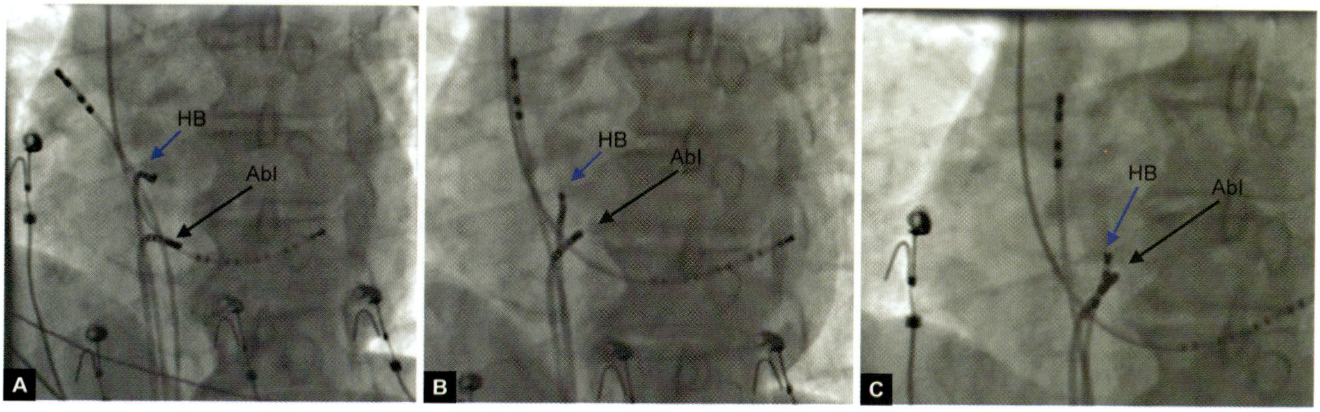

Figures 1.27A to C: Left anterior oblique projection showing ablation catheter locations used to ablate the slow pathway within the Koch's triangle, in presence of an interatrial septum that is more convex into the right atrium as compared to that in Figure 1.26 such septal curvatures are exaggerated in the presence of a dilated aortic root

Abbreviations: HB, His bundle; Abl, ablation catheter

by a 0.014" coronary wire introduced into the coronary arteries, and insulated up to the tip by an over-the-wire coronary balloon. Direct and extensive epicardial mapping and ablation is usually done via subxiphoid percutaneous epicardial access, using a technique first described by Sosa et al.[5] Percutaneous subxiphoid epicardial access may be obtained with the patient under deep conscious sedation, or under general anesthesia. The pericardial space is accessed using a Tuohy needle; the bevel at the tip of the needle reduces tissue injury and directs the guidewire appropriately. A endocardial catheter placed in the right ventricular apex aids in anatomical guidance during pericardial access. The fibrous pericardial reflection that extends onto the thoracic wall is punctured in the paraxiphoid angle between the left border of the xiphoid process and the inferior margin of the left thoracic cage to gain access to the space between the fibrous and visceral pericardial layers without puncturing the diaphragm. This entry point is superior to the xiphisternal attachment of the parachute—like dome of the diaphragm. In order to reach the pericardium at this point, the skin entry is made a few centimeter below this point; the depth of the subcutaneous tissue decides the distance between the point of skin entry and pericardial entry. A small nick is initially made in the skin, and the needle is introduced through this nick. Subsequent navigation is done under fluoroscopic guidance. Directing the needle just medial to the left shoulder in the 30 to 40° left anterior oblique projection grants access to the left posterolateral area of the pericardial sac few centimeters superior to the left ventricular apex. This is the most commonly used needle orientation during pericardial access, as most areas of the pericardium can be accessed through this entry. Alternatively, the needle may be directed more horizontally (more parallel to the skin) in the 30 to 40° left anterior oblique or the 20 to 30° right anterior oblique projection to access the anterior areas of the ventricles. The needle is introduced through the subcutaneous tissue without removing the inner trocar from the needle lumen. Once the needle is felt to abut a structure offering resistance, either by tactile feel or by fluoroscopy, the trocar is removed. A small amount of contrast material may now be injected through the needle to stain the tissue that abuts the needle tip. The spread of this contrast defines the position of the needle tip as abutting the fibrous pericardium (contrast tenting the pericardium), or in the case of an unintended, abdominal needle course below the diaphragm, as contrast layering the subdiaphragmatic space. A short, sharp forward movement of a needle tip abutting the fibrous pericardium should allow access to the pericardial space, with a distinct "give" in the resistance as the pericardium is punctured. Needle movement should immediately be halted. Injection at this point should show the contrast layering the pericardial space and describing the cardiac silhouette **(Figures 1.28A and B)**. If inadvertent ventricular puncture has occurred by too much advancement of the needle, the contrast will clear rapidly from the ventricles. Contrast in the pericardial space takes time to clear; therefore it is important to not inject more than 1 or 2 cc of contrast into the pericardial space to prevent obscuring of the pericardial space by contrast. Once the pericardium is accessed with the needle, a 0.035" wire is introduced through the needle. A wire looping around the heart in both right anterior oblique and left anterior oblique views confirms a pericardial as

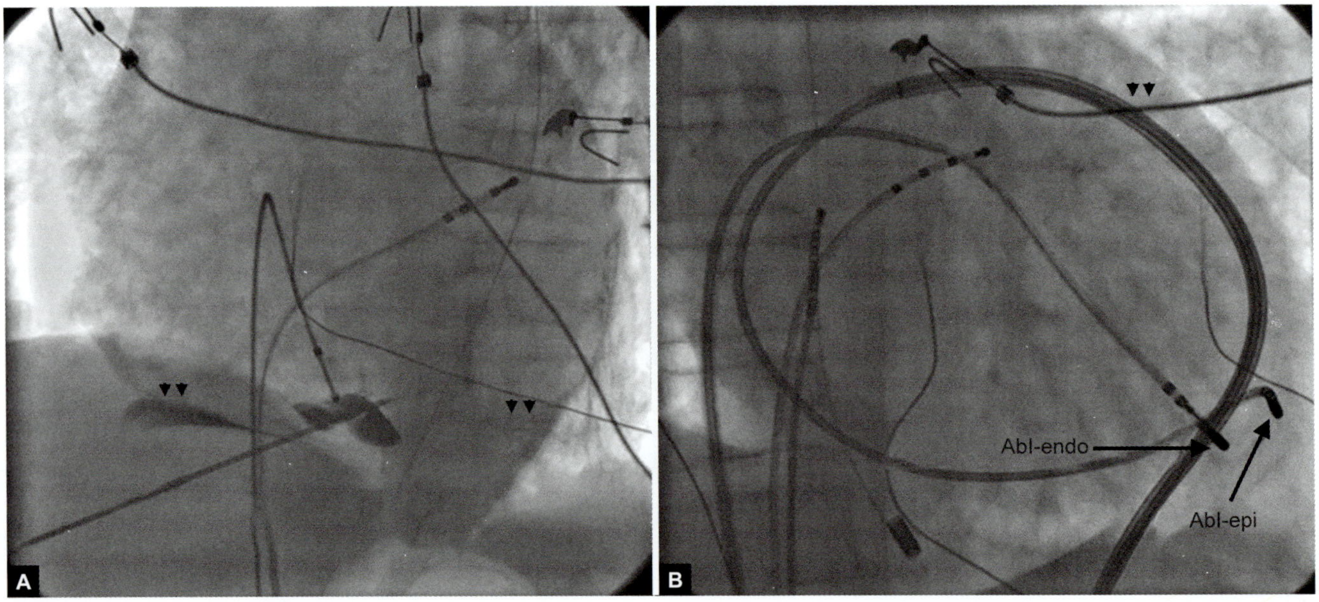

Figures 1.28A and B: (A) Contrast injection through the epicardial puncture needle shows contrast defining the cardiac silhouette following entry into the pericardial space (arrowheads); (B) The epicardial ablation catheter (Abl-epi), introduced through a deflectable sheath (arrowheads), is initially directed posterior to the heart, and passes anteriorly after coursing through the transverse sinus of the pericardium. This catheter has reached the epicardial aspect of the anterior apical area of the left ventricle at the site corresponding to the endocardial ablation catheter (Abl-endo). Such a catheter course gives more stable access to the apical area without risk of exiting back out of the pericardium, as compared to directly deflecting towards the apex

opposed to an intracardiac location of the wire. Once the pericardial location of the wire is confirmed, a sheath is introduced into the pericardium over this wire; either a standard length femoral sheath, or a longer length deflectable soft-tipped pericardial sheath (Agilis Epi™, St. Jude Medical, USA) may be used **(Figures 1.28A and B)**. Standard length femoral sheaths sometimes tend to get pushed back out of the pericardium during cardiac pulsations; hence longer sheaths are preferable. The catheter is introduced into the sheath after confirming absence of significant bleeding few minutes after pericardial access. When the catheter enters the pericardial space posteriorly, stable access to the anterior areas can be obtained by flexing and advancing the catheter and/or deflectable sheath around the heart.

In order to avoid damage to major coronary vessels during ablation, a coronary angiogram should be performed when it is suspected that the area to be ablated may contain such blood vessels. The phrenic nerve courses on the parietal aspect of the pericardium. As the two layers of the pericardium are apposed to each other in many regions, the ablation catheter may contact the pericardium at the region of the phrenic nerve during energy delivery, resulting in injury to the phrenic nerve. This complication may be avoided by high output pacing from the ablation catheter to check for phrenic nerve stimulation prior to ablation at the expected site/s of the phrenic nerve. If phrenic nerve stimulation occurs at the intended site of ablation, several techniques are described to avoid this complication. One of them involves introduction of a saline-inflatable long balloon through another pericardial access adjacent to the original access. Inflation of the balloon often separates the visceral and parietal pericardium at the site of the ablation catheter **(Figure 1.29)**.

During mapping and ablation, periodic aspiration of fluid through the side port of the sheath serves to check for pericardial bleeding, and may be required for adequate catheter-tissue contact if irrigated catheters are used. At the completion of the mapping and/or ablation procedure, the catheter is preferably replaced by a pigtail catheter which is left in situ for several hours to check for bleeding.

This section describes the various fluoroscopic correlates used for catheter positioning. An experienced operator will also know the precise amount of pushing force and torque that may be used safely at each of these locations in an individual case to achieve the crucial balance between efficacy and safety. This awareness, in conjunction with precise catheter manipulation, is critical to the success or otherwise of any electrophysiology procedure.

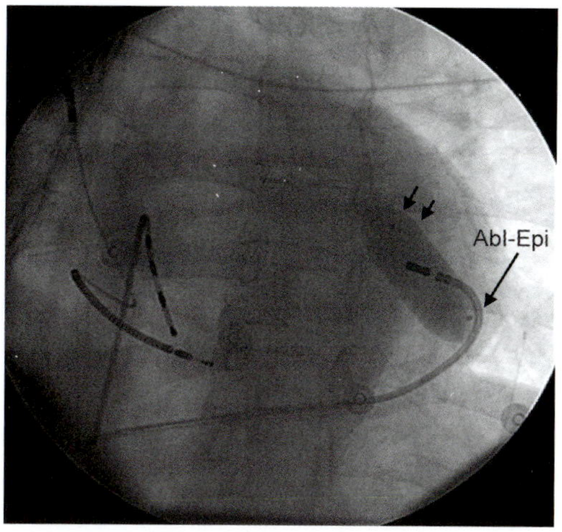

Figure 1.29: The epicardial ablation catheter (Abl-Epi) lies at the intended site of ablation, which is near the phrenic nerve. A Tyshak -II™ balloon (arrowheads) introduced through another epicardial access, has been inflated to separate the phrenic nerve-containing parietal pericardium from the visceral pericardium at this site

REFERENCES

1. Zipes DP, DiMarco JP, Gillette PC, Jackman WM, Myerburg RJ, Rahimtoola SH, Ritchie JL, Cheitlin MD, Garson A, Jr., Gibbons RJ, et al. Guidelines for clinical intracardiac electrophysiological and catheter ablation procedures. A report of the American College of Cardiology/American Heart Association Task Force on Practice Guidelines (Committee on Clinical Intracardiac Electrophysiologic and Catheter Ablation Procedures), developed in collaboration with the North American Society of Pacing and Electrophysiology. J Am Coll Cardiol. 1995;26:555-73.
2. Lehrmann H, Schneider J, Jadidi AS, Park CI, Schiebeling-Romer J, Allgeier J, Arentz T, Weber R. Transseptal access for left atrial ablation: the catheter-probing techniques are not without risk. J Cardiovasc Electrophysiol. 2014;25:479-84.
3. Smelley MP, Shah DP, Weisberg I, Kim SS, Lin AC, Beshai JF, Burke MC, Knight BP. Initial experience using a radiofrequency powered transseptal needle. J Cardiovasc Electrophysiol. 2010;21:423-7.
4. Kalavakolanu S, Rao HB, Kumar DN, Calambur N. Successful ablation of aortic cusp tachycardia from right ventricle outflow tract using a superior approach. J Interv Card Electrophysiol. 2006;16:187-9.
5. Sosa E, Scanavacca M, d'Avila A, Pilleggi F. A new technique to perform epicardial mapping in the electrophysiology laboratory. J Cardiovasc Electrophysiol. 1996;7:531-6.

EDITORS' SUMMARY

The principles of electrophysiology whether learning our field for the first time as a beginning student or trying to tackle a complex arrhythmia for the most experienced and advanced electrophysiologist comes down to a mastery of the fundamentals. These fundamentals are the pillars of anatomy, electrophysiology, and biophysics. In this introductory chapter, Dr Thachil provides a surprisingly broad but comprehensive overview of some of these basic skills. A careful study of the fluoroscopic images, diagrams of catheters and sheaths, along with the electrograms will be an excellent first introduction or a revision for students of electrophysiology. When used in conjunction with the other chapters and references on electrogram recordings (Chapters 2 and 8), pacing maneuvers for rhythm diagnosis (Chapters 14 to 16) and biophysics (Chapter 10), coupled with instruction, experienced teacher, and practice, the necessary fundamentals will be there to be used in the lifetime of the invasive electrophysiologist (*See* also, Asirvatham SJ. Introduction to the Electrophysiology Manual: Fluoroscopic Views, Electrograms, and Relevant Anatomy. In: Asirvatham SJ, Friedman PA, Cha YM. Mayo Clinic Electrophysiology Manual. 2014:3-64).

1. ***The fluoroscopic views***: Anatomic fluoroscopic views, specifically the use of the right and left anterior oblique projections are a prerequisite for safe and effective catheter manipulation. Once mastered, fluoroscopy can be used minimally and in some ablations not at all. However, for the beginner, carefully correlating these views with anatomy is a huge step towards successful practice.
2. ***The tools that we use***: The electrograms obtained, stability and contact of the catheters being used to ablate, and avoidance of complications, such as perforation, are largely dependent on completely understanding our tools. How close are the bipoles with a multielectrode catheter? What is the stiffness of the catheter, particularly the distal portions, and how is this affected by the curve we place, the additional sheath we use, and features, such as contact force assessment, irrigation, and deflection capabilities, added to a catheter that we may otherwise be familiar with?
3. ***Access***: Dr Thachil reviews both common, as well as complex, access in a straightforward and practical manner with illustrations that can serve as a backdrop for practical experience and instruction.

CHAPTER 2

Katherine Duello, KL Venkatachalam

Electrophysiology Study: Technical Details, Electrograms, Noise and Filtering

LIST OF ABBREVIATIONS

CMRR	Common-mode Rejection Ratio	HPF	High Pass Filter
DC	Direct Current	LPF	Low Pass Filter
DSP	Digital Signal Processing	RF	Radiofrequency
ECG	Electrocardiogram	RMS	Room Mean Squared
EP	Electrophysiology	WCT	Wilson Central Terminal

INTRODUCTION

Successful mapping and ablation in the electrophysiology (EP) laboratory is dependent on the acquisition of multiple, low amplitude intracardiac signals obtained amidst numerous sources of electrical noise and interference, presenting a significant engineering challenge. Knowledge of the challenges and ability to optimize the electronic data acquisition system can ensure that signals are presented in an uncomplicated and clinically relevant fashion with minimal artifact.

This chapter will present information on approaches to amplification and filtering of the electrocardiogram (ECG) and intracardiac signals in a typical EP lab, minimization of noise and interference, and clinical relevance of unipolar and bipolar signals. With this background we will discuss possible errors in mapping from artifact or inappropriate filtering.

In all of the electrogram illustrations, the following abbreviations are used:
P1 ART: arterial pressure tracing, II and V1: surface ECG leads, RVa and RVa d: proximal and distal right ventricular apex signals, HRA and HRA d: high right atrial catheter proximal and distal signals, His 4 to His 1: His bundle signals from an octapolar catheter with His 1 being most distal, Lasso 1,2 to Lasso 10,1: Circular catheter signals, ABL and ABL d: proximal and distal ablation catheter signals, CS 19,20 to CS1,2: coronary sinus catheter signals with CS1,2 being most distal.

DIFFICULTIES WITH SIGNAL ACQUISITION

The patient in the EP lab is connected to many pieces of equipment which can interfere with intracardiac signals; these may include an ECG machine, pulse oximeter, external defibrillator, intracardiac catheters and an electro-anatomic mapping system. Safety standards require the total current from patient connections via the patient to earth (the reference point), or "leakage current,"[1] to be less than 10 microamperes for each attached device. With multiple devices connected, there is a total leakage current of several tens of microamperes flowing through the patient at a fundamental frequency of 50 or 60 Hz, with significant harmonics extending to several thousand hertz (Hz). While most patients safely tolerate this leakage current without significant risk of ventricular fibrillation, it can produce artifact on intracardiac signals. This artifact is exacerbated as the patient is coupled capacitively and inductively to the line voltage wiring in the EP lab (120–240V) and also picks up radiofrequency interference from wireless headsets, mobile phones and wireless monitors near the lab. The patient's body may have interference voltages of 1–3 V RMS (root mean squared, a mathematical approach to calculate the effective heating capacity of a complex signal), encompassing a wide frequency spectrum from 50 Hz to several tens of megahertz (MHz).

Signal to noise ratio (SNR) is an extremely important parameter in signal processing, which defines the clarity with which signals can be measured or visualized. In general, a minimum SNR of a factor of 10 (20 decibels) is required to distinguish small changes in signal in the presence of noise. Ideally, this number should be a factor of 1000 (60 decibels) or more, but this is very hard to achieve in a real-life EP lab. Intracardiac electrograms, typically ranging in amplitude from 25 microvolts to 5 millivolts, need to be accurately amplified and displayed ignoring any previously described interference, while delivering RF ablation energy (at about 500 KHz) with amplitudes of up to 100 V RMS (100 W maximum into a 100 ohm impedance). In this setting, a high SNR is not always possible. With smaller signals, such as 25 microvolts, a SNR of 10 may be sufficient, which corresponds to a total noise at the input of the amplification system of 2.5 microvolts in the bandwidth of interest.

Attention to detail in electronic design can overcome many of these challenges. **Figure 2.1** shows typical connections to the patient in the EP lab. "Noise" is used to describe sources intrinsic to the electronic system and "interference" to describe external sources. The capacitance (which is the ability of an object to store electrical charge) is caused by the proximity of the patient to grounded objects in the environment, and is a path for leakage current from the devices attached to the patient.

POSSIBLE APPROACHES TO ARTIFACT-FREE SIGNAL ACQUISITION

Ideally, interference in the EP lab is minimized by eliminating sources before electronic processing, as additional signal processing may add to a data-acquisition system's intrinsic artifact. Some methods used to decrease interference include shielding of cables, appropriate grounding of equipment, balancing signal inputs and outputs, filtering, electrical isolation, physical separation and perpendicular orientation, lowering circuit impedances and frequency- or time-domain-based cancellation or enhancement techniques.[1] The following discussion will address some of these methods.[2]

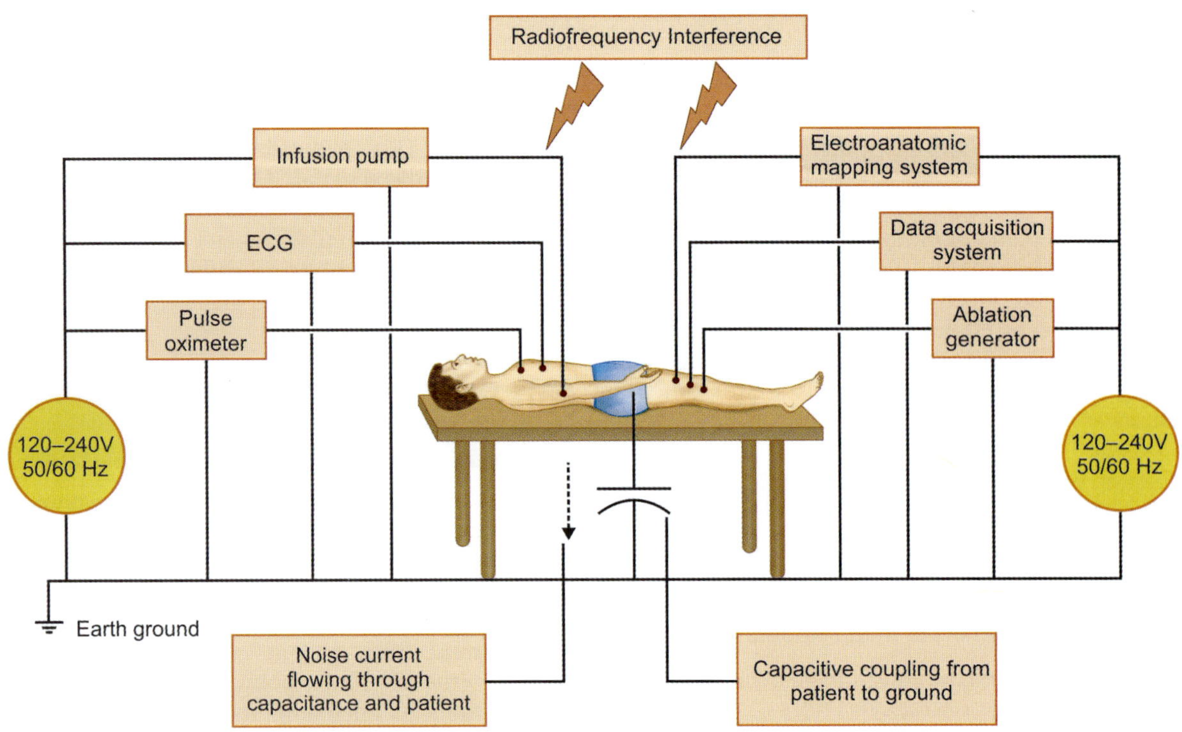

Figure 2.1: Typical sources of electrical interference in EP lab

Shielding and Grounding

Through electrical or magnetic coupling, line frequency interference may affect the signal processing system. Extensive shielding surrounding the EP lab prevents X-rays from exiting the lab and potential outside electromagnetic fields from entering the lab. Lab power sources should be routed away from the patient and kept as far away as possible from the cables carrying sensitive intracardiac signals. If in close proximity, minimizing the length of cables running parallel (which increases coupling and crosstalk), running groups of cables perpendicular to each other (optimizing rejection of coupled signals by the amplifiers) and minimizing coiling of cables (decreasing coupling) will decrease interference. Bundling cables together, as is frequently done for esthetic purposes, will increase crosstalk and interference. High-density braiding provides cable shielding that helps to shunt capacitively and inductively coupled interference to the ground reference of the electronic system. Special nickel-iron alloys such as Mumetal may also be used to shield sensitive circuits exposed to magnetic interference. To meet the leakage current requirements for patient safety, the electronic circuit ground reference (to which the cable shields are usually attached) needs to "float" with respect to the earth, which may also reduce the efficacy of cable shielding. Faulty shield connections are a common cause of interference, and replacing the interconnect cable between the catheter and connector block (junction box) may improve the signal. To minimize cable length, preamplifiers and amplifiers should be placed close to the patient, and may be replaced with fiber optic cables with subsequent conversion to electrical signals if needed.

Isolation

It is a mandatory safety requirement to electrically isolate patient connected equipment from the wall outlet. This has the additional effect of reducing circulating current at 50/60 Hz, which may cause interference. Most safety standards committees have a 10 microamperes "leakage current" limit that results in an effective coupling capacitance at 120 V/60 Hz of 220 pF (picofarads, a measure of capacitance) to earth ground. Equipment is usually designed to isolate instruments connected to the patient with coupling capacitances of less than 100 pF, reducing circulating currents at line frequencies.

To minimize the effects of interference between equipment, the EP lab staff can try to plug each of them into wall sockets as far apart as possible, but even this can cause interference occasionally. The signal quality may be improved with empiric trial of various sockets in the room. Keeping unused equipment off and unplugged from wall sockets also can minimize interference.

Balancing and Differential Amplification

Both balancing and differential amplification are additional approaches to minimizing interference.[3] Differential amplifiers possess the ability to reject signals common to both their inputs while also amplifying the difference. This property is called common-mode rejection ratio (CMRR). Typically, two adjacent electrodes on an intracardiac catheter are connected to the two inputs of the differential amplifier. Most amplifiers have CMRR around 100 dB (decibels) at low frequencies which decreases at higher frequencies. This means that in a data acquisition system with 1 V of interference at 60 Hz, the interference will be attenuated to 10 microvolts (100 dB or 100,000 times smaller than the original signal). At the same time, the required intracardiac signal is amplified by a factor of 100 or more depending on the circuit design. This will enhance the signal-to interference ratio. Using a tightly twisted pair of wires to deliver a bipolar signal as input to such an amplifier increases the chances of coupling equal amounts of interference to both inputs. This allows the amplifier's CMRR to effectively reject the interference.

"Balancing" the inputs requires maintaining similar impedances between each input and the circuit ground. Imbalances between the two inputs will affect the CMRR causing increased interference. This can be seen in the EP lab during ablation with RF energy while trying to observe electrograms on the distal pair of electrodes. If the pacing function on the distal pair of electrodes is enabled during ablation, noise on the distal electrogram is often noted due to the minor imbalance produced by attaching the pacing current source to the two electrodes, even if no pacing energy is being delivered. In this case, the electrogram appearance will be restored by turning off the pacing function. By lowering the input impedance of the differential amplifier, the interference may be reduced by decreasing coupled signals. However, very low input impedances will also reduce the amplitude of required signals, lowering the overall SNR. To ensure adequate transfer of signals, the input impedance of any voltage amplification system should be generally at least 10 times higher than the impedance of the signal source it is attached to.

Filtering

Filtering enhances portions of the frequency spectrum and rejects unwanted portions. It can be utilized at several stages in the electronic system including combinations of passive (only resistors, capacitors and inductors) and active (operational amplifiers) filters along with digital filters using digital signal processing (DSP) hardware and software algorithms.

ECG signals of diagnostic quality require a processing bandwidth of 0.05 Hz–100 Hz, while monitor quality ECGs are limited to 0.5 Hz–40 Hz. The lower frequency cutoff of 0.05 Hz results in better reproduction of the ST segments, but also results in increased baseline drift. With an upper cutoff frequency of 100 Hz, any rapid changes in QRS complexes are well represented with the tradeoff of increased susceptibility to interference at the power line frequency of 50/60 Hz. Using a combination of high- and low-pass filters (HPF and LPF), most filters in electronic systems in the EP lab achieve a band-pass response that allows certain bands of frequencies through the filter and rejects frequencies on either side. For example, a HPF with a cut off frequency of 0.05 Hz will block DC voltages (which have a frequency of 0 Hz), but pass any frequencies above 0.05 Hz. An LPF with a cutoff of 100 Hz will reject all frequencies above 100 Hz and pass all from DC up to 100 Hz. Adjusting the cutoff frequencies of the filters in the EP lab is analogous to using a tone control in a home stereo system to accentuate bass or treble frequencies. In the EP lab, data acquisition systems may also utilize digital filtering to improve deficiencies in traditional hardware filters.

By passing the amplified ECG voltage through both the HPF and LPF sequentially, a band-pass response from 0.05 Hz to 100 Hz is achieved **(Figure 2.2)**. If a diagnostic quality ECG is to be obtained, interference at 50 to 60 Hz could be a problem in this passband and most systems provide an optional notch filter to reject such interference. This notch (or band-reject) filter suppresses line-related noise by passing all frequencies on either side of a narrow band of frequencies centered on 50 or 60 Hz.

Depending on their design, these filters may also add noise into the system (usually at high frequencies). However, another significant disadvantage of the notch filter is that certain EP signals, such as near-field pulmonary vein deflections or rapidly varying fractionated potentials, can also be attenuated making it difficult to locate a good signal even with appropriate catheter position or effective ablation **(Figures 2.3A and B)**.

Due to differences in frequency content, intracardiac electrograms require a different passband from ECG signals. A lower cutoff frequency of 30 Hz is commonly used to ensure good rejection of baseline drift **(Figures 2.4A and B)**.

In such a system the fundamental frequency being amplified is low (only 5 Hz at a heart rate of 300 beats per minute). Individual electrograms such as His bundle electrograms, pulmonary vein potentials and Purkinje potentials can have components with very rapid deflection with more energy content at higher frequencies (also implying near-field information). An upper cutoff frequency of 500 Hz will typically reproduce signals with minimum distortion **(Figures 2.5A and B)**.

While a higher cutoff frequency (1000–2000 Hz) may improve accuracy by minimizing phase shifts (different signal delays in various parts of the frequency spectrum), it may also increase the overall noise and interference since the intrinsic noise of an electronic system increases by the square root of bandwidth (frequency range of the system). Distinguishing near-field signals with higher frequency energy content from far-field signals with low frequency content can be compromised with lower cutoff frequencies for the LPF. Selection of appropriate filters is further complicated when analyzing unipolar versus bipolar signals.

As most catheter signals are routed through the mapping system, filter selection also must be performed within the

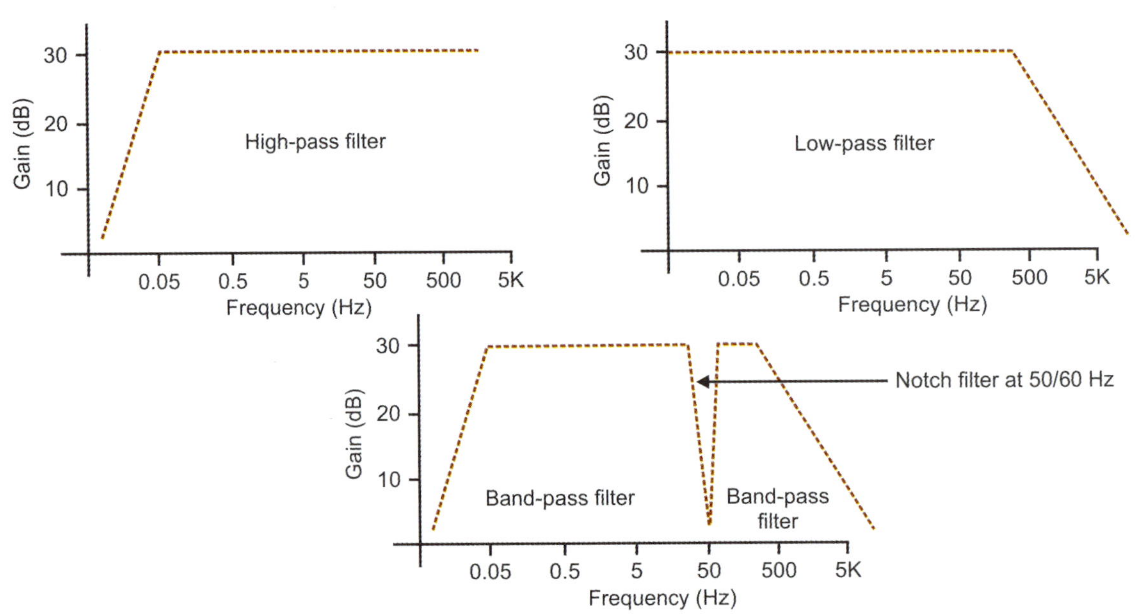

Figure 2.2: Combining a high-pass filter, low-pass filter and a notch filter to produce the composite frequency response

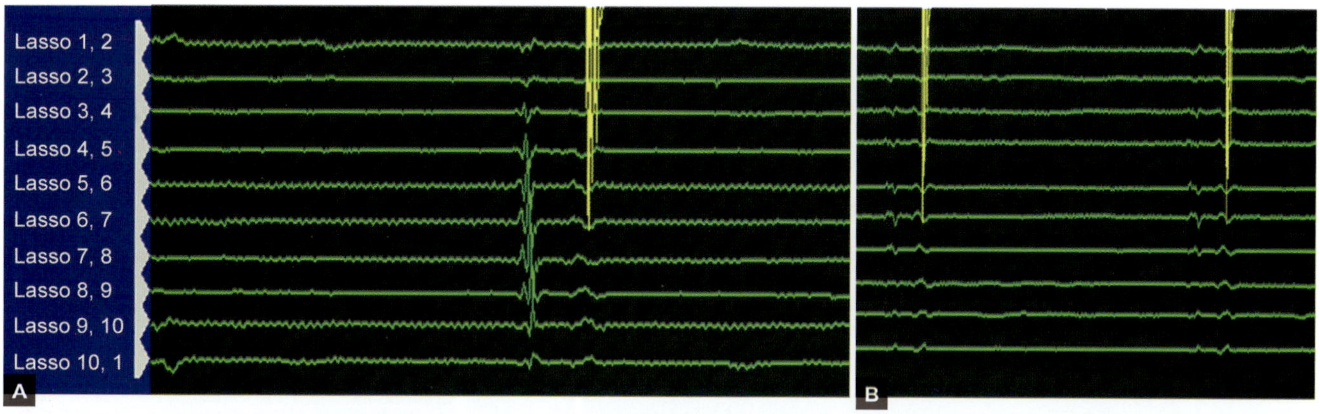

Figures 2.3A and B: Pulmonary vein potentials on a lasso catheter (A) are greatly attenuated when the 50/60 Hz notch filter is turned ON (B)

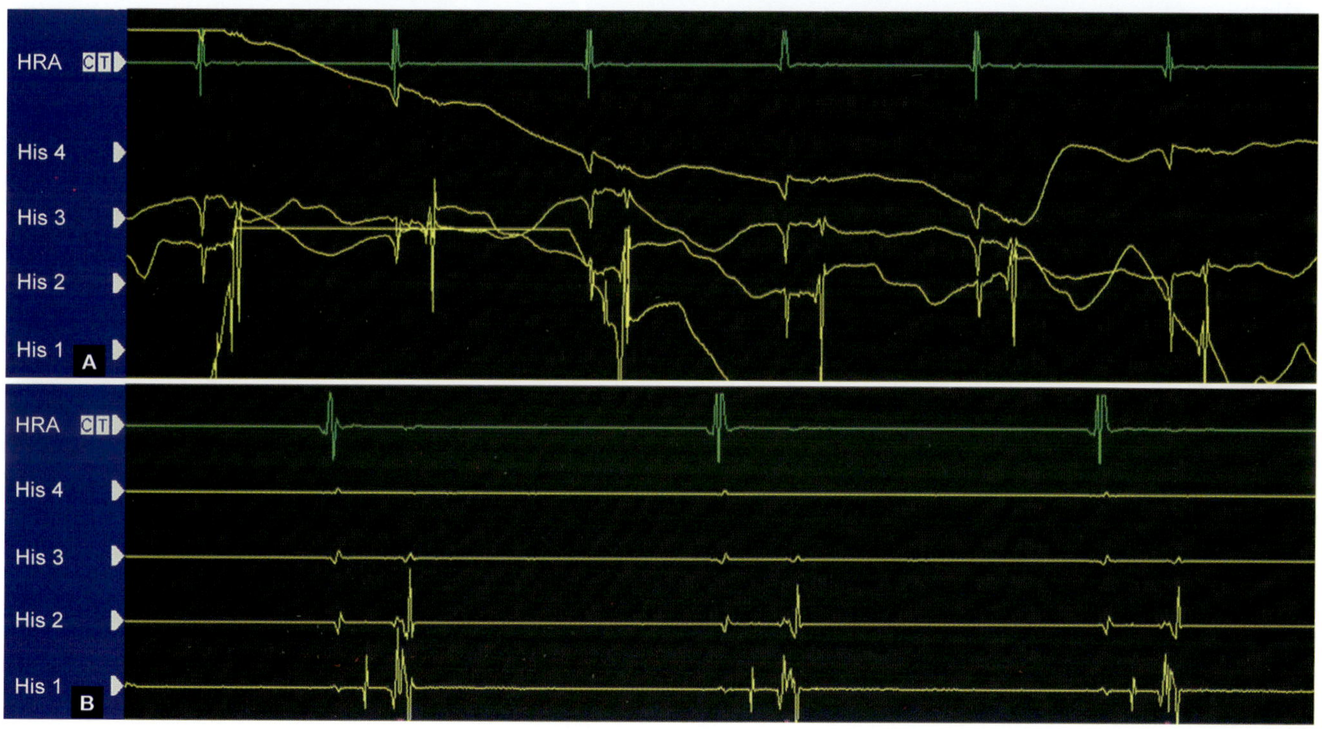

Figures 2.4A and B: Changing the high-pass filter cutoff frequency from 0.05 Hz (A) to 100 Hz (B) substantially reduce baseline drift in the His catheter signals

mapping system. This is in addition to the filter setting in the signal acquisition system. For optimization of signal acquisition with appropriate noise rejection, most mapping systems suggest specific frequency ranges for intracardiac electrograms.

Given the significant sources of noise and interference, the minuteness of the signals being amplified and the inherent imprecision of localizing signals in the moving heart, great care has to be taken during set-up and interpretation of the EP study to avoid being misled. Several sources of artifact will be discussed next.

ARTIFACT

Saturation Artifact

Amplifier saturation can occur when an input signal is amplified at such a high gain that the amplified signal exceeds the power supply voltage of the electronic system. If a 2 mV peak signal is being amplified at a gain of 5000, the final output will be 10,000 mV or 10 V. However, if the system supply voltage is limited to 5 V, the overall signal amplitude would be limited to about 4.5 V (slightly below the

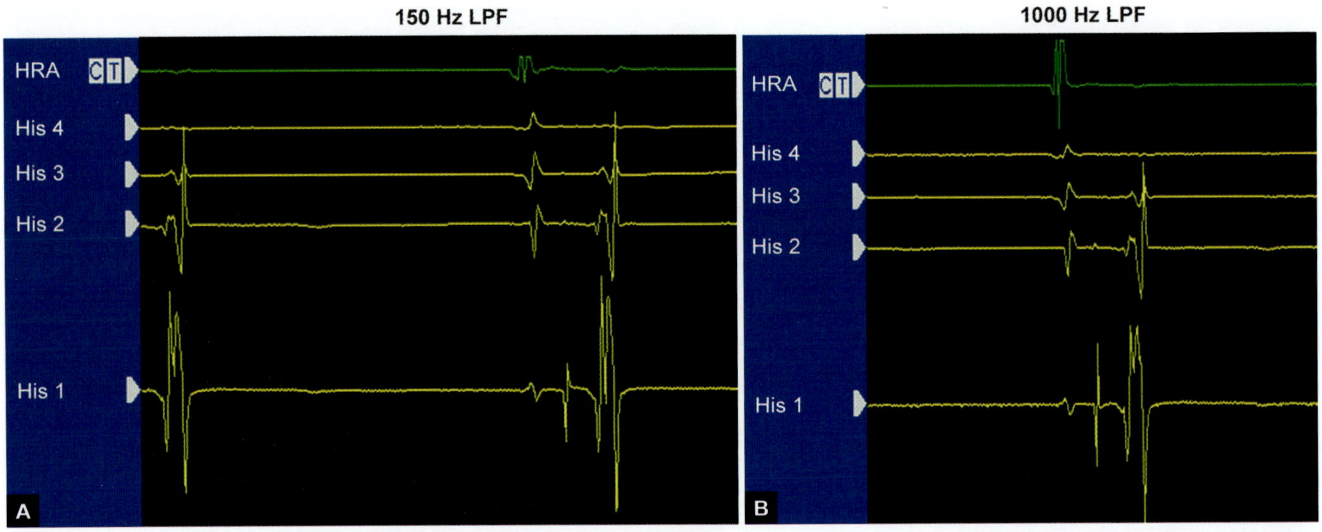

Figures 2.5A and B: The amplitude of the His deflection in His 1 is increased by increasing the low-pass filter cutoff frequency from 150 Hz (A) to 1000 Hz (B)

supply voltage). The signal would simply be cutoff above 4.5 V, although the amplifiers would attempt to drive themselves up to the required 10 V output unsuccessfully. The amplifiers remain "saturated" during this time and the peak of the signal remains unresponsive to changes in amplitude (flat top) until the signal amplitude decreases to below 4.5 V, when it can be tracked with fidelity once again. This is a form of distortion and can only be avoided by reducing the gain of the system (in this numerical example, to less than about 2000). When amplifiers saturate, they can take several milliseconds to recover, further delaying the time to faithful reproduction of signals. This is exacerbated with extremely large signals, such as pacing signals, which are typically 3 orders of magnitude larger than the electrograms. In this case, the signal recovery time for the paced electrodes as well as adjacent electrodes can be long enough that the artifact envelops a substantial portion of electrogram information immediately following the pacing spike. This can be a vexing problem when attempting to measure post-pacing intervals after entraining a tachycardia. Despite this artifact, the operator must make every effort to use the paced electrode signals for this measurement, as using more distant electrodes may produce artifactually longer postpacing intervals.

Clipping Artifact

One problem with using high-gain settings on multiple electrodes is that signals can overlap on the display. This is often circumvented by artificially "clipping" the signals of interest. The advantage of clipping (usually done at the software level although it can be done in hardware also) is that it can limit the numerical voltage displayed on-screen without the prolonged signal recovery times associated with amplifier saturation **(Figure 2.6)**. This allows the electrophysiologist to see a small electrogram that immediately follows a very large clipped electrogram without overlapping the displayed signals on adjacent channels.

However, the significant disadvantage of clipping is that one could get easily misled when looking at fused waveforms (pathway potentials during an accessory pathway ablation, for instance) if the selected clipping level by the software prevents visualization of two discrete, fused signals, and instead represents them as a single, wide signal **(Figure 2.7)**.

The operator usually cannot control the clipping level as this is programmed into the software in most systems. In this setting, one is almost always better off deliberately running the amplifiers at a low gain in order to prevent amplifier saturation and not require clipping (to avoid adjacent channel signal overlap). The only problem with this approach is that great care has to be taken to look at every nuance of the signals to not miss small potentials (such as pulmonary vein potentials or accessory pathway potentials), which are difficult to see at low gain settings, especially when the operator is several feet away from the display screen. In general, it is preferable to observe signals closely at low gain to minimize the deleterious effects of saturation and clipping.

Phantom Signals

Signals that appear real but are artifactual can also be seen due to the less than perfect properties of the input amplifiers, especially at higher frequencies.[1,3] An ideal differential amplifier would be able to reject equally coupled interference at both its inputs (such as from the distal and 2nd electrodes of a mapping catheter). At high-gain settings, even if a catheter is only partially in a sheath or is not even in the body, unequal coupling of large signals such as pacing spikes may occur. This can mimic real signals at

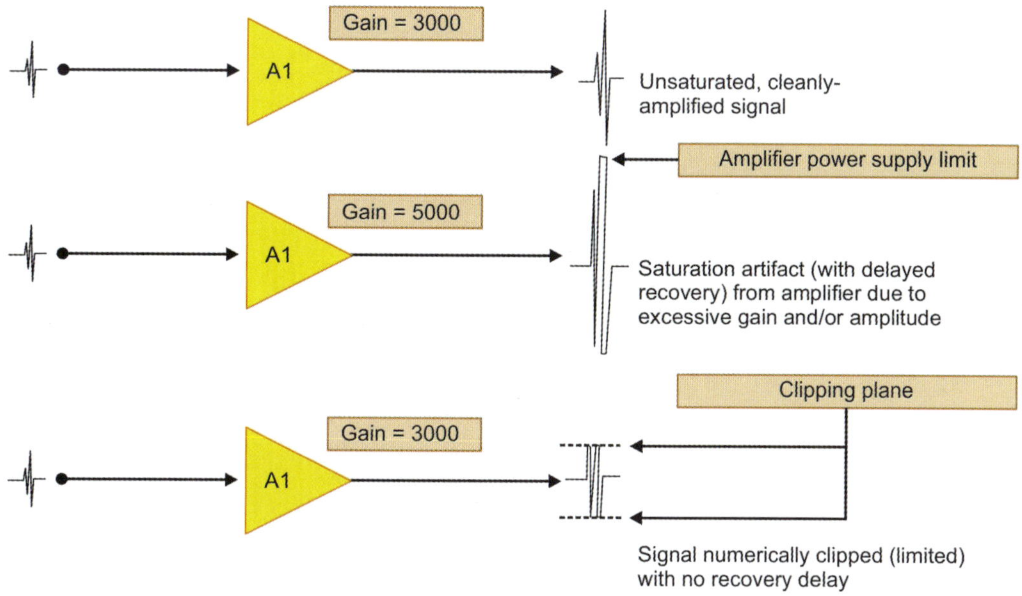

Figure 2.6: Saturation and clipping artifact

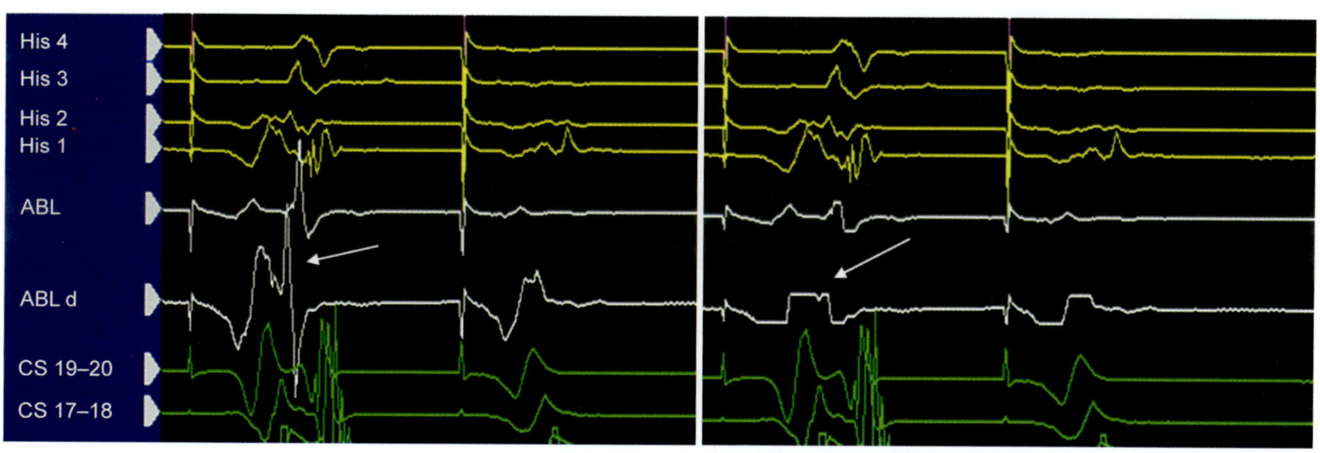

Figure 2.7: Clipping causing fusion of accessory pathway potential (on ABL d on right), compared to unclipped signal on left (arrow)

the pacing rate, especially after filtering smooths out the interference and makes it look like a far-field signal. This problem can be minimized by programming the output currents of the pacing stimulator to twice the diastolic threshold at a fairly narrow pulse width, confirming that all catheters are well extended out of the sheath tips and making good contact between tissue and tip. RF ablation noise can also be coupled into the system this way.

Electrode Contact Artifact

Intermittent contact between electrodes on different catheters or electrodes on the same catheter (such as a variable diameter lasso catheter with overlapping electrodes or contact between an ablation catheter and mapping catheter) can produce misleading signals. In the case of a lasso catheter, one could be misled into diagnosing pulmonary vein exit block due to noise on several overlapping electrodes that would produce sharp, near field signals reminiscent of pulmonary vein potentials, which do not get transmitted to the atrium. This may also be seen with a fixed diameter lasso catheter that has been pushed into a pulmonary vein ostium with consequent overlap of electrodes. Correlation of the location of these "potentials" with fluoroscopic electrode information reveals the true nature of these signals **(Figure 2.8)**.

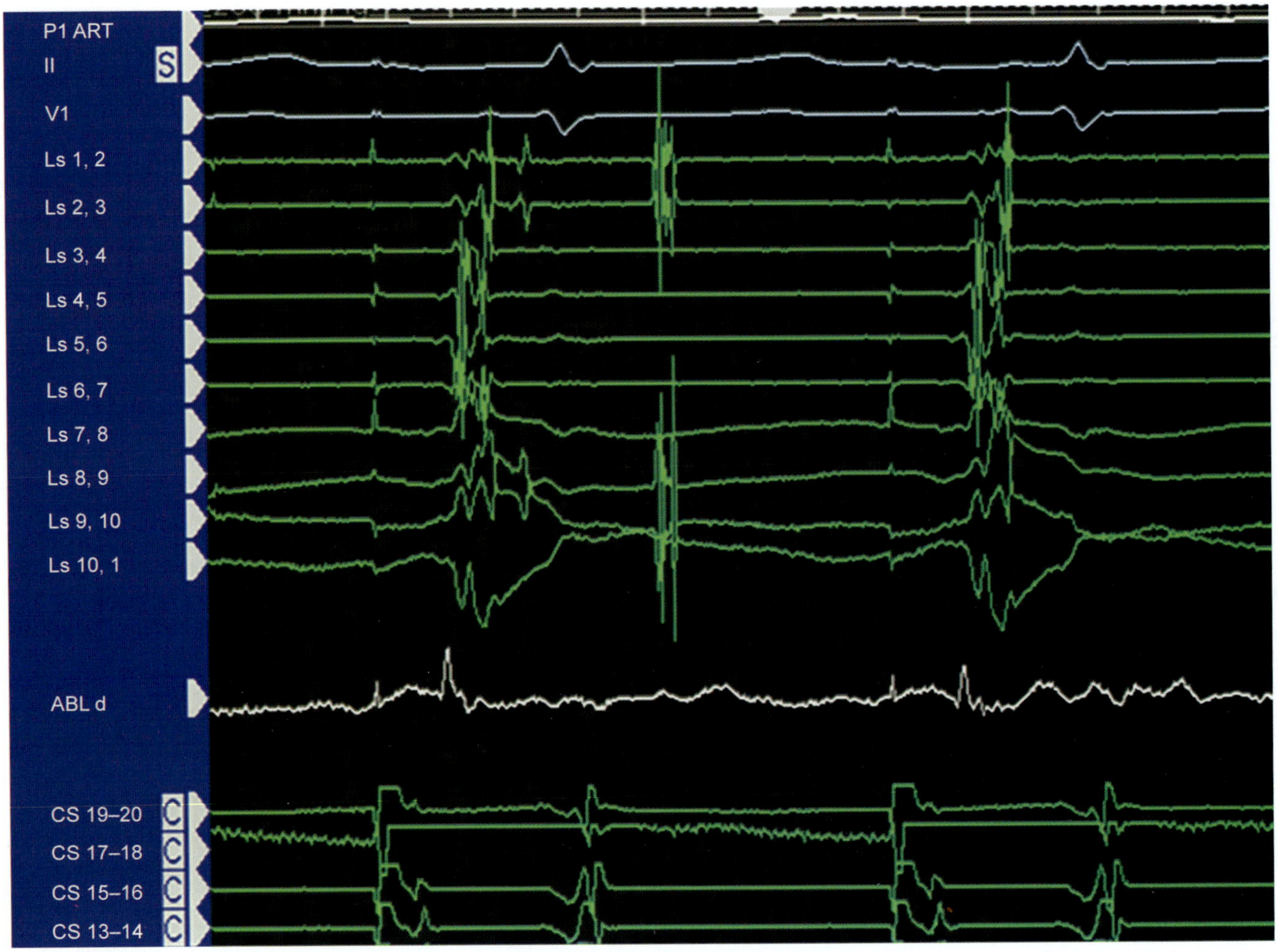

Figure 2.8: Mechanical artifact on lasso catheter mimicking pulmonary vein firing with exit block

UNIPOLAR AND BIPOLAR ELECTROGRAMS

Unipolar Electrograms

All recorded signals in the EP lab are bipolar since they are measured as a voltage difference between two electrodes. However, when one of the electrodes is some distance from the cardiac structures (ideally several inches away), the voltage difference between the exploring electrode and the distant electrode (indifferent electrode) is referred to as a unipolar signal.[4] On the 12-lead ECG, precordial leads V_1 through V_6 record voltages between each of the precordial wires and the indifferent electrode, which is the Wilson Central Terminal (WCT). WCT is assumed to be at the center of a triangle with the three limb wires at the apices **(Figure 2.9)**. The vector sum of currents entering WCT is theoretically zero, and this is considered to be a simplified electrical center of the heart.

When intracardiac electrograms need to be displayed in unipolar fashion, WCT may be used as the reference with the exploring electrode being the distal electrode of a mapping catheter. The mapping system can be configured to display these unipolar signals directly. Electroanatomic mapping systems generate their own WCT and display an independent unipolar electrogram on their dedicated displays.

A wavefront of depolarization that approaches a unipolar exploring electrode generates a positive deflection on the display. As this wavefront moves away from the electrode, a negative deflection is displayed. The steepest negative slope of the signal occurs when the wavefront is below the exploring electrode. This approach works best when the low-frequency cutoff for the amplifier channel is kept suitably low (DC or 0.5 Hz maximum instead of the usual 30 Hz cutoff used for bipolar channels). The instantaneous amplitude of the voltage is directly proportional to the area of the wavefront of depolarization and inversely proportional to the square of its distance from the exploring electrode.[5, 6] Directionality

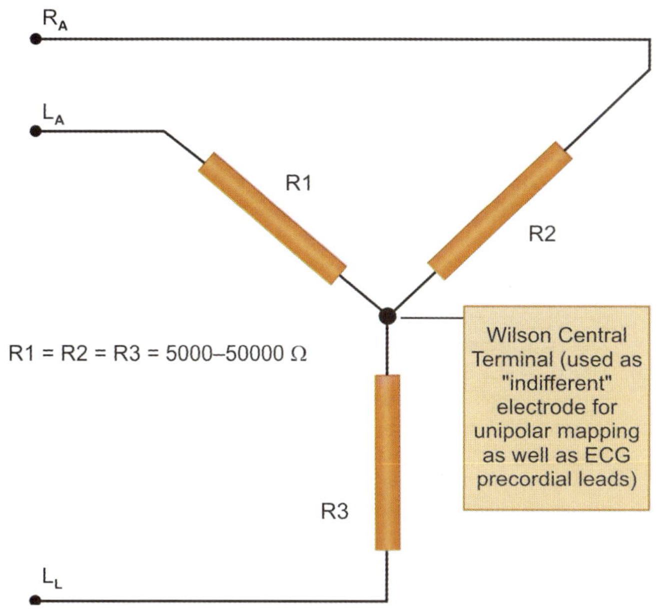

Figure 2.9: Wilson Central Terminal, used as reference electrode for unipolar mapping and ECG pre-cordial leads
Abbreviations: R_A, right arm; L_A, left arm; L_L, left leg; $R_{1,2,3}$, summing resistors

(superior, inferior, lateral, medial) is lost with this mapping approach.

If the wavefront of depolarization originates immediately below the exploring electrode, it spreads away from this electrode in all directions simultaneously, producing a negative deflection (QS waveform). This is usually a site of successful ablation of a focal tachycardia. A very small R wave may be present in this location since the origin of the ectopic focus could be intramyocardial, some distance away from the electrode. Poor electrode contact (or no electrode contact, as is seen if the electrode is floating in the cardiac chamber) manifests as a slow (low rate-of-change) signal instead of the expected rapid positive-to-negative polarity change. Using the unipolar signal to locate accessory pathways and ablate successfully has also been described, with the best results being obtained with a P-QS pattern (the atrial signal fused to the unipolar QS signal) on an "unfiltered" (no high pass filtering) signal.[7]

When mapping diseased tissue, far-field high-amplitude signals from healthy tissue may obscure the effects of low-amplitude local signals. Increasing the cutoff frequency of the high-pass filter to 10–30 Hz minimizes the far-field contribution.[4] A disadvantage of unipolar signals is the increased susceptibility to noise due to the differential coupling of interfering signals to the two widely spaced electrodes. This can be particularly troublesome when using WCT as the indifferent electrode due to surface electrode polarization and contact noise. Using an internal, indifferent electrode in the IVC instead may ameliorate this problem.

Bipolar Electrograms

When two narrowly spaced electrodes (less than 2–3 mm apart) in contact with myocardium are attached to the inputs of an instrumentation amplifier, the difference between the two signals produces a bipolar electrogram. Successive pairs of closely spaced electrodes on a multipolar catheter (1-2, 3-4, 5-6, etc.) produce reasonable bipolar signals as long as the electrode spacing is small. The same bipolar information may be obtained by subtracting one unipolar signal from another unipolar signal as long as the two unipolar electrodes are close to each other and in contact with myocardium. These signals are a good indicator of local electrical activity immediately beneath the two closely spaced electrodes, and so can provide information on timing of local activation.[8] Local activation is denoted by the time of maximum deflection of the electrogram. Reducing the distance between the two electrodes of the bipole can further reduce the sensitivity to distant activation events.[9] The amplitude of these signals in healthy ventricular myocardium (measured with a 10 mm electrode spacing) ranges from 3 mV to 10 mV with durations of less than 70 msec.[10] These amplitudes are reduced substantially with smaller spacing. Also, a lot of the far-field information present in a unipolar signal is removed from the bipolar signal because each electrode of the bipolar pair "sees" a similar (or identical) far-field voltage, and these similar signals are canceled out by the amplifier. Thus, it is reasonable to use a high pass filter with a higher cutoff frequency, such as 30 Hz, for bipolar signals since this will help minimize baseline drifts/shifts with no loss of information.

With close electrode spacing, changes in polarity on the bipolar signals correlate with changes in direction of activation, such as may occur during creation of conduction block during radiofrequency ablation. In the extreme case, this could be a disadvantage since a wave of depolarization that is perpendicular to the two electrodes would be canceled.[11] Conversely, a wave of depolarization that is parallel to the two electrodes would be picked up sequentially by both, resulting in maximum amplitude. The time of peak amplitude in a bipolar signal is the equivalent of the fastest negative downslope of the unipolar signal. Furthermore, if both minimally-filtered unipolar signals and standard-filtered (30–500 Hz) bipolar signals are obtained simultaneously, the time between onset of unipolar electrogram and first peak of bipolar electrogram is usually very short (less than 15 msec) at the site of successful ablation of an automatic tachycardia.[11]

Given the difference in size between the tip electrode and the more proximal electrode of a bipole pair, and the fact that the tip is usually in contact with the tissue with perpendicular orientation (leaving the proximal electrode offset from the tissue by several millimeters), it is not clear if the voltage on the bipolar electrogram is truly representative of the "quality of tissue" beneath the catheter tip.

This uncertainty becomes particularly significant when creating voltage maps of ventricular myocardium, and using absolute amplitude cutoffs to differentiate scar from viable tissue. This is of somewhat lower concern during epicardial mapping since both electrodes are usually making contact with the tissue due to the more parallel orientation of the catheter "trapped" between epicardium and pericardium. During epicardial mapping, however, areas with more than 5 mm of epicardial fat thickness (near the base of the heart) tend to have lower bipolar voltages (less than 1.5 mV, possibly being misclassified as scar) compared to other areas.[12]

Another significant point is that bipolar electrograms on the distal pair of electrodes of the ablation catheter do not always decrease during ablation, which is the usual indicator of ablation success. Since the amplifier is calculating the difference between the distal electrode and proximal electrode potentials to generate the electrogram, as the tissue below the distal electrode is ablated this difference could decrease (as we would expect) or even increase with reverse polarity, since the proximal electrode may have a larger signal now due to its sampling of more healthy, unablated tissue compared to the desiccated tissue beneath the distal electrode. However, a true unipolar electrogram of the distal electrode would decrease unequivocally as the tissue is ablated effectively.

CONCLUSION

With a combination of high-quality hardware and software design, careful management of lab wiring, appropriate filter settings and knowledge of the limitations of the system, it is possible to effectively map and ablate cardiac arrhythmias in the electrically noisy environment of the EP lab.

REFERENCES

1. Ott H. Noise reduction techniques in electronic systems, 2nd edition, 1988.
2. Venkatachalam KL, Herbrandson JE, Asirvatham SJ. Signals and signal processing for the electrophysiologist. Part I and Part II: Electrogram acquisition. Circulation: Arrhythmia & Electrophysiology. 2011;4:965-81.
3. Horowitz P, Hill W. The art of electronics, 2nd edition. Cambridge University Press, 1989.
4. Stevenson WG, Soejima K. Recording techniques for clinical electrophysiology. J Cardiovasc Electrophysiol. 2005;16: 1017-22.
5. Miyamoto N, Shimizu Y, Nishiyama G, Mashima S, Okamoto Y. On the potential of the wilson central terminal with respect to an ideal reference for unipolar electrocardiography. J Electrocardiol. 1995;28:336-7.
6. Daniel TM, Boineau JP, Sabiston DC, Jr. Comparison of human ventricular activation with a canine model in chronic myocardial infarction. Circulation. 1971;44:74-89.
7. Haissaguerre M, Dartigues JF, Warin JF, Le Metayer P, Montserrat P, Salamon R. Electrogram patterns predictive of successful catheter ablation of accessory pathways. Value of unipolar recording mode. Circulation. 1991;84:188-202.
8. Kupersmith J. Electrophysiologic mapping during open heart surgery. Prog Cardiovasc Dis. 1976;19:167-202.
9. Ideker RE, Smith WM, Blanchard SM, Reiser SL, Simpson EV, Wolf PD, Danieley ND. The assumptions of isochronal cardiac mapping. Pacing Clin Electrophysiol. 1989;12:456-78.
10. Cassidy DM, Vassallo JA, Marchlinski FE, Buxton AE, Untereker WJ, Josephson ME. Endocardial mapping in humans in sinus rhythm with normal left ventricles: Activation patterns and characteristics of electrograms. Circulation. 1984;70:37-42.
11. Delacretaz E, Soejima K, Gottipaty VK, Brunckhorst CB, Friedman PL, Stevenson WG. Single catheter determination of local electrogram prematurity using simultaneous unipolar and bipolar recordings to replace the surface ECG as a timing reference. Pacing Clin Electrophysiol. 2001;24:441-9.
12. Reddy VY, Wrobleski D, Houghtaling C, Josephson ME, Ruskin JN. Combined epicardial and endocardial electroanatomic mapping in a porcine model of healed myocardial infarction. Circulation. 2003;107:3236-42.

EDITORS' SUMMARY

In this chapter, Duello and Venkatachalam provide an insightful and practical approach to maximize the value of the recorded electrograms during our ablation procedures. Through the remainder of this textbook, several key maneuvers and techniques that define mechanism of arrhythmia and identify the appropriate substrate for ablation will be explained. However, the value of such maneuvers is greatly minimized when we cannot trust or do not know whether we can trust the electrograms we are interpreting.

Duello and Venkatachalam identify for us the fundamental issue of signal-to-noise ratio that defines our ability to record actual but sometimes small and fragmented signals that may be the key to successful ablation.

While there includes in this chapter an excellent discussion of filtering, clipping, gaining, and postprocessing signals to better identify the signals of interest, the authors emphasize the importance of excluding noise at the outset. For this, we make simple and practical suggestions that should form a checklist for every electrophysiology laboratory—identifying and varying the external output, avoiding coiling of cables from electronic equipment, and when necessary, braiding or placing cable perpendicular to each other.

With outstanding illustrative examples, the authors demonstrate the effect of clipping of both analog and digital signals that can exclude, as well as newly place apparent true signals that can obscure the true electrical phenomena occurring in a complex case. The use and limitations of a notch-filter, including an example where pulmonary vein potentials that were obscured because of the frequency of these signals falling within the filtered range.

While several of the limitations involved with optimizing the signal-to-noise ratio are theoretical and difficult to eliminate even in future iterations of mapping systems, the authors point out that improved sampling frequency and the dynamic range for processing signals are likely probable with improved computing power available and the recognized need for find mapping, specifically for supravalvar arrhythmia and identifying fragmented signals and late potentials for substrate-based ventricular tachycardia mapping.

Finally, we revisit the sum of the principles outlined by Duello and Venkatachalam in the subsequent sections that look at optimal techniques for 3-dimensional mapping and integrating analysis of recorded electrograms with complex maneuvers and the underlying pathological substrate.

CHAPTER 3

B Hygriv Rao

Measurements of Basic Intervals, Refractory Periods and Programmed Electrical Stimulation

LIST OF ABBREVIATIONS

AT	Atrial Tachycardia	FRP	Functional Refractory Period
AVNERP	Atrioventricular Nodal Effective Refractory Period	ICD	Implantable Cardioverter-Defibrillator
AVNRT	Atrioventricular Nodal Reentrant Tachycardia	PES	Programmed Electrical Stimulation
AVRT	Atrioventricular Reciprocating Tachycardia	RA	Right Atrium
BBR	Bundle Branch Reentry	RRP	Relative Refractory Period
CS	Coronary Sinus	RV	Right Ventricle
EP	Electrophysiology	SVT	Supraventricular Tachycardia
EPS	Electrophysiology Study	VT	Ventricular Tachycardia
ERP	Effective Refractory Period	WPW	Wolff-Parkinson-White

INTRODUCTION

Electrophysiological study (EPS) is performed most frequently as a part of ablative therapy for cardiac arrhythmias. In this context, an EPS is used to induce suspected or documented clinical arrhythmias, define the electrophysiological substrate and design a strategy for ablation. In patients with asymptomatic pre-excitation, EPS may help to define the need for ablative therapy. Some patients presenting with syncope may merit an EPS to assess the need for a pacemaker or an implantable cardioverter defibrillator (ICD). In selected subset of patients, particularly in the presence of structural heart disease, it is one of the tools used to stratify the risk of sudden death. The procedure is performed in a cardiac catheterization lab and needs the standard fluoroscopic equipment. Additional electrophysiology (EP) lab equipment including an oscilloscopic recorder, junction box, and a stimulator for delivering stimuli are also needed. Multipolar catheters are used to record the cardiac electrical activity.

THE BASIC ELECTROPHYSIOLOGY STUDY

The protocol and sequence of stimulation in the EP lab is dictated by the indication for which the EP study is being done. The study typically begins with the recording of a 12-lead ECG and intracardiac electrograms from the high right atrium, His bundle region, coronary sinus (CS) and the right ventricle. The CS catheter may not be needed in patients who are undergoing the study for syncope evaluation, bradycardia assessment or risk stratification of sudden death. During the study, right atrial (RA) signals are recorded from high RA, while right ventricular (RV) signals are recorded from the RV apex. A typical His bundle electrogram

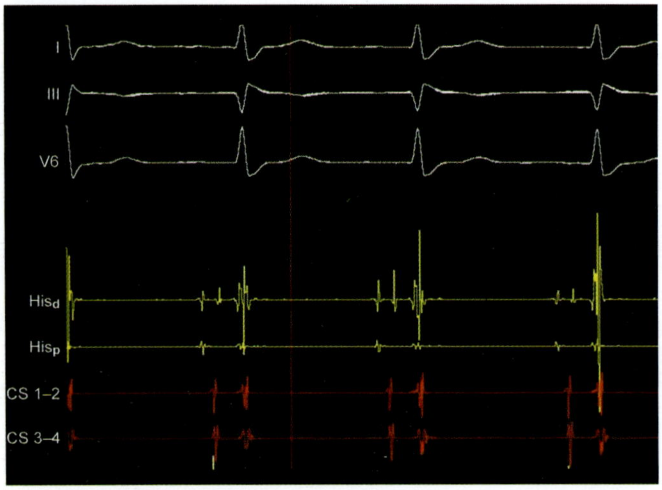

Figure 3.1: Baseline recording showing surface ECG leads, His bundle and CS recordings

during sinus rhythm has an "A" (atrial electrogram), a "V" (ventricular electrogram) and a biphasic or triphasic "H" (His deflection) in between. The decapolar CS catheter records left atrial and ventricular electrograms along the AV groove. The first step in all cases is the measurement of baseline intervals from the electrograms recorded from these appropriately placed catheters. These include the standard measurements on surface ECG and intracardiac recordings **(Figure 3.1)**. Systematic baseline interval recording on the 12-lead ECG comprise the P-P, R-R intervals, P-wave, QRS durations, PR interval, and QT/QTc intervals. The measurement of intracardiac signals include the PA, AH and HV intervals in addition to H deflection duration. These measurements are made using electronic calipers at a sweep speed of 200 mm/s or higher. The standard baseline measurements and corresponding intracardiac events are summarized in **Table 3.1**. Certain facts need to be remembered while recording the His signal. Pre-excitation can be missed unless HV interval is measured from the earliest V signal whether on surface ECG or intracardiac **(Figure 3.2)**. If the His catheter is placed too distally, one may mistake a right bundle potential for a His deflection and may erroneously record a short HV interval. A fractionated "A" signal may be mistaken for a short A-H interval **(Figures 3.3A and B)** and its differentiation may sometimes require pacing maneuvers.

PROGRAMMED ELECTRICAL STIMULATION

Programmed electrical stimulation (PES) is defined as cardiac stimulation by a pulse of electrical current delivered by a stimulator through an electrode catheter that is in contact with tissue of a cardiac chamber using prespecified protocols. A programmable stimulator delivers stimuli at precisely timed intervals. The impulse depolarizes the cardiac tissue

Table 3.1: Baseline intervals

Interval	*Measurement*	*Intracardiac event*	*Values*
ECG			
P-P	Beginning of P-wave to next P-wave	Atrial rate	
PR	Beginning of P-wave to beginning of QRS complex	Atrial depolarization, intranodal and infra-Hisian conduction	120–200 ms
R- R	Beginning of QRS complex to beginning of next QRS complex	Ventricular rate	
QRS duration	Beginning of Q-wave to end of S-wave	Ventricular depolarization	80–120 ms
QT interval	Beginning of Q-wave to end of T-wave	Ventricular depolarization +Repolarization	QTc Men: ≤450 ms Women: ≤470 ms
P-wave duration	Beginning of earliest P-wave to end of latest P-wave in a simultaneously recorded 12 lead ECG	Intra-atrial conduction	
Intracardiac measurements			
A-H	Beginning of A-wave to beginning of H deflection in low right atrial (His bundle electrogram) signal	Intranodal conduction	55–125 ms
H-wave duration	Beginning of H to end of H deflection in His bundle electrogram	Intra-Hisian conduction	< 30 ms
H- V	Beginning of H deflection to beginning of earliest V in ECG or intracardiac electrograms	Infranodal conduction	35–55 ms
PA	Beginning of earliest recorded atrial activity to beginning of A wave in the His bundle electrogram	Right atrial conduction	25–55 ms

in contact with the electrode and propagates through the conducting system and the myocardium. Pacing by different protocols in atria/ventricles is delivered either by continuous pacing or extrastimuli.

Continuous Pacing

Continuous pacing can be overdrive where pacing stimuli are delivered at a constant rate faster than that of the baseline rhythm. This is used to terminate induced or spontaneous tachyarrhythmias and is also known as antitachycardia pacing. In burst pacing, stimuli are delivered for a short duration but at constant rate (or cycle length). Ramp pacing implies a gradual decrease of pacing cycle length with each interval. The pacing protocols differ among different labs and operators and any of these can be used.

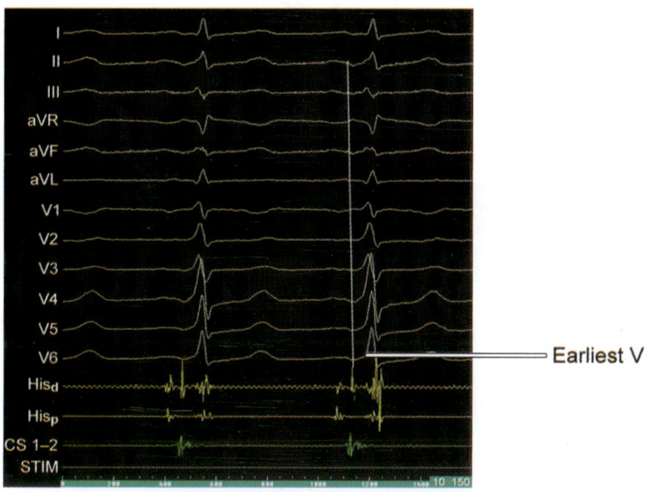

Figure 3.2: Electrogram of a patient with manifest pre-excitation. Vertical line from His deflection shows HV interval measured from H to earliest V in V6 is Zero, demonstrating ventricular pre-excitation

Generally for a supraventricular tachycardia (SVT) study, the protocol begins with a decremental ventricular pacing, though one can start with atrial pacing as well. The advantage of starting with ventricular pacing is rapid identification of a left sided accessory pathway if eccentric atrial activation is noted in the coronary sinus during ventricular pacing. More importantly, atrial pacing may inadvertently result in induction of nonclinical sustained atrial arrhythmias which cause a hindrance to studying the clinical arrhythmias and may require electrical cardioversion. This can be avoided to a large extent by initiating the EPS with ventricular pacing. The words incremental or decremental are interchangeably used to denote increasing pacing rate (in beats/minute) or decreasing cycle length (in milliseconds) respectively. Both however, mean that the chamber is being paced at progressively rapid rates. The relation between heart rate and cycle length is given by the formula heart rate = 60,000/ pacing cycle length. For SVT studies, ventricular pacing is begun at a cycle length shorter that the sinus cycle length and progressively decreased by 10 ms until VA conduction no longer occurs or a cycle length of 200 ms is reached. It is to be remembered that presence of VA conduction is not universal **(Figure 3.4)**. The complete absence of VA conduction in a patient with easily inducible arrhythmia rules out the diagnosis of orthodromic reciprocating tachycardia using the usual atrioventricular accessory pathway and makes the diagnosis of atrioventricular nodal re-entrant tachycardia (AVNRT) very unlikely. In contrast, atrial tachycardia can be induced and can continue irrespective of the presence of VA conduction. Interestingly, complete absence of antegrade AV conduction does not necessarily mean absence of retrograde conduction as VA conduction has been documented in 40%

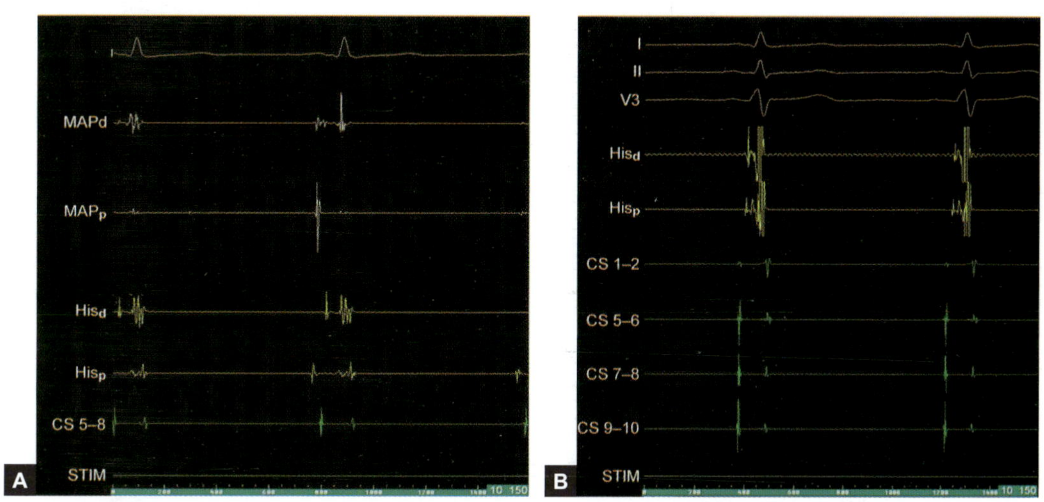

Figures 3.3A and B: (A) Split atrial signal can be mistaken for a His deflection. The timing of His bundle deflection in the His catheter confirms that the deflection in the mapping catheter is not true His bundle deflection; (B) Distally positioned His catheter records a right bundle potential which should not be mistaken for His deflection

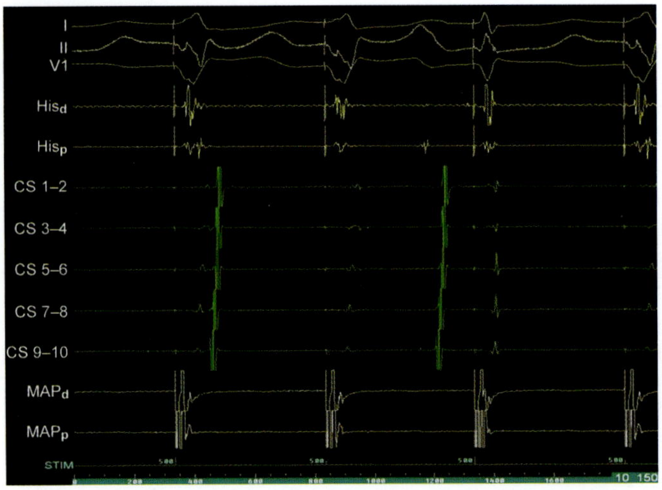

Figure 3.4: Ventricular pacing shows absence of VA conduction and VA dissociation

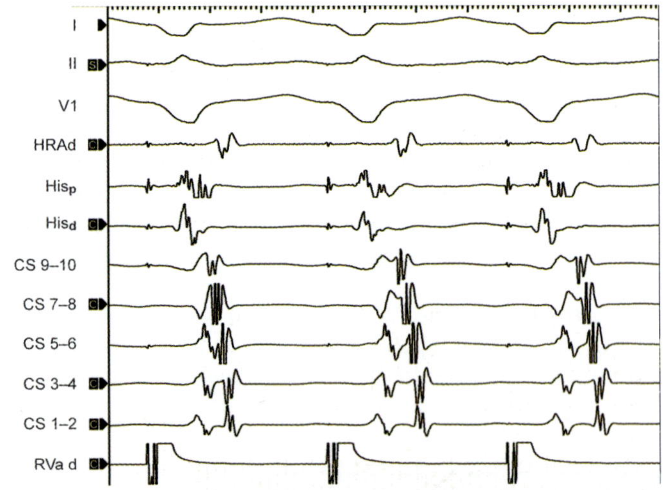

Figure 3.6: Concentric atrial activation where the earliest atrial signal is seen in His catheter and retrograde atrial activation in CS is proximal to distal during right ventricular pacing

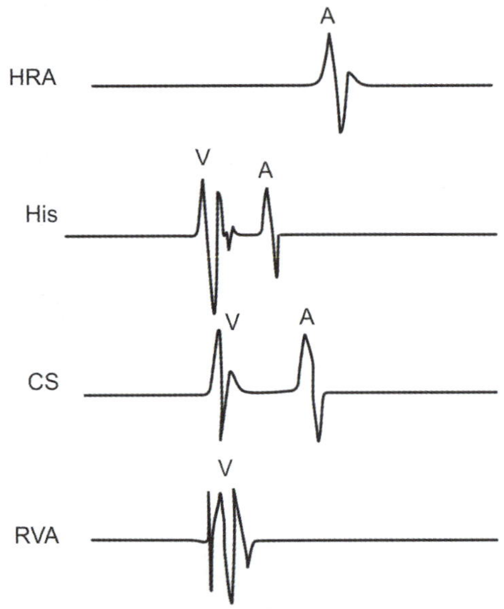

Figure 3.5: Normal VA conduction during ventricular pacing. Note that the earliest atrial signal in recorded in His catheter

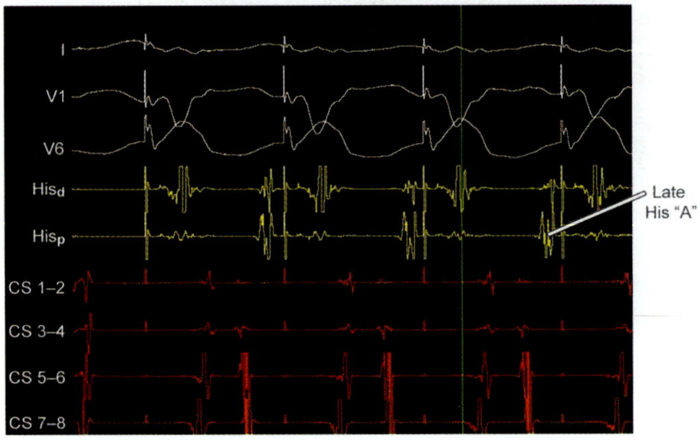

Figure 3.7: Eccentric atrial activation in a patient with retrogradely conducting left sided accessory pathway where the earliest atrial signal is in the distal CS (CS 1–2) which precedes the atrial signal in His catheter

of patients with infra-Hisian block.[1] When VA conduction is present, normally the earliest atrial activation is seen in the His bundle region followed by progression from CS proximal to distal. This normal activation sequence is called concentric atrial activation **(Figures 3.5 and 3.6)**. The distal to proximal atrial activation in CS electrodes during retrograde atrial activation is defined as eccentric atrial activation and usually denotes the presence of a retrogradely conducting left lateral accessory pathway **(Figure 3.7)**. Atrial activation that is later in His bundle region than in CS is also suggestive of extranodal VA conduction. The clue to location of an accessory pathway is provided by the CS channel recording the earliest atrial electrogram. When the distal CS records the earliest A, it denotes the presence of a left sided pathway. An earliest "a" signal in proximal CS indicates conduction through a posteroseptal pathway. Presence of concentric atrial activation does not rule out the presence of retrogradely conducting accessory pathways like right sided pathways and anteroseptal pathways. Sometimes during ventricular pacing, fusion between nodal and extranodal conduction can be seen that becomes purely extranodal over the accessory pathway as the AV node blocks at a faster pacing rate **(Figure 3.8)**.

Atrial pacing can be delivered from a dedicated catheter positioned in the right atrium or from any of the CS poles. Pacing the distal CS stimulates the left atrium while pacing the proximal CS stimulates right atrium. Decremental atrial pacing is performed to assess AV nodal conduction which depends on the integrity of the conduction system, the autonomic tone and medications being used. Normally with progressively increasing atrial rates, the AH interval gradually lengthens, before resulting in AH block which is the AV Wenckebach point. The HV interval throughout atrial pacing normally remains constant. Normal AV conduction is denoted by consistent AV conduction at least until 400 ms (150 bpm heart rate) with AH block occurring at the Wenckebach point. Atrial pacing can be done by ramp method (as described above) or by stepwise decremental atrial pacing wherein each paced cycle length is maintained for 15–60 seconds before reducing it sequentially. There are a few clinically relevant observations that can be made during atrial pacing. Pre-excitation may become manifest with progressive widening of QRS and corresponding shortening of the HV interval **(Figures 3.9A and B)**. Arrhythmias that may be induced are the clinical SVT and sometimes nonclinical atrial fibrillation which is undesirable. Sometimes ventricular tachycardia (VT) particularly idiopathic left ventricular tachycardia may be induced by atrial pacing **(Figure 3.10)**.

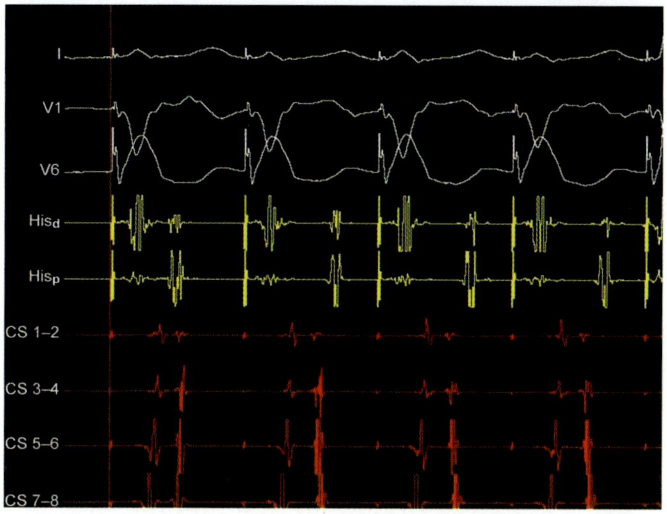

Figure 3.8: Change in retrograde atrial activation during ventricular pacing. The first beats shows fused atrial activation pattern whereas the subsequent beats show an eccentric atrial activation with earliest atrial activation in distal coronary sinus (CS 1–2)

Refractory Periods

During a cardiac cycle, once an action potential is initiated, the cardiac tissue is unexcitable to stimulation for some duration of time. This period is termed as refractory period. Refractory periods are generally determined during PES as response of the cardiac tissue to extrastimuli. Progressively premature extrastimuli are delivered scanning the diastole and their timing with respect to the action potential determines their conduction/capture or failure to achieve this (refractory). This is shown in **Figure 3.11**. There are 3 types of refractory periods:

1. *Effective refractory period (ERP)*: The ERP is the longest premature coupling interval (S1-S2) that results in failure of propagation or conduction through the tissue (Failure to capture or conduct). In practice, ERP is the one most often used in clinical electrophysiology. This period includes phases 0, 1, 2 and a part of phase 3 of the action potential. While assessing the ERP, one must be aware of the *Gap phenomenon*, wherein an atrial extrastimulus

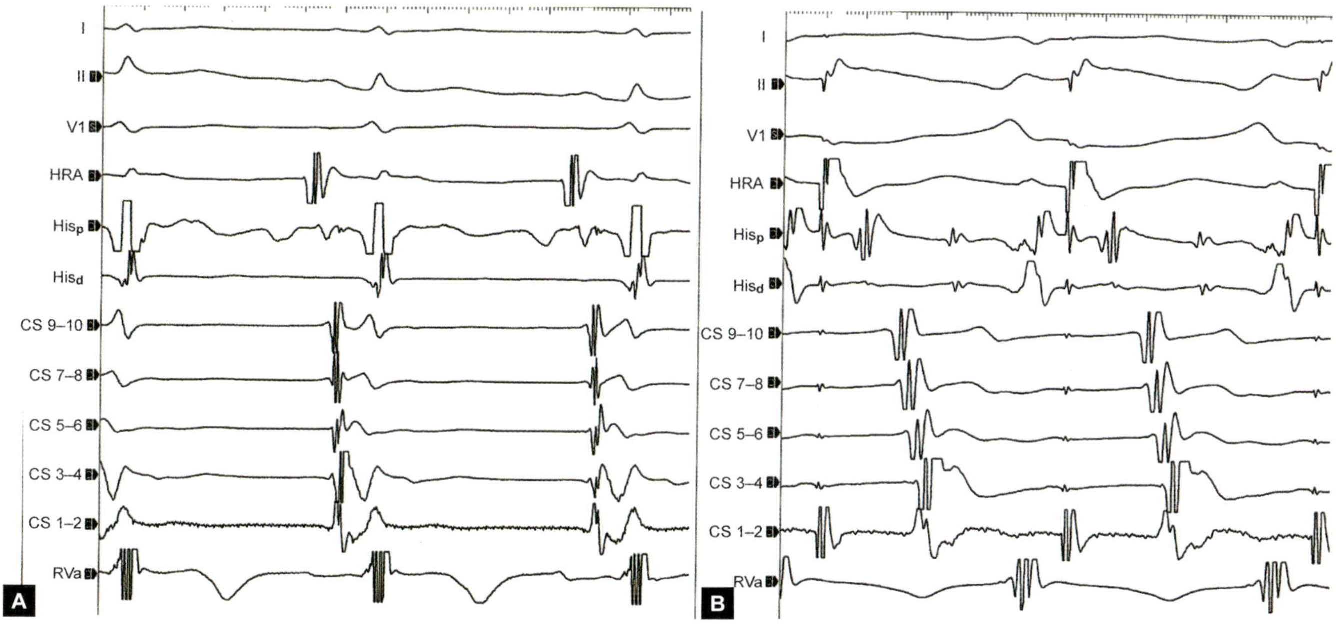

Figures 3.9A and B: (A) Ventricular preexcitation; (B) High atrial pacing is shown to cause widening of QRS complex with further shortening of HV interval demonstrating increasing preexcitation

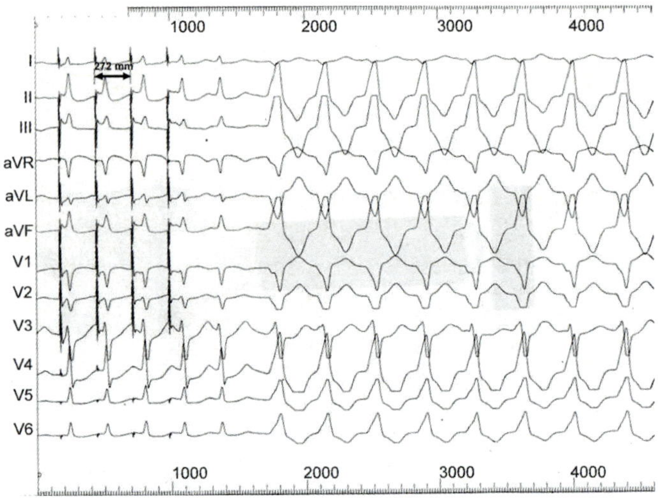

Figure 3.10: Atrial pacing inducing a sustained monomorphic VT of outflow tract origin

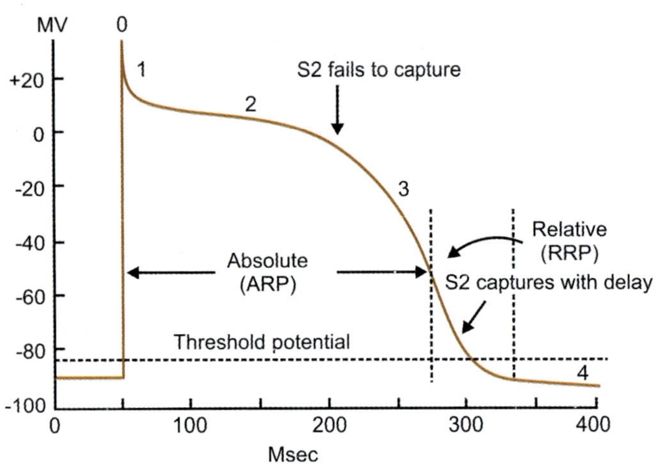

Figure 3.11: Figure showing the relation of extrastimuli to the action potential. As the extrastimulus is delivered more prematurely, it transits from relative refractory period to absolute refractory period. This is seen as transiting from conduction delay to loss of capture

causes a block in AV node but a more premature atrial extrastimulus conducts to the ventricle. This phenomenon is a normal response occurring due to differing refractory periods and conduction velocities at two different levels in the AV conduction system.[2] An atrial extra-stimulus may reach the His bundle when it is refractory causing an intra-Hisian block but with increased prematurity, this impulse conducts with a delay in the AV node, and reaches His bundle when it has recovered hence facilitating conduction. Though described as an illustrative example in the AV node, this phenomenon can occur anywhere in the conduction system antegradely or retrogradely.

2. *Relative refractory period (RRP):* The RRP is defined as the longest premature coupling interval (S1-S2) that results in prolonged conduction of the premature impulse. The RRP is generally slightly longer than ERP due to slowing or decremental conduction called as latency period. RRP extends over middle and late parts of the action potential.
3. *Functional refractory period (FRP)*: FRP is the shortest output interval that can result from any 2 consecutive input impulses into that tissue.

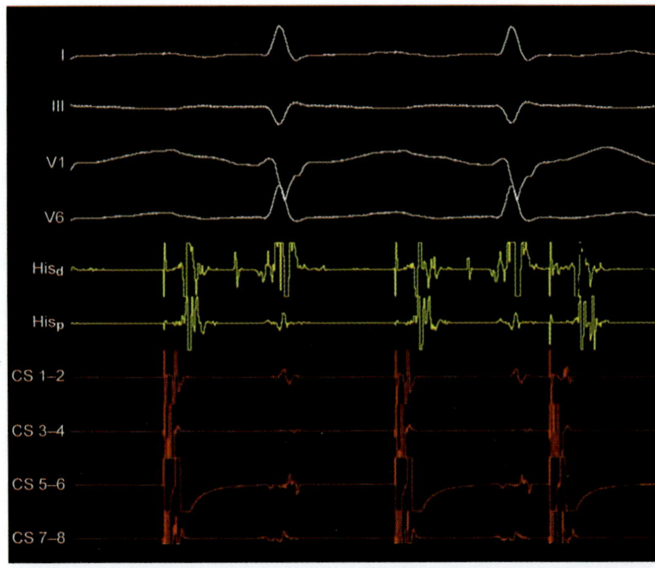

Figure 3.12: AVNERP. The first 2 pacing stimuli delivered in right atrium capture the atrium and conduct to the ventricle while the 3rd stimulus captures the atrium but does not conduct to ventricle. It blocks in the AV node as shown by the absence of H and V following the atrial electrogram in the His bundle electrograms

Examples of refractory periods are shown in **Figures 3.12 to 3.17**.

PROGRAMMED ELECTRICAL STIMULATION: MECHANISTIC INSIGHTS

Electrophysiology study involves 2 types of pacing—the incremental/decremental pacing, which has been described earlier and the extrastimulus technique. The extrastimulus technique involves pacing from chamber of interest (atrium/ventricle) at a constant drive train (S1) of 6–8 impulses followed by a single extrastimulus (S2). The cycle length of the drive cycle is shorter than the sinus cycle length and is typically 600 or 500 ms. The time interval between S1 and S2 is the coupling interval which is gradually decremented by 10 ms until it is not conducted further or fails to capture. The physiology of EP study with extrastimuli is closely related to the static and dynamic refractory periods of the cardiac tissue. To understand this, we can use the example of PES from right atrium. A basic drive train achieves a constant refractory period and conduction times through the AV node, His bundle and distal conduction system. As the premature

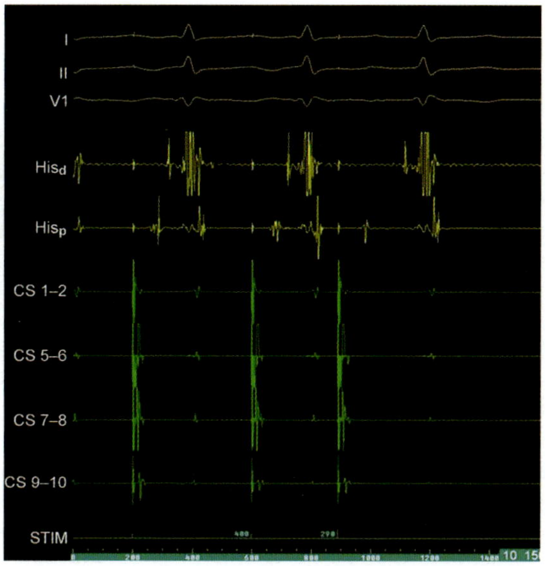

Figure 3.13: The 1st 2 beats show conduction of a captured atrial impulse to the ventricle with a constant AH interval. With the introduction of an atrial extrastimulus there is a sudden increase in the AH interval, demonstrating transition of nodal conduction from fast to slow pathway

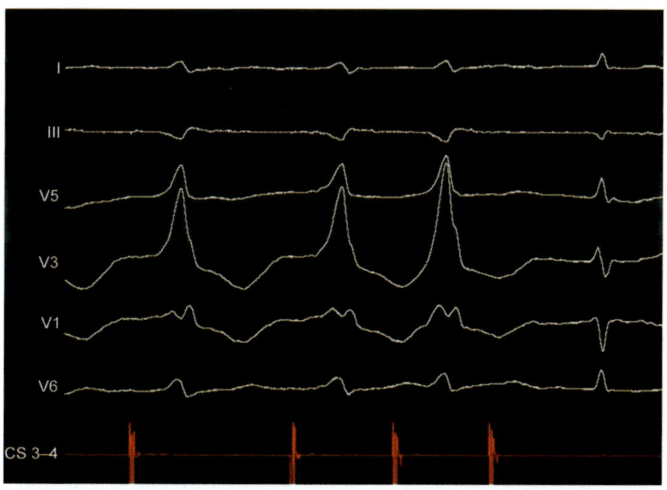

Figure 3.14: Accessory pathway ERP. Loss of pre-excitation with the second atrial extrastimulus, shown by narrowing of QRS complex

impulse (S2) is introduced with progressively decreasing coupling intervals, initially it may be conducted with no perceptible delay but as coupling interval becomes shorter, the relative refractory period of AV node is reached which is seen by progressive prolongation of AH interval followed by AH block. The coupling interval at which conduction blocks in AV node is the AV nodal effective refractory period (AVNERP). In the situation where there are dual AV nodal pathways, AV conduction continues through the slow pathway when the fast pathway ERP is reached. This is shown

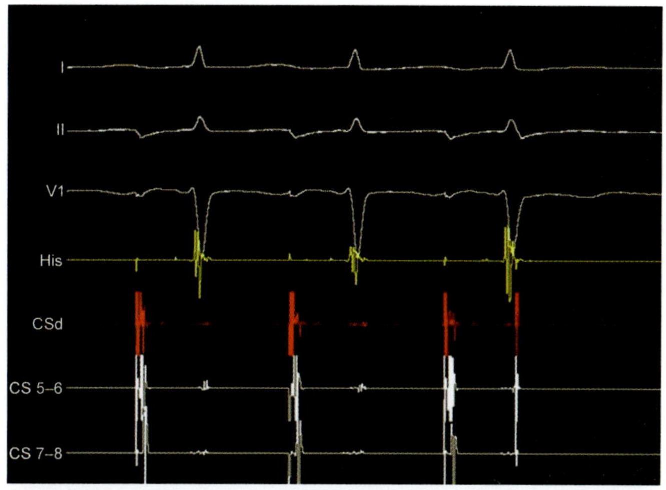

Figure 3.15: Atrial ERP. The drive cycle (1st 3 beats) captures the atrium but the extrastimulus does not, indicating that the atrium has become refractory

in **Figure 3.13**. In this case, the AH interval gradually prolongs but instead of blocking, the AH suddenly prolongs markedly (AH jump) due to a sudden shift of conduction from the fast pathway to the slow pathway. Once conduction begins in the slow pathway, the AH again progressively lengthens with decreasing coupling intervals and finally blocks. The AVNERP is in this case is hence the ERP of the slow pathway. At cellular level the concept of the extrastimulus can be understood by appreciating that the delivered premature impulse gradually scans the phase 3 of the action potential before it blocks (reaches ERP). In the presence of a slow pathway, the premature impulse shifts to RRP of slow pathway instead of blocking and progressively ascends up until it reaches the steep potion of phase 3, when it blocks. In a patient with distally diseased conduction system, this normal physiology may not occur and extrastimuli may result in prolongation of HV interval and block distal to the His bundle. This indicates pathology (most commonly degenerative) of the infra-Hisian conduction system necessitating implantation of a pacemaker.

Extrastimuli in Tachycardia Induction

The era of PES with extrastimuli began with the paper from Wellens' lab where EP study was performed in 4 patients with Wolff-Parkinson-White (WPW) syndrome and tachycardia was induced in 2 of them.[3] The same group subsequently published their observations on the relation of extrastimuli to induction of ventricular tachycardia (VT) in the lab.[4] Josephson et al demonstrated the safety and feasibility of using multiple extrastimuli and performing stimulation protocols from the left ventricle.[5] Currently PES technique using extrastimuli is used to induce tachyarrhythmias like AVNRT, AVRT, reentrant VT, AT and atrial flutter. In all these reentrant arrhythmias, the basic underlying substrate is the presence of two pathways having differing refractory periods and conduction velocities—limb A having a faster conducting velocity with a longer refractory period and limb B having a slower conducting velocity with a shorter refractory period. These two limbs are connected proximally and distally to form a reentrant circuit. In addition, at least one of the limbs should be capable of retrograde conduction. The basic drive cycle impulses conduct through the limb A of the reentrant circuit. The premature impulse (the extrastimulus) arrives at a time when the faster conducting limb A is refractory due to the previous impulse, hence conducts through the slower conducting limb B. This impulse reaches the distal end of the circuit when the limb A has recovered to accept this impulse and conduct retrogradely to reach the proximal end of the circuit. By this time the limb B has also recovered and conducts antegradely resulting in initiation of the reentrant tachycardia. As progressively premature extrastimuli are delivered, tachycardia continues to get initiated until ERP of limb B is also reached. The zone of coupling intervals between ERP of limb A and ERP of limb B is the tachycardia zone, and wider this zone, the easier it is to initiate the tachycardia. It can be appreciated that drugs that increase the ERP of cardiac tissue result in narrowing the tachycardia zone and make it difficult for tachycardia to get initiated or sustain. Tachycardia induction may necessitate introduction of double or triple extrastimuli. In these situations, the first extrastimulus shortens the ERP facilitating the conduction of the 2nd extrastimulus (S3). This shortening of ERP occurs at coupling intervals of S2, 50–100 ms above the ERP determined during the basic drive cycle length. For example, if ERP is 400/210 ms the next sequence of stimulation begins from 400/260/260 ms. Induction protocols are performed with at least two drive cycles as the refractory periods of the conducting system, atrial and ventricular tissue depends on the basic drive cycle length—the shorter the drive cycle, the shorter is the ERP. AV node behaves differently as ERP increases with increasing cycle lengths due to fatigue phenomenon.[6]

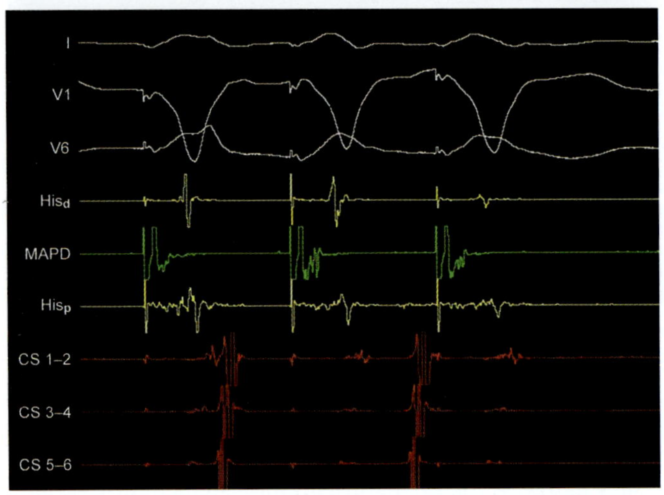

Figure 3.16: Ventriculoatrial Effective Refractory Period (VAERP). The ventricular extrastimulus captures the ventricle but does not conduct to atrium due to refractoriness or block in the AV node

The Technique of Ventricular Extrastimuli

Programmed electrical stimulation (PES) in ventricle is usually performed to induce ventricular tachycardia. Standard stimulation protocol involves pacing from two different sites of right ventricle (RV apex and RVOT), and with two different basic drive cycles. Less commonly left ventricle is used for pacing if VT is not induced with RV pacing.

- *Single extrastimulus (S1–S2)*: The first technique involves 6–8 ventricular paced beats at a constant drive cycle

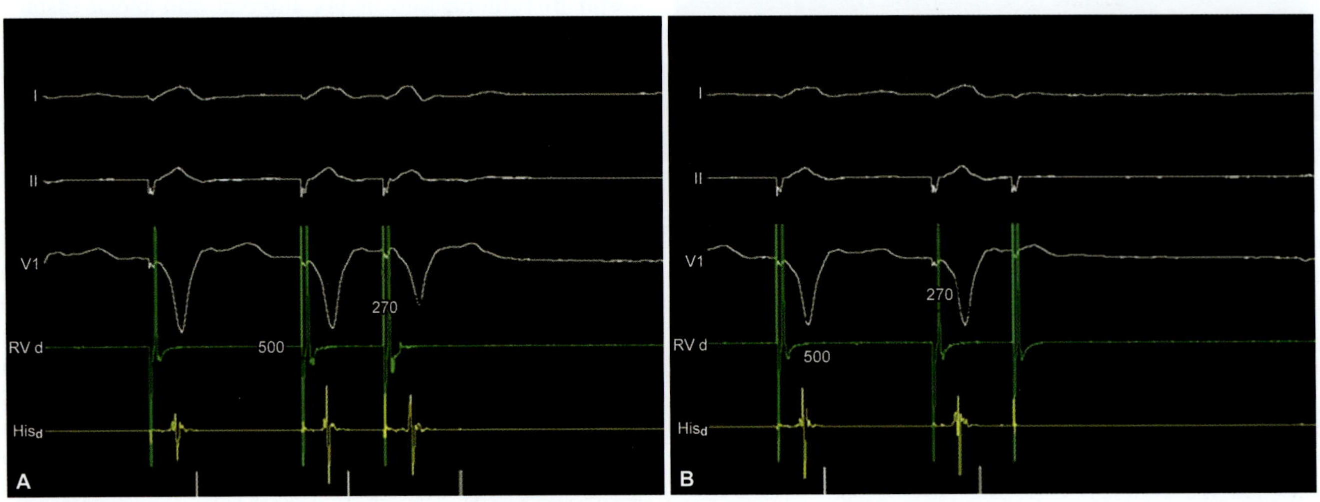

Figures 3.17A and B: Decrement of ventricle extrastimulus by 10 ms (270–260 ms) from A to B causes loss of capture demonstrating Ventricular Effective Refractory Period (VERP)

(usually 500, 400 or 350 ms) followed by a premature ventricular stimulus S2. S2 is gradually moved closer to S1 by intervals of 10–20 ms until arrhythmia is induced or the refractory period of ventricle is reached. Each cycle is followed by a 3–5 second pause to assess the response to stimulation.

- *Double extrastimuli (S1, S2, S3)*: This technique involves 6–8 ventricular paced beats at a constant drive cycle followed by premature double extrastimuli. The value of S2 and S3 is obtained by adding approximately 50 ms to ERP. For example, if the ERP is 250 ms, S2 and S3 are initiated at 300 ms. During stimulation, S3 is gradually brought closer to S2 by decrements of 10 ms until S3 no longer captures. Then S2 is brought closer to S1 by decrements of 10 ms until S3 captures again. Gradually S1 S2 and S2 S3 are decremented. These cycles are repeated until S2 reaches refractory period of ventricle **(Figure 3.18)**.

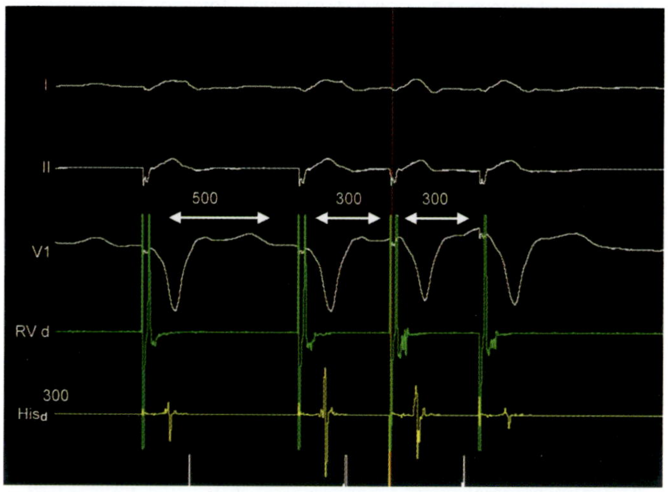

Figure 3.18: An example of ventricular double extrastimuli at a drive cycle of 500 ms with 2 extrastimuli delivered at coupling intervals of 300 and 300 ms

- *Triple extrastimuli (S1, S2, S3, S4)*: The introduction of a 3rd extrastimulus is sometimes needed to induce arrhythmia. This technique increases sensitivity of induction at the cost of specificity. The starting value of S3 and S4 is 50 ms greater than the ERP obtained by double extrastimuli. S4 is gradually brought closer to S3 until S4 no longer captures. S2 S3 are then decremented, so that S4 captures again. S1 S2 and S2 S3 are decremented. Diastole is scanned by these premature stimuli until S2 reaches refractory period of ventricle or arrhythmia is induced.
- *Burst pacing*: Burst is a sequence of 8–10 paced ventricular beats which are progressively decremented by 20–50 ms until ERP is reached. Generally one does not pace below 200 ms to avoid induction of nonclinical arrhythmias like ventricular fibrillation.
- *Use of drugs*: When PES at baseline fails to induce clinical arrhythmia, drugs like isoproterenol or phenylephrine may be used to provoke and facilitate the induction of arrhythmia. These drugs are infused at 1–2 μg/minute. Isoproterenol increases heart rates by 15–25 beats/minute and facilitates arrhythmia induction by increasing conduction, decreasing refractory periods and increasing automaticity. Phenylephrine causes increase in blood pressure and decrease in heart rates. Sometimes an AV nodal blocking drug like diltiazem may be used to uncover retrograde accessory pathway conduction **(Figures 3.19A and B)**.

Long-short sequence: The relation of drive cycle to the refractory periods of atria, ventricles and His-Purkinje system

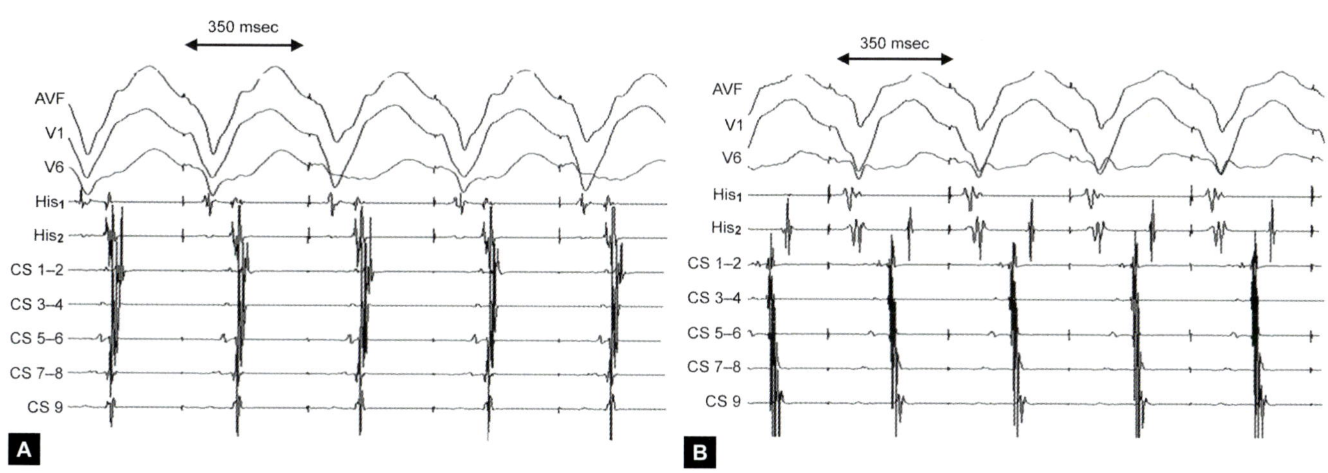

Figures 3.19A and B: Presence of a very robust nodal VA conduction may not reveal a retrograde accessory pathway during V pacing. Use of intravenous Diltiazem shows eccentric VA conduction due to slowing of nodal VA conduction. (A) V pacing at 350 ms demonstrating concentric VA conduction; (B) V pacing at the same cycle length on IV Diltiazem infusion shows VA conduction through a left accessory pathway with His A being later and distal CS (CS 1–2) being earliest

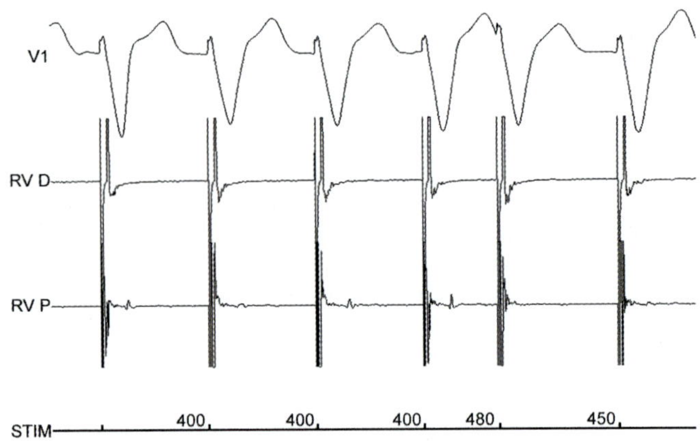

Figure 3.20: Long-short-long pacing sequence

is fairly predictable, that is, the ERP decreases with shorter cycle lengths. However, the abrupt changes in the drive cycle length or premature impulses may have differential effects on the refractory periods of the His-Purkinje system and ventricular myocardium. These observations have resulted in specific ventricular pacing protocols to induce VTs like bundle branch reentry VT (BBR VT). It has been shown that decreasing the drive cycle length shortens the refractory period of His-Purkinje system and ventricular myocardium similarly, but increasing the drive cycle length lengthens the ERP of the His-Purkinje system but not the ventricular muscle.[7] When an extrastimulus is delivered after a basic drive cycle, it shortens the ERP of His-Purkinje system and ventricle but if such an extrastimulus is followed by a pause equal to basic drive cycle, delivery of next drive cycle after this pause will show that the refractory period of the ventricular muscle has recovered to baseline but that of the His-Purkinje system has markedly lengthened.[8] A short-long or a long-short-long sequence of paced ventricular stimuli is sometimes helpful in induction of BBR VT where the underlying electrophysiological abnormality is the infra-Hisian conduction delay **(Figure 3.20)**.

Response to Ventricular Stimuli

The primary objective in ventricular stimulation protocol is induction of VT. It is necessary to be conversant with various responses observed during PES.

- *Repetitive ventricular responses*: 2–5 nonstimulated ventricular beats in response to paced premature beat/beats. These should be recognized as normal variants. These are commonly due to bundle branch reentry and less often due to reentry in AV node or in the ventricular myocardium.[9] **(Figure 3.21)**.
- *Nonsustained VT*: VT lasting from 6 beats to 30 seconds, terminating spontaneously and not requiring any intervention **(Figure 3.22)**.

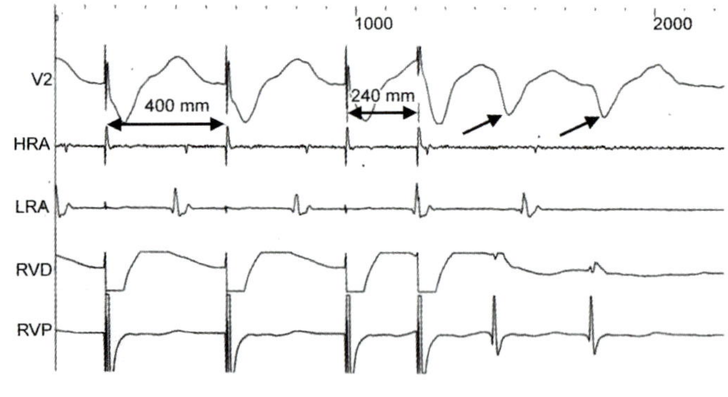

Figure 3.21: Repetitive ventricular beats

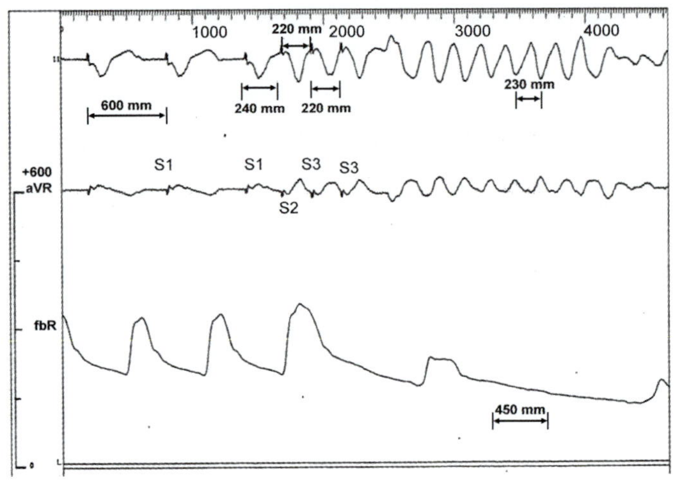

Figure 3.22: Induction of nonsustained VT by triple extrastimuli

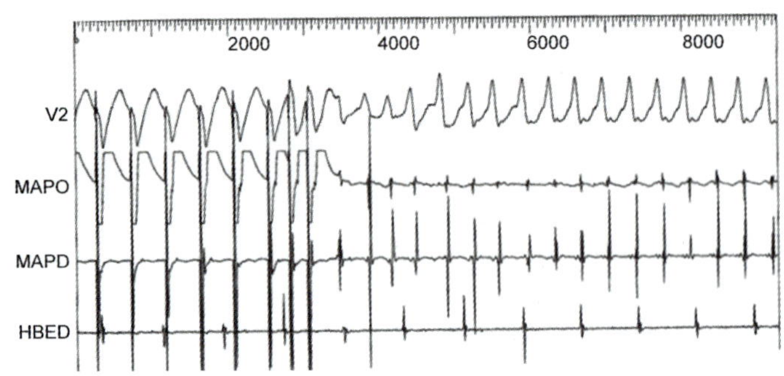

Figure 3.23: Sustained monomorphic VT induced by ventricular double extrastimuli

- *Sustained VT*: VT lasting more than 30 seconds or clinically requiring intervention to terminate arrhythmia **(Figure 3.23)**. Sustained monomorphic VT is the most important response to ventricular stimulation as it has the highest predictive value for sudden death.

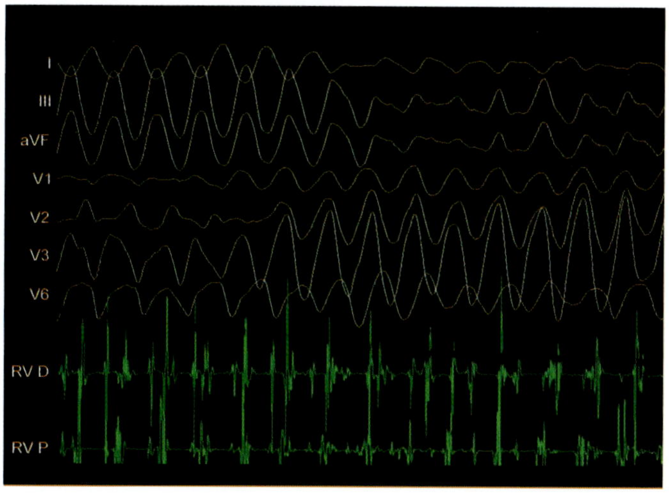

Figure 3.24: Induced polymorphic VT

- *Monomorphic VT*: VT with a stable configuration of QRS complexes in at least 3 simultaneously recorded ECG leads.
- *Polymorphic VT*: VT with continuously varying QRS complex configuration in any recorded ECG lead **(Figure 3.24)**.
- *Ventricular fibrillation*: Ventricular arrhythmia with absence of clearly defined QRS complexes in the ECG.

REFERENCES

1. Schuilenburg RM. Patterns of VA conduction in the human heart in the presence of normal and abnormal AV conduction. In: Wellens HJJ, Lie KI, Jane MJ (Eds). The conduction system of the heart. Philadelphia; Lea and Febiger; 1976.pp.485-503.
2. Josephson ME. Miscellaneous phenomenon related to atrioventricular conduction. In: Josephson ME (Ed). Clinical Cardiac Electrophysiology, 4th edn. Philadelphia. Lippincott Williams and Wilkinson; 2008.pp.145-59.
3. Durrer D, Schoo L, Schuilenburg RM, Wellens HJ. The Role of Premature Beats in the Initiation and the Termination of Supraventricular Tachycardia in the Wolff-Parkinson-White Syndrome. Circulation. 1967;36:644-62.
4. Wellens HJ, Düren DR, Lie KI. Observations on mechanisms of ventricular tachycardia in man. Circulation. 1976;54:237-44.
5. Michelson EL, Spielman SR, Greenspan AM, Farshidi A, Horowitz LN, Josephson ME. Electrophysiologic study of the left ventricle: indications and safety. Chest. 1979;75:592-6.
6. Simson MB, Spear JF, Moore EN. Electrophysiologic studies on atrioventricular nodal Wenckebach cycles. Am J Cardiol. 1978;41:244-58.
7. Denker S, Lehmann MH, Mahmud R, Gilbert C, Akhtar M. Divergence between refractoriness of His-Purkinje system and ventricular muscle with abrupt changes in cycle length. Circulation. 1983;68:1212-21.
8. Denker S, Shenasa M, Gilbert CJ, Akhtar M. Effects of abrupt changes in cycle length on refractoriness of the His-Purkinje system in man. Circulation. 1983;67:60-8.
9. Roy D, Brugada P, Bar FW, Wellens HJ. Repetitive responses to ventricular extrastimuli: incidence and significance in patients without organic heart disease. Eur Heart J. 1983;4:79-85.

EDITORS' SUMMARY

This chapter taken along with that on signals, signal processing, and artifacts (Chapter 2), is the foundation for all the complex mapping and technical maneuvers performed in the EP and ablation laboratory. Beyond the definitions that are well-explained by Dr Rao, the importance of exact measurements and recognizing incorrectly made measurements or executed maneuvers has been outlined.

Well-illustrated in this chapter are the basic differences in extrastimulus versus incremental or decremental pacing, particularly the responses to such pacing maneuvers during arrhythmia and related to AV node and infra-Hisian conduction.

The information provided in this chapter would be a prerequisite to reading the chapter on 3-dimensional mapping (Chapter 9) as well as the interpretation of pacing maneuvers done to elucidate the differential diagnosis of narrow and wide complex tachycardias.

CHAPTER 4

Watchara Lohawijarn, Negar Salehi, Vini Singh, Aravdeep S Jhand, Ranjan K Thakur

Sinus Node Function Evaluation and Abnormalities

LIST OF ABBREVIATIONS

AF	Atrial Fibrillation	IHR	Intrinsic Heart Rate
AFl	Atrial Flutter	IST	Inappropriate Sinus Tachycardia
AT	Atrial Tachycardia	POTS	Postural Orthostatic Tachycardia Syndrome
CL	Cycle Length	SA	Sinoatrial
CSNRT	Corrected Sinus Node Recovery Time	SN	Sinus Node
EP	Electrophysiology	SND	Sinus Node Dysfunction
HRA	High Right Atrium	SNRT	Sinus Node Recovery Time

INTRODUCTION

The sinus node (SN) is the primary cardiac pacemaker. While numerous abnormalities in SN function can be identified, including rare genetic mutations resulting in sinus node dysfunction in young patients, this chapter will focus on the most common abnormalities encountered in practice and their clinical evaluation.

Structurally, the SN is a complex, crescent-shaped structure, located subepicardially at the junction of the superior vena cava and the right atrium, measuring about 1 to 2 cm in length and 2 to 3 mm in width and thickness.[1,2] The SN receives its blood supply from the sinus node artery, which arises either from the right coronary artery or the left circumflex artery in nearly equal proportion. The SN is richly innervated by sympathetic and parasympathetic nerves, which play a key role in heart rate regulation.[1,3]

The pacemaking nodal cells in the SN are widely distributed within the structure, but they discharge synchronously, giving rise to 2 or 3 individual wavefronts, which merge to form a single, dominant wavefront.[4] The nodal cells are isolated electrically from the surrounding atrial myocardium by perinodal, dense connective tissue. The dominant wavefront exits the sinus node via limited number of exit sites located at the periphery, consisting of nodal cells intermingled with ordinary atrial myocytes.

Heart rate is determined by a complex interplay between sinus node automaticity, determined by the slope of phase 4 depolarization, autonomic influences via vagal and adrenergic inputs and hormonal factors. Changes in physiologic parameters, such as blood pressure, respiration and posture influence heart rate via autonomic modulation. There is an anatomical correlate of heart rate and site of impulse formation within the SN – faster heart rates originate in the superior portion of the SN, whereas slower rates originate more inferiorly in the SN.[5] Furthermore, detailed mapping studies have shown spontaneous variation in P-wave morphologies related to atrial exit site from the SN.[6]

Major clinically relevant sinus node abnormalities may be classified as tachycardias or bradycardias **(Table 4.1)**.

Table 4.1: Common forms of sinus node dysfunction

Tachycardias—rare
• Sinus node reentry • Inappropriate sinus tachycardia
Bradycardias—common
• Intermittent bradycardia – Bradycardia—pauses - Sinus bradycardia - Sinus pause or sinus arrest - Sinoatrial exit block First-degree Second-degree—type I and type II Third-degree – Tachycardia-bradycardia syndrome • Persistent bradycardia Chronotropic incompetence

Clinically, tachycardias due to sinus node abnormalities are rare and bradycardias predominate. Intermittent bradycardias are more common and add to the complexity of documenting electrocardiographic findings and correlating them with symptoms, which may be very nonspecific. The most common persistent bradycardia is chronotropic incompetence.

Bradycardia due to sinus node dysfunction (SND) may result from idiopathic degeneration of the nodal cells (associated with aging), ischemia or fibrosis/infiltrative processes. Recently, a reversible form of SND due to atrial tachyarrhythmias has been identified. Since the advent of catheter ablation, reversible SND (postconversion pauses and abnormal sinus node function during electrophysiologic testing) has been identified in patients undergoing ablation for atrial fibrillation (AF) or atrial flutter (AFl)[7] **(Figures 4.1 and 4.2)**. The mechanism of SND is thought to be due to

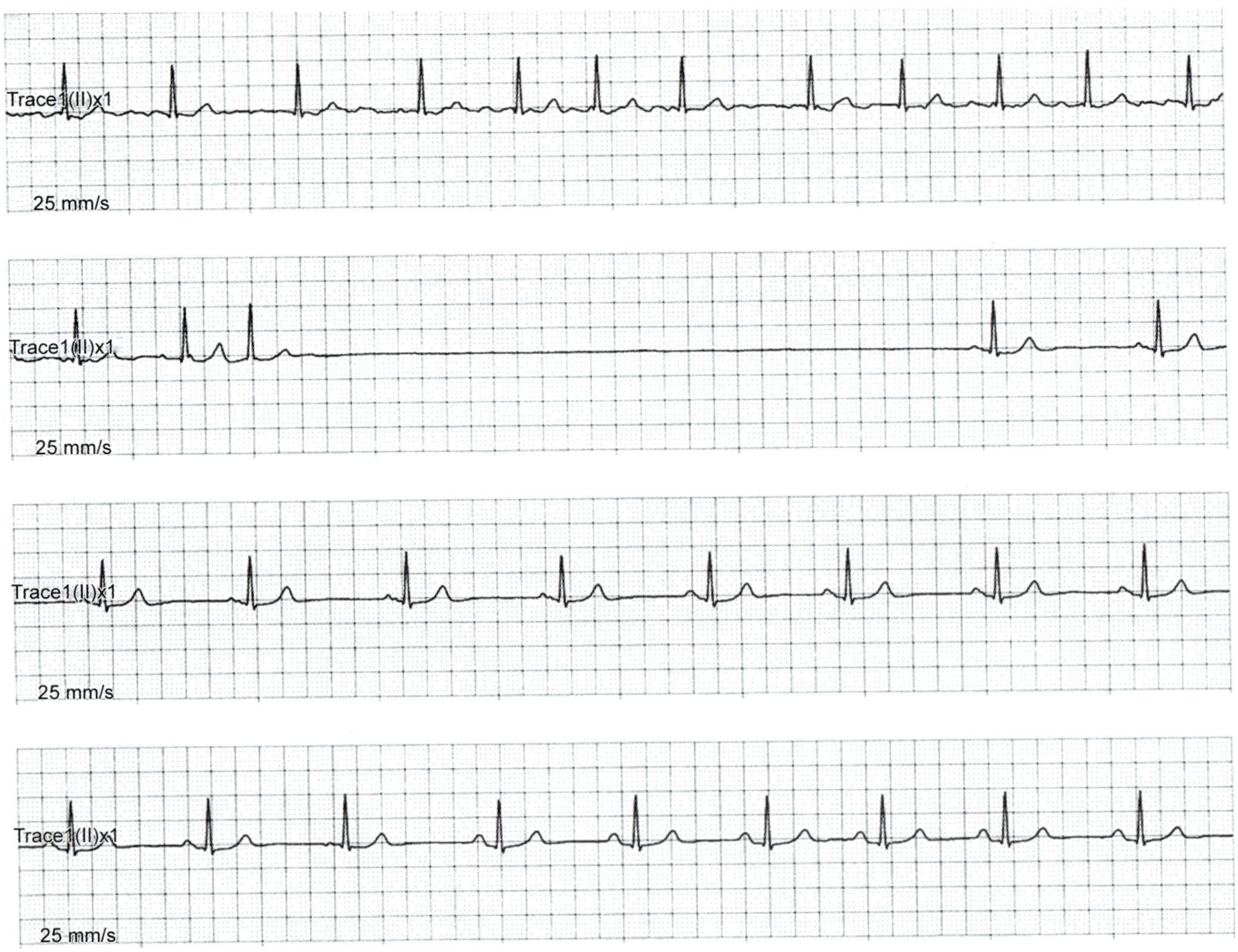

Figure 4.1: A 78-year-old man with atrial fibrillation is shown. After AF terminates, a long pause follows and then sinus node function returns. Atrial fibrillation caused suppression of the sinus node, resulting in a pause at its termination

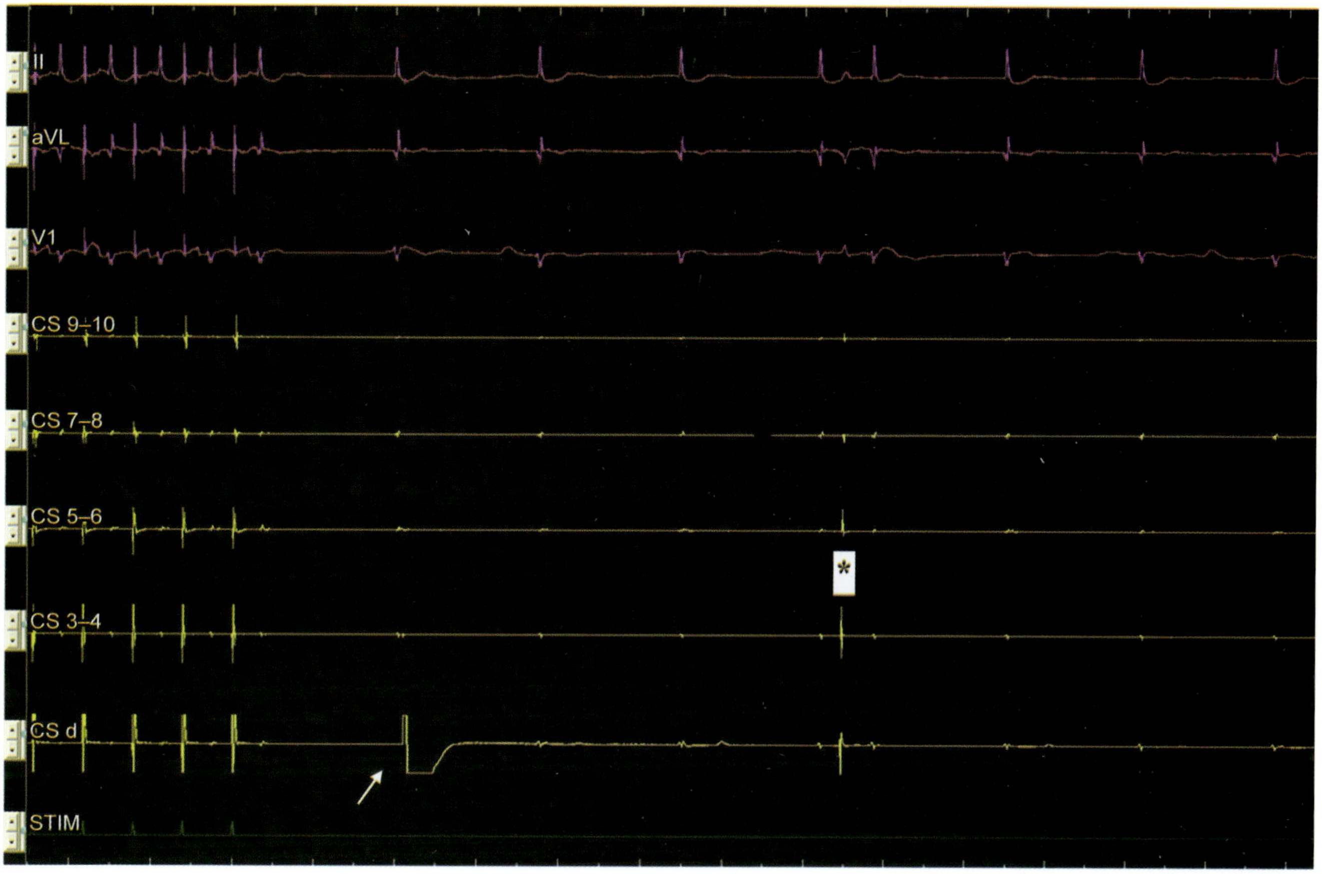

Figure 4.2: After AF ablation in a 48-year-old woman, sinus node recovery time is tested at a drive cycle length of 600 ms. After atrial pacing terminates, sinus node recovers nearly 7 seconds later (*). Arrow marks an artifact

tachycardia-induced ionic remodeling in the SN.[8,9] However, for the majority of patients, the exact mechanism of SND cannot be identified with any certainty and is subject to conjecture.

SINUS NODE ABNORMALITIES: TACHYCARDIAS

- *Sinus node reentry tachycardia:* Sinus node reentry as the mechanism of a paroxysmal tachycardia can be a difficult diagnosis to establish with certainty. A point of contention is that reentry strictly limited to the SN has never been demonstrated unequivocally. Sinus node reentry was originally described to have the following electrophysiologic features: 1) inducibility and termination by programmed stimulation, 2) P-wave morphology during tachycardia identical to sinus P-waves and 3) tachycardia cycle lengths (CL) 350 to 550 ms.[10] Differentiation from atrial tachycardias (AT) can be difficult because ATs may have the same electrophysiologic features and often originate from the crista terminalis, which is anatomically adjacent to the SN leading to similar P-wave morphology.
- *Inappropriate sinus tachycardia (IST):* IST is a poorly characterized condition that may be due to multiple mechanisms. Salient clinical features of IST include a persistently elevated resting heart rate (>90 bpm), associated with an exaggerated response to minimal exertion or postural change (>25 bpm).[11] Postural orthostatic tachycardia syndrome (POTS) and physiologic factors that may contribute to tachycardia, such as hyperthyroidism or drug effect, need to be excluded before reaching this diagnosis.[11] To a large extent, IST is a diagnosis of exclusion. Many potential mechanisms have been postulated for IST, the most widely quoted being: 1) abnormality of the sympathovagal balance in the sinus node, evidenced by elevated intrinsic heart rate (IHR) determined after autonomic blockade (intravenous atropine 0.04 mg/kg and propranolol 0.2 mg/kg),[12] 2) hyper-responsiveness to adrenergic influences, evidenced by an exaggerated response to infusion of isoproterenol[13] and 3) a channelopathy involving the

adenosine-sensitive potassium channel, evidenced by a blunted response to intravenous adenosine.[14]

SINUS NODE ABNORMALITIES: BRADYCARDIAS

SND and resultant bradycardia is correlated with advancing age. Symptoms can vary from being asymptomatic to having recurrent syncope. Significant hemodynamic symptoms or syncope are usually due to prolonged sinus pauses resulting in cerebral hypoperfusion. Arrhythmias associated with SND usually occur intermittently.

Intermittent Bradycardias

Bradycardia–Pauses

SND may manifest as sinus bradycardia as well as a variety of arrhythmias leading to pauses.

- *Sinus bradycardia:* Sinus bradycardia is arbitrarily defined as a heart rate less than 60 bpm. Most patients with sinus bradycardia do not have SND. In fact, most are due to physiologic condition or medications; systemic disease such as hypothyroidism or electrolyte abnormalities are uncommon causes of sinus bradycardia. Persistent sinus bradycardia without a reversible cause, associated with blunted response to an increasing metabolic demand, is known as chronotropic incompetence (discussed below) and it should be considered a form of SND. The clinical manifestations of sinus node dysfunction are diverse and nonspecific, such as exercise intolerance, fatigue, malaise, lassitude, dyspnea on exertion, dizziness, lightheadedness or syncope. It is believed that these symptoms are caused by an inadequate cardiac output due to the slow heart rate relative to the metabolic demand of the body.

  ECG: Sinus bradycardia is defined as a rate less than 60 beats per minute with normal P-wave axis (upright P-waves in leads II, III and aVF) **(Figure 4.3)**. The P-wave morphology may be atypical at slow rates, possibly related to the wavefront exiting from a different exit site in the sinus node.
- *Sinus pause or sinus arrest:* Sinus pause or sinus arrest manifests as a pause > 2 seconds in duration and the pause is not a multiple of the preceding PP interval **(Figure 4.4)**.[15] Like sinus bradycardia, sinus pause may be caused by physiologic conditions rather than sinus node dysfunction. Most episodes may be due to high vagal tone, for example, associated with nausea, vomiting, pain or in well-trained athletes.
- *Sinoatrial exist block:* In sinoatrial (SA) exit block, the impulse is generated normally in the SN but fails to conduct to the atrium because of delay in conduction or block in the perinodal connective tissue called the sinoatrial junction. It is classified by severity into three categories:

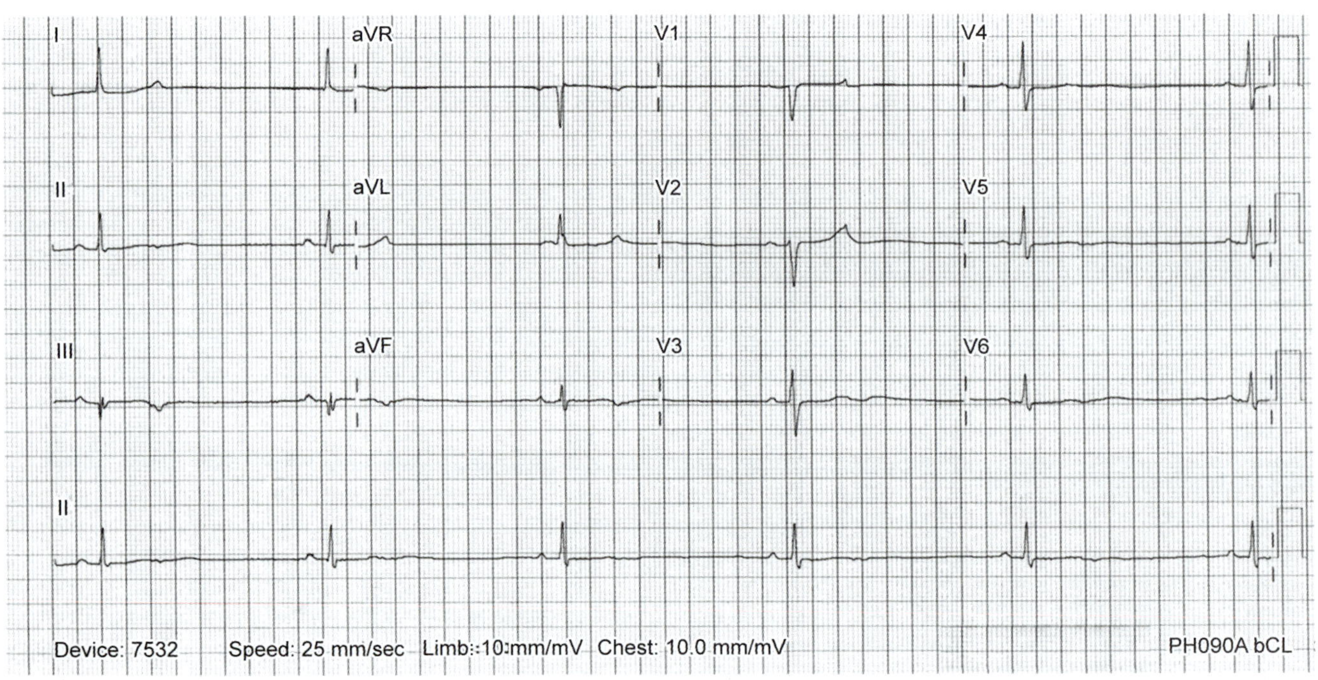

Figure 4.3: 12-lead ECG showing marked sinus bradycardia at a rate of 32 beats per minute

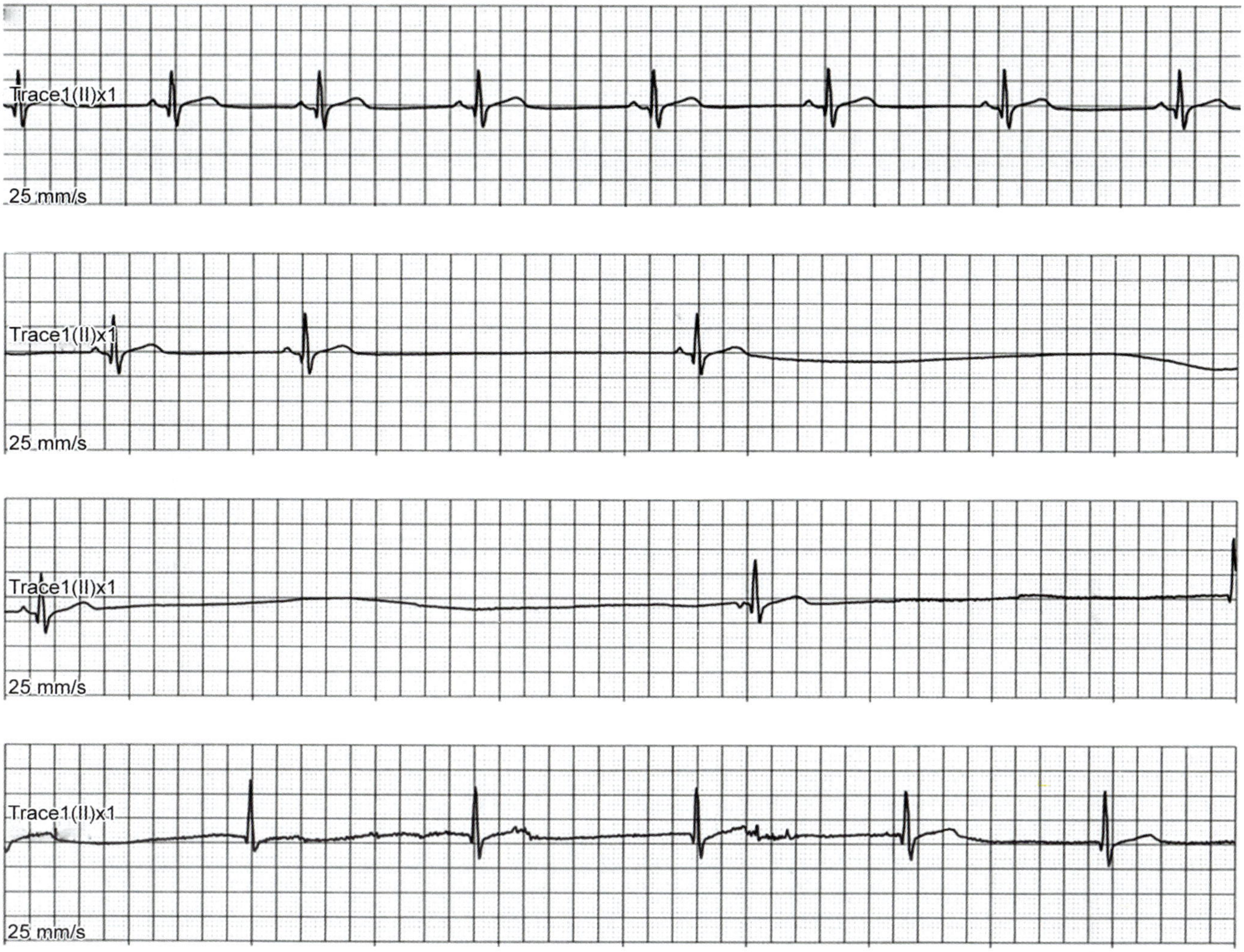

Figure 4.4: Continuous telemetry monitor strip showing sinus bradycardia followed by first sinus pause of 3.16 seconds, second sinus pause 4.72 seconds and sinus arrest with junctional escape rhythm

First-degree sinoatrial exit block: Every impulse formed within the SN can conduct to the atria with a delay but with no changes in the PP interval **(Figure 4.5)**. This condition cannot be detected on a surface ECG as the origin of the impulse from sinus node is not depicted on the ECG. It can only be diagnosed by an electrophysiology (EP) study to measure the sinoatrial conduction time.

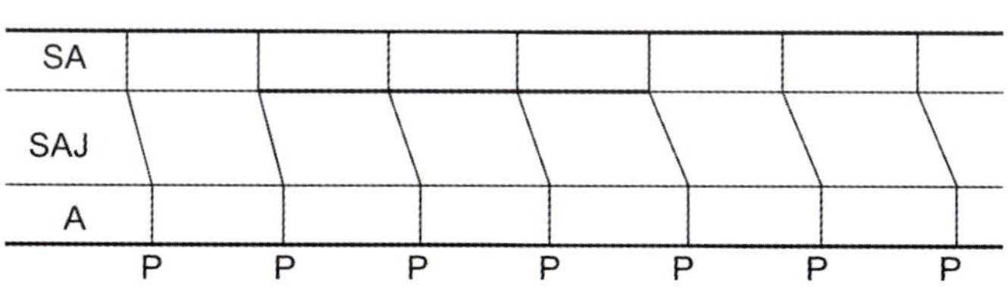

Figure 4.5: Ladder diagram showing activation sequence in first degree sinoatrial block

Abbreviations: SA, SA node; SAJ, sinoatrial junction; A, atria; P, P-wave

Second-degree sinoatrial exit block: Second-degree sinoatrial exit block can be divided into Type I and Type II.[15] Mobitz Type I sinoatrial exit block **(Figure 4.6)** is characterized by:

- Normal P-wave morphology/axis with pauses without visible P-waves

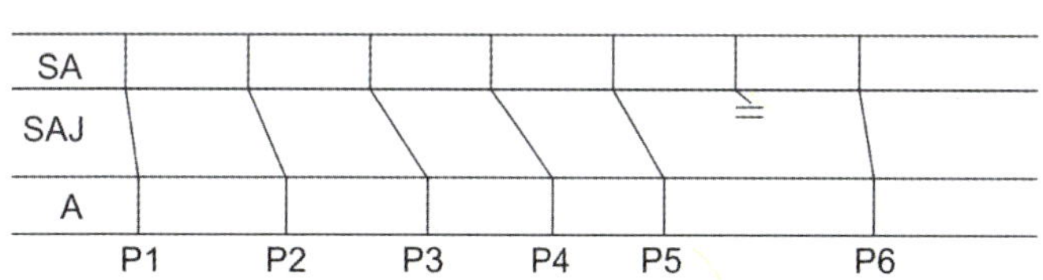

Figure 4.6: A ladder diagram showing activation sequence in second degree, Mobitz Type I sinoatrial block

Abbreviations: SA, SA node; SAJ, sinoatrial junction; A, atria; P, P-wave; P1P2 > P2P3 > P3P4 > P4P5

- Progressive decrease in PP interval before pause
- Constant PR intervals
- PP interval of pause less than twice the PP interval preceding the pause
- PP interval following the pause greater than twice the PP interval preceding the pause

Mobitz Type II sinoatrial exit block **(Figure 4.7)** is characterized by:

- Normal P-wave morphology/axis with pauses without P-waves
- Constant PP interval before and after pause
- Pause is an integral multiple (within 100 ms) of normal PP interval

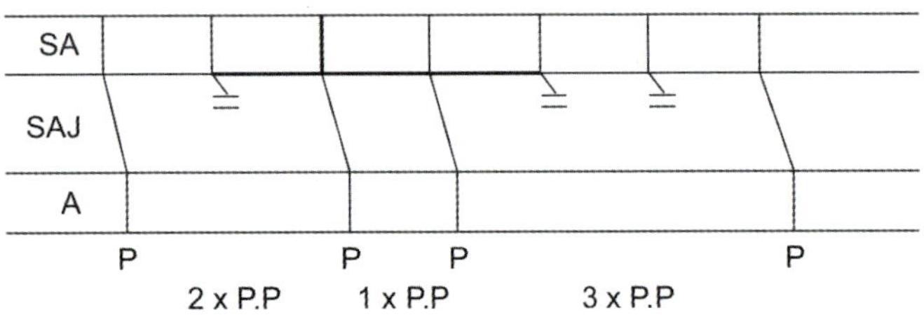

Figure 4.7: A ladder diagram showing activation sequence in second degree, Mobitz Type II sinoatrial exit block
Abbreviations: SA, SA node; SAJ, sinoatrial junction; A, atria, P, P-wave; PP, P to P interval Note absence of P-waves

Third-degree sinoatrial exit block: Every impulse formed within the SN is completely blocked at the sinoatrial junction **(Figure 4.8)**. No impulse is conducted to the atria, resulting in sinus pause on surface ECG. The ventricular rhythm is maintained by a junctional escape rhythm. This cannot be differentiated from sinus arrest on ECG and needs an EP study for its diagnosis. The finding on surface ECG cannot differentiate between problems with sinus node impulse formation and sinoatrial conduction abnormalities.

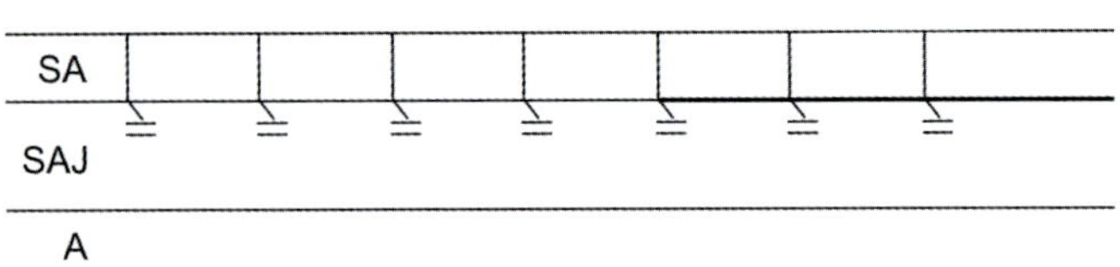

Figure 4.8: A ladder diagram showing activation of the conduction system in third degree sinoatrial exit block. Note absence of P-waves
Abbreviations: SA, SA node; SAJ, sinoatrial junction; A, atria

Tachycardia-bradycardia Syndrome

In tachycardia-bradycardia syndrome, paroxysmal atrial arrhythmias, primarily atrial fibrillation, alternate with sinus pause or sinus bradycardia **(Figure 4.9)**.[16-18] This is the most commonly encountered form of symptomatic sinus node dysfunction and it is associated with the highest incidence of syncope.[17,19] Although AF is the most common associated tachyarrhythmia, it is not unusual to see AFl or nonsustained atrial tachycardia.

Persistent Bradycardias

Chronotropic Incompetence

Patients with chronotropic incompetence may have normal or near normal resting heart rate or sinus bradycardia but the heart rate is not able to accelerate normally with exertion. While definitions are numerous, a reasonable definition of chronotropic incompetence may be inability to achieve 75% of age-predicted maximum heart rate (220–age) or 100 bpm with maximal exertion. The diagnosis can be made definitively during a graded exercise stress test.

ELECTROPHYSIOLOGY STUDY

Electrophysiology (EP) study may be necessary if patients present with nonspecific symptoms or syncope and SND is suspected. If clinically significant abnormalities of sinus node function are discovered or provoked, an implantable permanent pacemaker may be indicated (Class IIa).[18]

Sinus node depolarization can be recorded directly by placing an EP catheter precisely at the SA node, located at the superior vena cava-right atrial junction and recording an unfiltered electrograms at high gain settings.[17] This method is rarely used in clinical practice due to difficulty with catheter positioning. Practically, in most EP laboratories, sinus node function is assessed using the sinus node recovery time (SNRT).

The sinus node recovery time (SNRT) assessment is performed by pacing in the high right atrium (HRA), close to the SA node, at different cycle lengths starting just below the baseline sinus cycle length for at least 30 seconds.[20] Usually, pacing is performed at 2–3 different cycle lengths. It is imperative that at least 1 minute elapse between pacing drives to let the sinus node recover to baseline condition.[16] The time interval from the last pacing stimulus to the first returned sinus atrial electrogram recorded in HRA channel is the SNRT for that paced cycle length. The SNRT is composed of both impulse formation time (basic sinus cycle length) and impulse conduction time in and out of the SA node. In order to make sure that the returned atrial electrogram originates from the SA node, there should be at least two catheters simultaneously recording high and low atrial electrograms and the returned P-wave morphology should be similar to sinus P-wave morphology.[17] In clinical practice, this is rarely done; usually, SNRT is measured in the catheter placed in the high right atrium. However, it is important to ensure that the return atrial electrograms originates in the sinus node by ensuring high-to-low atrial activation, evidenced by upright P-waves in leads II, III and aVF. The maximal SNRT

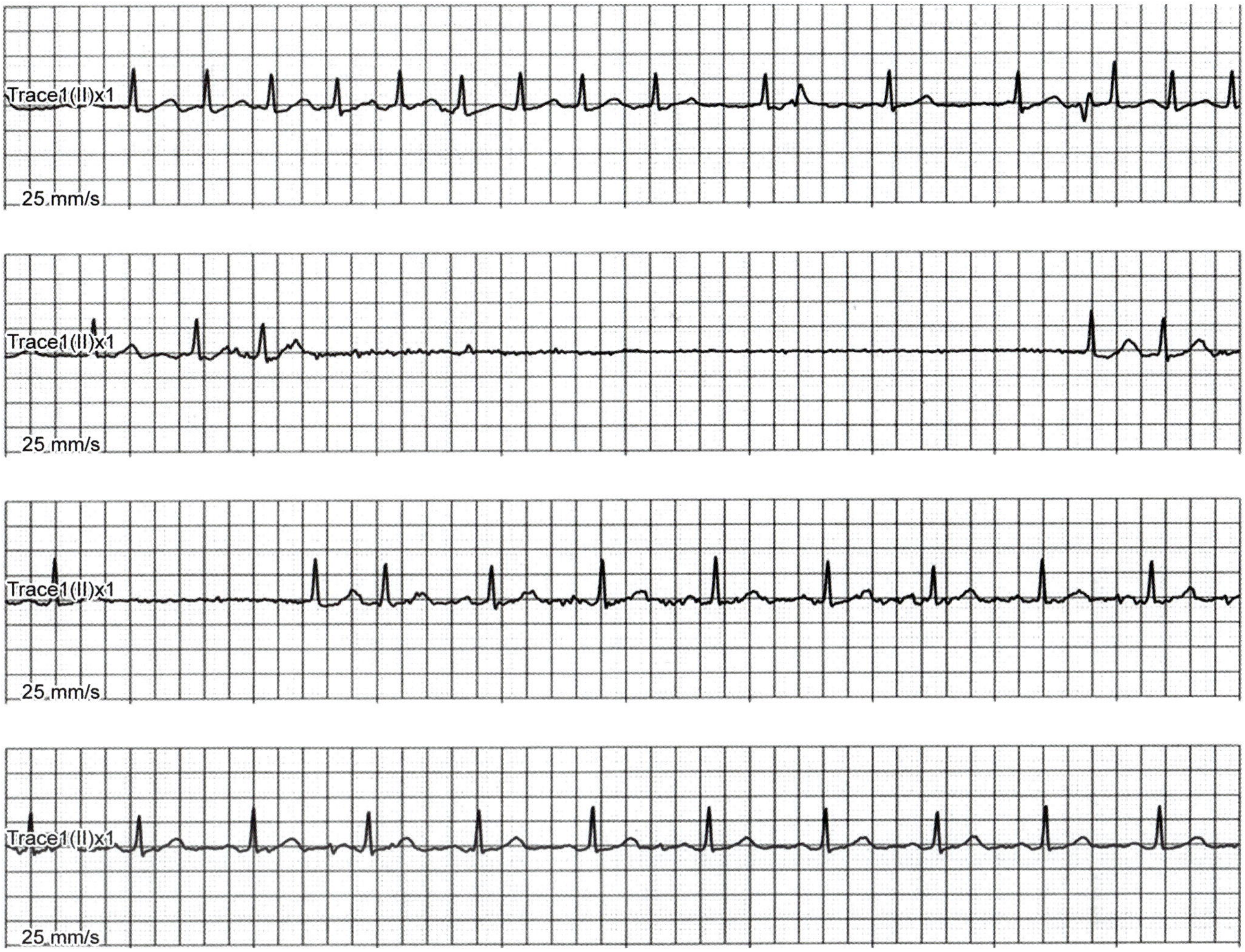

Figure 4.9: Continuous telemetry strip showing spontaneous termination of atrial fibrillation followed by 6.7 second sinus pause, followed by junctional escape beats and then, resumption of sinus rhythm

at any paced cycle length is used for assessment of sinus node function. The corrected SNRT (CSNRT) obtained by subtracting the baseline sinus cycle length from the maximal SNRT may be used as a standard to correct for intra- and interindividual differences. The normal value of CSNRT is less than 550 ms.[17]

In patients with documented pauses on an ECG, electrophysiology study may be normal, suggesting that the EP study has a low sensitivity.[21] Therefore, if symptoms are suspected to be due to SND and the EP study is normal, the detection of arrhythmias and their correlation with symptoms may require prolonged continuous monitoring with an event monitor for up to 30 days or an implantable loop recorder **(Figure 4.10)**.

CONCLUSION

Bradyarrhythmias are the most common form of sinus node dysfunction. Invasive electrophysiologic testing has low sensitivity in detecting actionable evidence and if bradyarrhythmias are suspected as the underlying cause of a patient's symptoms, prolonged electrocardiographic monitoring should be considered.

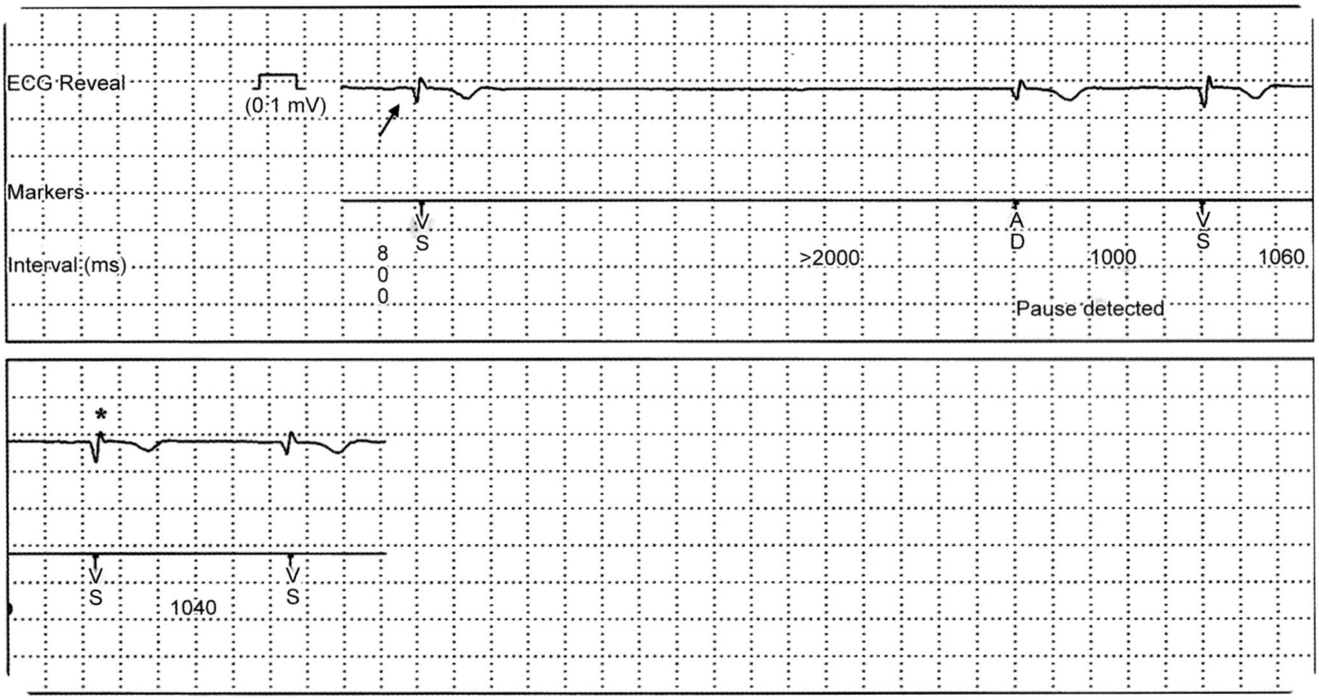

Figure 4.10: A typical bradycardia event documented by an implantable loop recorder from a 77-year-old man with recurrent episodes of dizziness and two syncopal episodes. Baseline ECG and hospital telemetry were normal. Electrophysiology study showed normal intervals and maximum CSNRT of 480 ms. The implanted monitor showed recurrent episodes of sinus pauses > 3 seconds in duration (last sinus beat marked with an arrow), ending with 2 junctional escape beats and then, resumption of sinus rhythm (*)

REFERENCES

1. Strauss HC, Prystowsky EN, Scheinman MM. Sino-atrial and atrial electrogenesis. Prog Cardiovasc Dis. 1977;19:385-404.
2. Lau DH, Roberts-Thomson KC, Sanders P. Sinus node revisited. Curr Opin Cardiol. 2011;26:55-9.
3. Levy MN, Zieske H. Autonomic control of cardiac pacemaker activity and atrioventricular transmission. J Appl Physiol. 1969;27:465-70.
4. Sinus Node Dysfunction. In Issa ZF, Miller JM, Zipes DP. Clinical Arrhythmology and Electrophysiology, 2nd edn. Elsevier, Philadelphia; 2012. p. 164.
5. Boullin J, Morgan JM. The development of cardiac rhythm. Heart. 2005;91:874-5.
6. Stiles MK, Brooks AG, Roberts-Thomson KC, Kuklik P, John B, Young GD, Kalman JM, Sanders P. High-density mapping of the sinus node in humans: Role of preferential pathways and the effect of remodeling. J Cardiovasc Electrophysiol. 2010; 21:532-9.
7. Hocini M, Sanders P, Deisenhofer I, Jaïs P, Hsu LF, Scavée C, Weerasoriya R, Raybaud F, Macle L, Shah DC, Garrigue S, Le Metayer P, Clémenty J, Haïssaguerre M. Reverse remodeling of sinus node function after catheter ablation of atrial fibrillation in patients with prolonged sinus pauses. Circulation. 2003; 108:1172-5.
8. Yeh YH, Burstein B, Qi XY, Sakabe M, Chartier D, Comtois P, Wang Z, Kuo CT, Nattel S. Funny current downregulation and sinus node dysfunction associated with atrial tachyarrhythmia: A molecular basis for tachycardia-bradycardia syndrome. Circulation. 2009;119:1576-85.
9. Joung B, Lin S-F, Chen Z, Antoun PS, Maruyama M, Han S, Piccirillo G, Stucky M, Zipes DP, Chen P-S, Das MK. Mechanisms of sinoatrial node dysfunction in a canine model of pacing-induced atrial fibrillation. Heart Rhythm. 2010;7: 88-95.
10. Josephson ME. Supraventricular tachycardias. In: Josephson ME (Ed): Clinical Cardiac Electrophysiology, 4th edn. Lippincott Williams and Wilkins, Philadelphia; 2008. pp. 175-284.
11. Olshansky B, Sullivan RM. Inappropriate sinus tachycardia. J Am Coll Cardiol. 2013;61:793-801.
12. Morillo CA, Klein GJ, Thakur RK, Li H, Zardini M, Yee R. Mechanism of 'inappropriate' sinus tachycardia. Role of sympathovagal balance. Circulation. 1994;90:873-7.
13. Line D, Callans D. Sinus rhythm abnormalities. In: Zipes D, Jalife J (Eds): Cardiac electrophysiology: from cell to bedside, 4th edn. Philadelphia, Saunders, 2004. pp. 479-84.
14. Still AM, Huikuri HV, Airaksinen KE, Koistinen MJ, Kettunen R, Hartikainen J, Mitrani RD, Castellanos A, Myerburg RJ, Raatikainen MJ. Impaired negative chronotropic response to adenosine in patients with inappropriate sinus tachycardia. J Cardiovasc Electrophysiol. 2002;13:557-62.
15. Buxton AE, Calkins H, Callans DJ, DiMarco JP, Fisher JD, Greene HL, Haines DE, Hayes DL, Heidenreich PA, Miller JM, Poppas A, Prystowsky EN, Schoenfeld MH, Zimetbaum PJ, Goff DC, Grover FL, Malenka DJ, Peterson ED, Radford MJ, Redberg

RF. ACC/AHA/HRS 2006 key data elements and definitions for electrophysiological studies and procedures: A report of the American College of Cardiology/American Heart Association Task Force on Clinical Data Standards (ACC/AHA/HRS writing committee to develop data standards on electrophysiology). Circulation. 2006;114:2534-70.
16. Rubenstein JJ, Schulman CL, Yurchak PM, DeSanctis RW. Clinical spectrum of the sick sinus syndrome. Circulation. 1972;46:5-13.
17. Josephson ME. Sinus node function. In: Josephson ME (Ed). Clinical Cardiac Electrophysiology, 4th edn. Lippincott Williams and Wilkins, Philadelphia; 2008. pp. 67-92.
18. Epstein AE, DiMarco JP, Ellenbogen KA, Estes NA, 3rd, Freedman RA, Gettes LS, Gillinov AM, Gregoratos G, Hammill SC, Hayes DL, Hlatky MA, Newby LK, Page RL, Schoenfeld MH, Silka MJ, Stevenson LW, Sweeney MO. 2012 ACCF/AHA/HRS focused update incorporated into the ACCF/AHA/HRS 2008 guidelines for device-based therapy of cardiac rhythm abnormalities: A report of the American College of Cardiology Foundation/American Heart Association Task Force on Practice Guidelines and the Heart Rhythm Society. Circulation. 2013;127:e283-352.
19. Short DS. The syndrome of alternating bradycardia and tachycardia. Br Heart J. 1954;16:208-14.
20. Reiffel JA, Kuehnert MJ. Electrophysiological testing of sinus node function: Diagnostic and prognostic application-including updated information from sinus node electrograms. Pacing Clin Electrophysiol. 1994;17:349-65.
21. Fujimura O, Yee R, Klein GJ, Sharma AD, Boahene KA. The diagnostic sensitivity of electrophysiologic testing in patients with syncope caused by transient bradycardia. New Engl Journal Med. 1989;321:1703-7.

EDITORS' SUMMARY

The sinus node remains one of the least understood and most difficult structures to study in the invasive EP laboratory. Although the authors state and reference the possibility of directly measuring the sinus node electrogram (with wide open filtering and enhanced gain) of the sinus impulse, in practice, the dynamic range and frame rates with present systems make this very difficult to do. As a result, the sinus node function has to be evaluated indirectly, and the authors explain the correct execution of the most common method to do so—the sinus node recovery time. They reference but do not cover other methods to assess sinus node function that are rare to perform in the EP laboratory.

Two ailments described, namely, inappropriate sinus tachycardia and sinus node reentry, are most likely not disorders of the sinus node itself but generally common to the differential diagnosis of sinus node related disorders. The anatomical substrate for sinus node reentry, if such an entity can actually be differentiated from microreentry near the sinus node, remains unexplained. Similarly, inappropriate sinus tachycardia is likely a primary problem that involves inputs to the sinus node, while the sinus node itself is normal both anatomically and physiologically.

The arterial input to the sinus node is important for invasive electrophysiologists to be thoroughly conversant with. Ablation in distant structures such as the left atrial endocardial ridge, the vein of Marshall region, and the roof of the left atrium may result in irreversible sinus node dysfunction because of damage to a predominate sinus node artery originating from the left circumflex coronary artery.

The authors provide outstanding examples for the electrocardiographic manifestations of severe sinus node dysfunction. The rhythm monitor including implanted devices is the only clinically relevant tool for diagnosing sinus node and other bradyarrhythmias given the difficulty with provocative maneuvers and electrophysiology study-based diagnosis.

CHAPTER 5

Kartikeya Bhargava

Atrioventricular Conduction and Block

LIST OF ABBREVIATIONS

APC	Atrial Premature Contraction	HB	His Bundle
ARP	Absolute Refractory Period	HPS	His-Purkinje System
AV	Atrioventricular	ICD	Implantable Cardioverter-Defibrillator
AVN	Atrioventricular Node	JPB	Junctional Premature Beat
AVNRT	Atrioventricular Nodal Reentrant Tachycardia	MI	Myocardial Infarction
AWP	Alternating Wenckebach Periods	RBBB	Right Bundle Branch Block
BBB	Bundle Branch Block	RRP	Relative Refractory Period
CCAVB	Congenital Complete Atrioventricular Block	SAN	Sinoatrial Node
ECG	Electrocardiogram	VA	Ventriculoatrial
EP	Electrophysiology	VPC	Ventricular Premature Contraction
ERP	Effective Refractory Period	VT	Ventricular Tachycardia
FRP	Functional Refractory Period		

INTRODUCTION

The normal coordinated cardiac function needs the electrical impulse to travel from its site of origin, i.e. the sinoatrial node (SAN) in the right atrium to the ventricles. It is interesting to note that though the atria and the ventricles lie adjacent to each other, they are electrically insulated from each other by the presence of a fibrous framework or annulus. The only electrical connection normally between these structures is through the atrioventricular node (AVN). The atrioventricular (AV) conduction system consists of the atrial myocardium, the AVN, the bundle of His, the left and right bundle branches and the Purkinje system network. The His-Purkinje system (HPS) conducts the electrical impulse rapidly leading to rapid spread of excitation with simultaneous activation of both the right and the left ventricles. This is in contrast to the normally sequential activation of the two atria—first the right and then the left, due to the normal location of the SAN in the right atrium. The AVN not only conducts the electrical impulse from the atria to the ventricles, it also does so with a sufficient delay so as to allow the relaxation and optimal filling of the ventricles before the next atrial contraction. Moreover, the AVN also has a filtering action such that during situations with rapid rates in the atria like atrial fibrillation or flutter, some of the atrial impulses are blocked by the AVN so that the ventricular rate does not become dangerously fast.

AVN or the AV junction (term that includes both the AVN and the bundle of His) also has the property of automaticity, meaning that it can spontaneously generate an electrical impulse in conditions with slow or absent incoming impulses to these regions; for example, during sinus arrest.

The AVN, thus, acts as a transmitter of electrical impulse from the atria to the ventricles, provides the necessary delay in conduction to enable optimal ventricular filling, acts as a filter during rapid atrial rates and can act as a subsidiary pacemaker in times of need.

Many disorders and disease processes can affect the transmission of impulses through the AV conduction system and result in what is known as AV block. The present chapter discusses the normal AV conduction system, various types and degrees of AV block, ECG-EP correlation of these situations and also few other associated phenomena.

ATRIOVENTRICULAR CONDUCTION SYSTEM

The AV conduction system consists of all the structures that participate in the transmission of the electrical impulse from its origin in the sinus node to its destination in the ventricular myocardium.

Internodal Tracts

AV conduction system includes the atrial myocardium in which certain preferential pathways have been described that transmit the electrical impulse from the SAN to the AVN.[1,2] Although, these anterior, middle and posterior internodal "tracts" have never been proven to be histologically distinct from the other atrial myocardium;[3,4] the fiber orientation and arrangement, cellular properties, and packing of muscle fibers have been used to explain possible rapid propagation of the impulse from the SAN to the AVN. The anterior internodal pathway starts at the anterior margin of the SAN, traverses anteriorly around the superior vena cava and enters the superior margin of the AVN. During its course it also gives rise to a muscle bundle called the Bachmann's bundle that preferentially conducts the impulse from the right to the left atrium. The middle internodal pathway or tract originates at the posterior and superior margins of the SAN, passes inferiorly and medially around the inferior vena cava to enter the interatrial septum to join the superior end of the AVN. The posterior internodal tract begins at the posterior margin of the SAN, passes inferiorly through the crista terminalis to the interatrial septum above the os of the coronary sinus to join the posterior surface of the AVN.

Atrioventricular Junction

The AV junction is a term used to describe a structure in the normal heart that can be divided into three regions—(a) the transitional cell zone, (b) the compact AVN and (c) the penetrating part of the His bundle (HB).[5] The AVN is a collection of specialized cells discovered and described by Tawara.[6] The AVN and the perinodal area are composed of three distinct cell types—atrionodal (AN), nodal (N) and nodal-His (NH) cells located in two zones—the transitional and compact. The transitional zone comprises of transitional cells—cells whose morphology and function is intermediate between compact nodal cells and the atrial myocytes. The transitional zone envelopes the compact portion of the AVN and connects it to the surrounding atrial myocardium.[3] The compact AVN is located at the base of the atrial septum in the mid portion of the triangle of Koch.[7] The triangle of Koch is seen on the right side of the endocardial surface of the atrial septum, and is bounded anteriorly by the insertion of the septal leaflet of the tricuspid valve and posteriorly by the tendon of Todaro. The apex of the triangle is formed by junction of these two boundaries and the base is formed by the superior lip of the os of coronary sinus.[8] The tendon of Todaro runs in the Eustachian ridge and inserts into the central fibrous body—a thickened area of fibrous continuity where the leaflets of the aortic, mitral and tricuspid valves meet. The compact AVN lies anterior to the coronary sinus os and is adjacent to the central fibrous body on the right side but is contiguous with the atrial myocardium on the other sides. It gives rise to three extensions—one along the tricuspid annulus in the direction of the coronary sinus (rightward posterior extension or the *slow pathway*), second in the anterior portion of the triangle of Koch (rightward anterior extension or the *fast pathway*) and the third in the direction of the mitral annulus (leftward extension or the *left atrial extension*).[9]

The blood supply of the AVN is through the AV nodal artery that arises from the right coronary artery in 85% and from the left circumflex artery in 15%. The AVN is richly innervated by the sympathetic adrenergic and parasympathetic cholinergic nerve fibers. The AV nodal conduction time and refractoriness is shortened by sympathetic stimulation and prolonged by parasympathetic stimulation.

His Bundle and the Bundle Branches

The distal part of the compact AVN continues as the penetrating bundle of His. Although, it is difficult to define the exact point where the AVN ends and His bundle (HB) begins, the HB is said to begin anatomically where the AV nodal tissue enters the central fibrous body. The penetrating bundle continues as the non-branching portion in the central fibrous body and then exists this body into the membranous ventricular septum as the branching portion. It then branches into the right and the left bundle branches. The cells of the HB from the penetrating region are heterogeneous and are like those of the compact AVN whereas those from the distal branching portion are larger and resemble those from the proximal bundle branches and ventricular myocytes.

Though, the HB does not have any specific branch supplying blood to it, it receives dual blood supply from the branches of the anterior and posterior descending coronary arteries. It is also innervated by both sympathetic and parasympathetic nerves though lesser than as compared to the AVN.

The bundle branches rapidly branch out into a network of Purkinje fibers that lie in the subendocardium of the ventricles. These Purkinje fibers have highly specialized tissue with cells that contain numerous mitochondria and voltage-gated sodium channels and fewer myofibrils than surrounding ventricular myocardium. These structural peculiarities enable these fibers to conduct electrical impulses very rapidly and efficiently leading to rapid spread of excitation simultaneously to different parts of both the ventricles.

ATRIOVENTRICULAR JUNCTION: STRUCTURAL AND FUNCTIONAL CORRELATIONS

It is somewhat interesting that despite more than a century since the AVN was discovered by Tawara,[6] the fascinating electrophysiological behavior of this structure still perplexes the scientists and electrophysiologists. The normal AV nodal delay and decremental conduction, the dual AV nodal physiology and consequent perplexing rhythms, the anatomic and functional substrate for atrioventricular nodal reentrant tachycardia (AVNRT) and concealed conduction are some of these features that have always been a point of discussion and debate. Many research studies using the rabbit and other mammalian models that included histology,[10,11] immunohistochemistry, microelectrode studies[12-15] and more recently fluorescent imaging and optical coherence tomography[16-18] apart from electrophysiological studies in animals and humans[19] have attempted to solve these issues and complexities. The following discussion tries to summarize and simplify these issues for the clinical electrophysiologist.

The AV junction is a heterogeneous structure consisting of the nodal extensions and approaches within the triangle of Koch, along with the compact AVN and the penetrating bundle of His enclosed in the central fibrous body. There is not only morphological but also marked electrophysiological heterogeneity in these structures with different electrical responses at various sites. Histologically, AVN is a three layered structure with each layer responsible for a distinct electrophysiological response in the AV junction. The three distinct regions of the AVN have been identified based on the action potential morphology recorded with microelectrodes:[14,20] the atrionodal (AN), true nodal (N) and nodo-His (NH). The transitional region (AN) includes cells that act as a bridge that transmits atrial depolarizations to the compact AVN through discrete AV nodal approaches or extensions. These are not insulated from the surrounding atrial myocardium but have a distinct action potential different from the atrial cells as well as the cells of the compact AVN. Classically, there are two such approaches—the right posterior extension (slow pathway) that lies in the inferoseptal right atrium and the right anterior extension (fast pathway) that lies near the apex of the triangle of Koch. A third group of transitional cells—left sided extension has also been identified that connects the left atrium with the compact AVN.[21]

The action potential of the N response is characteristically of slow amplitude with a relatively slow rate of rise during upstroke and has a longer duration. This characteristic has been held largely responsible for the typical AV nodal delay and decremental conduction and is mainly a property of the typical N cells found in the compact AV node, though this fact is debated by many researchers. Billette et al.[22] identified six different electrophysiological cell types based on the action potential morphology, excitability and refractoriness from their microelectrode mapping studies of the AV junction and showed them to be present throughout the entire triangle of Koch. There is morphological and electrophysiological evidence of the presence of the nodal and transitional cells in the right posterior extensions (putative slow pathway) which can reach the coronary sinus and sometimes connect to the far away crista terminalis indicating presence of these cells at sites distant from the compact AVN. The fast AV nodal pathway conduction through the AVN bypasses many of the N cells of the compact AVN, but the slow pathway conduction passes through the entire compact AVN. Also, for reasons still not completely understood, the slow pathway recovers excitability much faster than the fast pathway after conduction of an impulse.[23]

The NH region refers to the distal nodal cells that connect to the insulated penetrating bundle of His.

Molecular and Ionic Mechanisms

The different areas of the AVN show nonuniform expression of sodium and potassium channels that correlates with the differences in function of these areas.

The cells of the N zone have been shown to have (a) lower density of sodium ion channels (I_{Na})[24] that explains the slow rising upstroke of their action potential; (b) presence of both the L-type ($I_{Ca,L}$)[25] and the T-type[26] of the calcium channels, the former being primarily responsible for the upstroke of action potential and hence essential for impulse transmission and also responsible for the positive dromotropic action in response to sympathetic stimulation; (c) prominent "funny" current type of potassium channels (I_F) that explains their pacemaking ability;[27,28] (d) scarce expression of I_{to} potassium channels.

In contrast, the transitional cells of AN and NH types have (a) abundant expression of I_{Na}[29] explaining the fast upstroke in their action potential and higher speed of conduction; (b) prominent expression of the potassium channels of the transient outward current type (I_{to}).[25]

The negative dromotropic action of the AVN to vagal stimulation is mediated by the inwardly rectifying potassium channels (I_{KACh}).[30,31] The effects of activation of these channels include hyperpolarization and action potential shortening in the cells of the AVN, decrease in action potential amplitude and increase in conduction time.

Gap Junctional Channels

The gap junctional channels have been shown to play an important role in AV conduction and three major proteins —connexins Cx43, Cx40 and Cx45 have been found to be expressed in the triangle of Koch. The Cx43 isoform is responsible for cell to cell communication in the entire atrial and ventricular myocardium but is scarcely expressed in the compact AVN (N region).[32,33] The transitional layers of the AVN (AN and NH cells) show much higher levels of expression of this isoform. In fact, spatial heterogeneity of expression of Cx43 isoform has been proposed to explain the dual AV nodal physiology[18] based on the immunohistochemical studies using neurofilament 160 (NF160) staining.

ATRIOVENTRICULAR BLOCK: CLASSIFICATION, SITE AND DEGREE OF BLOCK—ECG AND EP CORRELATION

AV block is said to be present whenever there is delay or block in conduction from the atria to the ventricles. As can be gathered from the earlier discussion, the various sites where this delay or block in conduction can occur include the atria, the AV node, the bundle of His and the bundle branches. The various degrees of AV block and possible sites of block in each degree are presented in **Table 5.1**.

The surface electrocardiogram (ECG) is usually diagnostic of the degree of AV block and often helps in deciphering the site of block as well. However, it must be realized that the entire AV conduction on the surface ECG is depicted within the PR interval. The PR interval is measured from the onset of atrial depolarization (P-wave, typically the region of SAN in the normal state) to the onset of ventricular depolarization (QRS). An electrophysiology study that by virtue of recording the HB electrogram can classify the delay or block in AV conduction into that occurring above, in or below the HB. This classification is of prognostic importance as well since the block occurring in or below the HB can have serious outcomes even in the absence of symptoms compared to that occurring above the HB. Hence, the major usefulness of EP study in assessing AV block is to precisely localize the anatomic site of block.

It will be useful at this point to clarify a few terms used in reference to the site of AV block that are self-explanatory but often are a cause of confusion among students.

Nodal: Pertains to block at the level of the AV node.

Infranodal: Indicates block below the level of AV node, that is, either in the His bundle or bundle branches.

Suprahisian: Refers to the block above the bundle of His that is in the AV node or rarely atria.

Intrahisian: Indicates the block is in the His bundle itself.

Infrahisian: Indicates that the site of block is below the bifurcation of the bundle of His and hence in the bundle branches, left or right bundle branch or both.

Another fact that should always be remembered is that block or delay in conduction can occur at multiple sites in the same patient.

First Degree AV Block

Definition

Any increase of PR interval from the normal upper limit of 200 ms in adults on the surface ECG with one to one AV conduction qualifies to be called AV block of the first degree. As indicated in **Table 5.1**, the first degree AV block can occur at any site, though AVN is the most common location especially when associated with a narrow QRS.

Site of Block

First degree AV block at the atrial level can be due to intra- or interatrial delay and is seen in patients with marked left

Table 5.1: Sites and degrees of atrioventricular block

Degree	*Subtypes*	*Definition*	*Possible sites*
First degree		Prolonged AV conduction	Atrium, AVN, HB, BB
Second degree		Intermittent conduction	
	Mobitz type 1		AVN, rarely HB or BB
	Mobitz type 2		HB or BB
	Two to one AV block		AVN, HB, BB
	Advanced or high grade AV block		HB, BB
Third degree or complete AV block		No AV conduction	AVN, HB, BB

Abbreviations: AV, atrioventricular; HB, His bundle; BB, bundle branches; AVN, atrioventricular node (e.g. mitral valve disease) or right (e.g. Ebstein's anomaly) atrial enlargement. Interatrial delay may be responsible for first degree AV block in some patients with coronary artery disease or heart failure and its recognition indicates a worse prognosis.[34] A prolonged PA interval on an EP study suggests intraatrial first degree AV block.

AVN is the most common site of first degree AV block and can be suggested on the surface ECG by a very long PR interval (> 300 ms) or marked variability in PR interval. A prolonged AH interval (> 125 ms) during an EP study confirms AV nodal first degree AV block.

Intrahisian first degree AV block is uncommon but needs to be recognized since it may portend a worse prognosis if left untreated especially in those with symptoms. It can only be diagnosed on an EP study wherein a markedly fragmented or split His potential is seen **(Figures 5.1 and 5.2)** with a prolonged His bundle duration (> 30 ms). It should always be suspected in patients with first degree AV block with narrow QRS who have marked mitral annular or aortic valve calcification. Bharati et al. were among the first authors to describe intrahisian block secondary to calcific aortic stenosis.[35]

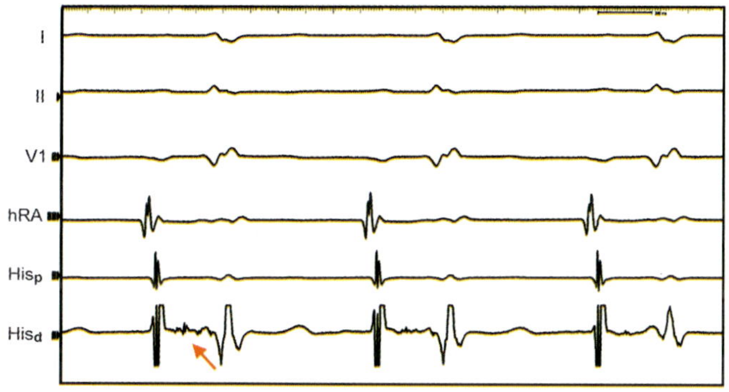

Figure 5.1: Fragmented His potential (red arrow) in a patient with first degree AV block and right bundle branch block on ECG. The markedly prolonged His bundle duration is the cause of first degree AV block in this patient. From top to bottom are surface ECG leads I, II and V1, high right atrium (HRA), His bundle proximal (His_p) and His bundle distal (His_d) recordings

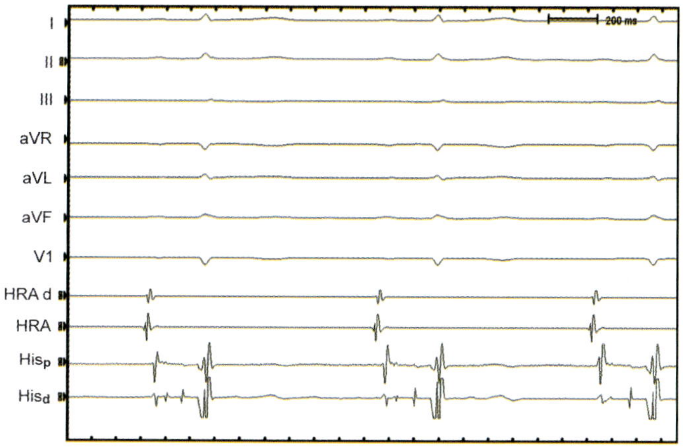

Figure 5.2: Split His bundle electrogram in a patient with first degree AV block and narrow QRS complex. The HH' interval was 60 ms in this patient with first degree intrahisian block. From top to bottom are surface ECG leads I, II, III, aVR, aVL, aVF, V1, high right atrium distal (HRA d), and proximal (HRA), His bundle proximal (His_p) and distal (His_d) recordings

Infrahisian first degree AV block can occur only with associated bundle branch block (BBB) with either total block in conduction in one bundle branch with delayed conduction in the other or with marked conduction delay in both bundle branches. In case of latter, the QRS morphology is that of BBB of the side with worse conduction. For example, first degree AV block with right bundle branch block (RBBB) indicates either complete block in right bundle branch and delayed conduction in left bundle or marked delay in conduction in both bundle branches with worse conduction in the right bundle branch **(Figures 5.3 to 5.5)**. It should be understood by the students of electrophysiology that equal degree of conduction delay (only theoretical, not usually seen clinically) in both bundle branches will result in a narrow QRS complex. Hence, first degree AV block associated with narrow QRS can exist with conduction delay at atrial, AV nodal or intrahisian level. On the other hand, first degree AV block associated with BBB can be due to conduction delay at any level, as, e.g. a patient with RBBB may have AV nodal delay in addition. Infrahisian first degree block is diagnosed when the HV interval is prolonged above its normal upper limit of 55 ms and can exist even if the PR interval on surface ECG is within normal limits. Also, it should be realized that even with HPS disease, the HV interval can sometimes be normal at baseline, but may prolong when stressed in the laboratory with atrial pacing **(Figures 5.6A to C)** or drugs like procainamide. A prolonged HV interval in the presence of chronic BBB in patients with symptoms due to bradycardia is an indication for pacing.

Clinical Implications

First degree AV block occurs with an incidence of 0.5–1.6% in asymptomatic individuals[36] who may not warrant any evaluation or treatment. Symptoms due to first degree AV block are unlikely except when the PR interval is markedly prolonged approaching the RR interval, when symptoms similar to pacemaker syndrome may occur.[37] Though, first degree AV block has been generally considered to be benign, a recent subsidy of Framingham cohort has shown it to be associated with increased risk of atrial fibrillation, increased risk of requirement of pacemaker and moderately increased risk of death over long-term.[38]

Second Degree AV Block

Definition

Second degree AV block implies that some of the atrial impulses are conducted to the ventricles whereas some

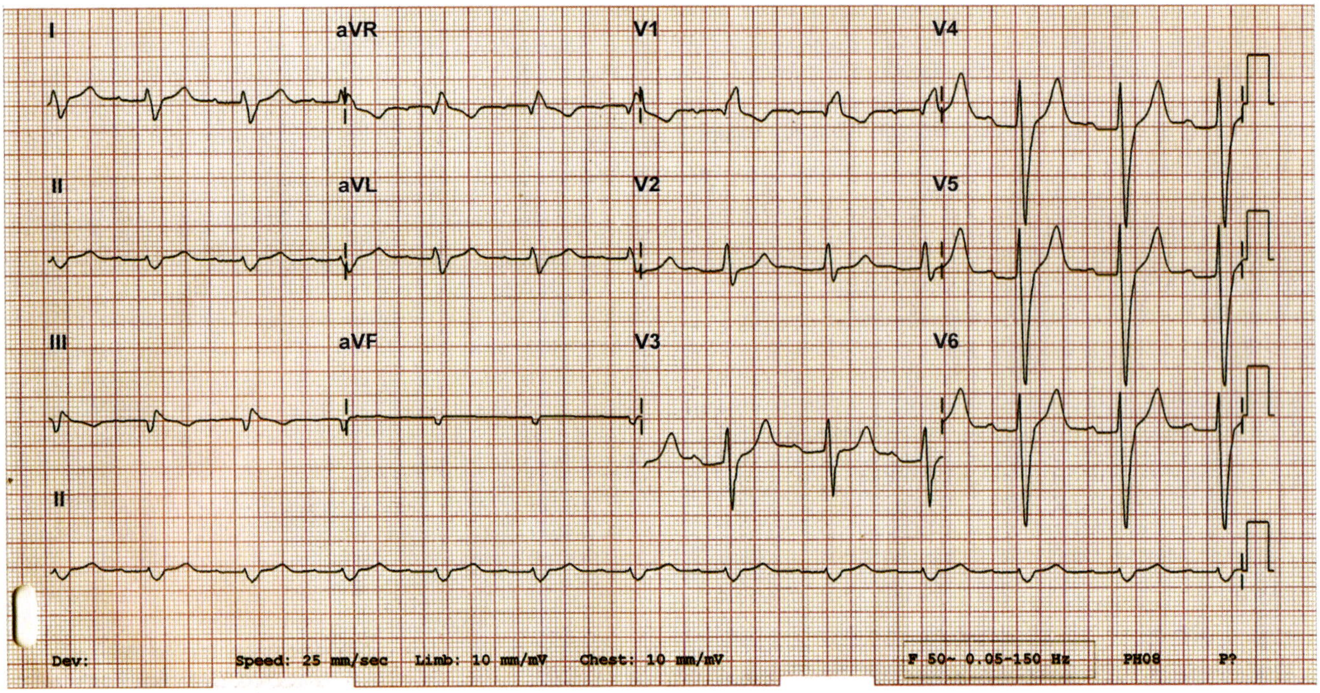

Figure 5.3: Surface ECG showing first degree AV block with right bundle branch block in a patient with recurrent syncope. With wide QRS complex the site of first degree AV block can be anywhere and cannot be deciphered from the surface ECG alone

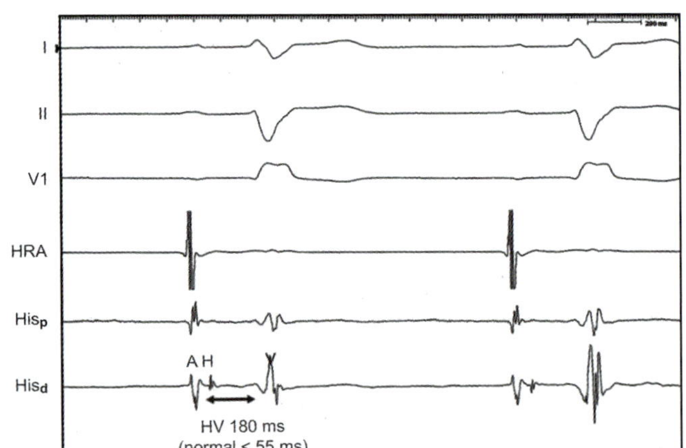

Figure 5.4: Intracardiac tracing of the same patient as in Figure 5.3 showing markedly prolonged HV interval of 180 ms. Hence, this is an example of infrahisian first degree AV block and suggests significant His-Purkinje system disease. From top to bottom are surface ECG leads I, II and V1, high right atrium (HRA), His proximal (His_p) and distal (His_d) recording

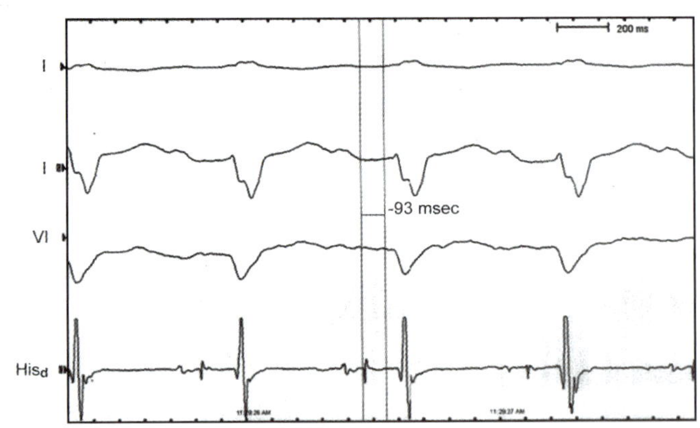

Figure 5.5: Left bundle branch block with prolonged HV interval of 93 ms indicating infrahisian first degree AV block. Note that infrahisian location of first degree AV block can exist only with wide QRS, though the location of first degree AV block in wide QRS can be anywhere. From top to bottom are surface ECG leads I, II and V1, and His bundle distal (His_d) recording

are blocked, i.e. intermittent failure of AV conduction. It is classified into at least four types **(Table 5.1)** based on the ECG patterns. If a single P-wave fails to conduct during a sequence, it is either Mobitz type 1 or type 2 second degree AV block that can be differentiated based on the variability of PR intervals of the conducted beats. A block of every alternating P-wave during a regular atrial rhythm (2 to 1 AV block) cannot be classified into type 1 or 2 and hence is classified separately.

Woldemar Mobitz, a German internist is credited with classifying second degree AV block in to type 1 and 2 based on his publication in 1924.[39,40] However, it was Karel Frederik

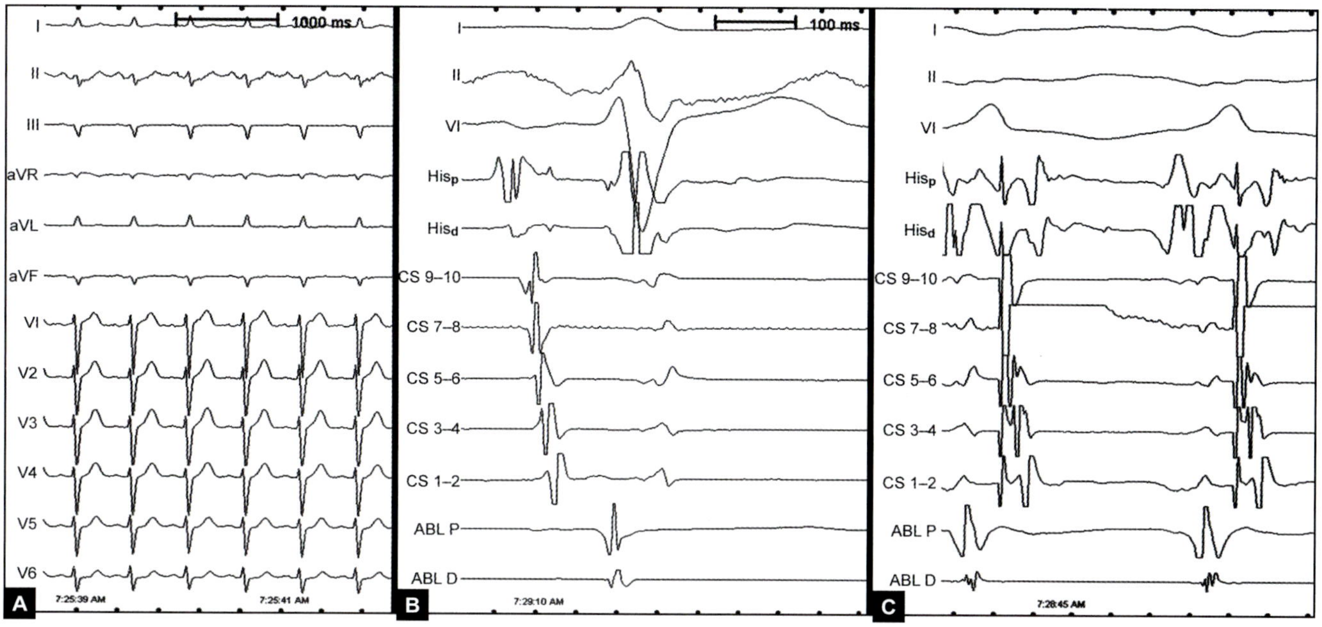

Figures 5.6A to C: Atrial pacing induced prolongation of HV interval with development of RBBB in a patient with syncope. A narrow QRS was present during sinus rhythm (A) with baseline HV interval of 52 ms (B). The HV interval increased to 68 ms with atrial pacing from the proximal coronary sinus (C) with development of RBBB. Note that development of RBBB with or without HV prolongation on atrial pacing can sometimes be due to functional infrahisian delay and may not indicate underlying HPS disease. (A) Surface ECG leads at 25 mm/s, (B and C) are recorded at 200 mm/s and show from top to bottom surface ECG leads I, II and V1, His proximal (His_p) and distal (His_d), coronary sinus proximal (CS 9–10) to distal (CS 1–2) and right ventricular apex proximal (ABL P) and distal (ABL D) recordings

Wenckebach, a Dutch physician who in 1889 (even before the discovery of SAN, AVN or the invention of ECG) had recorded and published the type 1 conduction pattern based on his observation of the carotid artery and jugular venous pulsations in a patient.[41] So, type 1 AV block is also known as Wenckebach AV block and the pattern of conduction, Wenckebach phenomenon.

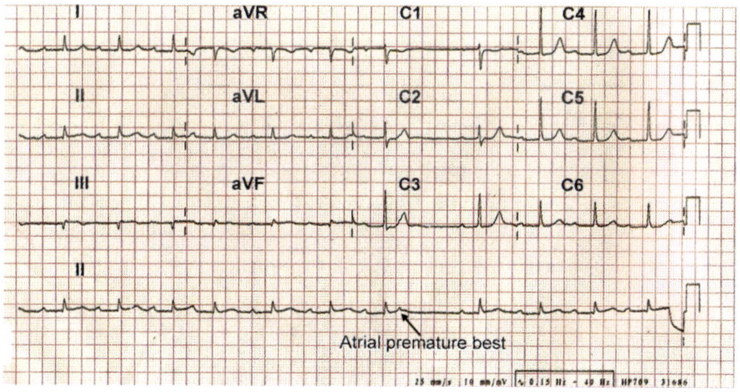

Figure 5.7: A nonconducted atrial premature beat during a background of sinus rhythm with first degree AV block gives a deceptive impression of Wenckebach AV block

Mobitz Type 1 AV Block

Type 1 second degree AV block presents as progressive prolongation of the PR interval till a P-wave is blocked. The PR interval returns to the baseline in the next beat. Hence, the PR intervals of the beats encompassing the blocked P-wave are markedly different and should be the ones to diagnose this kind of AV block. It should be remembered that the blocked P-wave should not be a premature atrial beat **(Figure 5.7)** and the atrial rhythm should be regular before labeling a sequence as type 1 AV block. In a Wenckebach sequence, as the PR interval progressively increases, the RR interval decreases.

The features of classical Wenckebach phenomenon are—(a) Progressively increasing PR intervals throughout the sequence; (b) The first increment in the PR interval is the highest, as the PR intervals progressively increase, the increment in the PR interval progressively shortens; (c) Progressive decrease in the RR intervals as a result of above; (d) The P-wave preceding the blocked P-wave has the longest PR interval in the sequence; (e) The RR interval in the beats encompassing the blocked P-wave is less than the sum of two PP intervals; (f) The PR interval of the beat following the blocked P-wave is shortest in the sequence. More often than not, the clinically seen Wenckebach sequences do not follow all of these classical features and hence are atypical. Sometimes, atypical Wenckebach AV block may be inappropriately diagnosed as Mobitz type 2 AV block.

Mechanisms

The underlying mechanism of Wenckebach AV block relates to the decremental conduction property of AVN. To simplify the understanding of Wenckebach block, it can be considered that the AVN has a relatively long relative refractory period (RRP) during which any incident impulse (P-wave) takes longer than the usual time to propagate through the AVN.[42] The earlier the incoming impulse, longer is the time it requires to pass through the AVN. An impulse arriving much earlier that is in the absolute refractory period (ARP) gets blocked in the AVN and fails to conduct. Thus, Wenckebach periodicity develops because each successive atrial impulse arrives earlier and earlier in the RRP of the AVN, resulting in progressively increasing conduction delay until one impulse arrives during the ARP and blocks resulting in a pause. The next impulse after the pause finds the AVN totally nonrefractory and conducts with a normal or baseline interval.[42] The shorter the RP interval, longer is the ensuing PR interval in this sequence till a very short RP interval leads to failure of conduction of the corresponding P-wave **(Figure 5.8)**. This also explains the features of the typical or classical Wenckebach phenomenon.

Although, a lot of discussion has been done in the literature on Wenckebach periodicity, whether delays in the AV node are due to conventionally accepted slow propagation of the impulse through the entire level that takes place during the relative refractory period, or due to the existence of "step" delays at the corresponding level is not entirely clear.[43] Rosenbleuth in 1958 first postulated that the Wenckebach periods were not due to progressive impairment of propagation but rather due to arrest of conduction at a barrier (representing step delay) with resumption of conduction after a delay **(Figure 5.9)**.[44] Young et al. later expanded this

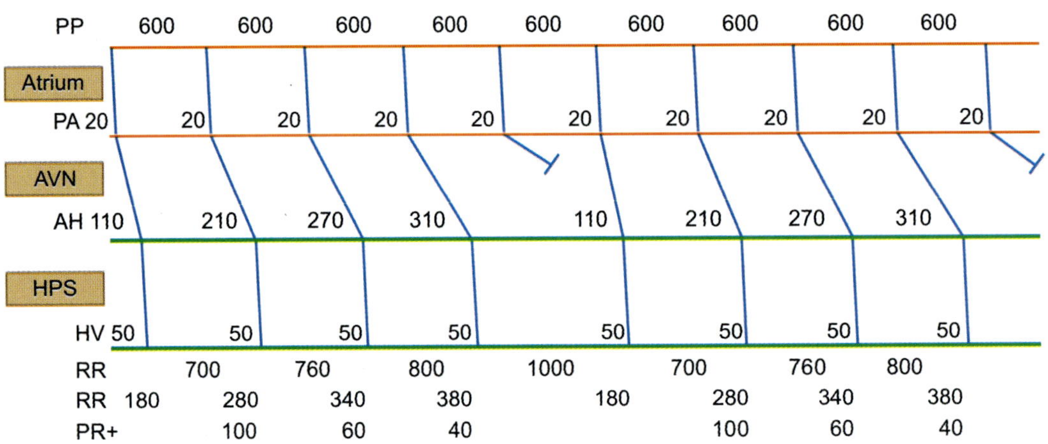

Figure 5.8: Schematic diagram showing sinus rhythm (at 100 beats per min) and 2nd degree type 1 AV block at the level of the AV node. The Wenckebach periodicity shows a 5:4 block pattern. Note that the AH interval shows progressive increase whereas the PA, and HV intervals remain fixed. The PR interval is the sum of PA, AH and HV intervals. See text for details. All the numbers are in milliseconds. PP, AH, HV, PR and RR indicate corresponding intervals in ms. PR+ indicates the increment in PR interval from the previous PR interval in ms

Abbreviations: AVN, atrioventricular node; HPS, His-Purkinje system

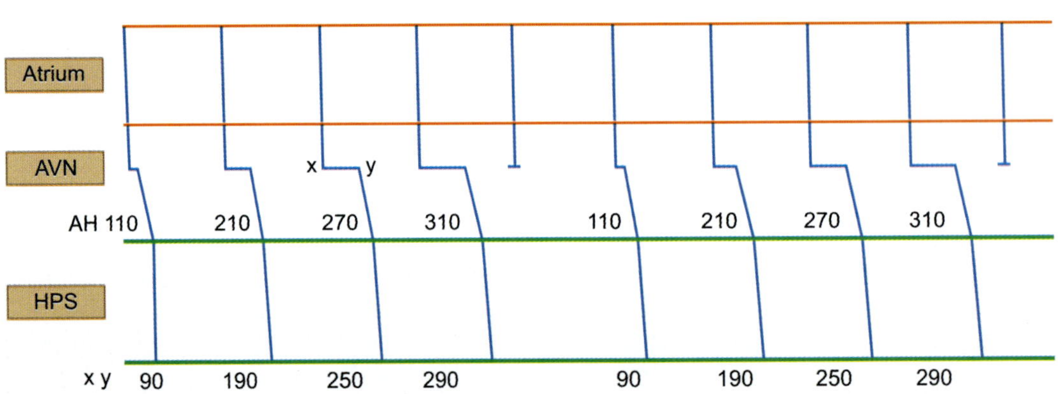

Figure 5.9: Schematic representation of same Wenckebach periodicity as in Figure 5.8, with progressive PR prolongation explained by "step delays" due to presence of a barrier in the AV node where every impulse gets arrested for a period that progressively prolongs. This is in contrast to the explanation with progressive delay in the AV node as shown in Figure 5.8

Abbreviations: AVN, atrioventricular node; HPS, His-Purkinje system hypothesis and explained that in Wenckebach periods the successively appearing atrial impulses are delayed at a barrier for increasing periods of time, propagation not being able to resume until the distal tissues recover enough to respond.[45] This explanation of Wenckebach periods using "step delays" is compatible with the physiologically demonstrable features of transmission in the relative refractory cardiac tissue.[46]

Site of Block

The Wenckebach periodicity is a feature of AVN just like decremental conduction and hence 2nd degree type 1 AV block occurs most commonly at this site. However, rarely it may occur at the His bundle or infrahisian levels. Progressive lengthening of AH interval (with constant HV intervals) till the atrial signal is not followed by HB signal (during blocked P-wave) is confirmatory of AV nodal type 1 block on EP study.

With a narrow QRS complex, type 1 block almost always lies in the AV node, though rarely intrahisian block may be responsible. In intrahisian type 1 AV block, the His bundle recording shows progressive delay in first (H) and second (H') components of the HB electrogram till the H is not followed by H' during the blocked P-wave. Narula and colleagues were the first to describe electrophysiologically documented intrahisian AV block in man.[47]

Even when wide QRS (BBB) is present in a patient with type 1 AV block, AV node is still the most common site **(Figures 5.10 and 5.11)**, but the block may be localized in (intrahisian) or below the His bundle (infrahisian). An infrahisian type 1 AV block is characterized by progressive lengthening of the HV interval on EP study till the HB electrogram is not followed by ventricular signal during blocked P-wave. A very long baseline PR interval in the beat after the blocked P-wave usually suggests AV node as the site of block even with a wide QRS complex. Small increments in PR interval during type 1 AV block with a wide QRS suggest HPS disease and possibly infrahisian block. Apart from baseline PR interval, QRS width and degree of PR interval increment, effect of exercise and atropine may also help in localizing the site of block, both causing improvement in conduction if the block is AV nodal. Infranodal block is likely to worsen with exercise or atropine.

Clinical Implications

Second degree type 1 AV block at the AVN level can sometimes occur normally due to high vagal tone as in athletes or during sleep. In such situations, it does not require any treatment and is not likely to result in any symptoms. Asymptomatic individuals with type 1 block especially with narrow QRS complex usually do not require any treatment. Patients with symptomatic bradycardia or in whom the block is localized to intra- or infrahisian locations usually warrant pacemaker implantation.

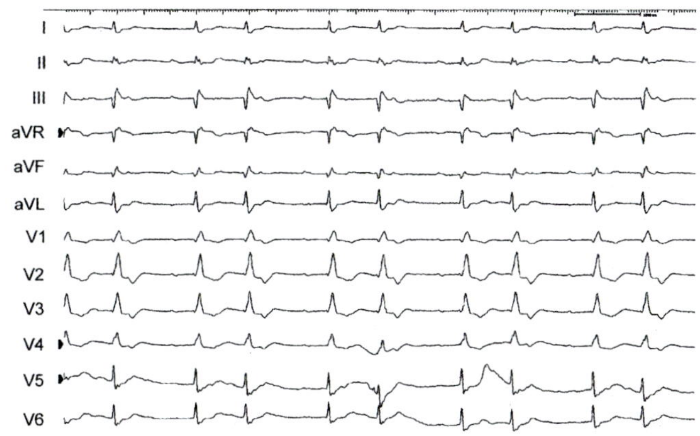

Figure 5.10: Twelve-lead ECG showing sinus rhythm with 2nd degree type 1 (Wenckebach) AV block with RBBB. Though, the site of Wenckebach AV block with wide QRS can be anywhere in the AVN-HPS, AV node is still the most common location of this kind of block as was confirmed later by EP study in this example

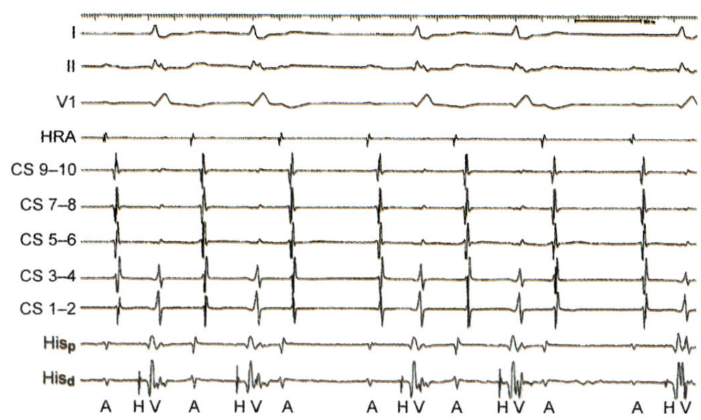

Figure 5.11: Second degree type 1 AV nodal block with RBBB with 3:2 conduction pattern of the same patient whose ECG is shown in Figure 5.10. The intracardiac atrial (A), His bundle (H) and ventricular (V) electrograms in the His bundle tracing show progressive prolongation of AH interval terminating with an A not followed by H indicating AV node as the site of block. From top to bottom are surface ECG leads I, II and V1, high right atrium (HRA), coronary sinus proximal (CS 9–10) to distal (CS 1–2) and His bundle proximal (His$_p$) and distal (His$_d$) recordings

Mobitz Type 2 Block

In this type of block, the PR interval of the conducted beat remains constant and there is abrupt block of one nonpremature P-wave. Thus, the pause encompassing the blocked P-wave is twice the PP interval **(Figure 5.12)**. The way to recognize is to look at and compare the PR intervals of the beats spanning the blocked P-wave, which are the same in 2nd degree type 2 AV block (viz-a-viz type 1 AV block).

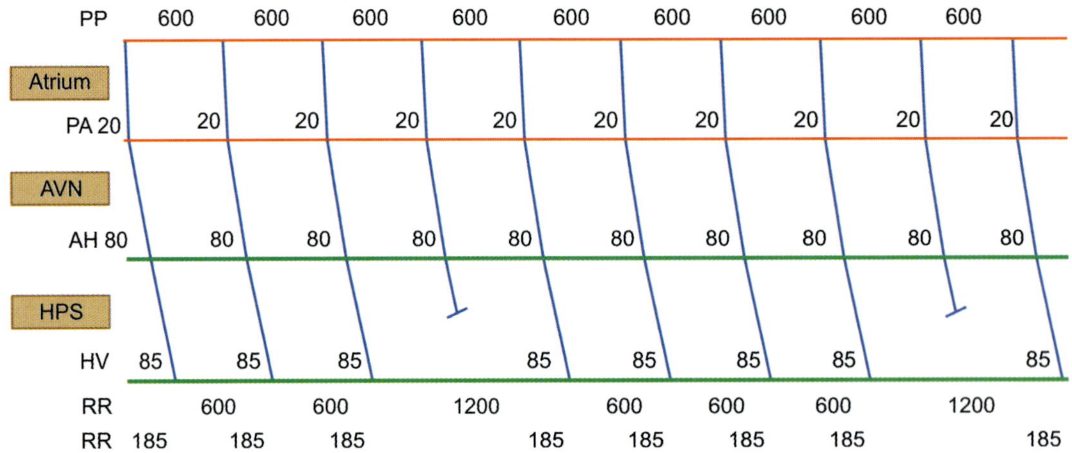

Figure 5.12: Schematic diagram showing sinus rhythm (at 100 beats per min) and 2nd degree type 2 AV block at the level of the His-Purkinje system (HPS). The AH, HV and PR intervals remain constant and there is abrupt block of one P-wave. The RR interval of the pause due to the blocked P-wave is twice the basic RR interval. Also, the PR intervals of beats spanning the blocked P-wave are the same. All the numbers are in milliseconds. PP, AH, HV, PR and RR indicate corresponding intervals in ms

Abbreviations: AVN, atrioventricular node; HPS, His-Purkinje system

Site of Block

Mobitz type 2 AV block does not occur in the AV node and is always infranodal. Usually it is infrahisian and hence is associated with BBB **(Figures 5.13 and 5.14)**. It is diagnosed during EP study by presence of atrial and His electrogram that is not followed by ventricular signal in the His bundle catheter recording during the blocked P-wave. A prolonged but constant HV interval during times of one to one AV conduction is also usually present. True type 2 AV block occurring with narrow QRS complex can only occur at the level of the His bundle but is uncommon. The His bundle recording during an EP study will show a split or a fragmented His signal with at least some component present during the blocked P-wave and associated narrow QRS complex. In the series by Narula et al,[47,48] only three of the 12 patients with type 2 block had narrow QRS complexes and the site of block in all three was localized to the His bundle. Apparent type 2 second degree AV block with narrow QRS is sometimes seen during Holter monitoring in young asymptomatic persons especially during sleep. This is not true type 2 block and can be explained either by concealed junctional ectopic[49] or AV nodal Wenckebach with non-measureable variations in PR intervals.[50]

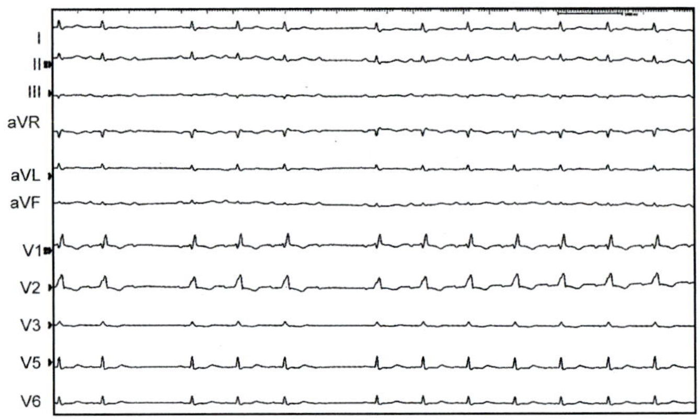

Figure 5.13: Second degree type 2 AV block with RBBB. The PR interval remains constant indicating type 2 block

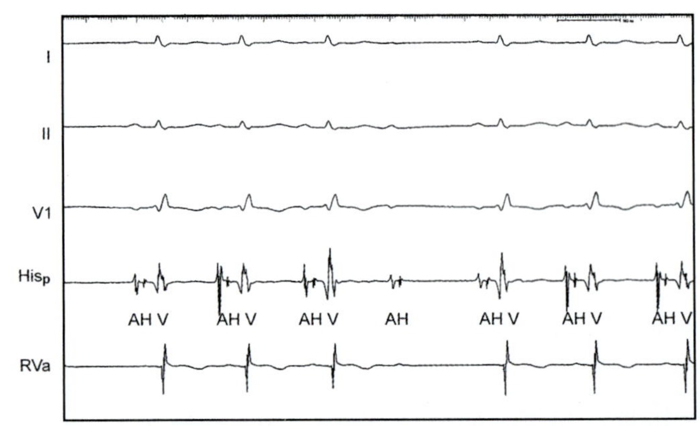

Figure 5.14: Intracardiac electrograms of the same patient whose ECG is shown in Figure 5.13 demonstrating Mobitz type 2 infrahisian AV block. The HV intervals remain constant and some A and H complexes are not followed by V characteristic of infrahisian type 2 block. From top to bottom are surface ECG leads I, II and V1, His proximal (His_p) and right ventricular apex (RVa) recordings

Clinical Implications

The second degree type 2 AV block indicates severe HPS disease and is usually not seen in normal healthy individuals. It has a high risk of progression to more advanced or complete AV block that may at times be sudden, unexpected and life threatening. Hence, pacemaker implantation should be considered in these patients even in the absence of bradycardia-related symptoms. Even among patients with chronic intrahisian block of second (type 1, type 2 or 2 to 1)

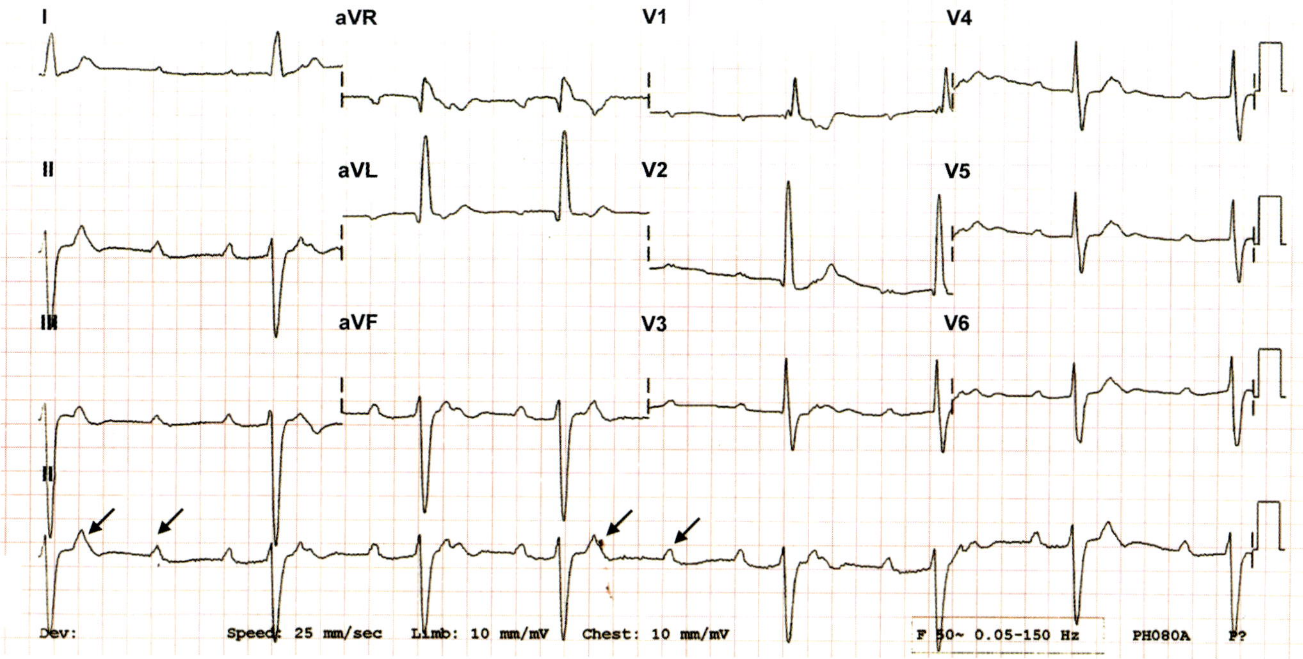

Figure 5.15: Twelve-lead ECG showing sinus tachycardia with mostly 2 to 1 block with prolonged PR interval and RBBB in the conducted beats with intermittent advanced AV block as indicated by two consecutively blocked P-waves (marked by arrows). Note that though, there is some variation in the PR intervals of the conducted beats, this is not an example of complete AV block since the ventricular rhythm is irregular

or third degree, pacemaker implantation was required in almost all patients in one series.[51]

Advanced or High Grade AV Block

When two or more consecutive P-waves fail to conduct to the ventricles during a rhythm which otherwise has some AV conduction, advanced or high grade AV block is said to be present **(Figure 5.15)**. Sometimes, a fixed pattern of block that is more than 2 to 1, that is either 4 to 1 or 3 to 1 **(Figure 5.16)** during a stable regular atrial rhythm is also classified as high grade AV block.

Site of Block

Advanced or high grade AV block is usually associated with wide QRS complexes in the conducted beats that suggest infrahisian location of block. Rarely, it may occur at the level of AVN or HB when the QRS complexes in the conducted beats are narrow.

Clinical Implications

Patients with advanced or high grade AV block are usually symptomatic and require pacemaker implantation. Asymptomatic patients will also need pacing if associated with wide QRS complexes and/or demonstrated to be infrahisian or intrahisian in location.

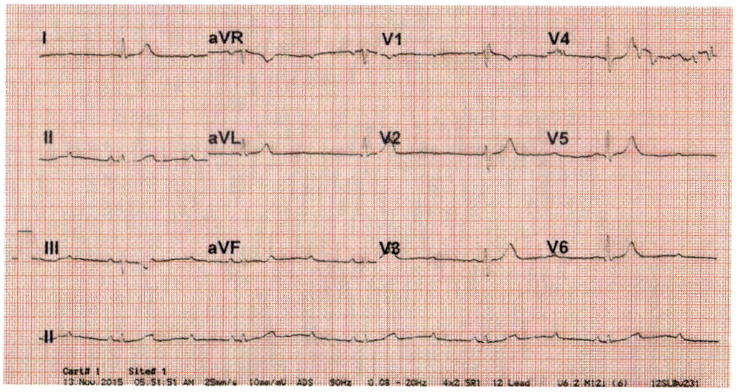

Figure 5.16: Twelve lead ECG of a patient with sinus rhythm, 3 to 1 AV block with RBBB in the conducted beats. Note that the fixed PR interval in the conducted beats helps us in identifying it as 3 to 1 block and not complete AV block

Two to One AV Block

AV block wherein only alternate P-waves are conducted resulting in a 2 to 1 ratio of atrial and ventricular events is classified as 2 to 1 AV block. The QRS complex of the conducted beats could be narrow or wide. Also, the PR interval of the conducted beats can be normal or prolonged but is usually constant. This type of block cannot be classified into type 1 or type 2 and hence is classified separately. It is incorrect to classify 2 to 1 AV block as type 1, if nodal and type 2, if infranodal on EP testing as it is a violation of the appropriate definitions.[52] It is important to remember that 2 to 1 block is a pattern diagnosed on the basis of ECG irrespective of the anatomical location of block.

Site of Block

A fixed pattern of 2 to 1 AV block can occur at the level of AVN or HB or bundle branches. An EP study is diagnostic with His bundle catheter recording during the blocked P-wave showing only atrial signal, atrial and partial or first component of His signal and both atrial and His signal in AV nodal, intrahisian and infrahisian 2 to 1 AV block respectively. However, certain features on the ECG like QRS width, PR interval of the conducted beat; response to maneuvers like carotid sinus massage and exercise; and effect on AV conduction of vagolytic drug atropine can help in suggesting the location of block during 2 to 1 AV block with fair accuracy **(Table 5.2)**.

A narrow QRS complex in the conducted beat during 2 to 1 AV block almost excludes infrahisian location of block and makes AV nodal block most likely, though uncommonly intrahisian block **(Figures 5.17A and B)** may occur. However, it is important to look at all the 12-leads before labeling a QRS as narrow since QRS width during BBB especially RBBB may appear narrow in some leads **(Figure 5.18)**. In the series by Narula, 35% of patients with 2 to 1 AV block and narrow QRS had intrahisian level of block.[48]

If the QRS during 2 to 1 AV block is wide, the block is likely to be located in the bundle branches, though it can be in the AVN or HB as well **(Figures 5.19A and B)**. The PR interval of the conducted beats may help in suggesting the location of block in such cases. A PR interval of less than 160 ms in

Table 5.2: Localization of block during 2 to 1 AV block

Site of block	*AV node*	*His bundle*	*Bundle branches*
QRS width	Narrow or wide	Narrow or wide	Wide
PR interval of conducted beat	> 280 ms	< 160 ms	< 160 ms
Carotid sinus massage	Conduction worsens	Conduction improves	Conduction improves
Exercise	Conduction improves	Conduction worsens	Conduction worsens
Atropine	Conduction improves	Conduction worsens	Conduction worsens

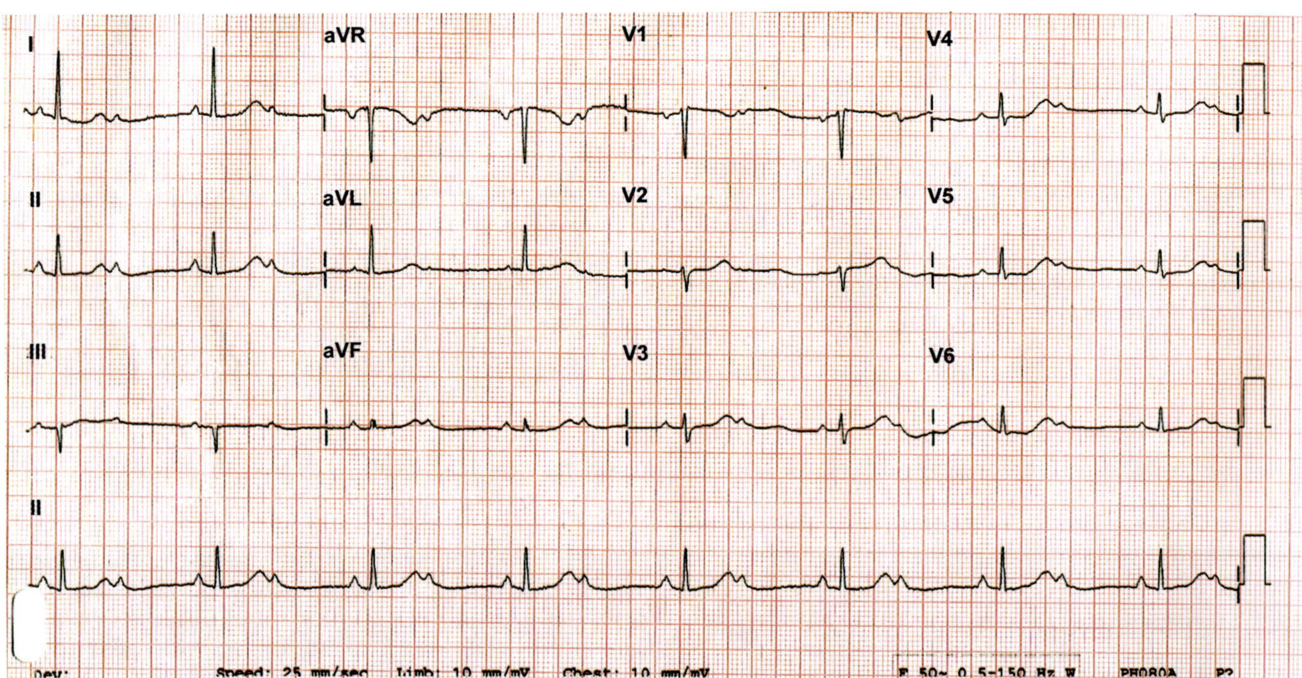

Figure 5.17A: Twelve-lead ECG showing sinus rhythm with 2 to 1 AV block and narrow QRS complexes in the conducted beats. The presence of normal narrow QRS excludes infrahisian location and leaves with AV node and His bundle (intrahisian) as the possible locations. Note, that the PR interval is normal and hence does not help in differentiating the AV nodal versus intrahisian location

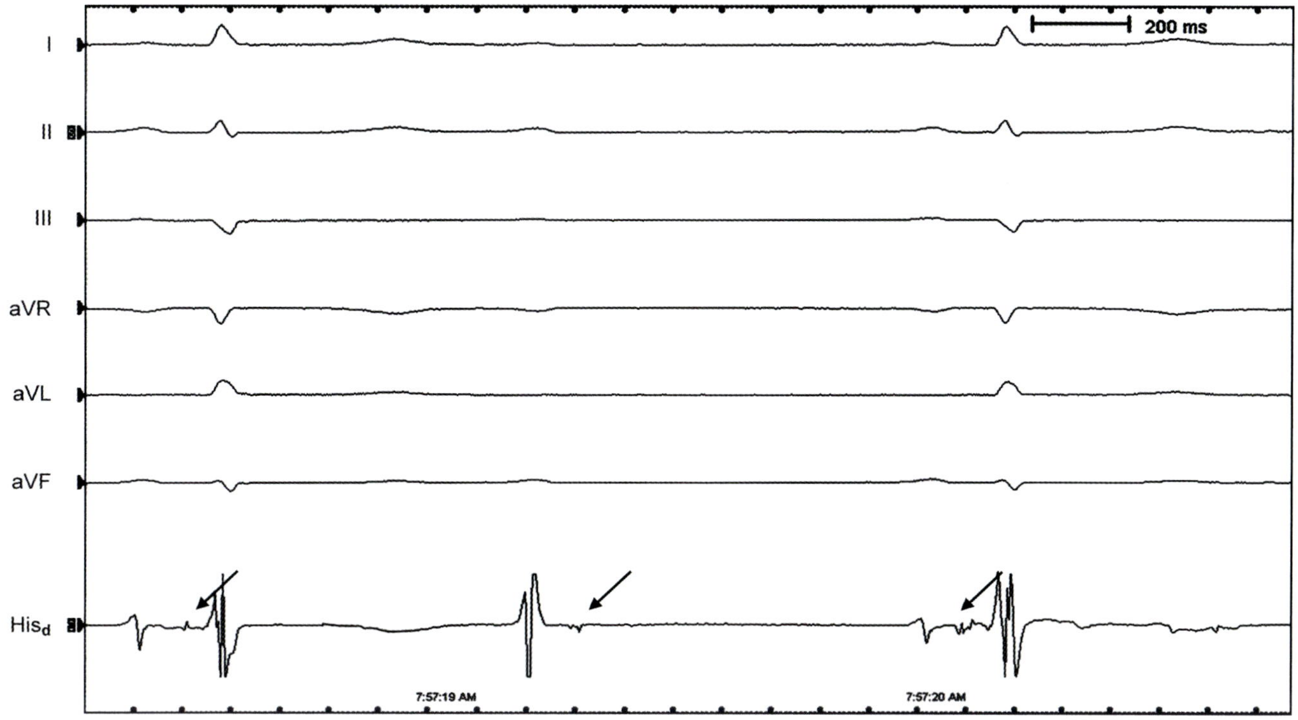

Figure 5.17B: Intracardiac electrograms of the patient whose ECG is shown in Figure 5.17A. The blocked P-wave shows an atrial signal followed by small, incomplete His bundle deflection suggesting intrahisian level of 2 to 1 block. Also note the fragmented His bundle signal in the conducted beats again suggesting diseased His bundle

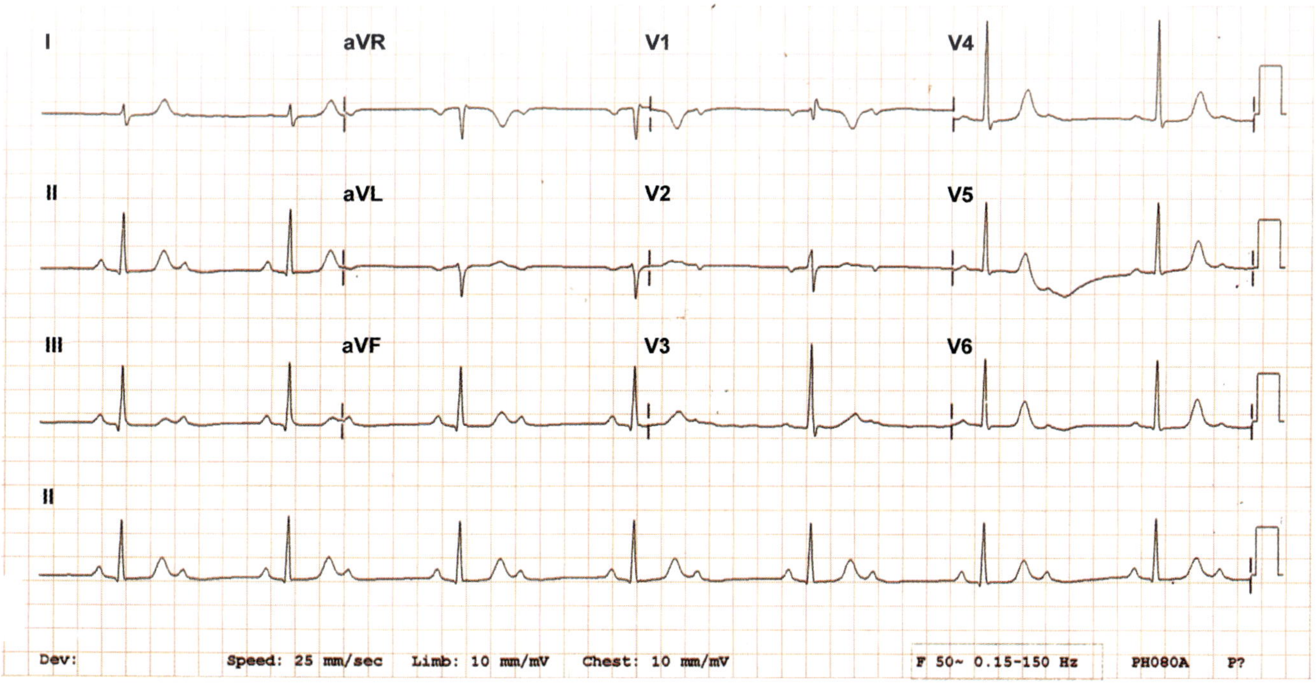

Figure 5.18: Surface ECG of sinus rhythm with 2 to 1 AV block with apparently narrow QRS complexes. Only V1 shows rsR′ pattern suggesting RBBB. This example shows the importance of looking at all the 12 leads before labeling QRS as narrow. Invasive EP study confirmed infrahisian 2 to 1 AV block (not shown)

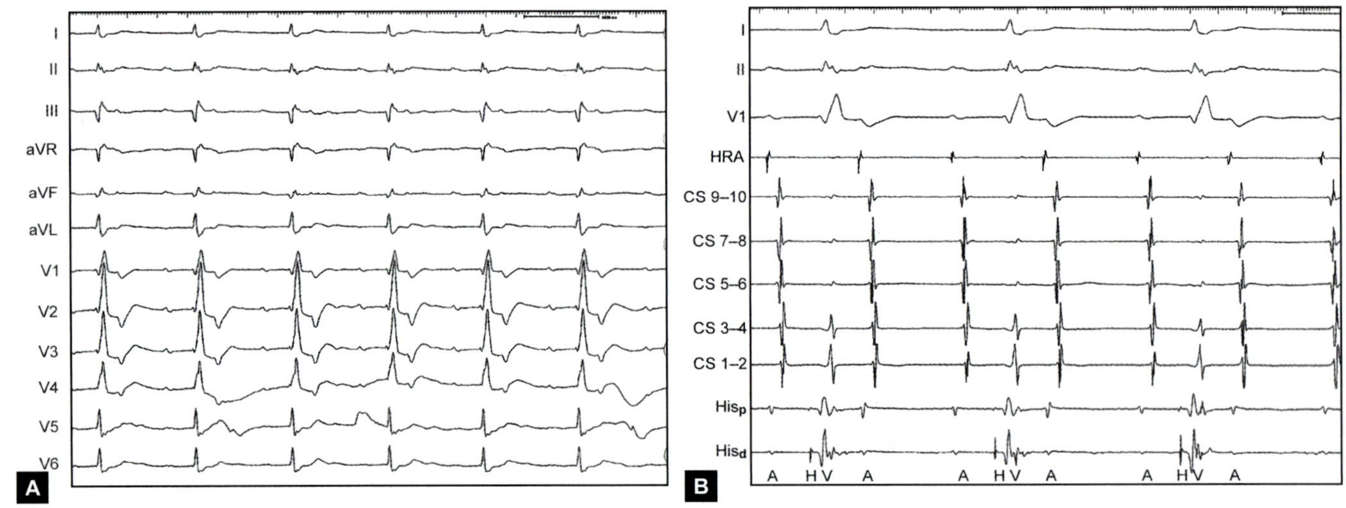

Figures 5.19A and B: Sinus rhythm with 2 to 1 AV nodal block and RBBB. (A) Surface ECG with prolonged PR interval in the conducted beats and RBBB; (B) Intracardiac electrograms with His bundle recording demonstrating atrial signal (A) not followed by His (H) or ventricular (V) signal in the blocked P-wave indicating AV nodal location of the block. Note that bundle branch block in the conducted beats during 2 to 1 AV block suggests infrahisian location of block but does not exclude AV nodal or intrahisian location. (B) From top to bottom, surface ECG leads I, II and V1; high right atrium (HRA), coronary sinus proximal (CS 9–10) to distal (CS 1–2) and His bundle proximal (His_p) and distal (His_d) recordings

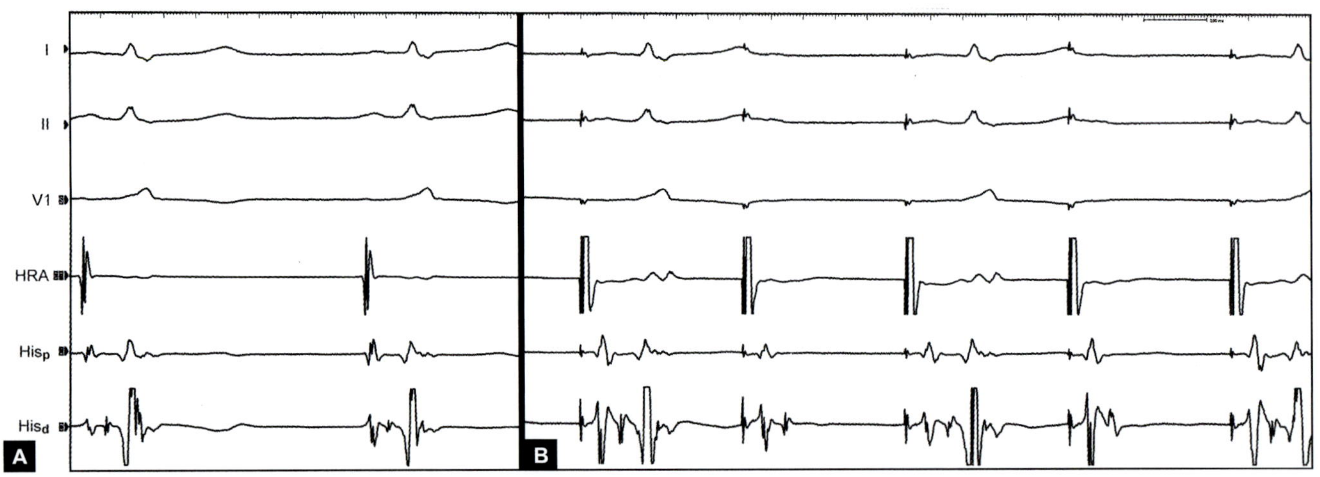

Figures 5.20A and B: Atrial pacing induced 2 to 1 infrahisian AV block is seen in (B) in a patient with chronic bifascicular block and recurrent syncope. (A) baseline intracardiac electrograms during sinus rhythm. From top to bottom are surface ECG leads I, II and V1, high right atrium (HRA), His bundle proximal (His_p) and distal (His_d) recordings

the conducted beats during 2 to 1 AV block suggests infranodal (intra- or infrahisian) location of block whereas a PR interval of 300 ms or more suggests AV nodal block.[53] A PR interval between 160 and 300 ms does not help in localization of site of block. Exercise results in sympathetically mediated increase in AV conduction and hence likely to show improvement in conduction in a patient with AV nodal 2 to 1 AV block to either type 1 block or 1 to 1 conduction. Similar response is seen with atropine in AV nodal 2 to 1 block. Both exercise and atropine have no direct affect on infranodal conduction, but increase the sinus rate that results in worsening of AV conduction to higher degrees of block in patients with infranodal 2 to 1 AV block. Sometimes atrial pacing induced 2 to 1 infrahisian block may be seen in patients with bifascicular block undergoing EP study for evaluation of syncope **(Figures 5.20A and B)**. However, it should be remembered that atrial pacing induced infrahisian block can also be physiological and may not warrant any treatment in the absence of symptoms.

Carotid sinus massage, on the other hand, reduces the sinus rate and with reduction in input the AV conduction improves in infranodal block. However, direct negative effect of carotid massage on AV nodal conduction results in worsening of conduction during AV nodal 2 to 1 block.

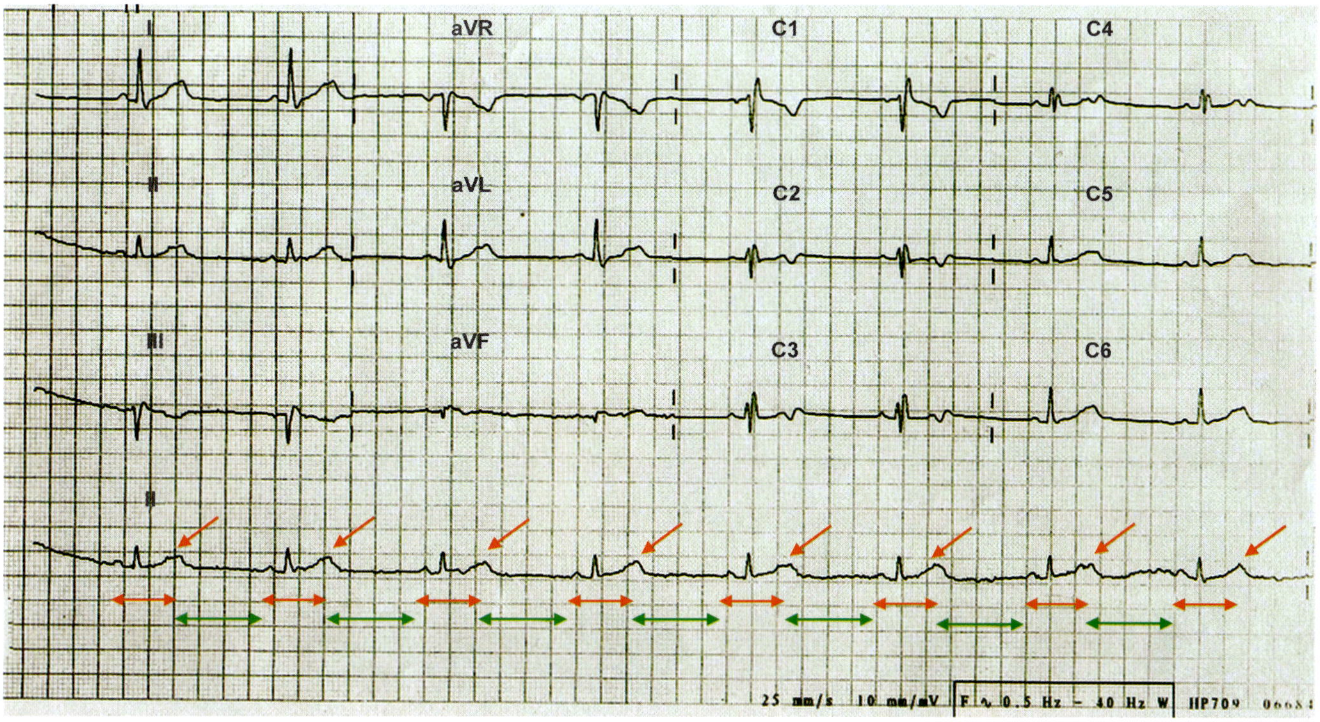

Figure 5.21: Atrial bigeminy with nonconducted atrial premature beats falling on the previous T-waves (arrows) during RBBB simulating 2 to 1 AV block. The red horizontal lines denote the coupling intervals of the premature beats. Remember that hump or deformation or undue peaking of a T-wave may indicate presence of an ectopic P-wave

The site of block during 2 to 1 AV block can also be suggested by the company it keeps.[52] Occurrence of type 1 AV block before or after episodes of 2 to 1 AV block suggests AV node as the site of block. Likewise, presence of episodes of Mobitz type 2 block at other times suggests infrahisian location of block in a patient with 2 to 1 AV block and wide QRS in the conducted beats.

It is important to recognize 2 to 1 block on surface ECG in any patient with bradycardia by carefully looking for alternate nonconducted P-waves that may be hidden on the preceding T-waves. Similarly, one should make certain that 2 to 1 block is not due to nonconducted atrial premature beats during atrial bigeminy **(Figure 5.21)** that is likely a physiological AV block and does not warrant pacemaker therapy.

Clinical Implications

The presence of symptoms and the location of block guide the need for pacemaker implantation in patients with 2 to 1 AV block. Symptomatic patients with 2 to 1 block need permanent pacemaker implantation irrespective of the site of block. Also, pacemaker therapy is reasonable in patients with infranodal 2 to 1 AV block even if asymptomatic.[54]

Atropine should not be used in stable patients with 2 to 1 AV block and wide QRS, which is likely to be infrahisian, since it can cause worsening of AV conduction and induce instability.[55]

Complete or Third Degree AV Block

Definition

Complete or third degree AV block refers to complete absence of conduction of atrial or supraventricular impulses to the ventricles. The ventricular rhythm is maintained by an escape rhythm that originates at a site distal to the location of the block. Hence, the atria (P-waves) and ventricles (QRS complexes) are dissociated from each other—AV dissociation; and a dual rhythm exists at any point of time. The atrial rate is greater than the ventricular rate. Complete AV block can at times be intermittent with resultant intermittent symptoms due to bradycardia.

Site of Block

Complete AV block can exist at any level, i.e. AV node, His bundle or the bundle branches. The ventricular rhythm originates in an escape focus that is distal to the block and occurs at a rate intrinsic to that focus. For example, in complete AV nodal block, the AV junctional area distal to the block forms the escape focus resulting in narrow QRS slow ventricular rhythm that is dissociated from the faster P-waves. Similarly, in infrahisian complete AV block, the escape rhythm arises from the ventricles and hence is quite slow, unreliable and has a widened QRS complex **(Figure 5.22)**. It is quite apparent that a narrow QRS escape

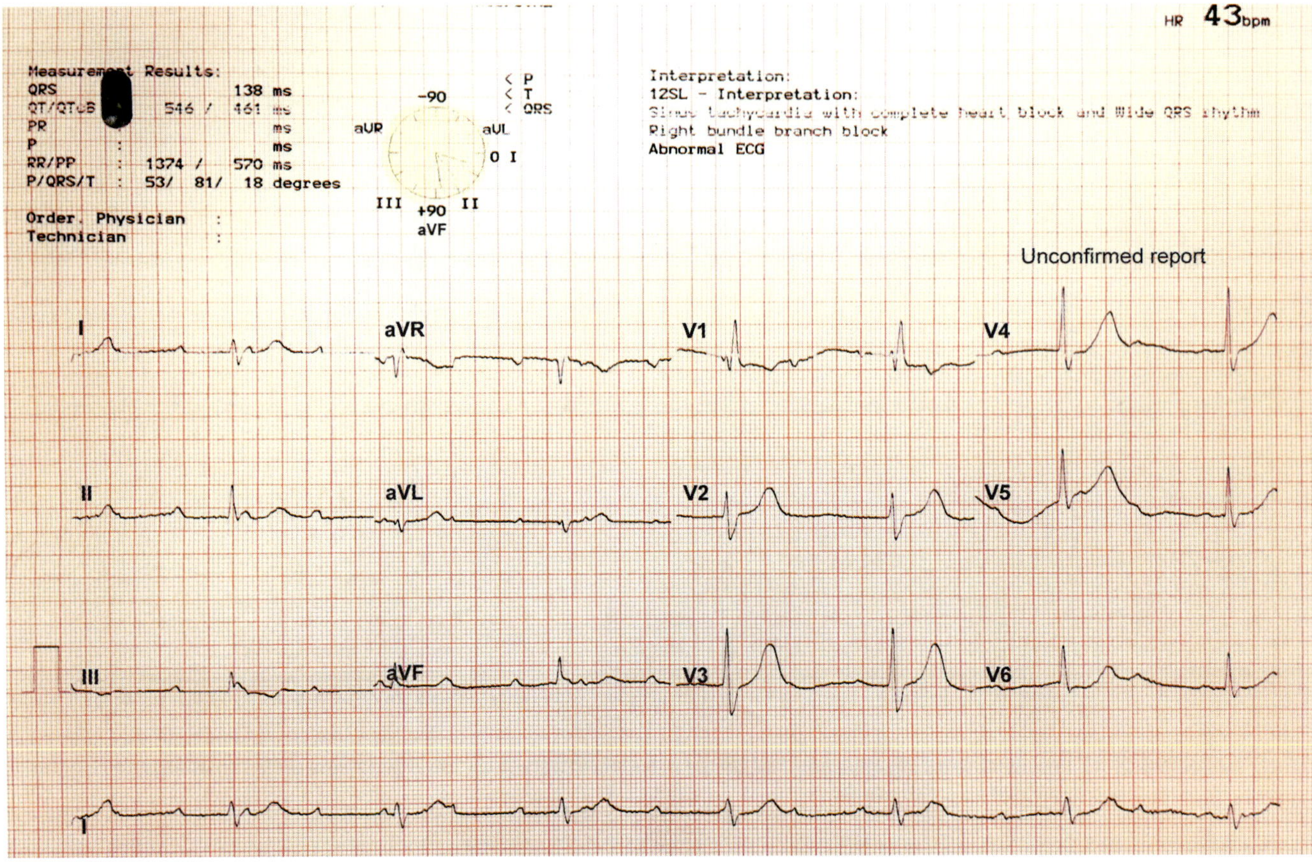

Figure 5.22: Sinus tachycardia with complete AV block and wide QRS (RBBB morphology) ventricular escape rhythm in an 80-year-old gentleman. The P-waves occur regularly at an atrial rate of 110 beats per minute and have no relationship with the QRS complexes that also occur regularly though at a much slower rate of 43 beats per minute. Note that the apparent PR intervals are highly variable. The slow wide QRS escape rhythm suggests infrahisian location of block—most common site in adults with degenerative heart block

rhythm during complete AV block implies block at the level of AV node or His bundle. On the other hand, a wide QRS escape rhythm indicates infrahisian location of block, though rarely it can be AV nodal or intrahisian with additional BBB. The latter is commonly seen with postoperative AV nodal block in children after corrective surgery for congenital heart disease where the RBBB is due to ventriculotomy **(Figure 5.23)**.

The acquired degenerative complete AV block in adults is usually infrahisian whereas the congenital complete AV block is usually AV nodal with junctional escape rhythm **(Figure 5.24)**. Intrahisian 3rd degree AV block can occur in older patients especially in those with calcific aortic stenosis and was seen in 16% of patients with complete heart block and narrow QRS in Narula's series.[48]

Although, the site of block in a patient with complete AV block can be suggested by the clinical setting (congenial complete AV nodal block in a child, AV nodal block after ablation for AVNRT, infrahisian in old age), ventricular rate (faster with junctional escape rhythm in nodal block, slower with ventricular escape rhythm in distal block) and QRS width (narrow with nodal or intrahisian, wide with infrahisian block) on surface ECG; an invasive EP study can precisely localize the site of block. An AV nodal complete AV block will reveal atrial signals at a rate faster than ventricular rate that are dissociated with His and ventricular signals. His signal precedes each ventricular electrogram with normal HV interval indicating junctional escape rhythm that exists at a rate of 50–60 per minute. On the other hand, His signal following each atrial electrogram with a fixed AH interval with dissociated slower ventricular rhythm with a wide QRS confirms infrahisian complete AV block **(Figure 5.25)**.

In intrahisian complete AV block, each atrial signal is followed by the first component of His electrogram (H) and these AH complexes are dissociated with slower H′V complexes comprising of second component of His (H′) and ventricular electrograms. The H′V interval is usually shorter than normal HV interval and the surface ECG shows narrow QRS; all these features indicating lower junctional escape rhythm **(Figures 5.26 and 5.27)**.

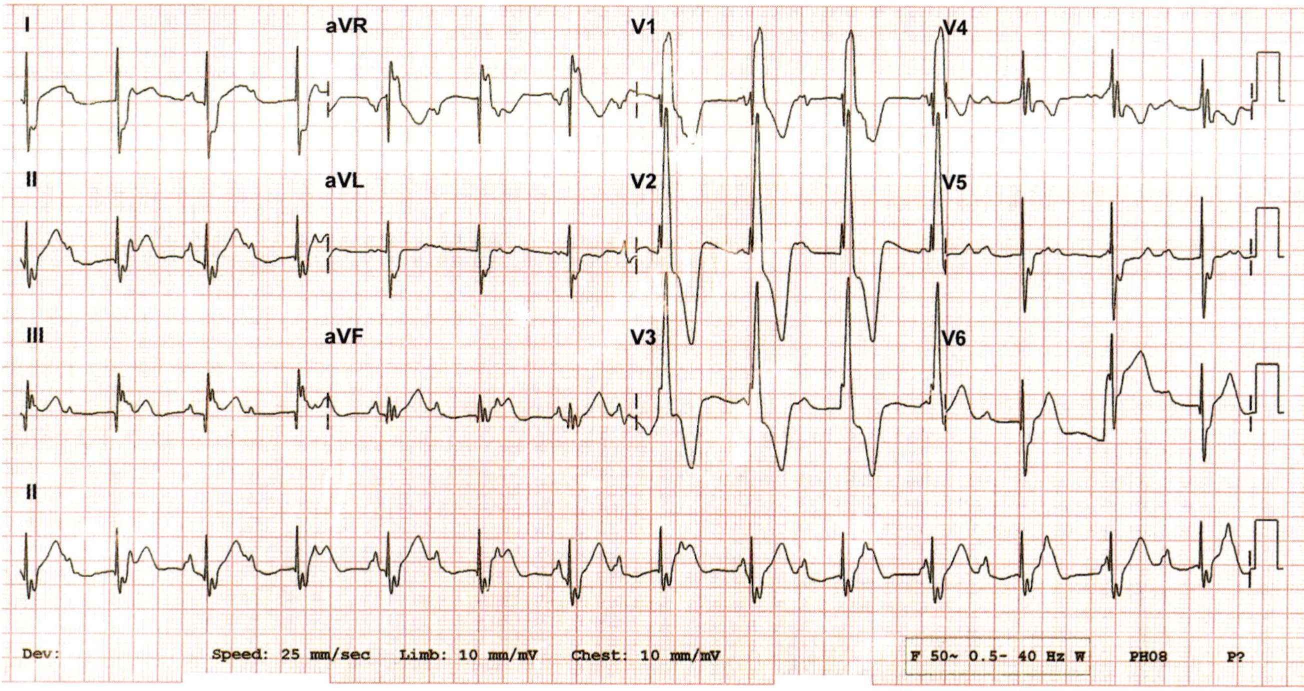

Figure 5.23: AV nodal complete AV block after corrective surgery for tetrology of Fallot's in a child. Note that the RBBB is due to distal block in the right bundle branch as a result of ventriculotomy. A fast ventricular escape rate of 108 bpm suggests junctional origin of the escape rhythm. An identical QRS morphology during 1 to 1 AV conduction three days later (not shown) confirmed that the block is not infrahisian

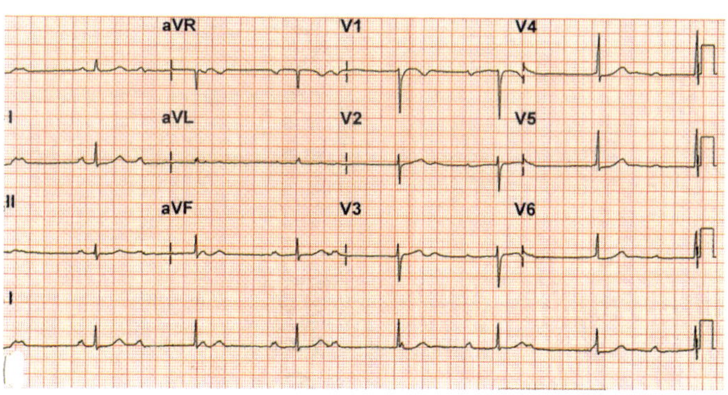

Figure 5.24: Sinus rhythm with complete AV block and narrow QRS escape rhythm in an asymptomatic adult with structurally normal heart. Congenital complete AV block is usually AV nodal and has a narrow QRS junctional escape rhythm

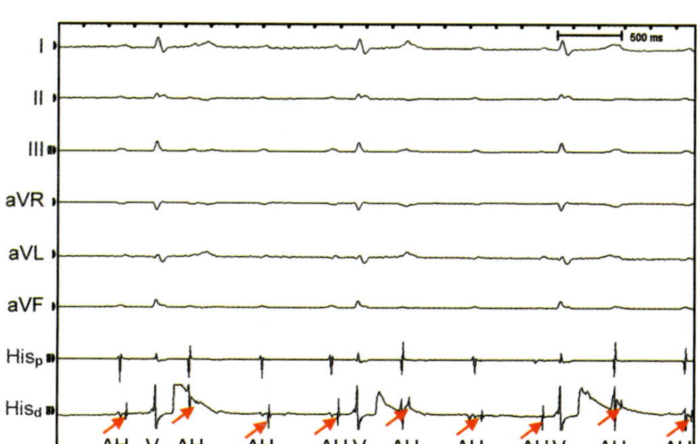

Figure 5.25: Intracardiac tracing of the patient whose ECG is shown in Figure 5.22 showing infrahisian location of the complete AV block. The His distal recording shows that each atrial (A) signal is followed by His signal (H) with normal and constant AH interval. The ventricular signal (V) is dissociated from the A and H signals and occurs at much slower rate. Note that the diagnosis of infrahisian AV block is already clear from the ECG and EP study usually has no role to play. It may be done for academic reasons or to check for inducibility of ventricular tachycardia in patients who also have left ventricular dysfunction. From top to bottom are surface ECG leads, I, II, III, aVR, aVL and aVF, His proximal (His_p) and distal (His_d) recordings

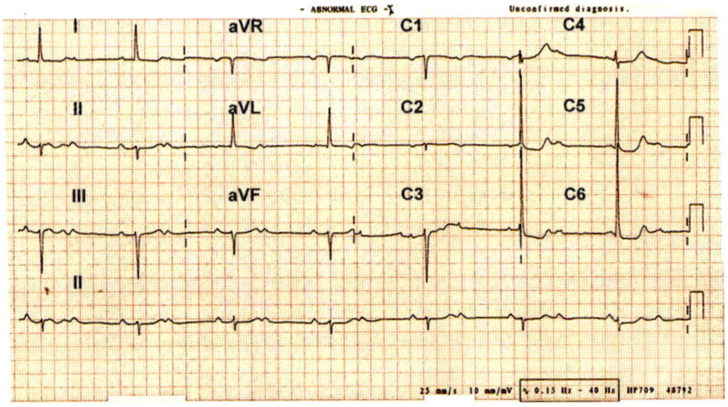

Figure 5.26: Sinus rhythm with complete AV block and narrow QRS escape rhythm in a 75-year-old patient with mitral annular calcification. A narrow QRS escape rhythm excludes infrahisian location, and with findings of mitral annular calcification makes intrahisian block quite likely

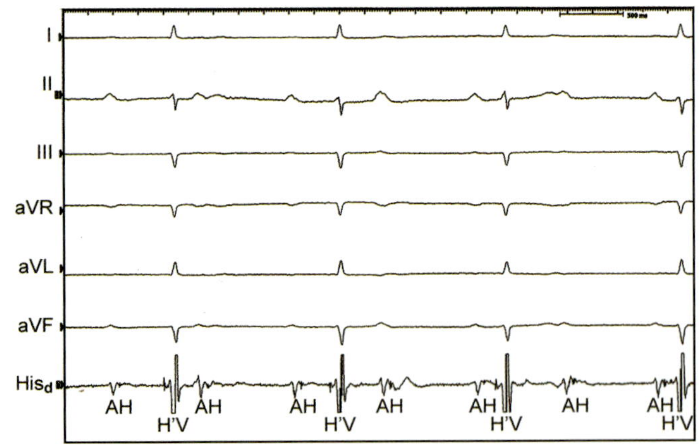

Figure 5.27: Intracardiac recording of the patient whose ECG is shown in Figure 5.26 confirming intrahisian complete AV block with junctional escape rhythm. The His bundle recording shows split His with its initial component (H) associated with atrial signal (A) and dissociated from its second component (H')

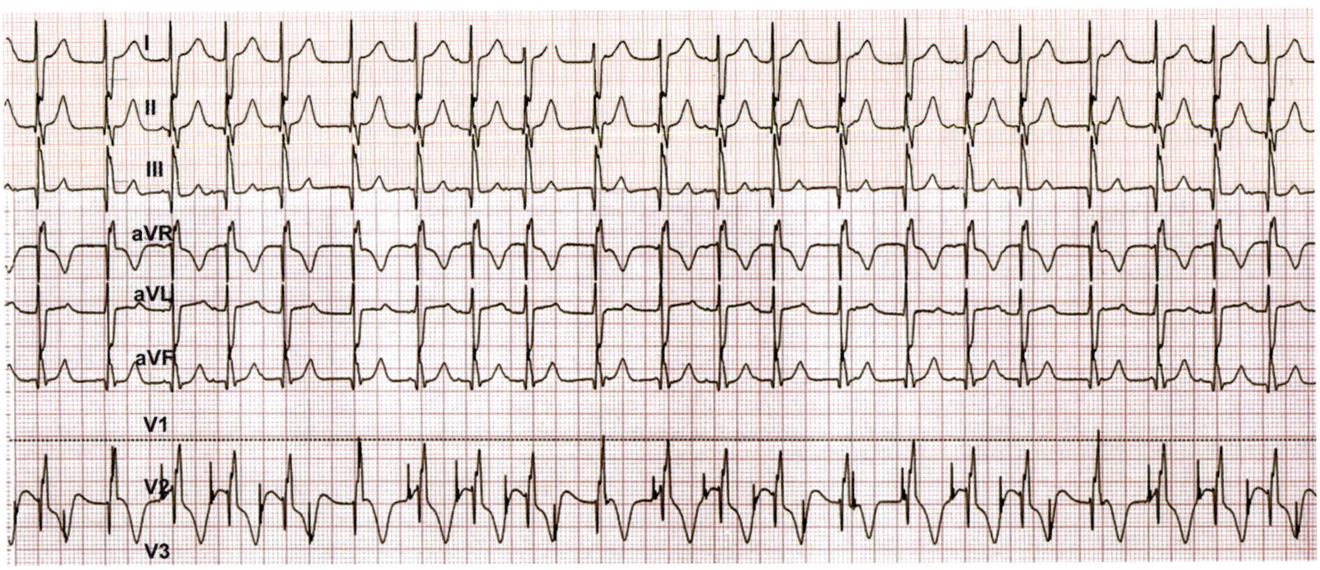

Figure 5.28: A-wire study in a child after corrective surgery for cyanotic congenital heart disease using epicardial pacing wire connected to lead V2. The atrial event or P-wave is depicted as a sharp spike in V2 clearly demonstrating a faster atrial rate and AV dissociation due to complete AV block

In postoperative patients especially after congenital heart disease surgery, an A-wire ECG using the epicardial pacing wires can be helpful if there is confusion in diagnosis with the surface ECG. In complete AV block, a faster atrial rhythm can be seen dissociated from the slower ventricular rhythm that usually shows RBBB **(Figure 5.28)**.

Clinical Implications

Most patients with complete AV block that is not due to reversible causes (like acute myocardial infarction, or hyperkalemia) or not likely to recover (immediate postsurgery) will require permanent pacing. Even asymptomatic patients especially with infrahisian or intrahisian complete AV block usually require pacing therapy. One exception can be asymptomatic patients with congenital complete AV block with stable narrow QRS escape rhythm and adequate rate who can be followed clinically and may not require pacing.

It is important to realize that a slow regular rhythm during atrial fibrillation suggests a diagnosis of complete AV block since the ventricular rhythm with intact AV conduction should be irregular and rapid **(Figure 5.29)**. This scenario used to be common in patients with digitalis toxicity but is rarely seen nowadays. Similarly, a slow regular rhythm due

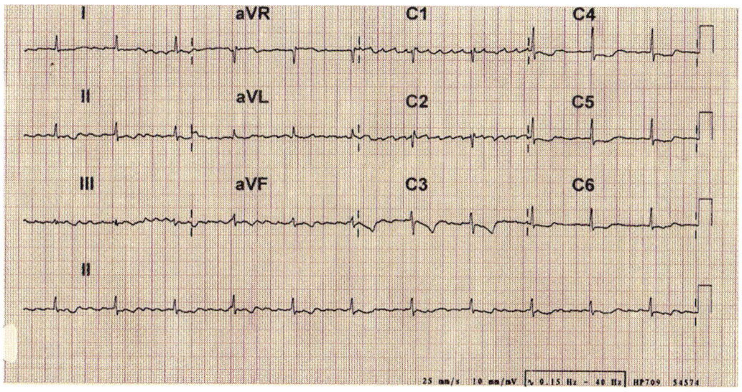

Figure 5.29: Atrial fibrillation with complete AV block and slow regular ventricular escape rhythm arising from AV junction

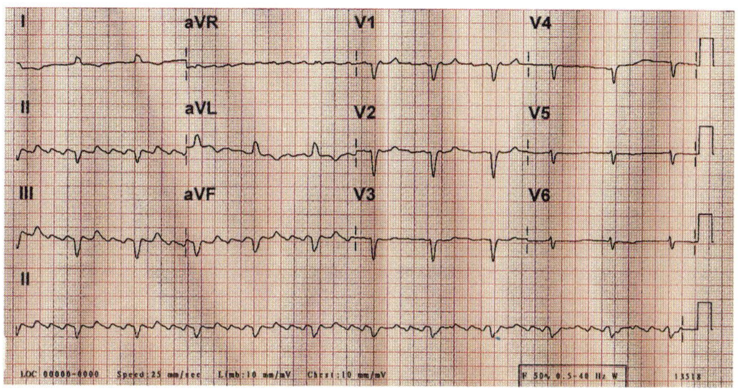

Figure 5.30: Atrial flutter with complete AV block and regular wide QRS ventricular escape rhythm. The clue to the presence of complete AV block lies in the observation that the apparent PR intervals are not constant. The simplest way is to compare the PR intervals of the first and the last QRS in the rhythm strip. In a fixed 4:1 AV conduction during atrial flutter, the PR intervals during conducted beats should be constant

to complete AV block during atrial flutter can be mistaken for physiological 4 to 1 (or higher degree) AV conduction unless the apparent PR intervals are carefully examined. During complete AV block, the apparent PR interval is likely to be variable, but is constant in atrial flutter with fixed AV conduction **(Figure 5.30)**.

SPECIAL CATEGORIES OF ATRIOVENTRICULAR BLOCK

Pseudo AV Block

Pseudo AV block refers to occurrence of apparent first and second degree AV block in the absence of primary impairment in the AV conduction system and is usually ascribed to concealed junctional premature beats (JPBs). It was way back in 1947, when Langendorf et al. first reported cases of nonconducted JPBs imitating first and second degree AV block.[56] Many different but interesting ECG phenomena were explained by these concealed JPBs using deductive electrocardiography in subsequent years. Later, Langendorf and Pick suggested the term "pseudo AV block" for this phenomenon.[57] Rosen et al. in 1970 confirmed the presence of these concealed (neither propagated antegradely to ventricles nor retrogradely to atria) JPBs using His bundle recordings as the cause of apparent AV block.[58]

Mechanism

A JPB, recognized as premature His bundle depolarization on EP study, can block antegradely as well as retrogradely and hence remain "concealed" on the surface ECG. The block is due to physiological refractoriness of the AV conduction axis proximal and distal to the origin of the premature impulse. Though concealed, it effects the conduction of the subsequent P-wave by prolonging the refractoriness of the AV conduction system resulting in either prolonged PR or complete block of the next P-wave, thus enabling its recognition on the ECG. This is visible on the surface ECG as either unexpected prolonged PR interval in one beat or single nonconducted P-wave **(Figures 5.31A and B)**.

Although, one should suspect concealed JPB as a cause of unexplained rhythms including pseudo AV block, this assumption assumes more strength if a similar sequence of events is recorded when the JPBs conduct to the ventricles. The concealment of a JPB is more likely after a longer preceding cycle and this longer cycle can in fact be as a result of compensatory pause after any premature beat including a conducted JPB. Whether a JPB will be conducted or remain concealed depends on its coupling interval and the length of the preceding RR interval.[49,58]

Diagnosis

Pseudo AV block is usually seen in individuals who do not have symptoms of bradycardia and have unexplained AV block recorded on ECGs or Holter tracings. The diagnosis of pseudo AV block secondary to concealed JPB should be suspected in the presence of unusual ECG findings like:

- Sudden appearance of unexplained PR prolongation
- Occurrence of type 1 and apparent type 2 AV block in the same patient
- Apparent type 2 AV block with narrow QRS in a patient not likely to have conduction system disease or brady-related symptoms
- Antegradely conducted JPBs seen at other times.

The diagnosis can be confirmed during an EP study wherein the His bundle recording during a JPB shows a premature His deflection (H') with a polarity same or different from normally occurring His deflections. The JPB may be conducted antegradely (H' followed by V), retrogradely (H' followed by retrograde A), both or may be blocked (H' not followed by A or V). The effect of a nonconducted H' on conduction of subsequent sinus P-wave in the form of AH prolongation or block can be readily seen.

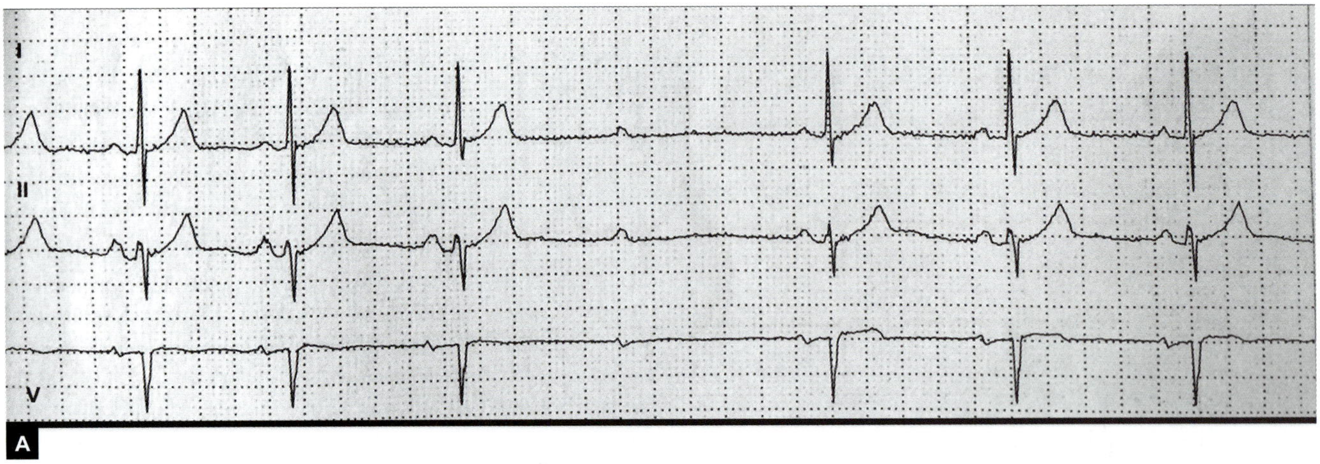

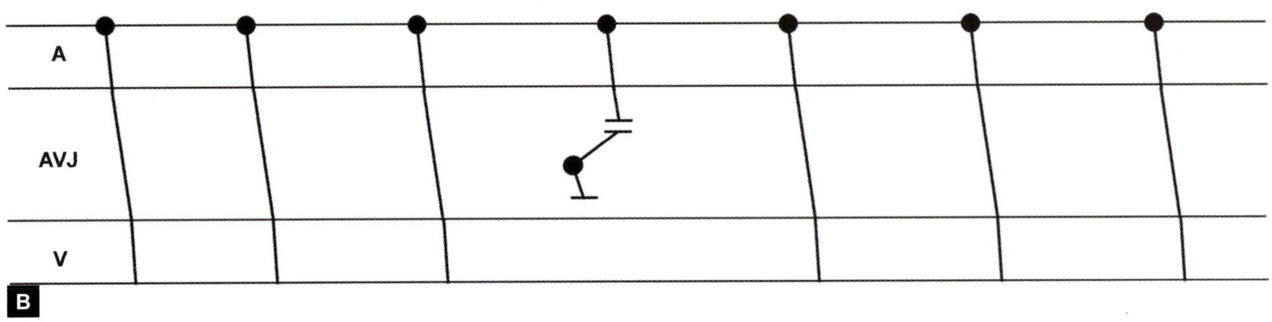

Figures 5.31A and B: Pseudo-AV block. The Holter tracing of an asymptomatic individual shows episodes of apparent 2nd degree Mobitz type 2 AV block with narrow QRS complexes (A). This can be explained by the presence of concealed junctional premature beat that makes the AV node refractory to the subsequent P-wave resulting in its block. The mechanism is well-explained in the ladder diagram (B)
Abbreviations: A, atrium; AVJ, atrioventricular junction; V, ventricle

Clinical Implications

The importance of recognition of pseudo AV block lies in preventing unnecessary pacemaker implantation in usually asymptomatic patients with no primary impairment of AV conduction. In fact, suppression of JPBs using drugs can sometimes help in reducing or eliminating episodes of pseudo AV block especially relevant in patients who have palpitations secondary to pauses due to this phenomenon.

Multilevel AV Block

The AV conduction disturbances discussed so far have assumed that the block resides only at one level. However, various complex ECG patterns are sometimes seen that cannot be explained by a single level block. Many phenomena have been used to explain these and AV block at multiple levels is one of them. Multilevel block is more commonly seen during physiological block in AV conduction during times of rapid atrial rhythms like atrial flutter or during rapid atrial pacing in the EP lab, however, it can sometimes be seen occurring spontaneously during sinus rhythm as well.[59,60]

Mostly, the AV block is at two levels but can be at three or more levels also and occurs due to horizontal dissociation in the AV conduction axis. Though, higher level block at the AV node, and lower level block at the His bundle or bundle branches has been most commonly described, both levels of block can occur in the AV node itself.[60] The explanation of blocks at multiple levels was based mostly on deductive electrocardiography initially; invasive EP study has confirmed their presence in many case studies published later.

Types

Kosowsky et al. in their case series of multilevel AV block, mostly in patients with atrial flutter, classified multilevel AV block into two types based on the pattern of conduction at the upper and lower levels.[60]

Type A multilevel block: The upper level of block has an integral conduction ratio mostly 2 to 1 whereas Wenckebach block occurs at the lower level. The lower level block may also progress to 2 to 1 resulting in 4:1 AV block. In fact, the authors suggested that two level block is usually the mechanism in patients with atrial flutter and 4:1 AV conduction pattern.[60] Since the lower level shows Wenckebach block which is known to be most common in the AV node, both levels of block in type A multilevel block may occur in the AV node itself. During atrial flutter with type A multilevel block, the ECG shows classic Wenckebach periodicity in alternate

P (flutter) waves and the sequence terminates with three blocked P-waves **(Figure 5.32)**. This pattern of conduction has also been termed as Alternate Wenckebach Periods (AWP) that is alluded to below:

Type B multilevel block: The upper level of block has a non-integral conduction ratio (usually Wenckebach block) with either 2:1 or Wenckebach block at the lower level **(Figure 5.33)**. The conduction in this type of block display a diversity of patterns that is dependent on length of the Wenckebach sequence at the upper level, type of block at lower level, and the relationship of the sequences of block at the two levels. The usual site of upper level block is AV node, though lower level of block may be at the bundle branches, His bundle or AV node itself. Due to diverse conduction patterns in this type, the sequence may terminate with one, two or more successively blocked P-waves.

Mechanisms

Multilevel AV block has been used to explain the occurrence of alternating Wenckebach periods (AWP) that are episodes

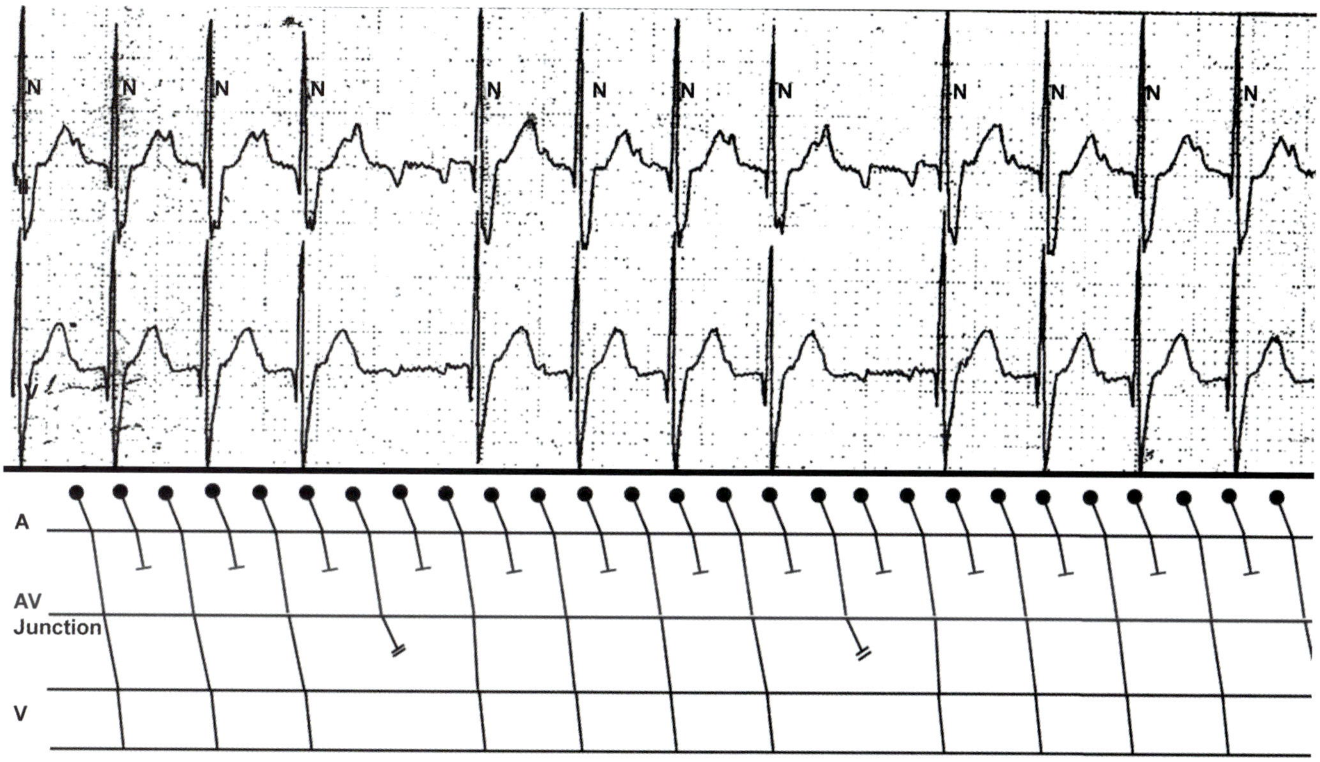

Figure 5.32: Atrial flutter with type A multilevel block in a 5-month-old child operated for large ventricular septal defect. The upper level of block is 2 to1 and lower level is Wenckebach (5:4). Since the lower level of block is Wenckebach, both levels may lie in the AV node itself. It is an example of alternate Wenckebach periodicity wherein the PR intervals of the conducted beats progressively increases till the sequence terminates. Note that the sequence typically ends with three consecutive blocked P-waves. Also, notice that if the alternate blocked P-wave is not recognised, it may be misdiagnosed as high grade AV block

Abbreviations: A, atrium; AVJ, atrioventricular junction; V, ventricle

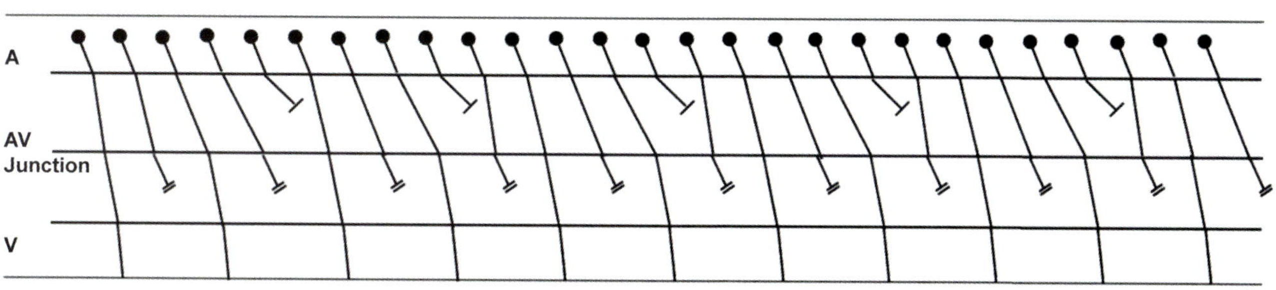

Figure 5.33: Schematic ladder diagram showing type B multilevel block during atrial flutter – 5:4 Wenckebach AV block at upper level and 2 to 1 block at lower level. It appears as 5:2 conduction pattern on the surface ECG with varying RR intervals. Mostly without deep analysis, it is referred to as atrial flutter with varying block

Abbreviations: A, atrium; AVJ, atrioventricular junction; V, ventricle

Table 5.3: Mechanisms of conduction in multilevel AV block

Observed rhythm	*Mechanisms of conduction*		
	Level 1	*Level 2*	*Level 3*
3:1	3:2	2:1	–
3:1	6:5	5:4	2:1
3:1	9:8	2:1	4:3
3:1	3:2	4:3	3:2
4:1	2:1	2:1	–
4:1	4:3	3:2	2:1
5:1	5:4	2:1	2:1
5:3	5:4	4:3	–
5:2	5:4	2:1	–
5:2	5:4	4:3	3:2
8:1	2:1	2:1	2:1

From Schindler et al.[61]

of 2 to 1 block with gradually increasing PR intervals in the conducted beats terminating in a greater degree of block (3:1, 4:1 or 5:1).[43] The mechanisms of Wenckebach block in one of the levels (usually AVN) remain same as discussed in the section on type 1 AV block and can also be extended to AWP.[60]

Whatever may be the mechanism, Schindler et al. empirically postulated based on their observations and deductive reasoning that only two patterns of conduction, i.e. 2 to 1 and Wenckebach, are needed to explain all types of integral and nonintegral high degree atrioventricular block sequences.[61] These possible mechanisms have been shown in **Table 5.3** and can help the reader to deduce the mechanism in a complex rhythm.

Clinical Implications

Many interesting complex rhythms and conduction patterns that are sometimes transient can be explained using multilevel AV block especially those occurring during physiological AV block with atrial flutter. Similarly, careful look at intracardiac electrograms obtained during atrial pacing can reveal that these phenomena are quite common, and though the block may be physiological with little prognostic value in most, their study can increase interest and improve understanding of clinical electrophysiology.

Paroxysmal AV Block

Paroxysmal AV block is a poorly described clinical condition that is characterized by sudden and abrupt transition from 1:1 AV conduction to complete AV block resulting in syncope and sometimes sudden cardiac death.[62] The importance of this entity lies in its potential to cause sudden death that can easily be prevented by pacemaker implantation provided the disease is diagnosed in time. Unfortunately, the problem lies in its detection since it often exists with no abnormality on usual investigations. Moreover, the entity is not widely known among physicians and cardiologists.

Mechanism

Though, the precise mechanism is not entirely known, local phase 4 block in the HPS is believed to be the underlying mechanism. The block is usually but not always precipitated by sudden lengthening of the PP interval (HH interval on EP study) that leads to abrupt spontaneous depolarization of the fibers of the HPS. Any supraventricular impulse that reaches these fibers during this phase 4 of action potential finds them nonresponsive due to sodium channel inactivation. Once such critical diastolic membrane potential is reached, conduction does not resume until an escape or ectopic or sinus beat arrives at an appropriate time to reset the membrane potential to its maximal resting value.[62] The PP interval lengthening can occur due to spontaneous slowing of sinus rate, though more commonly occurs due to pause after an atrial, junctional or ventricular premature beat. Similar to initiation, the resumption of 1:1 conduction is often brought about by a premature atrial or ventricular beat. Interestingly, a ventricular escape (or premature) beat can conduct retrogradely during antegrade block (a feature seen only in infranodal AV block), can reset and resume one to one AV conduction.

Clinical Features

This disease entity can occur at any age including children.[63] The baseline ECG can be entirely normal in about 28% patients, though some conduction abnormality is usually present with RBBB being the most common (45%), others being left bundle branch block (15%) and intraventricular conduction defect in 12%.[62,64,65] The patients usually present with recurrent syncope or presyncope and occasionally aborted sudden death. Routine investigations as a part of evaluation of syncope including ECG, Holter, and even an EP study may be entirely normal. Prolonged ECG monitoring can reveal the diagnosis **(Figures 5.34A to C)** and maneuvers to specifically reproduce paroxysmal AV block during an EP study can be rewarding **(Figure 5.35)**. Extra-stimulation testing with critically timed atrial or ventricular beats or rapid atrial or ventricular pacing can result in appropriate HH interval lengthening resulting in induction of paroxysmal AV block. The HV interval may be normal at baseline but may get prolonged on stressing with drugs like procainamide or ajmaline, though this provocative test is not specific to paroxysmal AV block and only suggests underlying HPS disease.

Salient Features

Some of the salient features of paroxysmal AV block include:

- Initiation with sudden and critical PP interval prolongation due to an atrial, junctional or ventricular premature beat.

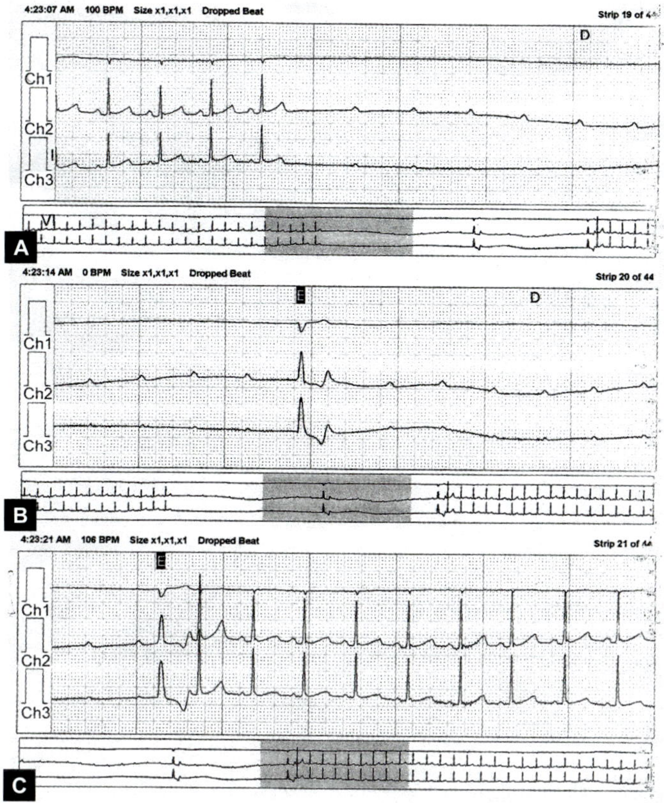

Figures 5.34A to C: Paroxysmal AV block seen during a Holter recording. Note that the initiation of block (A) occurs after PP lengthening likely due to a nonconducted atrial premature beat. Also, an escape beat occurring at a critical timing (C) leads to resumption of 1:1 AV conduction whereas another escape beat (B) is not able to do so. The narrow QRS complex with normal PR interval during 1:1 AV conduction (normal baseline ECG) and presence of hardly any escape beats typical of paroxysmal AV block are also well illustrated

- Unreliable or absent escape rhythm with unpredictable duration of asystole.
- PR interval prolongation at initiation is typically absent in contrast to vagal-mediated AV block.
- Site of block is infranodal and mechanism is local phase 4 block in the HPS.
- Baseline ECG is often shows RBBB, rarely LBBB and often has normal QRS.
- Important and easily treatable cause of sudden cardiac death.
- Clinical diagnosis is often elusive due to paroxysmal nature against a background of absent AV conduction disturbances.

Treatment

Though the diagnosis of paroxysmal AV block is difficult, the treatment once a diagnosis is made is straight forward. Permanent pacemaker implantation in these patients not only prevents episodes of syncope, but can also be lifesaving.

Congenital Complete AV Block

Congenital complete AV block (CCAVB) is present since birth and can often be diagnosed in utero and occurs with an incidence of 1 in 15000 to 1 in 22000 live births. It is associated with concomitant complex congenital heart disease (usually corrected transposition of great vessels or left isomerism) in one-third; though most cases (two-thirds) have structurally normal heart.[66] The other congenital heart diseases that can be associated with CCAVB include AV canal defects, tricuspid atresia, ventricular septal defect, and Ebstein's anomaly.[67]

The CCAVB is thought to result from embryonic maldevelopment of the AVN with fatty replacement of the AVN and its approaches.[23] Since the defect is usually suprahisian, the QRS complex of the escape rhythm is of narrow duration **(*see* Figure 5.24)**. The underlying cause in up to 90% of the cases is maternal lupus due to auto-antibodies. These antibodies cross the placenta and target the intracellular ribonucleoproteins of the fetal heart but do not affect the maternal heart.[68] Various studies on the use of agents like fluorinated steroids, intravenous immunoglobulin and hydroxychloroquine in the pregnant mothers at high risk for development of CCAVB in the fetus have showed conflicting results in prevention of CCAVB in the child. There are clear guidelines for indications of pacing in children and adolescents with CCAVB both with and without structural heart disease.[54]

AV Block in Acute Myocardial Infarction

AV block during acute myocardial infarction (MI) can occur due either to ischemia of the arteries supplying the conduction system or to heightened vagal tone and is seen in 12 to 25% of all infarctions, though its incidence is decreasing with increasing use of primary angioplasty. The incidence, degree and site of AV block depend on the area of infarction and the site of occlusion in the affected infarct-related artery.

During inferior wall MI, AV block can occur due to involvement of the AV nodal artery and thus affects the AVN with sparing of the HPS. First degree and 2nd degree type 1 AV block is more common with inferior MI, is usually due to vagotonia, occurs during the initial days of MI, and responds to atropine.[69] These AV blocks usually do not result in any symptoms, are transient, resolve spontaneously and do not require any treatment. Complete AV block in the setting of inferior wall MI is usually at the AV nodal level, with resulting narrow QRS junctional escape rhythm **(Figure 5.36)**. It also resolves spontaneously, though may require up to 2 weeks in some cases. Hemodynamic instability can occur in few cases especially in those with associated right ventricular involvement and may require fluid administration, atropine,

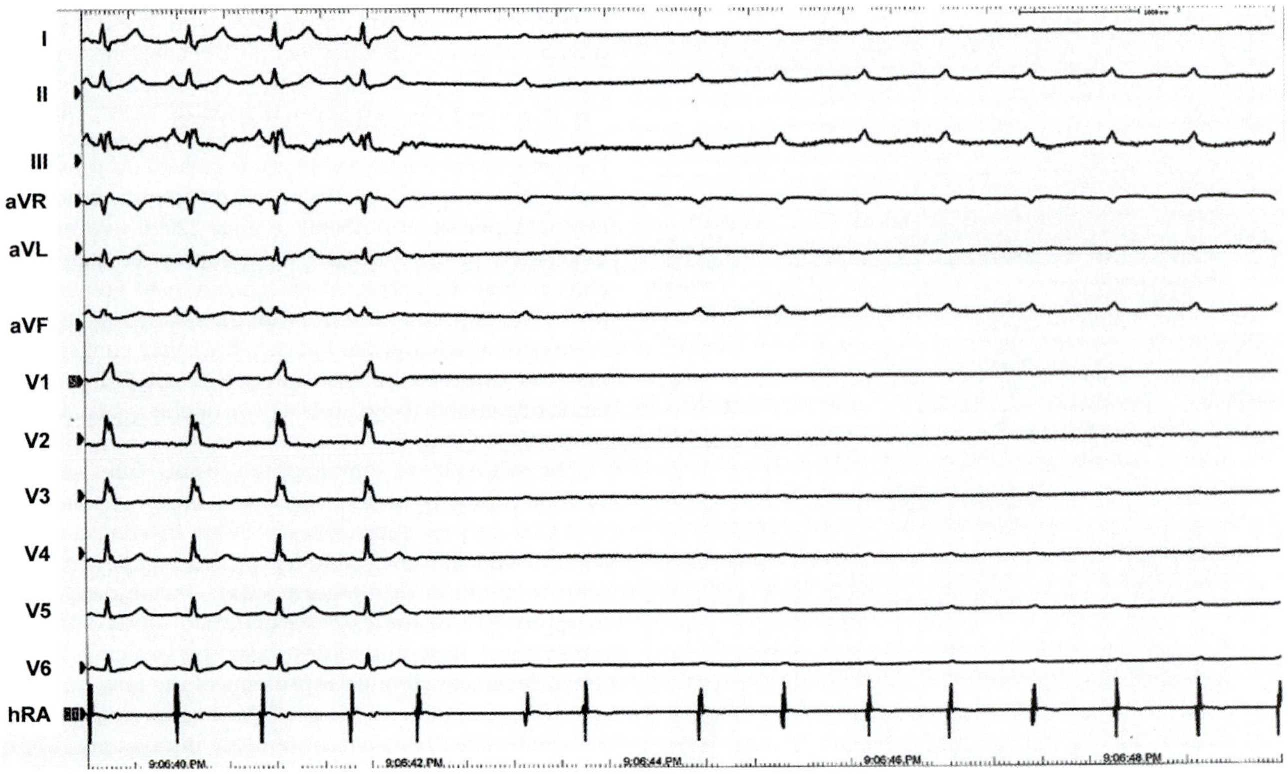

Figure 5.35: Paroxysmal AV block occurring spontaneously during an EP study in a patient with RBBB at baseline. Notice that an atrial premature beat during sinus rhythm leads to PP interval lengthening with initiation of AV block with absence of escape rhythm. In patients suspected with this diagnosis, atrial stimulation should be attempted in order to induce AV block with a critically timed extrastimulus

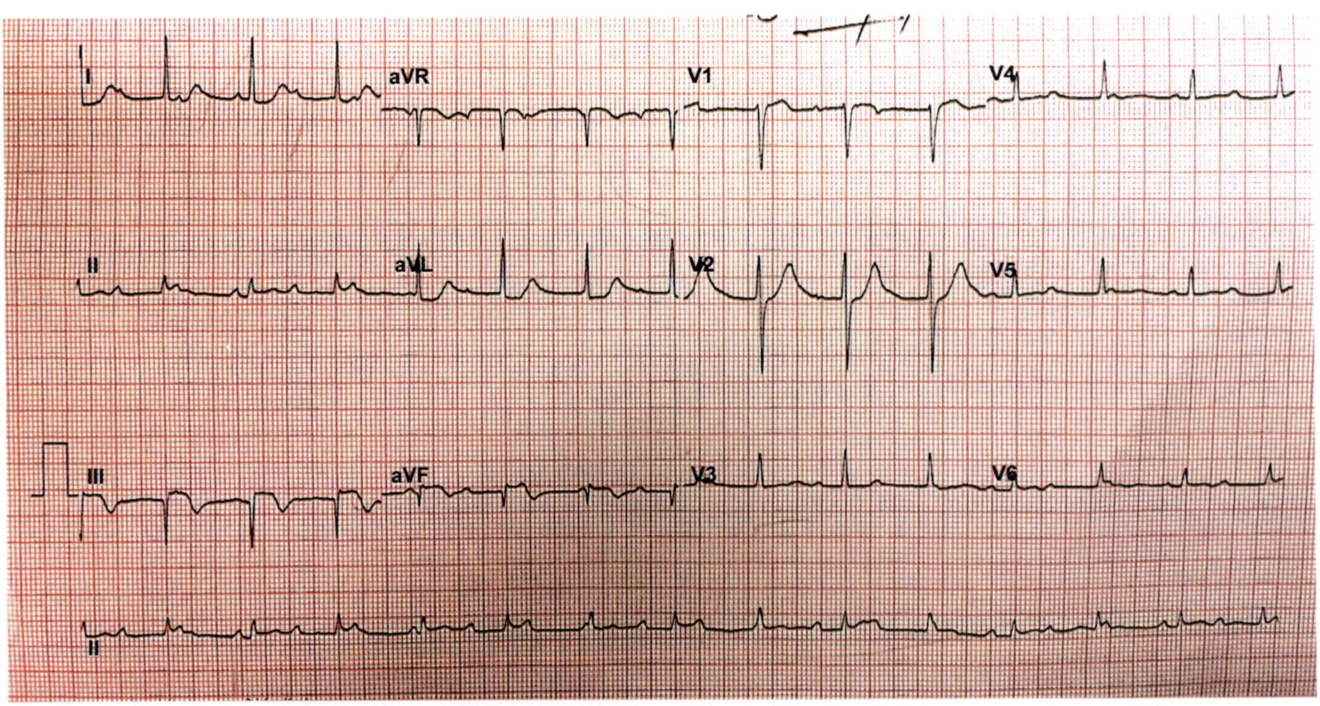

Figure 5.36: Sinus tachycardia with complete AV block with junctional escape rhythm during acute inferior wall myocardial infarction

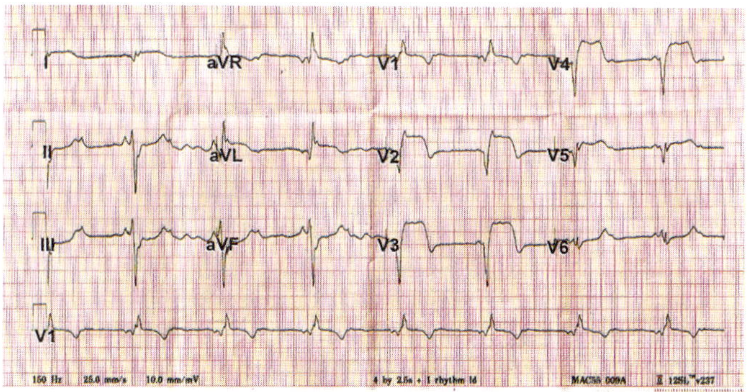

Figure 5.37: Two to one AV block with RBBB and left anterior hemiblock during acute anterior wall myocardial infarction. Note that a short PR interval of 120 ms in the conducted beats along with wide QRS complexes suggests infrahisian location of the block

catecholamines, and sometimes AV sequential temporary pacing. AV block occurring or resolving late in the course of inferior infarction is due to edema and local accumulation of adenosine in the conduction tissue.[70] Permanent pacing is almost never required for complete AV block occurring in acute inferior wall MI.

Type 2 second degree AV block or 2:1 AV block with wide QRS in the conducted beats **(Figure 5.37)** is uncommon, more often seen with anterior (compared to inferior) MI, is associated with ischemia of HB and bundle branches, has a worse prognosis and often progresses to complete AV block.

AV conduction disturbances during anterior MI are usually associated with proximal left anterior descending artery occlusion, are due to necrosis of the infranodal conduction tissue (HPS) in the septum, and carry a worse prognosis. The development of complete AV block during anterior wall MI is often preceded by bifascicular block with or without PR prolongation or second degree type 2 block; is often sudden and unpredictable and can be life threatening.[71] The higher mortality associated with complete AV block in anterior MI is largely related to progressive pump failure due to extensive myocardial necrosis and higher risk of ventricular tachyarrhythmias.[72] Though, temporary pacing is useful during anterior MI in the presence of complete AV block, or in those at high risk of its development like patients with bifascicular block; in the long-term most of such patients need implantable cardioverter defibrillator device rather than permanent pacemaker due to high risk of sudden arrhythmic death.

ATRIOVENTRICULAR CONDUCTION AND RELATED PHENOMENA

AV Dissociation

The students of cardiology and electrophysiology sometimes have confusion about the term AV dissociation and often use it interchangeably with complete AV block which is incorrect. Hence, it's important to understand the difference between the two.

Normally, only one pacemaker—the SAN controls both the atria and the ventricles. AV dissociation means that the atria and ventricles depolarize independently of each other. The atria are controlled by one pacemaker and the ventricles by some other pacemaker and a dual rhythm is controlling the heart. On the other hand, complete AV block is a type of AV dissociation in which the atrial impulse is not able to conduct to the ventricles. AV dissociation is never a primary diagnosis; in fact it is always secondary to another primary rhythm disturbance, complete AV block being one of them. In complete AV block the atrial rate is faster than the ventricular rate. The atrial rhythm is usually sinus but can be anything else like atrial fibrillation or flutter; however, none of the atrial impulses conduct to the ventricles. The ventricular rhythm is controlled by an escape focus that is below the level of block like AV junction or ventricles itself and is slower and typically regular. In fact, a slow regular ventricular rhythm during atrial fibrillation points towards a diagnosis of complete AV block (*see* **Figure 5.29**).

AV dissociation can also occur when the atrial rate is nearly same as the ventricular rate—*isorhythmic AV dissociation*. The best example is sinus bradycardia with junctional escape rhythm occurring at nearly the same rate **(Figure 5.38)**. Also, note that if the junctional escape rhythm shows retrograde conduction **(Figure 5.39)** to the atria, there is no AV dissociation. In this example of AV association, there is only one pacemaker—in the AV junction that is controlling both atria and the ventricles.

Ventricular tachycardia (VT) with retrograde ventriculoatrial (VA) block is the most common example of AV dissociation in which the ventricular rate is higher than the atrial rate. It should be remembered that VA conduction may or may not be present normally. VT can therefore, occur with retrograde VA conduction and hence absence of VA or AV dissociation does not rule out VT.

Table 5.4 lists a few examples of situations with AV association and dissociation with different A and V ratios to help the reader understand the fundamentals of AV dissociation.

AV dissociation is often also labeled as incomplete or complete. None of the atrial impulses conduct to the ventricles in complete AV dissociation, and the atrial and ventricular rates remain constant. In incomplete AV dissociation, some of the atrial impulses conduct to the ventricles. For example, in capture beats during VT, A and V are associated, indicating incomplete AV dissociation.

Gap Phenomenon

Gap phenomenon refers to a situation wherein premature impulses (atrial) fail to conduct (to the ventricles) but conduction resumes with even more premature impulses

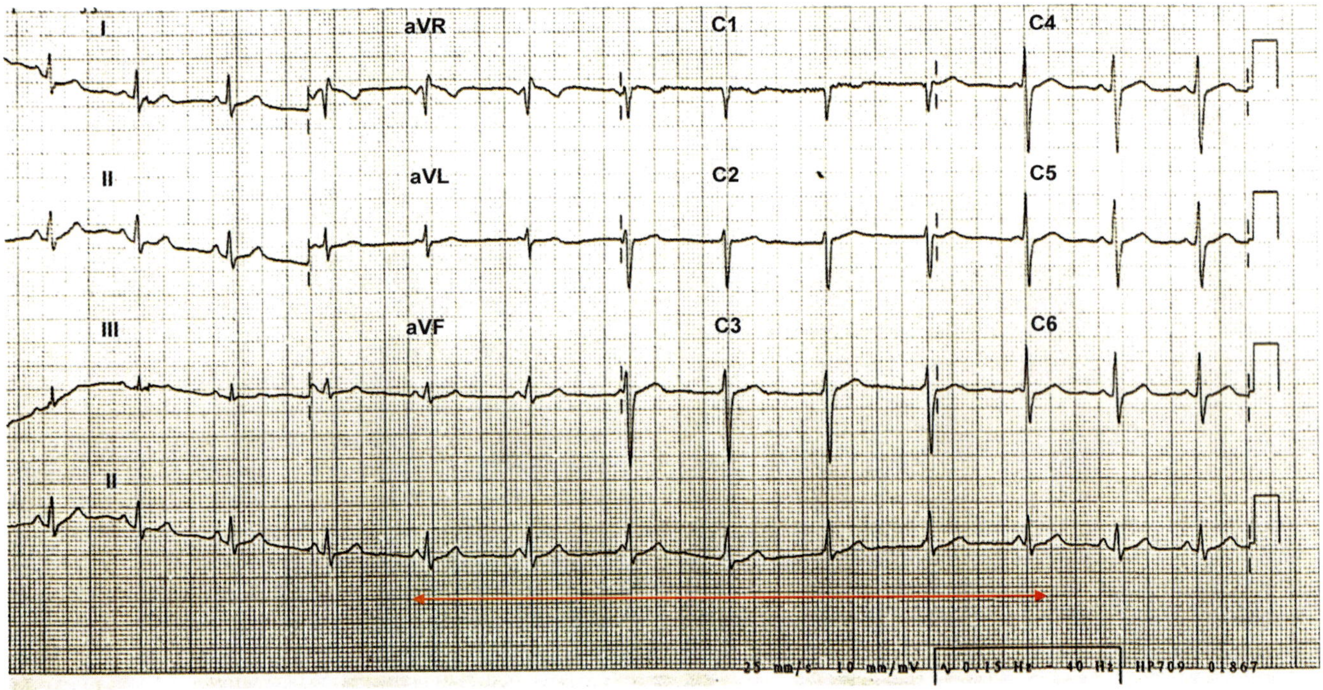

Figure 5.38: Isorhythmic AV dissociation during the interval indicated by red line in a child with relative bradycardia. Note that the junctional escape beats (a faster rate is commensurate with the age of the patient) control the ventricular rhythm and are dissociated with the sinus P-waves that control the atrial contraction. The P-waves seem to march into the QRS complexes and the atrial and ventricular rates are nearly equal

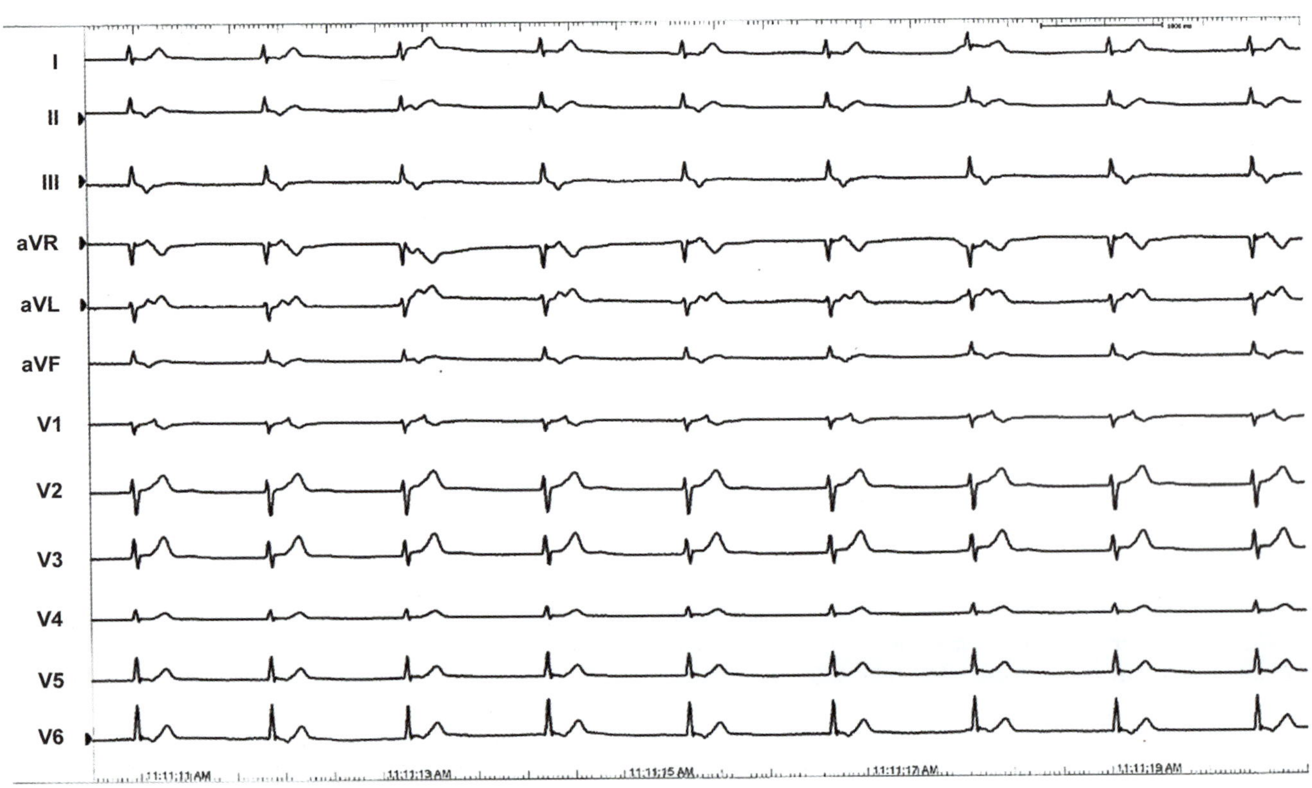

Figure 5.39: Junctional escape rhythm with retrograde 1:1 conduction to the atria. Note the narrow P-waves, inverted in inferior leads immediately following the QRS complexes that are typical of retrograde atrial activation

Table 5.4: Examples of rhythms with AV association and dissociation classified according to ratio of atrial and ventricular events

A and V ratio	AV (or VA) dissociation	AV association
A > V	• SR with CHB with junctional/ventricular escape rhythm • AF or AFL with CHB with junctional/ventricular escape rhythm	• AF with rapid ventricular rate • AFL with 2:1 or 4:1 AV conduction • AT with variable AV conduction • AVNRT with 2:1 AV block
A = V	• Accelerated junctional rhythm with isorhythmic AV dissociation • Sinus bradycardia with junctional escape rhythm with isorhythmic AV dissociation	• Sinus rhythm with 1:1 AV conduction • AVNRT • AVRT • AT with 1:1 AV conduction • Junctional rhythm (or tachycardia) with 1:1 retrograde VA conduction
A < V	• VT with retrograde VA block and sinus rhythm • AIVR with retrograde block • Junctional ectopic tachycardia with retrograde VA block and sinus (slower) rhythm	• VT with Wenckebach or 2:1 or any other non 1:1 VA conduction • Junctional tachycardia with Wenckebach or 2:1 or any other non 1:1 retrograde conduction

Abbreviations: A, atrial; V, ventricular; AV, atrioventricular; VA, ventriculoatrial; SR, sinus rhythm; CHB, complete heart block; AF, atrial fibrillation; AFL, atrial flutter; VT, ventricular tachycardia; AIVR, accelerated idioventricular rhythm; AT, atrial tachycardia; AVNRT, atrioventricular nodal reentrant tachycardia; AVRT, atrioventricular reciprocating tachycardia

resulting in a "gap" in conduction. The gap refers to the zone in the cardiac cycle during which the premature atrial impulses fail to conduct to the ventricles, though atrial impulses with greater or lesser prematurity show conduction. This was first described in dogs by Moe in 1965,[73] and later in humans by Durrer[74] and other researchers.[75,76] Akhtar et al. described the same phenomenon during retrograde conduction in humans.[77] Though, it is not considered to be true supernormal conduction by some authors, others consider it as one type of supernormal conduction. Gap phenomenon occurs due to functional differences in refractory periods and conduction in two or more sites in the AV conduction axis. A premature atrial impulse can block in the distal conduction site as it reaches its refractoriness. However, a more premature impulse may lead to delayed conduction in the proximal conducting site resulting in arrival of the impulse at the distal conducting site after a delay facilitating its conduction to the ventricles. The occurrence of gap phenomenon depends on two conditions. The first requires that the effective refractory period (ERP) of the distal site must be longer than the functional refractory period (FRP) of the proximal tissue, so that during a critical coupling interval there is block in the distal site. Second, the RRP of the proximal tissue at closer coupling interval should permit enough proximal delay so that the initially blocked distal tissue can recover.

The gap phenomenon has been classified depending on the sites of block initially into two types by Gallagher et al.[76] and later into many more types[78,79] **(Table 5.5)**.

The clinical significance of gap phenomenon lies in understanding the conduction and refractoriness of various conducting tissues of the AV conduction axis and in interpretation of difficult to understand tracings while performing atrial stimulation in the EP laboratory.

Table 5.5: Types of antegrade gap phenomena based on the proximal and distal sites of conduction delay or block

Type	Proximal site	Distal site
Type 1	AVN	HPS
Type 2	HPS proximal	HPS distal
Type 3	HB	HPS
Type 4	Atrium	AVN or HPS
Type 5	AVN proximal	AVN distal
Type 6	HPS proximal	HPS distal

In type 6, there is no conduction delay or block at proximal site compared to type 2, where the proximal site shows block in conduction.

Abbreviations: AVN, atrioventricular node; HB, His bundle; HPS, His-Purkinje system

Supernormal Conduction

Supernormal conduction is defined as a conduction pattern that is more rapid than expected or presence of conduction when block is anticipated.[80] It should not be thought of as conduction that is more rapid than normal. True supernormal conduction is occurrence of better conduction than expected and occurs during a period of supernormal excitability and conduction associated with altered membrane potential. This phenomenon has always been controversial since some researchers believe that most if not all the examples of supernormal conduction including those that do not occur during the period of supernormal excitability can be explained by other more common phenomena like gap phenomena, dual AV nodal physiology, "peeling back" of refractoriness, diastolic phase 4 depolarization and summation of subthreshold responses. The details of this phenomenon are beyond the scope of this chapter and interested readers are advised to read the case reports and reviews published in the literature.[80-82]

Concealed Conduction

Concealed conduction refers to the effects caused by penetration and block of an impulse into the cardiac conduction tissue on the conduction or formation of the subsequent impulse. The effect on the conduction of the subsequent impulse may be either delay or block and on impulse formation is either delay or failure of the discharge of an expected subsidiary pacemaker tissue. The concept underlying this phenomenon was enunciated by Engelmann[83] (9 years before the invention of electrocardiogram!) and Erlanger,[84] though its mechanism was investigated much later by many researchers.[85-87] The phenomenon is extremely common in clinical scenarios and has been used to explain many simple and complex arrhythmias, to interpret conduction disturbances that occur as a result of premature impulses, to decipher unexplained disturbances in AV conduction axis including aberrant conduction during many arrhythmias, to understand the normal response of the AV node and AV conduction in rhythms like atrial fibrillation and last but not the least to interpret apparent irregularities of the junctional pacemaker in AV dissociation in the presence or absence of AV block.[88]

A simplistic explanation of this phenomenon is that any impulse that arrives at the conduction tissue at a time that is the transition of ARP into the RRP (phase of interference[89] or phase of concealed conduction[88]) penetrates into the tissue, but fails to conduct. This penetration causes refractoriness in the conducting tissue resulting in delay or block in the conduction of a subsequent impulse or a delay or failure of expected impulse formation in the conducting tissue. The subsequently blocked impulse may itself cause penetration and concealment resulting in repetitive concealed conduction. The phenomenon has been demonstrated in almost every specialized conduction tissue, i.e. SAN, atria, AVN, HB, and the bundle branches and in the accessory pathways. Moreover, this can occur both in physiological as well pathological circumstances. The interested readers are advised to read excellent cited reviews for detailed information,[88,90,91] however, a few examples are provided below to enhance the understanding and application of this phenomenon in common rhythm disturbances one may encounter in clinical practice.

- The sinus impulse following an interpolated ventricular premature contraction (VPC) conducts with a prolonged PR interval. The penetration and block of the VPC into the AVN, results in increased refractoriness of the AVN with resultant prolongation of PR interval in the subsequent sinus beat.
- Block of a number of consecutive atrial premature contractions (APC) in the AVN occurs because repetitive concealed conduction of each APC prolongs the refractory period of AVN resulting in physiological block of the subsequent APC.
- An AV conduction ratio that is less than 2:1 (that is 3:1 or higher) during atrial flutter is also explained by concealed conduction. A 2:1 conduction can be easily explained by protective physiological refractoriness in the AVN, but unusual ratios like 3:1 need to be explained by concealed conduction of the first blocked P-wave (second P of 3:1 sequence) resulting in block of the next P-wave.
- The irregularity of ventricular response during atrial fibrillation is also explained in part by varying penetration and concealed conduction of atrial impulses in the AVN altering its refractoriness to subsequent impulses.[92]
- In preexcited atrial fibrillation, the ventricular rate and conduction over the accessory pathway (with a very short refractory period) though faster is still limited by retrograde concealment in the accessory pathway from the impulses conducted over the AVN-HPS and traveling retrogradely. The impulse that enters the ventricles through AVN-HPS travels retrogradely to the ventricular insertion site of the accessory pathway; penetrates it, increasing its refractoriness resulting in block in the accessory pathway of the subsequent atrial impulse. This retrograde concealed conduction also occurs in the AVN with impulses that conduct antegradely over the accessory pathway to the ventricles. This accounts for the peculiar grouping of beats with normal conduction and preexcitation during atrial fibrillation in such patients. More important clinically, AV nodal block by drugs like adenosine removes this retrograde concealment in the accessory pathway leading to potentially disastrous increase in conduction over the accessory pathway and very high ventricular rate.
- The perpetuation of aberrant bundle branch block during a supraventricular tachycardia is due to transseptal conduction of the impulse in the ventricles and retrograde concealed conduction in the bundle branch that is blocked. Though, the bundle branch aberrancy is initiated (1st beat) due to phase 3 block in the bundle branch, its perpetuation is due to repetitive retrograde concealed conduction into the bundle branch.
- In second degree AV block, occasional concealed discharge of the subsidiary AV junctional pacemaker by a penetrating but blocked atrial impulse may result in long RR interval that is terminated by a conducted P-wave. It may appear that the subsidiary pacemaker is unstable, though failure of its discharge occasionally can often be explained by concealed conduction.

PRINCIPLES OF MANAGEMENT OF ATRIOVENTRICULAR CONDUCTION DISTURBANCES

The patients with marked bradycardia-related symptoms or hemodynamic instability due to AV block need acute therapy with either drugs or preferably with temporary pacing. The latter can be achieved via either transcutaneous patches, transvenous pacing leads or epicardial pacing wires in postsurgery patients with AV block. The aim of temporary pacing is to prevent ventricular asystole or achieve better hemodynamics. The patients with reversible causes usually do not require conversion to permanent pacing. However, some temporarily paced patients and some other with stable AV block may need permanent pacemaker implantation as a part of long-term therapy. The indications and type of pacing mode has been discussed in detail in the published guidelines[54] and will not be described here. However, a few principles that guide pacing therapy in a patient with AV block are mentioned below:

- Transient and reversible causes like acute inferior wall MI, hyperkalemia, drug-induced AV block or infections like Lyme disease[93] should be identified and treated. These patients most often do not require permanent pacing if the offending cause can be removed or treated successfully.
- Among patients with AV block due to nonreversible causes, symptoms of bradycardia especially if they correlate with ECG documentation of AV block-related bradycardia, indicate need for permanent pacing.
- HPS disease that is intrahisian or infrahisian AV block may be an indication of pacing even among asymptomatic patients since these can progress suddenly and unexpectedly. The site of block can be suggested by QRS width, PR interval, and response to carotid massage, exercise or atropine and confirmed by invasive EP study.
- Patients with possibly intermittent AV block-related symptoms with or without baseline conduction abnormalities like bundle branch block may need evaluation by tests like Holter recording, event monitors, exercise testing or invasive EP study with or without provocative drugs to arrive at a conclusive diagnosis.
- Asymptomatic patients like those with congenital complete AV block can sometimes do well without pacing since long-term right ventricular pacing can cause left ventricular dysfunction in some patients. Various variables like low rate or broad QRS of the escape rhythm, QT prolongation **(Figure 5.40)**, complex ventricular

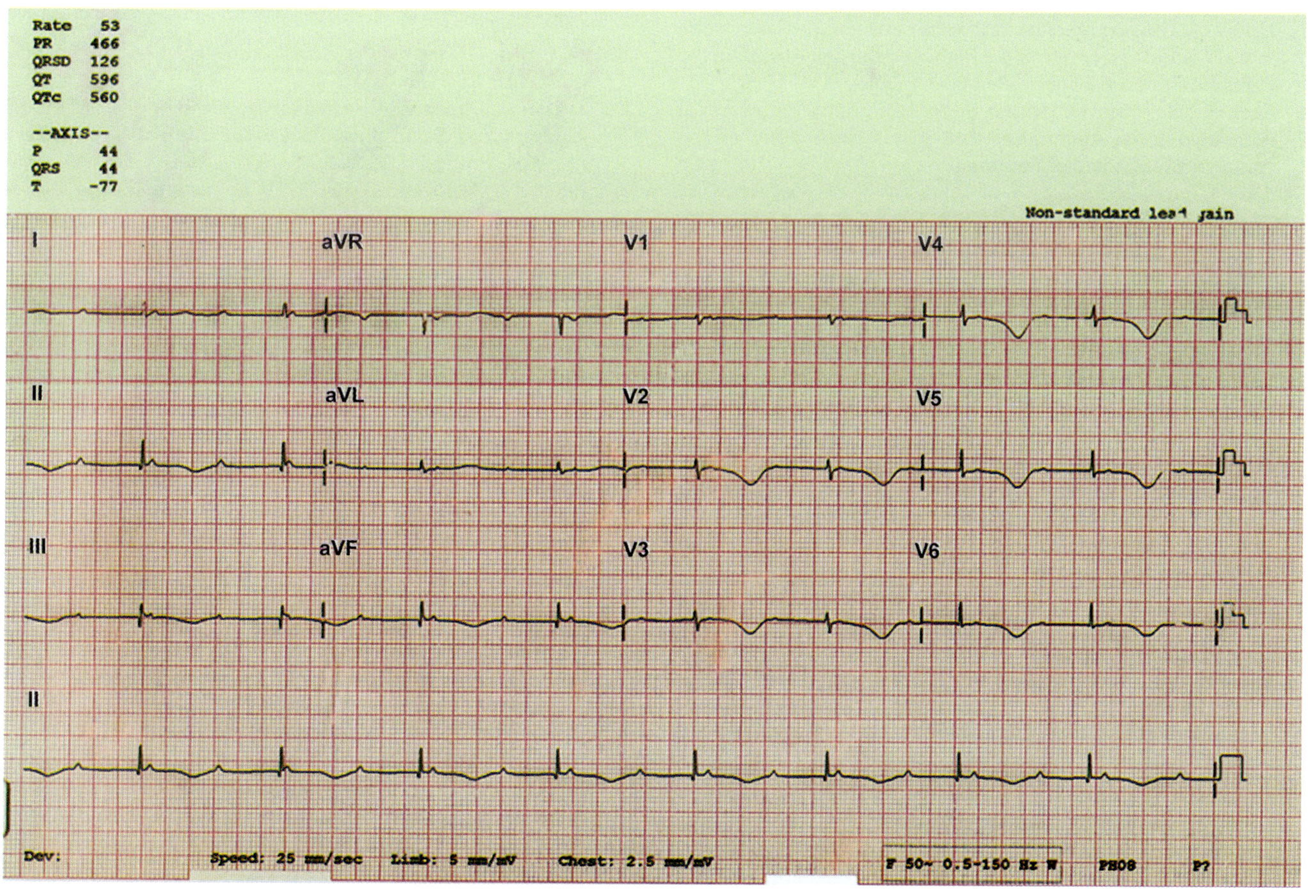

Figure 5.40: Sinus rhythm with congenital complete AV block in a child. Notice a markedly prolonged QT interval. Also, note that the apparent low voltages are due to a nonstandard gain settings (half-one-fourth)—one half voltage in the limb leads and one-fourth voltage in the precordial leads. The marked QT prolongation makes this child vulnerable to life-threatening ventricular arrhythmias and indicates need for pacemaker implantation

ectopy or development of left ventricular dysfunction or dilatation may guide towards the need for pacing in such situations. It is important to realize that many such patients develop syncope not due to bradycardia but rather due to ventricular tachyarrhythmias.

- Certain etiologies of AV block like neuromuscular disorders (myotonic dystrophy, Emery-Dreifuss muscular dystrophy, Kearns Sayre syndrome, limb-girdle muscular dystrophy), cardiac sarcoidosis, amyloidosis and post-surgical AV block have been shown to demonstrate sudden and unexpected worsening. Hence, pacing may be warranted in these patients with lower degrees of AV block even with absence of symptoms.
- The patients who also have high risk of sudden cardiac death due to ventricular tachyarrhythmias like ischemic or nonischemic cardiomyopathy or cardiac sarcoidosis should be evaluated for need for implantable cardioverter-defibrillator (ICD) implantation even if they have documented or symptomatic complete AV block, before deciding for pacemaker therapy.

REFERENCES

1. James TN. The Connecting Pathways between the Sinus Node and a-V Node and between the Right and the Left Atrium in the Human Heart. Am Heart J. 1963;66:498-508.
2. Racker DK. Atrioventricular node and input pathways: a correlated gross anatomical and histological study of the canine atrioventricular junctional region. Anat Rec. 1989;224: 336-54.
3. Anderson RH, Yanni J, Boyett MR, Chandler NJ, Dobrzynski H. The anatomy of the cardiac conduction system. Clin Anat. 2009;22:99-113.
4. Anderson RH, Ho SY. The architecture of the sinus node, the atrioventricular conduction axis, and the internodal atrial myocardium. J Cardiovasc Electrophysiol. 1998;9:1233-48.
5. Luc Pasquie J. Common form of atrioventricular nodal reentrant tachycardia: do we really know the circuit we try to ablate? Heart Rhythm. 2007;4:711-2.
6. Tawara S. Die Topographie und Histologie der Bruckenfasern. Ein Beitrag zur Lehre von der Bedeutung der Purkinjeschen Faden (Vorlaufige Mitteilung). Zbl Physiol. 1905;19:70-6.
7. Koch W. Weiter mitteilungen uber den Sinusknoten der Herzens. Verhandlungen der Deutschen.
8. Sanchez-Quintana D, Yen Ho S. [Anatomy of cardiac nodes and atrioventricular specialized conduction system]. Rev Esp Cardiol. 2003;56:1085-92.
9. Lee PC, Chen SA, Hwang B. Atrioventricular node anatomy and physiology: implications for ablation of atrioventricular nodal reentrant tachycardia. Curr Opin Cardiol. 2009;24: 105-12.
10. Anderson RH. The disposition and innervation of atrioventricular ring specialized tissue in rats and rabbits. J Anat. 1972;113:197-211.
11. Bharati S. Anatomic-morphologic relations between AV nodal structure and function in the normal and diseased heart. In: Mazgalev TN, Tchou PJ (Eds). Atrial-AV nodal electrophysiology: a view from the millennium. Armonk: Futura; 2000. pp. 25-48.
12. Scher AM. Direct recording from the A-V conducting system in the dog and monkey. Science. 1955;121:398-9.
13. Van Der Kooi MW, Durrer D, Van Dam RT, Van Der Tweel LH. Electrical activity in sinus node and atrioventricular node. Am Heart J. 1956;51:684-700.
14. Hoffman BF, De Carvalho AP, De Mello WC. Transmembrane potentials of single fibres of the atrio-ventricular node. Nature. 1958;181:66-7.
15. Hoffman BF, De Carvalho AP, Mello WC, Cranefield PF. Electrical activity of single fibers of the atrioventricular node. Circ Res. 1959;7:11-8.
16. Efimov IR, Fahy GJ, Cheng Y, Van Wagoner DR, Tchou PJ, Mazgalev TN. High-resolution fluorescent imaging does not reveal a distinct atrioventricular nodal anterior input channel (fast pathway) in the rabbit heart during sinus rhythm. J Cardiovasc Electrophysiol. 1997;8:295-306.
17. Efimov IR, Mazgalev TN. High-resolution, three-dimensional fluorescent imaging reveals multilayer conduction pattern in the atrioventricular node. Circulation. 1998;98:54-7.
18. Nikolski VP, Jones SA, Lancaster MK, Boyett MR, Efimov IR. Cx43 and dual-pathway electrophysiology of the atrioventricular node and atrioventricular nodal reentry. Circ Res. 2003;92: 469-75.
19. Medkour D, Becker AE, Khalife K, Billette J. Anatomic and functional characteristics of a slow posterior AV nodal pathway: role in dual-pathway physiology and reentry. Circulation. 1998;98:164-74.
20. de CA, de AD. Spread of activity through the atrioventricular node. Circ Res. 1960;8:801-9.
21. Kurian T, Ambrosi C, Hucker W, Fedorov VV, Efimov IR. Anatomy and electrophysiology of the human AV node. Pacing Clin Electrophysiol. 2010;33:754-62.
22. Billette J. Atrioventricular nodal activation during periodic premature stimulation of the atrium. Am J Physiol. 1987;252:H163-77.
23. Basso C, Ho SY, Thiene G. Anatomical and histopathological characteristics of the conductive tissues of the heart. In: Gussak I, Antzelevitch C (Eds). Electrical diseases of the heart: genetics, mechanisms, treatment, prevention. London: Springer; 2008. pp. 37-51.
24. Petrecca K, Amellal F, Laird DW, Cohen SA, Shrier A. Sodium channel distribution within the rabbit atrioventricular node as analysed by confocal microscopy. J Physiol. 1997;501(Pt 2): 263-74.
25. Munk AA, Adjemian RA, Zhao J, Ogbaghebriel A, Shrier A. Electrophysiological properties of morphologically distinct cells isolated from the rabbit atrioventricular node. J Physiol. 1996;493(Pt 3):801-18.
26. Liu Y, Zeng W, Delmar M, Jalife J. Ionic mechanisms of electronic inhibition and concealed conduction in rabbit atrioventricular nodal myocytes. Circulation. 1993;88:1634-46.
27. Paes de Carvalho A, de Mello W C, Hoffman BF. The specialized tissues of the heart. Amsterdam: Elsevier; 1961.
28. Noma A, Irisawa H, Kokobun S, Kotake H, Nishimura M, Watanabe Y. Slow current systems in the A-V node of the rabbit heart. Nature. 1980;285:228-9.
29. Petrecca K, Shrier A. Spatial distribution of ion channels, receptors, and innervation in the AV node. In: Mazgalev TN, Tchou PJ (Eds). Atrial-AV nodal electrophysiology: a view from the millennium. Armonk: Futura; 2000. pp. 89-105.
30. Clemo HF, Belardinelli L. Effect of adenosine on atrioventricular conduction. I: Site and characterization of adenosine action

in the guinea pig atrioventricular node. Circ Res. 1986;59: 427-36.
31. Mazgalev T, Dreifus LS, Michelson EL, Pelleg A. Vagally induced hyperpolarization in atrioventricular node. Am J Physiol. 1986;251:H631-43.
32. Gourdie RG, Severs NJ, Green CR, Rothery S, Germroth P, Thompson RP. The spatial distribution and relative abundance of gap-junctional connexin40 and connexin43 correlate to functional properties of components of the cardiac atrioventricular conduction system. J Cell Sci. 1993;105(Pt 4): 985-91.
33. Coppen SR, Severs NJ. Diversity of connexin expression patterns in the atrioventricular node: vestigial consequence or functional specialization? J Cardiovasc Electrophysiol. 2002;13:625-6.
34. Spodick DH, Ariyarajah V. Interatrial block: the pandemic remains poorly perceived. Pacing Clin Electrophysiol. 2009;32:667-72.
35. Bharati S, Lev M, Wu D, Denes P, Dhingra R, Rosen KM. Pathophysiologic correlations in two cases of split His bundle potentials. Circulation. 1974;49:615-23.
36. Averill KH, Lamb LE. Electrocardiographic findings in 67,375 asymptomatic subjects. I. Incidence of abnormalities. Am J Cardiol. 1960;6:76-83.
37. Kim YH, O'Nunain S, Trouton T, Sosa-Suarez G, Levine RA, Garan H, Ruskin JN. Pseudo-pacemaker syndrome following inadvertent fast pathway ablation for atrioventricular nodal reentrant tachycardia. J Cardiovasc Electrophysiol. 1993;4: 178-82.
38. Cheng S, Keyes MJ, Larson MG, McCabe EL, Newton-Cheh C, Levy D, Benjamin EJ, Vasan RS, Wang TJ. Long-term outcomes in individuals with prolonged PR interval or first-degree atrioventricular block. JAMA. 2009;301:2571-7.
39. Mobitz W. Über die unvollständige Störung der Erregungsüberleitung zwischen Vorhof und Kammer des menschlichen Herzens [On the partial block of impulse conduction between atrium and ventricle of human hearts]. Z Gesamte Exp Med. 1924;41:180-237.
40. Silverman ME, Upshaw CB, Jr., Lange HW. Woldemar Mobitz and His 1924 classification of second-degree atrioventricular block. Circulation. 2004;110:1162-7.
41. Cooper J, Marriott HJ. To Wenckebach: a centenary salute. Tex Heart Inst J. 1999;26:8-11.
42. Atrioventricular Conduction Abnormalities. In: Issa ZF, Miller JM, Zipes DP (Eds). Clinical Arrhythmology and Electrophysiology: Companion to Braunwald's Heart Disease. Philadelphia: Saunders; 2009 .p. 179.
43. Castellanos A, Interian A, Jr., Cox MM, Myerburg RJ. Alternating Wenckebach periods and allied arrhythmias. Pacing Clin Electrophysiol. 1993;16:2285-300.
44. Rosenblueth A. Mechanism of the Wenckebach-Luciani cycles. Am J Physiol. 1958;194:491-4.
45. Young ML, Wolff GS, Castellanos A, Gelband H. Application of the Rosenblueth hypothesis to assess cycle length effects on the refractoriness of the atrioventricular node. Am J Cardiol. 1986;57:142-5.
46. Zipes DP, Mendez C, Moe CK. Some examples of Wenckebach periodicity in cardiac tissues, with an appraisal of mechanisms. In: Rosenbaum MB, Elizari M (Eds). Frontiers of Cardiac Electrophysiology. Boston, MA: Nijoff Publishers; 1983. pp. 357-76.
47. Narula OS, Samet P. Wenckebach and Mobitz type II AV block due to block within the His bundle and bundle branches. Circulation. 1970;41:947-65.
48. Narula OS. Current concepts of atrioventricular block. In: Narula OS (Ed). His bundle electrocardiography and clinical electrophysiology. Philadelphia: FA Davis Co; 1975. pp. 139.
49. Fisch C, Zipes DP, McHenry PL. Electrocardiographic manifestations of concealed junctional ectopic impulses. Circulation. 1976;53:217-23.
50. Lange HW, Ameisen O, Mack R, Moses JW, Kligfield P. Prevalence and clinical correlates of non-Wenckebach, narrow-complex second-degree atrioventricular block detected by ambulatory ECG. Am Heart J. 1988;115:114-20.
51. Amat-y-Leon F, Dhingra R, Denes P, Wyndham C, Chuquimia R, Rosen KM. The clinical spectrum of chronic His bundle block. Chest. 1976;70:747-54.
52. Barold SS. 2:1 Atrioventricular block: order from chaos. Am J Emerg Med. 2001;19:214-7.
53. Josephson ME. Atrioventricular conduction. In: Josephson ME (Ed). Clinical cardiac electrophysiology, 4th edn. Philadelphia: Lippincott Williams and Wilkins; 2008. pp. 93-113.
54. Epstein AE, DiMarco JP, Ellenbogen KA, Estes NA, 3rd, Freedman RA, Gettes LS, Gillinov AM, Gregoratos G, Hammill SC, Hayes DL, Hlatky MA, Newby LK, Page RL, Schoenfeld MH, Silka MJ, Stevenson LW, Sweeney MO, Smith SC, Jr., Jacobs AK, Adams CD, Anderson JL, Buller CE, Creager MA, Ettinger SM, Faxon DP, Halperin JL, Hiratzka LF, Hunt SA, Krumholz HM, Kushner FG, Lytle BW, Nishimura RA, Ornato JP, Riegel B, Tarkington LG, Yancy CW. ACC/AHA/HRS 2008 Guidelines for Device-Based Therapy of Cardiac Rhythm Abnormalities: a report of the American College of Cardiology/American Heart Association Task Force on Practice Guidelines (Writing Committee to Revise the ACC/AHA/NASPE 2002 Guideline Update for Implantation of Cardiac Pacemakers and Antiarrhythmia Devices) developed in collaboration with the American Association for Thoracic Surgery and Society of Thoracic Surgeons. J Am Coll Cardiol. 2008;51: 1-62.
55. Kastor JA. Atrioventricular Block. In: Kastor JA (Ed). Arrhythmias, 2nd edn. Philadelphia: WB Saunders; 2000. pp. 509-65.
56. Langendorf R, Mehlman JS. Blocked (nonconducted) A-V nodal premature systoles imitating first and second degree A-V block. Am Heart J. 1947;34:500-6.
57. Langendorf R, Pick A. Concealed conduction in the A-V junction. In: Dreifus LS, Likoff W, Moyer JH (Eds). Mechanisms and therapy of cardiac arrhythmias. New York: Grune and Stratton, Inc; 1966. p. 395.
58. Rosen KM, Rahimtoola SH, Gunnar RM. Pseudo A-V block secondary to premature nonpropagated His bundle depolarizations: documentation by His bundle electrocardiography. Circulation. 1970;42:367-73.
59. Bhargava K, Shrivastava S, Singh B, Wellens HJ. AV block. Which type and where? J Electrocardiol. 2007;40: 358-9.
60. Kosowsky BD, Latif P, Radoff AM. Multilevel atrioventricular block. Circulation. 1976;54:914-21.
61. Schindler S, Albers W, Luria MH. A-V block. Circulation. 1977;56:689.
62. Lee S, Wellens HJ, Josephson ME. Paroxysmal atrioventricular block. Heart Rhythm. 2009;6:1229-34.

63. Silver ES, Pass RH, Hordof AJ, Liberman L. Paroxysmal AV block in children with normal cardiac anatomy as a cause of syncope. Pacing Clin Electrophysiol. 2008;31: 322-6.
64. Rosenbaum MB, Elizari MV, Levi RJ, Nau GJ. Paroxysmal atrioventricular block related to hypopolarization and spontaneous diastolic depolarization. Chest. 1973;63:678-88.
65. Shohat-Zabarski R, Iakobishvili Z, Kusniec J, Mazur A, Strasberg B. Paroxysmal atrioventricular block: clinical experience with 20 patients. Int J Cardiol. 2004;97:399-405.
66. Al-Ahdab M. Complete heart block-third degree heart block. In: Macdonald D (Ed). Clinical cardiac electrophysiology in the young. New York: Springer Science+Business Media; 2006. pp. 173-81.
67. Walsh EP. Interventional electrophysiology in patients with congenital heart disease. Circulation. 2007;115:3224-34.
68. Friedman DM, Rupel A, Buyon JP. Epidemiology, etiology, detection, and treatment of autoantibody-associated congenital heart block in neonatal lupus. Curr Rheumatol Rep. 2007;9:101-8.
69. Feigl D, Ashkenazy J, Kishon Y. Early and late atrioventricular block in acute inferior myocardial infarction. J Am Coll Cardiol. 1984;4:35-8.
70. Bertolet BD, McMurtrie EB, Hill JA, Belardinelli L. Theophylline for the treatment of atrioventricular block after myocardial infarction. Ann Intern Med. 1995;123:509-11.
71. Hindman MC, Wagner GS, JaRo M, Atkins JM, Scheinman MM, DeSanctis RW, Hutter AH, Jr., Yeatman L, Rubenfire M, Pujura C, Rubin M, Morris JJ. The clinical significance of bundle branch block complicating acute myocardial infarction. 1. Clinical characteristics, hospital mortality, and one-year follow-up. Circulation. 1978;58:679-88.
72. Zimetbaum PJ, Josephson ME. Use of the electrocardiogram in acute myocardial infarction. N Engl J Med. 2003;348: 933-40.
73. Moe GK, Mendez C, Han J. Aberrant a-V Impulse Propagation in the Dog Heart: A Study of Functional Bundle Branch Block. Circ Res. 1965;16:261-86.
74. Durrer D. Electrical aspects of human cardiac activity: a clinical-physiological approach to excitation and stimulation. Cardiovasc Res. 1968;2:1-18.
75. Wit AL, Damato AN, Weiss MB, Steiner C. Phenomenon of the gap in atrioventricular conduction in the human heart. Circ Res. 1970;27:679-89.
76. Gallagher JJ, Damato AN, Caracta AR, Varghese PJ, Josephson ME, Lau SH. Gap in A-V conduction in man; types I and II. Am Heart J. 1973;85:78-82.
77. Akhtar M, Damato AN, Caracta AR, Batsford WP, Lau SH. The gap phenomena during retrograde conduction in man. Circulation. 1974;49:811-7.
78. Agha AS, Castellanos A, Jr., Wells D, Ross MD, Befeler B, Myerburg RJ. Type I, type II, and type 3 gaps in bundle-branch conduction. Circulation. 1973;47:325-30.
79. Wu D, Denes P, Dhingra R, Rosen KM. Nature of the gap phenomenon in man. Circ Res. 1974;34:682-92.
80. Moore EN, Spear JF, Fisch C. "Supernormal" conduction and excitability. J Cardiovasc Electrophysiol. 1993;4:320-37.
81. Elizari MV, Schmidberg J, Atienza A, Paredes DV, Chiale PA. Clinical and experimental evidence of supernormal excitability and conduction. Curr Cardiol Rev. 2014;10:202-21.
82. Rosenbaum MB, Levi RJ, Elizari MV, Vetulli HM, Sanchez RA. Supernormal excitability and conduction. Cardiol Clin. 1983;1:75-92.
83. Engelmann TW. Beobachtungen und Versuche am suspendirten Herzen. Archiv für die gesamte Physiologie des Menschen und der Tiere. 1894;56:149-202.
84. Erlanger J. On the physiology of heart-block in mammals, with especial reference to the causation of Stokes-Adams disease. J Exper Med. 1905;7:676-724.
85. Ashman R. Conductivity in compressed cardiac muscle. I. The recovery of conductivity following impulse transmission in compressed auricular muscle of the turtle heart. Am J Physiol. 1925;74:121-39.
86. Ashman R. Electrocardiographic studies of conductivity in cardiac muscle. Proc Soc Exp Biol Med. 1927;24:292-3.
87. Lewis ST, Drury AN. Revised views of the refractory period, in relation to drugs reputed to prolong it, and in relation to circus movement. Heart. 1926;13:95-100.
88. Langendorf R, Pick A. Concealed conduction further evaluation of a fundamental aspect of propagation of the cardiac impulse. Circulation. 1956;13:381-99.
89. Lewis T, Master AM. Observations upon conduction in the mammalian heart A-V conduction. Heart. 1925;12:209-69.
90. Langendorf R. Concealed A-V conduction; the effect of blocked impulses on the formation and conduction of subsequent impulses. Am Heart J. 1948;35:542-52.
91. Fisch C. Concealed conduction at the AV nodal level. Prog Clin Biol Res. 1988;275:287-300.
92. Soderstrom N. What is the reason for the ventricular arrhythmia in cases of auricular fibrillation? Am Heart J. 1950;40: 212-23.
93. Forrester JD, Mead P. Third-degree heart block associated with lyme carditis: review of published cases. Clin Infect Dis. 2014;59:996-1000.

SECTION B

Fundamentals of Cardiac Anatomy, Imaging, Mapping and Ablation

CHAPTER 6

José Angel Cabrera, Sergio Castrejón,
Damián Sánchez-Quintana

Cardiac Anatomy for Electrophysiologists

LIST OF ABBREVIATIONS

AF	Atrial Fibrillation	LV	Left Ventricle
AV	Atrioventricular	LVOT	Left Ventricular Outflow Tract
CFB	Central Fibrous Body	OVM	Oblique Vein of Marshall
CRT	Cardiac Resynchronization Therapy	PV	Pulmonary Vein
CS	Coronary Sinus	RA	Right Atrium
CT	Terminal Crest or Crista Terminalis	RAA	Right Atrial Appendage
GCV	Great Cardiac Vein	RAO	Right Anterior Oblique
IAS	Interatrial Septum	RV	Right Ventricle
IVC	Inferior Vena Cava	RVOT	Right Ventricular Outflow Tract
LA	Left Atrium	SMT	Septomarginal Trabeculation
LAA	Left Atrial Appendage	SN	Sinus Node
LAO	Left Anterior Oblique	SVC	Superior Vena Cava
LOM	Ligament of Marshall	VT	Ventricular Tachycardia

INTRODUCTION

Studies conducted during the last three decades have unraveled anatomical, architectural and histological details of the heart enlightening the substrate of tachycardias and their ablation procedures. In this chapter, we provide the basic anatomic information of various cardiac regions and their neighboring landmarks needed to understand mapping and ablative procedures for the cardiac interventional electrophysiologist. The pericardial space, the autonomic innervations of the atria as well as the anatomic relations between the cardiac chambers with extracardiac structures are also described.

SPATIAL LOCATIONS OF THE CARDIAC CHAMBERS DURING AN ELECTROPHYSIOLOGICAL STUDY

Effective and safer catheter-based procedures have to come from a correct understanding of the attitudinally-oriented position and spatial relationships of the different cardiac structures. Viewed from the frontal aspect of the chest, the right ventricle (RV) is not only a right-sided chamber but also the most anteriorly situated cardiac chamber since it is located immediately behind the sternum. Owing to the obliquity of the interatrial septum (IAS) plane (approximately at an angle of 65° from the sagittal plane) and due to the different levels of the mitral and tricuspid valve orifices, the left atrium (LA) is turned posterior and superior to the right atrium (RA). Only the tip of the left atrial appendage (LAA) contributes to the left cardiac silhouette in a frontal view of the body.[1-3]

Most interventional arrhythmologists currently utilize nonfluoroscopic navigational tools capable of reconstructing a computer-based surrogate of the endocardial surface of the heart chambers. Computed tomography and magnetic resonance imaging studies of the cardiac chambers conducted before the ablation can be merged with these virtual cardiac anatomy reconstructions to correctly interpret the gross morphology and attitudinal position of the cardiac chambers during the course of a mapping and ablation procedure. Some endocardial structures such as the oval fossa or terminal crest can also be visualized using intracardiac echocardiography.

Under the guidance of simple fluoroscopy, two or more fluoroscopic views are usually needed to define the anatomic position in the heart and to more accurately estimate the location of the exploring electrode. The right anterior oblique (RAO) projection defines what is anterior, posterior, superior and inferior. The left anterior oblique (LAO) defines the superior, inferior, anterior and posterior locations for both the right and left AV grooves **(Figures 6.1A and B)**. The LAO is also useful to define what is septal, permitting the differentiation between the complex right and left paraseptal regions. It is the preferred projection to catheterize the coronary sinus and its continuation along the epicardial aspect of the posteroinferior region.[1-3]

THE COMPONENTS OF THE ATRIA

From a gross anatomical viewpoint, each atrium comprises of a venous component, a vestibule, and an appendage and shares the IAS with the other atrium.[4] Both atria also possess a body; this is best seen in the LA, and represents the smooth walled component interposed between the vestibule and the venous component **(Figures 6.2A to C)**. The body of the RA is much smaller, and represents the space between the left venous valve, when this structure can be recognized, and the IAS. The venous component of the RA is located posterolaterally and receives the systemic venous return from the superior vena cava (SVC), the inferior vena cava (IVC); and the coronary venous return from the coronary sinus (CS). The venous component of the LA is located posterosuperiorly and receives the pulmonary veins (PV) at the four corners, enclosing a prominent atrial dome. The vestibule on both atria represents the smooth muscular wall around the atrioventricular (AV) valve orifices that supports the leaflets of the tricuspid or mitral valves.[3-5]

Structures of the Right Atrium Relevant for the Electrophysiologist

The Right Atrial Appendage

The RA consists of a flat-walled posterior venous portion and a trabeculated anterolateral sector that is the pectinated right atrial appendage (RAA). The anterolateral portion of the RA is dominated by its appendage, a roughly triangular-shaped offshoot whose apex generally points upwards and overlaps the aortic root; its inferior margin lies over the anterosuperior aspect of the right AV groove. The RAA contains multiple pectinate muscles, which arise from the terminal crest or crista terminalis (CT) and extends all round the smooth vestibule of the tricuspid valve **(Figures 6.2 and 6.3)**.[3-5]

The Crista Terminalis and the Region of the Sinus Node

The CT is a significant structure in several forms of atrial tachyarrhythmias, acting as a natural barrier to conduction in isthmus-dependent atrial flutter, and been the origin of many focal atrial tachycardias. The CT is a large muscular ridge that separates the smooth-walled venous part (venous component) from the extensive trabeculated (pectinated) RAA. Thus, the C-shaped crest extends laterally and inferiorly, turning in beneath the orifice of the IVC to ramify as a series of trabeculations in the area between the IVC and the tricuspid valve **(Figures 6.2A to C)**. The pectinate muscles, originating from the crista and extending along the wall of the appendage towards the vestibule of the tricuspid valve, show a nonuniform trabecular pattern in most hearts. It is relevant for the confluence between the CT at its origin in the interatrial groove and the origin of another important muscular fascicle, the interatrial Bachmann's bundle, which extends into the left atrium. It is also relevant for the presence of myocardial extensions over the wall of the SVC because spontaneous onset of ectopic beats and initiation of atrial fibrillation (AF) from this vein has been described. The electrical disconnection of the SVC from the RA is feasible.[6]

The sinus node (SN) is the source of the cardiac impulse. It is usually localized in the superior part of the terminal groove, close to the junction between the SVC and the RAA. The SN is a 13.5 ± 2.5 mm long crescent-like formation with an extensive longitudinal axis **(Figures 6.3A to E)**. Notably, it is not insulated by a sheath of fibrous tissue and varies in position and length along the terminal groove, gradually penetrating through the thickness of the CT to terminate

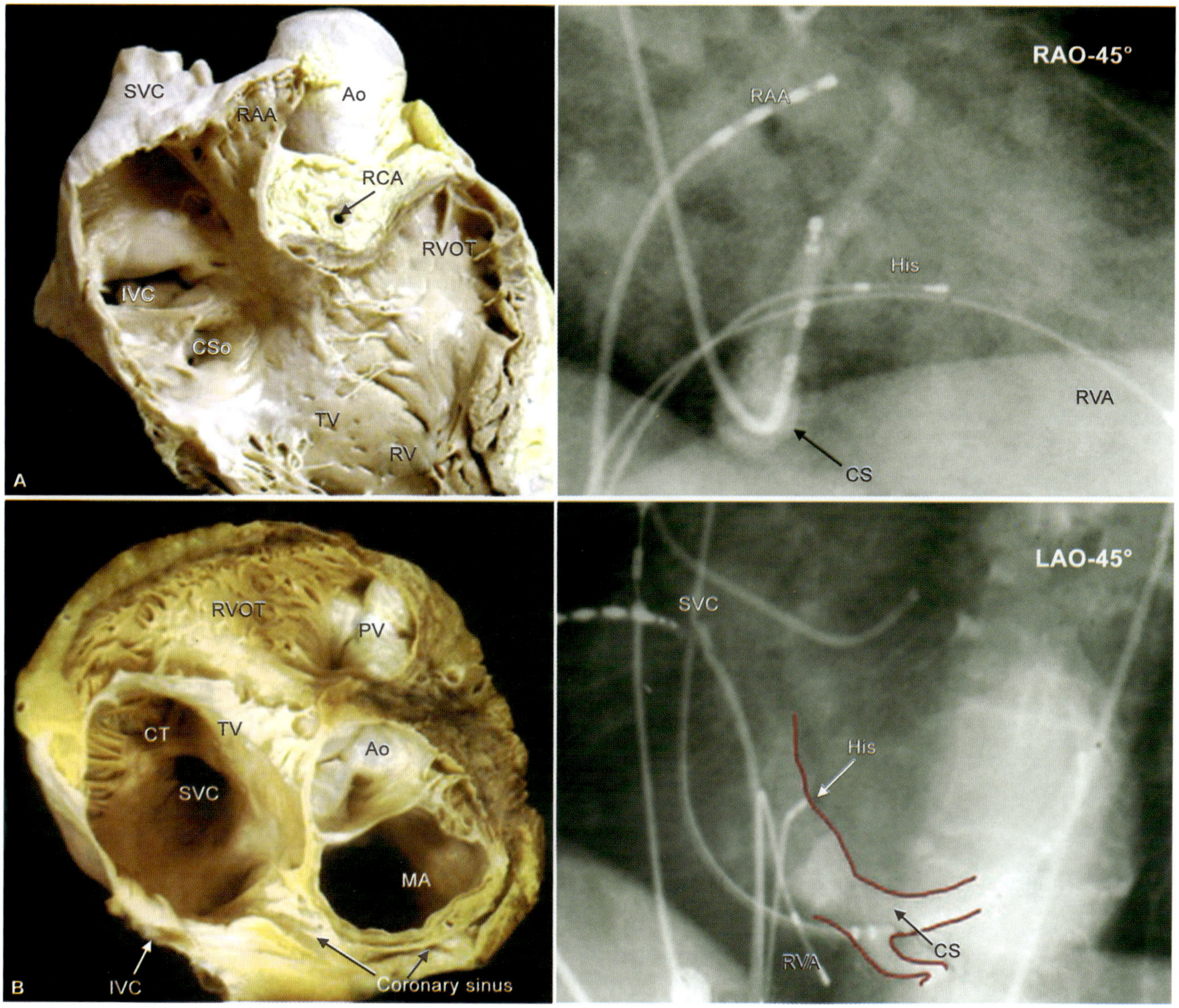

Figures 6.1A and B: Simulated (gross human specimens) and fluoroscopic right anterior oblique (RAO) projection (A) and left anterior oblique (LAO) projection (B) showing electrode catheters placed at the right atrial appendage (RAA), bundle of His (His), right ventricular apex (RVA) and coronary sinus orifice (CSo). The coronary sinus runs on the atrial side of the mitral annulus (MA) along the inferior wall of the left atrium towards the posterior border of the heart. Both RAO and LAO projections define what is anterior, posterior, superior and inferior. The LAO view serves to demonstrate in an attitudinal orientation the septal location permitting the differentiation between the right and left atrioventricular grooves

Abbreviations: Ao, aorta; IVC, inferior vena cava; LV, left ventricle; MCV, mid cardiac vein; PV, pulmonary valve; RAA, right atrial appendage; RCA, right coronary artery; RV, right ventricle; RVOT, right ventricular outflow tract; SVC, superior vena cava; CT, crista terminalis; TV, tricuspid valve; MA, mitral annulus

in a tail that is buried deep in the myocardium of the CT **(Figure 6.3B)**. The SN is usually arranged around a prominent artery originating from the right or left circumflex coronary artery and running along the interatrial groove. A paranodal area composed of loosely packed myocytes in the CT adjacent to the SN has been described, but its role is unclear and may be a persistent part of the primary myocardium shown experimentally in the mouse.

While in 72% of the hearts the location of the nodal body is subepicardial, in the other 28% the inner aspect of the nodal body is more subendocardial. Its margin is irregular with multiple extensions interdigitating into the neighboring working atrial myocardium.[7]

Both inappropriate sinus tachycardia and sinus nodal reentrant tachycardia are arrhythmias arising from the sinoatrial area. Endocardial radiofrequency catheter ablation is

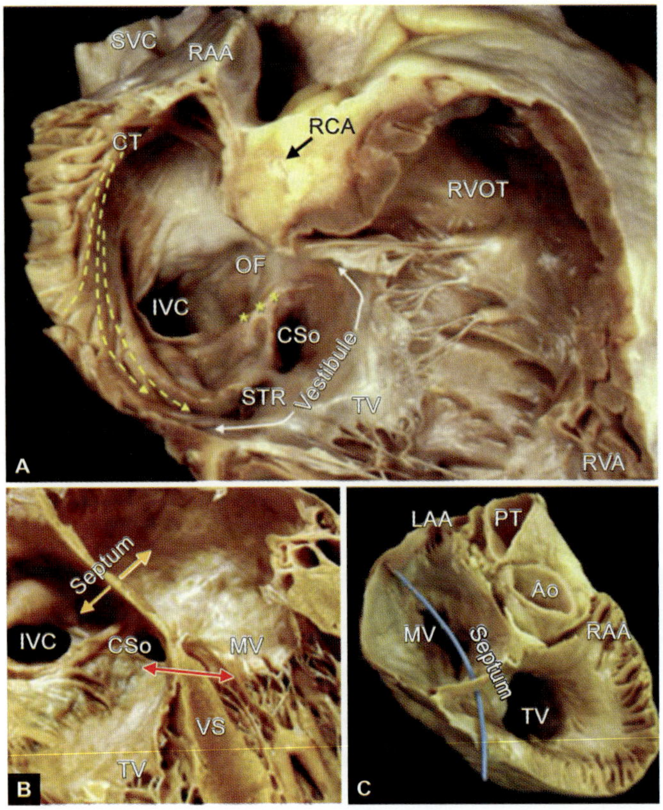

Figures 6.2A to C: (A) Opened right atrium in simulated right anterior oblique view to show the crista terminalis (CT) (dotted lines). The crest arches anterior to the orifice of the superior vena cava (SVC) and extends to the area of the anterior interatrial groove. Inferiorly, the crest turns in beneath the orifice of the inferior vena cava, breaking up into a series of pectinate muscles which reach to the vestibule. The asterisks mark the level of attachment of Eustachian crest; (B) Four-chamber section through the heart showing the atrial septum in profile. The floor of the oval fossa (arrows) is the true septum. Note the offset arrangement of the mitral valve and tricuspid valve which produces the so-called muscular atrioventricular septum (double red arrow in panel); (C) Short-axis section across the atrial chambers through the flap valve of the oval fossa. A probe is passed through the oval fossa and its end is placed in the lateral wall of the left atrium next to the left atrial appendage

Abbreviations: Ao, aorta; CSo, coronary sinus orifice; IVC, inferior vena cava; LAA, left atrial appendage; MV, mitral valve; OF, oval fossa; PT, pulmonary trunk; RAA, right atrial appendage; RCA, right coronary artery; RVA, right ventricular apex; RVOT, right ventricular outflow tract; SVC, superior vena cava; STR, sub-Thebesian recess; CT, crista terminalis or terminal crest; TV, tricuspid valve; VS, ventricular septum

less effective for multiple reasons: (1) most of the sinus node is a subepicardial structure, relatively distant from the RA endocardium, (2) the constantly present central sinus node artery exerts a cooling effect on the node, (3) a significant mass of the node is separated from the RA endocardium by the thick CT, (4) it is an extensive structure not amenable to a focal complete injury, and (5) the nodal cells are packed in a dense matrix of connective tissue.

The Region of the Triangle of Koch and AV Node

The triangle of Koch is the inferior paraseptal right atrial region containing the AV node and its inferior rightward and leftward extensions, as well as the transitional fibers approaching the compact AV nodal area. It is bordered posteriorly by a fibrous extension from the Eustachian valve and by a ridge called the tendon of Todaro. The anterior border is demarcated by the attachment of the septal leaflet of the tricuspid valve **(Figure 6.3C)**. The AV component of the membranous septum forms the anterosuperior apex of the triangle, the area of the central fibrous body (CFB) where the His bundle penetrates. The base of the triangle is the orifice of the CS, and the vestibular region immediately anterior to it **(Figures 6.3A to E)**.

The area of the triangle is targeted for ablation of the slow nodal pathway. In addition, it is commonly the seat of the atrial insertions of midseptal and some paraseptal AV accessory pathways and certain forms of atrial tachycardia. This right atrial region may have different sizes and configurations. In some patients is more vertically oriented while in others it has a more horizontal display which is clinically relevant in the case of catheter ablation procedures largely guided by anatomic landmarks **(Figures 6.4A to E)**. The site of recording of the largest His bundle deflection does not always coincide with the anterosuperior vertex of the triangle. This has implications regarding the position of the compact node that is just proximal to the His bundle. The compact AV node is an unprotected structure, very sensitive to the application of radiofrequency current. The node becomes the His bundle as the AV conduction axis enters the membranous septum and is encircled by fibrous tissue. The penetrating His bundle can readily be distinguished from the compact node at the point where the conduction axis itself becomes completely surrounded by tissues of the CFB. Thus, the bundle of His is better protected than the compact node against radiofrequency energy **(Figures 6.3D and E)**.[8-11]

The Inferior Right Cavotricuspid Isthmus

The inferior right atrial cavotricuspid isthmus, is a critical link for the macroreentrant circuit of isthmus-dependent atrial flutter. Anatomical and imaging studies have shown a wide range of morphologies and architectural factors at the isthmus level that may influence the feasibility to obtain a complete, transmural and permanent ablation line across this anatomic landmark.

The inferior isthmus is limited posteriorly by the Eustachian valve, and anteriorly by the annular insertion of the septal leaflet of the tricuspid valve **(Figures 6.5A to C)**. The isthmus consists of three areas: a posterior region which is mainly membranous, an intermediate pouch that is muscular and trabeculated, and an anterior smooth region, also muscular, that is the vestibule. This pouch-like formation

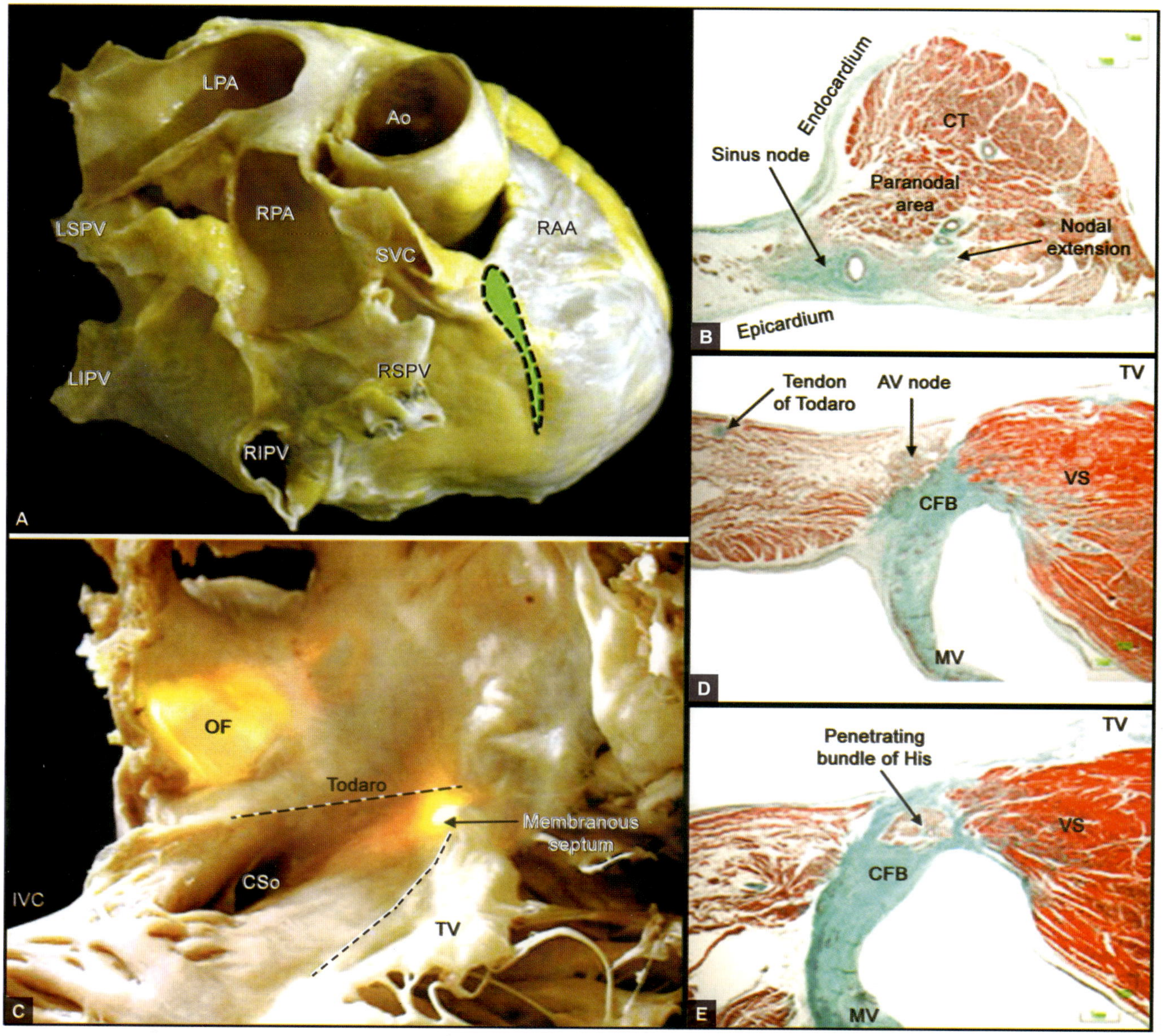

Figures 6.3A to E: (A) Superior view of the heart showing the location of the sinus node (fusiform green color). The sinus node is usually localized in the superior part of the terminal groove, close to the junction between the superior vena cava and the right atrial appendage; (B) Histological section of the sinus node (Masson trichrome stain) within a dense matrix of connective tissue (green color) and showing a nodal extension to the terminal crest; (C) Transillumination of the septal and paraseptal walls of the right atrium showing the limits of the triangle of Koch. The vestibule of the right atrium and the coronary sinus orifice form the lower limit. The apex of the triangle is the membranous septum; (D) and (E) Sagittal sections stained with Masson trichrome through the compact part of the AV node (D), and penetrating bundle of His (E) embedded in fibrous tissue of the central fibrous body

Abbreviations: Ao, aorta; CSo, coronary sinus orifice; IVC, inferior vena cava; LPA, left pulmonary artery; LSPV, left superior pulmonary vein; LIPV, left inferior pulmonary vein; MV, mitral valve; OF, oval fossa; RAA, right atrial appendage; RIPV, right inferior pulmonary vein; RPA, right pulmonary artery; RSPV, right superior pulmonary vein; SVC, superior vena cava; CT, crista terminalis; TV, tricuspid valve; VS, ventricular septum; CFB, central fibrous body

and the vestibule of the tricuspid valve are clearly depicted in the RAO projection by injecting contrast into the IVC. The degree of development of the pouch and its angiographic demarcation in relation to the tricuspid vestibule varies from patient to patient.

With the heart in an attitudinal orientation, we identified three levels of the isthmus: paraseptal (24 ± 4 mm), inferior (19 ± 4 mm), and inferolateral (30 ± 3 mm). The paraseptal isthmus forms the base of the triangle of Koch. The inferior isthmus is also known as the "central isthmus" owing to

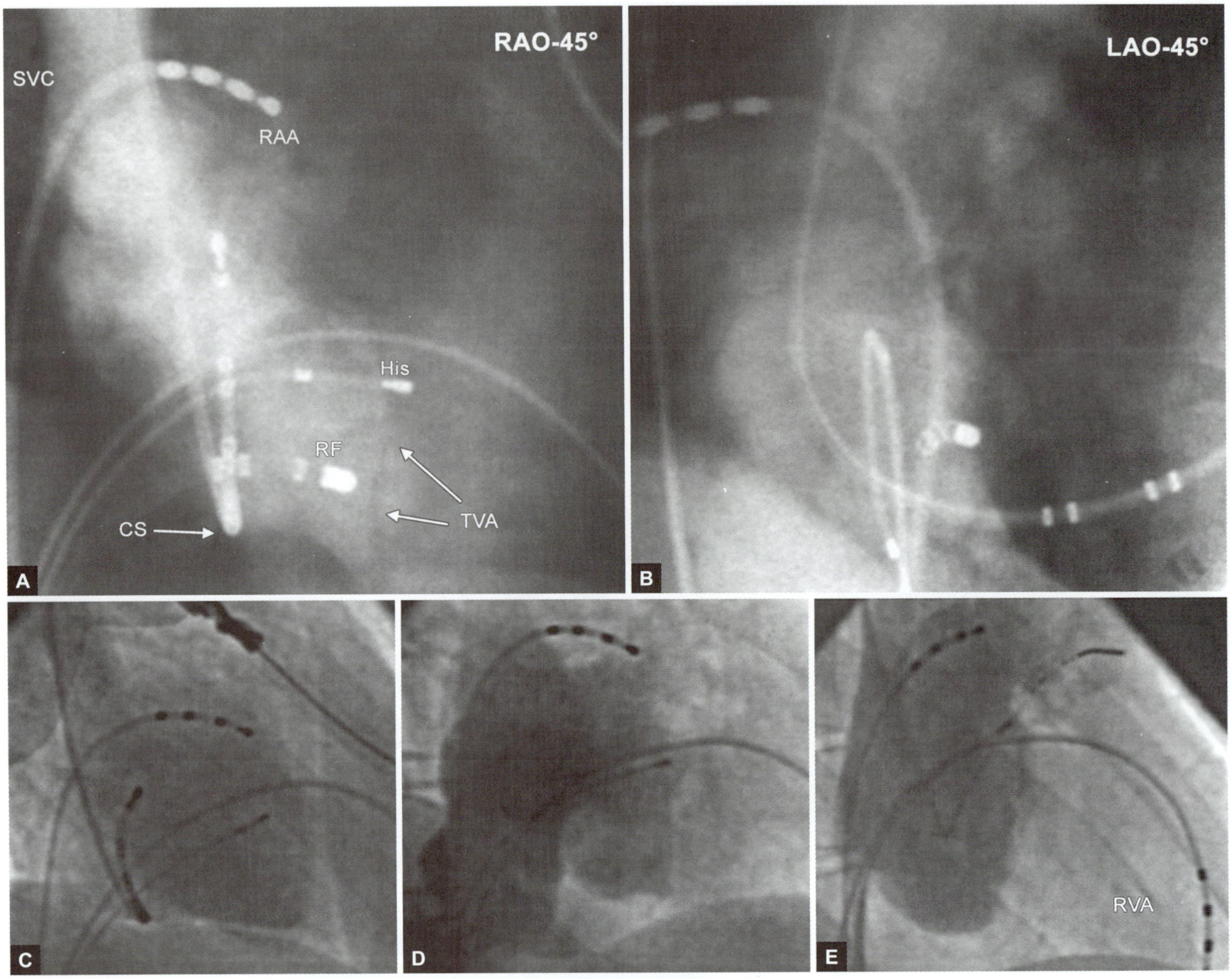

Figures 6.4A to E: Right atrial angiograms in 45° right (RAO) and left anterior oblique (LAO) projection showing the tricuspid valve annulus (TVA) plane. The position of the ablation catheter at the site of radiofrequency (RF) application during slow pathway is also shown. Note the variable dimension of the triangle of Koch in the three inferior panels
Abbreviations: CS, coronary sinus; SVC, superior vena cava; RAA, right atrial appendage; RVA, right ventricular apex

its location between the other two isthmuses. The inferior isthmus represents the optimal target for linear ablation since this is the site where 1) the orifice of the IVC is closer to the tricuspid valve insertion, 2) the wall thickness is minimal, and 3) there is a larger distance to the right coronary artery and the atrioventricular node or its arterial supply **(Figures 6.5A to C)**. Fluoroscopically, the 6 or 7 O'clock position in the LAO view correlates with the preferred site for ablation.[12-16]

The Paraseptal Region and the Inferior Pyramidal Space

The inferior paraseptal region represents the confluence of all four chambers (the so-called inferior pyramidal space) and the coronary sinus. The pyramidal space is an area whose superior vertex is the central fibrous body, the lateral sides are formed by the convergence of the left and right atria and whose floor is the muscular ventricular septum and left ventricle. The coronary sinus limits the base of this area, which has a pyramidal configuration. Tissues that are continuous with the inferior epicardial AV groove occupy the pyramidal space together with the AV nodal artery and the proximal coronary sinus with the middle cardiac vein and posterior coronary vein.[17]

The traditionally called right and left posteroseptal accessory pathways are in fact inferior and paraseptal, because this region is inferior to the true atrial septum. Inferior paraseptal accessory pathways can be ablated from the right side of the heart, outside or inside the coronary

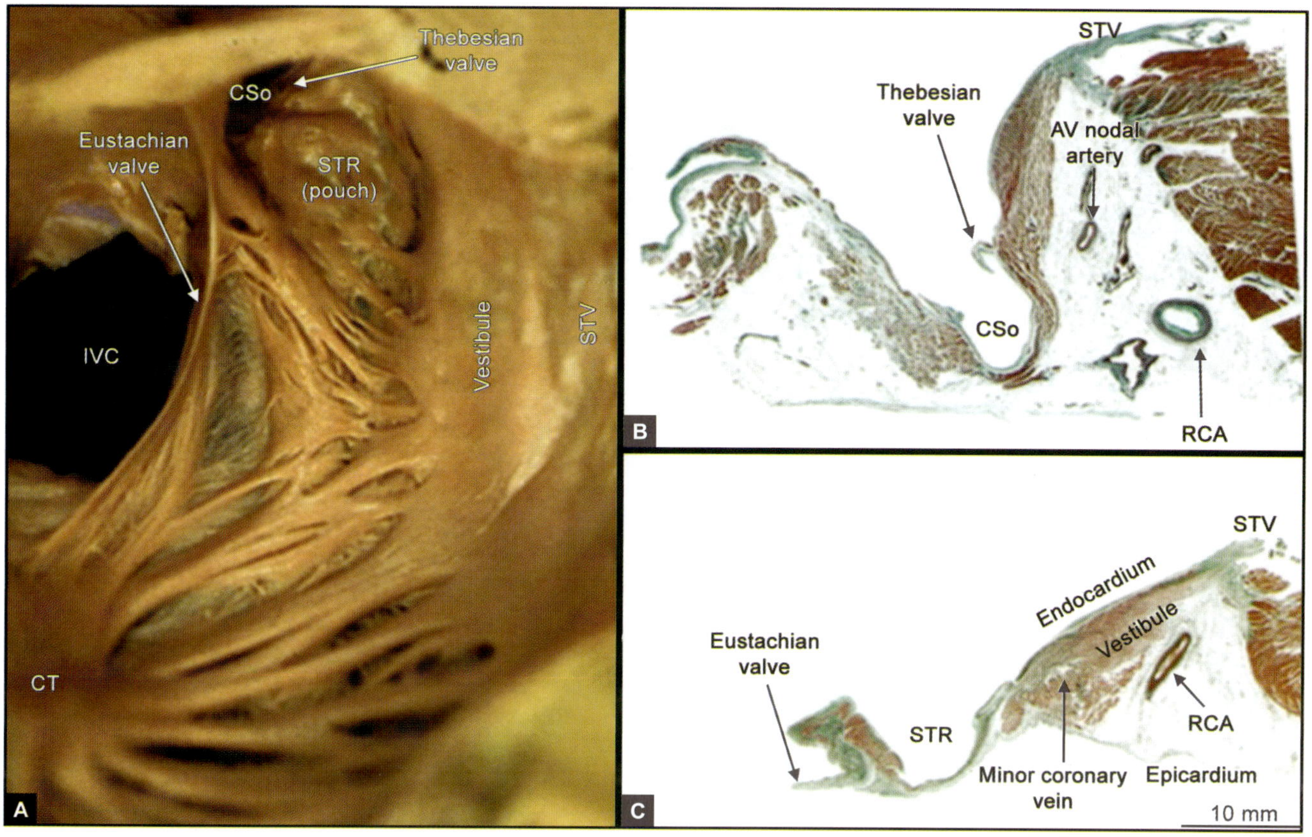

Figures 6.5A to C: (A) The right inferior cavo-tricuspid isthmus is a quadrilateral area in the floor of the right atrium bounded by the inferior vena cava and the Eustachian valve posteriorly and by the septal attachment of the tricuspid valve anteriorly. Note in this specimen the complex endocardial topography of the isthmus with thicker trabeculations from the terminal crest and a deep sub-Thebesian recess (pouch); (B) and (C) Histological sections (Masson's trichrome stain) at the level of the paraseptal (B) and central (C) isthmus illustrating its different myocardial thickness and relationships

Abbreviations: CSo, coronary sinus orifice; IVC, inferior vena cava; RCA, right coronary artery; STR, sub-Thebesian recess; STV, septal tricuspid valve; CT, crista terminalis; AV, atrioventricular

sinus, or in the middle cardiac vein, and from the left side of the heart. The midseptal region (mid-septal accessory pathways) correspond to the floor of Koch´s triangle between the His recording location and the anterior portion of the CS ostium. In this region, owing that the tricuspid valve is displaced apically and inferiorly in relation with the mitral annulus, there is an opposition between the inferomedial right atrium and the posterior region of the left ventricle **(Figures 6.6A and B)**. In addition there is no atrial septum in the region of the His bundle at the apex of Koch's triangle (former anteroseptal). Thus, this area is more properly regarded as superoparaseptal.[1-3]

The True Interatrial Septum the Oval Fossa

The true IAS is the oval fossa, which is seen as a relative depression in the right atrial aspect of the area traditionally considered to be the IAS. The floor of the oval fossa is formed by the embryonic septum primum, which, in most individuals, is completely adhered to the periphery (rim or limbus) of the oval fossa. On the left atrial side of the IAS, the floor of the oval fossa is usually indistinguishable from the rest of atrial wall except for a small crescent-like edge that marks the free margin of the septum primum **(Figures 6.7A to E)**. The rim of oval fossa at anterosuperior and postero-inferior margins is formed by the infolded muscular right atrial wall and is not considered a true septum. This atrial muscular fold is filled with the epicardial fibrofatty tissues and termed the "interatrial groove" (also known as the 'Waterston groove' to the cardiac surgeons). The antero-inferior rim, which anchors the flap valve of the oval fossa into the atrioventricular junctions, is also a septal structure which continues into the atrial vestibules on both sides of the septal component and into the Eustachian ridge (sinus septum) on the right atrial side. The anteroinferior rim is separated from ventricles by the fat-filled inferior pyramidal space, through which passes the AV nodal artery.[18-20]

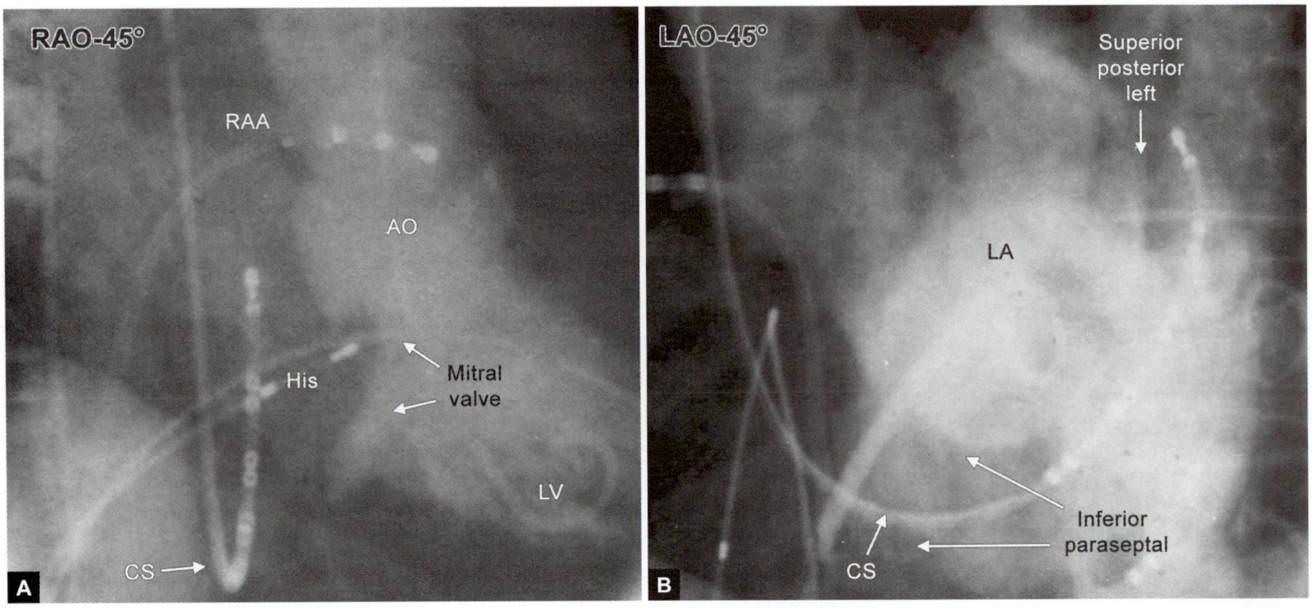

Figures 6.6A and B: (A) Fluoroscopic 45° right anterior oblique (RAO) projection showing the angiographic display of the mitral valve during the injection of radiographic contrast into the left ventricle (LV); (B) Left atrial angiography through a trans-septal puncture in the left anterior oblique projection (LAO). Note in both RAO and LAO projections the anatomic relation of the coronary sinus (CS) catheter with the mitral valve annulus and the endocardial aspect of the left atrium (LA)
Abbreviations: AO, aorta; CS, coronary sinus; LA, left atrium; LAO, left atrial oblique; LV, left ventricle; RAA, right atrial appendage; RAO, right anterior oblique

It is important to perform the transseptal puncture through the oval fossa. An accidental puncture throughout the interatrial groove (the muscular IAS) may result in hemopericardium in an anticoagulated patient because blood will dissect the vascular fibrofatty tissue that is sandwiched between the right and left atrial myocardium at this level.

Also relevant is the spatial relationship between the anterior atrial wall or the plane of the atrial septum and the root of the aorta **(Figures 6 and 7E)**.[3]

Anatomy and Muscular Architecture of the Left Atrium

Although initial catheter ablation approaches were aimed at obtaining an electrical disconnection of the PVs so as to isolate the LA from the venous triggers, ablation techniques for AF and left atrial flutter have evolved from rather limited initial approaches to quite extensive atrial interventions. Modification of the atrial substrate by targeting structures of the LA that are thought to maintain AF appears to increase success rate in patients with persistent and permanent atrial fibrillation. In addition, non-PV triggers in patients with AF can be found in nonpulmonary thoracic veins such as caval veins, the oblique vein of Marshall, or the musculature lining the coronary sinus.

The major part of the LA, including the septal component, is smooth-walled except the ostium of the atrial appendage and its neighboring structures. The walls of the LA can be described as superior, posterior, left lateral, septal (or medial), and anterior. The anterior wall that is immediately inferior to the Bachmann's bundle, located just behind the aorta can be very thin, and measures approximately 1-2 mm in thickness transmurally. The superior wall, or dome, is thicker compared with the posterior and postero-inferior walls, measuring 3.5-6.5 mm **(Figures 6.8A to E)**.[18-22]

The Pulmonary Veins and the Venoatrial Junction

When assessed in a correct attitudinal orientation, the left PVs are located more superiorly than the right sided veins. The superior PVs run cranially and more anteriorly whereas the inferior veins have a more posterior and lateral course. The right superior PV runs near the posterior aspect of the right atrium immediately behind the SVC. The right PVs are also related to the right pulmonary artery that passes close to the roof of the LA. The left superior PV lies superiorly and posteriorly to the mouth of the LAA, both separated endocardially by a lateral ridge that, epicardially, is a fold that frequently extends to the origin of the left inferior PV. The orifices of the right PVs are directly adjacent to the plane of the atrial septum **(Figures 6.7 and 6.8)**. The most common anatomic variants (30-35%) of the PVs ending into the LA include a conjoined homolateral ostia of the left PVs (25% of specimens) and a supernumerary or additional right PV. The distance between the

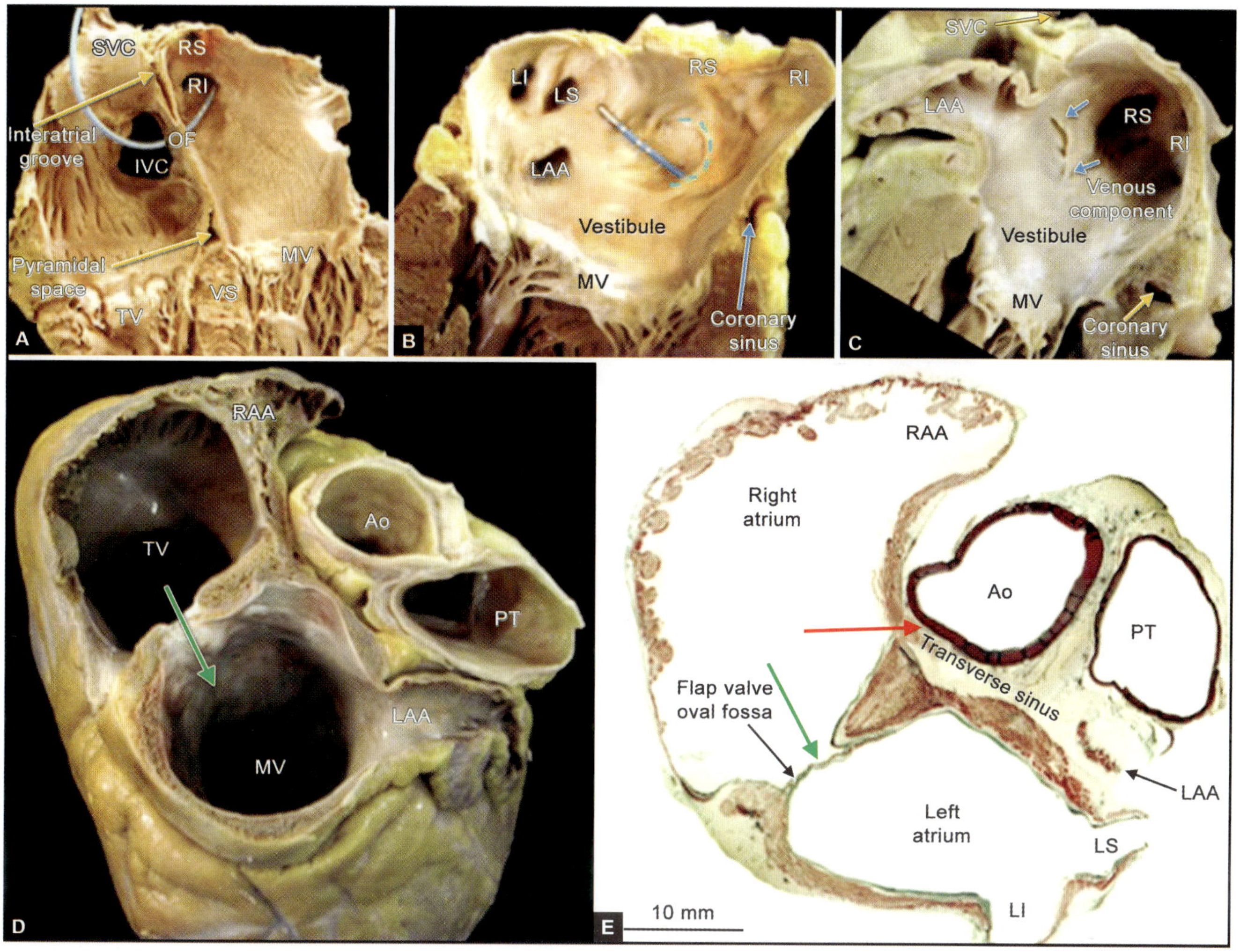

Figures 6.7A to E: (A) Four-chamber view of dissected heart to show the superior rim of the oval fossa. The infolded wall between the superior vena cava and the right pulmonary veins is known as interatrial groove (Waterston´s groove). Anteriorly and inferiorly, the rim and its continuation into the atrial vestibules overlie the inferior pyramidal space. A probe is passed through the oval fossa and its end is placed into the right inferior pulmonary vein; (B) Dissection of the posterior wall of the left atrium next to the posterior interatrial groove. The smooth walled venous component of the left atrium is the most extensive. The septal aspect of the LA shows the crescentic line of the free edge of the flap valve (blue dotted line) against the rim of the oval fossa. The orifices of the right superior and inferior pulmonary veins are adjacent to the plane of the septum; (C) Sagittal section through the left atrial appendage showing the orifices of the right pulmonary veins. Note the relation of the superior vena cava to the right superior pulmonary vein; (D) Short-axis through the interatrial septum (green arrow). The dome or roof of the left atrium has been removed and the left atrial side of the septum can be seen. Note the nonuniform thickness of the left atrial wall (red arrow); (E) Histological section with Masson trichrome taken through the short-axis of the heart to show the thin flap valve and the muscular rim of the fossa (green arrow). Note the close relationship of the anterior wall of the atria with the transverse sinus and aorta (red arrow)
Abbreviations: Ao, aorta; IVC, inferior vena cava; LAA, left atrial appendage; LS, left superior pulmonary vein: LI, left inferior pulmonary vein; MV, mitral valve; OF, oval fossa; PT, pulmonary trunk; RAA, right atrial appendage; RI, right inferior pulmonary vein; RS, right superior pulmonary vein; SVC, superior vena cava; TV, tricuspid valve; VS, ventricular septum

orifices of the right PVs ranged from 3 to 14 mm (mean 7.3 ± 2.7 mm), and in the left PVs were 2 to 16 mm (mean 7.5 ± 2.8 mm).[21-23]

Anatomic studies and clinical imaging investigations have shown that the PV ending in the LA is (a) not perfectly cylindrical but ovoid with a funnel-shaped morphology and (b) the transition from the atrial endocardium to the venous endothelial layer is smooth with an unclear anatomic border, thus making identification of the true PV ostium difficult. Discounting the common ostia of the PVs, the diameter of the venous orifices at the venoatrial junction ranged in our anatomic specimens from 8 mm to 21 mm (12.5 ± 3 mm). The transverse diameter of the common vestibule is longer than its superoinferior diameter (19.5 ± 3 mm vs 13.5 ± 1 mm).[41]

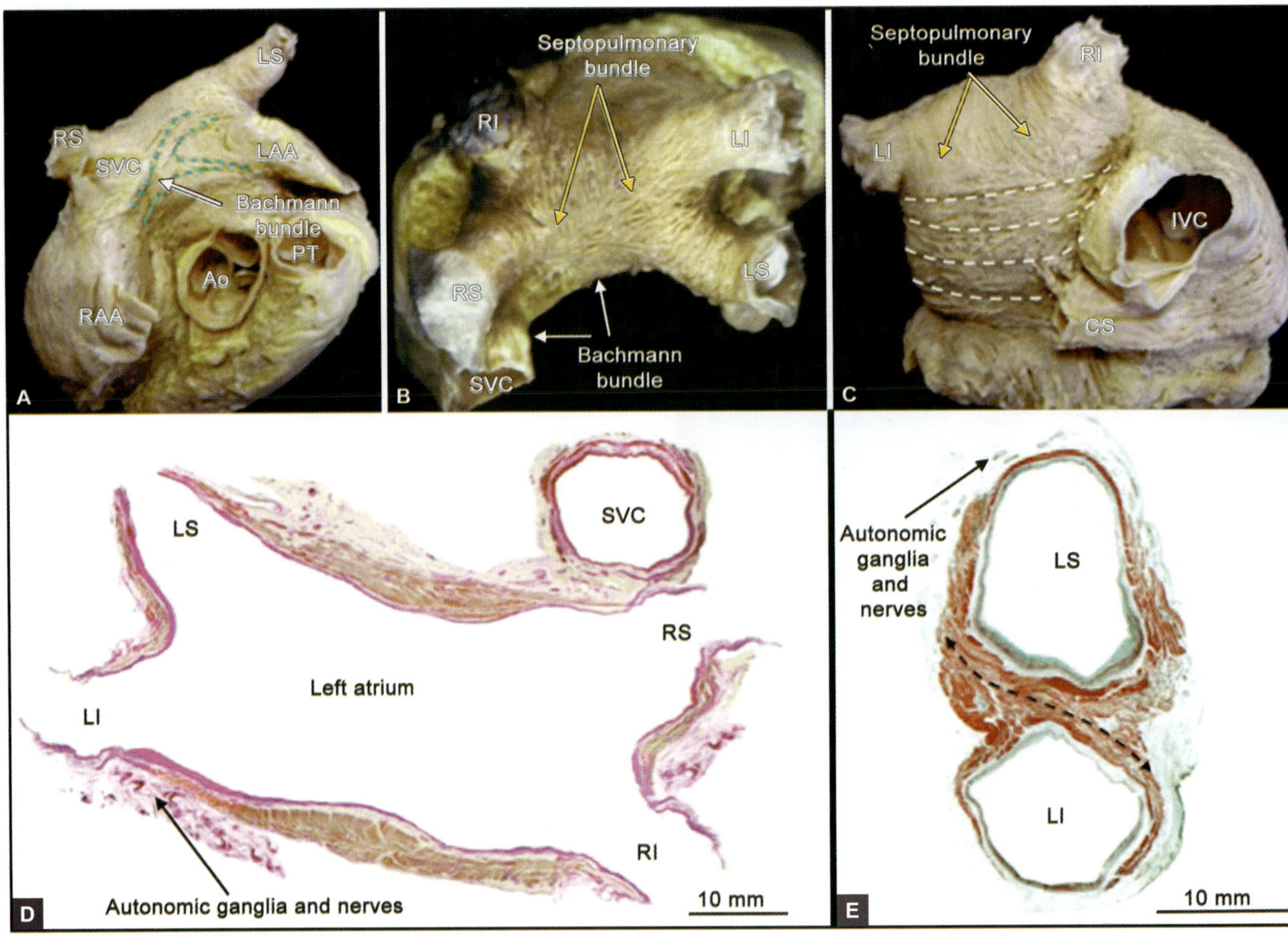

Figures 6.8A to E: (A to C) Serial dissections to display the subepicardial atrial myoarchitecture in a normal human heart; (A) and (B) Anterior and superior views to show the Bachmann bundle (blue dashed lines) crossing the anterior interatrial groove and branching towards the left atrial appendage. Note also the longitudinal fibers of the septopulmonary bundle, that arises from the interatrial groove underneath Bachmann's bundle, fanning out to line the pulmonary veins and to pass longitudinally over the dome and in the posterior wall of the left atrium; (C) On the posterior wall, the septopulmonary bundle often crossing the circumferential myocytes (white dashed lines) coming from the lateral wall which show an abrupt change of fiber orientation in the posterior wall of the left atrium. Note the highly variable anatomic orientation of the myocardial fibers making up the sleeves. The myocyte sleeves are mainly composed of circularly orientated bundles; oblique and longitudinally oriented fibers are also common; (D) Cross histological section, stained with elastic van Gieson, of the left atrium, pulmonary veins and the superior vena cava. Note the epicardial location of vegetative nerves and ganglia; (E) Cross histological section of the left pulmonary veins stained with Masson trichrome. Note the interpulmonary myocardial connections (black dotted line in panel) between the superior and inferior veins

Abbreviations: Ao, aorta; CS, coronary sinus; IVC, inferior vena cava; LAA, left atrial appendage; LS, left superior pulmonary vein: LI, left inferior pulmonary vein; PT, pulmonary trunk; RAA, right atrial appendage; RI, right inferior pulmonary vein; RS, right superior pulmonary vein; SVC, superior vena cava

The venous wall in humans shows an innermost layer formed by a thin endothelium overlying an irregular media of connective tissue and smooth muscle cells, and a thick outer layer of fibrous adventitia. At the pulmonary vein-atrial junction, the endocardium of the LA is in continuity with the endothelial lining of the vein. The transition from the venous media to the left atrial subendocardial region is represented by a gradual decline in the number of smooth muscle cells. In most PVs, the smooth muscle of the venous wall overlaps with a layer of myocardial bundles extending over the inner layer but is separated from it by a thin plane of fibrofatty tissue. This intermediate myocardial layer, between the adventitia and the venous media, is the myocardial continuity from the left atrial wall (so-called myocardial sleeves) in a fine matrix composed of collagen, elastic fibers and blood vessels. Therefore, as seen in longitudinal sections, the extension of left atrial musculature lies external to the venous wall and within the epicardium/adventitia **(Figures 6.8A to E)**.

The PV sleeves are thickest at the venoatrial junction, (1.88 ± 0.45, range 1.2–2.8 mm) and then tapered toward the lung hilum, but the decrease in thickness is not uniform circumferentially. The atrial myocardial sleeves in the superior veins are thickest inferiorly (at 6 O'clock), and thinnest superiorly (at 12 O'clock), whereas an opposite pattern is found in the inferior veins. Bridges of atrial myocardium and crossing strands have been observed connecting the superior and inferior PV, occurring more frequently between the left veins than between the right veins **(Figure 6.8E)**.[21-23]

The Lateral Ridge of the Left Atrium

The LA lateral ridge actually is a fold of the posterolateral left atrial wall protruding into the endocardial LA surface as prominent crest or ridge **(Figures 6.9A to E)**. Epicardially, this broad bundle is in continuity with the uppermost and distal part of the interatrial band (Bachmann bundle). Endocardially, the myocardial content is the prolongation of leftward fibers from the septoatrial bundle that run towards the orifices of the left-sided PVs and the mouth of the LAA **(Figures 6.8 and 6.9)**. The shape and size of this postero-lateral LA ridge is of relevance during catheter ablation of AF when encircling the orifices of the left PVs or during ablation of extrapulmonary vein triggers arising around or inside the LAA. The ridge extends along the lateral wall of the LA from the anterosuperior to the posteroinferior region.

The left lateral ridge is more than a simple endocardial fold of the lateral LA wall that influences the stability of the contact of the tip of the catheter with the endocardium during an ablation procedure. The oblique vein of Marshall courses obliquely above the left atrial appendage and can be traced laterally to the left superior PV bundle in the epicardial aspect of the left atrial fold that forms the left lateral ridge. The vein of Marshall is part of the ligament of Marshall (LOM), formed by the venous element and fibrofatty tissue, muscular bundle and autonomic nerves, all forming a vestigial fold of the pericardium.

The Marshall ligament is richly innervated by sympathetic nerve fibers. Adrenergic sensitivity of the myocardial tissues within the LOM may be responsible for atrial tachyarrhythmias arising from the LA. Both focal sources arising from Marshall structures and muscular connections with the epicardial interatrial Bachmann bundle and the inner septoatrial bundle may have implications in the fibrillatory process and spread of AF activity between both atria. Recent reports have shown that left to right interatrial conduction occurs predominantly through the Bachmann bundle and that sinus impulses propagated through this interatrial bundle could excite the Marshall musculature and the nearby left atrium simultaneously.[22]

The Left Atrial Appendage and the Mitral Isthmus

The LAA is characteristically a tubular extension of the LA with one or several bends resembling a little finger. On the endocardial aspect a narrow oval-shaped mouth marks the junction between the LAA and the venous component of the left atrium with a mean long diameter of 17.4 ± 4 mm and short diameter of 10.9 ± 4.2 mm. The myocardial ridge and an inflection of the endocardial surface bounded the ostial borders of the appendage **(Figures 6.7 to 6.9)**.

Reinforced superficially by the interatrial bundle, circumferential fibers that arise from the anterosuperior part of the septal raphe pass to either side of the neck of the left appendage to form broad bundles of muscular connections between the appendage and the body of the left atrium. In some patients, longer RF pulses are required to electrically disconnect the LAA, that gradually change the activation sequence, thus suggesting a dense circumferential connection of the appendage to the LA. In the LA, the pectinate muscles are mostly confined within the appendage. They form a complicated network of muscular strips lining the endocardial surface. In between the muscle bundles, the wall is paper-thin. In some specimens (28%), muscular trabeculations can be found extending inferiorly from the appendage to the vestibule of the mitral valve **(Figure 6.9B)**. These extra-appendicular myocardial bands correspond to the small posterior set of pectinate muscles originating from the septoatrial bundle to embrace the LAA. In those hearts with extra-appendicular posterior pectinate muscles, the areas in between the muscular trabeculae had the thinnest muscular wall (0.5 ± 0.2 mm) increasing the risk of cardiac perforation during ablation in this region. In other specimens (15%), remnants of pectinate muscles between the ostium of the left inferior PV and vestibule of the mitral annulus can be found ("small isthmus crevices"). The left circumflex coronary artery runs epicardially in the fat-filled AV groove, related with the smooth anterior vestibule and in close proximity with the inferior border of the orifice of the LAA (<3–5 mm in 80% of our unselected human heart necropsy specimens) **(Figures 6.9A to E)**. The previous anatomic detail should be considered when ablating inside or around the orifice of the LAA or during percutaneous occlusion of the LAA.[24-27]

Linear ablation connecting the inferior margin of the ostium of the left inferior PV to the mitral annulus appears to increase the success rate of catheter ablation in some patients with AF especially persistent AF. This posteroinferior wall of the left atrium has been named by electrophysiologists as left atrial isthmus or mitral isthmus. In this region, the vestibule directly opposes the wall of the great cardiac vein (GCV) and its continuation, the coronary sinus **(Figures 6.9A to E)**. In cases where the wall at the transition of vein to sinus is particularly muscular, it adds to the thickness of the isthmus. Frequently, the venous/sinus musculature is

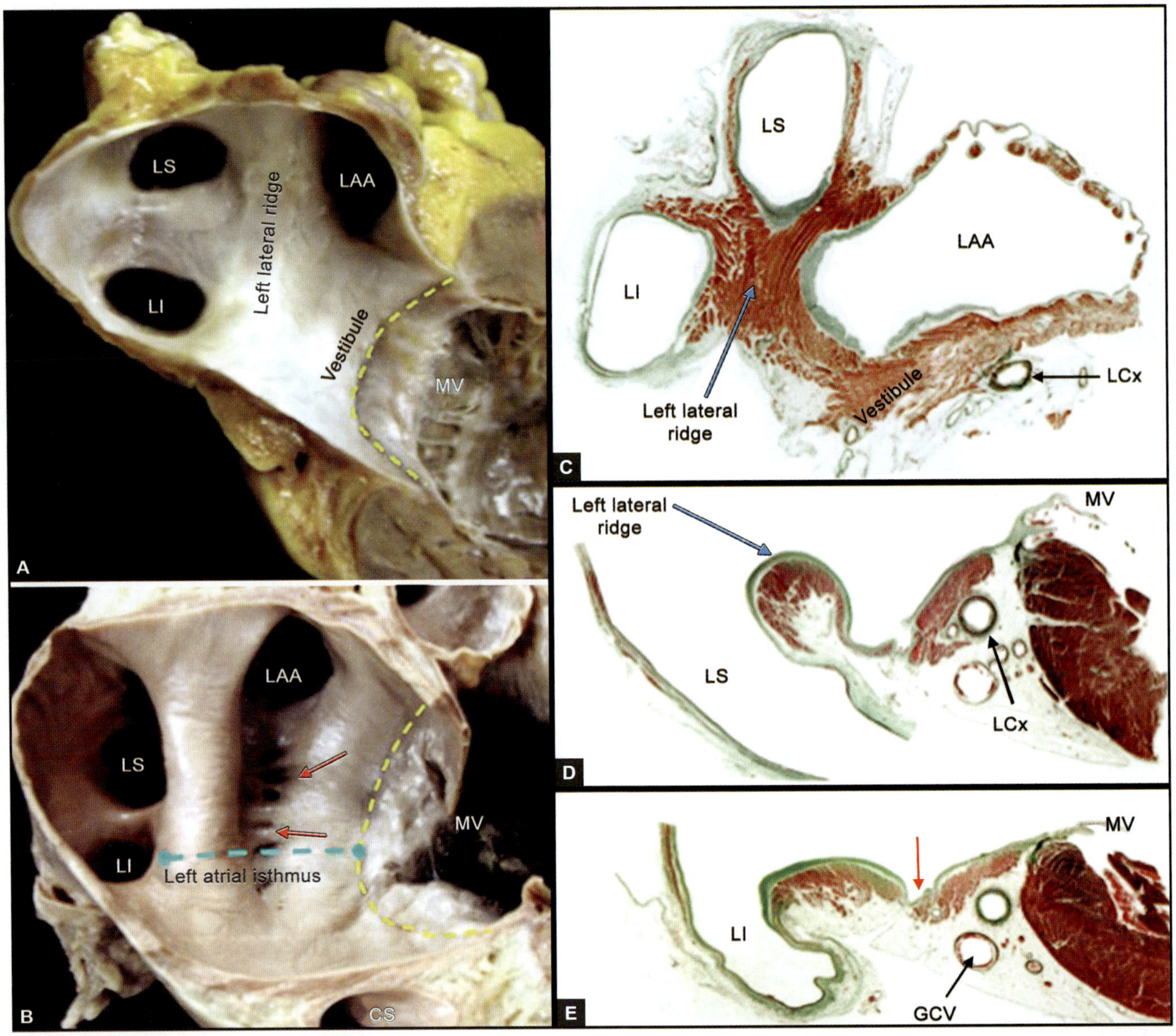

Figures 6.9A to E: (A) and (B) Longitudinal sections of two hearts through the roof of the left atrium illustrating endings of the pulmonary veins into the left atrium; (A) An individualized ending of the left superior and the left inferior pulmonary veins into the left atrium. Note the prominent left lateral ridge between the ostium of the left atrial appendage and the orifice of the left superior pulmonary vein; (B) This specimen showing a common vestibule for both left pulmonary veins, and extra-pectinate muscle trabeculations are extending inferiorly from the mouth of the appendage to the vestibule of the mitral valve (red arrows). Note the line (blue dotted line) connecting the inferior margin of the ostium of the left inferior pulmonary vein to the mitral valve called the left atrial isthmus or mitral isthmus; (C) Cross-histological sections of the left lateral wall of the left atrium stained with Masson's trichrome. Note the myofiber arrangement in the left lateral ridge and left pulmonary veins; (D) and (E) Histological sections (Masson's trichrome stain) of a specimen showing a pointed profile of the endocardial left lateral ridge (D) extending to the inferior margin of the left superior pulmonary vein. The vestibule overlies the left circumflex artery and great cardiac vein; (E) The histological section shows a flattened profile of the fold that forms the ridge extending to the inferior margin of the left inferior pulmonary vein. Note the space between the pectinate muscles where the left atrial wall becomes thinner (red arrow)

Abbreviations: CS, coronary sinus; GCV, great cardiac vein; LAA, left atrial appendage; LCx, left circumflex artery; LS, left superior pulmonary vein: LI, left inferior pulmonary vein; MV, mitral valve

continuous with the left atrial wall. The muscle sleeve around the coronary sinus and the close anatomic proximity of the circumflex artery are the two major anatomic determinants for the creation of complete mitral isthmus conduction block. Also relevant is the presence of small crevices or extra-appendicular posterior pectinate muscles, close to the base of the LAA, that may entrap the tip of the ablation catheter also increasing the risk of perforation.[22,24]

THE CORONARY SINUS AND INTERATRIAL MUSCLE CONNECTIONS

Gross Morphology and Muscular Architecture of the Coronary Sinus

The CS, which is the continuation of the great cardiac vein, runs on the atrial side of the true annulus along the postero-inferior wall of the LA. This separation from the annulus is more pronounced in the proximal 20 mm of the CS **(Figure 6.10)**. The ostium of the CS abuts the superior margin of the right atrial-left ventricular sulcus and the inferior paraseptal mitral annulus in the pyramidal space. The Thebesian valve demarcates the distal end of the CS. It can be seen in 80% of specimens and is highly variable in size and morphology. A complete circular valve is seen in 20%–30% of specimens and is absent in 20%. In most cases, a groove or depression is seen on the outer surface of the CS ostium, which can localize the atrial end of the CS in the absence of a CS valve. The oblique vein of Marshall (OVM) is the best landmark for localizing the origin of the CS. The oblique vein of Marshall (diameter 0.4–1.8 mm), located between the LAA and the left upper and lower PVs, runs inferiorly along the posteroinferior atrial wall to join the CS. In most hearts (70%), the oblique vein is <3 mm from the endocardium of the LA and has muscular connections to the left PVs **(Figure 6.10).** Because the CS and IVC valves share the same embryonic origin, both can be affected in congenital heart disease. A large "windsock" CS is seen in patients with a persistent left SVC. The CS length is 30–50 mm in 75% of anatomic sections. A short CS is defined as being less than 2 cm in length.

Cannulation of the oblique vein of Marshall can be used to analyze electrical activity for ablation of paroxysmal AF. Three anatomic landmarks are recognized for localization of the CS-GCV junction: the orifice of the oblique vein of Marshall, the valve of Vieussens, and the left margin of the myocardial sleeve of the CS, with the oblique vein of Marshall as the most constant landmark. These anatomic landmarks are not at the same level and are usually located within a 10 mm interval. The valve of Vieussens is present in 65%–85% of cadaveric heart specimens as a unicuspid or incomplete valve adjacent or proximal to the oblique vein of Marshall.[18,28-30]

Left ventricular lead placement in a suitable coronary vein branch along the dyssynchronous wall of the left ventricle is an important determinant of responsiveness to cardiac resynchronization therapy (CRT). Common target veins for

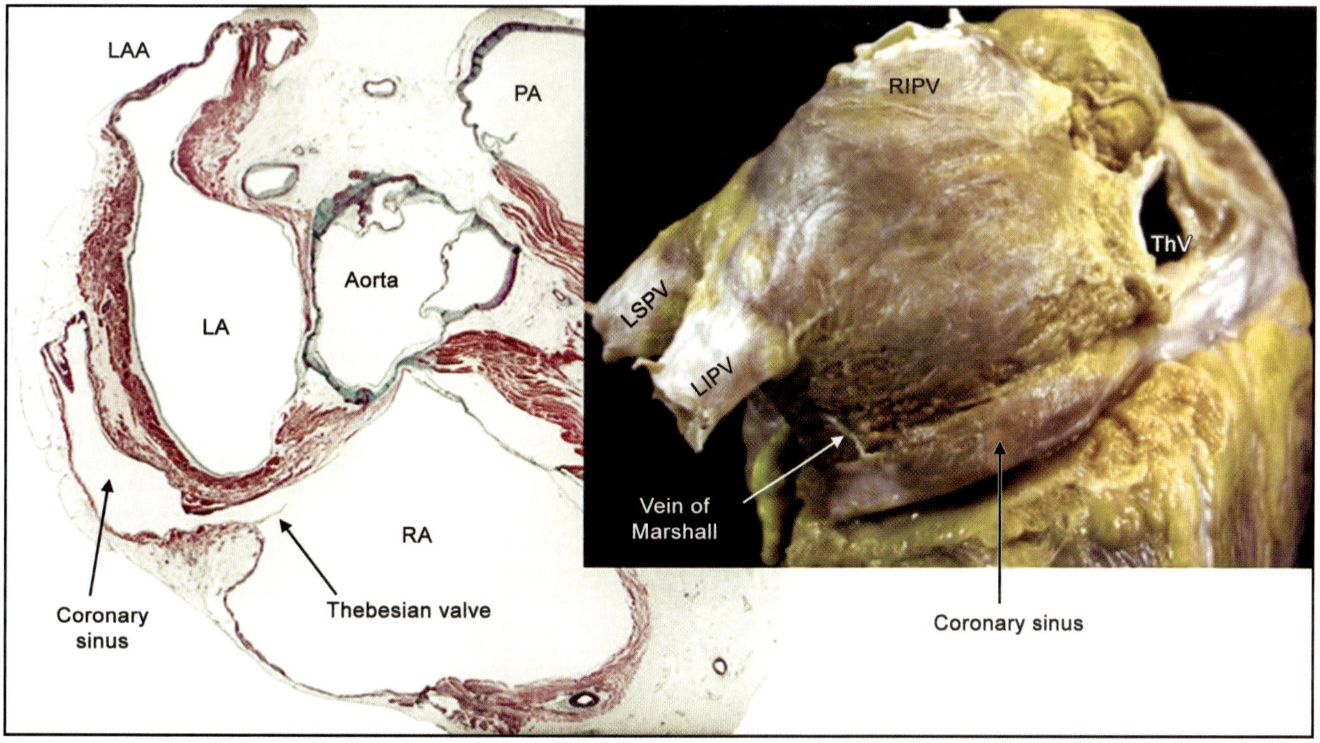

Figure 6.10: Histological section with Masson trichrome taken through the short-axis of the heart to show the muscular sleeves over the wall of the coronary sinus. The coronary sinus runs along the epicardial side of the left atrium next to the left AV junction with extensive myocardial connections to the left (LA) and right atrium (RA)

Abbreviations: LA, left atrium; LAA, left atrial appendage; LIPV, left inferior pulmonary vein; LSPV, left superior pulmonary vein: PA, pulmonary artery; RA, right atrium; RIPV, right inferior pulmonary vein; ThV, Thebesian valve placement of the lead are the left marginal vein or posterior veins of the left ventricle. In rare cases, the lead is placed in an anterolateral branch of the GCV. Implanting the electrode in a coronary vein can be difficult due to unfavorable anatomic factors. The observation that patients with previous posterolateral left ventricular infarction are frequently lacking the left marginal vein (27% in infarcted hearts vs 70% in normal hearts) has important implications for the selection of potential candidates for CRT. The absence of CS tributaries may be related to thrombosis and scar formation secondary to previous myocardial infarction in the region drained by these specific veins. Different reasons may also create anatomical difficulties during CRT: (1) morphological variants such as hypoplasia, absence, duplication, diverticulum, (2) level of CS insertion, (3) size of the CS and distance of target vein from the thebesian valve, (4) tortuosity and acute angle of target vein confluence (posterior and lateral veins have acute angle in 30% of cases).[28]

Coronary Sinus and Interatrial Muscle Connections

In all specimens, the venous wall of the coronary sinus was surrounded by a cuff of striated muscle extending 25–50 mm from the ostium **(Figure 6.10)**. Striated myocardial connections of varying number and morphology connected this coronary sinus muscle cuff to the left atrium. The coronary sinus musculature may also form extensions over the proximal portion of the middle cardiac vein and posterior cardiac vein.

The CS and the oblique vein of Marshall are both remnants of the sinus venosus, and their muscle sleeve can be an extension of the RA myocardium over the CS (CS-RA muscle continuity). Other fibers of varying thicknesses arise from this sleeve and connect to the LA myocardium along the inferior mitral annulus, providing the second-largest electrical continuity between the atria located posteroinferiorly (CS-LA muscle connections). Along with the Bachmann bundle (anterosuperior interatrial muscle bridge), these striated muscle connections ensure rapid interatrial conduction, leading to physiologic biatrial contraction. Electrophysiological studies have also demonstrated the electrical connection between the RA and LA through the musculature of the coronary sinus. Recent observations have identified focal sources of premature depolarizations originating within the coronary sinus that may trigger AF. It has been suggested that electrical disconnection of the two atria targeting the interatrial connections diminishes the electrophysiological substrate for perpetuation of AF.[28-30]

THE RIGHT AND LEFT VENTRICLES

In contrast to the conical morphology of the left ventricle (LV), the RV is more triangular in shape when viewed from the front and it curves over the LV **(Figures 6.11A to H)**. The geometry of the RV is also influenced by the convexity of the ventricular septum toward the RV in both systole and diastole under normal loading conditions. Both right and left ventricles have been described as having three components: the inlet (inflow tract), apical trabecular, and outlet portions (outflow tract). Morphologically, the RV is distinguished from the LV by having coarser trabeculae, a moderator band, and a lack of fibrous continuity between its inlet and outflow valves. The muscular trabeculations in the apical part of the RV are coarser than those in the LV **(Figures 6.11 and 6.12)**. The apical trabeculations of the LV are fine and display a criss-cross pattern. The inlets also differ markedly in the normal ventricles, as do the outlets. Thus, the tricuspid valve possessing inferior, septal and anterosuperior leaflets, has extensive chordal attachments to the ventricular septum, and is supported by markedly eccentric papillary muscles. The mitral valve possesses two leaflets, located anteriorly and posteriorly but positioned obliquely within the LV, and closing along a solitary zone of apposition. The anterior leaflet of the mitral valve is separated from the septum by the subaortic vestibule, having fibrous continuity with two of the leaflets of the aortic valve.[31-38]

Anatomy of the Outflow Tracts: Implication for Ablation of Ventricular Tachycardias

Premature ventricular contractions, ventricular tachycardia (VT) and initiating beats for ventricular fibrillation have all been localized at the level of the right and left ventricular outflow tracts (RVOT and LVOT). Absence of structural heart disease is the rule with these arrhythmias and most outflow tracts VTs originate in the perivalvular tissue.[34-37]

The majority of RVOT tachycardias originate in the superior, septal and anterior aspect of the infundibulum just underneath the pulmonary valve. The RVOT (outlet portion of the RV or the infundibulum) is a muscular structure of variable length (range 13–24 mm) that supports the semilunar leaflets of the pulmonary valve. Its posterior and inferior part consists of a prominent muscular crest, called supraventricular crest that separates the inflow and outflow components of the RV **(Figures 6.11A to H)**. The supraventricular crest is in contact with the posterior part of the LVOT, as it inserts in the interventricular septum. On the septal aspect, this crest inserts between the limbs of the septomarginal trabeculation (SMT), or septal band. This muscular strap reinforces the septal surface of the RV, breaking up at the apex to form the moderator band and the anterior papillary muscle. The moderator band incorporates the right bundle branch, as conduction tissue fibers move towards the apex of the ventricle before entering the anterior papillary muscle. The septoparietal trabeculations take origin from the anterior margin of the SMT and run round the parietal ventricular wall of the infundibulum.

These trabeculations showed a variable extension and thickness along the right and left septoparietal wall of the RVOT **(Figure 6.12)**.

All these structures are absent from the LV, where the outlet (LVOT) is much more reduced in size because of the fibrous continuity between two of the leaflets of the aortic valve and the aortic leaflet of the mitral valve. Therefore, in the LV, there is no muscular separation between inflow and outflow tracts **(Figures 6.11A to H)**.

Although the two ventricular outlets have important differences in their structure, they also have one feature in common, namely the semilunar attachment of their leaflets. Because of the semilunar shape of the pulmonary leaflets this valve does not have a ring-like annulus.

THE PERICARDIAL SPACE, AUTONOMIC NERVOUS SYSTEM AND THE EXTRACARDIAC ANATOMIC STRUCTURES RELEVANT FOR ABLATION

The close anatomic vicinity of the cardiac chambers to important structures and the regional distribution of the autonomic nervous system elements that may be affected by interventional maneuvers should also be understood by the electrophysiologist.[39-48]

The Pericardial Space

The heart and its adjoining great vessels are enclosed in a sac, the parietal (fibrous) pericardium. Superiorly, the fibrous pericardium is continuous with the adventitia of the great vessels. Within the fibrous pericardium, there is a delicate double-layered membrane known as the serous pericardium. One layer of the serous pericardium is fused to the fibrous pericardium while the other layer lines the outer surface of the heart and continues over the surfaces of the vessels as the visceral pericardium. Over the great vessels, the junctions between the two layers are the pericardial reflections. The pericardial cavity then is the space between the layers of the serous pericardium **(Figures 6.13A and B)**

There is a small area behind the lower left half of the body of the sternum and the sternal ends of the left fourth and fifth costal cartilages where the fibrous pericardium is in direct contact with the thoracic wall. This area does allow the pericardial space to be accessed. The pericardial cavity has two main sinuses and several recesses. These are

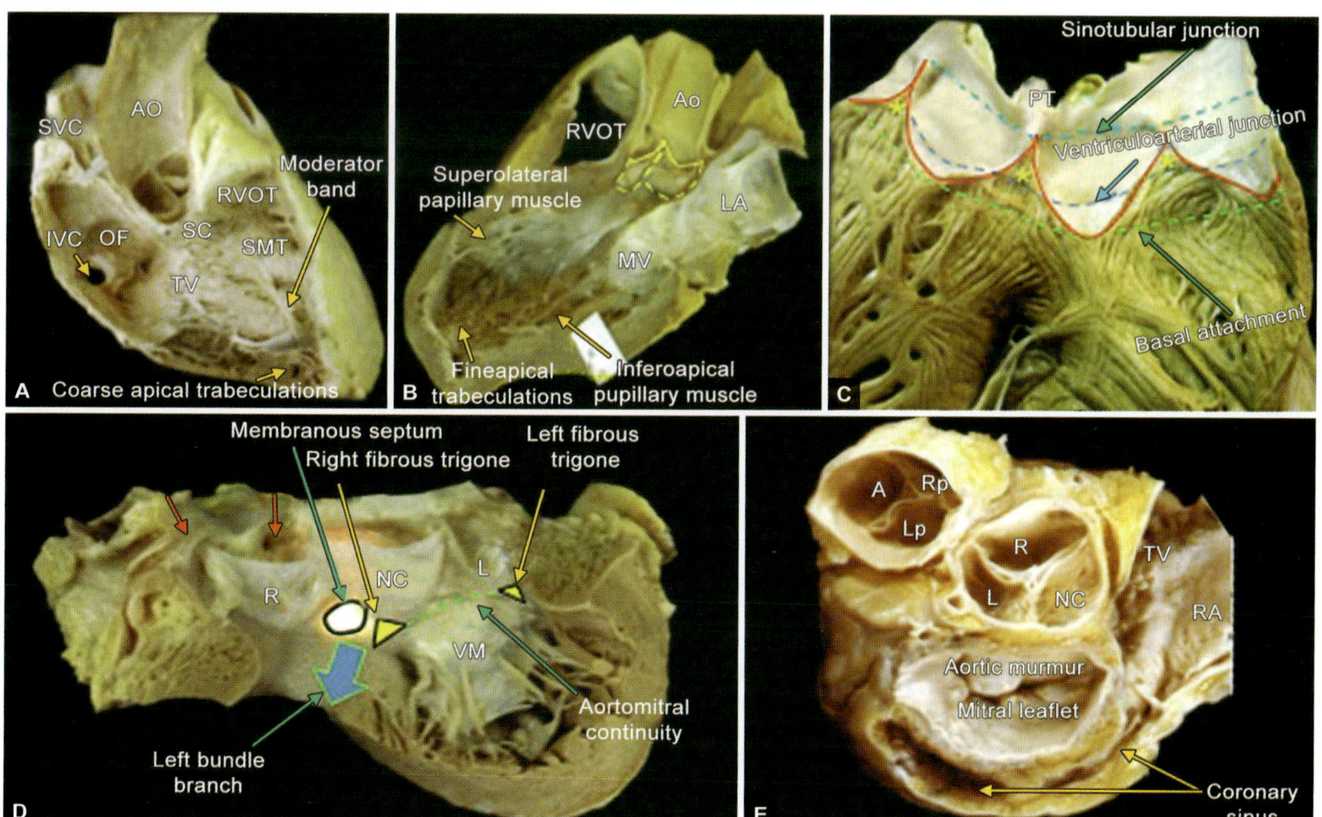

Figures 6.11A to E

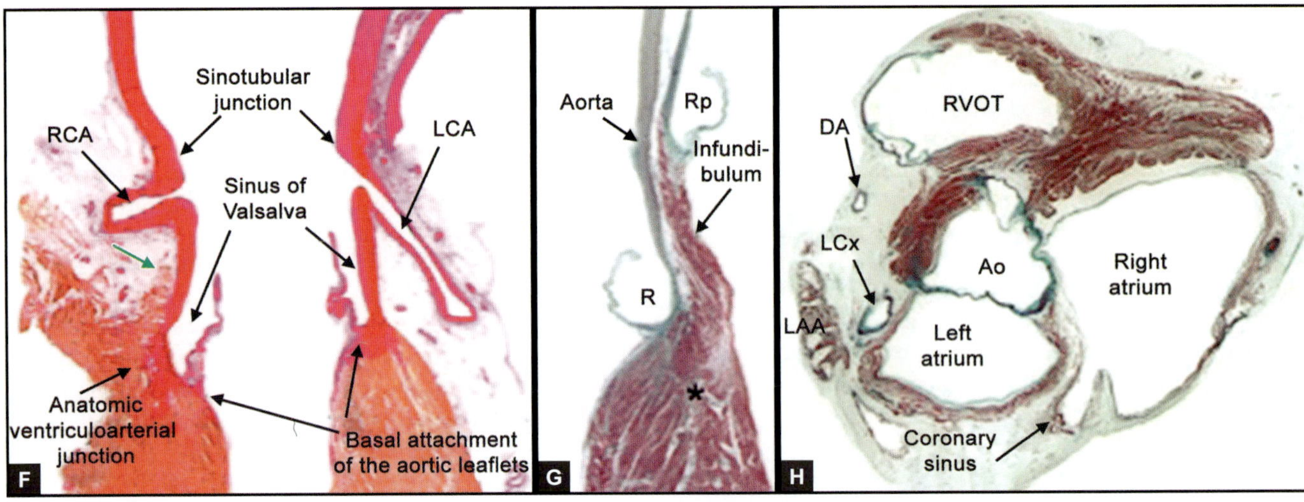

Figures 6.11F to H

Figures 6.11A to H: (A) Window dissection of a heart prepared by removing the anterosuperior wall of the right ventricle. The three components of the right ventricle are revealed: the inlet (tricuspid valve), apical trabecular, and right ventricular outflow tract or infundibulum. Note the location of the supraventricular crest and septomarginal trabeculation. The septomarginal trabeculation continues as an important muscular strand, the moderator band, to the anterior papillary muscle and the parietal wall of the right ventricle; (B) Window dissection into the left ventricle shows the inlet component surrounding the mitral valve, the ventriculoaortic junction tract, the papillary muscles, and the fine criss-crossing trabeculations at the apex; (C) Removal of the semilunar leaflets of the pulmonary valve and endocardial dissection of the right ventricle outflow tract. The sinotubular junction (blue dashed line), the anatomic ventriculoarterial junction (dark blue dashed line); intervalvular trigones (*); the semilunar attachments of the three arterial valvular leaflets (red line), and the virtual ring formed by joining basal attachment of semilunar leaflets (green dashed line), which correspond to the hemodynamic ventriculoarterial junction, are seen. No "annulus" is supporting the attachments of the leaflets; (D) The aortic root has been opened longitudinally to display the level of the sinotubular junction, orifices of the coronary arteries (red arrows), and the area of fibrous continuity (broken line) between aortic and mitral valves. The small black circle marks the membranous septum by transillumination; (E) Photograph of a heart shows the pulmonary and aortic valve sinuses. The kidney-shaped vestibule of the mitral valve is shown from the atrial side. Note the coronary sinus next to the atrioventricular groove surrounding the mitral valve from behind; (F) Histological sections at the level of the orifices of the coronary arteries stained with elastic van Gieson of a specimen shown the anatomic ventriculoarterial junction. Note that the basal attachment of the aortic valvar leaflets to the ventricular myocardium is proximal relative to the anatomic junction. Also note that the right coronary sinus frequently exhibits myocardial extensions to the vicinity of the coronary artery orifice (green arrow); (G) Histologic sagittal section of the right ventricular infundibulum, pulmonary valve root, left ventricle outflow tract, and aortic root stained with Masson trichrome. Note the contact area between both outflow tracts that there are connections (asterisk) between myocytes in the contact area between both outflow tracts; (H) Cross histological section stained with Masson trichrome through the left and the right atria. Note the anatomic relation of the right ventricle outflow tract with the subaortic outflow. Also note the close proximity to the epicardial coronary vessel, and the left atrial appendage, relevant during the epicardial approach for arrhythmia ablation

Abbreviations: A, anterior pulmonary sinus; Ao, aorta; CS, coronary sinus; DA, descending artery; IVC, inferior vena cava; L, left coronary sinus; LA, left atrium; LCx, left circumflex artery; LCA, left coronary artery; Lp, left posterior pulmonary sinus. LV, left ventricle; MV, mitral valve; NC, non-coronary sinus; OF, oval fossa; PT, pulmonary trunk; R, right coronary sinus; RA, right atrium; Rp, right posterior pulmonary sinus; RCA, right coronary artery; RVOT, right ventricle outflow tract; SC, supraventricular crest; SVC, superior vena cava; SMT, septomarginal trabeculation; TV, tricuspid valve; LAA, left atrial appendage

not complete compartments but represent extensions of the cavity. The transverse sinus is delineated anteriorly by the posterior surface of the ascending aorta and pulmonary trunk bifurcation and posteriorly by the anterior surface of the atria. The oblique sinus, a large cul-de-sac behind the LA is formed by the continuity between the reflections along the PVs and caval veins. The right and left pulmonary venous recesses are at the back of the LA between the superior and inferior PVs on each side, indenting the side walls of the oblique sinus to a greater or lesser extent. The pericardial reflections at the veins, particularly the PVs, are varied and they can restrict access around the veins. The inferior and superior aortic recesses are extensions from the transverse sinus. The superior recess lies between the ascending aorta and the RA, whereas the inferior recess between the aorta and the LA extends to the level of the aortic valve.[39-42]

The Autonomic Nervous System

Abundant nerves and ganglions of the autonomic nervous system are present at the junction between the PVs and the LA, and some more distally inside the vein. A regional

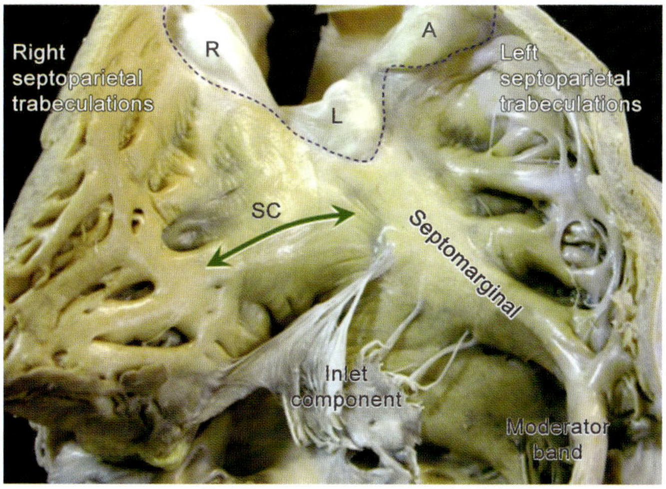

Figure 6.12: The anterior wall of the right ventricle (RV) is opened to show the three components of the ventricle: the inlet (tricuspid valve), apical trabecular and right ventricular outflow tract (RVOT) or infundibulum. The leaflets of the pulmonary trunk (PT) are mainly supported by the RVOT, however, at the level of their commissures the leaflets are attached to the pulmonary artery trunk. Note the location of the supraventricular crest (SC) and septomarginal trabeculation (SMT). The body of SMT continues as an important muscular strand, the moderator band to the anterior papillary muscle and the parietal wall of the RV. The septomarginal trabeculation (SMT) (septal band) consist of a body and two limbs anterior and posterior. The anterior limb extends along the infundibulum and the posterior limb runs toward the tricuspid valve (TV). The septoparietal trabeculations takes origin from the anterior margin of the SMT and extends along the parietal ventricular wall of the infundibulum

Abbreviations: A, anterior pulmonary sinus; L, left pulmonary sinus; R, right pulmonary sinus; SC, supraventricular crest

distribution of the cardiac nerves and differential patterns of innervation have been observed in mammalian hearts. In the human left atrium, ganglionated plexi were observed in the superior surface between the PVs and in the posterior aspect of the LA. Preganglionic parasympathetic and postganglionic sympathetic fibers come together in the fat pads on the epicardial surface of the posterior LA wall. Histochemical studies for acetylcholinesterase, have shown epicardial ganglionated nerves that extend through 3 neural pathways or subplexus in the left atrium; the left ventral, the left dorsal and the middle dorsal. Interestingly, the left dorsal subplexus extends over the area of the vein of Marshall along the epicardial aspect of the left posterolateral ridge.

A quantitative histological evaluation identified gradients of innervation in the LA and in the PVs. This study showed that the greatest nerve density was found in the left and posterior parts of the LA and at the antrum of the PVs. The left-sided PVs had a more dense nervous system elements content than the right-sided veins, and the density of innervation was higher at the orifices of the PVs than in their distal segments.[43-45]

Anatomic Risk of Esophagus, Vagus and Phrenic Nerves Injury during Ablation Procedure

The development of an atrioesophageal fistula after catheter ablation in the posterior wall of the LA is probably the most severe complication that has been encountered in patients subjected to an ablation procedure. Understanding the spatial relations between the esophagus and the LA is essential to reduce this risk. The esophagus descends in virtual contact with the posterior wall of the LA **(Figures 6.13C and D)**. Behind the posterior left atrial wall is a layer of fibrous pericardium and fibrofatty tissue of irregular thickness that contains esophageal arteries and the vagus nerve plexus.[19] These anatomic structures may be affected by ablative procedures. Radiofrequency may substantially elevate the temperature within the esophageal lumen resulting in subacute inflammatory reaction of the esophageal wall. Thus, it is strongly recommended to avoid excessively deep lesions by decreasing the power and duration of RF energy application in the posterior LA wall.[46]

Thermal injury may involve the periesophageal vagal nerves resulting in acute pyloric spasm and gastric hypomotility. The vagus nerves pass behind the root of the lungs and form right and left posterior pulmonary plexi. From the caudal part of the left pulmonary plexus, two branches descend on the anterior surface of the esophagus joining with a branch from the right pulmonary plexus to form the anterior esophageal plexus. The anterior esophageal plexus passes external to the pericardial sac but in very close proximity to the posterior and to the right and left venoatrial junctions. The posterior and anterior esophageal plexi enter the abdomen through the diaphragm to become the posterior and anterior vagal trunks that innervate the pyloric sphincter and the gastric antrum. Our anatomic observation in normal cadavers revealed a mean distance between the bundles of the anterior esophageal plexus and posterior left trial endocardium of 4.1 ± 1.4 mm (range: 2.5–6.5 mm).

The right phrenic nerve has a close anatomic relationship with the SVC and the right PVs **(Figures 6.13E and F)**. Consequently, catheter ablation techniques aimed at modifying the sinus node function at the lateral right atrium and AF ablation at the orifice and adjacent area of the right superior PV carry a certain risk of injuring the right phrenic nerve.[20] Our study on cadavers also revealed that the left phrenic nerve and its accompanying pericardiophrenic vessels in the fibrous pericardium were overlying the atrial appendage in majority of cases **(Figure 6.13F)**. On the other hand, the left phrenic nerve descends along the obtuse cardiac margin in relation with the left obtuse marginal vein (minimal distance 3.5 ± 0.5 mm) in 79% of our specimens. In the remaining specimens, its course was anterosuperior, passing over the main stem of the left coronary artery or the anterior descending artery and the great cardiac vein (minimal distance 1.4 ± 0.3 mm). These anatomic details

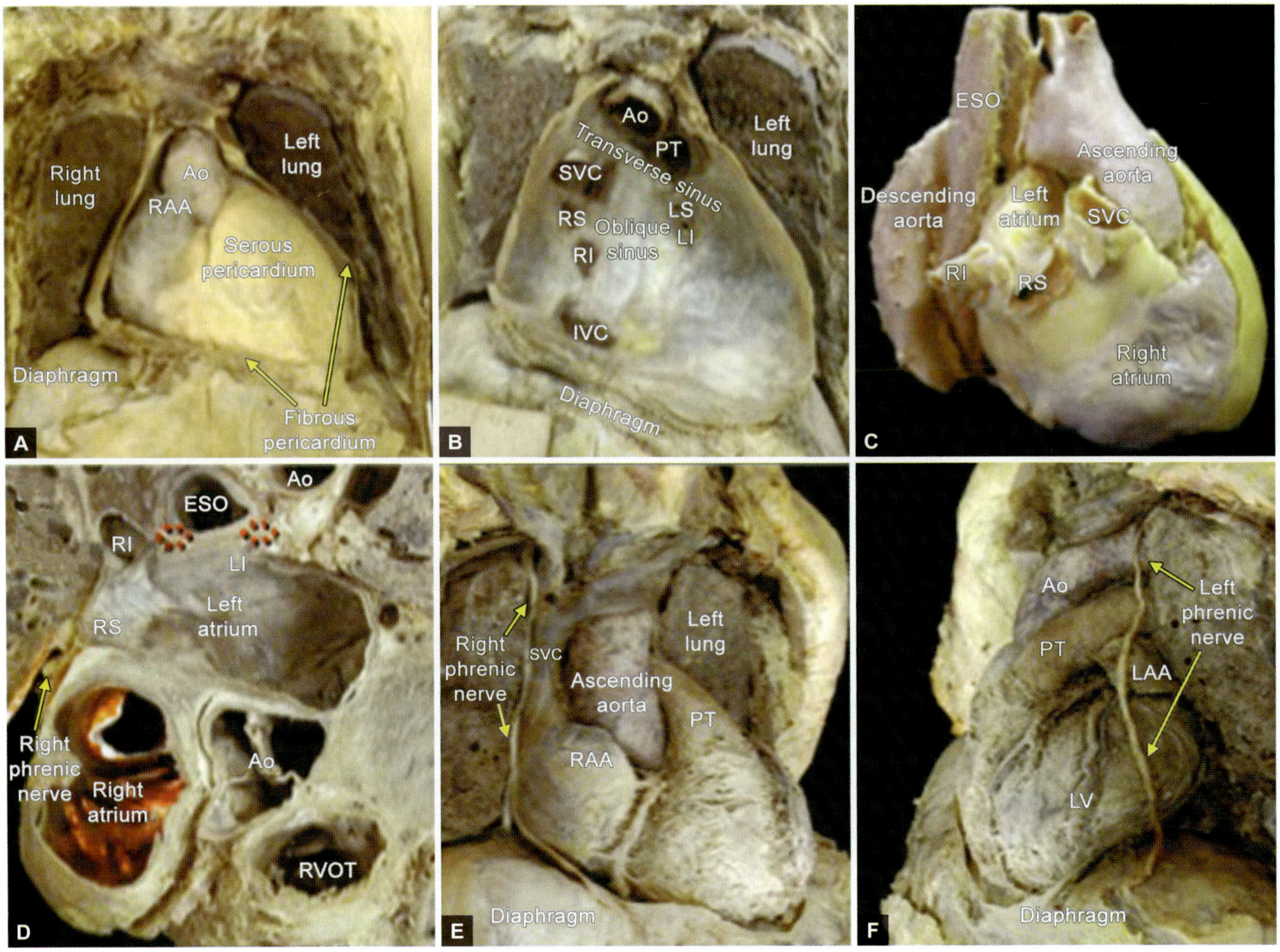

Figures 6.13A to F: (A) Pericardial surfaces of cadaveric heart photographed in attitudinal position to simulate the view as seen in living condition; (B) This dissection of a cadaver viewed from the front shows the sinuses (transverse and oblique) following removal of the heart; (C) Specimen viewed from a right posterolateral perspective to show the course of the esophagus and descending aorta relative to the left atrium; (D) An overview of a transthoracic section through a cadaver showing the locations of the esophagus, the descending aorta, the vagus nerves (red dashed circles) and right phrenic nerve. Note the minimal distance between the posterior endocardial surface of the left atrium and esophagus, and the right superior pulmonary vein to the phrenic nerve; (E) This dissection shows a right lateral view of the heart. The course of the right phrenic nerve is closely related to the superior cavo-atrial junction and the orifice of the right superior pulmonary vein; (F) Left lateral view of the heart showing the close anatomic relation of the left phrenic nerve with the left atrial appendage and the lateral wall of the left ventricle to penetrate into the left part of the diaphragm

Abbreviations: Ao, aorta; ESO, esophagus; IVC, inferior vena cava; LAA, left atrial appendage; LI, left inferior pulmonary vein; LS, left superior pulmonary vein; LV, left ventricle; PT, pulmonary trunk; RAA, right atrial appendage; RI, right inferior pulmonary vein; RS, right superior pulmonary vein; SVC, superior vena cava; RVOT, right ventricular outflow tract

are also relevant during pacing close to these areas during CRT to avoid phrenic nerve capture.[47-48]

REFERENCES

1. Cosío FG, Anderson RH, Kúck KH, Becker A, Borggrefe M, Campbell RW, Gaita F, Guiraudon GM, Haïssaguerre M, Rufilanchas JJ, Thiene G, Wellens HJ, Langberg J, Benditt DG, Bharati S, Klein G, Marchlinski F, Saksena S. Living anatomy of the atrioventricular junctions. A guide to electrophysiologic mapping. A Consensus Statement from the Cardiac Nomenclature Study Group, Working Group of Arrhythmias, European Society of Cardiology, and the Task Force on Cardiac Nomenclature from NASPE. Circulation. 1999;100:e31-7.
2. Farré J, Anderson RH, Cabrera JA, et al. Cardiac Anatomy for Catheter Mapping and Ablation of Arrhythmias. In: Huang SK, Wood MA (Eds). Catheter Ablation of Cardiac Arrhythmias, 2nd edn. Elsevier Inc. Philadelphia (USA); 2011. pp. 74-102.
3. Cabrera JA, Sámchez-Quintána D. Cardiac anatomy: What the electrophysiologist need to know. Heart. 2013;99:417-31.

4. Ho SY, Anderson RH, Sánchez-Quintana D. Gross structure of the atriums: more than an anatomical curiosity. Pacing Clin Electrophysiol. 2002;25:342-50.
5. Ho SY, Sánchez-Quintana D. The importance of atrial structure and fibers. Clin Anat. 2009;22:52-63.
6. Sánchez-Quintana D, Anderson RH, Cabrera JA, Climent V, Martin R, Farre J, Ho SY. The terminal crest: morphological features relevant to electrophysiology. Heart. 2002;88:406-11.
7. Sánchez-Quintana D, Cabrera JA, Farré J, Climent V, Anderson RH, Ho SY. Sinus node revisited in the era of electroanatomical mapping and catheter ablation. Heart. 2005;91:189-94.
8. Inoue S, Becker AE. Koch's triangle sized up: anatomical landmarks in perspective of catheter ablation procedures. Pacing Clin Electrophysiol. 1998;21:1553-8.
9. Sánchez-Quintana D, Picazo-Angelín B, Cabrera A, Murillo M, Cabrera JA. Koch's triangle and the atrioventricular node in Ebstein's anomaly: implications for catheter ablation. Rev Esp Cardiol. 2010;63:660-7.
10. Inoue S, Becker AE. Posterior extensions of the human compact atrioventricular node: a neglected anatomic feature of potential clinical significance. Circulation. 1998;97:188-93.
11. Medkour D, Becker AE, Khalife K, Billette J. Anatomic and functional characteristics of a slow posterior AV nodal pathway: role in dual-pathway physiology and reentry. Circulation 1998;98:164-74.
12. Ho SY, Anderson RH, Sánchez-Quintana D. Atrial structure and fibers: morphologic bases of atrial conduction. Cardiovasc Res. 2002;54:325-36.
13. Cabrera JA, Sánchez-Quintana D, Ho SY, Medina A, Anderson RH. The architecture of the atrial musculature between the orifice of the inferior caval vein and the tricuspid valve: the anatomy of the isthmus. J Cardiovasc Electrophysiol. 1998;9: 1186-95.
14. Cabrera JA, Sánchez-Quintana D, Ho SY, Medina A, Wanguemert F, Gross E, Grillo J, Hernandez E, Anderson RH. Angiographic anatomy of the inferior right atrial isthmus in patients with and without history of common atrial flutter. Circulation. 1999;99:3017-23.
15. Cabrera JA, Sánchez-Quintana D, Farré J, Rubio JM, Ho SY. The inferior right atrial isthmus: further architectural insights for current and coming ablation technologies. J Cardiovasc Electrophysiol. 2005;16:402-8.
16. Waki K, Saito T, Becker AE. Right atrial flutter isthmus revisited: normal anatomy favors nonuniform anisotropic conduction. J Cardiovasc Electrophysiol. 2000;11:90-4.
17. Sánchez-Quintana D, Ho SY, Cabrera JA, Farre J, Anderson RH. Topographic anatomy of the inferior pyramidal space: relevance to radiofrequency catheter ablation. J Cardiovasc Electrophysiol. 2001;12:210-7.
18. Cabrera JA, Farré J, Ho SY, et al. Anatomy of the left atrium relevant to atrial fibrillation ablation. In: Aliot E, Haïssaguerre M, Jackman WM (Eds). Catheter ablation of atrial fibrillation. Blackwell Futura. Oxford (UK); 2008. pp. 3-31.
19. Ho SY, Sánchez-Quintana D, Cabrera JA, Anderson RH. Anatomy of the left atrium: implications for radiofrequency ablation of atrial fibrillation. J Cardiovasc Electrophysiol. 1999; 10:1525-33.
20. Ho SY, Cabrera JA, Sánchez-Quintana D. Left atrial anatomy revisited. Circ Arrhythm Electrophysiol. 2012;5:220-8.
21. Ho SY, Cabrera JA, Tran VH, Farre J, Anderson RH, Sanchez-Quintana D. Architecture of the pulmonary veins: relevance to radiofrequency ablation. Heart. 2001;86:265-70.
22. Cabrera JA, Ho SY, Climent V, Sanchez-Quintana D. The architecture of the left lateral atrial wall: a particular anatomic region with implications for ablation of atrial fibrillation. Eur Heart J. 2008;29:356-62.
23. Cabrera JA, Ho SY, Climent V, Fuertes B, Murillo M, Sanchez-Quintana D. Morphological evidence of muscular connections between contiguous pulmonary venous orifices: relevance of the interpulmonary isthmus for catheter ablation in atrial fibrillation. Heart Rhythm. 2009;6:1192-8.
24. Becker AE. Left atrial isthmus: anatomic aspects relevant for linear catheter ablation procedures in humans. J Cardiovasc Electrophysiol. 2004;15:809-12.
25. Qamruddin S, Shinbane J, Shriki J, Fuertes B, Murillo M, Sanchez-Quintana D. Left atrial appendage: structure, function, imaging modalities and therapeutic options. Expert Rev Cardiovasc Ther. 2010;8:65-75.
26. Cabrera JA, Saremi F, Sánchez-Quintana D. Left atrial appendage: Anatomy and imaging landmarks pertinent to percutaneous transcatheter occlusion. Heart. 2014;100: 1636-50.
27. Su P, McCarthy KP, Ho SY. Occluding the left atrial appendage: anatomical considerations. Heart. 2008;94:1166-70.
28. Saremi F, Muresian H, Sánchez-Quintana D. Coronary veins: comprehensive CT-anatomic classification and review of variants and clinical implications. Radiographics. 2012;32: E1-32.
29. Chauvin M, Shah DC, Haïssaguerre M, Marcellin L, Brechenmacher C. The anatomic basis of connections between the coronary sinus musculature and the left atrium in humans. Circulation. 2000;101:647-52.
30. Noheria A, DeSimone CV, Lachman N, Edwards WD, Gami AS, Maleszewski JJ, Friedman PA, Munger TM, Hammill SC, Hayes DL, Packer DL, Asirvatham SJ. Anatomy of the coronary sinus and epicardial coronary venous system in 620 hearts: an electrophysiology perspective. J Cardiovasc Electrophysiol. 2013;24:1-6.
31. Ho SY, Nihoyannopoulos P. Anatomy, echocardiography, and normal right ventricular dimensions. Heart. 2006;92(Suppl 1): i2-13.
32. Hai JJ, Lachman N, Syed FF, Desimore CV, Asirvatham SJ. Tha anatomic basis for ventricular arrhythmia in the normal heart: what the student of anatomy need to know. Clin Anat. 2014;27:885-93.
33. Partridge JB, Anderson RH. Left ventricular anatomy: its nomenclature, segmentation, and planes of imaging. Clin Anat. 2009;22:77-84.
34. Saremi F, Ho SY, Cabrera JA; Sánchez.Quintana D. Right ventricular outflow tract imaging with CT and MRI: Part 1. Morphology. Am J Roengenol. 2013;200:w39-50.
35. Saremi F, Ho SY, Cabrera JA, Sánchez-Quintana D. Right ventricular outflow tract with CT and MRI: Part 2, Function. Am J Roentgenol. 2013;200:w51-61.
36. De Ponti R, Ho SY. Mapping of right ventricular outflow tract tachycardia/ectopies: activation mapping versus pace mapping. Heart Rhythm. 2008;5:345-7.
37. Gami AS, Noheria A, Lachman N, Edwards WD, Friedman PA, Talreja D, Hammill SC, Munger TM, Packer DL, Asirvatham SJ. Anatomical correlates relevant to ablation above the semilunar valves for the cardiac electrophysiologist: a study of 603 hearts. J Interv Card Electrophysiol. 2011;30:5-15.
38. Natale A, Raviele A, Al-Ahmad A, Alfieri O, Aliot E, Almendral J, Breithardt G, Brugada J, Calkins H, Callans D, Cappato R,

Camm JA, Della Bella P, Guiraudon GM, Haissaguerre M, Hindricks G, Ho SY, Kuck KH, Marchlinski F, Packer DL, Prystowsky EN, Reddy VY, Ruskin JN, Scanavacca M, Shivkumar K, Soejima K, Stevenson WJ, Themistoclakis S, Verma A, Wilber D. Venice Chart International Consensus document on ventricular tachycardia/ventricular fibrillation ablation. J Cardiovasc Electrophysiol. 2010;21:339-79.

39. D'Avila A, Scanavacca M, Sosa E, Ruskin JN, Reddy VY. Pericardial anatomy for the interventional electrophysiologist. J Cardiovasc Electrophysiol. 2003;14:422-30.
40. Akhter SA. The heart and pericardium. Thorac Surg Clin. 2011;21:205-17.
41. Scanavacca MI, Venancio AC, Pisani CF, Lara S, Hachul D, Darrieux F, Hardy C, Paola E, Aiello VD, Mahapatra S, Sosa E. Percutaneous transatrial access to the pericardial space for epicardial mapping and ablation. Circ Arrhythm Electrophysiol. 2011;4:331-6.
42. Macedo PG1, Kapa S, Mears JA, Fratianni A, Asirvatham SJ. Correlative anatomy for the electrophysiologist: ablation for atrial fibrillation. Part I: pulmonary vein ostia, superior vena cava, vein of Marshall. J Cardiovasc Electrophysiol. 2010;21:721-30.
43. Pauza DH, Skripka V, Pauziene N, Stropus R. Morphology, distribution, and variability of the epicardiac neural ganglionated subplexuses in the human heart. Anat Rec. 2000;259:353-82.
44. Vaitkevicius R, Saburkina I, Rysevaite K, Vaitkeviciene I, Pauziene N, Zaliunas R, Schauerte P, Jalife J, Pauza DH. Nerve supply of the human pulmonary veins: an anatomical study. Heart Rhythm. 2009;6:221-8.
45. Ho SY, Cabrera JA, Sánchez-Quintana D. Vagaries of the vagus nerve: relevance to ablationists. J Cardiovasc Electrophysiol. 2006;17:330-1.
46. Sánchez-Quintana D, Cabrera JA, Climent V, Farre J, Mendonca MC, Ho SY. Anatomic relations between the esophagus and left atrium and relevance for ablation of atrial fibrillation. Circulation. 2005;112:1400-5.
47. Sánchez-Quintana D, Cabrera JA, Climent V, Farre J, Weiglein A, Ho SY. How close are the phrenic nerves to cardiac structures? Implications for cardiac interventionalists. J Cardiovasc Electrophysiol. 2005;16:309-13.
48. Sánchez-Quintana D, Ho SY, Climent V, Murillo M, Cabrera JA. Anatomic evaluation of the left phrenic nerve relevant to epicardial and endocardial catheter ablation: implications for phrenic nerve injury. Heart Rhythm. 2009;6:764-8.

EDITORS' SUMMARY

The world's pioneering experts on correlating anatomy with the needs of invasive electrophysiology—Drs Cabrera and Sanchez-Quintana (partnering with Dr Castrejon) from Madrid and Badajoz—have provided for the readers of this textbook the clear pointed and organized information set that simplify for us a complex and highly nuanced subject. As with any anatomy-focused writing, this installment is studded with the incomparable dissections of Dr Sanchez-Quintana and collaborators to visually emphasize the needs and correlative reflexes required for the ablationist that the written word alone cannot provide.

We, as students of electrophysiology, are reminded that the purpose of being informed and mastering the anatomic subtext of our field is not to be experts in anatomy but rather to be able to correlate fluoroscopy, intraprocedural nonfluoroscopic imaging, and our primary visualization—the sensed electrograms with the underlying anatomy in a given patient. Without such detailed yet fundamental understanding, extrapolation to pathology and congenital anomalies become impossible. Specific areas where such correlation is essential and well-highlighted in this chapter include:

- The right atrium. Anatomic transitions abound in this chamber and include the pectinates as they become the crista terminalis with a near perpendicular anisotropy and thus resulting zones of slow conduction and double potentials along the long axes of this bundle, as well as the neighboring Eustachian ridge. Another example includes the transition between the remnants of the sinus venosus with both the primordial atrium and the pulmonary venous atrium.
- The pulmonary venous atrium and pulmonary veins. The authors, who have provided the bulk of our field's knowledge of these structures, outline the complexity of the venoatrial junction, as well as the veins themselves and the relationship with the left atrial appendage, as well as the externally developed remains of the left superior vena cava and the left horn of the sinus venosus.
- The ventricular outflow tract. Perhaps the most complex structures within and around which we routinely perform our ablation procedures are the ventricular outflow tracts. The left-to-right as well as anterior and posterior intertwining of the outflow tracts, their relationship to the semilunar valves and the junction with the right ventricular inflow (crista supraventricularis) and the left ventricular inflow (including the aortic mitral continuity) are both well-described and well-illustrated and will form a valuable bulwark for an interventional electrophysiologist mapping and ablating in this area.

CHAPTER 7

Gerard Loughlin, Karen Ordovas, Edward P Gerstenfeld

Imaging in Cardiac Electrophysiology

LIST OF ABBREVIATIONS

18-F-FDG	Flourine-18 Fluorodeoxyglucose	LSVC	Left Superior Vena Cava
AF	Atrial Fibrillation	LV	Left Ventricle
ARVC	Arrhythmogenic Right Ventricular Cardiomyopathy	LVEF	Left Ventricular Ejection Fraction
CMR	Cardiac Magnetic Resonance Imaging	MDCT	Multidetector Computerized Tomography
CRT	Cardiac Resynchronization Therapy	MI	Myocardial Infarction
CT	Computerized Tomography	MR	Magnetic Resonance
DE	Delayed Enhancement	MRI	Magnetic Resonance Imaging
EAM	Electroanatomical Mapping	PET	Position Emission Tomography
Gd	Gadolinium	PV	Pulmonary Vein
ICD	Implantable Cardioverter-Defibrillator	PVI	Pulmonary Vein Isolation
ICE	Intracardiac Echocardiography	RV	Right Ventricle
LA	Left Atrial	SCD	Sudden Cardiac Death
LAA	Left Atrial Appendage	SSFP	Steady State Free Precession
LGE	Late Gadolinium Enhancement	TEE	Transesophageal Echocardiography
		VT	Ventricular Tachycardia

INTRODUCTION

Early electrophysiology procedures targeted specific discrete electrophysiological targets such as an accessory atrioventricular pathway or the focal origin of an atrial tachycardia. However, over the past decade ablation procedures have been developed for more complex arrhythmias such as atrial fibrillation (AF) and scar-based ventricular tachycardia (VT). Treatment of these arrhythmias often involves sophisticated imaging, initially to guide diagnosis and understand the underlying substrate, and then for treatment which increasingly relies on anatomic targets such as the pulmonary veins for atrial fibrillation and heterogeneous scar for VT. This chapter will outline the contributions of each imaging modality to the management of specific arrhythmia syndromes.

CARDIAC MAGNETIC RESONANCE IMAGING

Atrial Fibrillation

AF is the most common sustained arrhythmia in the general population. Management options range from ventricular rate control to restoration and maintenance of sinus rhythm using antiarrhythmic drugs or catheter ablation. Catheter ablation is now a Class I indication for symptomatic, paroxysmal AF breaking through a single antiarrhythmic agent. The ablation approach has increasingly become an anatomically guided procedure, targeting circumferential electrical isolation of the pulmonary veins. Since up to 15% of patients may have variations in pulmonary vein anatomy, cardiac magnetic resonance imaging (CMR) is now widely used to evaluate left atrial anatomy prior to the procedure and also shows promise as a potential prognostic tool.

CMR as a Risk Stratification Tool in AF

Both animal models and human studies have shown that recurrent atrial fibrillation leads to atrial fibrosis. In turn, progressive atrial fibrosis represents the ideal substrate for arrhythmia recurrence and, eventually, for progression to persistent forms of atrial fibrillation.[1] Consequently, it has been proposed that the degree of atrial fibrosis could act as a marker of disease progression, and potentially aid in selection of patients more likely to benefit from a rhythm control approach.

Myocardial fibrosis is associated with substitution of normal myocytes with fibroblasts and collagen deposition. The resulting increase in extracellular matrix volume, with parallel reductions in capillary density, leads to altered Gadolinium (Gd) kinetics, whereby Gd washout from fibrous areas is impaired as compared to remote healthy myocardium. CMR images can then be obtained 10–15 minutes postcontrast administration, using an inversion recovery pulse to suppress the signal from normal myocardium resulting in enhancement of the signal from the gadolinium accumulated in fibrous areas.

Delayed enhancement CMR (DE-CMR) can thus be used to visualize the extent of atrial fibrosis, which has been shown to correlate with ablation outcomes in various studies[2,3] leading some authors to postulate that DE-CMR-derived data may aid in patient selection for AF ablation procedures. One such example of this tailored approach comes from Marrouche and colleagues,[4,5] who have proposed a 4 stage classification of AF patients according to the extent of late Gadolinium enhancement (LGE) relative to total LA wall volume ["Utah stages" I (defined as LGE < 10%), II (10–20%), III (20–30%) and IV (>30%)]. This group describes a significant increase in single-procedure recurrence rates with each stage, with as many as 71.4% of patients suffering AF recurrence within one year in stage IV.[5] Based on these findings, the authors recommend opting for PVI in patients with "Utah stage" I, II and certain stage III subjects with more focal fibrosis, while pursuing a more conservative approach for stage III patients with diffusely distributed LGE as well as stage IV patients **(Figure 7.1)**.

CMR-based assessment of atrial fibrosis may also have prognostic value regarding stroke risk, as shown by Daccarett et al.[6] In their series of AF patients referred for DE-CMR, those with prior stroke had significantly greater extent of atrial scar, and increasing thromboembolic risk (measured with the CHADS score) was associated with increasing degrees of atrial fibrosis. Further large prospective studies may clarify whether atrial fibrosis detected using DE-CMR increases the predictive value of established thromboembolic risk stratification schemes such as the CHADS-VASc score.

Preprocedural CMR

Episodes of AF are typically triggered by firing from sleeves of cardiac muscle that extend into the pulmonary veins.[7] Delivery of circumferential lesions around the pulmonary vein antra with the aim of electrical isolation (pulmonary vein isolation) has become an accepted treatment option for AF patients.

Contrast enhanced "gated" CMR is the method of choice for pulmonary vein assessment prior to catheter ablation, as it avoids exposing the patient to additional ionizing radiation. For patients in whom gadolinium contrast administration is undesirable (such as patients with advanced renal failure) 3D steady state-free precession (SSFP) sequences are a useful alternative.[8]

Key features to be assessed include left atrial size, anatomical relationships with relevant neighboring structures such as the left atrial appendage (in close proximity to the left superior pulmonary vein), superior vena cava (right superior pulmonary vein) and esophagus (posterior left atrial wall) and variations in pulmonary vein anatomy, most importantly their number and spatial orientation. Pulmonary vein anatomy is subject to a certain variability, with the most common pattern involving four distinct pulmonary vein ostia **(Figure 7.2A)**; however up to 10% of patients may have a large common left PV trunk, single or multiple mid-right pulmonary veins,[9] or more unusual anatomic variants such as an accessory pulmonary vein inserting into the left atrial roof **(Figure 7.2B)**. A CMR can also be registered with left atrial fiducial points acquired with intracardiac catheters to allow electrophysiologists to use the 3D CMR as a model and record ablation points **(Figure 7.3A)** or bipolar voltage **(Figure 7.3B)** directly on the CMR image.

Atrial fibrillation ablation entails the risk of mobilizing previously existing left atrial thrombi, and thus imaging techniques aimed at ruling out thrombus prior to the procedure are required in a large majority of patients. Although traditionally transesophageal echocardiography (TEE) has fulfilled this role, in a study by Rathi et al, contrast enhanced CMR was shown to be equivalent to TEE for the detection of left atrial thrombus in a population of low thromboembolic risk patients referred for PVI. In this patient series, a strategy of preprocedural CMR aimed both at providing anatomical information and ruling out thrombus proved to be cost-effective as compared to a combined

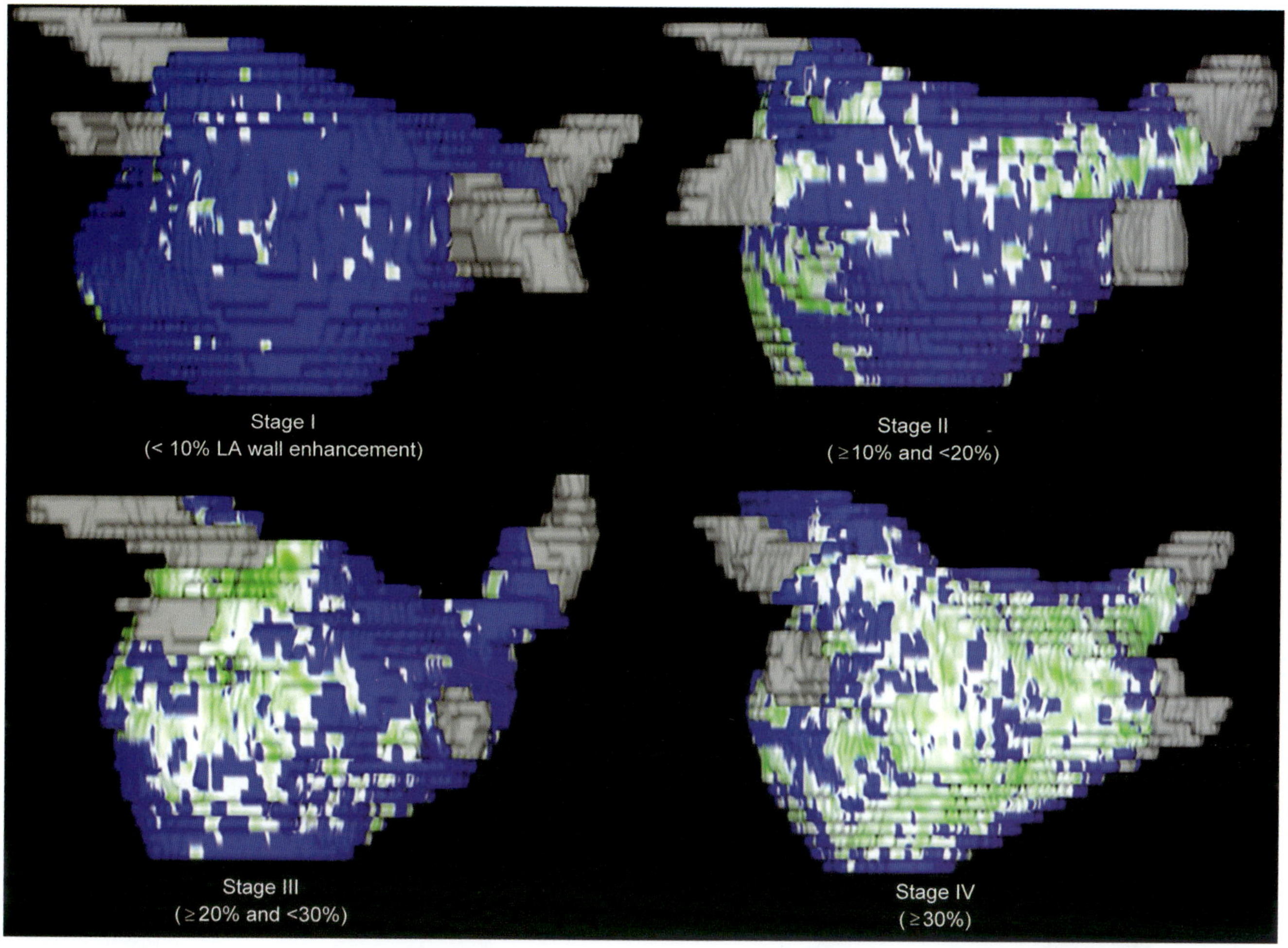

Figure 7.1: Four stages of left atrial (LA) structural remodeling based on 3-dimensional late gadolinium enhancement MRI scans. Representative examples from patients in each stage of LA remodeling in posterior–anterior views (above examples of stages I–IV are 3%, 13%, 26%, and 56%, respectively). Normal LA wall is displayed in blue with remodeling changes in green. The pulmonary veins are shown in gray
From: McGann C et al. Circ Arrhythm Electrophysiol. 2014;7:23-30, with permission

CMR-TEE approach, also avoiding the potential risks of a semi-invasive technique such as TEE.[10]

CMR for Postprocedural Assessment

Finally, CMR can be used to detect certain post-procedural complications associated with PVI. One such example is atrioesophageal fistula, an infrequent yet potentially lethal complication of PVI linked to delivery of high-power radiofrequency energy to the posterior left atrial wall. Although rare in clinical practice, small studies with systematic postprocedural CMR suggest that the incidence of subclinical damage to the esophagus (ascertained by the presence of delayed enhancement in the anterior esophageal wall) can be as high as 12%[11] whereas a complete left atrial-esophageal fistulae after ablation can be detected by the presence of air in the left atrium **(Figures 7.4A to C)**. CMR is also the diagnostic modality of choice for the detection of PV stenosis, an increasingly rare complication of PVI that can nevertheless be associated with limiting symptoms and morbidity if undiagnosed.

Ventricular Tachycardia

In patients suffering from ventricular tachycardia, CMR can not only aid in establishing the presence or absence of underlying structural heart disease, but also serve as a guide for ablation procedures. CMR can also be used with the objective of refining the risk of sudden death and establishing eligibility for implantation of an implantable cardioverter-defibrillator (ICD).

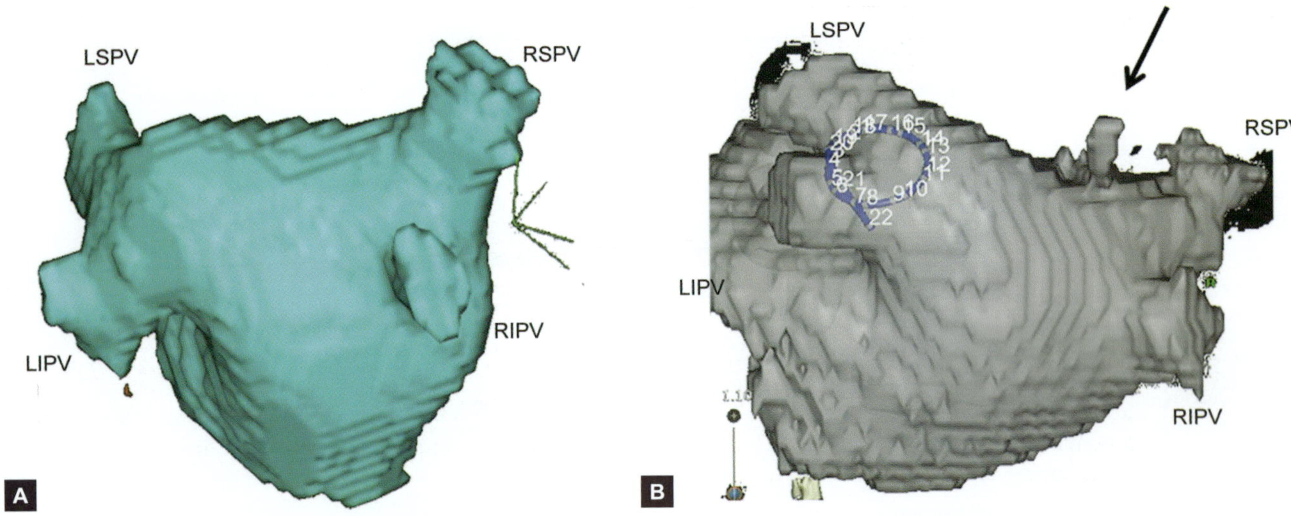

Figures 7.2A and B: (A) Normal cardiac MRI of the left atrium, after segmentation to remove surrounding structures, depicting four separate pulmonary veins; (B) Cardiac MRI in a patient with an accessory pulmonary vein inserting into the left atrial roof (arrow)

Abbreviations: RSPV, right superior pulmonary vein; RIPV, right inferior pulmonary vein; LSPV, left superior pulmonary vein; LIPV, left inferior pulmonary vein

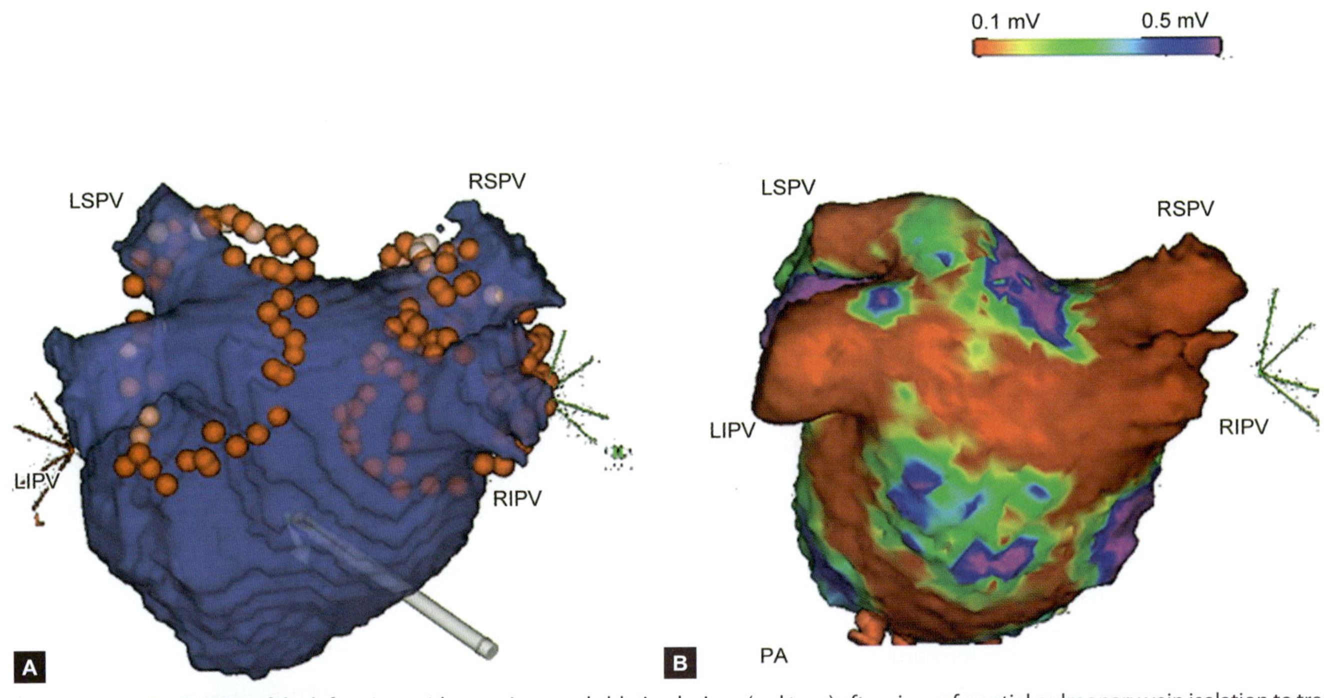

Figures 7.3A and B: (A) MRI of the left atrium with superimposed ablation lesions (red tags) after circumferential pulmonary vein isolation to treat atrial fibrillation; (B) Projection of bipolar voltage on the left atrium in a patient with multiple prior ablations and significant left atrial scarring. Normal voltage is >0.5 mV and depicted as purple (see color bar), while low voltage (scar) is <0.1 mV and depicted as red

Abbreviations: RSPV, right superior pulmonary vein; RIPV, right inferior pulmonary vein; LSPV, left superior pulmonary vein; LIPV, left inferior pulmonary vein

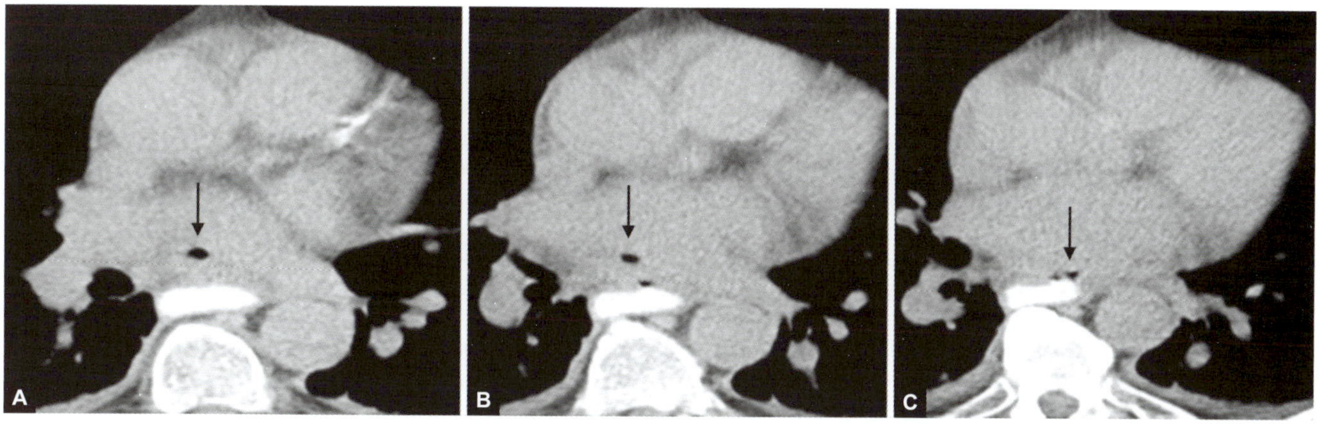

Figures 7.4A to C: LA-esophageal fistula: Axial CT images of the heart with oral contrast at three separate levels demonstrate a small air collection within the left atrium (arrows) which is contiguous with the contrast-filled esophagus

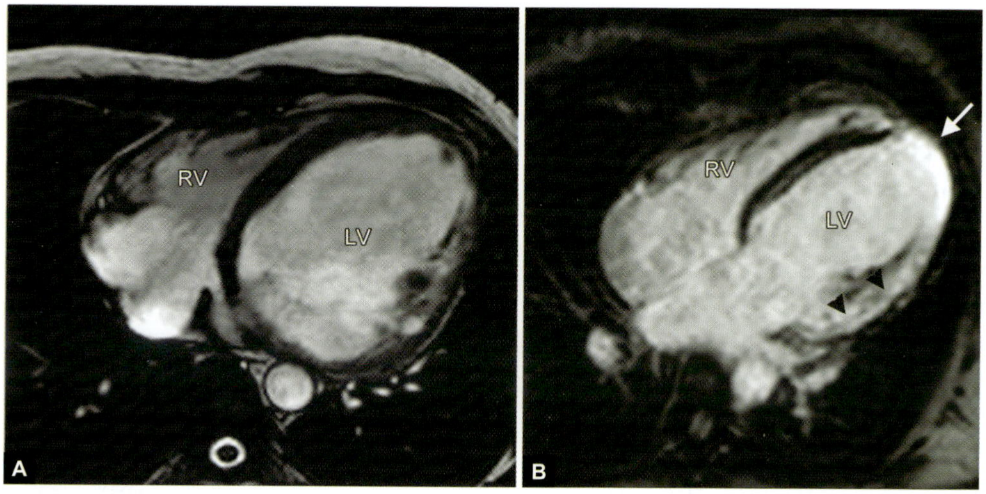

Figures 7.5A and B: Ischemic dilated cardiomyopathy: (A) Axial steady-state free precession cine images show left ventricular enlargement; (B) Delayed enhancement images in the horizontal long-axis plane demonstrate subendocardial hyperenhancement of the lateral left ventricular wall (arrowheads), and transmural hyperenhancement of the apex (arrow)
Abbreviations: LV, left ventricle; RV, right ventricle

Noninvasive Characterization of Myocardial Scar

Sudden cardiac death risk stratification

Post-Myocardial infarction (MI) patients are at risk for sudden cardiac death (SCD), due to ventricular arrhythmias. ICD implantation has been shown to reduce mortality in certain high risk patients,[12] nonetheless, current risk stratification for SCD based on left ventricular ejection fraction (LVEF) remains imperfect. There is general agreement that bundles of surviving myocytes within and in the border of the dense infarct scar lead to slow conduction necessary to sustain reentry,[13] which is in turn the mechanism of the vast majority of post-MI ventricular tachycardia.

DE-CMR can not only serve to asses LVEF and LV volumes, but can also provide insight into the extent and structure of myocardial scar, which has been associated with arrhythmic risk **(Figures 7.5A and B)**. In a small retrospective study, Scott et al. observed that both endocardial scar surface extension and the number of transmural scar segments determined by MRI were associated with appropriate ICD therapies independently of LVEF.[14] Additionally, some authors have proposed that SCD risk stratification may be further refined by quantifying the peri-infarct border zone. This area of heterogeneous tissue would include strands of viable myocardium that would serve as substrate for VT, and could be identified by delayed enhancement CMR as regions with intermediate late gadolinium enhancement (usually defined by a signal intensity between 2 and 3 standard deviations above reference remote healthy myocardium). Using this method Yan et al. described an association between the extent of the peri-infarct border zone and all-cause and cardiovascular mortality, after adjusting for LV ejection fraction and volume. Interestingly, in this study CMR-assessed total infarct size per se did not predict mortality.[15]

Despite differences in arrhythmogenic substrate (including less scar burden, more basal location of scar and greater epicardial involvement), CMR also has potential value for SCD risk stratification in nonischemic cardiomyopathy. In a prospective analysis of both ischemic and nonischemic patients undergoing evaluation for ICD implantation, Klem et al. described that myocardial scarring quantified with DE-MRI predicts adverse outcomes, with a marked increase in the risk of death or appropriate ICD therapy when scar extent is greater than 5%. In patients with LVEF lower than 30% but minimal or no scarring event rates were similar to patients with LVEF >30%, and conversely, in patients with LVEF greater than 30% and extensive scar outcomes were similar to patients with LVEF <30%.[16] CMR quantified replacement fibrosis and diffuse fibrosis have also been proposed as predictors of adverse outcomes in nonischemic cardiomyopathy patients.[17]

Procedure guidance and selection of the optimal approach

Preprocedural delayed enhancement CMR can provide an accurate characterization of myocardial structure in patients undergoing VT ablation, thus guiding the electrophysiologist towards regions of interest likely to harbor the arrhythmogenic substrate. Various studies in post-MI patients suffering from VT have shown that DE-CMR images can be obtained prior to an ablation procedure and successfully integrated with electroanatomical mapping (EAM) data in order to identify arrhythmogenic substrate and guide ablation **(Figures 7.6A to C)**. LGE dense scar has an excellent correlation with areas of low voltage in the EAM.[18,19] Additionally, a small study in nonischemic cardiomyopathy patients revealed that DE-CMR can identify two distinct patterns of scar distribution (one basal anteroseptal and the other basal inferolateral), which could have implications for the ablation strategy[20] **(Figure 7.7)**.

CMR can also be helpful in establishing the optimal approach for ablation, particularly in nonischemic cardiomyopathy where the scarring is often mid-myocardial or epicardial. The ability of CMR to identify and characterize scar holds promise as a means of selecting patients who may benefit from initial epicardial mapping. The extent of heterogeneous scar tissue and the presence of a "patchy" scar pattern have been associated with VT inducibility in a post-MI swine model.[21] Furthermore, in a series of 80 patients with VT and underlying structural heart disease, the presence of subepicardial late gadolinium hyperenhancement had 84% sensitivity and 100% specificity in predicting an epicardial origin of VT,[22] and in a series of nonischemic cardiomyopathy patients basal inferolateral scar frequently required an epicardial approach.[20]

Ventricular Tachycardia in the Setting of Cardiac Sarcoidosis

Sarcoidosis is a systemic disease of unclear etiology characterized by the formation of noncaseating granulomas that can appear in virtually any organ system, with pulmonary involvement being the most common. Sarcoidosis affects

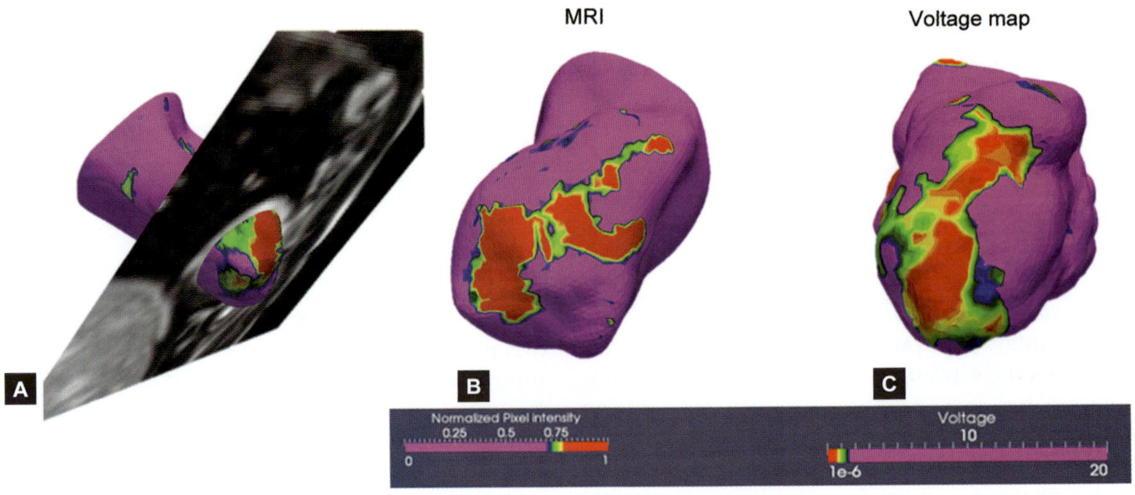

Figures 7.6A to C: (A) Level of delayed enhancement is superimposed on the left ventricular geometry acquired with CMR; (B) Delayed enhancement map of the left ventricle of a swine after creation of and anteroseptal myocardial infarction; red represents low voltage (scar). The scale is normalized to the maximum intensity of the delayed enhancement in the myocardial blood pool; (C) An electroanatomic bipolar voltage map corresponds well with the scar depicted by the processed CMR. For the voltage map, normal voltage (>1.5 mV) is depicted as purple and scar (<0.5 mV) is depicted as red

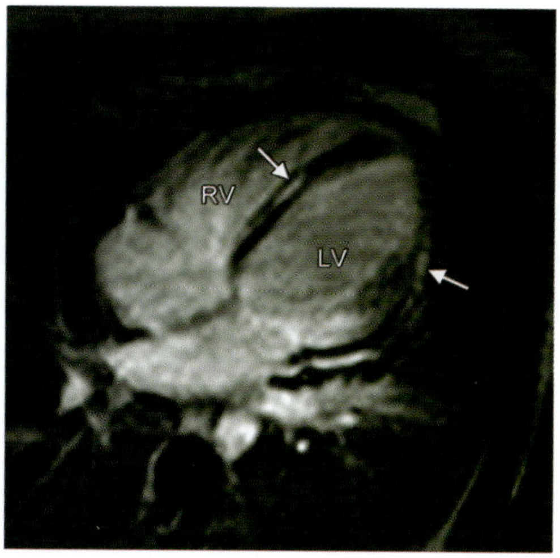

Figure 7.7: Dilated cardiomyopathy mid-wall DE: Delayed enhancement image in the horizontal long-axis plane shows hyperenhancement (arrows) in a mid-wall distribution, involving the septal and lateral left ventricular walls
Abbreviations: LV, left ventricle; RV, right ventricle

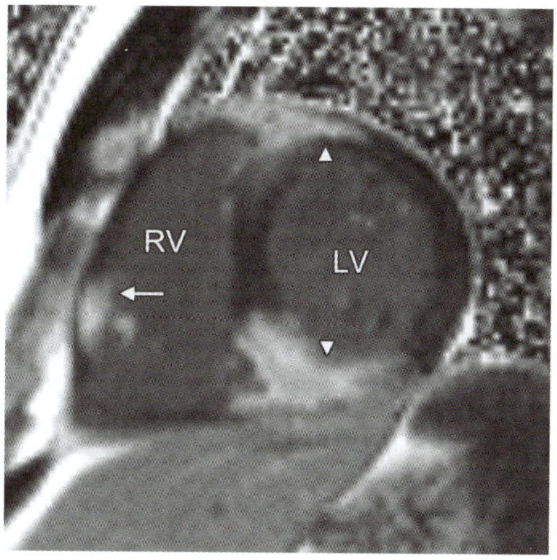

Figure 7.8: Sarcoid: Delayed enhancement image in the short-axis plane shows extensive hyperenhancement in the right ventricular free wall (arrow), and basal areas of the left ventricular septum (arrowheads)
Abbreviations: LV, left ventricle; RV, right ventricle

the heart in up to 25% of patients (with granulomas more often found in the subepicardium and the interventricular septum), leading to conduction abnormalities, ventricular arrhythmias and/or heart failure, and can thus present as sudden cardiac death. As such, sarcoidosis should be considered in the differential diagnosis of young patients presenting with sustained monomorphic VT or unexplained Mobitz II or third degree AV block.[23]

The Heart Rhythm Society has recently published an Expert Consensus Statement on the Diagnosis and Management of Arrhythmias in Patients with cardiac sarcoidosis (CS).[24] This document recognizes the utility of advanced imaging techniques (such as Positron Emission Tomography and CMR) in the work-up of patients suspected of cardiac sarcoid on the basis of initial screening (symptoms, echocardiography or ECG findings). Suspicious findings on MRI for cardiac sarcoidosis include nodular or "patchy" LGE with a distribution atypical for myocardial infarction, involving the mid-myocardium or the epicardium **(Figure 7.8)**. In the setting of acute active inflammation, myocardial thickening and an increased T2 signal suggesting edema can also be found.[25] Interestingly, these findings can be partially reversed with immunosuppressive therapy. It should also be noted that there is a certain overlap in the presentation and diagnostic findings of cardiac sarcoidosis and arrhythmogenic right ventricular cardiomyopathy (ARVC). In this sense, sarcoidosis should be suspected in the presence of interventricular septal late enhancement in CMR or LV dysfunction.[26]

Two additional areas in which CMR has a potential role include: 1) guidance of endomyocardial biopsy, in order to offset the limited diagnostic yield of "blind" unguided biopsy (alternative guidance may be provided by voltage mapping) and 2) sudden cardiac death risk stratification, especially in patients with LVEF > 35%, as it has been proposed that CS patients with normal left ventricular systolic function, absence of conduction abnormalities, no history of either documented or induced ventricular arrhythmias and no LGE on CMR are at low risk for SCD.[24]

Arrhythmogenic Right Ventricular Cardiomyopathy

Arrhythmogenic right ventricular cardiomyopathy (ARVC) is characterized by replacement of right ventricular free wall myocardium with fibrous or fibroadipose tissue. ARVC patients may present with sustained monomorphic ventricular tachycardia originating in the right ventricle, and thus with a left bundle branch block morphology, with either a superior or an inferior axis.[27] In the latter case, differentiation from idiopathic outflow tract VT is fundamental, given the implications of ARVC on sudden death risk and familial screening. CMR is the diagnostic test of choice when excluding the presence of structural heart disease in patients with VT appearing to originate from the right ventricular outflow tract, and can additionally be of value in differentiating ARVC from different forms of right ventricular cardiomyopathy such as cardiac sarcoidosis[26] (see above).

Although, some studies have suggested DE-CMR could identify fibroadipose infiltration with acceptable correlation with histological findings,[28] later reports have highlighted the limited sensitivity and specificity of the identification of intramyocardial fat.[29] Currently, CMR-based tissue characterization is not part of diagnostic criteria for

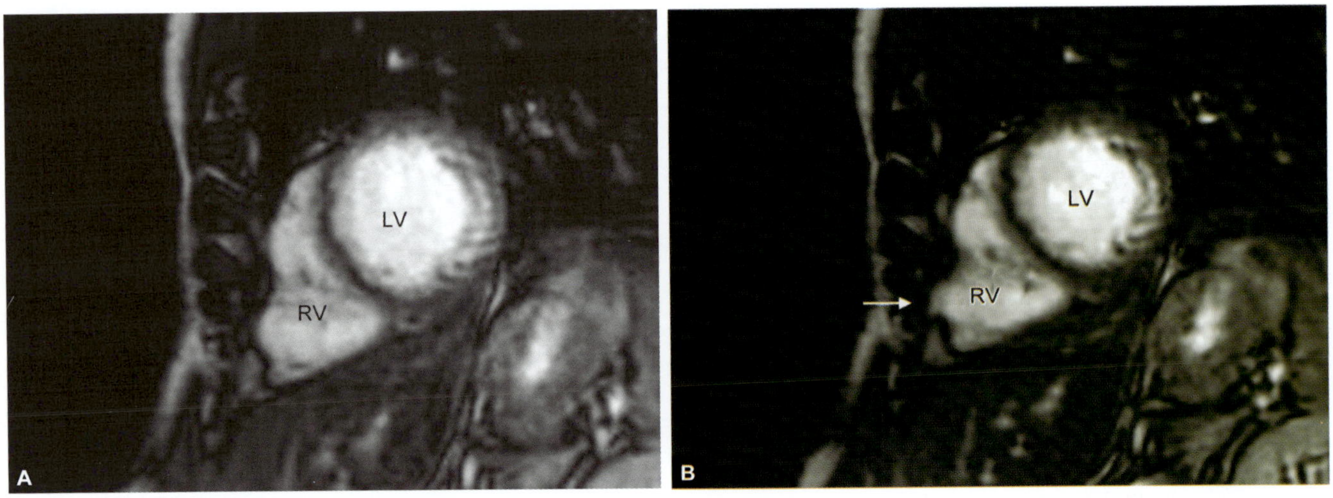

Figures 7.9A and B: ARVC: Short-axis steady-state free precession cine images in the end-diastolic (A) and end-systolic; (B) phases are shown. Notice the focal dyskinetic segment of the right ventricular free wall (arrow)

ARVC, which include regional right ventricular akinesia or dyskinesia in the presence of increased RV dimensions or RV systolic dysfunction[30] **(Figures 7.9A and B)**.

The diagnostic yield of endomyocardial biopsy in ARVC is relatively low as tissue samples are usually obtained from the interventricular septum, which tends to be spared in ARVC. Nonetheless, analogous to cardiac sarcoidosis, CMR (or alternatively electroanatomical mapping) can guide endomyocardial biopsy increasing its sensitivity.

CMR in ICD Patients

With the expanding use of implantable cardioverter-defibrillators (ICD) and the increasing use of CMR, there is a growing likelihood of ICD patients requiring an MRI/CMR during the lifetime of their device. Furthermore, noninvasive scar characterization is an attractive tool in patients with post-ischemic VT, a large number of whom are ICD recipients. Potential complications in ICD patients undergoing thoracic/cardiac MRI include:[31] 1) lead and tissue heating, which in turn can cause tissue edema and damage leading to increased pacing thresholds, 2) vibration and movement of the device lead (usually minimal beyond 6 weeks postimplantation), 3) misinterpretation of radiofrequency pulses by the device as underlying electrical activity, leading to inappropriate withholding of pacing or delivery of antitachycardia pacing or shocks during the MRI, 4) changes in the device's sensing or pacing thresholds, 5) battery depletion or 6) programming changes or "electrical reset" (non-reprogrammable return to a back-up VVI mode with no therapies that may necessitate generator change). Although traditionally CMR has been considered absolutely contraindicated in ICD patients, it has been shown that MR of "non-MR conditional" cardiac devices can be performed safely in patients who are not device dependent and in whom no abandoned leads are present **(Figure 7.10)** when certain safety precautions are adhered to (including device interrogation before and after MR).[32,33] Additionally, more recent efforts have led to the development of "MR conditional" or "MR compatible" ICDs, that include hardware and software modifications that allow them to function normally during and after MR.

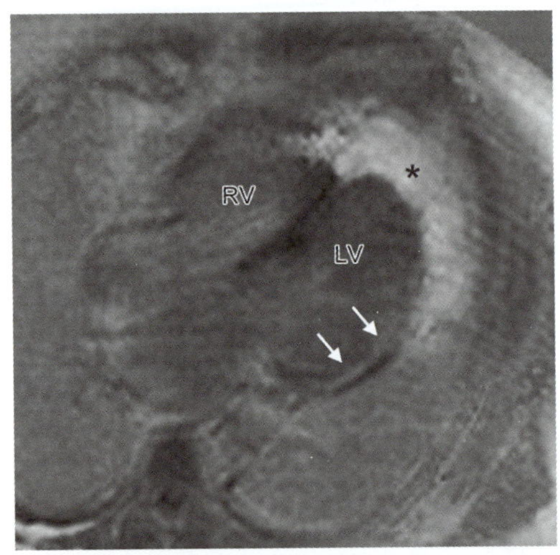

Figure 7.10: MRI scar in patient with implanted defibrillator: Horizontal long-axis delayed enhancement image from a patient with an implanted defibrillator is shown. Although the apical left ventricular regional is obscured by susceptibility artifact (*), it is still possible to identify mid-wall hyperenhancement of the lateral left ventricular wall (arrows)

Abbreviations: LV, left ventricle; RV, right ventricle

Even with dedicated "MR compatible" devices, ICD-related hyperintensity imaging artifacts (which can be mistaken for myocardial scar in LGE studies) remain a significant drawback, typically more prominent in the short-axis plane and affecting regions of the heart close to the device generator (mostly the left ventricular apex and anterior wall).[34] To overcome this limitation Rashid et al. have proposed modifying standard pulse sequences replacing nonselective conventional inversion pulses with a wide-band LGE inversion pulse, which in their study eliminated device hyperintensity image artifacts[35] allowing for diagnostic quality imaging in these patients.

CARDIAC COMPUTERIZED TOMOGRAPHY

The advent of multidetector (64–320 detectors) computerized tomography (MDCT) scanners capable of providing detailed high spatial and temporal (as low as 33 ms[36]) resolution images of the beating heart has had a large impact in the management of patients with structural heart disease, most importantly regarding coronary artery evaluation. The expanding indications of this imaging modality have reached arrhythmia patients, with cardiac computerized tomography (CT) now being performed in a number of different heart rhythm disorders.

Relative to CMR, cardiac CT involves shorter acquisition time (ranging seconds), higher spatial resolution and the possibility of safe use in cardiac device patients.[37] On the other hand, limitations of CT include patient exposure to radiation and iodine-based contrast agents as well as relatively low functional information as compared with CMR.

Atrial Fibrillation

Preprocedural imaging with cardiac computerized tomography (CT) or CMR has become widespread in patients undergoing pulmonary vein isolation for AF and its use has been associated with improved outcomes in retrospective studies.[38] As with CMR, cardiac CT provides information on left atrial size and anatomy, pulmonary vein branching pattern and size, and relations to neighboring structures such as the esophagus **(Figures 7.11A and B)**. This information can be fused with the electroanatomical map increasing spatial awareness and facilitating the ablation procedure. Preprocedural screening for left atrial thrombus with CT (obviating the need for transesophageal echocardiography) is also an attractive concept, yet findings in this regard have so far been mixed. In a study by Tang et al,[39] non-gated 64-detector CT failed to detect more than 50% of cases of left atrial/left atrial appendage thrombi. Conversely, Martinez et al. showed that nongated 64-detector CT had 100% sensitivity for the detection of thrombus. The authors defined thrombus on CT on the basis of incomplete opacification of the left atrial appendage (LAA), which can be caused by the presence of true thrombus as well as by slow flow and early image acquisition, leading to a positive predictive value of 23%.[40]

Traditionally, arrhythmia with rapid ventricular rate has been considered a contraindication for ECG gating, potentially limiting the use of CT prior to PVI in patients presenting for imaging in AF. Nevertheless, the pulmonary veins can be adequately imaged with 64 or greater multidetector

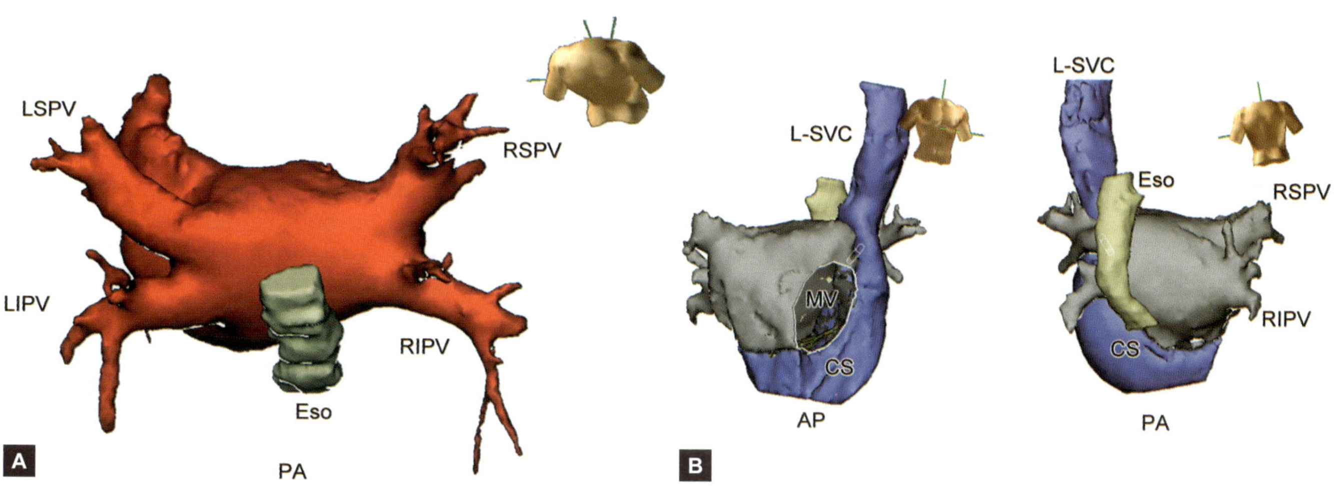

Figures 7.11A and B: (A) CT angiography of a normal left atrium with four distinct pulmonary veins in the posteroanterior (PA) view. The resolution of CTA is typically better than the CMR images, however it does expose the patient to ionizing radiation. With CT images the esophagus can also be depicted. This is important for the electrophysiologist to know as ablation near the esophagus can lead to a severe complication of left atrial-esophageal fistula; (B) CT angiography in a patient with a left sided superior vena cava (L-SVC) draining into a large coronary sinus (CS). This is important for the electrophysiologist to know as the L-SVC can serve as a source of atrial fibrillation triggers

Abbreviations: RSPV, right superior pulmonary vein; RIPV, right inferior pulmonary vein; LSPV, left superior pulmonary vein; LIPV, left inferior pulmonary vein; Eso, esophagus

CT scans with no need for ECG gating.[41] Without ECG gating, information on coronary anatomy is lost and slightly lower spatial resolution should be expected, on the other hand, radiation exposure is decreased with nongated CT. Use of preprocedural CT for AF patients can also be limited by impaired renal function, which would favor using CMR in subjects with significant chronic kidney disease.

Cardiac CT is also fundamental in diagnosing complications of atrial fibrillation ablation. Atrioesophageal fistula is a rare yet devastating complication of PVI that can present with a clinical picture suggestive of endocarditis as well as sepsis and upper gastrointestinal bleeding. When atrioesophageal fistula is suspected, endoscopic evaluation is contraindicated and contrast chest CT scanning can promptly detect the fistulous tract, usually located in the posterior-left atrial wall. Pulmonary vein stenosis is a much more prevalent complication of the procedure which can cause pulmonary hypertension, exertional dyspnea, cough and chest pain. Cardiac CT in these patients can reveal eccentric stenotic lesions extending between 0.5 and 23 mm into the pulmonary veins.[42]

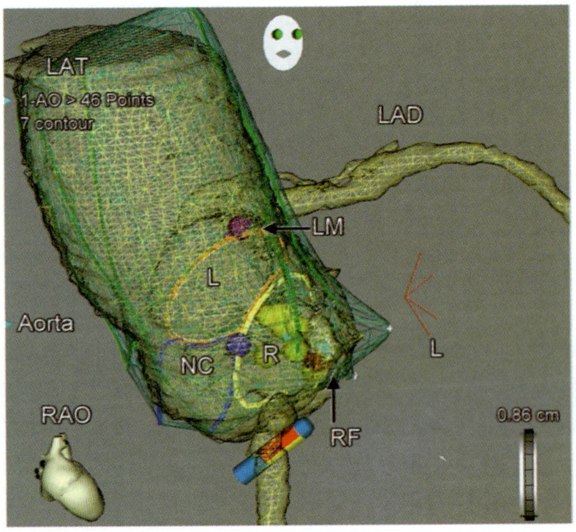

Figure 7.12: CT angiography of the aortic root, registered with an electroanatomic mapping system using landmarks identified using intracardiac echocardiography. The exact locations of the right coronary (RC), left coronary (LC), and noncoronary (NC) aortic cusps and the location of the left main (LM) and left anterior descending (LAD) coronary artery are also depicted. The ablation lesion (red tag) has been delivered to the region of the right coronary cusp; this can be guided by the registered CT angiogram without need for performing coronary angiography to assess proximity to the coronary arteries

Other Applications of Computerized Tomography

Epicardial ablation has become an option for patients with VT and unsuccessful endocardial ablation due to epicardial substrate, and is now performed regularly in certain high volume centers. One of the potential complications of this approach is damage to the epicardial coronary arteries. In order to avoid this, it has been recommended that delivery of radiofrequency energy should be performed from a distance of at least 5 mm from the closest coronary artery.[43] As a result, knowledge of coronary anatomy is fundamental in safely performing epicardial VT ablation. Multidetector CT coronary angiography is one of the options available to electrophysiologists for defining the coronary anatomy, and the images obtained can be merged with the electroanatomical map, providing a clearer real-time picture of the relationship between the tip of the ablation catheter and the coronary arteries **(Figure 7.12)**.

The coronary venous system is increasingly targeted both for placement of cardiac resynchronization leads and for application of radiofrequency energy in certain heart rhythm disorders such as for ablation of accessory pathways and atrial tachycardias. In a study including 100 patients scheduled for CRT implantation, 16-detector CT was successfully used to noninvasively assess coronary venous branch diameter, length and angulation.[44]

PET SCANNING IN CARDIAC SARCOIDOSIS

Diagnostic work-up in patients with suspected cardiac sarcoidosis includes 12-lead ECG, echocardiography and usually advanced imaging such as position emission tomography (PET) scanning, MRI or Gallium or Technetium scintigraphy. PET scanning can allow for evaluation of both myocardial perfusion and metabolic activity through the use of Fluorine-18-fluorodeoxyglucose (18F-FDG), which accumulates in inflammatory cells present in the affected tissue (including the myocardium) pointing towards region of active inflammation[45] **(Figures 7.13A and B)**. Compared to scintigraphy, PET involves less radiation and higher sensitivity. Relative merits of PET over CMR include the potential for use in cardiac device patients and in subjects with severely impaired renal function and the advantage of providing direct data on both cardiac and extracardiac inflammatory activity.

Regarding the prognostic value of PET, it has been shown in patients with suspected cardiac sarcoidosis that abnormal PET results and focal right ventricular FDG uptake are associated with an increase in the risk of death or sustained ventricular arrhythmias. Specifically, the presence of both abnormal perfusion and abnormal FDG uptake (which as indicated earlier is a correlate for increased metabolic activity and inflammation) conferred a 3-fold risk of death or ventricular arrhythmias.[46]

INTRACARDIAC ULTRASOUND

Ablation procedures for cardiac arrhythmias require knowledge of the position of diagnostic and ablation catheters

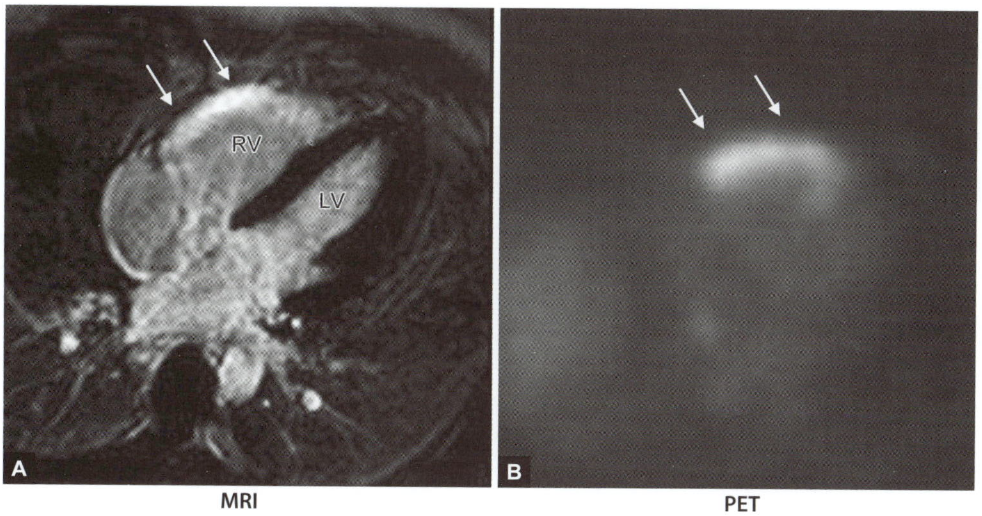

Figures 7.13A and B: Cardiac sarcoidosis: (A) Delayed enhancement image in the horizontal long-axis plane shows extensive transmural hyperenhancement in the right ventricular free wall; (B) FDG-PET CT image in the same plane shows corresponding abnormal FDG uptake in the same region

Abbreviations: LV, left ventricle; RV, right ventricle

within the heart as well as detailed information on intracardiac anatomy, with fluoroscopy and 3D electroanatomical mapping systems usually fulfilling this purpose. Intracardiac echocardiography (ICE) is an additional imaging modality that can also aid in invasive electrophysiology procedures, reducing fluoroscopy times[47] and increasing patient safety. Modern phased-array ICE catheters can be placed through a venous sheath into the right atrium, with sufficient penetration to visualize the left cardiac chambers as well as relevant neighboring structures (such as the pulmonary veins or the aortic root). ICE is valuable in a number of areas:

- *Transseptal access*: Ablation of atrial fibrillation and other left atrial arrhythmias requires access to the left atrium through transseptal puncture, a technique that can be guided by fluoroscopy or transesophageal echocardiography. ICE permits direct identification of the fossa ovalis, which appears as a thin-walled structure surrounded by a muscular rim **(Figure 7.14)**, and precise guiding of the transseptal needle to the posterior fossa along with a significant decrease in complications (including cardiac and aortic root perforation).
- *Anatomical information*: ICE can produce detailed anatomical information of cardiac structures beyond that provided by fluoroscopy and 3D electroanatomical mapping. Relevant landmarks that are usually assessed with ICE include the pulmonary veins **(Figure 7.14)**, the papillary muscles **(Figures 7.15A and B)** and the aortic root including the proximal coronary arteries. Although coronary angiography is usually required before ablation of ventricular arrhythmias originating in the aortic cusps, Hoffmeyer and colleagues report successful ablation in this setting using only ICE to delineate coronary anatomy.[48] ICE not only provides anatomic data but can also be used to establish adequate catheter positioning[49] and tissue contact in these and other settings. Additionally, data derived from ICE can be merged with electroanatomical maps, facilitating ablation procedures in anatomically complex regions such as in papillary muscle and left ventricular outflow tract/aortic root VT or premature ventricular contractions.

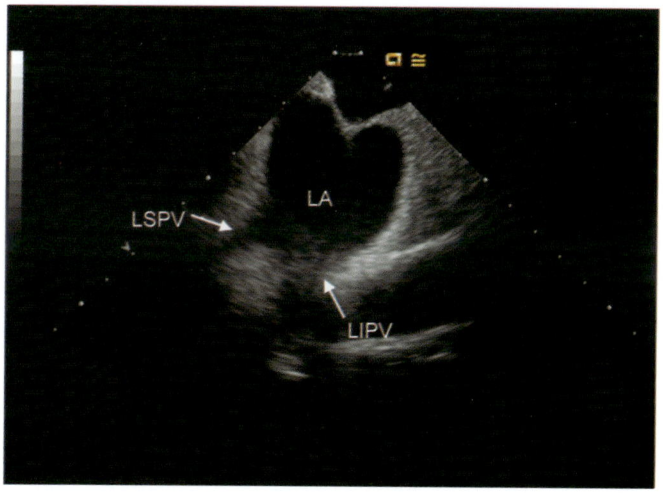

Figure 7.14: Phased-array intracardiac echocardiography view of the septum and left atrium, with the probe in the right atrium. "Tenting" of the fossa ovalis can clearly be seen, as a sheath is positioned prior to transseptal puncture

Abbreviations: LSPV, left superior pulmonary vein; LIPV, left inferior pulmonary vein; LA, left atrium

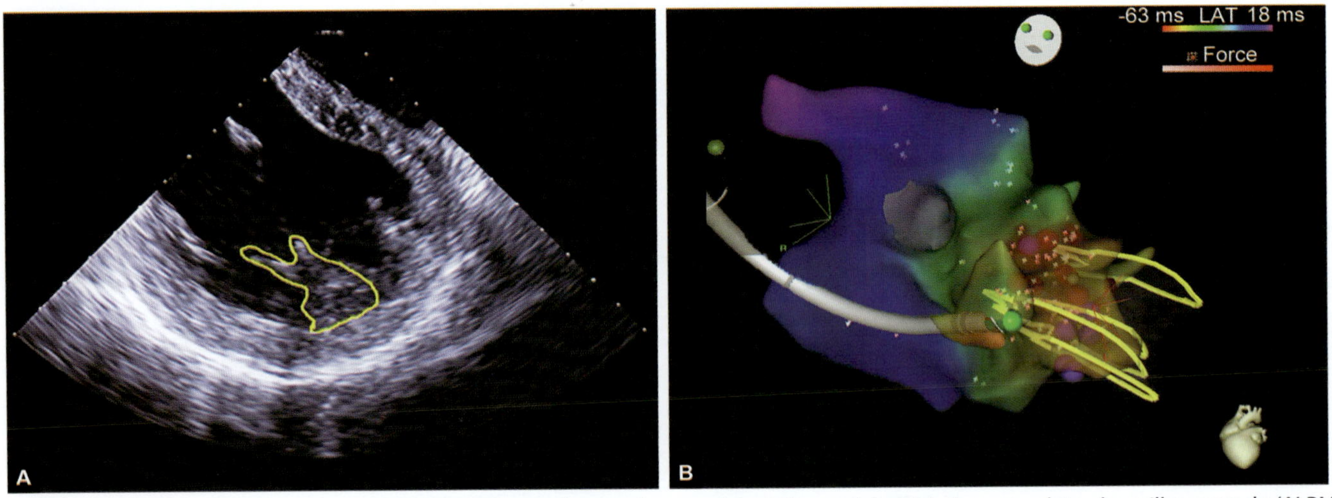

Figures 7.15A and B: (A) Phased array intracardiac echocardiogram image of the left ventricle, with the anterolateral papillary muscle (ALPM) highlighted in yellow; (B) The outline of the ALPM can then be superimposed on an electroanatomic map to guide ablation of ventricular arrhythmias originating from the ALPM. The imaging transducer is located in the right ventricle

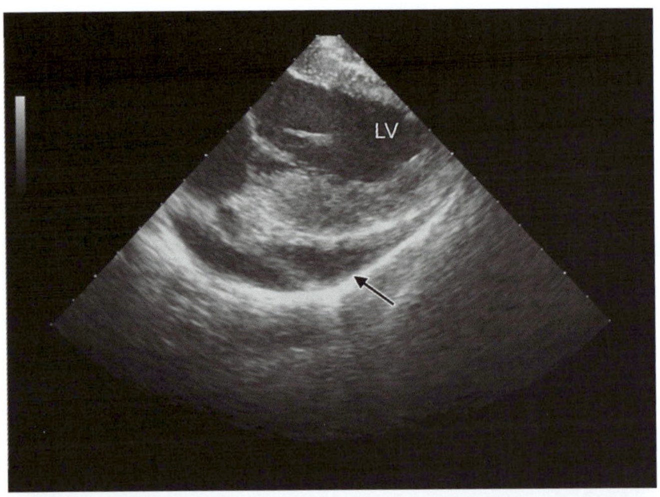

Figure 7.16: Phased array intracardiac echocardiogram (ICE) image of the left ventricle (LV). There is an "echo free" space inferiorly (arrow) identifying a pericardial effusion. One of the advantages of using ICE is early recognition of complications, such as pericardial effusion or tamponade

- *Detection of complications*: ICE affords the possibility of prompt detection of complications of ablation procedures. For instance, potentially life-threatening pericardial effusion, which can appear as a consequence of cardiac perforation **(Figure 7.16)**, can be identified before hemodynamic deterioration develops. Microbubble and microemboli formation at the catheter-tissue interface can also be detected with ICE. Pulmonary vein flow can potentially be assessed with color Doppler and pulsed-wave Doppler in order to reveal the presence and magnitude of pulmonary vein stenosis. Indeed, increases in PV velocity following PVI have been reported,[50] nonetheless, acute changes in pulmonary vein flow patterns immediately after ostial pulmonary vein isolation have not been clearly associated with later development of pulmonary vein stenosis.[51] This same concept can be applied to other locations, such as superior vena cava obstruction after sinus node modification for inappropriate sinus tachycardia.[52]
- *Detection of thrombus*: In a series of 76 patients, Baran et al. showed that ICE was as effective as transesophageal echocardiography for the detection of left atrial thrombus in patients undergoing PVI.[53] Interestingly, the left atrial appendage (LAA) could only be thoroughly assessed in its entirety by placing the ICE catheter in the pulmonary artery, with right atrial positioning affording only a limited view of the LAA.

CONCLUSION

Noninvasive imaging, including CMR, CT, PET and intracardiac echocardiography are critical tools for the electrophysiologist evaluating patients with cardiac arrhythmias. They now play a routine role in guiding diagnosis and treatment of many arrhythmia substrates, particularly atrial fibrillation and ventricular tachycardia. Such tools will continue to evolve in the future, and will play an increasingly important role in helping the electrophysiologist manage patients with cardiac arrhythmias and/or sudden death risk.

REFERENCES

1. Wijffels MC, Kirchhof CJ, Dorland R, Allessie MA. Atrial fibrillation begets atrial fibrillation. A study in awake chronically instrumented goats. Circulation. 1995;92:1954-68.

2. Marrouche NF, Wilber D, Hindricks G, Jais P, Akoum N, Marchlinski F, Kholmovski E, Burgon N, Hu N, Mont L, Deneke T, Duytschaever M, Neumann T, Mansour M, Mahnkopf C, Herweg B, Daoud E, Wissner E, Bansmann P, Brachmann J. Association of atrial tissue fibrosis identified by delayed enhancement MRI and atrial fibrillation catheter ablation: the DECAAF study. JAMA. 2014;311:498-506.
3. Oakes RS, Badger TJ, Kholmovski EG, Akoum N, Burgon NS, Fish EN, Blauer JJ, Rao SN, DiBella EV, Segerson NM, Daccarett M, Windfelder J, McGann CJ, Parker D, MacLeod RS, Marrouche NF. Detection and quantification of left atrial remodelling with delayed-enhancement magnetic resonance imaging in patients with atrial fibrillation. Circulation. 2009; 119:1758-67.
4. Han FT, Akoum N, Marrouche N. Value of magnetic resonance imaging in guiding atrial fibrillation management. Can J Cardiol. 2013;29:1194-202.
5. McGann C1, Akoum N, Patel A, Kholmovski E, Revelo P, Damal K, Wilson B, Cates J, Harrison A, Ranjan R, Burgon NS, Greene T, Kim D, Dibella EV, Parker D, Macleod RS, Marrouche NF. Atrial fibrillation ablation outcome is predicted by left atrial remodeling on MRI. Circ Arrhythm Electrophysiol. 2014;7: 23-30.
6. Daccarett M, Badger TJ, Akoum N, Burgon NS, Mahnkopf C, Vergara G, Kholmovski E, McGann CJ, Parker D, Brachmann J, Macleod RS, Marrouche NF. Association of left atrial fibrosis detected by delayed-enhancement magnetic resonance imaging and the risk of stroke in patients with atrial fibrillation. J Am Coll Cardiol. 2011;57:831-8.
7. Haïssaguerre M, Jaïs P, Shah DC, Takahashi A, Hocini M, Quiniou G, Garrigue S, Le Mouroux A, Le Métayer P, Clémenty J. Spontaneous initiation of atrial fibrillation by ectopic beats originating in the pulmonary veins. N Engl J Med. 1998;339: 659-66.
8. Hundley WG, Bluemke DA, Finn JP, Flamm SD, Fogel MA, Friedrich MG, Ho VB, Jerosch-Herold M, Kramer CM, Manning WJ, Patel M, Pohost GM, Stillman AE, White RD, Woodard PK. ACCF/ACR/AHA/NASCI/SCMR 2010 Expert Consensus Document on Cardiovascular Magnetic Resonance: A report of the American College of Cardiology Foundation Task Force on Expert Consensus Documents. J Am Coll Cardiol. 2010;55:2614-62.
9. Kato R, Lickfett L, Meininger G, Dickfeld T, Wu R, Juang G, Angkeow P, LaCorte J, Bluemke D, Berger R, Halperin HR, Calkins H. Pulmonary vein anatomy in patients undergoing catheter ablation of atrial fibrillation: lessons learned by use of magnetic resonance imaging. Circulation. 2003;107:2004-10.
10. Rathi VK, Reddy ST, Anreddy S, Belden W, Yamrozik JA, Williams RB, Doyle M, Thompson DV, Biederman RW. Contrast-enhanced CMR is equally effective as TEE in the evaluation of left atrial appendage thrombus in patients with atrial fibrillation undergoing pulmonary vein isolation procedure. Heart Rhythm. 2013;10:1021-7.
11. Badger TJ, Adjei-Poku YA, Burgon NS, Kalvaitis S, Shaaban A, Sommers DN, Blauer JJ, Fish EN, Akoum N, Haslem TS, Kholmovski EG, MacLeod RS, Adler DG, Marrouche NF. Initial experience of assessing esophageal tissue injury and recovery using delayed-enhancement MRI after atrial fibrillation ablation. Circ Arrhythm Electrophysiol. 2009;2:620-5.
12. Moss AJ, Zareba W, Hall WJ, Klein H, Wilber DJ, Cannom DS, Daubert JP, Higgins SL, Brown MW, Andrews ML. Multicenter Automatic Defibrillator Implantation Trial II Investigators. Prophylactic implantation of a defibrillator in patients with myocardial infarction and reduced ejection fraction. N Engl J Med. 2002;346:877-83.
13. de Bakker JM, van Capelle FJ, Janse MJ, Tasseron S, Vermeulen JT, de Jonge N, Lahpor JR. Slow conduction in the infarcted human heart. 'Zigzag' course of activation. Circulation. 1993;88:915-26.
14. Scott PA, Morgan JM, Carroll N, Murday DC, Roberts PR, Peebles CR, Harden SP, Curzen NP. The extent of left ventricular scar quantified by late gadolinium enhancement MRI is associated with spontaneous ventricular arrhythmias in patients with coronary artery disease and implantable cardioverter-defibrillators. Circ Arrhythm Electrophysiol. 2011;4:324-30.
15. Yan AT, Shayne AJ, Brown KA, Gupta SN, Chan CW, Luu TM, Di Carli MF, Reynolds HG, Stevenson WG, Kwong RY. Characterization of the peri-infarct zone by contrast-enhanced cardiac magnetic resonance imaging is a powerful predictor of post-myocardial infarction mortality. Circulation. 2006;114: 32-9.
16. Klem I, Weinsaft JW, Bahnson TD, Hegland D, Kim HW, Hayes B, Parker MA, Judd RM, Kim RJ. Assessment of myocardial scarring improves risk stratification in patients evaluated for cardiac defibrillator implantation. J Am Coll Cardiol 2012;60:408-20.
17. Ghosn M, Green P, Chaikriangkrai K, Birnbaum I, Nagueh S, Quinones M, Zoghbi W, Shah D. Non-invasive risk stratification in patients with non-ischemic cardiomyopathy using cardiac magnetic resonance imaging. J Am Coll Cardiol. 2014;63(12_S).
18. Andreu D, Berruezo A, Ortiz-Pérez JT, Silva E, Mont L, Borràs R, de Caralt TM, Perea RJ, Fernández-Armenta J, Zeljko H, Brugada J. Integration of 3D electroanatomic maps and magnetic resonance scar characterization into the navigation system to guide ventricular tachycardia ablation. Circ Arrhythm Electrophysiol. 2011;4:674-83.
19. Gupta S, Desjardins B, Baman T, Ilg K, Good E, Crawford T, Oral H, Pelosi F, Chugh A, Morady F, Bogun F. Delayed-enhanced MR scar imaging and intraprocedural registration into an electroanatomical mapping system in post-infarction patients. JACC Cardiovasc Imaging. 2012;5:207-10.
20. Piers SR, Tao Q, van Huls van Taxis CF, Schalij MJ, van der Geest RJ, Zeppenfeld K. Contrast-enhanced MRI-derived scar patterns and associated ventricular tachycardias in nonischemic cardiomyopathy: implications for the ablation strategy. Circ Arrhythm Electrophysiol. 2013;6:875-83.
21. Arenal A, Pérez-David E, Avila P, Fernández-Portales J, Crisóstomo V, Báez C, Jiménez-Candil J, Rubio-Guivernau JL, Ledesma-Carbayo MJ, Loughlin G, Bermejo J, Sánchez-Margallo FM, Fernández-Avilés F. Noninvasive identification of epicardial ventricular tachycardia substrate by magnetic resonance-based signal intensity mapping. Heart Rhythm. 2014;11:1456-64.
22. Andreu D, Ortiz-Pérez JT, Boussy T, Fernández-Armenta J, de Caralt TM, Perea RJ, Prat-González S, Mont L, Brugada J, Berruezo A. Usefulness of contrast-enhanced cardiac magnetic resonance in identifying the ventricular arrhythmia substrate and the approach needed for ablation. Eur Heart J. 2014;35:1316-26.
23. Kron J, Ellenbogen KA. Cardiac Sarcoidosis: Contemporary Review. J Cardiovasc Electrophysiol. 2015;26:104-9.

24. Birnie DH, Sauer WH, Bogun F, Cooper JM, Culver DA, Duvernoy CS, Judson MA, Kron J, Mehta D, Cosedis Nielsen J, Patel AR, Ohe T, Raatikainen P, Soejima K. HRS expert consensus statement on the diagnosis and management of arrhythmias associated with cardiac sarcoidosis. Heart Rhythm. 2014;11:1305-23.
25. Cummings KW, Bhalla S, Javidan-Nejad C, Bierhals AJ, Gutierrez FR, Woodard PK. A pattern-based approach to assessment of delayed enhancement in nonischemic cardiomyopathy at MR imaging. Radiographics. 2009;29:89-103.
26. Steckman DA, Schneider PM, Schuller JL, Aleong RG, Nguyen DT, Sinagra G, Vitrella G, Brun F, Cova MA, Pagnan L, Mestroni L, Varosy PD, Sauer WH. Utility of cardiac magnetic resonance imaging to differentiate cardiac sarcoidosis from arrhythmogenic right ventricular cardiomyopathy. Am J Cardiol. 2012;110:575-9.
27. Hoffmayer KS, Scheinman MM. Electrocardiographic patterns of ventricular arrhythmias in arrhythmogenic right ventricular dysplasia/cardiomyopathy. Front Physiol. 2012;3:23.
28. Tandri H, Saranathan M, Rodriguez ER, Martinez C, Bomma C, Nasir K, Rosen B, Lima JA, Calkins H, Bluemke DA. Noninvasive detection of myocardial fibrosis in arrhythmogenic right ventricular cardiomyopathy using delayed-enhancement magnetic resonance imaging. J Am Coll Cardiol. 2005;45: 98-103.
29. Tandri H, Macedo R, Calkins H, Marcus F, Cannom D, Scheinman M, Daubert J, Estes M 3rd, Wilber D, Talajic M, Duff H, Krahn A, Sweeney M, Garan H, Bluemke DA. Multidisciplinary Study of Right Ventricular Dysplasia Investigators. Role of magnetic resonance imaging in arrhythmogenic right ventricular dysplasia: insights from the North American arrhythmogenic right ventricular dysplasia (ARVD/C) study. Am Heart J. 2008;155:147-53.
30. Marcus FI, McKenna WJ, Sherrill D, Basso C, Bauce B, Bluemke DA, Calkins H, Corrado D, Cox MG, Daubert JP, Fontaine G, Gear K, Hauer R, Nava A, Picard MH, Protonotarios N, Saffitz JE, Sanborn DM, Steinberg JS, Tandri H, Thiene G, Towbin JA, Tsatsopoulou A, Wichter T, Zareba W. Diagnosis of arrhythmogenic right ventricular cardiomyopathy/dysplasia: proposed modification of the Task Force Criteria. Eur Heart J. 2010;31:806-14.
31. Ainslie M, Miller C, Brown B, Schmitt M. Cardiac MRI of patients with implanted electrical cardiac devices. Heart. 2014;100:363-9.
32. Nazarian S, Roguin A, Zviman MM, Lardo AC, Dickfeld TL, Calkins H, Weiss RG, Berger RD, Bluemke DA, Henry R. Halperin HR. Clinical utility and safety of a protocol for noncardiac and cardiac magnetic resonance imaging of patients with permanent pacemakers and implantable-cardioverter defibrillators at 1.5 tesla. Circulation. 2006;114:1277-84.
33. Roguin A, Schwitter J, Vahlhaus C, Lombardi M, Brugada J, Vardas P, Auricchio A, Priori S, Sommer T. Magnetic resonance imaging in individuals with cardiovascular implantable electronic devices. Europace. 2008;10:336-46.
34. Cronin EM, Wilkoff BL. Magnetic resonance imaging conditional pacemakers: rationale, development and future directions. Indian Pacing Electrophysiol J. 2012;12:204-12.
35. Rashid S, Rapacchi S, Vaseghi M, Tung R, Shivkumar K, Finn JP, Hu P. Improved late gadolinium enhancement MR imaging for patients with implanted cardiac devices. Radiology. 2014;270:269-74.
36. Bardo DM, Brown P. Cardiac Multidetector Computed Tomography: Basic Physics of Image Acquisition and Clinical Applications. Current Cardiology Reviews. 2008;4:231-43.
37. Hussein AA, Abutaleb A, Jeudy J, Phelan T, Patel R, Shkullaku M, Siddiqi F, See V, Saliaris A, Shorofsky SR, Dickfeld T. Safety of computed tomography in patients with cardiac rhythm management devices: assessment of the U.S. Food and Drug Administration advisory in clinical practice. J Am Coll Cardiol. 2014;63:1769-75.
38. Steinberg BA, Hammill BG, Daubert JP, Bahnson TD, Douglas PS, Qualls LG, Pokorney SD, Calkins H, Curtis LH, Piccini JP. Periprocedural imaging and outcomes after catheter ablation of atrial fibrillation. Heart. 2014;100:1871-7.
39. Tang RB, Dong JZ, Zhang ZQ, Li ZA, Liu XP, Kang JP, Yu RH, Long de Y, Ma CS. Comparison of contrast enhanced 64-slice computed tomography and transesophageal echocardiography in detection of left atrial thrombus in patients with atrial fibrillation. J Interv Card Electrophysiol. 2008;22: 199-203.
40. Martinez MW, Kirsch J, Williamson EE, Syed IS, Feng D, Ommen S, Packer DL, Brady PA. Utility of nongated multidetector computed tomography for detection of left atrial thrombus in patients undergoing catheter ablation of atrial fibrillation. JACC Cardiovasc Imaging. 2009;2:69-76.
41. Cronin P, Sneider MB, Kazerooni EA, Kelly AM, Scharf C, Oral H, Morady F. MDCT of the left atrium and pulmonary veins in planning radiofrequency ablation for atrial fibrillation: a how-to guide. AJR Am J Roentgenol. 2004;183:767-78.
42. Packer DL, Keelan P, Munger TM, Breen JF, Asirvatham S, Peterson LA, Monahan KH, Hauser MF, Chandrasekaran K, Sinak LJ, Holmes DR Jr. Clinical presentation, investigation, and management of pulmonary vein stenosis complicating ablation for atrial fibrillation. Circulation. 2005;111:546-54.
43. Aliot EM, Stevenson WG, Almendral-Garrote JM, Bogun F, Calkins CH, Delacretaz E, Della Bella P, Hindricks G, Jaïs P, Josephson ME, Kautzner J, Kay GN, Kuck KH, Lerman BB, Marchlinski F, Reddy V, Schalij MJ, Schilling R, Soejima K, Wilber D. European Heart Rhythm Association (EHRA); Registered Branch of the European Society of Cardiology (ESC); Heart Rhythm Society (HRS); American College of Cardiology (ACC); American Heart Association (AHA). EHRA/HRS Expert Consensus on Catheter Ablation of Ventricular Arrhythmias: developed in a partnership with the European Heart Rhythm Association (EHRA), a Registered Branch of the European Society of Cardiology (ESC), and the Heart Rhythm Society (HRS); in collaboration with the American College of Cardiology (ACC) and the American Heart Association (AHA). Heart Rhythm. 2009;6:886-933.
44. Sun J, Yang X, Lam Y, Garcia M, Yu C. Evaluation of Coronary Venous Anatomy by Multislice Computed Tomography, World Journal of Cardiovascular Surgery. 2012;2(4):91-5.
45. Soejima K, Yada H. The work-up and management of patients with apparent or subclinical cardiac sarcoidosis: with emphasis on the associated heart rhythm abnormalities. J Cardiovasc Electrophysiol. 2009;20:578-83.
46. Blankstein R, Osborne M, Naya M, Waller A, Kim CK, Murthy VL, Kazemian P, Kwong RY, Tokuda M, Skali H, Padera R, Hainer J, Stevenson WG, Dorbala S, Di Carli MF. Cardiac positron emission tomography enhances prognostic assessments of patients with suspected cardiac sarcoidosis. J Am Coll Cardiol. 2014;63:329-36.

47. Chu E, Fitzpatrick AP, Chin MC, Sudhir K, Yock PG, Lesh MD. Radiofrequency catheter ablation guided by intracardiac echocardiography. Circulation. 1994;89:1301-5.
48. Hoffmayer KS, Dewland TA, Hsia HH, Badhwar N, Hsu JC, Tseng ZH, Marcus GM, Scheinman MM, Gerstenfeld EP. Safety of radiofrequency catheter ablation without coronary angiography in aortic cusp ventricular arrhythmias. Heart Rhythm. 2014;11:1117-21.
49. Epstein LM, Mitchell MA, Smith TW, Haines DE. Comparative study of fluoroscopy and intracardiac echocardiographic guidance for the creation of linear atrial lesions. Circulation. 1998;98:1796-801.
50. Ren JF, Marchlinski FE, Callans DJ, Zado ES. Intracardiac Doppler echocardiographic quantification of pulmonary vein flow velocity: an effective technique for monitoring pulmonary vein ostia narrowing during focal atrial fibrillation ablation. J Cardiovasc Electrophysiol. 2002;13:1076-81.
51. Saad EB, Cole CR, Marrouche NF, Dresing TJ, Perez-Lugones A, Saliba WI, Schweikert RA, Klein A, Rodriguez L, Grimm R, Tchou P, Natale A. Use of intracardiac echocardiography for prediction of chronic pulmonary vein stenosis after ablation of atrial fibrillation. J Cardiovasc Electrophysiol. 2002;13:986-9.
52. Callans DJ, Ren JF, Schwartzman D, Gottlieb CD, Chaudhry FA, Marchlinski FE. Narrowing of the superior vena cava-right atrium junction during radiofrequency catheter ablation for inappropriate sinus tachycardia: analysis with intracardiac echocardiography. J Am Coll Cardiol. 1999;33:1667-70.
53. Baran J, Stec S, Pilichowska-Paszkiet E, Zaborska B, Sikora-Frąc M, Kryński T, Michałowska I, Łopatka R, Kułakowski P. Intracardiac echocardiography for detection of thrombus in the left atrial appendage: comparison with transesophageal echocardiography in patients undergoing ablation for atrial fibrillation: the Action-Ice I Study. Circ Arrhythm Electrophysiol. 2013;6:1074-81.

EDITORS' SUMMARY

Here Drs Gerstenfeld, Loughlin, and Ordovas provide a concise yet comprehensive review of cardiac imaging for the invasive electrophysiologist. Once the relevant anatomy has been mastered, we are required to fully appreciate the nuances of the commonly used imaging modality to visualize the anatomy and recognize variations and pathology when present.

The authors describe the primary modalities used today sequentially and in well-referenced detail. In addition, where appropriate, they emphasize specific disorders that may require multiple imaging techniques for visualization, such as with cardiac sarcoidosis.

This up-to-date review explains for us what we gain with the very latest techniques, including those related to gating and visualization of fibrosis even in difficult areas such as the left atrium. The reader is also provided with an outstanding discussion, again well-referenced, of intracardiac echocardiography with phased array imaging, particularly highlighting the value of this technology to allow rapid recognition of intraprocedural complications.

Finally, any imaging reference of value would not be complete without figures. The authors have chosen great examples that are meticulously annotated and by themselves will provide the reader an appreciation of the value of each technology as a standalone portion of this chapter.

CHAPTER 8

Daniel Pelchovitz, Rishi Arora

Conventional Mapping Techniques: Fundamentals

LIST OF ABBREVIATIONS

ARVC	Arrhythmogenic Right Ventricular Cardiomyopathy	RVOT	Right Ventricular Outflow Tract
EGM	Electrogram	TCL	Tachycardia Cycle Length
PPI	Postpacing Interval	VT	Ventricular Tachycardia
PVC	Premature Ventricular Contraction		

INTRODUCTION

This chapter will cover conventional mapping techniques, which are the foundation on which advanced techniques are based. Understanding conventional mapping is predicated on a detailed understanding of the derivation of electrograms and filtering and recording processes that are covered in previous chapters. The treatment of the vast majority of arrhythmias in the electrophysiology laboratory relies on accurate mapping of the tachycardia so that ablation can be performed in areas of the heart that are critical to the initiation and maintenance of the tachycardia while avoiding damage to surrounding normal structures, e.g. the conduction system.

In broad view, mapping in the electrophysiology lab is the method in which one uses physiologic and anatomic data obtained during the procedure to clarify mechanisms of tachycardia and obtain anatomic correlates of these mechanisms with the ultimate goal of providing information that may assist in the treatment of arrhythmias. These techniques, along with atrial and ventricular pacing maneuvers to be covered in other chapters, can define both the mechanism of tachycardia and identify critical areas of the tachycardia circuit in which ablation may be successful in terminating the arrhythmia. These maneuvers form the cornerstone of diagnosis of arrhythmia in the electrophysiology lab.

Conventional mapping techniques such as activation mapping, entrainment mapping, and pace mapping combined with anatomic information obtained from fluoroscopy is the foundation on which advanced 3-dimensional mapping techniques are based, and a clear understanding of the principles as well as pitfalls of these approaches is required to use the advanced techniques reliably. Mapping with the goal of finding a critical isthmus where tachycardia can be terminated or with the goal of finding the site of origin of tachycardia are the typical approaches when using these techniques in a therapeutic manner. Typically some combination of conventional mapping approaches is used, with the relative utility of each mapping technique varying from case to case. In cases where an arrhythmia can be readily induced, entrainment mapping and activation mapping are typically most useful. On the other hand, in cases where an arrhythmia cannot be induced or sustained, these approaches are less useful and more utility is found in alternate approaches such as pace mapping.

Mapping is typically performed with a multipolar catheter that is moved to various locations of the heart using fluoroscopy in order to evaluate the local activation and other electrical parameters of each anatomical site. Typically other stable multipolar catheters are used in various locations (high right atrium, His position, right ventricular apex, coronary sinus) to both provide a fluoroscopic reference for anatomical position and to provide additional relative electrophysiologic data. The roving catheter is used as the mapping catheter and in the setting of using an ablation catheter for mapping; it can also be used to deliver therapy. Traditionally, mapping performed in the electrophysiology lab is "contact" mapping, i.e. the mapping catheter is typically in contact with the endocardium. Many noncontact mapping techniques have been developed, however, these are beyond the scope of this chapter.

ACTIVATION MAPPING

The most commonly used conventional mapping approach is termed activation mapping. Activation mapping is a method that is designed to localize the origin of an arrhythmia by comparing the timing of a local electrogram on a mapping catheter to the global depolarization of interest, which is either a surface electrocardiographic marker or a surrogate intracardiac electrogram. The general principal that allows for activation mapping is the idea that a focal tachycardia originates from a single site and spreads radially away from this area with relatively uniform conduction. By finding the area with the local electrogram with the earliest activation compared to the global depolarization of interest one can infer that the origin of the tachycardia is the location with the earliest electrogram. For example, in mapping the origin of a premature ventricular contraction (PVC), the timing of the local electrogram in various areas of the ventricle can be compared to the onset of the surface QRS deflection. Activation of the ventricle should proceed in a radial manner provided there is a single area of origin. The area of origin should have the earliest temporal activation relative to the QRS complex, with areas further from the area of origin having later and later activation. By finding the earliest site that is pre-QRS, one can localize the origin of the PVC. In addition to finding the origin of the arrhythmia, activation mapping can be used to infer that the tachycardia does not originate from a chamber of interest. For example, in the case of an atrial tachycardia, finding that there is no site in the right atrium that is earlier than the onset of the P-wave, can suggest that the tachycardia originates from the left atrium. This may then indicate the need for a transseptal access.

Not all tachycardias can be evaluated by activation mapping. Activation mapping requires that the tachycardia of interest be inducible in the electrophysiology lab or spontaneously occurring with significant frequency as to perform a multipoint activation map during tachycardia. In addition, the tachycardia must be hemodynamically tolerated so mapping can be performed during tachycardia without adverse consequence to the patient. The typical mapping protocol begins with identification of a fiducial point, the point which will serve as the reference for timing for the remainder of the map. In mapping of ventricular arrhythmias this is typically the onset of the QRS complex as this can typically be readily and reliably identified on the surface ECG. In mapping of atrial arrhythmias, however, this can be difficult as the P-wave of interest often falls in the T-wave or QRS complex of the surface ECG, making reliable measurement of the onset of this deflection difficult. In instances similar to this, a stable intracardiac electrogram can be used to determine the relative timing of the surface P-wave. Oftentimes pacing the ventricle to dissociate the P-wave from the T-wave is required, after which the timing of the surface P-wave can be referenced to the intracardiac signal which can be used for the remainder of the intracardiac map. This, however, requires a very stable intracardiac electrogram which in practical experience is typically a coronary sinus signal as catheter position is often stable and reliable in this area. It is helpful to save a fluoroscopic marker of the reference catheter so that if the catheter changes position during activation mapping the catheter position can be reset.

Next, the mechanism of tachycardia needs to be elucidated. If the tachycardia is thought to be a focal tachycardia, the goal of mapping will be to localize the earliest electrogram that precedes either the P-wave or QRS complex of interest. Often this is 20–40 ms presurface depolarization as this is the time that transit from the area of onset to global depolarization. If the tachycardia is thought to be a reentrant tachycardia, mapping the earliest onset will not be fruitful as activation is by definition continuous. Instead, the goal is to localize an area of critical conduction that has mid-diastolic activity that may possibly be fractionated, indicating either diseased tissue or location within a protected isthmus. Understanding the mechanism of the tachycardia is important prior to creation of the map so that this pitfall can be avoided. Measuring the cycle length represented by tachycardias in the chamber of interest can be helpful. Reentrant tachycardias that are confined to the chamber of interest typically have significant diastolic activity and therefore, greater than 85% of the cycle length of the tachycardia can be represented by electrograms in the circuit. This is opposed to focal tachycardias that typically do not exhibit mid diastolic activity and a much lower percentage of the tachycardia cycle length is demonstrated with electrograms in the chamber of interest. What is thought to be an early site in a focal arrhythmia (up to 50 ms pre-surface) may not be an early site in a reentrant arrhythmia, and ablation in this region may not lead to termination of a tachycardia. Mid diastolic sites in reentrant arrhythmias are typically associated with the critical isthmus and ablation in these regions may be more successful in treating tachyarrhythmias. An isoelectric segment in a macroreentrant tachyarrhythmia typically results from slow conduction through a small critical isthmus of tissue that does not result in a large surface depolarization. These are the regions that are typically associated with mid-diastolic potentials and are the most successful targets of ablation. These mid-diastolic potentials are present during arrhythmia and most often are not present during sinus rhythm, and therefore identification of these sites often requires sustained tachycardia. These areas typically precede surface depolarization by up to several hundred milliseconds, suggesting a nonfocal origin of the arrhythmia. Mid-diastolic potentials should precede the QRS complex by the same interval of time for each beat in ventricular arrhythmias; otherwise these may represent artifact.[1] An example of mid-diastolic potentials during VT is shown in **Figure 8.1**. In this case of a VT originating from the basal right ventricular septum in a patient with arrhythmogenic right ventricular cardiomyopathy, mid-diastolic potentials are noted during tachycardia. Ablation in this site terminated the tachycardia and no further VT could be induced. This corresponded to areas of late potentials seen in sinus rhythm, likely demonstrating slow conduction.

Typically, the chamber in which the tachycardia is thought to originate is mapped in its entirety with the goal of finding the earliest activation. This is readily determined by careful analysis of the surface ECG. However, if the earliest activation does not sufficiently precede the surface ECG signal of interest, other chambers of the heart should be investigated. A prime example of this is mapping of presumed right ventricular outflow tract PVCs. If a significant pre-QRS electrogram cannot be identified in this area, structures in different chambers adjacent to the RVOT including the left ventricular outflow tract, coronary cusps, and possible epicardial areas adjacent to the anterior interventricular vein via the coronary sinus should be mapped in order to find the earliest local electrogram pre-QRS. In the case of some ventricular arrhythmias that cannot be localized endocardially this involves epicardial access and epicardial mapping to find the area of earliest activation. Rarely, there are equally early earliest areas of activation on each side of the ventricular septum suggesting an intramyocardial origin. In these cases, conventional ablation techniques may not eliminate the arrhythmia of interest.

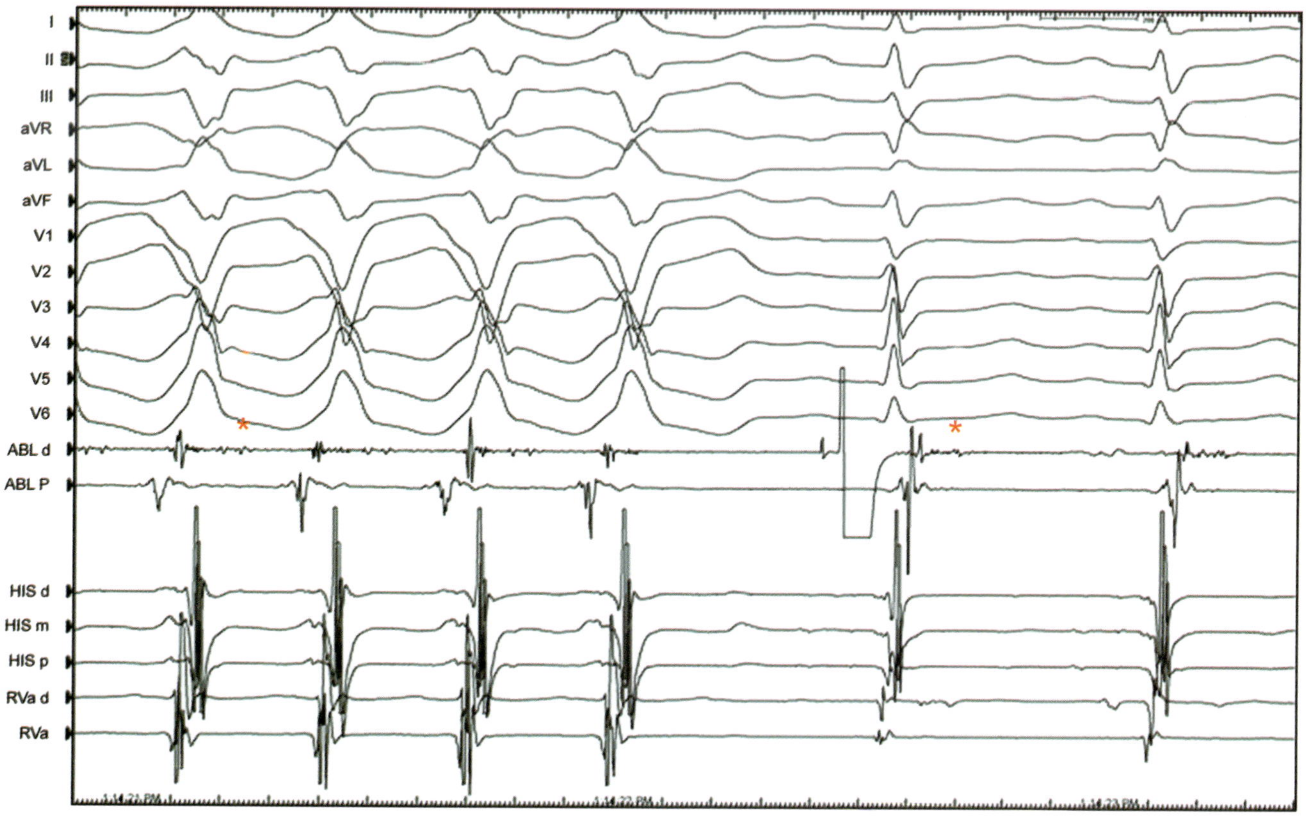

Figure 8.1: Mapping of a ventricular tachycardia circuit in the basal RV septum of a patient with ARVC demonstrated an area of significant mid-diastolic potentials during ventricular tachycardia (asterisks), signifying slow conduction in a critical isthmus for the tachycardia circuit. Ablation in this area terminated the tachycardia and rendered it noninducible. Late potentials are also seen in sinus rhythm signifying slow conduction

The mapping is then performed by moving the mapping catheter to various areas of the chamber of interest and measuring the local activation. Initially large catheter movements are made to determine an area of focus which can then be "micro-mapped" with very small catheter movements and deflections. The earliest site of activation is thought to represent the origin of the tachycardia. An example is shown in **Figure 8.2**. In a case of PVCs originating from the left coronary cusp, the bipolar electrogram at the site of origin is significantly pre-QRS and earlier than any other site in the heart. Ablation was successful in this area.

Several techniques are used to perform activation mapping. Both unipolar and bipolar recordings are used for activation mapping, and both have relative advantages and disadvantages. In most electrophysiology laboratories, bipolar mapping is performed with additional information gained from the unipolar map, particularly direction of activation, at the sites of earliest activation of the bipolar map.

Unipolar Mapping

The unipolar electrogram is generated as a far-field bipole between the distal electrode tip (by convention typically considered positive) and a remote negative electrode. This electrode may either be the Wilson central terminal or a distant catheter in the superior or inferior vena cava. There is considerable debate as to which component of the unipolar electrogram should be used for timing during activation mapping. Most often the maximum negative slope of the electrogram is used, however the onset of the electrogram and the maximum amplitude have also been used. Consistency throughout the mapping procedure is required for the operator to perform an accurate activation map.

The major advantage of unipolar mapping over bipolar mapping is the inherent directionality associated with the electrogram. As the catheter tip is by convention positive, the movement of electrical current towards the catheter tip will result in a positive deflection (i.e. an R-wave) and movement of current away from the catheter tip will result in a negative deflection (i.e. a QS wave). This is helpful in activation mapping as electrical signals that originate at the catheter tip will result in a QS electrogram, whereas sites remote from the origin will originate with an initial R-wave suggesting current towards the mapping catheter tip. An example is present in **Figure 8.2**. In this 18-year-old male patient, with symptomatic PVCs since age 9, a site in the left coronary cusp where

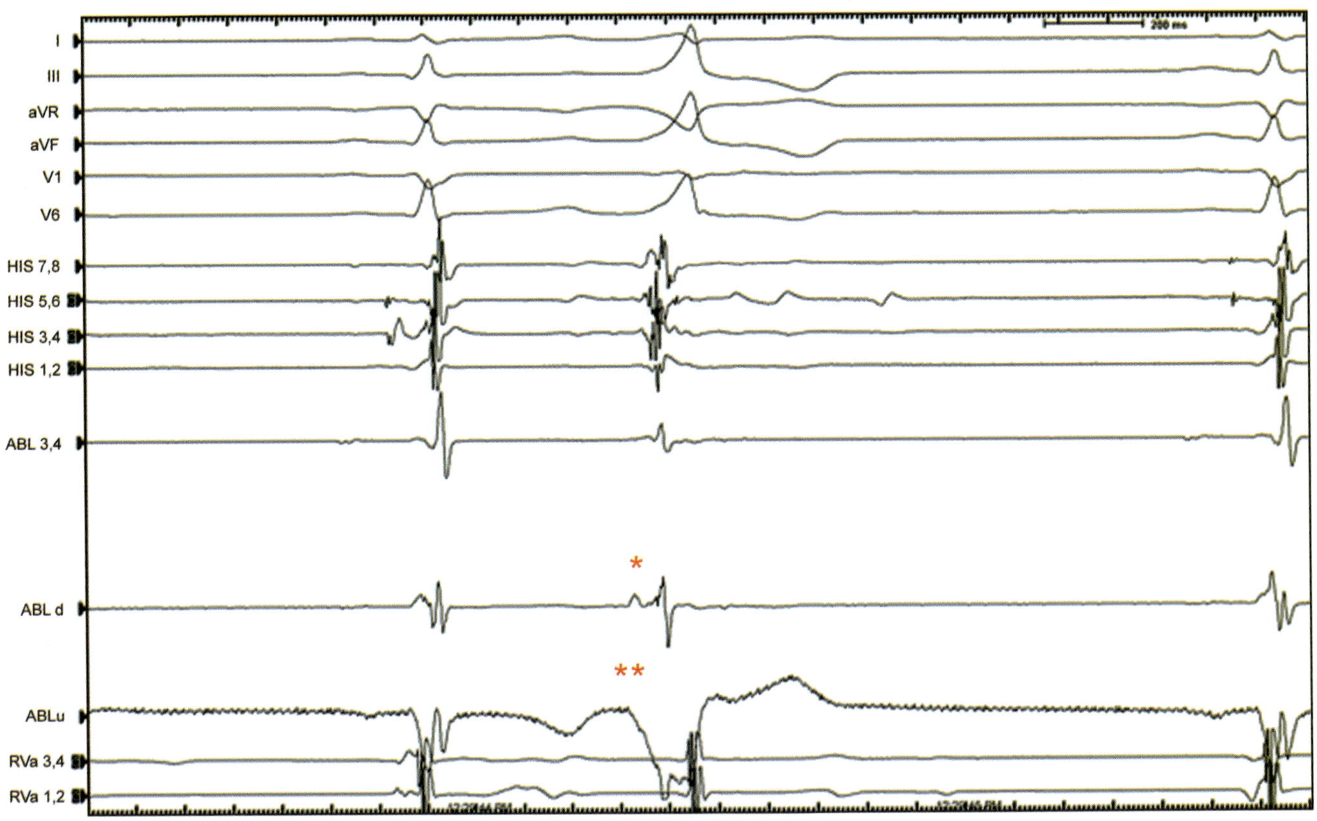

Figure 8.2: Activation mapping, both unipolar and bipolar, are demonstrated in this figure. The frequent PVCs in this 18-year-old male patient were found to be originating from a site in the left coronary cusp. There is a small prepotential noted on the bipolar electrogram (asterisk) that preceded the QRS by over 20 ms. This corresponds to the rapid downslope of the unipolar electrogram (double asterisk). This unipolar electrogram demonstrates a QS complex suggesting origin of the PVC from the catheter position

ablation was ultimately successful is shown. The unipolar electrogram shows a QS complex with no significant R-wave. Absence of a QS complex predicted a 92% of failure of an ablation lesion in a study of ablation of accessory pathways.[2] While the presence of a QS complex is a sensitive marker for a successful ablation site in a focal arrhythmia, it is very nonspecific as up to 70% of unsuccessful sites may exhibit a QS complex. In fact, QS complexes can be seen in a 1 cm^2 region, and in particular in one study 65% of subjects exhibited a QS complex over 1 cm from the site of impulse formation.[3] These complexes are also less reliable in diseased myocardium as there will be slowed conduction. In addition, as unipolar recordings only use the distal catheter tip electrode, both pacing and recording can be performed from the tip of the catheter perhaps allowing for higher fidelity mapping in several different modalities.

Disadvantages of the unipolar recordings for the most part involve the poor signal to noise ratio of unipolar recordings due to significant far-field effects of remote tissues involved in the unipolar circuit. This is particularly of issue in non-homogeneous tissues, such as areas of scar from either myocardial infarction or infiltrative cardiomyopathies. In these instances, it can be difficult to separate electrograms from local tissue versus fractionated tissues along the unipolar circuit. Filtering is often required which can affect slope data and decreases the accuracy of the unipolar electrogram.

Bipolar Mapping

Bipolar mapping involves recording of electrograms between two electrodes on the mapping catheter. With a quadripolar catheter, three sets of electrodes produce recordings at one time: distal (1,2), mid (2,3), and proximal (3,4). All three bipoles can be displayed on a recording system to provide a relative timing of activation based on the spatial location of the mapping catheter. Bipolar recording, as compared with unipolar recording, is more ambiguous as to the local activation time as the recording is by nature spread over an antenna that is separated by several millimeters. In particular, mapping with an ablation catheter can be fraught with error as the tip of the ablation catheter is often larger than a conventional ring electrode and therefore, the mapping bipole is often quite large. As opposed to unipolar recording, the initial deflection of a bipolar electrogram typically corresponds to local activation between the recording bipole. This is particularly true in normal tissues. However, in diseased tissues that result in fractionated electrograms the onset of the electrogram can be difficult to determine and the operator must use the information about the mechanism of the arrhythmia being mapped to determine the relative timing of this electrogram, specifically which component to select for creation of an activation map.

Directionality of the electrograms in a bipolar recording cannot be ascertained as reliably as unipolar recordings. In general, depolarizations that occur parallel to the orientation of the recording bipole create large signals and those that occur perpendicular to the bipole create no signals. Unlike a unipolar recording, the origin of a bipolar recording cannot be ascertained from a QS complex. Instead, pairs of electrodes that lie on a line of block can be used to determine directionality. For example, if a quadripolar catheter is placed perpendicular to a line of block, the electrogram on one side of the line may exhibit a prominent R-wave while the electrogram on the other side of the line may exhibit a prominent S-wave, and essentially these electrograms may be "mirror images" on each other.

The main advantage of bipolar electrograms is an optimal signal-to-noise ratio given the lack of far-field inputs on the electrogram.

PACE MAPPING

Pace mapping is also used to localize the origin of focal tachycardias as well as the exit sites of reentrant tachycardias. Pace mapping is a technique in which the origin of a tachycardia is elucidated by pacing from the site of interest and comparing the morphology of the resulting deflection (P-wave, QRS complex) on the ECG to a previously recorded ECG of the arrhythmia of interest, ideally which has been recorded in the electrophysiology lab with the ECG electrodes in the same position. Pacing from the site of origin of a focal tachycardia should result in an identical QRS complex or P-wave as the ECG appearance of the tachycardia.

Pace mapping is performed by pacing at the lowest output that results in capture at the site of interest, so as to capture the minimum amount of myocardium possible which limits the ECG appearance to the site of pacing. The resulting morphology can be used to guide the operator to different locations (i.e. if pace mapping a PVC, if the resulting QRS complex demonstrates an apical pacing morphology but the arrhythmia is more suggestive of a basal morphology, this would prompt the operator to move the mapping catheter to a more basal location).

Pace mapping during sinus rhythm may be less effective in situations associated with diseased myocardium. In these situations, the lack of functional barriers to conduction may lead to the avoidance of critical isthmuses that are present during tachycardia, and therefore, the resulting morphology may be completely different from that noted during tachycardia, even if pacing is performed very close to the tachycardia circuit.

Pace mapping should be performed at the cycle length of the tachycardia in order to avoid rate-related aberrancy or fusion with other electrocardiographic signals (P-wave, QRS complex, T-wave) that occur at different cycle lengths than the spontaneous or induced tachycardia.[4] If this is not employed in practice, then other factors that may change the QRS complex or P-wave independent of pacing site (which is the goal of this mapping modality) may affect the results of mapping.

Pace Mapping for Ventricular Arrhythmias

Pace mapping is perhaps most useful for mapping ventricular arrhythmias. This is because the surface QRS complex can be readily evaluated as it is less often fused with other deflections on the surface ECG. Pace mapping is most useful for determining the site of origin of infrequent or hemodynamically untolerated rhythms in which activation and entrainment mapping cannot be readily performed. Using either fluoroscopy or three dimensional mapping, a mapping catheter is moved to different areas of the ventricle, and pacing is performed at low output and with a similar coupling interval to the arrhythmia of interest. Low output pacing is performed to reduce the amount of ventricular myocardium that is captured and to increase the fidelity of the mapping. The QRS complex that is created by pacing at each location is analyzed in all twelve leads of the surface ECG. This paced ECG is compared to the ECG of the arrhythmia of interest, and movement of the mapping catheter is performed based on the difference between the pace map ECG and the arrhythmia PVC. For example, if the precordial transition of the arrhythmia is earlier than the precordial transition of the pacemap, a more basal position is sought. The goal of the pacemapping is to find an area with a 12/12 match to the surface ECG, that is that 12/12 of the surface leads from the pacemap are identical to the arrhythmia. An example of pacemapping is shown in **Figure 8.3**. In this case of a 32-year-old female with symptomatic palpitations due to PVCs, a pacemap obtained at the site of origin of the arrhythmia, the anteroseptal right ventricular outflow tract is shown. Ablation from this catheter position led to termination of the arrhythmia.

Even slight variations in the paced complex compared to the spontaneous complex are important, as investigators have reported that successful ablation sites typically arise from areas with at least 11/12 pacemaps, preferably pacemaps that match is each lead.[5,6] This area, however, can only provide an estimate of the origin of the tachycardia as a 1 cm^2 area surrounding the origin can have a 12/12 pacemap. However, the origin of a tachycardia is unlikely to be from an area that does not have a 12/12 pacemap. Therefore, if ancillary data such as activation information or entrainment are available these are very useful adjuncts in pace mapping. Investigators have demonstrated that under ideal conditions, using only minor differences in amplitude and configuration, a unipolar pace map may have a spatial resolution of less than 5 mm.[7] Unipolar pacing was used in this situation due to difficulties with localization of the paced impulse between electrodes in bipolar pacing. However, in practical

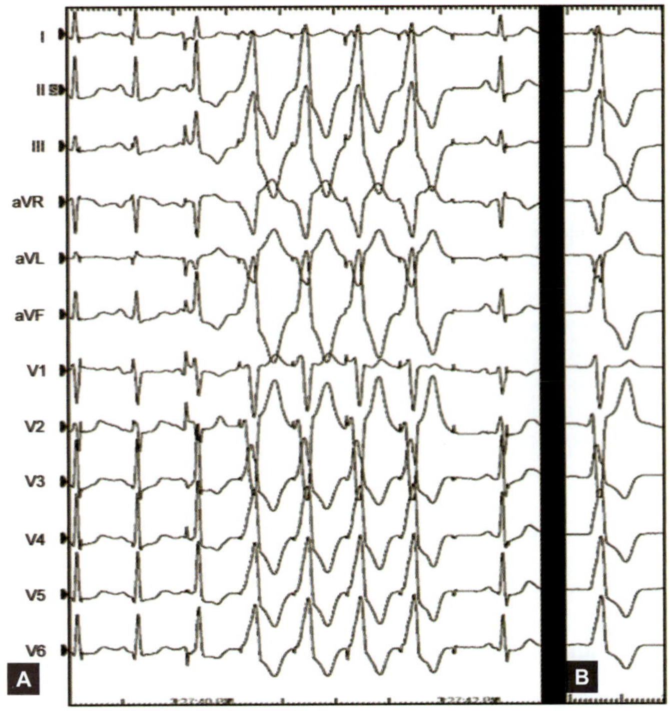

Figures 8.3A and B: Pacemapping is demonstrated in this figure. The patient, a 32-year-old female with frequent PVCs, was found to have PVCs from the anteroseptal right ventricular outflow tract. Here, pacing from the site of origin (A) creates a QRS complex that is nearly identical in morphology to the clinical PVC (B). Ablation in this region led to elimination of the PVCs

experiences this approach may not be possible to perform during a typical case in the electrophysiology lab due to time constraints. In addition, use of the stimulus to QRS time has been used in the setting of ventricular arrhythmias in peri-infarct regions.[8] Areas with a long stim-QRS time (>80 ms) were associated with slow conduction and were more likely to be successful ablation sites than times with no stim-QRS delay.

Pace Mapping for Atrial Arrhythmias

Pace mapping for atrial arrhythmias is inherently more difficult than pace mapping for ventricular arrhythmias based on the difficulty of analyzing the surface P-wave morphology for subtle differences. In addition, it is often difficult to have a clean, unperturbed P-wave for analysis as the P-wave during tachycardia is often affected by the T-wave and QRS complex. For these reasons pace mapping of atrial arrhythmias is not employed as often as for ventricular arrhythmias. That being said, one can use intracardiac electrograms to perform pace mapping of an atrial arrhythmia. This typically involves placing catheters in various locations in the atrium, typically including the high right atrium and coronary sinus. The intracardiac electrogram is then recorded for the tachycardia of interest, and this can be compared to the intracardiac electrograms recorded during pacing for an intracardiac pace map. Sites with the closest matches to the intracardiac electrogram recorded during tachycardia are thought to have the closest proximity to the tachycardia circuit.

ENTRAINMENT MAPPING

Entrainment is defined as constant resetting of a tachycardia by a train of premature stimuli. To understand entrainment one must understand the concept of resetting. A hypothetical tachycardia circuit with a partially excitable gap can be used to illustrate this concept. If an extrastimulus is late-coupled and arrives at the tachycardia once the tail is no longer excitable, this extrastimulus will not penetrate the tachycardia. If the extrastimulus is very early coupled, it will collide with both the antidromic and orthodromic wavefronts, thereby terminating the tachycardia. If an extrastimulus is timed such that it collides with the antidromic wavefront but advances the timing of the orthodromic wavefront, the tachycardia will emerge from the exit site at a time that is earlier than typical based on how early the extrastimulus arrives. In tachycardias with partially excitable gaps the decreased conduction time of the partially excitable tail can result is advancement by a lesser extent. Extrastimuli that collide with the antidromic wavefront but advance the orthodromic wavefront are said to reset the tachycardia. Entrainment is defined as continuous resetting of a tachycardia circuit by a pacing train.

In an entrained tachycardia, each stimulus both collides retrograde with the previous beat and conducts anterograde through the tachycardia circuit with the exception of the last stimulus which exits the tachycardia circuit without interference from a subsequent paced beat and therefore matches the morphology of the tachycardia at the pacing rate. After the pacing train ends, the tachycardia then resumes at the previous rate of the tachycardia with the same morphology as the tachycardia. Criteria have been established to determine if entrainment of the tachycardia has occurred.[9] These include fixed fusion at a single pacing rate between the paced complex and the tachycardia, progressive fusion with increased similarity to the pacing complex at faster pacing rates, and resumption of the initial tachycardia rate and morphology after cessation of pacing with the last entrained complex demonstrating no fusion. A fourth criterion has been proposed in which progressive fusion in the intracardiac electrograms can be demonstrated in the absence of progressive fusion on the electrocardiogram.[10] In clinical practice it is often difficult to document all of these criteria as pacing at a faster rate risks termination of the tachycardia. Entrainment with progressive fusion can only occur with reentrant tachycardias. Automatic or triggered tachycardias are not entrained with fixed fusion and instead often demonstrate variable fusion.

Entrainment can occur when the pacing site is not within the tachycardia circuit. Instead, one can use entrainment behavior to gage proximity of the pacing site to the circuit. With sites that are in close proximity to the circuit, fewer stimuli at less premature intervals are required to entrain the tachycardia. In contrast, if a pacing site is remote from the tachycardia circuit typically many stimuli are required at a shorter coupling interval. In practice, tachycardias are typically entrained in the electrophysiology lab at intervals 20 ms shorter than the tachycardia as this reliably produces entrainment of reentrant tachycardias without risk of terminating the tachycardia, which in the case of atypical flutters and indeterminate locations of macroreentrant circuits can make treatment of the clinical arrhythmia impossible. Entrainment is documented by measuring local capture in a site remote from the pacing site. During entrainment the local electrograms are advanced to the rate of the pacing train, and upon cessation of pacing there is a pause and then resumption of the original rate of the tachycardia. If the tachycardia rate increases or decreases after pacing, it is important to assess for termination and reinitiation of the same or a different tachycardia.

Entrainment can be used to map the circuit of a tachycardia.[11] This is most often employed by measuring the post-pacing interval (PPI) and comparing this with the tachycardia cycle length (TCL). If one is to imagine a hypothetical tachycardia circuit with an excitable gap, when a premature extrastimulus resets the tachycardia it travels from the origin of the extrastimulus and traverses the tachycardia circuit and then returns to the origin. If the post-pacing interval is defined as the time it takes the extrastimulus to return to the site of origin after resetting the tachycardia, then the post-pacing interval minus the tachycardia cycle length determines the time it takes for the extrastimulus to travel to and from the tachycardia circuit. Therefore, PPI-TCL is a surrogate for distance from the stimulus to the tachycardia circuit.[12] The PPI will always exceed the TCL. By measuring various PPI-TCL values, one can create a map of proximity to the tachycardia circuit. In general, in tissues with normal conduction properties, a PPI-TCL cutoff of 30 milliseconds is often used to determine if the pacing site is in circuit or remote from the circuit. PPI measurement should be made using near-field signals, not pacing stimuli, due to latency in tissues. Oftentimes near-field signals cannot be recorded from the pacing site due to saturation artifact from pacing. In these cases, one can use either adjacent electrodes on the mapping catheter or surface markers that establish local capture.

In addition to the PPI-TCL, evaluation of the surface electrocardiogram and intracardiac electrograms for fusion can be used to determine if the pacing site is in circuit or remote from the circuit. Specifically, evaluation for fusion on the ECG or intracardiac EGM is useful. If one imagines a hypothetical tachycardia circuit, fusion occurs when the pacing site is remote from the tachycardia circuit and the

QRS complex or P-wave generated by the tachycardia collides with that generated by the pacing site. The last paced beat that resets the tachycardia exits the exit site of the tachycardia without interference from the pacing site and therefore, the surface morphology is identical to the tachycardia but occurs at the pacing rate. With more rapid pacing from the pacing site, there is more and more of a contribution of the paced morphology to the overall QRS or P-wave morphology, until a critical rate at which the QRS complex or P-wave is identical to the paced morphology. This can only occur at site remote to the tachycardia, as entraining from sites within the critical isthmus of a tachycardia will not produce a fused complex, but instead will produce a similar complex morphology to that of the tachycardia. Therefore, if entrainment occurs with fusion (also known as manifest entrainment or entrainment with manifest fusion), one can infer that the pacing site is not located within the critical protected isthmus of the tachycardia. Typically, at sites of entrainment with manifest fusion, ablation lesions are not likely to terminate the tachycardia. In rare circumstances, the surface ECG does not demonstrate fusion but the intracardiac electrograms appear fused. This often occurs at pacing sites near, but not in, the tachycardia circuit. Sufficient myocardium is not captured by the pacing site to affect the surface ECG but fusion is apparent on the intracardiac electrograms. Fixed fusion cannot occur with focal arrhythmias, as the interaction between the pacing stimulus and the tachycardia is variable and variable degrees of fusion will therefore, be exhibited. When pacing at cycle lengths similar to the tachycardia, subtle morphology changes will be exhibited that can differentiate between reentrant and focal rhythms.

Entrainment with concealed fusion (also known as concealed entrainment) occurs when pacing is performed in a protected site within the tachycardia circuit.[9] In this case, the tachycardia is accelerated to the pacing rate but the surface ECG and intracardiac electrograms are identical to those of the tachycardia. This occurs when pacing is performed in a critical isthmus or protected bystander site within the tachycardia circuit. An example of entrainment with concealed fusion is present in **Figure 8.4**. In this case, mapping of a stable ventricular tachycardia circuit was performed in a patient with a large prior anterior myocardial infarction and a large left ventricular apical aneurysm. Entrainment is demonstrated by the fact that the tachycardia is accelerated to the pacing rate, however there is no difference between the entrained QRS morphology and the

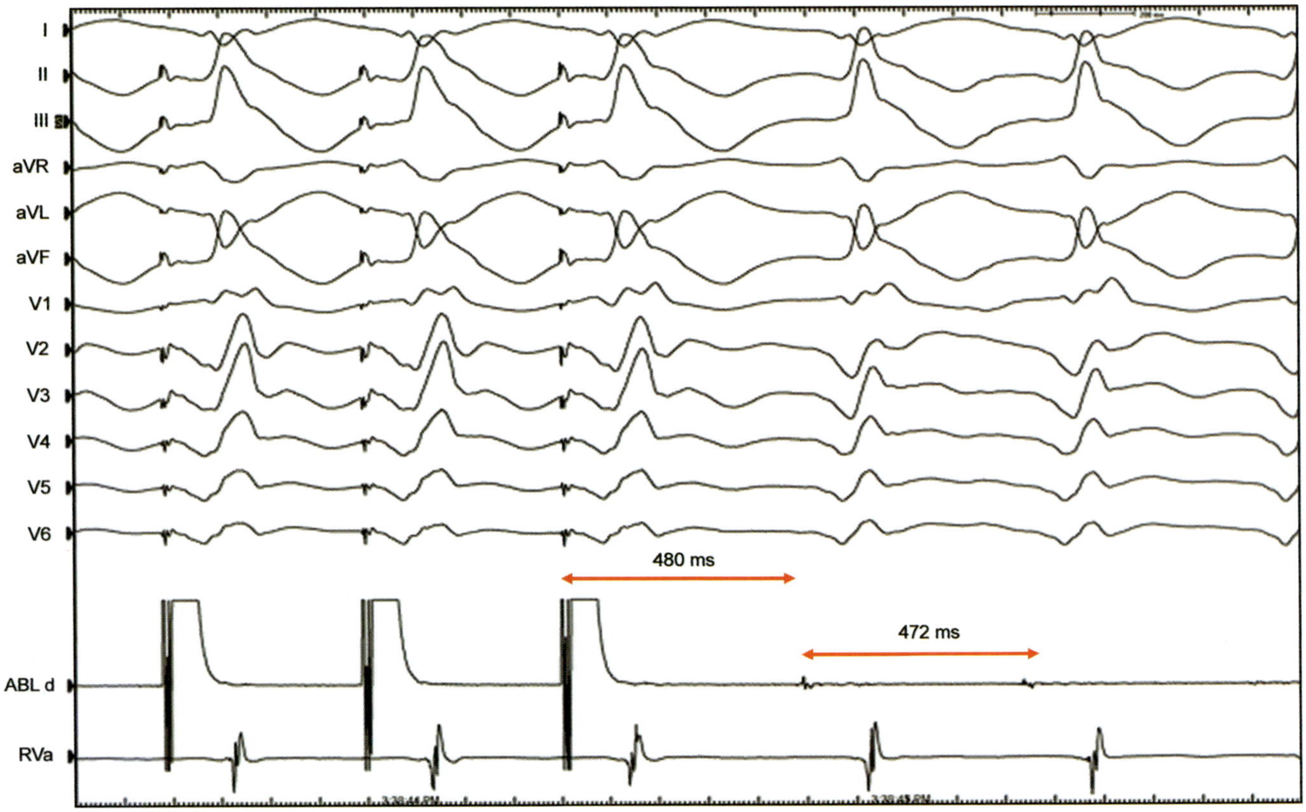

Figure 8.4: Entrainment mapping of ventricular tachycardia originating from an LV apical aneurysm in a patient with prior myocardial infarction and ischemic cardiomyopathy. Entrainment of the tachycardia from the distal ablation catheter demonstrated concealed entrainment, i.e. the QRS morphology of the entrained beats is a perfect match to that of the tachycardia beats. In addition, the post-pacing interval (480 ms) is almost equal to the tachycardia cycle length (472 ms). This suggests that the ablation catheter is located within the critical isthmus

VT QRS morphology. The PPI was nearly equal to the TCL in this site, suggesting that this was within a protected isthmus of the tachycardia.

During entrainment with concealed fusion, antidromic capture occurs but is not recorded as the electrograms within this critical isthmus are not apparent and do not contribute to the surface ECG. Entrainment with concealed fusion can occur in a critical isthmus in which ablation will likely terminate the tachycardia or can occur in protected bystander sites in which antidromic capture cannot be recorded but are not involved in the tachycardia and therefore, are unlikely to terminate the tachycardia with ablation. However, these areas are typically quite close to critical isthmuses that will be successful ablation sites.

One can compare the time between pacing stimulus and QRS production (Stim-QRS) and the time between local electrogram and QRS production (EGM-QRS) to determine if a site that demonstrates entrainment with concealed fusion is a critical isthmus site or if it is a protected bystander.[12] The EGM-QRS time represents the time from local activation at the mapping catheter site to the exit site (which results in QRS formation) during tachycardia. In contrast, the Stim-QRS time represents the time that a pacing stimulus takes to exit the tachycardia circuit and produce a QRS complex. In sites that are involved in tachycardia, the Stim-QRS time should equal the EGM-QRS time as both of these are activated in series. However, in protected bystander sites, the EGM-QRS time will be shorter than the Stim-QRS time. This is due to the fact that the local electrogram and the exit site are activated in parallel in bystander sites, whereas with pacing from the bystander, site the bystander site and exit site are activated in series and hence take a longer time. An example from the same patient as above is shown in **Figure 8.5**. From the site with concealed entrainment, the Stim-QRS was equal to the EGM-QRS, suggesting that the ablation catheter was located within the tachycardia circuit and not in a bystander region. Ablation in this area terminated the tachycardia, and no further VT could be induced.

Entrainment mapping is rarely used in isolation to map a reentrant tachycardia. Instead, activation mapping or pace mapping is typically performed to identify areas of interest, after which entrainment is performed to determine if the site is a suitable site for ablation or not. An example of this is shown in **Figures 8.6A and B**, in which case an activation map of an atypical left atrial flutter was created, with entrainment used to confirm the critical isthmus of the circuit. Use of

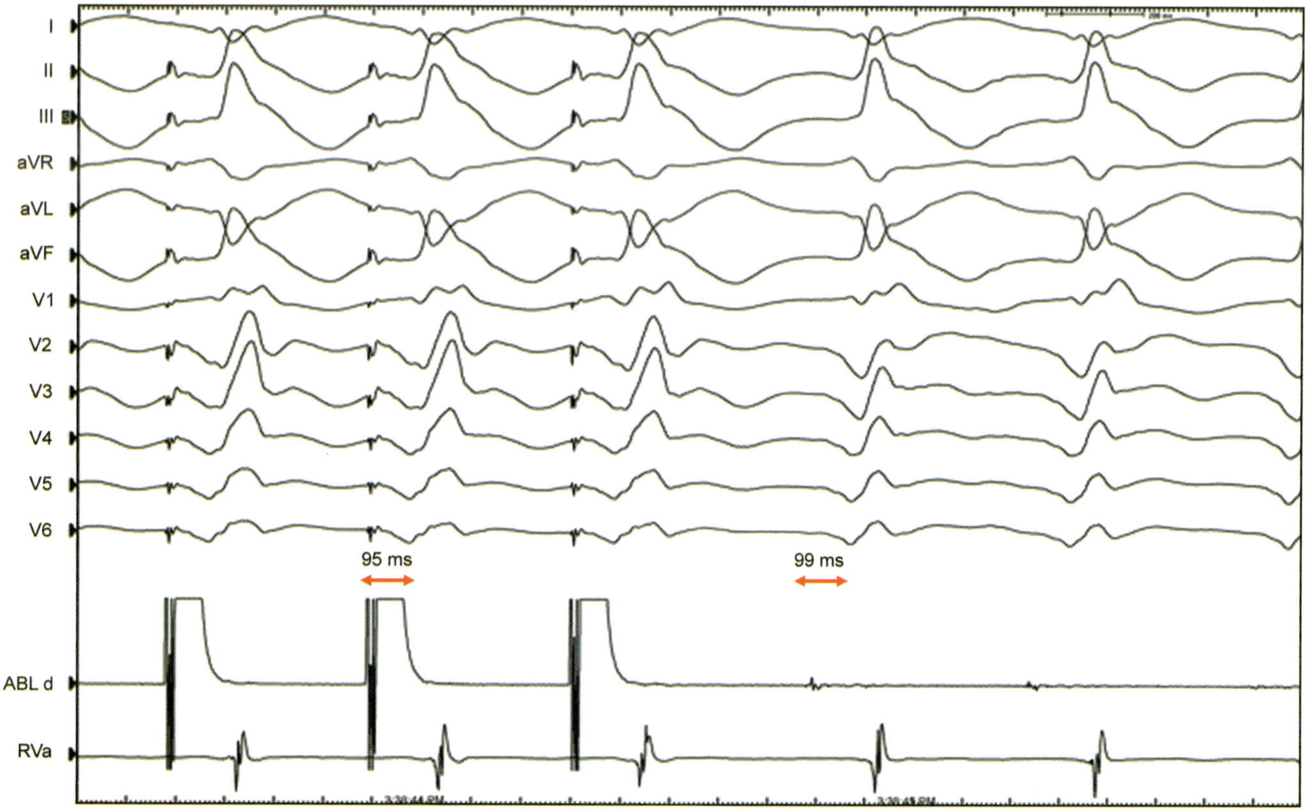

Figure 8.5: Further evaluation of the entrainment of the same patient demonstrates that the time from the pacing stimulus to the QRS complex (stim-QRS) is equal to the time from the electrogram to the QRS complex during tachycardia (EGM-QRS), suggesting that the location of the ablation catheter is part of the circuit, not a bystander. In addition, the time from stimulus to QRS was less than 30% of the tachycardia cycle length, suggesting that this was an exit site of the tachycardia. Ablation in this region terminated the tachycardia and rendered it noninducible

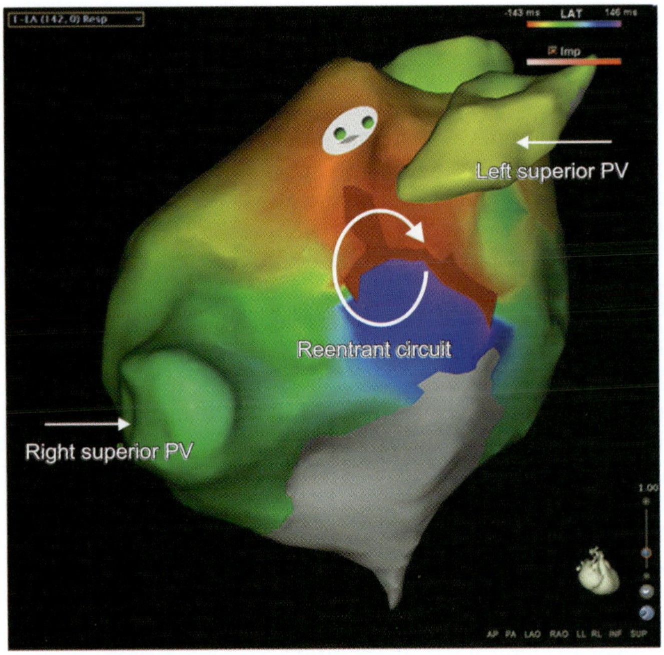

Figure 8.6A: Activation map of a post-Maze left atrial flutter created with the Carto 3 system. A macrorentrant tachycardia is noted around the left sided pulmonary veins

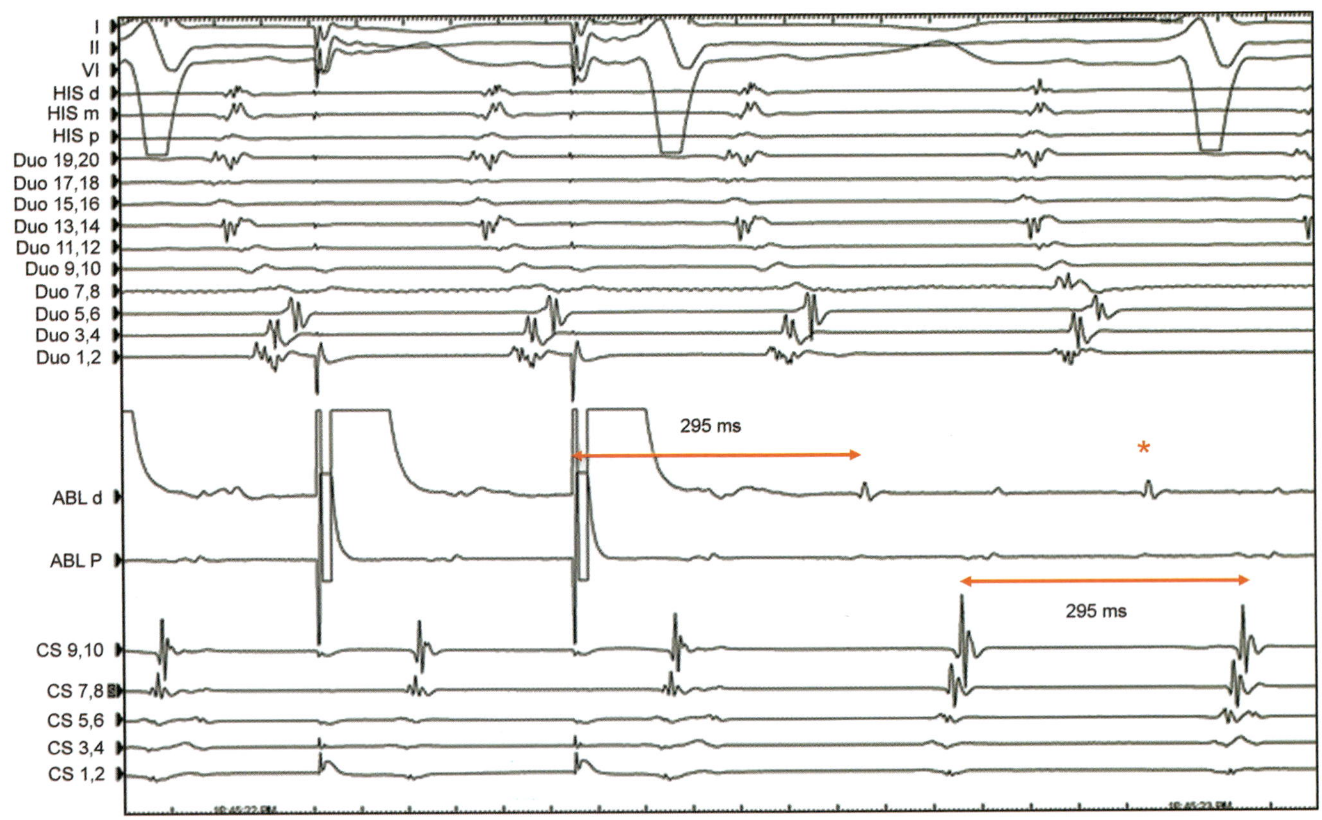

Figure 8.6B: Entrainment mapping can be used to confirm the tachycardia circuit as determined by activation mapping. The Halo catheter is around the right atrium. With entrainment, there is no change in the activation sequence of the Halo catheter. In addition, the post-pacing interval (295 ms) is equal to the tachycardia cycle length (295 ms). Entrainment also helped us to determine which of the electrograms on the mapping catheter was the electrogram of interest for mapping purposes (asterisk). These findings suggested that the area of the mapping catheter (outside the left superior pulmonary vein) was both in circuit and part of the critical isthmus. Ablation in this region led to termination of the tachycardia

entrainment mapping without other modalities of mapping is cumbersome and risks termination of the tachycardia by pacing too often. Entrainment mapping requires a tachycardia that is able to be entrained, i.e. not an automatic or triggered rhythm. In addition, entrainment requires that a tachycardia is inducible or present during the ablation procedure and is hemodynamically tolerated. Pacing and recording from the same area is required to measure the post-pacing interval with accuracy.

Areas of interest are identified, at which point the tachycardia is entrained by a pacing train that is around 20 ms faster than the tachycardia of interest. Before measuring a post-pacing interval, it is critical to determine if the tachycardia has in actuality been entrained. This is performed by evaluating electrograms within the tachycardia circuit and determining if they have been accelerated to the pacing rate in the presence of fixed fusion. Care should be taken to ensure that the tachycardia has not been terminated and reinitiated, mimicking entrainment. Measurement of the post-pacing interval when entrainment has not been documented lacks physiologic meaning and leads to mapping errors. After entrainment has been documented, one can evaluate for manifest fusion or concealed entrainment to gather more information related to the proximity of the pacing site to the tachycardia circuit. When the complex morphology cannot reliably be used to determine if there is manifest fusion or concealed fusion (i.e. in atrial arrhythmias), intracardiac electrograms can be used as a surrogate. An example of this is shown in **Figure 8.7**, in which a typical cavotri-cuspid isthmus dependent atrial flutter is mapped and entrained with concealed fusion based on the appearance of the intracardiac electrograms which are unchanged during entrainment.

In addition, as described above, Stim-QRS can be compared with EGM-QRS to evaluate if the pacing site is involved in the tachycardia or is a protected bystander. An endocardial or epicardial map can be created by measuring the PPI-TCL at various sites in the chamber of interest and

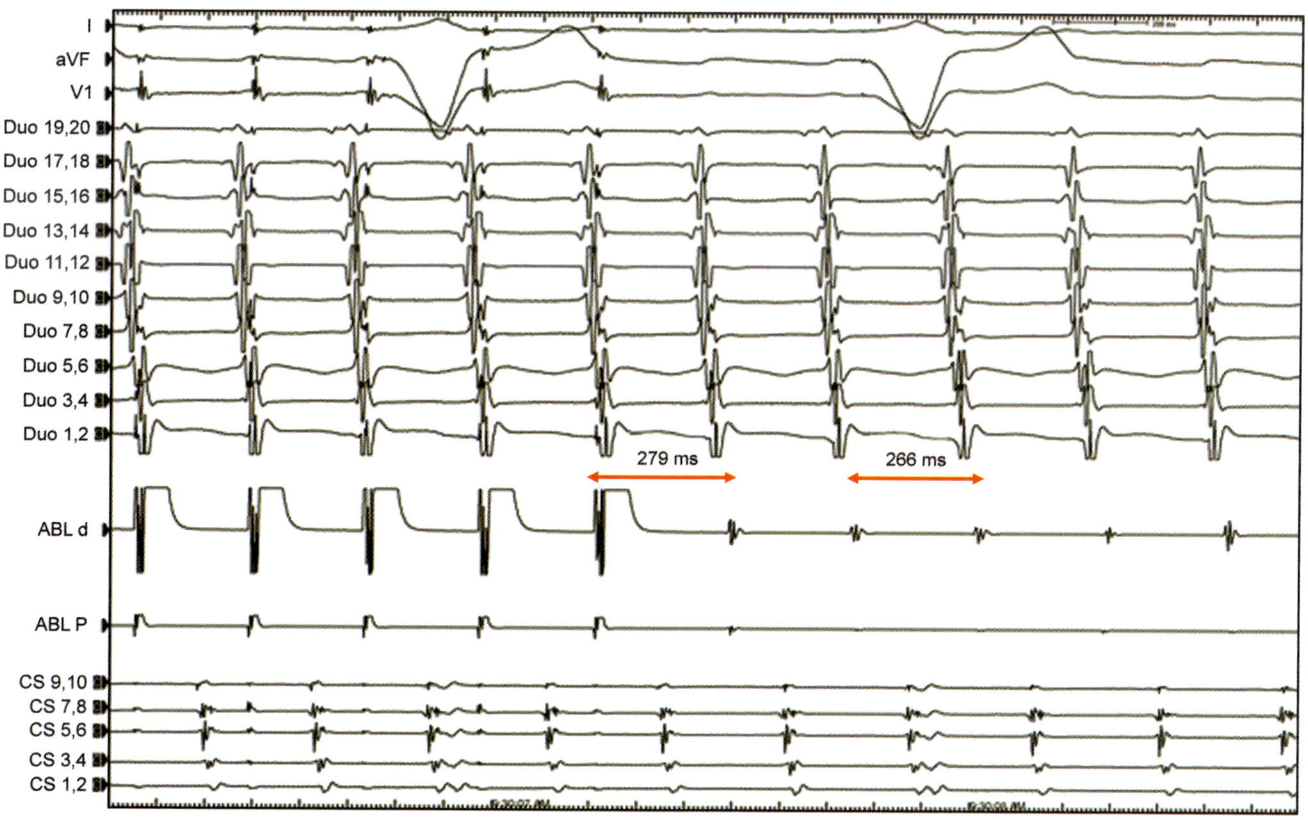

Figure 8.7: Entrainment mapping can also be performed using intracardiac electrograms when the surface depolarization is difficult to analyze, as is the case in this patient with typical cavotricuspid isthmus dependent atrial flutter. The Halo catheter is around the right atrium. With entrainment from the cavotricuspid isthmus, there is no change in the activation sequence in the Halo catheter, indicating intracardiac concealed fusion. In addition, the post-pacing interval (279 ms) is similar to the tachycardia cycle length (266 ms). These findings together suggest that the area of the mapping catheter (at the cavotricuspid isthmus) is both in the circuit and part of the critical isthmus. Ablation in this region led to termination of the tachycardia

creating a graphical map based on the values. Areas with the shortest PPI-TCL that also present entrainment with concealed fusion are likely to be in or near the protected isthmuses in which ablation may be successful in termination of tachycardia.

CONCLUSION

With a detailed understanding of the conventional mapping approaches of activation mapping, pace mapping, and entrainment mapping, arrhythmias can be reliably studied in the electrophysiology lab. These approaches are a necessary adjunct to pacing maneuvers in the identification of both the mechanism and anatomical basis of the arrhythmia of interest. Further chapters will delineate the advanced 3D mapping techniques that are based upon these conventional mapping techniques.

REFERENCES

1. Stevenson WG, Weiss JN, Wiener I, Rivitz SM, Nademanee K, Klitzner T, Yeatman L, Josephson M, and Wohlgelernter D. Fractionated endocardial electrograms are associated with slow conduction in humans: evidence from pace-mapping. J American Coll Cardiol. 1989;13:369-76.
2. Barlow MA, Klein GJ, Simpson CS, Murgatroyd FD, Yee R, Krahn AD, and Skanes AC. Unipolar electrogram characteristics predictive of successful radiofrequency catheter ablation of accessory pathways. J Cardiovasc Electrophysiol. 2000;11:146-54.
3. Man KC, Daoud EG, Knight BP, Bahu M, Weiss R, Zivin A, Souza SJ, Goyal R, Strickberger SA, and Morady F. Accuracy of the unipolar electrogram for identification of the site of origin of ventricular activation. J Cardiovasc Electrophysiol. 1997;8:974-9.
4. Goyal R, Harvey M, Daoud EG, Brinkman K, Knight BP, Bahu M, Weiss R, Bogun F, Man KC, Strickberger SA, et al. Effect of coupling interval and pacing cycle length on morphology of paced ventricular complexes. Implications for pace mapping. Circulation. 1996;94:2843-9.
5. Klein LS, Shih HT, Hackett FK, Zipes DP, and Miles WM. Radiofrequency catheter ablation of ventricular tachycardia in patients without structural heart disease. Circulation. 1992;85:1666-74.
6. Calkins H, Kalbfleisch SJ, el-Atassi R, Langberg JJ, and Morady F. Relation between efficacy of radiofrequency catheter ablation and site of origin of idiopathic ventricular tachycardia. American J Cardiol. 1993;71:827-33.
7. Kadish AH, Childs K, Schmaltz S, and Morady F. Differences in QRS configuration during unipolar pacing from adjacent sites: implications for the spatial resolution of pace-mapping. J American Coll Cardiol. 1991;17:143-51.
8. Brunckhorst CB, Stevenson WG, Soejima K, Maisel WH, Delacretaz E, Friedman PL, and Ben-Haim SA. Relationship of slow conduction detected by pace-mapping to ventricular tachycardia re-entry circuit sites after infarction. J American Coll Cardiol. 2003;41:802-9.
9. Waldo AL. Atrial flutter: entrainment characteristics. J Cardiovasc Electrophysiol. 1997;8:337-52.
10. Henthorn RW, Okumura K, Olshansky B, Plumb VJ, Hess PG, and Waldo AL. A fourth criterion for transient entrainment: the electrogram equivalent of progressive fusion. Circulation. 1988;77:1003-12.
11. Waldo AL, and Henthorn RW. Use of transient entrainment during ventricular tachycardia to localize a critical area in the reentry circuit for ablation. Pacing Clinical Electrophysiol. 1989;12(1 Pt 2):231-44.
12. Stevenson WG, Khan H, Sager P, Saxon LA, Middlekauff HR, Natterson PD, and Wiener I. Identification of reentry circuit sites during catheter mapping and radiofrequency ablation of ventricular tachycardia late after myocardial infarction. Circulation. 1993;88(4 Pt 1):1647-70.

EDITORS' SUMMARY

Perhaps the most fundamental skill, an electrophysiologist needs, is to accurately map a cardiac rhythm disturbance, yet this prerequisite and basic requirement is among the most difficult to execute well. In this chapter, Drs Pelchovitz and Arora review in a balanced yet highly instructive manner the limitations and correct execution of the main method we use in the EP laboratory to identify what needs ablation and where the most effective and safe area to deliver radiofrequency or other energy is. Although this chapter describes the basics of mapping, all advanced mapping techniques rely entirely on understanding the local electrogram characteristics, the normal rhythm, tachycardia, and the response to various pacing and entrainment maneuvers.

1. Mechanism of arrhythmia. The authors importantly emphasize the fact that the rationale and method for mapping is completely different when analyzing a reentrant versus a point-source or automatic tachycardia. While with point-source tachycardias the earliest recorded discrete electrogram relative to a fixed and reliable point of reference will readily identify a site for successful ablation, in reentrant arrhythmia the relative timing is irrelevant since the entire cycle length of the tachycardia will be present if a complete map of the cardiac chambers is done, i.e. there is no early or late site with reentrant arrhythmia. The authors point out that for reentry, not only does the entire circuit need to be mapped, but we need careful annotation and a strategy to deal with fragmented or fractionated electrograms and double potentials when present.
2. For both substrate mapping and identifying boundaries for reentrant arrhythmia, caution is required when defining or annotating scar. There is no absolute reliable "cut-off" electrogram amplitude (bipolar or unipolar) that distinguishes scar from viable myocardium or noise. The operator is required to correlate any electrogram with its timing and fixity with other portions of the cardiac cycle or surface ECG and the response to local pacing and capture.
3. The authors clearly delineate the pitfalls of "pace mapping" and the importance of varying the pacing output, size of the electrode tip and bipole used for local stimulation, and visualization that indeed only the tip electrode is making contact with only one cardiac structure (avoiding wedge green electrode contact between the papillary muscle and LV wall, for example).
4. The relative merits of bipolar and unipolar electrograms are clearly discussed, and a thorough study of these sections will be of great value, particularly for those early in their career in electrophysiology. Specifically avoiding annotation of far-field bipolar electrograms and recognizing that the unipolar electrograms can be deceiving when there is no contact with the tissue being mapped or when targeting areas where very small electrograms may represent the best site to target for eliminating the tachycardia (supravalvar signals, fascicular signals, etc).
5. Finally, within just a few pages, the authors have provided an outstanding and succinct review of entrainment mapping where the reader is taken through the entire rationale and pitfalls to avoid when performing this common maneuver.

CHAPTER 9

Freddy Del-Carpio Munoz, Samuel J Asirvatham

Three-dimensional Mapping of Cardiac Arrhythmias: Techniques, Principles and Application

LIST OF ABBREVIATION

3D	Three-dimensional

INTRODUCTION

The treatment of cardiac arrhythmias has experienced notable advancement in the last two decades. Among the most remarkable technological developments is the evolution of three-dimensional (3D) mapping techniques,[1,2] from relatively simple systems providing only localization of ablation catheters and simple catheter navigation features[3] to more sophisticated current systems that not only provide localization and navigation information, but also detailed information of the arrhythmic substrate as well as integration of mapping information with catheter contact force, more accurate activation mapping, fusion with other imaging modalities, and fast mapping techniques that can lead to a more efficient workflow and more accurate, high resolution 3D maps. These systems are important tools to guide invasive treatment of cardiac arrhythmias, and their use has now become routine to the point that in many electrophysiology laboratories worldwide it is difficult to conceive of catheter ablation of complex arrhythmic substrates, such as atrial fibrillation or ventricular arrhythmias without the support of 3D mapping systems. Therefore, it is critical for the modern practice of cardiac electrophysiology to be familiar with the currently available 3D mapping technology. The present chapter aims to review the basic principles of performing accurate 3D electroanatomic maps of cardiac arrhythmias, their interpretation, limitations, and some tips and flaws that any electrophysiologist should keep in mind when using these technologies to avoid misleading information that can potentially lead to an unsuccessful ablative procedure. It is important to mention that the use of advanced 3D mapping systems is complementary to the information obtained by analysis and correct interpretation of the electrophysiological characteristics of the arrhythmia under treatment, the knowledge of appropriate anatomical landmarks, the appropriate use of other adjunctive imaging modalities, etc., and that a 3D map can rarely stand alone to guide ablative therapies.

BRIEF REVIEW OF DIFFERENT MAPPING SYSTEMS

CARTO Mapping System (Biosense Webster, Diamond Bar, CA, USA)

The original system consists of a locator pad with three mounted coils on a triangular frame attached underneath the fluoroscopy table beneath the patient, a specialized catheter that has a magnetic sensor embedded in the tip, a skin patch adhered to the patient's back and a processor unit with a monitor where images can be displayed and electrical signals annotated. The three separate coils in the locator pad emit a low level electromagnetic field that is recognized by the specialized catheter tip sensor.[4,5] According to the location of the catheter, the strength of the magnetic field of each of the three coils as measured by the magnetic sensor is inversely proportional to the distance of the catheter tip to the coils. The mathematical calculation of this distance allows the system to locate the catheter tip in the 3D space. Roving the catheter and collecting multiple points allows the system to recreate the geometry of the mapped chamber. The signals recorded at the catheter tip are recorded and analyzed simultaneously with the location of the catheter tip and are then displayed in the 3D space relative to the location of the reference patch in the patient's back. For local activation timing, the collected signals are stored and compared to a timing reference signal that can be a stable intracardiac signal or surface electrocardiographic recording. The accrued points in the electrical activation map are assigned thus to isochronal color scales based on their respective activation times relative to the timing reference point; additionally, the system records voltage amplitude information and can also annotate the location of intracardiac signals of interest in the 3D map. This particular system is able to display only location of manufacturer-specific, sensor-embedded catheters. The most recent version of this system (CARTO® 3) includes two location technologies, the aforementioned and an advanced catheter location which displays location data from each electrode connected to the system. This latter location technology is based on the signals received from six patches attached to the patient; each electrode emits high-frequency, low-power current sensed by the patches, and an algorithm calculates the position of each electrode based on the relative measured current. The mean magnetic-based location accuracy is 1 mm while the advanced location technology mean accuracy is 3 mm. With the additional current-based location technology, the system can also recognize catheters without the embedded magnetic sensor.

The Carto system has a real-time integration module with intracardiac ultrasound called CartoSound® (Biosense Webster, Inc). This module is capable of obtaining 3D ultrasound-based geometry creation using an intracardiac ultrasound probe embedded with the magnetic sensor at the tip to allow tip location, origin, and direction of 2D echocardiographic images that are collated by the system to render 3D images of cardiac chambers.[6] Thus the ultrasound transducer generates and receives multiple rays of ultrasound. The system offers the option to acquire anatomical structures in real-time and relatively quickly. Once an anatomy is obtained, the 3D geometry map can serve to obtain electrophysiological data. In **Figure 9.1**, we show a map of four chamber geometries of both ventricles, including outflow tracts and the pulmonary artery and aortic roots, which were created with CartoSound for the catheter ablation of a ventricular tachycardia originating from the right coronary cusp.

Another commonly used module of the Carto-3 system is Fast Anatomical Mapping, which facilitates a rapid generation of anatomical 3D maps. The system collects anatomical location data continuously as the mapping catheter is displaced in the heart. Based on the recorded location data, a volume is construed, and using the outer surface of this volume, a geometrical 3D reconstruction is created after discarding the internal location data. The fast activation mapping module can be generated using a quadripolar catheter, but it can also be done more efficiently using multipolar catheters for simultaneous generation of large amounts of anatomical location points.

Further technological advancements in ablation catheters now permit direct measurement of catheter-tissue contact force.[7] Even though this is important to monitor good catheter-tissue contact while applying radiofrequency energy to achieve transmural ablation lesions, the technology can also be used during mapping in order to perform an accurate map by assuring good catheter-endocardial contact while electroanatomic mapping is obtained.

EnSite NavX Velocity System (St. Jude Medical, Minnetonka, MN, USA)

This is an updated version of the original EnSite NavX system (St Jude Medical). The system consists of two platforms: the EnSite Array, which enables noncontact mapping, and the EnSite NavX, which enables contact mapping and visualization of multiple catheters.[8] The 3D localization and navigation of catheters is based on the emission of external electrical fields from three pairs of patches orthogonally placed on the patient's thoracic surface. Electrodes in each catheter record voltage and impedance of the emitted electrical fields, and this information is used to locate the electrodes and catheters in the 3D space related to a reference electrode. By roving the mapping catheter, the geometry of the chamber of interest is generated. Then information about electrical activation, amplitude of electrical signals, and other electrogram characteristics are registered and displayed on a user interface monitor. The system's general principle of electrical-based intracardiac catheter visualization has been validated previously[8]; the system has a localization accuracy of 0.2 ± 1.7 mm, 0.1 ± 0.3 mm, and 0.2 ± 0.6 mm for the X, Y, and Z axes respectively.[3] The EnSite Velocity upgrade is able to perform faster sampling and yields more anatomical accuracy.[9] Importantly, the EnSite system is open to the localization of any type of electrophysiological catheter and is able to visualize and locate a total of 128 electrodes.

The non-contact mapping EnSite Array platform uses a 64-electrode mesh mounted over an ellipsoid inflatable balloon. In the catheter shaft there are two ring electrodes, 1 cm proximal and 1 cm distal to the balloon. A third electrode ring located more proximally in the catheter shaft serves

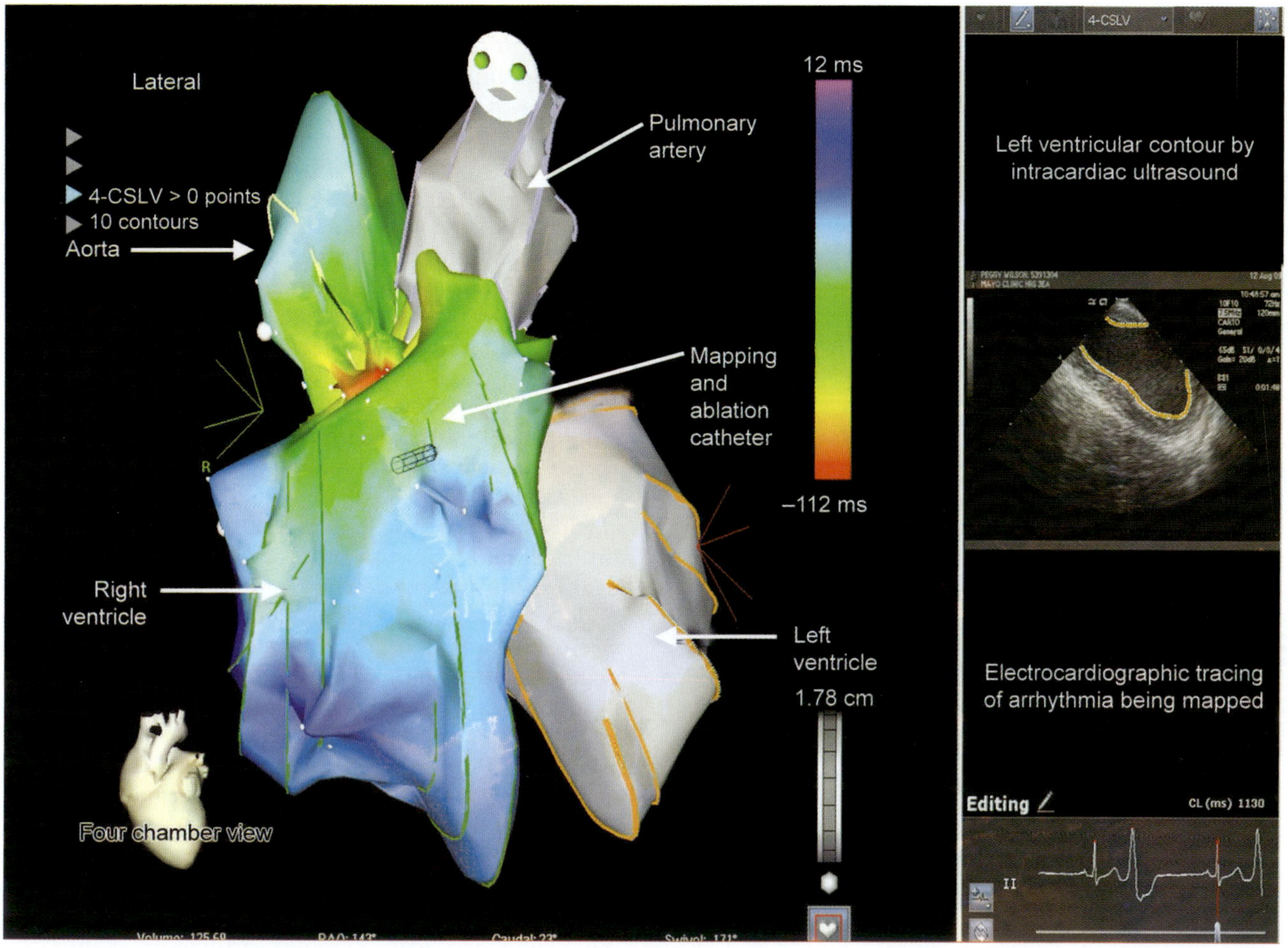

Figure 9.1: Intracardiac ultrasound-based imaging using the CARTO system to create anatomical geometries of cardiac chambers. In this case four chambers were created: aortic root and proximal pulmonary artery, right and left ventricles for mapping and ablation of frequent premature ventricular contractions originating in the right coronary cusp. Multiple intracardiac ultrasound contours of the endocardial surface of the chambers were collected using a magnetic-sensor embedded ultrasound probe. These contours are then collated for volume rendering. One of the contours of the left ventricle is shown in the right panel (orange contour). The system generates a quick anatomical map of the chambers in which an activation map is then obtained

as an indifferent electrode reference for virtual recording of unipolar electrograms by the array. Once the balloon is deployed and inflated inside a cardiac chamber of interest, a low-level electrical signal, which is sensed alternately by the electrode rings close to the balloon, is sent through a conventional or ablation catheter. A locator system localizes the tip of the mapping catheter relative to the array, and thus a 3D geometry is created. The 64-electrode array is able to sense far-field unipolar signals by galvanic contact with blood, generating an activation map using only one or a few cardiac cycles. The system is useful for mapping of nonsustained or hemodynamically unstable arrhythmias.[10] In **Figures 9.2A to C**, we show an activation map of the right atrium during a tachycardia originating in the superior part of the *crista terminalis*. The balloon-based non-contact mapping system has some limitations, including less accuracy when mapping large chambers or restricted balloon maneuverability in small ones.

MediGuide Technology (St. Jude Medical Inc, St Paul, MN)

It is not an electroanatomic system *per se*, but a real-time catheter tracking system that can guide nonfluoroscopic navigation of catheters. It is based on a novel, sensor-based electromagnetic tracking system, and uses very small sensors mounted over a sheath, diagnostic or ablation catheter, enabling real-time tracking of the catheter or

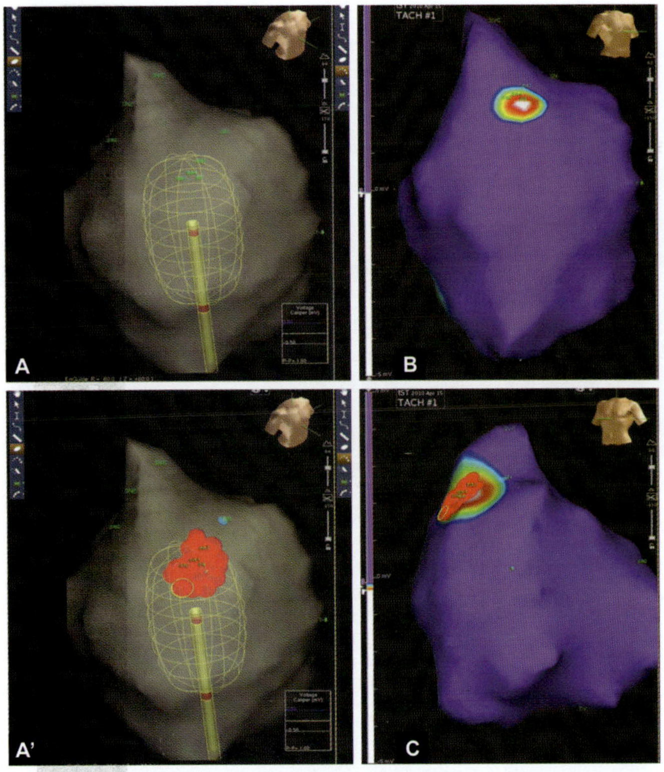

Figures 9.2A to C: Non-contact mapping. Using the EnSite Array mapping platform, activation of right atrium is shown. The balloon with a multielectrode array is placed in the right atrium to create an anatomical endocardial geometry (panels A and A'). Activation is coming around the sinus node (RAO view in panel B, LAO view panel C). Radiofrequency applications are displayed in panel A'. The activation map shows a centrifugal activation consistent with a focal tachycardia

Courtesy: Dr Gustavo Morales, University of Kentucky, Lexington, KY

sheath within a dynamic electromagnetic field provided by a transmitter unit installed over conventional flat-panel X-ray imaging system.[11] This system then enables 4D visualization and navigation of catheters within preacquired X-ray loops. The system is not able to handle electrophysiological data, but it can be used with an electroanatomic mapping system like the NavX system and can significantly reduce fluoroscopy exposure.[12]

Rhythmia (Boston Scientific, Inc, Cambridge, MA)

This system uses a hybrid technology based on impedance and magnetic localization technologies, a combination of principles of the CARTO and the EnSite systems. The magnetic location technology uses magnetic fields emitted by a generator placed under the patient table. A magnetic sensor inside the manufacturer-specific catheter measures the magnetic signals that are then processed to determine the spatial location of the catheter in relation to the location generator. Impedance location technology can track any catheter with electrodes connected to the system. Impedance tracking is based on driving small currents between multiple surface electrodes, including surface electrocardiography and a location reference patch attached to the patient's back. The system measures the voltage of each electrode on a tracked catheter to estimate its spatial location. The magnetic localization has accuracy of ≤ 1 mm and impedance localization of ≤ 2 mm. The system, for the use of impedance-based localization technology, is open, and the operator can choose diagnostic or ablation catheters from different manufactures. The system is capable of performing rapid and high-resolution anatomical, activation, voltage, and fractionated electrogram mapping using the manufacturer's IntellaMap Orion™ (Boston Scientific Inc.) mapping catheter, which consists of 64 simultaneously recording electrodes displayed on a mini-basket array with variable deployment features. The system is able to perform continuous mapping mode, which allows the acquisition of multiple points at a fast speed. The automatic acceptance criteria are based on cycle length stability, relative timing with a reference electrogram, electrode location stability, and respiratory gating; further, for cardiac signals with multiple components (fractionated), the system takes into consideration the timing of electrograms in the surrounding areas and can select the appropriate timing for annotation.[13,14] Alternatively a manual-mapping mode is also available, and the user can accept and annotate points individually. The system can then display anatomic, activation, voltage, and fractionation maps simultaneously.[15] The experience with complex arrhythmic substrates is limited, but the system appears to perform automatic, ultra-high-density mapping quickly and reproducibly identify activation sequences of right atrial substrates.[16] There is also limited experience to its use in pulmonary vein isolation and ventricular arrhythmias.[15]

It may seem redundant to mention that any electroanatomic mapping system is able to perform at least three different types of maps: purely anatomical, activation maps, and voltage or substrate maps. The first only provides the geometry of the anatomical structure; this can be used, for instance, when performing a pulmonary vein isolation procedure where the geometries of the left atrium and pulmonary veins are obtained. Then the ablation applications can be displayed over the anatomical map, as well as anatomical tagging of important anatomical landmarks that can alter the ablative strategy, such as the esophagus, phrenic nerves, the pulmonary vein-left atrium junction, the vein of Marshall, or the junction of the pulmonary vein and left atrial appendage. The activation map requires the annotation of the timing of the electrical signals in relation to a reference point. For a voltage map, the system automatically measures the peak-to-peak amplitude of the bipolar or unipolar recorded signals. There are several variations for activation mapping that can help in guiding ablative strategies. For instance in cases of severe intra-atrial or ventricular conduction delay, the interpretation of a map of a focal arrhythmia can be difficult and may mimic a reentrant mechanism. In some cases plotting a postpacing interval after entrainment maneuvers, as a user-defined map function can facilitate interpretation of the arrhythmia mechanism and guide the ablation plan.[17] In other instances the activation map can be used to confirm block when pacing across a presumptive line of block. Additionally, the systems can also display maps of complex fractionated electrograms.

In the following sections we will review the basic principles of performing accurate anatomical, activation, and substrate maps. Our discussion will be based mainly on the use of the CARTO system, but these principles are generally applicable to the other systems as well.

HOW TO OBTAIN AN ACCURATE ANATOMICAL MAP?

A good anatomical map is the critical foundation for obtaining an accurate 3D electroanatomic map, although its use as a stand-alone map was infrequent in the past. With the common implementation of catheter ablation for the treatment of atrial fibrillation, the use of a purely anatomical map has become also more frequent. The recreation of accurate geometries of the cardiac chambers now can be accomplished by different methods, from the relatively slow point-by-point approach to the use of fast anatomical maps using multielectrode catheters and to the use of hybrid methods including intracardiac ultrasound. Further, using company-specific software, the catheter-based anatomical maps can be merged with previously obtained computed tomography or cardiac magnetic resonance imaging to validate these maps.[18]

The placement of a stable anatomical or spatial reference patch is central to obtain an accurate anatomical map. Loosely placed patch or patches can lead to distortion of the anatomical map. The Carto 3® mapping system creates initial location reference according to the position of the three back patches in reference to each other and to the location pad. The system is able to monitor this initial location, and if any displacements (due to patient movement, patch dislodgement, location pad movement) occur, it can alert the operator. The system is able to compensate for slight movement of the locator pad, but in general, significant displacement of a single patch will not be compensated, and the accuracy of the anatomical map will be seriously affected. In many instances, it is better to restart a new anatomical map.

Another important aspect of obtaining an accurate anatomical map is to distinguish areas that are internal due to poor catheter contact from the true endocardial surface. In this case, the use of mapping catheters to record data with only the distal electrode can be less optimal and often more time consuming. It is important to keep in mind that the mapping system will process spatial data and interpolate points regardless whether the collected points are from different anatomical structures. For instance, by taking points of the left atrium and the pulmonary veins erratically as the same anatomical structure, the mapping system will interpolate points between both structures and obscure the details of the venoatrial junction. Therefore, it is better to obtain separate maps of these structures and to obtain more thorough information if the objective is to preserve the anatomical detail between neighboring geometries that can be important to guide a safe and successful ablation procedure.[19]

Perhaps one of the most recognizable limitations of current electroanatomic mapping systems is that the 3D maps are *static* representations of the heart chambers, which are *dynamic* anatomical structures. In this regard, the role of cardiac and respiratory movements can alter the anatomical reconstructs. Intrinsic cardiac motion due to the underlying cardiac rhythm is expected to lead to inconsistencies for accurate catheter localization and navigation according to: the cardiac rhythm during which the spatial data is collected and the rhythm when the ablation catheter is tracked (for instance, mapping during atrial fibrillation and applying ablation during sinus rhythm), the period of the mechanical cardiac systole or diastole (obtaining atrial points during ventricular contraction). In a similar manner, respiratory motion can significantly affect the anatomical reconstruction of cardiac chambers. In general it is advisable to acquire anatomical data at the end of expiration in a consistent manner to avoid potential cardiac positional distortion of the geometries processed by the mapping system.[20] This is more easily accomplished when the patient is mechanically ventilated, the inspiration/expiration ratio can be changed, and the system then can be programmed to acquire data only during expiration. When the patient is under conscious sedation, this can be more challenging, and even more so in patients with large intrathoracic pressure fluctuations due to obesity or obstructive sleep apnea.[21,22]

HOW TO OBTAIN AN ACCURATE 3D ACTIVATION MAP OF A CARDIAC ARRHYTHMIA?

In addition to appropriate clinical evaluation and review of previous cardiac history, including previous cardiac surgical interventions or ablative procedures, there are several basic principles that an experienced electrophysiologist should take into account in order to obtain an accurate 3D activation map of a cardiac arrhythmia. Familiarity with the system options is very important; since with recent technological advances there are new system-specific features that can facilitate the process, but if not known can be a hurdle for a smooth and efficient workflow. While obtaining a 3D map the operator should assure good catheter contact, (this can be guided and supported by fluoroscopy images, intracardiac ultrasound, and recently by assessment of the contact force between the catheter tip and endocardial surface), ensure complete mapping of the chamber of interest, confirm on a regular basis that the arrhythmia of interest has a stable tachycardia cycle length without variations of the activation sequences, and address issues regarding potential causes of distortion of the 3D anatomic shell, as previously stated.[23]

Before the accrual of the activation points, it is necessary to define an appropriate reference timing point. For the case of atrial arrhythmias, the timing reference point is commonly an intra-atrial electrogram, which has a stable morphology with minimal or no variation of the amplitude. Typically an electrogram from a multipolar catheter inside the coronary sinus is used, but in cases of complex congenital heart disease or inability to introduce a coronary sinus catheter, an active fixation intracardiac catheter can be temporarily placed in the atria. The operator or the assistant should guarantee that within the elected reference signal, the system picks the same point (initial peak, most negative deflection, etc.), so it is better to avoid electrograms with multiple deflections, low amplitude or with significant fractionation. Additionally, in cases of atrial electrograms it is preferable to choose a signal from an electrode that shows smaller or no ventricular electrograms. Hence the system will be able to take a consistent and reliable point as timing reference. For ventricular arrhythmias, the timing reference point is usually the QRS complex from a lead of the surface electrocardiogram, and the aforementioned considerations for atrial timing references are equally applicable. As shown in **Figure 9.3**, the reference signal has no morphology or amplitude variability, and the mapping system takes the same exact location of the electrogram (the peak of the positive deflection) consistently through all cycles.

Next, an appropriate mapping window or window of interest should be set up in the mapping system. The mapping window is a portion of the tachycardia cycle length that will be analyzed by the system to define the local activation time and the voltage amplitude of the signals that are collected. In general, for a presumptive focal cardiac arrhythmia, the window of interest should be programmed around 50–80 ms preceding the onset of the P wave or QRS complex for a focal atrial or ventricular tachycardia, respectively. If the arrhythmia to be mapped has a presumptive reentrant mechanism, then an appropriate window of interest should entail almost the entire tachycardia cycle length. It typically is 10 ms shorter than the tachycardia cycle length. One portion of this timing duration is set up before and the other portion after the timing reference point. For arrhythmias occurring in diseased hearts, care should be practiced to account for slow conduction even when the arrhythmia to be mapped has a focal mechanism. In cases of macro-reentrant arrhythmias, setting up too short of a window of interest will not map the entire tachycardia cycle length, while too long of a window of interest will lead to difficulties annotating all collected points.[23]

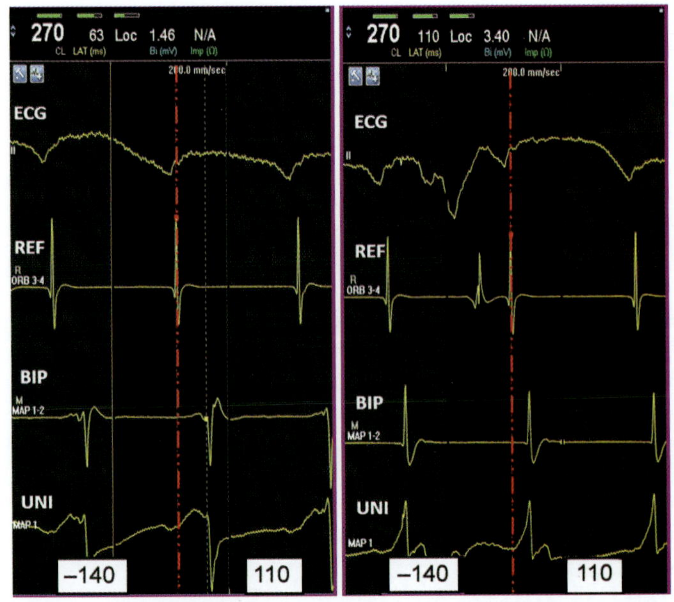

Figure 9.3: **Setting up the timing reference point and the mapping window or window of interest.** This is the case of an atrial tachycardia with a cycle length of 270 ms. In both panels from top to bottom the first channel is ECG lead II (ECG), followed by intracardiac signals from the mid to distal coronary sinus catheter (REF), the bipolar signal of the distal dipole of the mapping catheter (BIP), and the unipolar signal from the distal electrode of the mapping catheter (UNI). Observe that the chosen timing reference is a narrow signal with a single positive peak, minimal variation from cycle to cycle. The peak of the positive deflection has been elected (red vertical line) and the system consistently recognizes it even when there are ventricular electrograms (right panel). The window of interest is set up 140 ms before and 110 ms after the timing reference point for a total duration span of 250 ms (20 ms shorter than the tachycardia cycle length)

Annotation of Electrical Signals for an Accurate Activation Map

An accurate activation map will undoubtedly depend on an accurate annotation of the timing of the collected cardiac signals. First of all, it should be emphasized that the operator and assistant must have a consistent plan to avoid inaccuracies that can lead to misinterpretation of the mechanism of the arrhythmia under study and to acquire critical information that can be used to decide a catheter ablation approach.[23] The principle behind an accurate identification of the local activation timing is to annotate exactly when the activation wavefront is traversing at the site where the catheter is in contact with the heart. The original studies addressing how the intracardiac electrical signals are recorded with an exploring electrode in contact with myocardial fibers (indication of activity beneath an electrode on the surface of the heart) demonstrated that the timing when the activation wavefront passes underneath the exploring electrode is the onset of the intrinsic deflection of the signal. This point was defined as the longest, steepest, downward movement inscribed at or after the peak of the positive deflection of the recorded signal. However, localizing or estimating this point is not straightforward when the exploring electrode is in contact with the endocardium and depends on if the analysis is done with bipolar or unipolar signals.[24,25] It can even be more challenging in cases when the mapping catheter is at areas of diseased myocardium, and complex electrical signals are recorded. The recorded electrical signal will also vary according to the size of the recording electrodes, the spacing between electrodes, orientation of the catheter in relation to the surface of the heart and the activation front direction, use of the unipolar or bipolar signals, good catheter-tissue contact, etc. In general, the intracardiac signals displayed during activation mapping of an arrhythmia are bipolar signals from the distal dipole of the mapping/ablation catheter and also the unipolar signals of these two electrodes. There are several options where to annotate the timing of the recorded signals that we will develop in further detail.

Taking the Earliest Part of the Electrogram (Unipolar or Bipolar)

While in the setting of a focal atrial arrhythmia in an otherwise normal heart may not make a difference, taking the earliest part or the onset of the intracardiac electrogram can at times lead to error. For example, as shown in **Figures 9.4A and B**, a focal arrhythmia taking the onset of the electrogram when there is an initial far-field signal can be inaccurate. In the figure are shown opposite recording sites; the right panel shows the true origin of the arrhythmia characterized by a

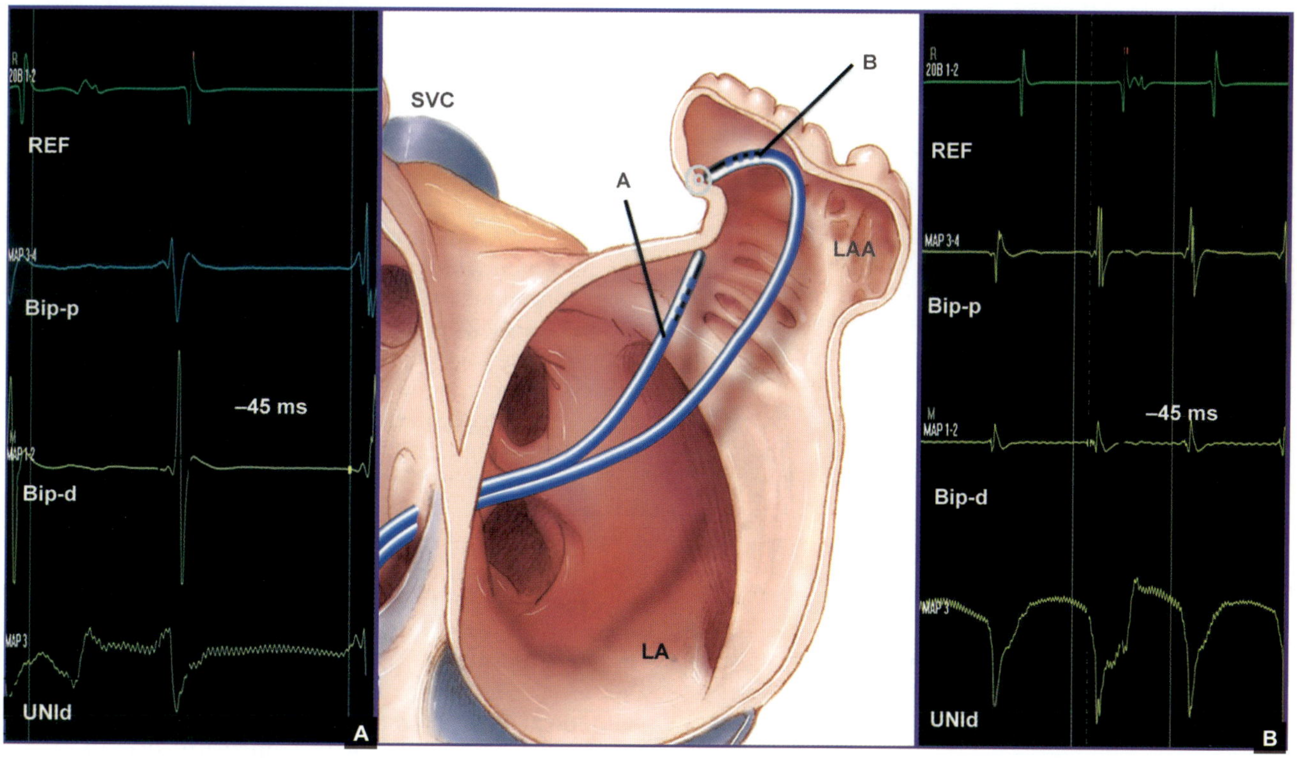

Figures 9.4A and B: Annotation of the local activation timing during a focal atrial tachycardia that presumptively originates inside the left atrial appendage (bulls' eye symbol). In panel A, the mapping catheter is placed at site close to the tachycardia origin but opposite, the catheter is able to record a far-field signal 45 ms preceding the timing reference. In panel B, the mapping catheter is placed on top the tachycardia site of origin also 45 ms preceding the timing reference. Taking the earliest onset of the bipolar signal regardless of the far-field morphology can lead to potential misinterpretation of the true site of the focal arrhythmia. Also observe the unipolar signals, at the nearby site in panel A there is a small positive initial deflection, while in panel B the unipolar signal is all negative with a rapid down sloping deflection

Abbreviations: REF, timing reference; Bip-p and Bip-d, bipolar signals at the proximal and distal electrodes of the mapping catheter; UNId, unipolar signal recorded at the distal electrode of the mapping catheter near-field signal preceding the timing reference by 45 ms. In the left panel, the recording site also records a signal 45 ms preceding the timing reference, but the signal is characterized by an initial far-field component. Similar scenarios can be observed for signals taken from sites where other nearby or surrounding structures are physically close (i.e. right pulmonary vein and the posterior right atrial wall; the posterior right ventricular outflow tract and the right coronary cusp).

Taking the First Peak of the Near-field Bipolar Electrogram

Differentiating a far-field from a near-field signal is at times not simple. But if possible, the near-field component of the signal should always be analyzed for an accurate activation map. In general, a near-field signal will have a sharper morphology compared to a far-field signal. If the signal is not clearly defined, analyzing the local activation timing of nearby points can help in appreciating better what component of the signal represents the near-field recording. In cases of complex multicomponent signals, pacing locally to find out what part of the signal is captured can be helpful in deciding what part of the local signal should be analyzed for the true activation time.

Taking the Steepest Downward Deflection of the Unipolar Signal

When activation passes beneath the recording electrode, a negative deflection (S wave) is inscribed in the unipolar recording. The earliest rapid down stroke of the unipolar signal approximates the local activation time of the myocardium in contact with the recording electrode. However, performing endocardial mapping of deep myocardial or epicardial sites or sites of slow conduction may lead to difficulties in obtaining an accurate determination of the steepest downward deflection of the unipolar signal.

Annotation of the Local Activation Timing of Complex Electrical Signals

While performing an activation 3D map, the handling of complex electrical signals, such as double potentials and fragmented or fractionated electrograms, can be challenging. One of the most important issues is the difficulty sorting out signals that are only bystanders (do not participate in the mechanism of the tachycardia) from signals that are critical parts of the arrhythmia mechanism. In many circumstances, annotation of the exact activation timing is not possible.

Double potentials represent the recording of an activation wavefront across a line of block.[26] The recording electrode is either on top of the line of block where two near-field signals will be registered, or it can be at one side of the line of block, in which case it will record a far-field and a near-field signal. The order will depend on the location of the catheter in relation to the line of block and the activation wavefront direction. Therefore, in most instances the annotation of the activation timing of double potentials should take into account the near-field signal over the far-field one.[27,28] There are many situations, however, when the interpretation of which signal represents a far- or near-field is not easy. In these circumstances, looking for the activation timing of surrounding or near-by points can aid in deciding where to annotate the activation timing. Alternatively performing pacing maneuvers and finding which of the two signals is captured can elucidate the true signal representing local activation at the site of the recording catheter.[29] If the operator is not able to make a definitive interpretation, it is better to tag the location of the double potentials without taking into account the activation timing of the signal; later on this information can be used to make an appropriate interpretation of the activation map.

Fractionated electrograms represent slow conduction most of the time due to areas of fibrosis embedded with surviving isolated myocardial fibers.[30] These bipolar signals have low amplitude, and determining the timing of the local activation can be very difficult. To further complicate the annotation, if the mapping catheter is positioned close to an endocavitary structure (papillary muscles in the ventricles or prominent pectinate muscles in the atria), the signals from these structures are also registered and can be of higher amplitude. Therefore, annotation of the accurate activation timing of these signals may not be possible to elucidate, even though similar maneuvers to sort out activation timing of double potentials can be used (pacing at the site, finding out what component of the electrogram is captured, and looking for nearby activation times). When determination of the activation timing is not possible, it is better to tag the complex signals as fractionated electrograms discarding the activation timing information but still using the anatomic location of these recordings. Further maneuvers (entrainment) can be used to clarify their participation in the reentrant mechanism of the tachycardia. To catalogue a complex fragmented signal as bystander, the operator can calculate the duration of the signal in relation to the tachycardia cycle length. As shown in **Figure 9.5**, intracardiac signals were recorded during a macroreentrant left atrial tachycardia in a patient who underwent multiple previous catheter ablation procedures for atrial fibrillation; the signals were obtained using a multipolar basket (64 electrodes simultaneously recording) catheter. At multiple sites, complex fragmented signals were recorded with the longest measuring 180 ms while the clinical tachycardia cycle length was 209 ms. The duration of the fragmented signal represents close to 90% of the tachycardia cycle length. Most of these signals represent bystander complex signals from previous ablative therapies; this was later on confirmed by entrainment maneuvers with no signal found to be in the reentrant circuit.

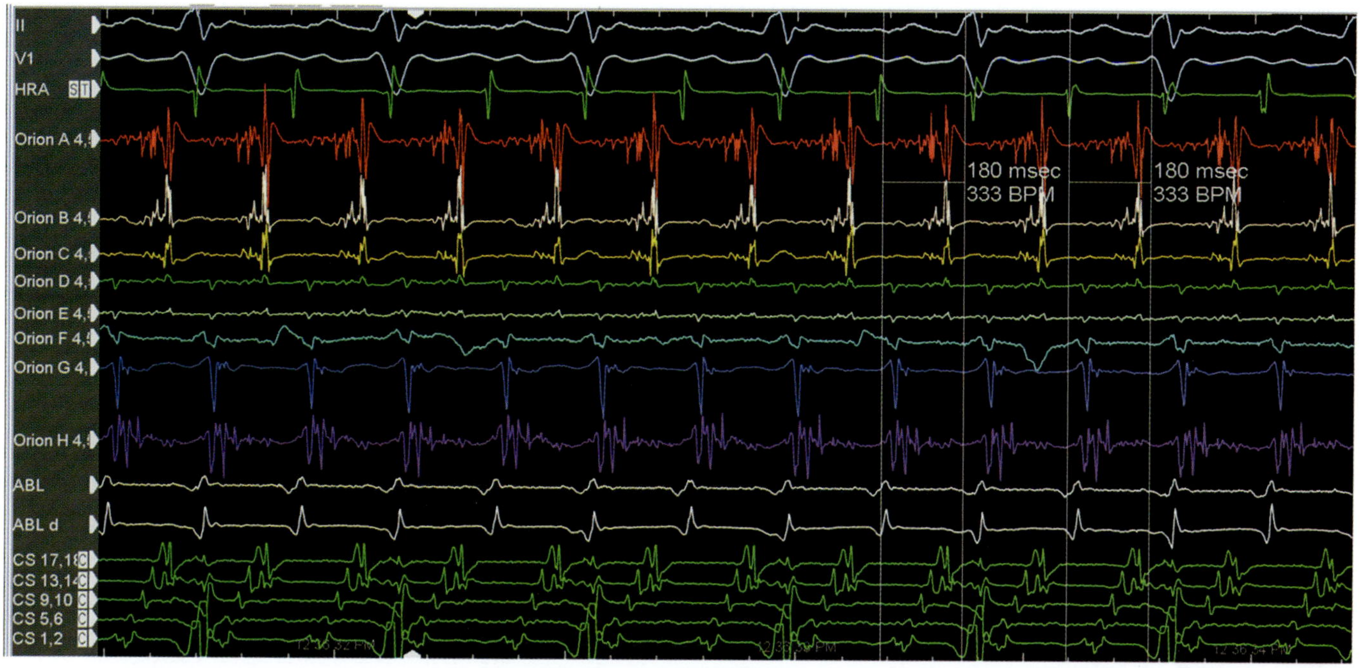

Figure 9.5: Mapping during an atypical left atrial flutter using a multielectrode array balloon catheter. Observe the significant fractionation of signals with long duration up to 180 ms. Tachycardia cycle length of 209 ms. Most of the recorded signals were catalogued as by-standers and not part of the reentrant circuit. See text for details

Interpretation of Activation Maps

Focal versus Macroreentrant Tachycardia

An activation electroanatomic map can support the diagnosis of a focal versus a macroreentrant tachycardia.[31] In a focal tachycardia, the origin of the arrhythmia is in a small area that spreads centrifugally to the rest of the atria or ventricles; therefore, the activation map shows a small activation segment that occurs earlier than the rest. On the other hand, in the case of a macroreentrant tachycardia there are no early or late points, since by definition during tachycardia there will always be electrical activation in different segments of the reentrant circuit. Typically, the total activation time of a focal arrhythmia will cover less than 50% of the tachycardia cycle length, while in a macroreentrant arrhythmia the total activation time embraces more than 90% of the tachycardia cycle length. In **Figure 9.6**, the left panel shows a focal atrial tachycardia originating close to the junction of the posterior left pulmonary veins. In relation to the reference timing point, the total activation time covers from –68 ms to +3 ms, for a total activation time of 71 ms out of the 210 ms of the tachycardia cycle length, representing approximately 30% coverage. The right panel is a right atrial flutter with a cycle length of 260 ms. The total activation time covers from –138 ms to +119 ms in relation to the timing reference point, for a total of 257 ms representing close to 100% of coverage of the tachycardia cycle length of 260 ms. When making this interpretation, it is important to realize that the map has been performed in the proper chamber and enough activation points have been accrued. An activation map of macroreentrant arrhythmia in an adjacent chamber can appear as a focal tachycardia, with the breakthrough activation simulating the focal origin of the tachycardia and the 'total' activation time accounting only partially for the tachycardia cycle length. Furthermore, in cases of focal arrhythmias in the setting of diseased myocardium with extensive areas of fibrosis, the activation map can look similar to a reentrant arrhythmia due to areas of slow conduction, which have no role in the mechanism of the arrhythmia but rather are simple bystanders.

What the Colors of an Activation Map Really Mean?

As activation mapping points are acquired and their timing is compared to the predetermined timing reference, the mapping system will assign a color scheme to different areas of the 3D chamber reconstruction. Regions of red color indicate sites that are of "early activation" versus hues of orange, yellow, green, blue, and purple. These colors correspond to an isochronal time bar located adjacent to the 3D map. In cases of focal tachycardias and in the absence of significant myocardial disease, the map will appear as a small area with the earliest activation in red color. In the case of a

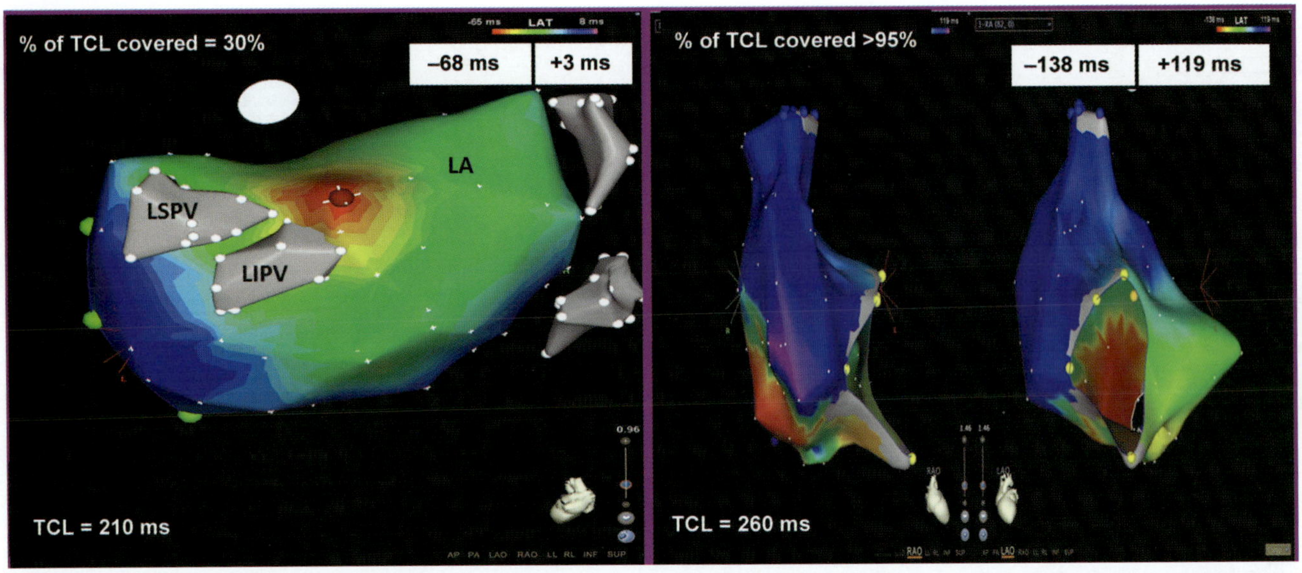

Figure 9.6: Activation mapping, accounting for the tachycardia cycle length. The left panel shows an electroanatomic activation map of a focal arrhythmia originating in the posterior left atrial wall close to the left sided pulmonary veins. The activation map accounts for approximately 30% of the tachycardia cycle length. The right panel shows a macroreentrant right atrial flutter. The activation map accounts for almost 100% of the tachycardia cycle length

Abbreviations: TCL, tachycardia cycle length; LSPV, left superior pulmonary vein; LIPV, left inferior pulmonary vein

macroreentrant arrhythmia, the value of the interpretation of "red color equals early" and "purple color equals late" is not accurate since by definition in a macroreentrant tachycardia there is no early and no late activation. The activation occurs continuously. This basic concept can easily be demonstrated in a 3D activation map by changing the reference timing point. In **Figures 9.7A to E**, we show the 3D activation map of a macroreentrant atrial tachycardia localized to the left atrium. Each panel shows a pair of maps representing the same view of the left atrium. The left-sided maps of each pair have the same reference timing point 120 ms earlier than the proximal electrodes of a coronary sinus catheter, while the right-sided maps of each pair have the reference point located in the proximal electrodes of the multipolar coronary sinus catheter. By selecting a different temporal reference point, the distribution of the colors assigned by the mapping system to the same reentrant tachycardia changes drastically. The interpretation of early or late activation would be an error. In a similar manner if the timing window or window of interest is modified, the system assignation of colors for the same tachycardia will also vary. This is illustrated in **Figures 9.8A to D**, where the window of interest has been modified while the temporal reference point remains unchanged. Finally, the mapping system feature of highlighting the area of activation as "early-meets-late" is based on the color assignation. According to the aforementioned concepts, the anatomical location of "early-meets-late" assignation by the mapping system will also change location; this is illustrated in **Figures 9.9A to E**.

Therefore, the analysis of the colors of an activation map requires careful interpretation. It can be a source of valuable information regarding conduction velocity. If the entire spectrum of the color scale is evident over a small anatomical area, this can be indicative of a region of slow conduction. In order to delineate areas of slow conduction, however, the point acquisition has to be dense enough for the mapping system to substantiate the construct. Additionally, care should be taken when modifying the system's feature called "fill threshold." This feature allows the user to modify how aggressive the system will interpolate data among the acquired points. For instance, an aggressive "fill threshold" will construct the anatomy of a chamber with only a few acquired points, the color range can become distorted and may not represent a true display of conduction velocity, activation sequence, or even anatomical map. For a map with densely obtained points, a low "fill threshold" will suffice to have an accurate 3D representation of an electroanatomic map.

Lastly, we arrive to the question of how many points are necessary to obtain an accurate activation map. The straightforward answer would be as many as safely and efficiently possible. This certainly is more proficiently achieved with the recent multielectrode fast activation systems. But it will depend on the underlying mechanism of the arrhythmia and the presence or absence of myocardial disease as well as anatomical variants. In cases, when the first mapped chamber does not yield reasonable results, for instance there is a relatively large area of early activation,

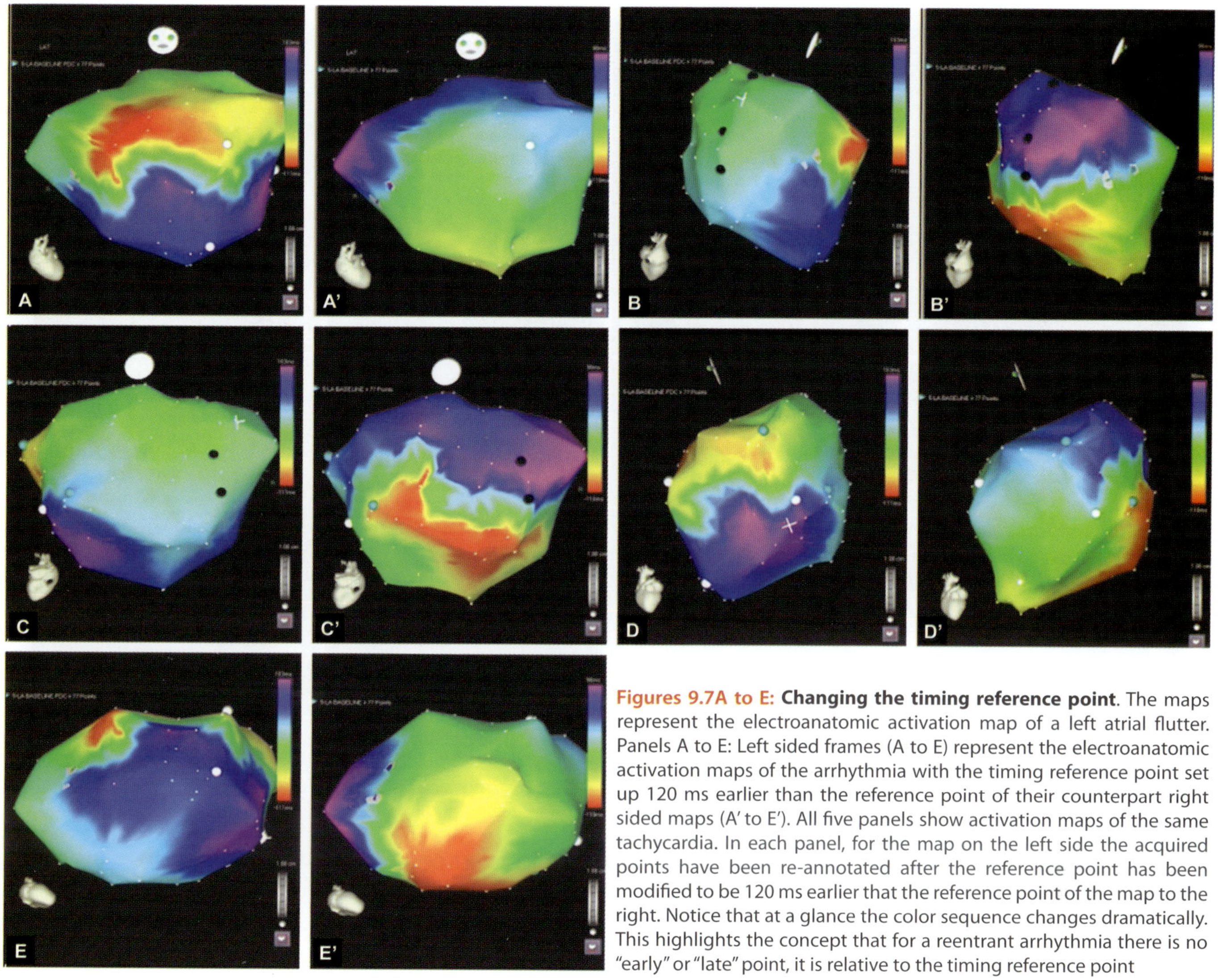

Figures 9.7A to E: Changing the timing reference point. The maps represent the electroanatomic activation map of a left atrial flutter. Panels A to E: Left sided frames (A to E) represent the electroanatomic activation maps of the arrhythmia with the timing reference point set up 120 ms earlier than the reference point of their counterpart right sided maps (A' to E'). All five panels show activation maps of the same tachycardia. In each panel, for the map on the left side the acquired points have been re-annotated after the reference point has been modified to be 120 ms earlier that the reference point of the map to the right. Notice that at a glance the color sequence changes dramatically. This highlights the concept that for a reentrant arrhythmia there is no "early" or "late" point, it is relative to the timing reference point

it is possible that breakthrough activation is coming from adjacent chambers. This is illustrated in **Figure 9.10**. A focal ventricular arrhythmia was initially mapped in the right ventricle, and a large area of earlier activation is localized to the superior and leftward outflow tract; then after mapping the neighboring left ventricular outflow tract, the area of earlier activation changes marginally. Subsequent mapping of the supra-valvar part of the pulmonary artery identifies a small area as the focal origin of the arrhythmia, leading to a successful ablation procedure.

Interpretation of Propagation Maps

All the available 3D electroanatomic mapping systems have a feature called propagation maps. Based on collected activation time, the data are arranged by isochrones, and then the system is able to reproduce a motion picture of the possible activation sequence pattern of the mapped arrhythmia. The user is able to define the timeframe of the isochrones (a portion of the cycle length) and get a sense of the course of the activation sequence. The same observations for the interpretation of activation map apply for a propagation map. For cases of focal arrhythmias in otherwise normal hearts, the propagation map can depict the centrifugal sequence of activation. For macro-reentrant arrhythmias and in the presence of significant conduction delays, the propagation map can reveal confusing activation sequences.

SUBSTRATE MAPPING

Substrate or voltage mapping is a commonly used technique to define plausible areas of myocardial fibrosis or scarring.

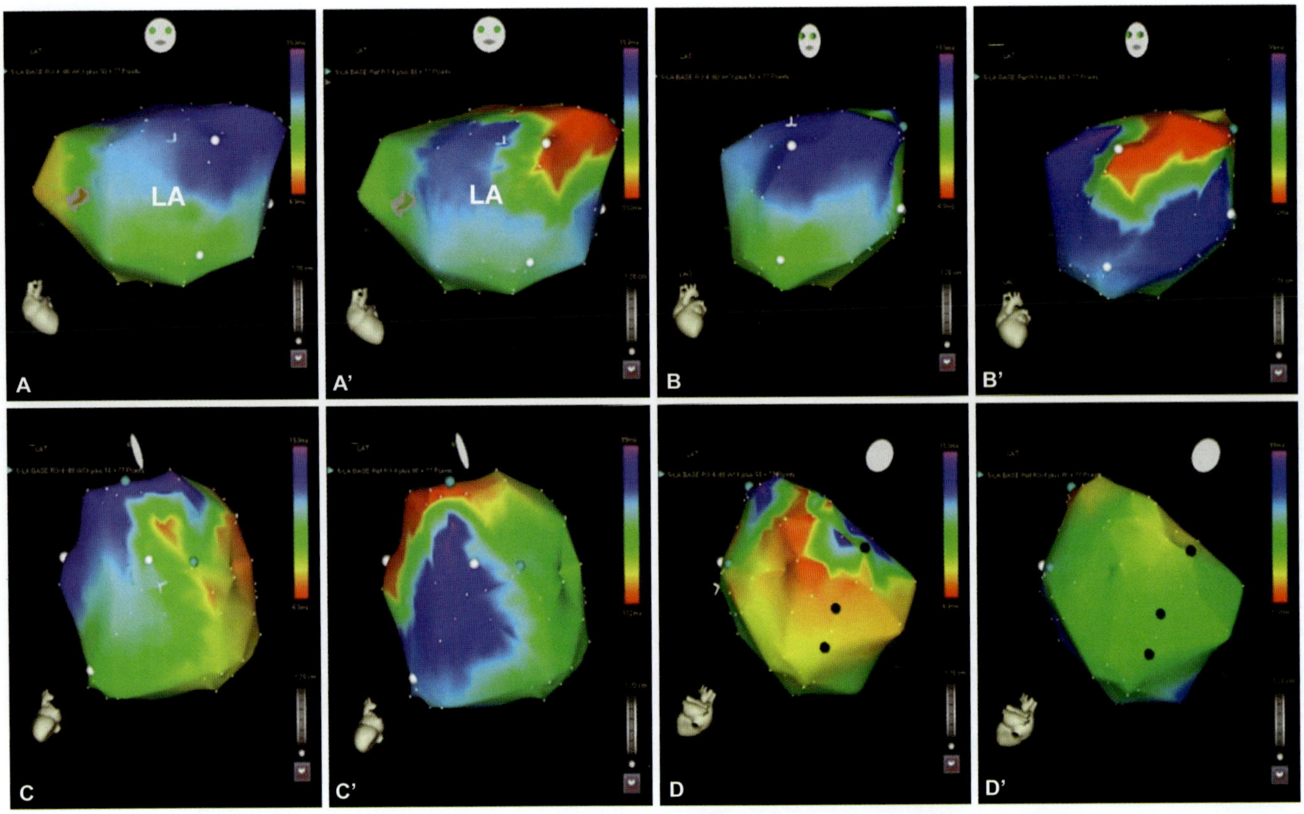

Figures 9.8A to D: Changing the mapping window or window of interest. Electroanatomic activation maps of a Left Atrial Reentrant tachycardia showing changes in the activation sequence as depicted by the Electroanatomic Mapping system after changing in Window of Interest Settings. Panels A to E: Left sided frames (A to D) represent the electroanatomic activation maps of the arrhythmia with the window of interest encompassing a timing range 62 ms before to 155 ms after the reference point. Right sided maps in each panel (A' to D') have the window of interest encompassing an interval 112 ms before to 105 ms after the reference point. The reference point in all cases remain the same. All panels represent activation map of the same tachycardia and both frames in each panel are the exact same view of the left atrium (LA). Notice that by making this change the "color sequence" of the activation map has been modified, however it is the representation of the same arrhythmia

These areas are the arrhythmogenic basis for scar-related arrhythmias.[32] For different reasons (unstable or non-sustained arrhythmias, multiple activation sequences) an arrhythmia may not always be mapped during tachycardia, and therefore an activation electroanatomic map is not possible. In these cases, performing a substrate map can be helpful to define potential arrhythmogenic channels that can be targeted with catheter ablation. Performing a substrate map consists of the collection of the unipolar and bipolar electrical signals by roving the mapping catheter in the chamber(s) of interest. The mapping system then, according to user-defined criteria, assigns different colors to different voltage amplitudes and displays them in the 3D anatomical map.

The areas of myocardial scarring have certain electrophysiological features. For instance in atrial macro-reentrant tachycardias due to previous surgical procedures (atrial incision for valvular surgeries or repair of congenital heart disease), cardiomyopathy, postsurgical, or catheter ablation procedures; surviving myocardial fibers are embedded in areas of myocardial fibrosis. In areas of dense fibrosis, no cardiac electrograms are encountered, and pacing at high outputs fails to capture myocardium locally. Areas of surgical incisions can lead to lines of block, while areas of extensive fibrosis with surviving myocardial fibers can lead to fragmented electrograms. In **Figure 9.11**, we depict the substrate for macro-reentrant tachycardias in subjects after a surgical MAZE procedure and after a surgical repair of an atrial septal defect. The areas of slow conduction act as the critical isthmuses of reentrant tachycardias. Something similar occurs for ventricular reentrant arrhythmias either post-infarct or in subject with nonischemic cardiomyopathies.

How to Perform an Accurate Substrate Map?

The basic general principles to perform accurate activation and anatomical maps also apply to perform an accurate substrate or voltage map. Importantly, appropriate catheter

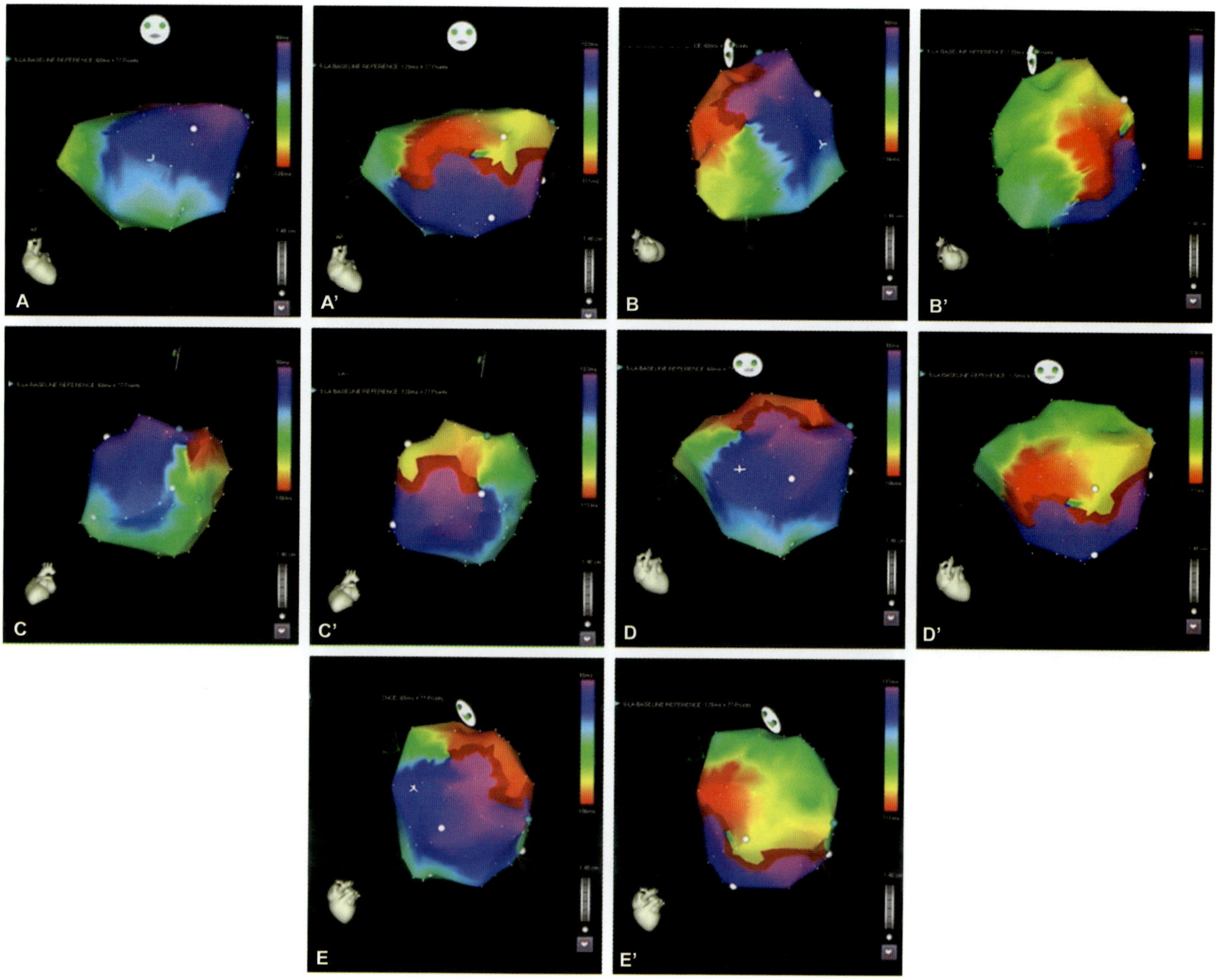

Figures 9.9A to E: Electroanatomic activation map of a left atrial flutter showing the "Early-meets-late" feature after changing the timing reference point. Panels A to E: Left sided frames (A to E) represent the electroanatomic activation maps of the arrhythmia with the reference point set up 60 ms later than the reference point of their counterpart right sided maps (A' to E'). All five panels show activation maps of the same tachycardia and each pair of frames represent the exact same view. The "Early-Meets-Late" feature of the system has been turned on and is seen as a solid red band with definite borders. As it can be appreciated even though the activation maps are electroanatomic representations of the same arrhythmia, by changing the timing reference point the "Early-Meets-Late" band changes position. This emphasizes that careful interpretation of the value of this feature. (In each panel, for the map on the left side the acquired points have been re-annotated after the reference point has been modified and is 60 ms later that the reference point of the map to the right.)

contact should be assured but catheter orientation and the presence of endocavitary structures should also be considered.

In this section is important to review the differences between bipolar and unipolar potentials. In general, bipolar potentials are produced by the subtraction of the two unipolar signals of the distal and proximal electrodes of the mapping catheter. Therefore, bipolar potentials inherently record fewer far-field signals, and their "recording antenna" is smaller. On the other hand, unipolar potentials have a wider "recording antenna"; the potentials are recorded as the difference of the potential of the exploring electrodes (distal or proximal) and an indifferent electrode that can be located in the inferior vena cava or the Central Terminal of Wilson. Thus, unipolar recordings include significant far-field signals. Additionally, bipolar signals are affected by the direction of

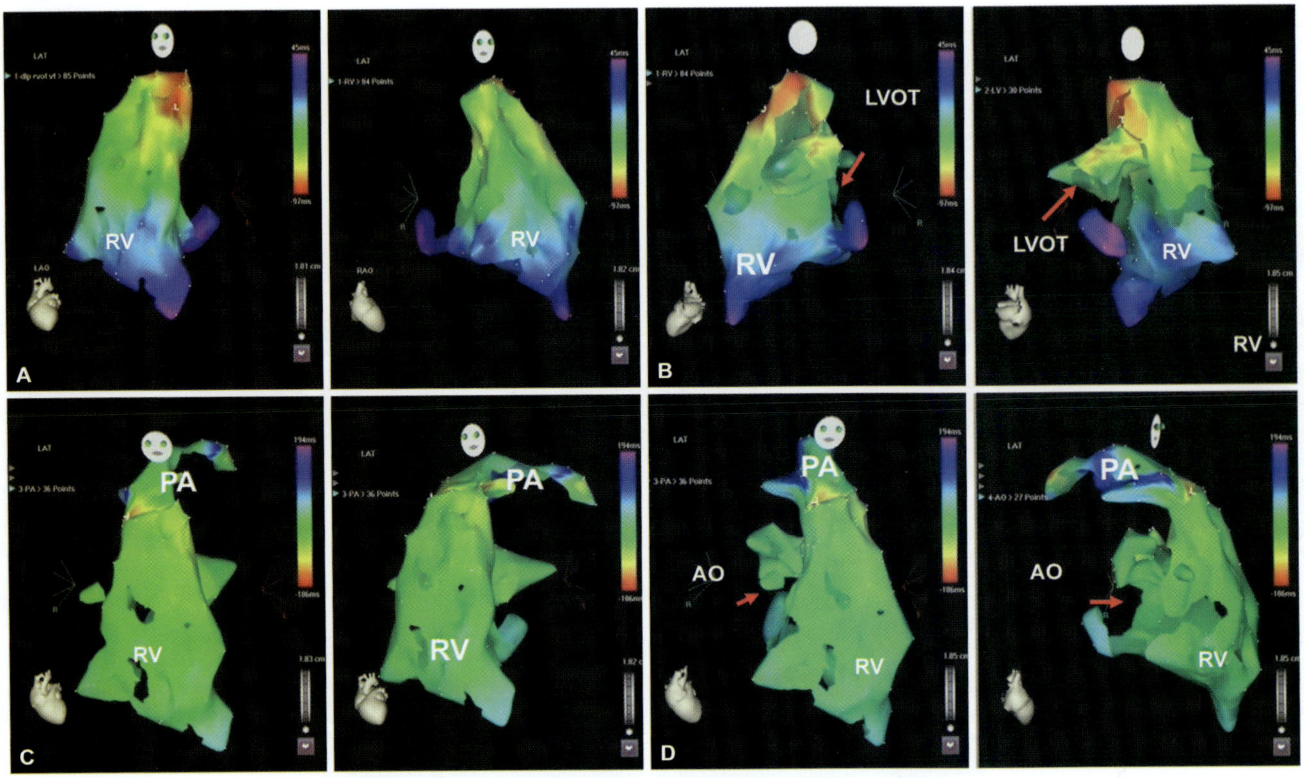

Figures 9.10A to D: Electroanatomic activation map of a focal ventricular tachycardia ablated at the supravalvar pulmonic area. Figures A to D: Each panel represents electroanatomic activation sequence of the same focal arrhythmia. (A) LAO (left) and RAO (right) views after mapping only the right ventricle showing earlier activation at the leftward and anterior outflow tract; but in a relatively large area that represents breakthrough activation from an adjacent chamber. (B) A limited portion of the left ventricular outflow tract was mapped and added to the map, no significant location change of the earlier activation point. (C) The proximal pulmonary artery then was mapped and added. Notice that now the earliest activation has shifted and pinpoints the origin to the supravalvar region. (D) Finally activation map of the aortic root is added, no further change in the earliest activation point. (From: Freddy Del Carpio Munoz et al. Circ Arrhythm Electrophysiol. 2011;4:e11-e14)

the activation wavefront relative to orientation of the pair of recording electrodes. If the wavefront is perpendicular to the dipole, the recorded signal will be diminished, compared to if the wavefront of activation is parallel to the dipole. Unipolar signals can indicate the direction of the impulse propagation, but they are less accurate to record low amplitude signals.

There exists histological validation in animal models of the electrophysiological characteristics of normal and abnormal myocardial substrate. In general, bipolar signals are more consistent for substrate definition. For endocardial ventricular substrate mapping in general, it is accepted that a bipolar voltage higher than 1.5 mV is consistent with healthy myocardium, a bipolar voltage less than 0.5 mV represent areas of significant myocardial fibrosis while bipolar voltages between 0.5–1.5 mV represent scar border zones.[33] These bipolar voltage thresholds to differentiate healthy myocardium from scar are less for right ventricular endocardial mapping. Also, in cases of epicardial mapping, the epicardial fat around the coronary arteries should be taken into account. In **Figures 9.12A to D**, we show a substrate endocardial and epicardial map from a patient with nonischemic cardiomyopathy and recurrent ventricular tachycardias. During the ablation procedure, multiple ventricular arrhythmias were induced, that were all unstable. Relatively preserved voltages were noted in the endocardial maps, while areas of low voltages are observed limited to the epicardial surface, something commonly observed in patients with non-ischemic cardiomyopathies. In terms of thresholds to define low voltage when performing substrate atrial mapping, there is no definitive consensus. For instance, in cases of reentrant atrial tachycardias in patients with prior surgical repair of congenital heart disease, dense scar is usually defined as voltages less than 0.03 mV or signals that are indistinguishable from electrical noise. Even small potentials < 0.1 mV should not be discarded and catalogued as dense scar, since many of those potentials are the critical isthmuses of macro-reentrant circuits where radiofrequency ablation can successfully treat these arrhythmias.[34,35]

The definition of low voltage areas as a surrogate of scar is a topic of debate. Even though in general, we use voltage thresholds as stated above to define abnormal myocardial substrate for atrial and ventricular arrhythmias, there

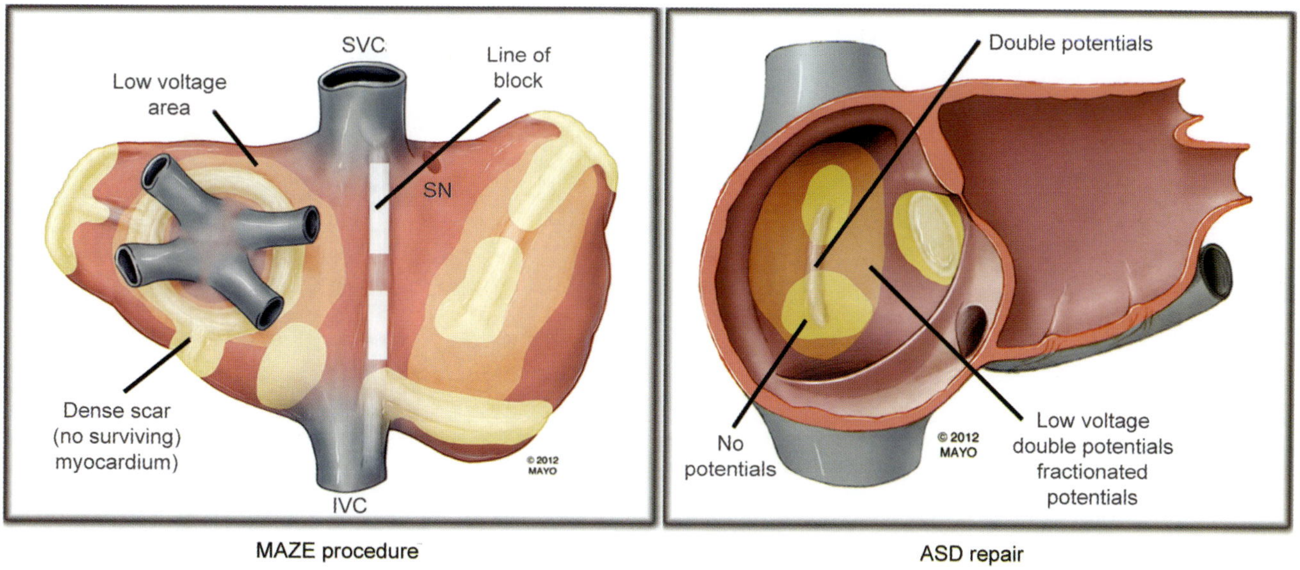

Figures 9.11: Anatomical substrate of macro-reentrant atrial arrhythmias. Left panel shows a posterior view of both atria and the scarring process after a surgical MAZE procedure. The right panel shows the scarring process after a surgical repair of an atrial septal defect. See text for details

Modified with permission from: Freddy Del-Carpio: "Flutter atipico", in book supplement "Flutter Auricular: Presente, Pasado y Futuro". Jorge Luis Salinas Arce, Editor. Grambs Corporacion Grafica, SAC, October 2015)

are several factors that determine the voltage amplitude during electroanatomic mapping. Low voltage areas are not necessarily equivalent to scarred or fibrotic myocardium. When performing a substrate map, it should be kept in mind that the following factors, among others, will determine the voltage amplitude of a bipolar signal and thus will determine how the mapping system will display the areas of low voltage as potential substrate of arrhythmias.[36] For instance, the orientation of the mapping catheter recording electrodes in relation to the direction of the activation wavefront and how the activation vector angle impacts with both recording electrodes; the size of the recording electrodes (larger electrodes will record signals from larger tissue areas and will generate larger voltage amplitudes, while the opposite occurs with smaller electrodes); interelectrode spacing, similar to the size of the electrodes the distance between the recording dipole also influences the "recording antenna" and the amplitude of the signal; tissue contact of the recording electrodes with the myocardial tissue; filtering of the signals; the mapping density, collecting fewer signals will allow the mapping system to interpolate data between points and lead to magnification of potential errors of the collected data, while a high density map will lead to less system interpolation and define better the extent of areas of normal and abnormal by myocardial substrate; mapping resolution similarly to what is stated for mapping density, the mapping system will fill in the gaps (the filling threshold). Therefore, in the interpretation of bipolar voltage maps all these factors should be taken into account.

A consistent plan for definition of dense scar is also important to perform an accurate substrate map. Dense scar ideally should be defined as areas when no surviving myocardial fibers exist and only fibrous tissue is present. In general, any consistent, albeit small, bipolar electrogram recorded in every cardiac cycle should be collected, annotated, and not be considered as dense scar. To validate a mapping area as dense unexcitable scar, failure to capture locally with high output pacing is an accepted maneuver, while good catheter-tissue contact is documented.[37] The limitation of this technique is that with high output pacing (at 10 mA) neighboring structures (endocavitary or adjacent chambers) can be captured and erroneously assign viable myocardium when capture is obtained in a zone of dense scar[38]; furthermore, pacing during tachycardia can terminate or induce a different tachycardia. Areas of dense scar can act as activation barriers and facilitate the reentrant mechanism of arrhythmias, therefore the accurate classification while performing a substrate map has important implications in planning the ablation strategy. In **Figure 9.13**, we show a bipolar voltage map in a patient with atypical atrial flutters and marked myocardial disease with areas of low voltage, unexcitable scar, and areas of slow conduction in between the dense scarring representing arrhythmogenic channels.

MULTIELECTRODE CATHETERS FOR FAST ANATOMICAL, VOLTAGE AND ACTIVATION MAPPING

Typically the 3D mapping systems have only been able to process the acquisition of data with a point-by-point

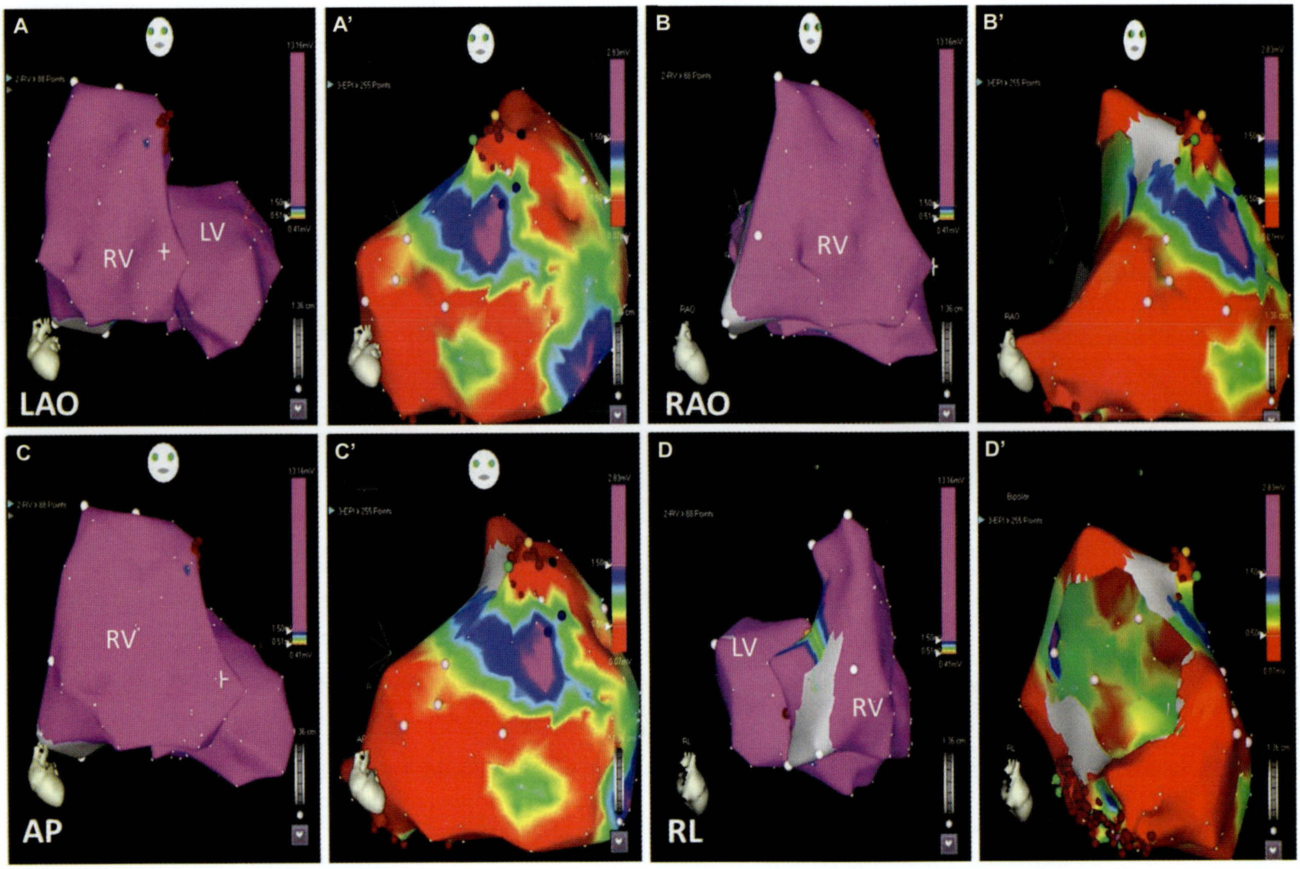

Figures 9.12A to D: Endocardial and epicardial ventricular voltage maps in a patient with nonischemic cardiomyopathy and recurrent ventricular tachycardias. The electroanatomic voltage map was obtained during sinus rhythm. Each pair of panels (A-A', B-B', etc.) represent the same views. The right panels (A to D) show the endocardial maps of both ventricles (RV and LV) and left panels (A' to D') show the corresponding view of the epicardial voltage map. Purple areas represent voltages higher than 1.5 mV and red areas less than 0.5 mV. The maps show a preserved voltage amplitudes in the endocardial maps, while the abnormal substrate is limited to the epicardial maps
Abbreviations: LAO and RAO, left and right anterior oblique; RL, right lateral; AP, anteroposterior views

approach, where the mapping/ablation catheter had to be roved around the chamber(s) of interest and one point at a time is acquired, annotated, and processed by the system. For activation mapping, first of all the tachycardia has to be stable and sustained over a long enough period to allow acquisition of a proper number of points to sustain a reasonable map upon which to make therapeutic decisions; but the process could be time-consuming and may not be possible in unstable or nonsustained arrhythmias. As we described at the beginning of the chapter, one of the systems developed a "noncontact" mapping system (EnSite) consisting of a multielectrode array mounted on a small balloon on a catheter that is inserted into the chamber of interest.[10] Using inverse-solution mathematics, the array allows reconstruction of 3360 electrograms, which are superimposed onto a computer model of the endocardium. The system uses a catheter localization system to obtain detailed information of the geometry of the chamber being mapped, except for endocavitary structures. The system offers the possibility to perform an activation map after only a few beats of the arrhythmia are observed and analyzed.

The Carto® 3 system has different multielectrode catheters to perform fast activation maps. The Pentaray® catheter (Biosense Webster, Inc.) has five flexible splines each with five 1 mm electrodes for a total of 20 electrodes that can quickly perform a multipoint acquisition of signals and produce a high density map. With similar properties, there is a circular catheter with 10 electrodes and another decapolar deflectable catheter. All these catheters are designed to perform high resolution and high density maps. The system also counts with software upgrades that can perform continuous mapping and automated acquisition of data according to prespecified operator-dependent criteria. The advantage of these multielectrode mapping systems is the relatively fast acquisition of signals allowing the operator to work more efficiently and providing the capability to map

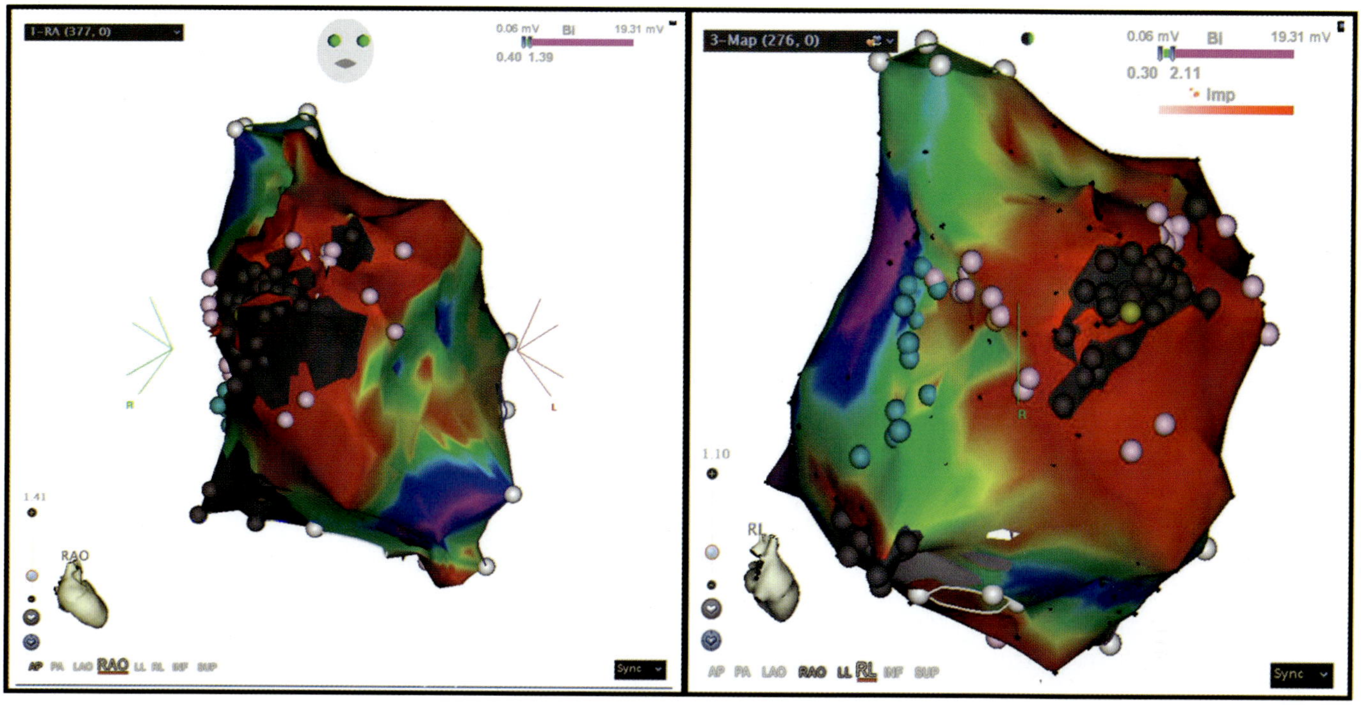

Figure 9.13: **Three dimensional bipolar voltage map of the right atrium in a patient with Myotonic Distrophy and atypical atrial flutters.** Right panel is a right anterior oblique and left panel a right lateral view. Unexcitable dense scar was defined as absence of bipolar potentials or potentials that could not be distinguished from noise and were assigned gray color (gray dots denote failure to local capture at high output). Areas of low voltage were defined as bipolar voltage amplitudes less than 0.3–0.4 mV. Areas colored purple denote bipolar voltages higher than 1.39 mV. Finally different hues of yellow, green, blue represent voltages in between dense scar and normal voltages. Pink dots represent areas of fractionated electrograms while blue dots represent double potentials. In the left panel observe that in between two areas of dense scar within the low voltage area there are points catalogued as fractionated potentials. This area was an arrhythmogenic channel for one of the clinical atrial flutters. Entrainment maneuvers from that area yielded concealed entrainment and a postpacing interval equal to the tachycardia cycle length. A short line of ablation joining the two areas of dense scar terminated the tachycardia. (Modified with permission from: Freddy Del-Carpio: "Flutter atipico", in book supplement "Flutter Auricular: Presente, Pasado y Futuro". Jorge Luis Salinas Arce, Editor. Grambs Corporacion Grafica, SAC, October 2015)

and potentially target several tachycardias in one session and also potentially to reduce fluoroscopy time and radiation exposure to patient and operators.

The Rhythmia™ system has a high resolution mapping deflectable catheter with a basket array of 64 electrodes in total (Intella Map Orion™, Boston Scientific) with 8 splines each with 8 electrodes and a 2.5 mm interelectrode spacing. The system can perform continuous data acquisition, and in a short timeframe it can acquire thousands of points compared to several hundred with the other multielectrode acquisition systems or few hundreds with a point-by-point approach. The system can perform anatomical, activation, voltage, and complex electrogram maps. **Figure 9.14** shows an ultra-high-density map of the left atrium in a patient with previous catheter ablations for recurrent persistent atrial fibrillation. The anatomical definition and the number of acquired points should be noted. Clinical experience with this system is just starting, and further studies are needed to validate its use with different arrhythmia mechanisms and substrates.

CONCLUSION

In summary, we have succinctly reviewed the most important features of the current 3D mapping technologies that guide modern catheter ablation therapies. We have reviewed tips on how to perform anatomical, activation, and substrate maps and how to obtain the most benefit from these important adjunctive tools. At the same time, it is important to recognize the limitations and keep in mind potential misinterpretations of maps that can misguide ablation therapies. The knowledge of the arrhythmia mechanism, as well as the simultaneous appropriate use of other imaging modalities, remains cornerstone for successful catheter ablation procedures. In spite of the availability of more sophisticated systems, for the experienced electrophysiologist, no mapping system

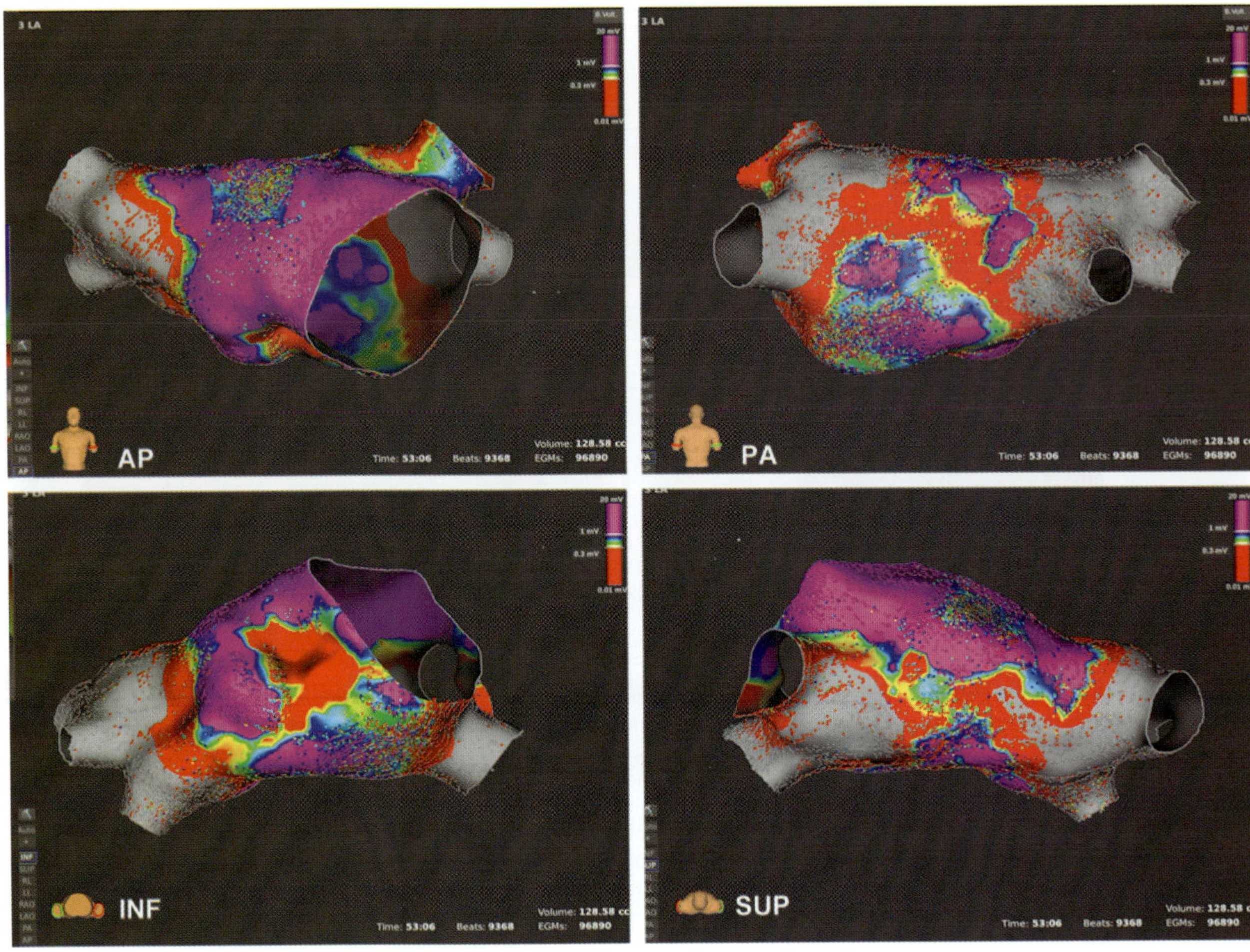

Figure 9.14: Ultra-high-density map of the left atrium using the Rhythmia™ mapping system. The 3D maps were obtained from a patient who had prior catheter ablations for atrial fibrillation. The voltage color scale indicates red for bipolar voltages <0.3 mV and purple for bipolar voltages > 1mV, other colors voltages in-between and gray for absent bipolar potentials. Observe that there are no potentials in all pulmonary veins, except the left superior which seems to be reconnected. The potentials displayed in this figure were collected from the roof of the left atrium

Abbreviations: AP, anteroposterior; PA, posteroinferior; INF, inferior; SUP, superior views. Total collected electrograms 96,890 from 9,368 beats analyzed

replaces an accurate interpretation of basic cardiac electrophysiology phenomena and cardiac anatomy.

REFERENCES

1. Packer DL. Evolution of mapping and anatomic imaging of cardiac arrhythmias. J Cardiovasc Electrophysiol. 2004; 15:839-54.
2. Packer DL. Three-dimensional mapping in interventional electrophysiology: techniques and technology. J Cardiovasc Electrophysiol. 2005;16:1110-6.
3. Wittkampf FH, Wever EF, Derksen R, Wilde AA, Ramanna H, Hauer RN, Robles de Medina EO. LocaLisa: new technique for real-time 3-dimensional localization of regular intracardiac electrodes. Circulation. 1999;99:1312-7.
4. Gepstein L, Hayam G, Ben-Haim SA. A novel method for nonfluoroscopic catheter-based electroanatomical mapping of the heart. In vitro and in vivo accuracy results. Circulation. 1997;95:1611-22.
5. Friedman PA. Novel mapping techniques for cardiac electrophysiology. Heart. 2002;87:575-82.
6. Okumura Y, Henz BD, Johnson SB, Bunch TJ, O'Brien CJ, Hodge DO, Altman A, Govari A, Packer DL. Three-dimensional ultrasound for image-guided mapping and intervention: methods, quantitative validation, and clinical feasibility of a novel multimodality image mapping system. Circ Arrhythm Electrophysiol. 2008;1:110-9.
7. Shah DC, Namdar M. Real-time contact force measurement: a key parameter for controlling lesion creation with radiofrequency energy. Circ Arrhythm Electrophysiol. 2015;8:713-21.
8. Krum D, Goel A, Hauck J, Hare J, Attari M, Dhala A, Cooley R, Akhtar M, Sra J. Catheter location, tracking, cardiac chamber geometry creation, and ablation using cutaneous patches. J Interv Card Electrophysiol. 2005;12:17-22.

9. Eitel C, Hindricks G, Dagres N, Sommer P, Piorkowski C. EnSite Velocity cardiac mapping system: a new platform for 3D mapping of cardiac arrhythmias. Expert Rev Med Devices. 2010;7:185-92.
10. Schilling RJ, Peters NS, Davies DW. Simultaneous endocardial mapping in the human left ventricle using a noncontact catheter: comparison of contact and reconstructed electrograms during sinus rhythm. Circulation. 1998;98:887-98.
11. Yamabe H. Utility of novel nonfluoroscopic 4D navigation technology for catheter ablation. Heart Rhythm. 2013;10: 1301-2.
12. Piorkowski C, Hindricks G. Nonfluoroscopic sensor-guided navigation of intracardiac electrophysiology catheters within prerecorded cine loops. Circ Arrhythm Electrophysiol. 2011;4:e36-8.
13. Nakagawa H, Ikeda A, Sharma T, Lazzara R, Jackman WM. Rapid high resolution electroanatomical mapping: evaluation of a new system in a canine atrial linear lesion model. Circ Arrhythm Electrophysiol. 2012;5:417-24.
14. Bollmann A, Hilbert S, John S, Kosiuk J, Hindricks G. Insights from preclinical ultra high-density electroanatomical sinus node mapping. Europace. 2015;17:489-94.
15. Anter E, Tschabrunn CM, Contreras-Valdes FM, Li J, Josephson ME. Pulmonary vein isolation using the Rhythmia mapping system: Verification of intracardiac signals using the Orion mini-basket catheter. Heart Rhythm. 2015;12:1927-34.
16. Bollmann A, Hilbert S, John S, Kosiuk J, Hindricks G. Initial experience with ultra high-density mapping of human right atria. J Cardiovasc Electrophysiol. 2015.
17. Ikeguchi S, Peters NS. Novel use of postpacing interval mapping to guide radiofrequency ablation of focal atrial tachycardia with long intra-atrial conduction time. Heart Rhythm. 2004;1: 88-93.
18. Tops LF, Bax JJ, Zeppenfeld K, Jongbloed MR, Lamb HJ, van der Wall EE, Schalij MJ. Fusion of multislice computed tomography imaging with three-dimensional electroanatomic mapping to guide radiofrequency catheter ablation procedures. Heart Rhythm. 2005;2:1076-81.
19. Markowitz SM, Lerman BB. How to interpret electroanatomic maps. Heart Rhythm. 2006;3:240-6.
20. Soejima K. How to troubleshoot the electroanatomic map. Heart Rhythm. 2010;7:999-1003.
21. Noseworthy PA, Malchano ZJ, Ahmed J, Holmvang G, Ruskin JN, Reddy VY. The impact of respiration on left atrial and pulmonary venous anatomy: implications for image-guided intervention. Heart Rhythm. 2005;2:1173-8.
22. Beinart R, Kabra R, Heist KE, Blendea D, Barrett CD, Danik SB, Collins R, Ruskin JN, Mansour M. Respiratory compensation improves the accuracy of electroanatomic mapping of the left atrium and pulmonary veins during atrial fibrillation ablation. J Interv Card Electrophysiol. 2011;32:105-10.
23. Del Carpio Munoz F, Buescher T, Asirvatham SJ. Teaching points with 3-dimensional mapping of cardiac arrhythmias: taking points: activation mapping. Circ Arrhythm Electrophysiol. 2011;4:e22-5.
24. Sodi-Pallares D, Barbato E, Delmar A. Relationship between the intrinsic deflection and subepicardial activation; an experimental study. Am Heart J. 1950;39:387-96.
25. Dower GE. In Defence of the Intrinsic Deflection. Br Heart J. 1962;24:55-60.
26. Morgan JM, Haywood G, Schirdewan A, Brugada P, Geelen P, Meyerfeldt U, Roberts P, Gibson C. "Double" potentials define linear lesion conduction block using a novel mapping/ linear lesion ablation catheter. J Cardiovasc Electrophysiol. 2003;14:236-42.
27. Shah D, Haissaguerre M, Jais P, Takahashi A, Hocini M, Clementy J. High-density mapping of activation through an incomplete isthmus ablation line. Circulation. 1999;99:211-5.
28. Tai CT, Haque A, Lin YK, Tsao HM, Ding YA, Chang MS, Chen SA. Double potential interval and transisthmus conduction time for prediction of cavotricuspid isthmus block after ablation of typical atrial flutter. J Interv Card Electrophysiol. 2002;7:77-82.
29. Tung S, Soejima K, Maisel WH, Suzuki M, Epstein L, Stevenson WG. Recognition of far-field electrograms during entrainment mapping of ventricular tachycardia. J Am Coll Cardiol. 2003;42:110-5.
30. de Bakker JM, van Capelle FJ, Janse MJ, Wilde AA, Coronel R, Becker AE, Dingemans KP, van Hemel NM, Hauer RN. Reentry as a cause of ventricular tachycardia in patients with chronic ischemic heart disease: electrophysiologic and anatomic correlation. Circulation. 1988;77:589-606.
31. Del Carpio Munoz F, Buescher TL, Asirvatham SJ. Teaching points with 3-dimensional mapping of cardiac arrhythmia: mechanism of arrhythmia and accounting for the cycle length. Circ Arrhythm Electrophysiol. 2011;4:e1-3.
32. de Bakker JM, van Capelle FJ, Janse MJ, Tasseron S, Vermeulen JT, de Jonge N, Lahpor JR. Slow conduction in the infarcted human heart. 'Zigzag' course of activation. Circulation. 1993;88:915-26.
33. Marchlinski FE, Callans DJ, Gottlieb CD, Zado E. Linear ablation lesions for control of unmappable ventricular tachycardia in patients with ischemic and nonischemic cardiomyopathy. Circulation. 2000;101:1288-96.
34. Nakagawa H, Shah N, Matsudaira K, Overholt E, Chandrasekaran K, Beckman KJ, Spector P, Calame JD, Rao A, Hasdemir C, Otomo K, Wang Z, Lazzara R, Jackman WM. Characterization of reentrant circuit in macroreentrant right atrial tachycardia after surgical repair of congenital heart disease: isolated channels between scars allow "focal" ablation. Circulation. 2001;103:699-709.
35. de Groot NM, Schalij MJ, Zeppenfeld K, Blom NA, Van der Velde ET, Van der Wall EE. Voltage and activation mapping: how the recording technique affects the outcome of catheter ablation procedures in patients with congenital heart disease. Circulation. 2003;108:2099-106.
36. Anter E, Josephson ME. Bipolar voltage amplitude: What does it really mean? Heart Rhythm; 2015.
37. Soejima K, Stevenson WG, Maisel WH, Sapp JL, Epstein LM. Electrically unexcitable scar mapping based on pacing threshold for identification of the reentry circuit isthmus: feasibility for guiding ventricular tachycardia ablation. Circulation. 2002;106:1678-83.
38. Madhavan M, Asirvatham SJ. The fourth dimension: endocavitary ventricular tachycardia. Circ Arrhythm Electrophysiol. 2010;3:302-4.

CHAPTER 10

Abhishek Deshmukh, Paul Friedman

Radiofrequency Ablation: Principles and Biophysics

LIST OF ABBREVIATIONS

AF	Atrial Fibrillation
ARVC	Arrhythmogenic Right Ventricular Cardiomyopathy
AV	Atrioventricular
CF	Contact Force
ICE	Intracardiac Echocardiography
LA	Left Atrium
LV	Left Ventricle
PVI	Pulmonary Vein Isolation
RF	Radiofrequency

INTRODUCTION

Treating arrhythmias through the disruption of arrhythmogenic tissues has made dramatic advancements since the initial report of surgical division of an accessory pathway by Dwight McGoon at Mayo Clinic in 1967.[1] Open surgical procedures were effective, but associated with prolonged recovery and surgical risk. Direct current ablation permitted percutaneous therapy, initially of the atrioventricular (AV) node to control rapid atrial fibrillation. However, complications included barotrauma, pain requiring general anesthesia, and difficult to control lesions that were often irregular in contour and at times arrhythmogenic themselves. The introduction of radiofrequency energy in the 500 kHz frequency range permitted creation of targeted lesions to disrupt arrhythmogenic substrates without causing pain via nerve stimulation or barotrauma, and revolutionized the percutaneous treatment of arrhythmias. The creation of lesions with smooth margins significantly mitigated the risk of ablation proarrhythmia.

Understanding of biophysics, innovation in catheter designs and delivery of energy and its clinical translation in improving efficacy and safety of electrophysiological procedures, has had a profound impact on the field. The radiofrequency (RF) catheter ablation indications for targeting cardiac and extracardiac structures continue to expand. Improvements in catheter design have continued to enhance the operator's ability to map and deliver effective energy to the arrhythmogenic substrate of interest. However, an understanding of the fundamental biophysics of RF energy delivery, monitoring lesion formation, and the mechanisms of tissue injury in response to ablation will help the clinician to optimize catheter ablation in order to enhance efficacy and safety of the procedure.

PHYSICS

Radiofrequency energy is a form of alternating electrical current that generates a lesion in the heart by electrically heating the myocardium. RF current is typically delivered in a unipolar fashion from an intracardiac electrode catheter to a dispersive grounding pad placed on the skin. Typically, an oscillation frequency of 500 kHz is selected. Lower frequencies can lead to stimulation of cardiac muscle and nerves, resulting in arrhythmias and pain. Higher frequencies will result in tissue heating; however, in the megahertz range, the mode of energy transfer changes from electrical (resistive) heating to dielectric heating (as observed with microwave energy), introducing antenna phenomena in the ablation catheters and challenges in energy control.

As per the first law of thermodynamics, the principle of catheter ablation with RF energy is to convert electromagnetic energy into thermal energy (heat) in the tissue effectively to obliterate the arrhythmogenic substrate by heating them to a threshold temperature. The mode of tissue heating by RF energy is resistive (electrical) heating or ohmic heating. As electrical current passes through a resistive medium, the voltage drops, and heat is produced. Due to significant difference between the surface area of ablation electrode vs. the dispersive electrode, current density is high at catheter tip, which functionally acts as a point source of energy. This results in resistive heating at the catheter tip-tissue interface and a small rim of surrounding tissue **(Figure 10.1)**. Deeper ablative lesions result from conductive heating of surrounding tissues.

Resistive heat production within the tissue is directly related to the RF power density, which is proportional to the square of the current density (I^2). When RF energy is delivered in a unipolar fashion, the current distributes radially from the source. The current density decreases in proportion to the square of the distance (r^2) from the RF electrode source. Thus, direct resistive heating of the tissue decreases in relation with the distance from the electrode to the fourth power.

In *resistive heating*, energy dissipated per unit time (W) is proportional to current and voltage, as described by the power equation:

$W = VI = (IR)I = I^2R$ (Watts) (V is voltage, I is current, R is resistance, and
$V = IR$ by Ohm's law)

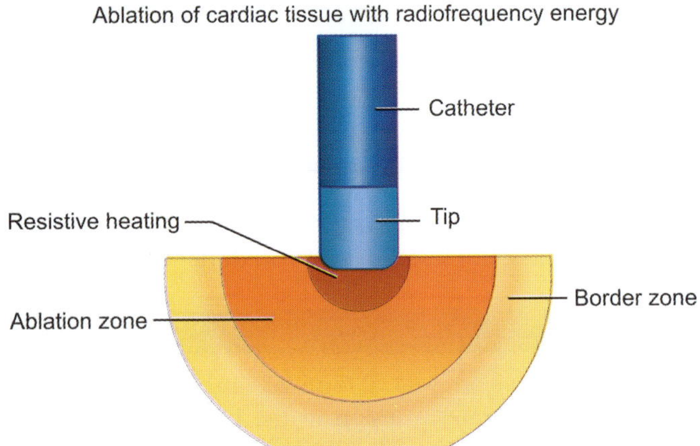

Figure 10.1: Transfer of thermal energy during ablation

Current disperses radially from the electrode tip and is inversely proportional to the square of the distance from the catheter tip. This is specified by the current density (Q) equation for a spherical electrode:

$Q = I/4r^2$ (amp/cm^2)

The heat generated per unit volume of tissue is inversely related to the fourth power of the distance from the catheter tip **(Figure 10.2)**. As the lesion size and volume decreases as a function of distance, lesions created by RF energy are typically small and well-circumscribed. Only a 1 to 2 mm rim of tissue directly adjacent to the catheter tip is heated resistively; deeper tissues are heated by passive thermal conduction. This *conductive heating* is responsible for most of the lesion volume from RF ablation catheters.[2]

The difference in heating mechanism between resistive heating and conductive heating is the construct for "thermal latency."[3] After 30–60 seconds applications, tissue temperatures have reached their maximum target and there is continual flow of heat from the tip electrode. Termination of RF application will then cause a direct but gradual decline in tissue temperatures instead of sudden temperature cut off. Early interruption of the application, e.g., in case of AV conduction block, therefore does not immediately terminate conductive heating.[4] Titration of RF power near a critical area like the AV node or esophagus/phrenic nerve should be standard practice. In addition, the relative rate of lesion formation is faster than the monitored physiological response such as junctional rhythm or loss of conduction or esophageal temperature monitoring. Thus, careful power titration should be considered in order to prevent irreversible damage to the bystander critical tissue. Alternatively, another source of energy whose effects are reversible such as cryoenergy should be considered in critical regions like while ablating midseptal pathways or areas in proximity to phrenic nerve.[5]

PATHOPHYSIOLOGY OF LESION FORMATION BY RADIOFREQUENCY ABLATION

The direct effects of energy delivery on the myocardial tissue are seen immediately and some evolve over weeks. The first change in the tissue surface (endocardial or epicardial) directly in vicinity with the electrode tip is tissue edema followed by pallor and a small indentation/deformation due to volume loss of the acute lesion. Pallor occurs because of denaturation of myocyte proteins (myoglobin) and subsequent loss of the red pigmentation. If high tissue temperatures are reached during ablation, there may be coagulum or char adherent to the ablation site, which introduces the potential for thromboembolism.[6] The lesion shape is a function of electrode size, contact force, catheter design (irrigation vs. non-irrigation), but with commonly used saline irrigated catheter typically has a teardrop shape

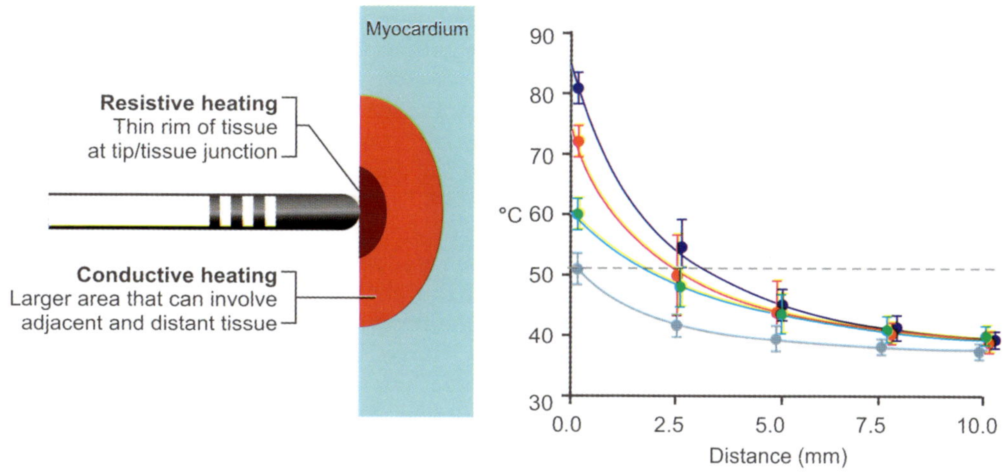

Figure 10.2: Heat mechanism as a function of distance
From: (A) Wittkampf FH et al. Control of radiofrequency lesion size by power regulation. Circulation. 1989;80:962-8. (B) Haines DE et al. Tissue heating during radiofrequency catheter ablation: a thermodynamic model and observations in isolated perfused and superfused canine right ventricular free wall. Pacing Clin Electrophysiol. 1989;12:962-76. (C) Wittkampf FH et al. RF catheter ablation: Lessons on lesions. Pacing Clin Electrophysiol. 2006;29:1285-97. (D) Bunch TJ et al. Insights into energy delivery to myocardial tissue during radiofrequency ablation through application of the first law of thermodynamics. J Cardiovasc Electrophysiol. 2009;20:461-5

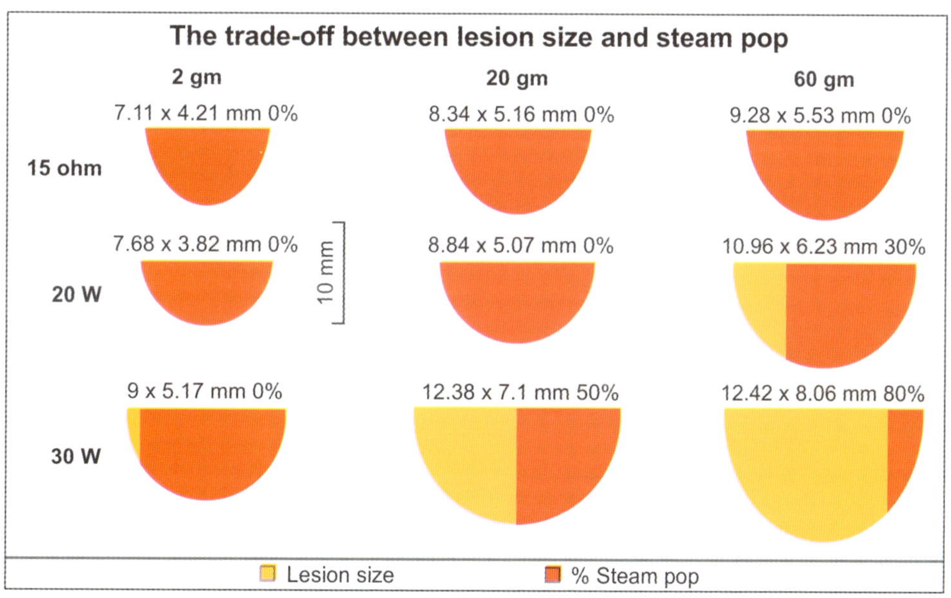

Figure 10.3: Ablation lesion size and safety data for the 9 different ablation groups
From: Thiagalingam A et al. J Cardiovasc Electrophysiol 2010;21:806-11

(Figure 10.3). The lesion frequently has a teardrop shape with a narrower lesion width immediately subendocardially and a wider width 2 to 3 mm below the endocardial surface. There is a band of hemorrhagic necrosis around the central pale zone. Beyond that border, the tissue appears relatively normal. The acute lesion border, as assessed by vital staining, correlates with the border between the hemorrhagic and normal tissue.

On sectioning, the central core of the RF ablation lesion shows desiccation, with surrounding areas of hemorrhagic and normal-appearing tissue. The acute assessment of the lesion border is dependent on the thermal inactivation of the enzymatic activity in the border zone region; however, the ultimate viability of the cell may depend on the integrity of more thermally sensitive organelles such as the plasma membrane.[7]

The most heat sensitive structures appear to be the plasma membrane and the gap junctions. The border zone accounts for documented effects of RF lesion formation well beyond the acute pathological lesion. The progression of the electrophysiological effects after cessation of energy delivery such as progression of block and delayed cure are due to further inflammatory injury and necrosis in the border zone region. Similarly, initial stunning and then early or late recovery can be demonstrated in the border zone, thus accounting for the recovery of electrophysiological properties after apparent successful catheter ablation in the clinical setting.[7] Damage to vasculature supplying myocardium may lead to lesion enlargement, whereas cooling introduced by blood flow in a vessel may limit lesion size. By 8 weeks the ablation lesion is comprised of fatty tissue, cartilage, and fibrosis and can be surrounded by chronic inflammation subsequently evolving into a uniform scar.[8]

Cellular Mechanisms of Thermal Injury

The responses of cellular components to varying degrees of hyperthermia determine the pathophysiologic response to ablation. Thermally sensitive cellular elements include the plasma membrane, the nucleus, cytoskeleton and gap junctions. Changes in these structures contribute to the ultimate cell death.

Hyperthermia leads to dramatic changes in the electrophysiological properties of myocardium. The heat sensitivity of myocytes has been tested in a variety of experimental systems and the mechanisms of the electrophysiologic responses to catheter ablation have been well described. In one of the classic in vitro experiments by Nath, isolated superfused guinea pig papillary muscles were subjected to 60 seconds of exposure to hyperthermic superfusate at temperatures varying from 38°C to 55°C.[9] Action potentials were recorded continuously during and after the hyperthermic pulse. The resting membrane potential was assessed in unpaced preparations, and the action potential amplitude, duration, dV/dt, and excitability were tested during pacing. The preparations maintained a normal resting membrane potential in the low hyperthermic range (<45°C).

In the intermediate hyperthermic range (45°C to 50°C), the myocytes developed a temperature-dependent depolarization that was reversible on return to normothermic superfusion. The high hyperthermic range (>50°C) resulted in irreversible depolarization, contracture, and cell death. There was a temperature-dependent decrease in action potential amplitude between 37°C and 50°C as well as an inverse linear relationship between temperature and action potential duration. Spontaneous automaticity was observed at a median temperature of 50°C. The occurrence of automaticity in unpaced preparations in the setting of hyperthermia-induced depolarization suggested abnormal automaticity as the mechanism. This may partly explain the presence of junctional rhythm during slow pathway ablation. At temperatures between 43°C and 51°C, there was reversible loss of excitability; irreversible loss of excitability (cell death) occurred only at temperatures of 50°C or higher. The construct of isotherm of reversible and irreversible thermal injury is based on specific electrophysiological changes across a temperature range **(Figure 10.4)**.

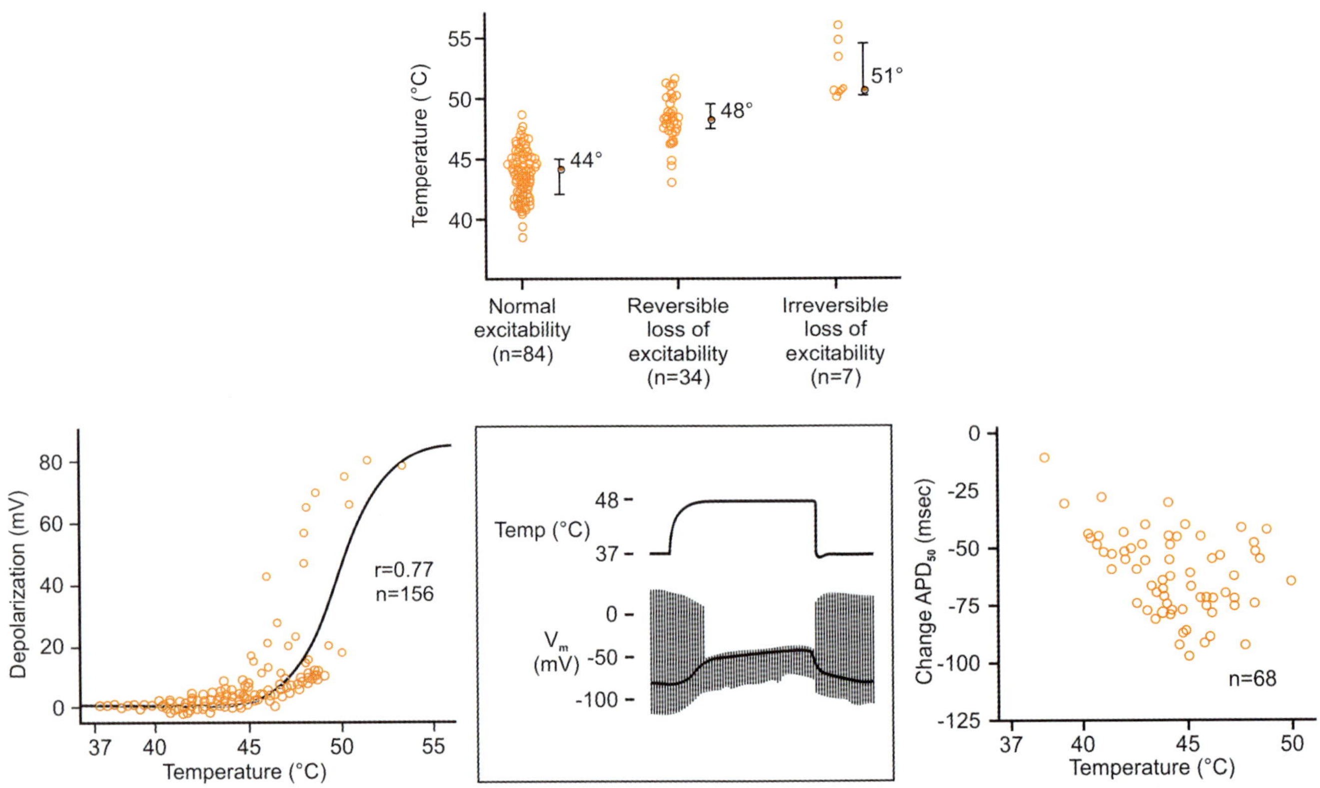

Figure 10.4: Impact of tissue heating on myocardial activity. (From reference 9)

Calcium Overload and Cellular Injury

Everett and colleagues studied the specific mechanisms of cellular depolarization and death in response to hyperthermia.[10] Isolated superfused guinea pig papillary muscles were attached to a force transducer to assess the pattern of contractility with varying hyperthermic exposure. There was a reversible increase in tonic resting muscle tension at temperatures between 45°C and 50°C. Above 50°C, the preparations showed evidence of irreversible contracture. This suggested that hyperthermia was causing calcium entry into the cell and ultimately calcium overload.

Conduction Velocity

Simmers and colleagues examined the effects of hyperthermia on impulse conduction in vitro in a superfused canine myocardium.[11] The average conduction velocity at baseline temperatures of 37°C was 0.35 m/second. When the superfusate temperature was increased, conduction velocity increased to 114% of baseline at 42.5°C. At temperatures above 45.4°C, conduction velocity slowed down. Transient conduction block was observed between 49.5°C and 51.5°C, and above 51.7°C permanent block was observed. The authors concluded that the sole effect of RF ablation on the electrophysiologic properties of the myocardium was related to hyperthermia. It is unknown whether these changes in conduction velocity are solely due to changes in intracellular ionic concentrations or whether thermal injury to gap junctions may also be implicated **(Table 10.1)**.

DETERMINANTS OF EFFECTIVE LESION FORMATION

Factors that affect lesion formation include tissue characteristics, electrical factors (power, temperature, and duration of energy delivery, ablation impedance, frequency and unipolar vs bipolar modality) and mechanical factors (contact force, convective cooling, catheter irrigation, electrode size, orientation, and material) **(Figure 10.5)**.

Table 10.1: Tissue effects of radiofrequency ablation

Temperature	*Effect*
Greater than or equal to 45°C	• Marked depolarization • ↑ rate of rise AP • ↓ AP amplitude and duration
48°C	Reversible loss of excitability
Greater than or equal to 50°C	Irreversible tissue injury
Greater than 45°C	Abnormal automaticity
50.3°C	Transient conduction block
53.6°C	Permanent conduction block

Abbreviation: AP, action potential

Tissue Composition

Lesion size is decreased in areas of dense scar due to heterogeneous channels of tissue capable for sustaining arrhythmia and presence of admix scar tissue. With epicardial ablation, an insulating layer of fat as thin as 2 mm overlying myocardium can act as a thermal insulator, preventing lesion formation with RF energy delivery. Similarly, ablation within a pouch or recess or over prominent ridge or pectinate muscle would have varied response compared to ablating on the smooth wall of the left atrium or right ventricular free wall.

Power

Lesion size is proportional to the power delivered **(Figure 10.6)**. Any method that allows greater power delivery into the tissue will result in more tissue heating and greater lesion size. Power delivery is limited by excessive heating at the electrode-tissue interface, denaturation of proteins that adhere to the electrode, reducing effective surface area and increasing current density. Temperature control, saline irrigation, impedance monitoring, and convective cooling all serve to mitigate excessive interface heating.

Electrode Temperature

The ablative electrode is passively heated by conduction of heat from the tissue during ablation. While electrode temperature parallels tissue temperature, lesion size increases directly with electrode temperature. However, many factors render this relationship invalid, so that electrode temperature is a poor surrogate for lesion size. Convective cooling and catheter motion in vitro confound the relationship between lesion size and electrode temperature, as does coagulum formation and impedance rise. The use of higher-power

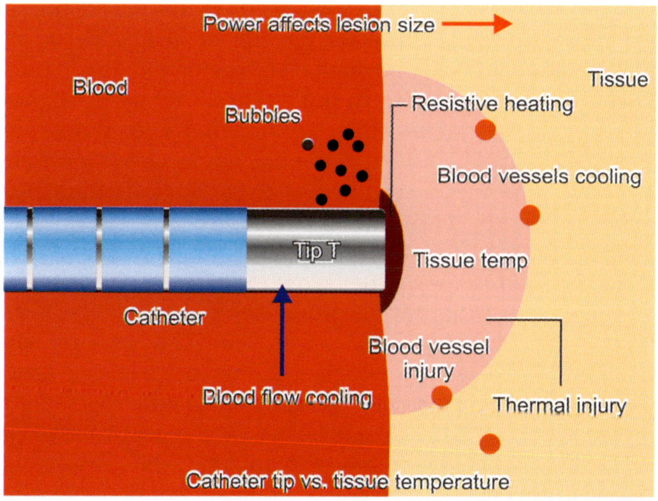

Figure 10.5: Potential factors affecting lesion size

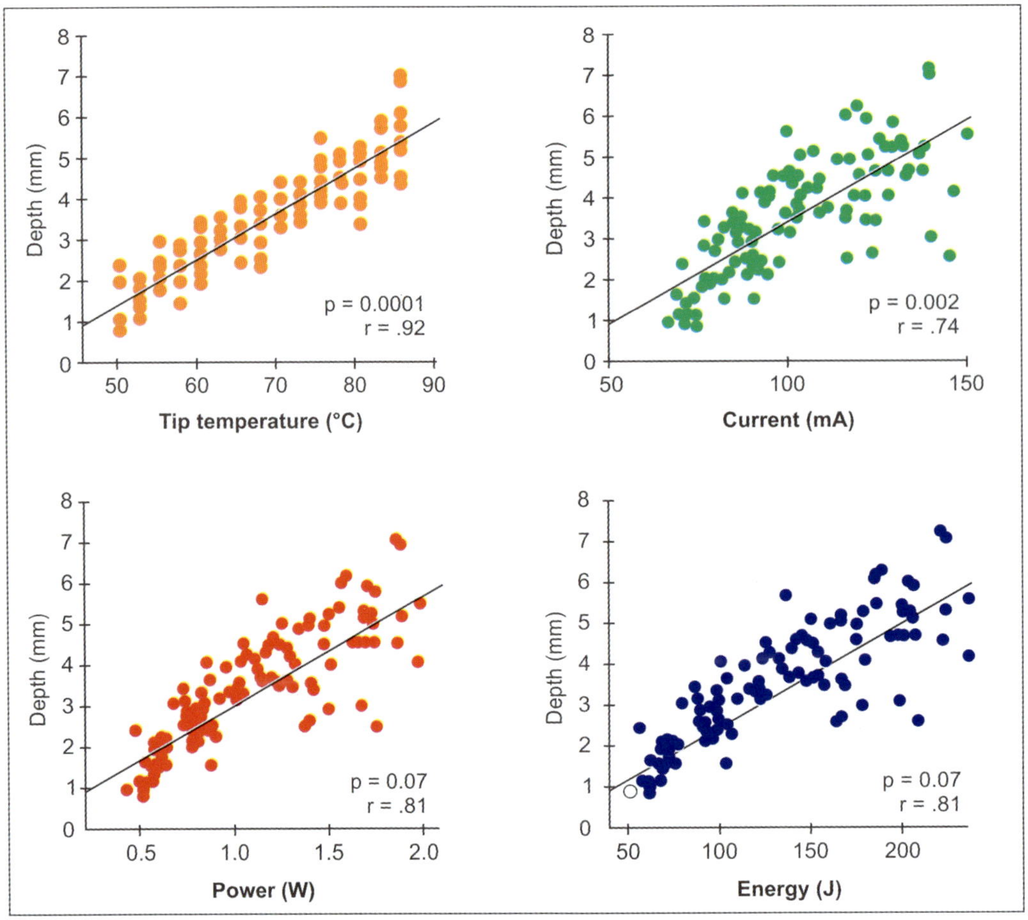

Figure 10.6: Relationship between lesion depth and tip temperature, current, power, and energy
From: Haines D. J Cardiovasc Electrophysiol 2004;15(10 Suppl):S2-S11

output to achieve higher tissue temperatures results in larger lesions by raising the temperature of the rim of resistively heated tissue to substantially more than 50°C so that a larger extent of deeper tissue reaches the 50°C threshold required for tissue necrosis. However, the rim of heated tissue in direct contact with the ablating electrode conducts not only to deeper tissue but also to the electrode tip itself. Higher electrode temperatures either limit further energy delivery (in temperature-controlled power delivery mode) or increase electrode impedance as a result of coagulum formation (see below), or both; these effects potentially limit lesion size. It is important to understand the fundamental principle that the amount of RF power delivered to the tissue determines lesion size, and that the recorded catheter tip temperature is poorly correlated with lesion size. The catheter tip temperature is always lower than the superficial tissue temperature due to convective cooling by blood flow.

Ablation can be delivered either in a power-controlled mode (operator adjusts power manually, while observing temperature or impedance) or a temperature-controlled mode (operator selects temperature target, and power is titrated by the system to maintain the target), discussed further below. In non-irrigated catheters, with good contact between catheter tip and tissue in a wedged position (such as a sub-Eustacian pouch, between pectinate muscles, or in a coronary vein), the target temperature can be reached with very little power since there is no convective cooling of the electrode by blood, resulting in small lesions despite a high catheter tip temperature. Saline irrigation permits additional power delivery by avoiding overheating of the electrode-tissue interface. Similarly, if the irrigation pores of an open irrigation catheter are occluded with tissue/char/coagulum, cooling may be impaired and higher tip temperature recorded at lower delivered power. Inspecting the pores and re-flushing the catheter outside the body mitigates this issue. In contrast, a low catheter tip temperature can be caused by poor contact or a high level of convective cooling. High blood flow areas permit a higher amount of RF power to be delivered to the tissue (because it is no longer limited by temperature rise of the ablation electrode) and yields relatively large lesions. This is best illustrated with active cooling of the ablation electrode using

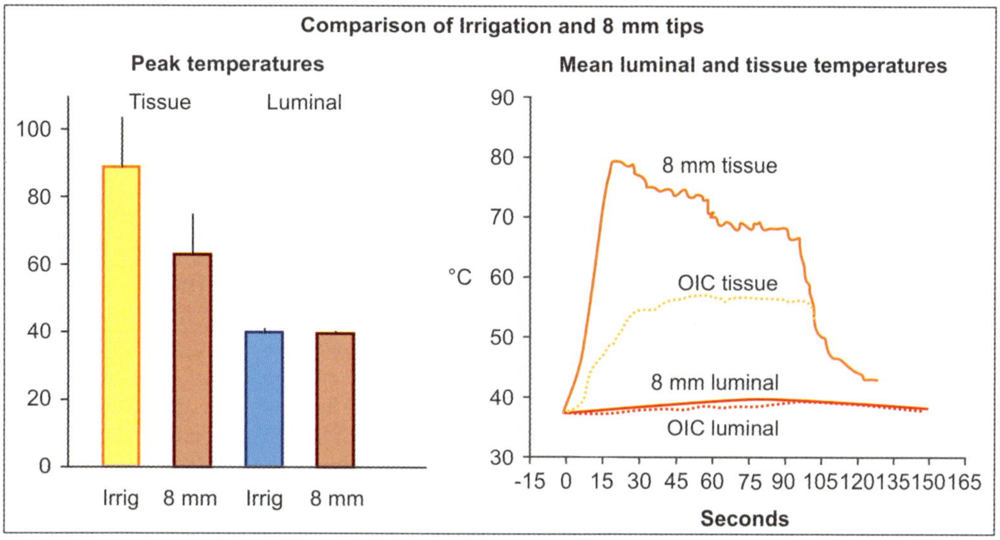

Figure 10.7: Discrepancy between tissue temperature and catheter tip temperature. (From Cummings JE, Natale A et al. J Cardiovasc Electrophysiol 2008;19:641-4)
Abbreviations: OIC, open irrigated catheter; Irrig, irrigated catheter

irrigation during RF energy delivery; the tip temperature is usually less than 40°C, which allows the application of high-power output for longer durations. This again illustrates that tip temperature is not an effective marker for tissue heating. Moreover the tip temperature is also dependent on location of temperature sensor (thermistor vs. thermocouple) **(Figure 10.7)**.

Peak Tissue Temperature

Peak tissue temperature is closely correlated with effective power delivery and lesion size, but is not measurable with current ablation systems. Because of convective cooling, electrode temperature underestimates peak tissue temperature—the real determinant of lesion size. Stevenson et al. have investigated a novel catheter with a needle tip for accurate mapping, recording intramural cardiac electrograms, pacing, and measuring tissue temperature that can create deep myocardial lesions.[12] The addition of intramyocardial saline infusion from the needle, likely creates an interstitial virtual electrode facilitating creation of large, deep myocardial lesions. Intracardiac echo has been used to visualize lesion. Future sensors such as infrared, microwave, or ultrasound detectors may allow the operator to monitor actual lesion growth. Real-time MRI may guide ablation and provide real-time thermography or imaging of lesion formation.

Electrode Contact Pressure

Contiguous transmural lesions over a wide region are challenging and often limited by cardiac and respiratory motion, catheter sliding and suboptimal catheter contact leading to dissipation of radiofrequency energy to the blood pool. Recently approved contact force-sensing catheters allow direct measurement of contact force, improving the efficacy and safety of ablation. Two different contact force-engineering platforms have emerged as commercially available open-irrigation contact force catheters. The first catheter uses a small spring connecting the ablation tip electrode to the catheter shaft, with sensors to measure microdeflections of the spring (Thermocool Smartouch CF, Biosense Webster Inc., Diamond Bar, California, USA). The second uses three optical fibers to measure microdeformation of a deformable body in the catheter tip (TactiCath, Endosense/St Jude Medical, St. Paul, Minnesota, USA). TOCCATA study explored the relationship between contact force parameters during acute pulmonary vein isolation (PVI) and atrial fibrillation (AF) ablation outcome at 12 months in 34 patients referred for ablation of paroxysmal AF. Analysis of the contact force during ablation revealed that 35% of lesions were performed with a low contact force (<10 g), and 52% of lesions were delivered with contact force between 10 and 30 g. At 12 months, all patients (100%) treated with an average contact force <10 g had recurrent AF, whereas 80% of the patients treated with an average contact force more than 20 g were free of AF or had persistent PVI (P = 0.01).[13] SMART-AF trial highlighted the contribution of real-time contact force (CF) sensing to the ablation outcome as demonstrated by the significantly higher success rate (probability of freedom from recurrence of 81% vs. 66%) in patients where the investigators stayed within their selected CF range ≥80% of the time during radiofrequency application, suggesting that consistent and stable catheter-tissue contact is necessary for effective ablation results. There was a trend toward greater percentage of time in higher CF

(≥40 g) for all the tamponade cases suggesting importance of monitoring contact force to minimize complications[14] **(Figure 10.8)**.

Greater electrode-tissue contact pressure increases lesion size by improving electrical coupling with the tissue, resulting in more delivery of energy in the tissue and reducing the shunting of current to the blood pool. In addition, greater contact pressure may prevent the electrode from sliding with cardiac motion. However, the operator should be mindful of the risk of the catheter being wedged in especially with steerable sheaths. The optimal electrode contact pressure is believed to be 20 to 40 grams forces. Excessive contact that buries the electrode in the tissue, however, may prevent convective cooling of the electrode, increase electrode tip temperature and reduce current delivery.[15]

Convective Cooling and Catheter irrigation

Role of Convective Cooling

Ultimately, lesion size is a function of tissue heating, and tissue heating is a function of the magnitude of RF power that is converted into heat in the tissues. The greater the magnitude of power delivered to the tissue, the greater the lesion size. Convective cooling at the electrode-tissue interface, either active or passive, will allow the operator to increase safely the power amplitude before impedance rises.

However, if the ablation is power limited (i.e., the maximal available power is delivered throughout the ablation), greater degrees of convective cooling will draw heat from the tissue resulting in a smaller lesion size. Factors that affect passive cooling at the electrode-tissue interface include the magnitude of regional blood flow, the stability of the electrode catheter on the tissue surface, electrode size, electrode orientation, and contact force. Catheter motion over the tissue greatly increases the loss of heat to the blood pool. Intramyocardial blood flow draws heat from the tissue and not from the electrode, and therefore, decreases lesion size.

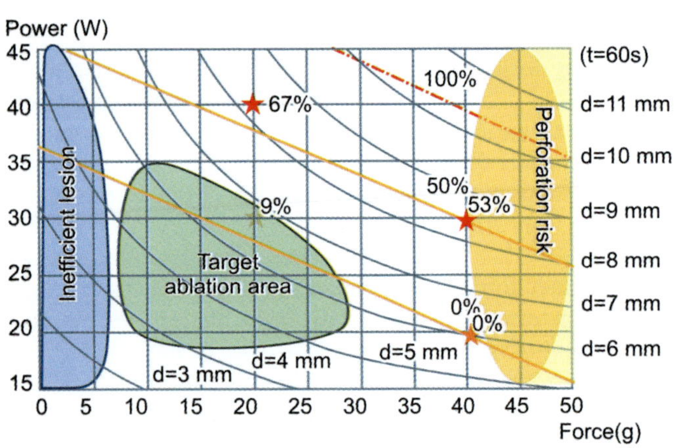

Figure 10.8: Relation of contact force, lesion depth, power and complications

Catheter Irrigation

The concept of irrigation and catheter design has come along a long way **(Figure 10.9)**.

Three catheter designs for tip cooling have been investigated at length. The first type, perhaps the low tech version and not in use, used a long sheath of slightly larger diameter than the ablation catheter. The ablation catheter is advanced through the sheath and saline flows externally around the ablation catheter and bathes the tip-tissue interface and surrounding tissue. This was an open system in which saline was continuously infused and emptied into the blood pool. A disadvantage of this system was the sheath itself, the presence of which limits potential sites on which it may be used. The second type of system is a method of internal irrigation through the catheter tip, also an open system. Saline is conducted down the body of the catheter and is forced out of holes in the porous catheter tip. This has been described as a showerhead or sprinkler design (Cordis Webster/Medtronic). The third also involves internal perfusion of the catheter tip. Saline is perfused via a pump mechanism through the catheter tip, turns around within the catheter tip, and returns back to the pump. This represents a closed system because no saline is infused into the blood pool (Chilli®, EPT/Boston Scientific).

The principle of irrigation of the catheter tip reduces excessive heating of the tissue and blood at the catheter tip and prevents the occurrence of thrombus and char formation. Due to the potential dramatic consequences, the prevention of thromboembolic events is of particular importance for left-sided procedures. As thrombus and char generate additional impedance and impair energy transfer to the tissue, the avoidance of thrombus and char formations would allow continuous energy transfer and lesion formation. A number of factors can be potentially manipulated to adjust ablation with saline-irrigated catheters. The flow rate of the irrigant determines the degree of cooling. Faster flow rates would likely allow greater power application without impedance rises, increase the difference between tissue and electrode temperature, and thereby potentially increase the risk of steam pops if temperature is used to guide ablation.

The impact of different irrigation catheter flow on the development of lesion dimension and thrombus formation has been investigated in a thigh muscle preparation in sheep. RF ablations (30 s, 30 W) were performed with three different irrigation flow rates (5 mL/min, 10 mL/min, and 20 mL/min) and a perpendicular position with constant contact pressure of the irrigated ablation catheter (Sprinkler, Medtronic, Inc.,

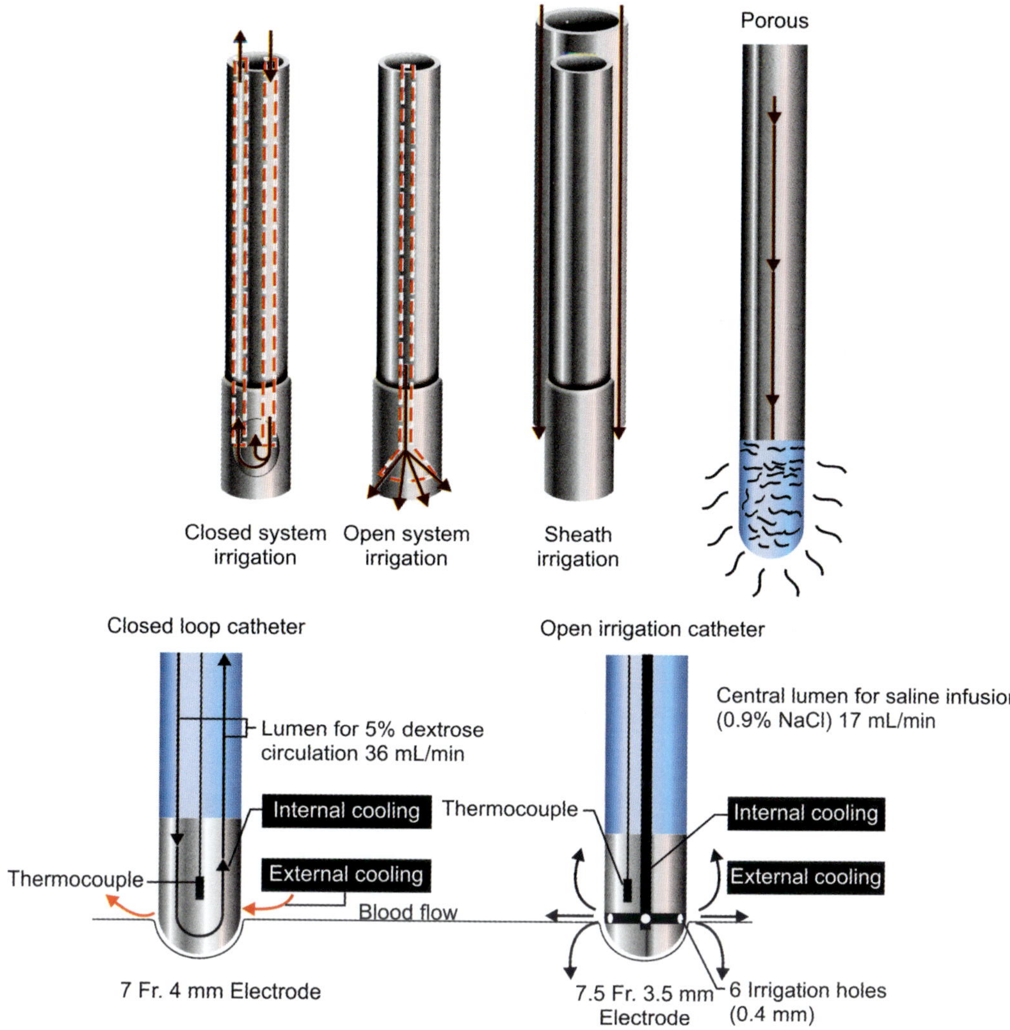

Figure 10.9: Irrigated catheter design (From EP Lab Digest)

Minneapolis, MN, USA).[16] Cross-sections of the lesions were investigated with regard to maximal depth and maximal diameter at and below the surface. During high flow irrigation (20 mL/min) the surface diameter was significantly smaller compared to irrigation flow rates of 5 mL/min and 10 mL/min. There was no significant difference in lesion depth with different flow rates. Thrombus formation was not observed during any RF application. Thus, lesion diameter does not increase with high irrigation flow rates. Minimal irrigation seems to be sufficient to warrant effective ablation and to prevent thrombus and char formation. However, ablation with more than 30 W in anatomic locations with low blood stream might warrant higher flow rates than 20 mL/min and/or "intelligent" catheter design in order to prevent clot formation and to enable sufficient lesion size. Depending on catheter design and company recommendations power settings with up to 50 W at irrigation rates between 15 and 30 mL/min are used in clinical practice.

With the internally irrigated ablation system (Chilli catheter; Boston Scientific, Natick, MA) the approved flow rate is fixed at 36 mL/min and is not presently manipulated.[17]

The temperature of the irrigant can also potentially be manipulated. Cooling the irrigant may also allow power delivery to be increased without coagulum formation. The cooled irrigant is warmed as it passes through the tubing to reach the catheter, and through the length of the catheter. The impact of cooling the irrigant has not been well studied. Demazumder studied irrigation with iced saline versus room temperature saline in vitro and found no difference in lesion size.[18] In most studies, the irrigant that enters the catheter is at room temperature.

The use of dextrose was found to impede power delivery, resulting in smaller lesions. The use of saline did not prevent tissue boiling. Boiling, however, did not prevent lesion growth.[18] Hypertonic saline used in canine prostate tissue was shown to increase lesion size. This was thought to be due to its greater conductivity than blood, thus, resulting in lowering of impedance at the catheter tip. Applicability with the human population in an EP lab setting is probably limited, however, due to potential for hypertonic saline causing volume overload in heart failure and other compromised patients.

Irrigated, flexible tip catheters such as Therapy Cool Flex (St. Jude Medical, St. Paul, MA, USA) have been designed to increase the contact surface and to improve the cooling effect. By directing up to 70% of the irrigation flow toward the tip-to-tissue interface the average tip temperature is approximately 5°C cooler in comparison to rigid tip catheters, with the possibility of reduced thrombus, char formation and steam pops. A larger number of irrigation channels are supposed to serve the same purpose. This concept has been successfully applied in the irrigated tip catheters ThermoCool SF Catheter (Biosense Webster, Diamond Bar, CA, USA).[19]

Electrode Size

In non-irrigated systems, larger electrodes permit creation of larger lesions since they increase convective cooling and permit the delivery of higher total power without excessive current density at the electrode-tissue interface. Thus, coagulum formation with a sudden rise in electrical impedance can be avoided despite high total power delivery. The higher power delivery to the tissue increases the depth of direct volume heating and, in turn, increases the size of the virtual heat source. This translates directly into a larger lesion. As is the case with cooled electrodes, a large electrode will only result in larger lesion formation only if it is accompanied by higher power delivery. If a large electrode is used with lower power, a larger endocardial surface area may be ablated, but the lesion will not be as deep. An increased electrode size reduces current density. Thus, if a 4 mm and 8 mm tip ablation catheters are used at the same power setting, the lesion volume and depth may be smaller with an 8 mm tip catheter. Consequently, an 8 mm electrode may require a 1.5 to 4 times higher power level than a 4 mm electrode to create an equivalent lesion size, and with additional power delivery will result in a larger lesion. With the use of catheter irrigation with large electrode, the advantages of larger electrode size are mitigated, and the limitations (effect of orientation, lower mapping resolution) become more manifest **(Figure 10.10)**.

Duration of Energy Delivery

Tissue temperature follows a monoexponential rise during RF delivery until steady state is achieved. The half-time for lesion formation is 5 to 10 seconds for conventional ablation. Therefore lesion formation is assumed to be nearly complete after 45 to 60 seconds (five half-lives). Simmers et al. evaluated the relation between RF duration and lesion size.[11] They applied a constant power of 25 W for 5, 10, 20, 30 and 60 seconds using a 7F, 4-mm tip electrode catheter (Mansfield-Webster, Watertown, MA, USA) in left and right ventricle in dogs. They found that the lesion is predominantly generated within the first 10 seconds of energy delivery and reaches a maximum after 30s. Further extension of RF delivery during power controlled RF delivery does not seem to further increase the lesion size, however,

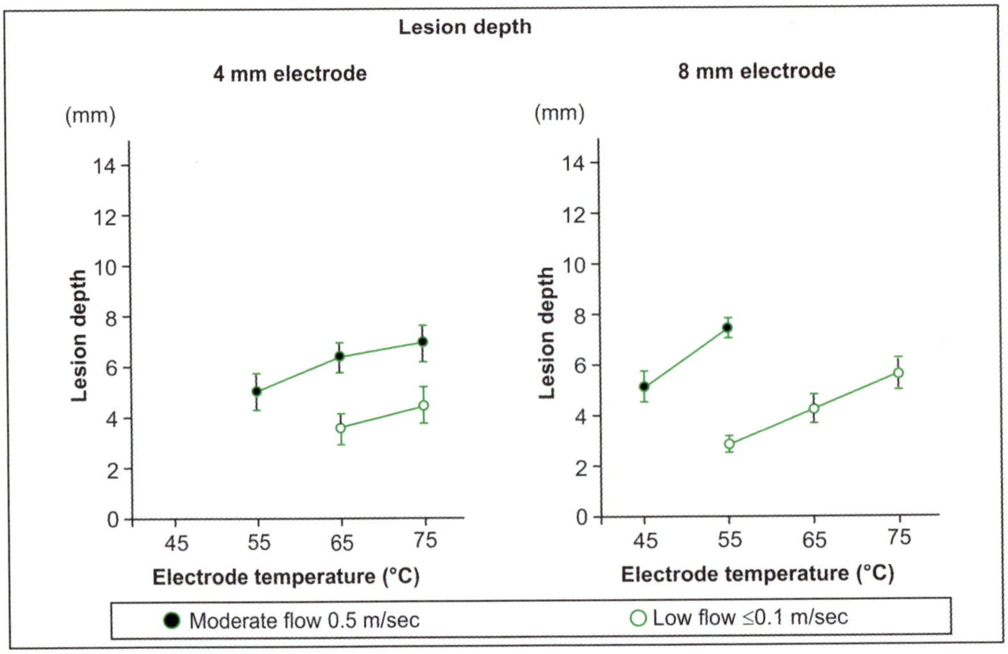

Figure 10.10: Relationship between lesion depth and electrode temperature

may cause harm due to collateral damage. This is especially important while ablating on the posterior wall of left atrium in order to prevent atrioesophageal fistula. Instead of a predefined duration for each ablation lesion, other characteristics as described in following sections should be used for effective and safe ablation **(Figure 10.11)**.

Ablation Circuit Impedance

The RF current path and skin grounding electrode interface present significant impedance for the ablation current flow, thereby dissipating part of the power. Increasing patch size (or using two patches) reduces patch impedance, providing for increased heating at the electrode-endocardium interface and thus increases tissue heating. The position of the dispersive electrode (on the patient's back or thigh) has little effect on the size of the resulting lesion. During prolonged procedures, if consistent high impedance develops, the dispersive electrode should be checked. The partial dislodgement of the dispersive electrode due to excessive sweating can lead to increase in ablation circuit impedance and impede energy delivery.

Electrode Orientation

When the catheter tip is perpendicular to the tissue surface, a much smaller surface area is in contact with the tissue (versus that exposed to the cooling effect of blood flow) than when the catheter electrode tip is lying horizontal. Clinically, perpendicular electrode orientation yields larger lesion volumes and uses less power than parallel electrode orientation. However, if the RF power level is adjusted to maintain a constant current density, lesion size will increase proportionally to the electrode-tissue contact area, which is larger with parallel tip orientation. Lesion depth is only slightly affected by catheter tip orientation using 4-mm-long tip catheters, but lesions are slightly longer in the parallel orientation as compared with the perpendicular orientation. For non-irrigated electrodes with unrestricted power, an orientation parallel to the tissue generally results in larger lesions because of a larger electrode area in contact with the tissue and less current shunting to the blood pool. For irrigated electrodes delivering high-power outputs, the parallel electrode orientation results in smaller lesion sizes because of a greater magnitude of tissue cooling.[20,21]

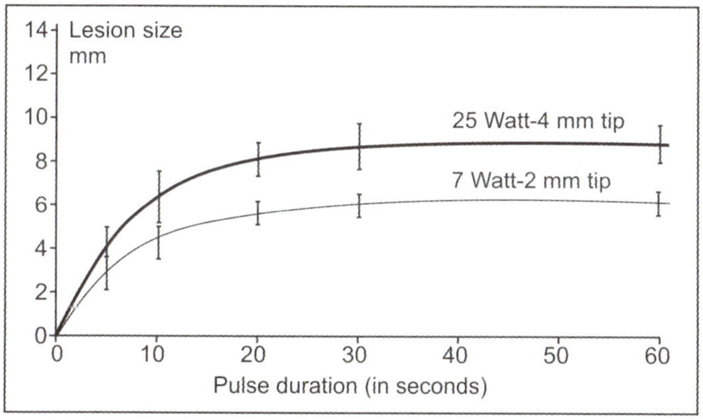

Figure 10.11: Impact of power and duration of energy delivery on lesion size. (From reference 2)

Electrode Material

Platinum-iridium electrodes have been the standard for most RF ablation catheters. Gold exhibits excellent electrical conductive properties, as well as a more than four times greater thermal conductivity than platinum. The higher thermal conductivity of gold can potentially lead to a higher mean rate of power because of better heat conduction at the tissue-electrode interface and, in turn, also facilitates increased passive cooling as a result of heat loss to the surrounding blood with this electrode material.[22]

Characteristics of RF Energy

Very high frequencies of alternating current lead to less efficient tissue heating, and lower frequencies may result in tissue stimulation causing pain and arrhythmias. Pulsed RF current may allow for electrode cooling than unmodulated RF, and, therefore, increase power delivery. Due to thermal latency, the temperature continues to accumulate within the tissue while surface temperature drops at the electrode tissue interface. With multielectrode ablation arrays, phased RF among the electrodes allows for more continuous linear lesions. Most RF lesions are created by applying energy in a unipolar fashion between an ablating electrode touching the myocardium and a grounded reference patch electrode placed externally on the skin. The unipolar configuration creates a highly localized lesion, greater depth but less lesion surface area than bipolar ablation endocardially.

When electrodes are placed on either side of target tissue, bipolar RF limits collateral injury and permits higher current density through the target. The effect of bipolar versus unipolar epicardial ablation on lesion size was compared in an ex vivo animal model with excised pig hearts. Bipolar ablation was performed between a 4 mm saline irrigated tip electrode on the left ventricular (LV) epicardium and an opposing 10 mm non-irrigated-tip electrode on the LV endocardium. Epicardial lesion width did not differ between unipolar and bipolar ablation, but lesion depth was significantly greater and transmural lesions were achieved more often with bipolar compared to unipolar ablation. It has been surmised that bipolar ablation of the LV free wall is highly effective at creating an appropriately deep epicardial and intramural lesion.[23] As expected, due to higher temperature achieved, steam pop occurred more often with bipolar ablation.[24] Bipolar ablation also created a narrower, deeper lesion than unipolar ablation across the interventricular septum of excised swine hearts. Thus, after accurate mapping and assessment of true location of the substrate, bipolar ablation may have a role in selective situations.

MONITORING AND TITRATION OF RADIOFREQUENCY ENERGY DELIVERY

The goal of optimizing RF ablation is to create an adequate-sized lesion while reducing collateral damage to the neighboring structures, coagulum formation at the electrode itself and steam formation within the tissue. As discussed previously, for ablation to be effective in causing tissue death, power must be increased sufficiently to achieve temperatures substantially higher than 50°C at the tissue directly in contact with the ablating electrode. The determinants of lesion formation (i.e., the temperature per Watt of applied power) is dependent on several variables, including catheter stability, electrode-tissue contact pressure, electrode orientation relative to the endocardium, effective electrode contact area, convective heat loss into the blood pool, and target location. Thus, applied energy, power, and current are poor indicators of the extent of lesion formation, and the actual electrode-tissue interface temperature remains the only predictor of the actual lesion size. The others at best could be surrogates for tissue heating.

Impedance Monitoring

Impedance monitoring has emerged as an important surrogate for tissue heating. Ablation circuit impedance reflects the resistance to current flow through the patient, from the tip of the ablation catheter to the dispersive pad. As the tissue is heated, ions in the tissue become more mobile, resulting in a fall in local resistivity, measured as a fall in ablation circuit impedance. Therefore, impedance provides a useful qualitative assessment of tissue heating; however, it does not correlate well with lesion size. Advantage with impedance measurement is that it does not require any specific catheter-based sensor circuitry and can be performed with any catheter designed for RF ablation. Larger dispersive electrodes and larger ablation electrodes result in lower impedance. Significant tissue heating is associated with a predictable fall in impedance, usually in the range of 5 to 10 Ω.[25]

As tissue is heated at the beginning of an RF application, a fall in local resistance occurs and a decrease in impedance measured at the catheter tip is observed. A decrease of greater than 5 Ohms observed during the first 5 seconds of RF energy delivery correlates with the force applied by the catheter tip.

Absence of an impedance fall may reflect inadequate energy delivery to the tissue, poor catheter–tissue contact, or catheter instability. A 5-to 10 Ω reduction in impedance is usually observed in clinically successful RF applications, it correlates with a tissue temperature of 55° to 60°C, and it is rarely associated with coagulum formation. Larger decrements in impedance are noted when coagulum formation is imminent. Once a coagulum is formed, an abrupt rise in impedance to more than 250 Ω may be observed **(Figure 10.12)**.

Impedance monitoring has several pitfalls. When blood flow rates are low, blood can also be heated, and electrode impedance drops accordingly. Moreover, a large rise in tissue temperature at a small contact area and a smaller rise with better tissue contact can result in a similar drop in impedance. Although coagulum formation is usually accompanied by an abrupt rise in impedance, the absence of impedance rise during ablation does not guarantee the absence of blood clot formation on the tissue contact site, which can unnoticeably be created on the lesion surface. In addition, as noted, with large ablation electrodes, formation of blood clots may only minimally affect electrode impedance by covering a much smaller part of the electrode surface. Any increase in impedance during RF application can, however, indicate the beginning of thrombus formation or unintended catheter movement either away from the tissue or in a low flow area (coronary sinus/pouch/pulmonary vein); in either case, RF application should be discontinued.

Particular situations when the impedance is suddenly high will include ablating inside the sheath, ablating inside the vein/coronary sinus, starting to ablate even before the catheters capacitors have had a chance to discharge. Repositioning of the catheter and a small waiting period to ensure capacitor discharge before coming on should solve these issues. However, in certain situations when the catheter is wedged inside a vein which is the site for ablation such as middle cardiac vein for accessory pathway or distal anterior interventricular vein for premature ventricular complexes (PVCs), it helps to increase the flow rate or adding another dispersive electrode.

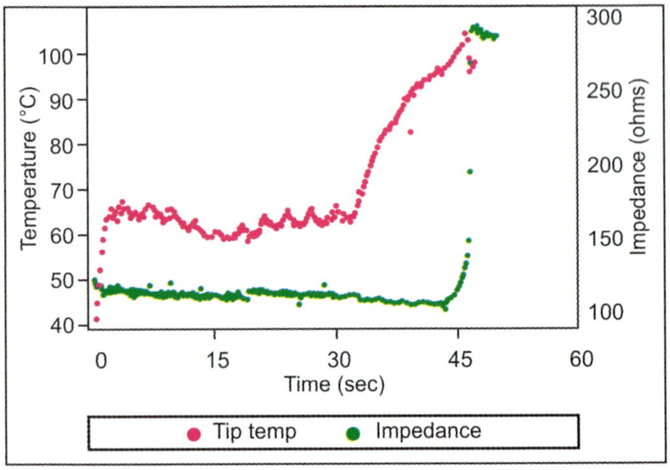

Figure 10.12: Sudden impedance rise during RF ablation

Temperature Monitoring

Multiple factors introduce challenges in temperature monitoring to identify lesion creation. A thermistor or thermocouple is located in the electrode, and its distance to the tissue (the heat source) is a function of catheter design and electrode tissue orientation; convective cooling lowers electrode temperature more than tissue temperature; maximum temperature is not at the tissue surface but deep to it; thermal latency differs for the electrode and for tissues at various depths. Thus, temperature is generally a poor surrogate for lesion size. In addition, direct tissue heating as compared to conductive electrode heating results in a totally different profile of temperature rise: while tissue temperature rise at the electrode tissue interface is very fast, it is rather slow deeper in the tissue[26] **(Figure 10.13)**. However, temperature control ablation monitoring of catheter tip temperature with closed-loop control of power output is useful to avoid excessive heating at the tissue surface to minimize the risk of coagulum formation, particularly when using non-irrigated catheters.

During power controlled ablation, the power titration is manually adjusted and directed by temperature and impedance monitoring. The power initially is set to 20 to 30 W and then is gradually increased until the target temperature is achieved. With both manual (power control ablation) and automatic power titration (temperature controlled ablation), change in power output is frequently required throughout the RF application to maintain the target temperature.

Temperature and impedance are used to determine whether an ablative lesion is ineffective due to energy delivery constraints or due to inadequate mapping. If within 5–10 seconds of ablation the electrophysiologic endpoint (e.g. pathway elimination) does not occur, the failed application is attributed to inadequate mapping if the temperature increased to the desired range, and impedance dropped 5–10 Ohms. If the target temperature or impedance is not achieved with maximum generator output within 20 seconds, the time it takes to achieve subendocardial steady-state temperature, the RF application can be terminated, and catheter adjustment should be considered to prevent tissue edema and obtain better tissue contact or a better mapping site. True tissue-temperature control, as opposed to electrode-tip temperature control, has been tested in vitro.[27]

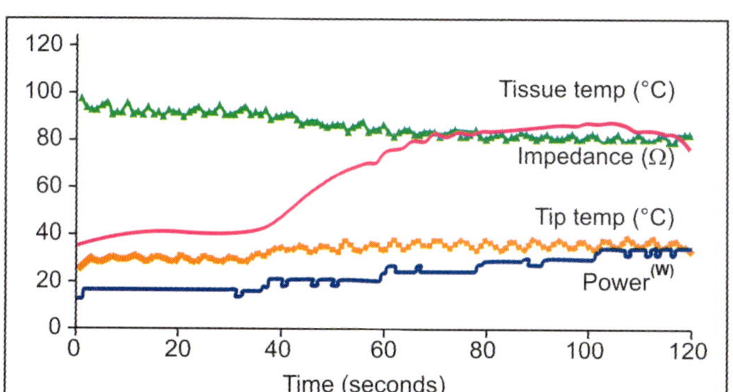

Figure 10.13: Discrepancy between tip and tissue temperature. (From reference 26)

RF energy delivery was titrated using a thermocouple needle extending 2 mm from the catheter tip into the myocardium. This achieved adequate lesions without excessive rise in intramyocardial temperature and prevented steam pops. In theory, tissue temperature-guided power titration would result in more predictable lesion size, reducing variability because of differences in catheter contact and convective blood-flow cooling. However, significant engineering obstacles must be overcome, including demonstrating the safety of inserting a needle into the beating human heart.

Electrogram Amplitude-titrated Energy Delivery

With this strategy, power and duration are titrated using reduction in electrogram amplitude as a physiologic marker of effective ablation. During RF application, local electrogram amplitude typically falls as tissue heating causes loss of excitability. However, the magnitude of this amplitude reduction varies, and the exact myocardial volume sensed by ablation catheter electrodes (field of view) is a function of recording electrode size, orientation recoding modality (unipolar vs. bipolar), and is difficult to know in the clinical setting. In a prospective evaluation using a 90% reduction in bipolar electrogram amplitude to titrate energy delivery, many lesions were small and not transmural.[28] Concerns about efficacy and procedure time have prevented this method of energy titration from being widely adopted. Analyses of bipolar signals are fraught with challenges. The bipolar signals are influenced by both the ablative electrode and a proximal ring electrode, which may be adjacent to viable myocardium not modified by an effective lesion at the tip. The orientation of the proximal electrode and myocardium is altered with catheter motion. Thus, a successful lesion may have no significant electrode diminution, leading to additional ablation and potential complication. The initial slope of unipolar electrogram may be a marker for adequate tissue destruction, although experience with its use is limited.

Ultrasound Imaging

Intracardiac echocardiography (ICE) permits assessment of tissue heating and steam pops (discussed below). The presence of microbubbles on intracardiac or transesophageal echocardiography is typically associated with a tissue temperature higher than 60°C and increased lesion size, and continued RF application after the appearance of the bubbles is usually followed by an increase in impedance.[29]

Moreover, pops are not always audible but can be seen well on ultrasound, often with a sudden explosion of echocardiographic contrast. Microbubble formation, however, is not a straightforward surrogate for tissue heating. The absence of microbubble formation clearly does not indicate that tissue heating is inadequate or that the power level should be increased, nor does the presence of scattered microbubbles indicate safe tissue heating. This marker is fairly specific for tissue heating as judged by tissue temperatures but is not routinely sensitive. Specifically, scattered microbubbles can occur over the entire spectrum of tissue temperatures, whereas dense showers of microbubbles appear only at tissue temperatures higher than 60°C. Scattered microbubbles can represent an electrolytic phenomenon, whereas dense showers of microbubbles suggest steam formation, with associated tissue disruption and impedance rises.[29]

COMPLICATIONS AND THEIR PREVENTION

Coagulum Formation

Coagulum is formed by excessive heating of blood near the electrode–endocardial interface, denaturating proteins in blood cells and serum.[6] This results in soft thrombus or char that initially anneals to the endocardium at the electrode–tissue interface, the site with the highest temperature. Coagulum is not formed by activation of clotting factors as seen during normal hemostasis and its formation is not prevented by heparin or other anticoagulants. As proteins denature at temperatures well below the interfacial boiling temperature, probably around 60° C, coagulum can form even in the absence of impedance rise or steam pop.[30] Coagulum annealing to tissue rather than to the electrode tip may fail to affect electrode temperature or impedance, yet may form the nidus for an embolus. Embolic complications have been reported even in patients undergoing relatively short ablation procedures when few lesions were created and no abrupt increases in impedance were observed. Limiting the RF power level and/or open irrigation are important safety measures for left-sided applications **(Figure 10.14)**.

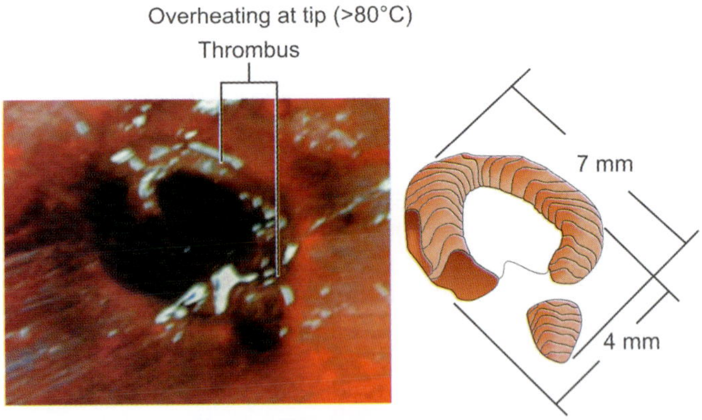

Figure 10.14: Coagulum formation. (From reference 17)

Myocardial Boiling (Steam Pop)

When tissue temperature exceeds 100°C, boiling of water in the myocardial tissue can cause a sudden buildup of steam, released at times with an audible steam pop. This is often associated with a shower of microbubbles on intracardiac echocardiography, composed of steam. When intra-tissue fluid vaporizes due to elevated tissue temperature, the tissue volume expands to approximately 1700 times that of the initial volume. The mechanism underlying this degree of tissue volume expansion is as follows: when 1 mol (18 mL) of water turns into gas at a standard temperature, pressure and dry, its volume increases to 22.4 L, which is 1244.4 times the volume of water. Assuming that the steam temperature is 373 K, the volume can be estimated by accounting for the increase in volume due to temperature with the following formula: 1244.4 times × 373 K/273 K = 1700 times. The escaping gas can cause barotrauma, and dissection along tissue planes as it escapes into the ablated chamber, or uncommonly, into the pericardial space. Damage ranging from superficial endocardial craters to full-thickness myocardial tears resulting in cardiac perforation and tamponade can occur. The consequences of a steam pop vary widely depending on location, myocardial thickness, and proximity to vulnerable structures such as the AV node. Temperature-controlled ablation with a conventional 4-mm-tip catheter carries a low risk of steam pop because tissue and electrode temperature do not diverge widely, and temperature is limited to well below 100°C (usually 50–65°C). However, this is not necessarily true in regions with brisk blood flow, in which convective cooling can cause significant discrepancy between tissue and electrode temperature. Steam pops are more likely to occur with newer technologies aimed at creating larger lesions, such as large-electrode ablation catheters (8- to 12-mm tips) and internally or externally irrigated ablation catheters. A common feature of these large-lesion catheters is that tissue temperature greatly exceeds electrode temperature, sometimes by as much as 40°C. Therefore, steam pops can occur even when electrode temperature is limited to ostensibly safe levels **(Figure 10.15)**.

Steam pops are at times associated with an impedance rise. This occurs since the accumulation of gas (steam), may act as an electrical insulator along the electrode surface. If gas is not trapped by intimate myocardial contact, but instead dissipated by brisk blood flow or open irrigation, the overall circuit impedance may not change despite interfacial boiling. The high temperatures associated with steam pops also promote coagulum formation, which may also increase impedance. Limiting RF power to achieve an impedance decrease of <18 ohms is a feasible method of reducing the likelihood of a pop when perforation risk is of concern.[31]

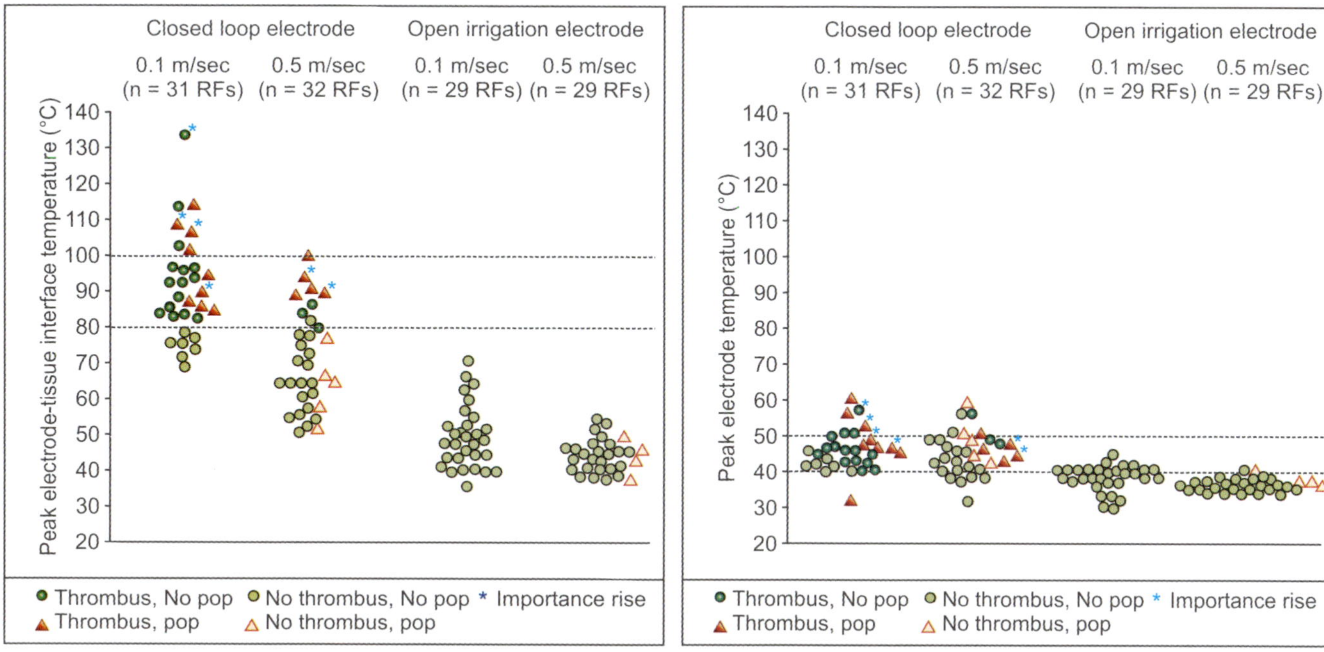

Figure 10.15: Comparison of thrombus, steam pop and impedance rise

Cardiac Perforation

Radiofrequency energy delivery can cause perforation even without steam pop. This is more likely in a thin-walled chamber such as the left atrium, especially with high power and excessive contact force. Long deflectable sheaths allow extremely effective contact with myocardium. Unless caution is exercised (e.g., by limiting power), this may increase the chances of cardiac perforation during delivery of RF energy. Some structures are particularly prone to perforation, including the thin-walled left atrial appendage and the coronary sinus. Left atrial ablation for atrial fibrillation is often performed with an irrigated catheter through a long sheath and carries a particularly high risk of cardiac perforation, effusion, and tamponade—over 1% in a worldwide survey and 3% from a more contemporary data.[32,33] Titrating energy delivery down to the minimal level required to achieve the procedural endpoint reduces the risk of local complications, including coagulum, steam pops, and perforation.

Collateral Damage

Collateral injury to extracardiac structures occurs when lesion depth exceeds myocardial wall thickness. Depending on the ablation target, damage to lung tissue, coronary arteries, phrenic nerves, aorta, or esophagus may be incurred. Although specific strategies have been developed to protect these structures, limiting power to the minimum required to achieve the physiologic objective lowers the risk.

Temperature monitoring of extracardiac structures has been used to screen for extracardiac heat. During posterior left atrial ablation, esophageal temperature monitoring detects heating of its lumen, permitting discontinuation of RF energy delivery at that site (discussed further below). Due to the juxtaposition of the right phrenic nerve and the ostium of the right superior pulmonary vein and the right atrial free wall, phrenic nerve injury can occur during ablation near these regions. Symptoms of dyspnea range from transient and mild to permanent and disabling. To avoid this complication, many operators avoid RF application at sites with phrenic nerve capture on high-output (10–20 mA) pacing. Another option is ablation at lower power during continuous pacing just above phrenic capture threshold, interrupting energy delivery if diaphragmatic stimulation is lost. Several methods of phrenic nerve protection have been developed to allow safer ablation at a critical site in which phrenic nerve injury is otherwise likely.[5, 34]

Atrioesophageal Fistula

The formation of an atrioesophageal fistula is the most feared and dreaded complication of catheter ablation of AF.[35] Although rare (with an incidence estimated at 0.03% to 0.2%), this complication is highly fatal, accounting for 15.6% of AF ablation fatalities, second only to cardiac tamponade. The risk of esophageal injury is directly related to local tissue heating (i.e., the total ablation energy (power x time) delivered to cardiac tissue near the esophagus), which is related to catheter tip size, contact pressure, catheter orientation, and power output and duration. Factors that increase the likelihood of ablation over the esophagus or increase mechanical pressure on the esophagus increase its risk. These include extensive ablation at the LA posterior wall, persistent as opposed to paroxysmal AF, the use of nasogastric tubes, and general anesthesia. Limitation of power and duration of RF applications along the posterior atrium may limit the risk of fistula formation, although due to the infrequent nature of the complication, the value of preventative maneuvers is not clear. During ablation near the esophagus, the RF power is typically reduced to 20 to 30 W and 55°C for no more than 20 seconds. Also, direct perpendicular orientation of the ablating electrode and forward pressure against the posterior left atrial (LA) wall is avoided, particularly, if an 8-mm or irrigated tip electrode is used. It is preferable to maintain frequent movements of the ablation catheter when RF energy is applied at the posterior LA wall in the vicinity of the esophagus. Open irrigation RF ablation may be associated with less risk of esophageal injury compared with standard RF ablation using an 8-mm-tip catheter. When using open-irrigated RF ablation, lower energy outputs (15 W compared with 25 W) were found to be associated with a decreased rate of esophageal ulcerations. The mechanism is thought to be injury to the blood supply of the esophagus, creation of an inflammatory milieu, erosion of the esophageal contents through the pericardium into the oblique sinus and left atrium **(Figures 10.16 and 10.17)**. Absence of pericardial fat that acts as a thermal insulator may also be a risk factor. Recording of intraluminal esophageal temperature is likely of incomplete utility, since by the time the esophageal lumen temperature increases, the LA posterior wall and esophageal

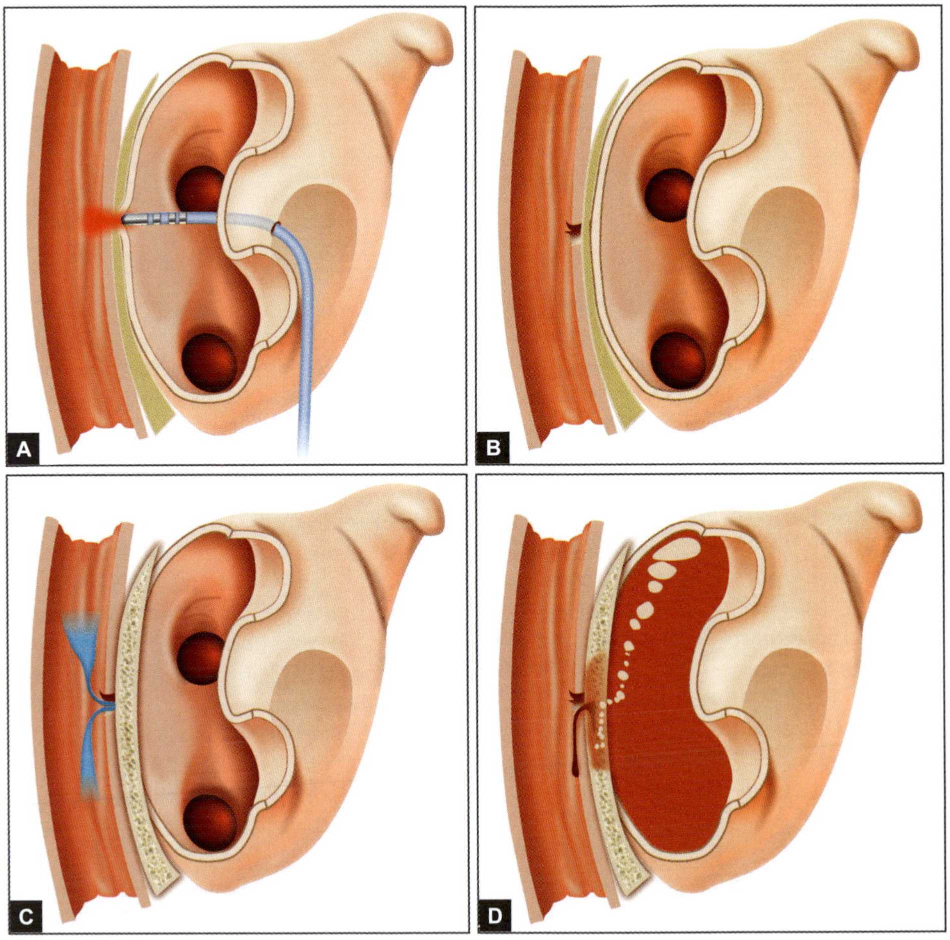

Figures 10.16A to D: Natural history of esophageal injury and late atrial-esophageal fistula formation. (A) Right lateral view of atrial esophageal junction with intervening oblique sinus. Ablation is done on the posterior wall with possible thermal injury to the anterior esophageal wall; (B) In some instances, this leads to esophageal ulcer formation and perforation; (C) Development of pneumopericardium. Digestion of the oblique sinus parietal layer results in communication between the esophagus and the pericardial space with resulting pneumopericardium and effusion; (D) Presumably over time the digestive/injury process will involve the posterior wall of the left atrium giving rise to late atrial-esophageal fistula

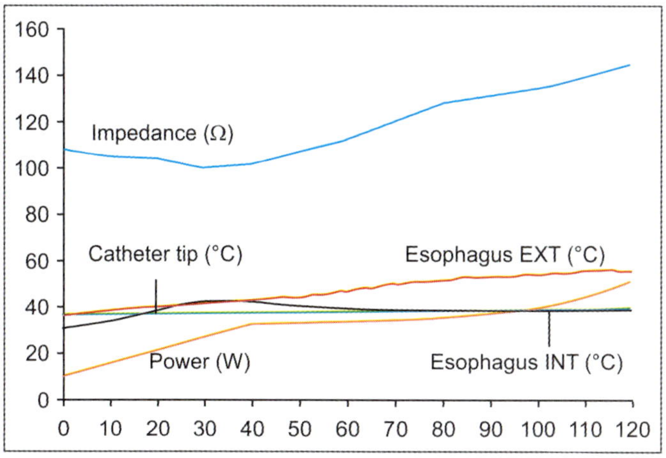

Figure 10.17: Irrigated tip catheter ablation at posterior left atrium

anterior wall have already been heated. Additionally, due to the potential distance between the temperature probe and ablative location over another region of esophagus, intraluminal probes underestimate esophageal RF ablation exposure.

ENERGY DELIVERY IN SPECIFIC ANATOMICAL LOCATIONS

Power Titration during Epicardial Ablation

Percutaneous epicardial ablation, introduced in 1996 by Sosa and co-workers to treat epicardial ventricular tachycardia in patients with Chagas disease, has been increasingly adopted to managing ventricular tachycardia in dilated cardiomyopathy, arrhythmogenic right ventricular cardiomyopathy (ARVC) and coronary artery disease especially after failed endocardial ablation.[36]

Due to the lack of blood flow in the pericardial space, convective cooling is absent. As a result, conventional non-cooled ablation catheters reach high tip temperature at relatively low power (<10 W), limiting energy delivery and resulting in small lesions. Intervening epicardial fat may also prevent effective ablation of targeted myocardial tissue. However, internally or externally irrigated catheters allow higher RF power (25 to 50 W) without temperature rise; larger lesions are created, even when ablating over epicardial fat. Most operators begin at 20 to 30 W and titrate up to a maximum of 50 W, maintaining adequate irrigation rate to keep tip temperature below 45°C. Indicators of lesion formation are similar to those used in irrigated endocardial ablation, including fall in impedance and local electrogram amplitude.

Special precautions should be taken when ablating within the pericardial space. When using externally irrigated ablation, the epicardial sheath must be periodically aspirated to prevent excess accumulation of fluid. Acute tamponade is rare in the absence of bleeding, but blood pressure tends to drift down over 5–10 minutes, with recovery following sheath aspiration. Coronary arteries are epicardial structures, and care must be taken not to deliver RF energy near them. Although in theory, the coronary arteries are somewhat protected by the cooling effect of intraluminary blood flow and the overlying fat, coronary complications of epicardial RF ablation have been described, including coronary thrombosis, vessel wall damage, and vasospasm. Smaller vessels and associated coronary disease may be at particularly high risk due to less flow and thus less heat sink effect. Real-time coronary angiography is generally necessary to delineate the course of the arteries. RF application is usually avoided within 5 to 10 mm of a coronary artery, although no absolute safe distance has been defined. There is suggestion that infusion of chilled saline into the coronary artery may help protect the endothelium, but this strategy is not yet widely used, and may promote spasm. The phrenic nerves are adherent to the pericardium, so that pacing maneuvers to confirm absence of diaphragmatic activation are performed at 10–20 mA. If an epicardial target is adjacent to the phrenic nerve, balloon inflation in the pericardium has been reported to displace the nerve away from the ablative electrode permitting safe ablation.

Power Titration during Ablation within the Coronary Sinus

Subepicardial accessory pathways, premature ventricular complexes, atypical atrial flutter, and atrial fibrillation have been successfully treated with RF ablation within the coronary sinus. One common reason for ablation in the coronary sinus is completing a mitral isthmus line as part of left atrial ablation for persistent atrial fibrillation. However, despite using relatively high power, successful creation of a mitral isthmus line remains technically challenging, even after combined endocardial and coronary sinus ablation. Some investigators hypothesize that this is due to coronary venous blood flow acting as a heat sink, carrying RF energy away and preventing adequate lesion formation.[37]

In an animal study, D'Avila and co-workers tested a device that occluded the coronary sinus ostium to prevent blood flow during ablation. They were able to achieve transmural lesions from endocardial ablation only when flow was prevented by balloon occlusion.[38] Care must be taken during ablation in the coronary sinus, because the left circumflex coronary artery also runs within the AV groove. Occlusion of the circumflex artery/posterior descending artery has been described during ablation. Ablation within CS is often performed with an irrigated ablation catheter with flow rate, 17 to 30 mL/minute; maximal temperature, 45°C to 50°C; and power, 20 to 30 W, as there may be low flow in the coronary sinus, particularly with an ablation catheter within it. Increasing the flow rate to 60 mL may mitigate excessive temperature elevation.

Table 10.2: Types of radiofrequency ablation catheters, their features and typical uses

	Standard catheter	*Irrigated catheter*	*Large-tip catheter*
Electrode length	4–5 mm	3.5–4 mm	6–10 mm
Power delivery	Up to 50 W	Up to 50 W	Up to 150 W
Power titration	Temperature control	Power control monitoring temperature and impedance	Usually temperature control monitoring impedance ± microbubble formation
Lesion size limited by	Electrode temperature and impedance rise	Power setting	Electrode temperature, current shunting, impedance rise
Coagulum risk	Present	Low (especially open irrigation)	Present (possibly highest)
Steam pop risk	Low	Present	Present
Typical uses	Atrioventricular node reentry Accessory pathways Atrial tachycardias Ventricular tachycardia with normal heart Atrioventricular junctional ablation	Ventricular tachycardias with structural heart disease Atrial flutter Atrial fibrillation Coronary sinus ablation Epicardial ablation	Atrial flutter Possibly atrial fibrillation Possibly epicardial

CONCLUSION

The introduction of radiofrequency catheter ablation revolutionized the therapy of arrhythmias. The technology has a high success rate, low complication rate and can be performed in a lightly sedated patient.

Current methods of RF energy titration allow safe and effective catheter ablation for the treatment of cardiac arrhythmias. A thorough understanding and appreciation of the biophysics and pathophysiology of RF energy heating of myocardium during catheter ablation will help the operator to make the proper adjustments to optimize ablation safety and success. "One size fits all" for ablation sources, catheter and energy outputs is not prudent. It is crucial to have the right catheter for the right patient for the right substrate **(Table 10.2)**. Contact force sensing has been an important advance in guiding lesion formation. In the future, technologies and techniques for titrating RF power and tissue response will continue to evolve, further improving the results of catheter ablation procedures. Finally a full understanding of the biophysics of catheter ablation, and the anatomy and physiology of the arrhythmogenic substrate will allow the operator to select the optimal ablation approach.

REFERENCES

1. Burchell HB, Frye RL, Anderson MW, McGoon DC. Atrioventricular and ventriculoatrial excitation in Wolff-parkinson-white syndrome (type b). Temporary ablation at surgery. Circulation. 1967;36:663-72.
2. Wittkampf FH, Nakagawa H. RF catheter ablation: Lessons on lesions. Pacing Clin Electrophysiol. 2006;29:1285-97.
3. Wittkampf FH, Nakagawa H, Yamanashi WS, Imai S, Jackman WM. Thermal latency in radiofrequency ablation. Circulation. 1996;93:1083-6.
4. Langberg JJ, Harvey M, Calkins H, el-Atassi R, Kalbfleisch SJ, Morady F. Titration of power output during radiofrequency catheter ablation of atrioventricular nodal reentrant tachycardia. Pacing Clin Electrophysiol. 1993;16:465-70.
5. Dib C, Kapa S, Powell BD, Packer DL, Asirvatham SJ. Successful use of "cryo-mapping" to avoid phrenic nerve damage during ostial superior vena caval ablation despite nerve proximity. J Interv Card Electrophysiol. 2008;22:23-30.
6. Haines DE, Verow AF. Observations on electrode-tissue interface temperature and effect on electrical impedance during radiofrequency ablation of ventricular myocardium. Circulation. 1990;82:1034-8.
7. Huang SK, Bharati S, Lev M, Marcus FI. Electrophysiologic and histologic observations of chronic atrioventricular block induced by closed-chest catheter desiccation with radiofrequency energy. Pacing Clin Electrophysiol. 1987;10:805-16.
8. Avitall B, Urbonas A, Urboniene D, Millard S, Helms R. Time course of left atrial mechanical recovery after linear lesions: Normal sinus rhythm versus a chronic atrial fibrillation dog model. J Cardiovasc Electrophysiol. 2000;11:1397-1406.
9. Nath S, Lynch C, 3rd, Whayne JG, Haines DE. Cellular electrophysiological effects of hyperthermia on isolated guinea pig papillary muscle. Implications for catheter ablation. Circulation. 1993;88:1826-31.
10. Everett THt, Nath S, Lynch C, 3rd, Beach JM, Whayne JG, Haines DE. Role of calcium in acute hyperthermic myocardial injury. J Cardiovasc Electrophysiol. 2001;12:563-9.
11. Simmers TA, De Bakker JM, Wittkampf FH, Hauer RN. Effects of heating on impulse propagation in superfused canine myocardium. J Am Coll Cardiol. 1995;25:1457-64.
12. Sapp JL, Beeckler C, Pike R, Parkash R, Gray CJ, Zeppenfeld K, Kuriachan V, Stevenson WG. Initial human feasibility of

infusion needle catheter ablation for refractory ventricular tachycardia. Circulation. 2013;128:2289-95.

13. Reddy VY, Shah D, Kautzner J, Schmidt B, Saoudi N, Herrera C, Jais P, Hindricks G, Peichl P, Yulzari A, Lambert H, Neuzil P, Natale A, Kuck KH. The relationship between contact force and clinical outcome during radiofrequency catheter ablation of atrial fibrillation in the toccata study. Heart Rhythm. 2012;9:1789-95.
14. Natale A, Reddy VY, Monir G, Wilber DJ, Lindsay BD, McElderry HT, Kantipudi C, Mansour MC, Melby DP, Packer DL, Nakagawa H, Zhang B, Stagg RB, Boo LM, Marchlinski FE. Paroxysmal af catheter ablation with a contact force sensing catheter: Results of the prospective, multicenter smart-af trial. J Am Coll Cardiol. 2014;64:647-56.
15. Hoffmayer KS, Gerstenfeld EP. Contact force-sensing catheters. Curr Opin Cardiol. 2015;30:74-80.
16. Weiss C, Antz M, Eick O, Eshagzaiy K, Meinertz T, Willems S. Radiofrequency catheter ablation using cooled electrodes: Impact of irrigation flow rate and catheter contact pressure on lesion dimensions. Pacing Clin Electrophysiol. 2002;25: 463-9.
17. Yokoyama K, Nakagawa H, Wittkampf FH, Pitha JV, Lazzara R, Jackman WM. Comparison of electrode cooling between internal and open irrigation in radiofrequency ablation lesion depth and incidence of thrombus and steam pop. Circulation. 2006;113:11-9.
18. Demazumder D, Mirotznik MS, Schwartzman D. Biophysics of radiofrequency ablation using an irrigated electrode. J Interv Card Electrophysiol. 2001;5:377-89.
19. Guerra JM, Jorge E, Raga S, Galvez-Monton C, Alonso-Martin C, Rodriguez-Font E, Cinca J, Vinolas X. Effects of open-irrigated radiofrequency ablation catheter design on lesion formation and complications: In vitro comparison of 6 different devices. J Cardiovasc Electrophysiol. 2013;24:1157-62.
20. Otomo K, Yamanashi WS, Tondo C, Antz M, Bussey J, Pitha JV, Arruda M, Nakagawa H, Wittkampf FH, Lazzara R, Jackman WM. Why a large tip electrode makes a deeper radiofrequency lesion: Effects of increase in electrode cooling and electrode-tissue interface area. J Cardiovasc Electrophysiol. 1998;9:47-54.
21. Wood MA, Goldberg SM, Parvez B, Pathak V, Holland K, Ellenbogen AL, Han FT, Alexander D, Lau M, Reshko L, Goel A. Effect of electrode orientation on lesion sizes produced by irrigated radiofrequency ablation catheters. J Cardiovasc Electrophysiol. 2009;20:1262-8.
22. Lewalter T, Bitzen A, Wurtz S, Blum R, Schlodder K, Yang A, Lickfett L, Schwab JO, Schrickel JW, Tiemann K, Linhart M, Zima E, Merkely B, Luderitz B. Gold-tip electrodes--a new "deep lesion" technology for catheter ablation? In vitro comparison of a gold alloy versus platinum-iridium tip electrode ablation catheter. J Cardiovasc Electrophysiol. 2005;16:770-2.
23. Nagashima K, Watanabe I, Okumura Y, Ohkubo K, Kofune M, Ohya T, Kasamaki Y, Hirayama A. Lesion formation by ventricular septal ablation with irrigated electrodes: Comparison of bipolar and sequential unipolar ablation. Circ J. 2011;75:565-70.
24. Nagashima K, Watanabe I, Okumura Y, Sonoda K, Kofune M, Mano H, Ohkubo K, Nakai T, Kunimoto S, Kasamaki Y, Hirayama A. Epicardial ablation with irrigated electrodes: effect of bipolar vs. Unipolar ablation on lesion formation. Circ J. 2012;76:322-7.
25. Harvey M, Kim YN, Sousa J, el-Atassi R, Morady F, Calkins H, Langberg JJ. Impedance monitoring during radiofrequency catheter ablation in humans. Pacing Clin Electrophysiol. 1992;15:22-7.
26. Bruce GK, Bunch TJ, Milton MA, Sarabanda A, Johnson SB, Packer DL. Discrepancies between catheter tip and tissue temperature in cooled-tip ablation: Relevance to guiding left atrial ablation. Circulation. 2005;112:954-60.
27. Wittkampf FH, Simmers TA, Hauer RN, Robles de Medina EO. Myocardial temperature response during radiofrequency catheter ablation. Pacing Clin Electrophysiol. 1995;18:307-17.
28. Schwartzman D, Michele JJ, Trankiem CT, Ren JF. Electrogram-guided radiofrequency catheter ablation of atrial tissue comparison with thermometry-guide ablation: Comparison with thermometry-guide ablation. J Interv Card Electrophysiol. 2001;5:253-66.
29. Stevenson WG, Cooper J, Sapp J. Optimizing rf output for cooled rf ablation. J Cardiovasc Electrophysiol. 2004;15:S24-7.
30. Demolin JM, Eick OJ, Munch K, Koullick E, Nakagawa H, Wittkampf FH. Soft thrombus formation in radiofrequency catheter ablation. Pacing Clin Electrophysiol. 2002;25:1219-22.
31. Seiler J, Roberts-Thomson KC, Raymond JM, Vest J, Delacretaz E, Stevenson WG. Steam pops during irrigated radiofrequency ablation: Feasibility of impedance monitoring for prevention. Heart Rhythm. 2008;5:1411-6.
32. Cappato R, Calkins H, Chen SA, Davies W, Iesaka Y, Kalman J, Kim YH, Klein G, Natale A, Packer D, Skanes A, Ambrogi F, Biganzoli E. Updated worldwide survey on the methods, efficacy, and safety of catheter ablation for human atrial fibrillation. Circ Arrhythm Electrophysiol. 2010;3:32-8.
33. Deshmukh A, Patel NJ, Pant S, Shah N, Chothani A, Mehta K, Grover P, Singh V, Vallurupalli S, Savani GT, Badheka A, Tuliani T, Dabhadkar K, Dibu G, Reddy YM, Sewani A, Kowalski M, Mitrani R, Paydak H, Viles-Gonzalez JF. In-hospital complications associated with catheter ablation of atrial fibrillation in the united states between 2000 and 2010: Analysis of 93, 801 procedures. Circulation. 2013;128:2104-12.
34. Kimura T, Takatsuki S, Fukumoto K, Nishiyama N, Sato Y, Aizawa Y, Fukuda Y, Sato T, Miyoshi S, Fukuda K. Electrical isolation of the superior vena cava using upstream phrenic pacing to avoid phrenic nerve injury. Pacing Clin Electrophysiol. 2012;35: 1053-60.
35. Nair GM, Nery PB, Redpath CJ, Lam BK, Birnie DH. Atrioesophageal fistula in the era of atrial fibrillation ablation: A review. Can J Cardiol. 2014;30:388-95.
36. Sosa E, Scanavacca M, d'Avila A, Pilleggi F. A new technique to perform epicardial mapping in the electrophysiology laboratory. J Cardiovasc Electrophysiol. 1996;7:531-6.
37. Wong KC, Qureshi N, Jones M, Rajappan K, Bashir Y, Betts TR. Mitral isthmus ablation using steerable sheath and high ablation power: A single center experience. J Cardiovasc Electrophysiol. 2012;23:1193-1200.
38. D'Avila A, Thiagalingam A, Foley L, Fox M, Ruskin JN, Reddy VY. Temporary occlusion of the great cardiac vein and coronary sinus to facilitate radiofrequency catheter ablation of the mitral isthmus. J Cardiovasc Electrophysiol. 2008;19:645-50.

EDITORS' SUMMARY

Drs Friedman and Deshmukh provide a comprehensive review as well as a ready reference for anyone who is involved with catheter ablation procedures. They primarily review the biophysics of radiofrequency ablation with an emphasis on how to maximize safety and enable efficacy.

Radiofrequency energy by itself does not produce an ablation lesion but rather serves as a means to generate heat by way of ohmic resistance heating at the electrode-tissue interface. The authors point out that for a lesion to be created, catheter tissue contact must be present, and optimized and adequate energy, as estimated by power in Watts, needs to be delivered. They provide an informative table comparing the differential characteristics of commonly used catheter electrode size and design with or without saline irrigation.

This chapter also provides an introduction on how to use currently available contact monitoring systems and to know what to expect in terms of correlation with other techniques that tell us whether we are creating a lesion, such as impedance monitoring or electrogram change. Students, carefully reviewing this chapter, will strengthen their understanding of how best to eliminate an arrhythmogenic target once established, but future studies are needed to establish a practical online method for assessing adequacy of lesion creation, tissue temperature, and a foolproof way of avoiding collateral damage, including to the coronary arteries.

CHAPTER 11

Sampath Gunda, Moustapha Atoui,
Dhanunjaya Lakkireddy

Non-Radiofrequency Sources of Ablation

LIST OF ABBREVIATIONS

AEF	Atrioesophageal Fistula	MW	Microwave Energy
AF	Atrial Fibrillation	PAF	Paroxysmal Atrial Fibrillation
AV	Atrioventricular	PNP	Phrenic Nerve Palsy
AVNRT	Atrioventricular Nodal Reentrant Tachycardia	PV	Pulmonary Vein
EP	Electrophysiology	PVI	Pulmonary Vein Isolation
HIFU	High Intensity Focused Ultrasound	RF	Radiofrequency
LASER	Light Amplification by Stimulated Emission of Radiation	RFA	Radiofrequency Ablation
LICU	Low Intensity Collimated Ultrasound	RIPV	Right Inferior Pulmonary Vein
LSPV	Left Superior Pulmonary Vein	RSPV	Right Superior Pulmonary Vein
		VGLA	Visually Guided Laser Ablation

INTRODUCTION

Radiofrequency ablation (RFA) is the highly effective, most studied and commonly used energy source for ablation of cardiac arrhythmias.[1] Typically, it is delivered through a metallic electrode mounted at the tip of the ablation catheter. While it serves a great purpose in ablating an arrhythmia focus, it has its short comings when it comes to ablating wide areas of tissue and isolating larger anatomic structures like the pulmonary veins (PVs) for atrial fibrillation (AF). Similarly, RFA in critical anatomic locations that are very close to atrioventricular (AV) node could sometimes result in collateral damage causing AV nodal blocks. Especially in the realm of AF ablation, the effectiveness of RFA is to some degree dependent on expertise of the operator as it requires fine catheter manipulation skills to navigate the complex PV antra, tedious process as it involves point by point lesions, and disruption of endothelial barrier with formation of coagulum potentially contributing to some of the compli cations associated with this modality.[1] Improved peri-procedural anticoagulation protocols, improving experience in gaining trans-septal access, open irrigated platforms, contact force enabled ablation catheters and overall improvement in the operator learning curve has dramatically leveled the playing field.

The scientific field has continued to experiment with non-RF sources of energy for ablation. Some were introduced to circumvent some of the procedural complications associated with RFA using older ablation platforms. New technologies are being invented claiming to reduce these complications and improve the efficacy of the ablation success. The purpose of this chapter is to review the current state of alternative energy sources of ablation. **Figure 11.1** depicts the electromagnetic spectrum and the different frequencies of the energy sources.[2]

CRYOENERGY

The application of cryoenergy as a source of ablation was first described by Klein and colleagues for the ablation of accessory pathways.[3] They became increasingly popular for the ablation of slow pathways and septal accessory pathways. Single-tipped cryoablation catheter failed miserably when used for cavotricuspid isthmus and pulmonary vein ablation with a significantly higher recurrence rates.[4] Since then it took many years for the first generation of cryoballoon catheters (Arctic Front™) to be available for clinical use to overcome some of the practical limitations of the point by point RFA. It subsequently went through a few iterations to settle at the current form.

Catheter Anatomy

The first generation single tipped cryoablation catheter (CryoCath technologies, Inc. Montreal Quebec, Canada) was a 10.5 Fr quadripolar steerable catheter with a 10 mm tip. The device has an outer shaft and an inner injection tube **(See Figures 11.2A and B)**. The inner tube emanates liquid nitric oxide (N_2O) or argon-based or helium-based coolant from the tip into the lumen around the outer shaft and evaporates, resulting in cooling of the tip by Joule-Thompson effect.[5] The outer shaft is maintained in constant suction to clear the N_2O which is finally drained into the reservoir outside of the body. The tip of the catheter has the temperature sensor and ring electrodes for recording and pacing purposes.

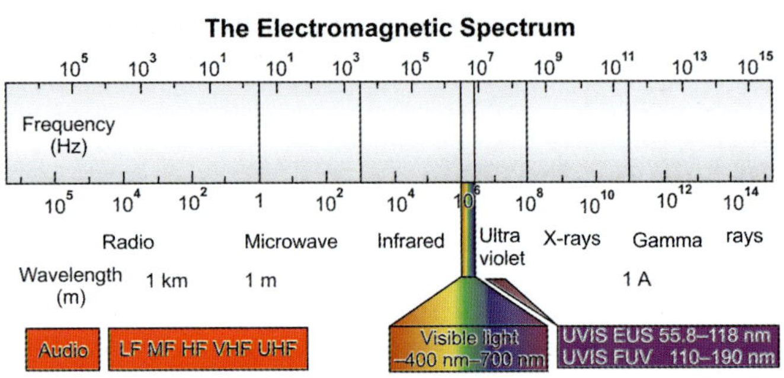

Figure 11.1: The electromagnetic spectrum

Abbreviations: EUV, extreme ultraviolet; FUV, far ultraviolet; HF, high frequency; LF, low frequency; MF, mid frequency; UHF, ultrahigh frequency; UVIS, ultraviolet imaging spectrum; VHF, very high frequency) (Reproduced from reference 2)

The second generation of cryoballoon (Arctic Front advance™®, Medtronic) that was released into the market in 2012 has 8 refrigerant ports on the injection coil instead of 4 in the earlier version and also the injection coil itself has been moved 4.5 mm distally to allow uniform freezing zone across the entire half of the distal balloon.

The control console has two modes of temperature settings, cryomapping and cryoablation. In the cryomapping mode, the temperature tip is maintained at or above –30°C and the cooling is halted for 80 seconds. In the cryoablation mode, the temperature is less than or equal to –68°C and the cooling is halted for up to 4 min.[4]

Mechanism of Tissue Injury

Freezing of the cells to –30°C causes reversible cell damage with near to complete recovery of function upon normalization of the temperature. This forms the basis for cryomapping mode. Freezing of the cells to –80°C causes irreversible cell damage with loss of Z and I lines, disruption of mitochondria, microfilaments with increased permeability of cytoskeletal membranes. This concept is the basis for the cryoablation mode. Cryoablation makes the surrounding tissue frozen, creating ice crystals within the cell that disrupts the cell membranes and interrupts cellular metabolism, electrical activity and vascular flow leading to cellular death.[6] There is minimal disruption of the endothelium and consequently less thrombus formation with preservation of myocardial architecture followed by minimal replacement with fibrous tissue.[7, 8]

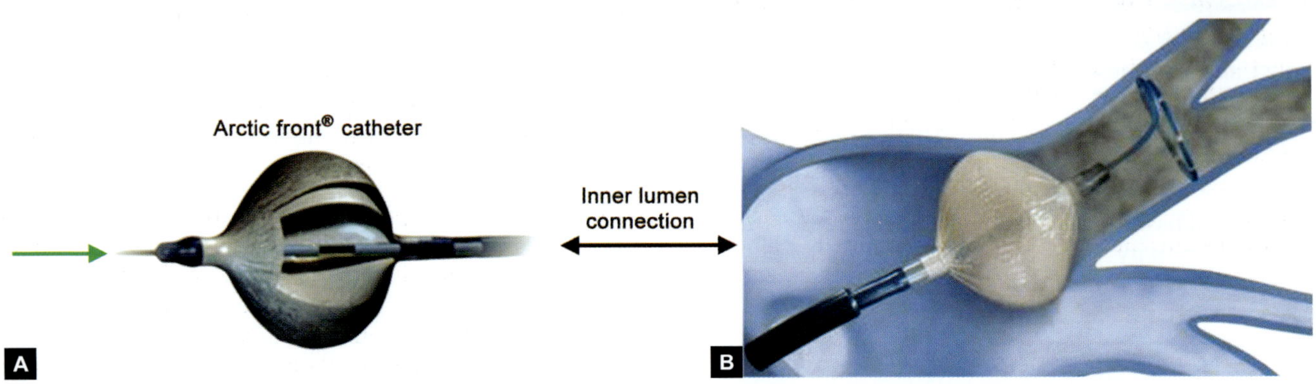

Figures 11.2A and B: (A) Cryoballoon catheter with inner and outer tube; (B) Cryoballoon catheter placed over the ostium of the pulmonary vein with the contrast being injected to look for the leak (Reproduced from Medtronic)

Histologically, the cryothermal lesions consist of central uniform coagulation necrosis surrounded by a peripheral zone, which consists of mixture of cells with irreversible and reversible damage.

Cryoballoon Ablation Procedure

After placement of standard transvenous catheters, a double trans-septal puncture is performed using the modified Brockenbrough technique. Su et al. recommend a low anterior transseptal puncture near or on the limbus of the septum for accessing right inferior pulmonary vein (RIPV).[9] Heparin is continuously administered to maintain thromboplastin time between 250–350 msec. A lasso catheter (Biosense-Webster, Inc., Diamond Bar, CA, USA) is inserted in the RIPV via the trans-septal puncture to identify the PV potentials. The cryoballoon is inserted using the sheath through the other trans-septal puncture guided by the mapping catheter to avoid the trauma. When parking the cryoballoon in the PV antrum, proper precautions are taken to avoid deep seating into the branch or ostium of PVs. Pulmonary vein isolation (PVI) is best achieved through the application of forward pressure to have optimal balloon to tissue contact. The leak can be detected by injecting the contrast before application of cryoenergy. If no leak is detected, apply the cryoenergy once or twice for 3–4 minutes. Monitoring of the right phrenic nerve with pacing and premature termination of cryoapplication in case of loss of capture is a standard protocol. Luminal esophageal monitoring can also be used to prevent unnecessary thawing of the tissue. However, this strategy was proven to be ineffective in preventing the esophageal lesions as the injury is mainly in the outer layers. The cryoballoon is then sequentially placed in the other three pulmonary veins and cryoenergy applied to achieve complete PVI.

Factors Affecting the Cryoablation and Other Ablation Systems

Multiple factors affect creation of optimal lesion.

- *Good contact*: Good contact is very important for creation of optimal lesion.
- *Time and number of applications*: A 3–4 min of application of cryoenergy will yield optimal results but repeat application may be necessary. Multiple applications may be necessary to accomplish the end points.
- *Blood flow*: Continuous blood flow around the balloon and also at the lesion dissipates the cryoenergy and decreases the chance of achieving an optimal lesion.

Advantages of Cryoablation

The advantages of using cryoenergy over RFA include:

- Possibly low risk for thrombus formation compared to RFA as the degree of endothelial disruption, and platelet activation is low which is mainly beneficial near the coronary blood vessels or in the veins.[7]
- Possibly low risk of pulmonary vein stenosis.
- Preservation of the architecture of the left atrium and also the pulmonary veins.
- As the effects of cryoenergy application can be reversed, Cryomapping technology allows focal tachycardia and reentrant circuit mapping by interrupting their activation and confirming the source of arrhythmia mainly in the region near the AV node or His bundle. This can potentially reduce the risk of ablation induced AV block or other collateral damage.
- No need for 3D-mapping especially for anatomic ablations like PV antral isolation.

Disadvantages of Cryoablation

- High incidence of PNP.
- Difficulty in manipulating the cryoballoon mainly near the right inferior pulmonary veins.
- Application of cryoenergy over a period of minutes compared to seconds with RFA.
- More expensive. The cryoballoon system is a lot more expensive than the RF system.
- Cannot be used for focal or linear ablation if patients were to develop focal or reentrant atrial arrhythmias after PV isolation using cryoballoon. This necessitates the use of a single-tipped catheter.

Efficacy and Outcomes of Cryoablation

Despite being relatively recent technology, cryoablation has gained popularity and is being used most commonly for ablation near the normal conduction pathways, difficult cases of atrioventricular nodal reentrant tachycardia (AVNRT) and for pulmonary vein isolation.

Atrioventricular nodal reentrant tachycardia (AVNRT): So far, cryoablation has been extensively used for treatment of AVNRT with good success.[10,11] In the study by Kimman et al. cryoablation was safe, as effective as RFA with fewer applications and comparable procedure times. A total of 63 patients, 30 in cryoablation group and 33 in RFA group were enrolled. The acute procedural success was 93% and 91% in cryo versus RFA group respectively. At a median follow up of 12.9 and 11.7 months, 3 patients in each group had recurrence of arrhythmia.[10]

Paroxysmal atrial fibrillation (PAF): The STOP-AF trial, the first generation cryoballoon catheters were compared with the antiarrhythmic drug therapy. A total of 163 patients were randomized to cryoablation and 82 patients were randomized to antiarrhythmic medications. It was found that the cryoablation is safe and an effective alternative to antiarrhythmic medications for patients with symptomatic paroxysmal AF who had failed at least one antiarrhythmic medication.[12] In the SUPIR study by Reddy et al., 21 patients underwent repeat EP study to look for reconnections after achieving PVI in 100% of veins during the first procedure with the newer second generation cryoballoon. PVI was present in 91% veins at a median of 3.4 months of follow up compared to 88% of veins at 2.5 months of follow up with the first generation cryoballoon in STOP AF study. Moreover, the number of cryoapplications were significantly lower with the second generation cryoballoon compared to first generation (8.7 ± 1.1 per patient in SUPIR study compared to 13 ± 2 per patient in STOP AF study, p<0.001). Reconnection of the inferior pulmonary veins was seen in most of the patients during the follow up in both the studies.[13] Mean procedure time was around 132 ± 25 min in a study by Reddy et al. A meta-analysis of 23 studies by Andrade et al., reported an acute procedural success of 98.8% in isolating PVs. Ablation with cryoballoon catheter alone without focal ablation resulted in PVI in 92.64% of targeted veins and complete PVI in 77.81% of patients. One year freedom from recurrent AF was achieved in 72.83% patients.[14] Similar findings were observed by Straube et al. in the FREEZE study.[6] Brugada et al. retrospectively compared RFA with the first generation of cryoablation in patients with paroxysmal AF. In their study, 260 patients had RFA and 136 patients had cryoablation. At a mean follow-up of 23 ± 13.4 months, there was no significant difference in the long term success rate between two energy sources (57.3% vs. 63.3%, p = 0.25). The peri-procedural complications were similar in both the groups. However, the procedure time was shorter with cryoablation.[15]

Complications and Adverse Events

Complications rates have varied widely from study to study.

Phrenic nerve palsy (PNP): PNP is more common with cryoenergy compared with RFA and almost always occurring on the right side. In the meta-analysis of 22 studies, the incidence of PNP was 4.7%, ranging from 1.6% to 15%.[15] However, most of these patients showed delayed recovery and at one year, only 0.37% of patients had persistent PNP. In STOP AF study, the incidence of PNP was 11.2%. However, persistent PNP was seen in only 3.1% of patients as the rest of the patients had complete resolution of palsy.[12] In a study by Furnkranz et al., persistent PNP occurred more commonly with second generation cryoballoons compared to first generation of cryoballoons (2.8% vs. 1.9%).[16] To mitigate the injury to phrenic nerve, its function should be actively monitored during the ablation and cryoapplication should be terminated at the first sign of PNP.[17]

Pulmonary vein stenosis: The incidence of significant pulmonary vein stenosis was 0.2% with a range from 0 to 3.1%, in some case series.[12,14,15] The incidence rises exponentially with the repeat cryoablation. It may not be much different than PVI using RF energy.

Esophageal lesions and atrioesophageal fistula (AEF): The esophageal lesions, ranging from mild erythematous lesions to abrasions to ulcerations have ranged from 3.2% to 19% in published reports. AEF has ranged from 0.1 to 0.25%. Metzner et al recommend an esophageal temperature cut-off of 10°C, while Furnkranz et al recommend a cut-off of 12°C for preventing esophageal injury during cryoballoon ablation.[18,19] The 2012 HRS expert consensus statement recommends monitoring esophageal temperature, limiting duration of energy application with reduced contact force, use of barium swallow to delineate the pathology in case of suspected injury and use of proton pump inhibitors post-procedurally.[20]

Other complications: Incidence of other vascular complications, cardiac tamponade and thromboembolic complications is usually around 1.8%, 1.5% and 0.6% respectively.[14] Stroke was also reported to occur during the cryoablation procedure with incidence being 2.2% in the study by Packer et al.[12] This probably related to clot formation on the sheaths in the left atrium.

Post Ablation Care

Standard practices including groin checks, monitoring for bleeding and hematomas, proper sheath care and anti-coagulation management should be in place.

Bottomline

Even though cryoballoon ablation for AF is perceived to be safer, the overall complication profile is not much different from RFA. The overall efficacy may be slightly lower or equivalent to RFA. More studies are needed to prove the efficacy and safety of cryoablation to become the standard of care for management of patients with PAF. The data on the use of cryoballoon for non-paroxysmal AF and VT is still not existent.

HIGH INTENSITY FOCUSED ULTRASOUND

Ultrasound waves are sound waves with a frequency of more than 20,000 Hz **(Figure 11.1)**. Using the ultrasound lens, these sound waves can be focused deep in the tissues. Sound waves at a frequency of 500 kHz to 20MHz were produced by passing the electricity through the piezoelectric crystals. The high intensity focused ultrasound (HIFU) (ProRhythm, Inc. Ronkonkoma, NY, USA) ablation system was first studied in humans by Nakagawa et al. in 2007 after some encouraging results from animal studies.[21] This particular energy source was used in balloon platform only.

Catheter Anatomy

The HIFU balloon catheter has two attached noncompliant balloons forming a 24, 27 and 32 mm ring to make a circumferential transmural left atrial lesion **(See Figure 11.3)**. The distal balloon is filled with water-contrast media which incorporates the 8–9 MHz ultrasound transducer crystal. The proximal balloon when filled with carbon dioxide covers the proximal portion of the distal balloon thus causing the 2–6 mm forward reflection of the emitted ultrasound rays from the transducer in 360°. The water contrast mixture in the distal balloon is used to cool and maintain the balloon surface below the required temperature, usually ≤42°C and the proximal balloon is maintained at 8 PSI pressure to maintain the parabolic shape. The catheter central lumen has a guidewire which is used to position over the entrance of the pulmonary veins and also for angiography of pulmonary veins. The catheter also has separate lumens to access the distal and proximal balloons.

The epicardial HIFU system, Epicor® (St. Jude Medical, Maple Grove, MN) was developed to perform the ablations during the off-pump surgeries as a part of mitral valve replacement or coronary artery bypass grafting surgery. The advantage of Epicor® is isolation of pulmonary veins from epicardial surface without need for atriotomy.

Mechanism of Tissue Injury

Several mechanisms have been postulated of which thermal effect is believed to be the main mode of tissue injury. The propagation of these high frequency ultrasound waves through the myocardial tissue raises the temperature of the tissue resulting in tissue injury. Unlike the diagnostic ultrasound which operates at a higher frequency, therapeutic ultrasound operates at a lower frequency such as (0.5 to 5 MHz) and uses higher acoustic energy to cause irreversible tissue damage. However, other mechanisms of tissue injury has been proposed by Laughner et al. which include, acoustic radiation force, acoustic cavitation or gas body activity and discontinuous linear lesions.[22] Like "steam pops" produced with RFA, acoustic cavitation occurs because of rapid creation and collapse of gas bubbles within the tissue from high acoustic pressures and high temperature induced by HIFU.

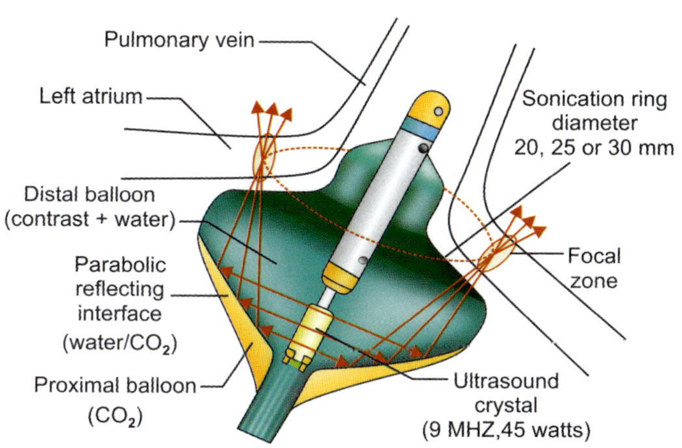

Figure 11.3: Schematic representation of high intensity focused ultrasound (HIFU) catheter ablation system (Reproduced from reference 23)

Ablation Procedure

After placement of standard transvenous catheters, a double trans-septal puncture is performed using the modified Brockenbrough technique. Heparin is continuously administered to maintain aPTT of between 250 and 350 msec. A lasso catheter (Biosense-Webster, Inc., Diamond Bar, CA, USA) is inserted via the trans-septal puncture to identify the PV potentials. The other transseptal sheath is exchanged for the HIFU balloon catheter over a guidewire. The distal balloon is inflated with water-contrast media and positioned at the ostium of the PV so that the sonicating ring abuts the antrum. However, firm contact is not needed for creation of a definitive lesion. Contrast in injected to confirm the position of the sonicating ring. Then the proximal balloon is inflated following which the ultrasound energy is applied for 40 seconds, if 24 mm balloon is used and 40–90 seconds, if bigger balloon sizes are used. One or two ultrasound applications are enough to create a durable lesion. This process is repeated for all the PVs and until no more PV potentials are recorded. Standard monitoring for esophageal temperature and phrenic nerve capture should be in place to prevent procedural complications.

Advantages

- Contact is not required for creation of lesions.
- Point by point ablation is not necessary.
- The lesion formation is not affected by the blood flow.
- No risk of thrombus formation as there is no endothelial disruption and the intervening tissue is not being heated.
- No need for 3D mapping.

Disadvantages

- Limited navigational properties of the catheter.
- Titration of energy delivery is not possible, if the power modulation is not available. So the ablation power cannot be regulated leading to potential risk of significant complications.

Efficacy and Outcomes of HIFU

In the first clinical study by Nakagawa et al. involving 27 patients, 19 with PAF and 8 with persistent AF, isolation of pulmonary veins was successful in 74% of targeted veins.

The success rate was higher on the right sided pulmonary veins compared to left side due to the left atrial ridge obstructing manipulation of HIFU catheter. At 12 months, 59% of patients were free from AF.[23] In an another follow up study by Neven et al. at a median follow up of 738 days, 22 (79%) out of 28 patients were free from AF.[24] In a study by Metzner et al., the acute success rate in isolating PVs with second generation of HIFU balloons was 87%. During a median follow-up 1400 days, 56% of patients remained free from AF.[25] With the use of third generation HIFU balloon catheters, the acute success rate in isolating PVs was 81% in a study by Schmidt et al. During a median follow up 342 days, 71% patients remained in sinus rhythm. The mean time to PVI was 166 ± 77 min in the study by Schmidt et al.[26]

The initial studies using the Epicor® surgical HIFU system revealed that the lesion formation was not complete or perhaps complete PVI was not possible. In a study by Garcia et al. the success rate of PVI during the cardiac surgery was 38%. However at six months, 64% of paroxysmal AF patients were free from AF.[27]

Complications

Esophageal lesions are the most common complication from HIFU.

Esophageal lesions and atrioesophageal fistula (AEF): Given deep penetration of ultrasound waves without raising the temperature of intervening tissue, they have a high propensity to cause esophageal ulcerations. In the study by Neven et al. the incidence of esophageal thermal lesions was 8% and one patient developed AEF.[24,28] They also illustrated that use of esophageal temperature measurement did not prevent development of these lesions as the injury was in the outer esophageal layers. Metzner et al. did not notice any AEF in their study.[25]

PNP: PNP is less common with HIFU than the RFA and Cryoablation and the incidence ranged from 14% to 21% in the previous studies. Metzner et al. reported 2 out of 32 patients with persistent PNP.[24,25,28]

Pulmonary vein stenosis: No significant pulmonary vein stenosis was noticed in most of the studies.

Bottomline

Given high occurrences of complications, especially the esophageal lesions, the clinical use of HIFU for cardiac arrhythmia ablations has been put on hold. Currently, this ablation energy is not under use clinically on any platform.

VISUALLY GUIDED LASER ABLATION (VGLA)

Light Amplification by Stimulated Emission of Radiation (LASER) is a monochromatic phase coherent beam with a specific wavelength. The Laser beam can be directed and focused on to a tissue at a distance of several millimeters. Laser energy decays as it passes through the medium due to absorption of part of the energy. Different types of Laser energy sources are in place with the neodymium : yttrium-aluminium-garnet (Nd:YAG) laser source having the most efficient transmission. This energy source has been studied on a balloon platform.

Catheter Anatomy

The visually guided laser ablation system (CardioFocus Inc, Marlborough, Massachusetts) has two components, the delivery sheath and the ablation system within the balloon **(Figures 11.4 and 11.5)**. The ablation system consists of optical fiber shaft which consists of two parts, the endoscope and the arc generator which are fixed within the balloon. The endoscope allows for visualization of 110°–150° field. The arc generator at the end of optical fiber can deliver an arc of varying sizes of laser energy to the tissue for creation of the lesions. The arc features different light source which enables the operator to visualize where the energy source is being focused. Red light is reflected by tissue and blood, the green light by tissue only. The arc can be advanced and retracted within the shaft of the optical fiber. The compliant balloon size comes in 20, 25 and 30 mm to match with the size of pulmonary vein ostium. An internal cooling fluid, deuterium oxide is being circulated from console to the balloon to prevent excessive heating of the tissue in contact.[29]

Mechanism of Tissue Injury

The lesion formation is mainly due to thermal injury. A high intensity beam of Laser energy is focused on to the medium or tissue to excite the electrons. These excited electrons release light energy of specific wavelength upon relaxation. Absorption of this Laser energy results in heating of the tissue resulting in thermal injury and tissue necrosis.

Ablation Procedure

After placement of standard transvenous catheters, a double transseptal puncture is performed using the modified Brockenbrough technique. Heparin is continuously administered to maintain a PTT of between 250–350 ms. A lasso catheter (Biosense-Webster, Inc., Diamond Bar, CA, USA) is inserted via the trans-septal puncture to identify the PV potentials. Through the other trans-septal puncture the balloon catheter is inserted and inflated to position at the PV ostium. Upon visualization of the left atrium-PV junction, energy delivery is performed with different power modulations available for 60 seconds to create an arc of ablation. Multiple applications need to be performed to create circumferential lesions around the PVs by connecting each arc.

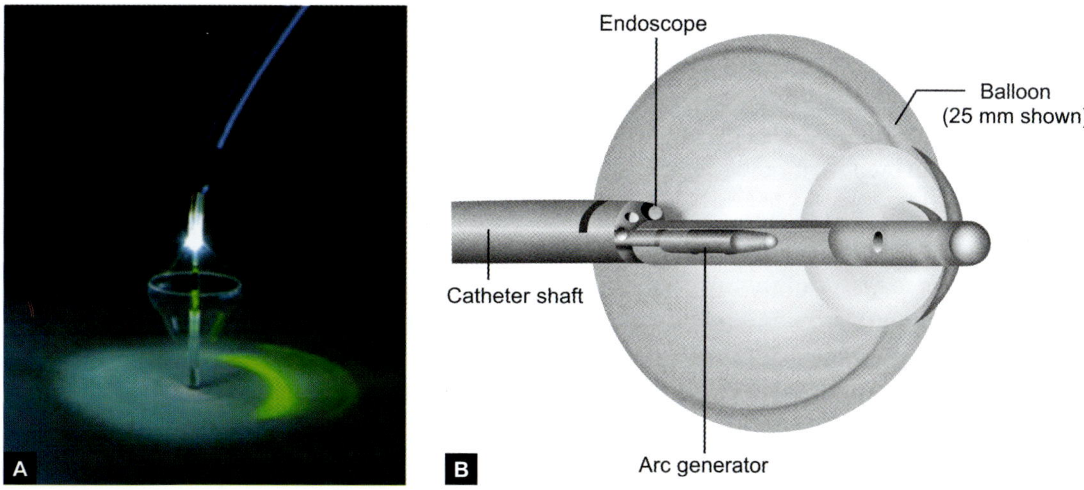

Figures 11.4A and B: Visually guided laser ablation catheter showing the projected arc in green (A) and inner structures at the end of the ablation catheter with balloon (B) (Reproduced from reference 29)

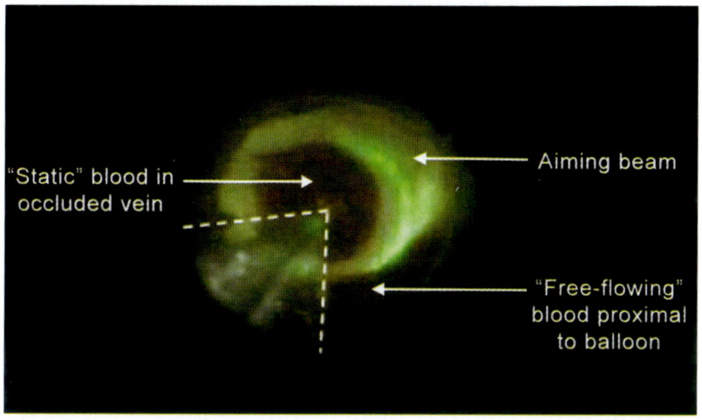

Figure 11.5: The area of the balloon in contact with the tissue blanches to white while not in contact with the tissue turns red which visually guides the ablation process (Reproduced from reference 29)

Advantages

- Endoscopic visualization of the left atrium-PV junction using the endoscope.
- Visualization of focus point of laser energy with the use of different light sources.
- Application for a short term creates enough lesions. The lesions could be overlapped to minimize the gaps and accomplish a more complete PV isolation. The lesions set has a memory that can be visualized very easily.
- Easy to control catheters.
- No need for contact with the tissue for creation of lesions.

Disadvantages

- Theoretically, a high risk of thrombus formation due to heating of the tissue. However, this has not been found to be an issue in the clinical trials
- Absorption of the laser energy and consequently lesion formation depends on the homogeneity of the tissue properties.
- Data in non-paroxysmal AF ablation is scanty.
- Additional lesion sets involving focal and reentrant arrhythmias cannot be created with this system.

Efficacy and Outcomes

In a small prospective feasibility study by Reddy et al. 30 patients with PAF who had failed at least one class I or class III antiarrhythmic medication were enrolled. Acute PVI was achieved in 86–100% depending upon the vein being isolated. At a mean follow-up of 12 months, 67% of patients were free from AF.[29] In an another study by Dukkipati et al. enrolling 200 patients with PAF and who failed at least one antiarrhythmic medication, acute PVI was achieved in 98% of patients with the use of second generation of VGLA balloons and 71.2% patients were free from AF at 12 months of follow up. The mean laser and ablation times has ranged from 64 ± 15 min and 113 ± 38 min respectively.[30,31] In a study by Sediva et al. in 194 patients with 12 patients being persistent AF, 99.2% of veins of the 698 vein targets were acutely isolated using the laser balloon system.[32] At the end of 12 and 48 months, 82.3% and 75% patients respectively were free from AF. Bordignon et al. enrolled 140 patients and compared the cryoballoon versus laser balloon technology in their prospective study. PVI was successful in 99.6% in cryoballoon versus 98.9% of patients in laser balloon group.[33] Cryoballoon group had significantly longer mean procedural time and higher incidence of PNP. However, the incidence of vascular complications were higher in the laser balloon group. At a median follow up of 393 days, 63% of patients in the cryoballoon group and 73% of patients in the laser balloon group were free from AF after a single procedure.

This success rate increased to 82% and 80% after the multiple procedures respectively. In a study by Gal et al. 58% of the patients were free from AF at a median follow up of 17.3 months.[34] The United States pivotal study, HeartLight® results are underway and will help us to better understand the efficacy and complication rates.

Complications

The major complications were PNP and vascular injuries as described below.

Phrenic nerve palsy: In the study by Reddy et al. the incidence of temporary PNP was around 3% and the similar rates were observed by Sediva et al.[32]

Vascular injuries: Vascular injuries accounted for around 3% of the complications.

Pulmonary vein stenosis: There were no occurrences of significant pulmonary vein stenosis in these studies.

Bottomline

Visually guided laser ablation (VGLA) technology offers an innovative approach for ablation of cardiac arrhythmia. However, the first randomized controlled pivotal study has just completed and will be anticipating the results any time now. This seems to be a solid technology for PAF ablation involving just PV isolation alone.

MICROWAVE ENERGY

Microwave energy (MW) has an electromagnetic spectrum with frequencies ranging from 900 to 2450 MHz and uses dielectric properties to heat the tissue. MW energy offers a potential for ablation of deeper tissues with larger lesion formation. It has been increasingly utilized intraoperatively during the surgical maze procedure.

Catheter Anatomy

The microwave ablation system (AFx Inc., Fremont, CA) consists of a surgical ablation probe (FLEX 2) and a microwave generator, connected by coaxial cable. The probe has a 25 mm long monopole antenna which is the actual ablation element. The microwave generator delivers a continuous energy flow (2.45GHz) with variable power output ranging from 35W to 75W. The ablation element, the antenna increases the tissue temperature up to 40°C to cause an irreversible tissue injury without raising the surface temperature.

Mechanism of Tissue Injury

Microwave propagates through the tissue, creating an electromagnetic field and provokes the vibration and rotation of the dipoles of water molecules thus, generating heat by friction. The propagation of the MW is not hindered by the coagulum formation at the tip of the antenna as seen with RFA. Moreover MW is capable of heating the deeper tissue without raising the surface temperature.[35] Also, for the same amount of rise of surface temperature, MW cause larger and deeper lesions than RFA.[36] The size and depth of the lesion formation depends on the frequency of MW that is generated, antenna design and the dielectric properties of the tissue. Thus, MW energy produces thermal cell necrosis with transmural damage, and foci of coagulation necrosis in the central part of the lesion.

Advantages

- Creation of larger, deeper and transmural lesions.
- Low risk for surface heating and coagulum formation.
- Tissue contact is not necessary for the creation of lesions.

Disadvantages

- Antenna design plays a critical role in creation of transmural lesion.
- No consistency and reliability in creation of fixed size lesions.

Efficacy and Literature Review

In a preclinical study by Wang et al. MW was safe and efficacious in creating durable and fixed size lesions in the ventricles of the mongrel dogs.[37] Most of the experience and literature on MW was with creating the lesion set as a part of Cox-maze procedure during the surgery for mitral valve repair. Wisser et al. compared MW ablation with RFA in patients undergoing Cox-maze procedure as a part of the mitral valve surgery. A total of 23 patients with permanent AF were enrolled in each group. Freedom from AF was seen in 80% and 81.2% of patients undergoing MW ablation and RFA respectively at a median follow up of 12 months. The procedure time was significantly less in patients with RFA compared to MW due to bulky catheters and technical difficulty with the manipulation of MW catheters.[38] Schuetz et al. studied 43 patients with long-standing AF undergoing open-heart surgery in a prospective randomized study that compared 24 patients in the treatment group that underwent MW ablation for creation of Cox-maze lesion set with 19 patients in the control group. Immediately after surgery, 91.7% of patients in the treatment group converted to sinus rhythm compared to only 31.5% in the control group. Even at a median follow up of 12 months, 80% of patients in the MW ablation group were free from AF compared to only 33.3% in the control group.[39] In another analysis, at a median follow up of 5.37 ± 0.91 years, 39.3% of patients were in sinus rhythm in microwave ablation group. However, 13 patients were lost to follow up and authors concluded that the left atrial endocardial MW ablation for long-standing AF after

Cox-maze lesion during valve surgery is not a reliable method of achieving long-term conversion to sinus rhythm.[40] Lin et al. conducted a prospective trial comparing MW versus RFA in patients undergoing valve surgery and enrolled 94 patients in MW ablation group and 93 patients in RFA group. At a median follow up of 24 months, freedom from AF was seen in 71.2% and 88.7% in MW ablation group and RFA respectively. The authors have concluded that RFA is superior to MW ablation in patients with permanent AF undergoing valve surgery.[41]

Complications

Very limited data exists regarding the complications associated with the MW ablation system.

Stroke and bleeding: Compared to other energy sources, microwave energy is associated with increased incidence of stroke and bleeding, mainly postoperative. In a study by Schuetz et al. the incidence of stroke was 6% in postoperative period.[39]

Bottomline

MW for catheter ablation has been slow to develop because of the difficulty in designing the successful catheters and inconsistency in formation of size and depth of the lesions.

THERMAL BALLOON CATHETER SYSTEM

The first thermal balloon system was developed by Toray-Satake industries, Tokyo, Japan. In this balloon catheter system, the RF energy is not used directly but is used to produce thermal energy which in turn is used as an energy source for ablation.

Catheter Anatomy

The thermal balloon system consists of an RF catheter, an RF generator which can deliver a current of up to 1.8 MHz, a deflectable sheath and the suction pump **(Figure 11.6)**.

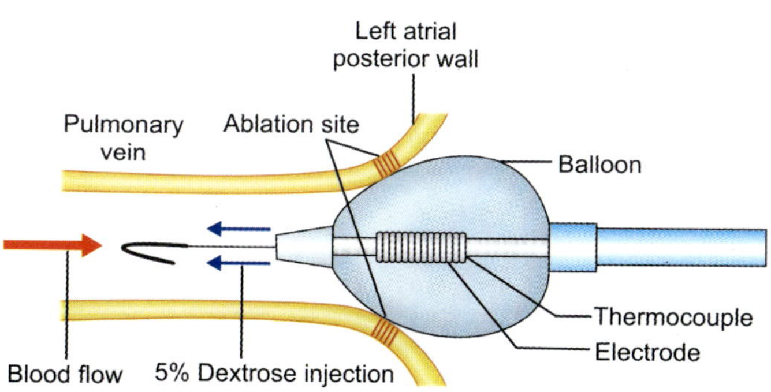

Figure 11.6: Thermal balloon catheter system (Reproduced with permission from Toray-Satake Technologies)

The RF catheter is a 12F outer flexible shaft with two lumens, a main lumen for an inner tube, a central lumen for the guidewire and balloon at the tip. Contrast is injected through the central lumen for angiography of pulmonary veins. Between the balloon and the inner tube, there are Teflon-coated leads which are connected to the RF current generator and also to a temperature sensor. The inner tube has a coil at the distal end for the delivery of RF energy. Balloon is dilated with ionized contrast medium (Iopamidol) through central lumen to different sizes to match the pulmonary vein ostial size.[42] The balloon temperature can be maintained up to 80°C and can be modulated depending on the tissue parameters. The agitation system within the balloon delivers vibratory waves to stir the balloon fluid to keep the temperature of the balloon even throughout the tube. The newer generation thermal balloons are more elastic and compliant so as to fit different shapes of the PVs.

Mechanism of Tissue Injury

The injury occurs due to capacitive heating of the tissue from the thermal energy generated within the balloon secondary to RF energy. The lesion formation and the properties are similar to the RFA.

Advantages

- Creation of definitive circumferential lesions.
- Temperature within the balloon can be controlled and maintained by delivering specific amount of RF energy.
- A compliant balloon with a membrane thickness as thin as 20 µm.

Disadvantages

High risk of esophageal mucosal ulcerations and PNP. The obvious limitations of any other balloon-based ablation systems also apply to this technology as well.

Efficacy and Literature Review

In the preclinical study by Tanaka et al. 15 of 18 PVs (83%) were successfully isolated. Also, there were no acute complication noticed.[42] In the first clinical study by Satake et al. where they enrolled 20 patients with paroxysmal AF, they were able to successfully isolate 95% of LSPV and 100% of RSPVs. The mean coil temperature rise was 68 ± 5°C. The mean fluoroscopy time was 22 ± 7 min. At a follow up of 8 months, 17 out of 20 patients were free from AF. Besides mild pericardial effusions, there were no other complications noticed. In this study, Inferior PVI was not attempted.[43] In a study by Sohara et al. using the newer generation of radiofrequency thermal balloon catheter, they were able to acutely isolate all the PVs. The mean RF time was 10 ± 2.7 min. At a mean follow up of 11 ± 4.8 months, 92 (60 paroxysmal and 32 persistent) of 100 (63 paroxysmal, 37 persistent) patients were free from AF.[44]

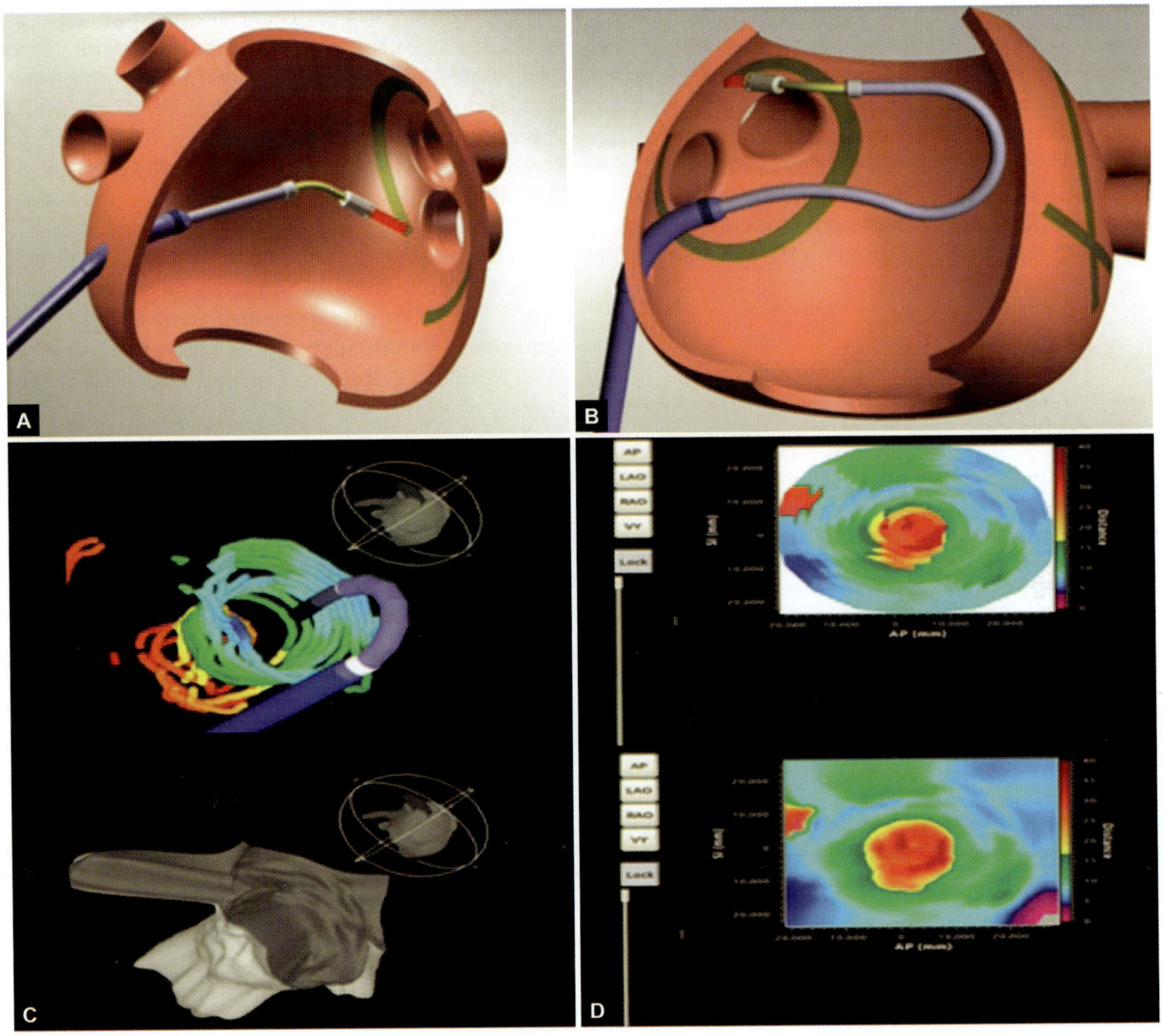

Figures 11.7A to D: Low intensity collimated ultrasound (LICU). (A and B) Using the M mode to define the anatomy of LA and predefine the linear lesion path; (C) Mapping with the robotically controlled catheter; (D) Pulmonary orifice in red and yellow on mapping (Reproduced from reference 46)

Complications

The most common complications include esophageal ulceration and PNP.

Esophageal ulcerations: In the study by Sohara et al., there were 4 (4%) patients who had esophageal ulcerations out of 100 patients who underwent the ablation procedure. However, three patients had these findings during the early experience when the esophageal cooling system was not used routinely.[44] In a follow-up study by Sohara et al. the incidence of esophageal ulcerations was found to be 10.1%. All these ulcerations were seen close to the left pulmonary veins. The esophageal damage can be reduced by introducing cooling solution in to the esophagus via a gastric tube when the esophageal temperature rises above 39°C during the hot balloon catheter ablation.[45] No patients had atrioesophageal fistula in the above studies.

PNP: In the study by Sohara et al. the incidence of PNP was found to be 1%.[44]

Bottomline

Thermal balloon catheter system has a potential to offer a reliable and efficacious catheter balloon ablation technology for management of patients with AF. However, randomized studies are needed to prove their effectiveness. This technology still has a long way to go.

LOW INTENSITY COLLIMATED ULTRASOUND

Low intensity Collimated Ultrasound (VytronUS, Inc) is a novel, noncontact, robotically controlled catheter system which emits low intensity collimated ultrasound (LICU) using the M mode for mapping and creating continuous lesions. Koruth et al. studied the feasibility of PVI using a robotically driven LICU system in a preclinical porcine model that showed promising results.[46,47] A clinical study (ClinicalTrials.gov Identifier: NCT01900678) is underway and enrolling participants to confirm the efficacy and safety of the LICU technology. However, at this stage, this technology merits additional developments before it can be released for clinical use **(Figures 11.7A to D)**.

REFERENCES

1. Calkins H, Reynolds MR, Spector P, Sondhi M, Xu Y, Martin A, Williams CJ, Sledge I. Treatment of atrial fibrillation with antiarrhythmic drugs or radiofrequency ablation: two systematic literature reviews and meta-analyses. Circ Arrhythm Electrophysiol. 2009; 2:349-61.
2. Cesario D, B.N., Shivkumar K, Cardiac Electrophysiology: From Cell to Bedside, 5th edn. 2009: Saunders. 1184.
3. Klein GJ, Guiraudon GM, Perkins DG, Jones DL, Yee R, Jarvis E. Surgical correction of the Wolff-Parkinson-White syndrome in the closed heart using cryosurgery: a simplified approach. J Am Coll Cardiol. 1984;3:405-9.
4. Friedman PL, Dubuc M, Green MS, Jackman WM, Keane DT, Marinchak RA, Nazari J, Packer DL, Skanes A, Steinberg JS, Stevenson WG, Tchou PJ, Wilber DJ, Worley SJ. Catheter cryoablation of supraventricular tachycardia: results of the multicenter prospective "frosty" trial. Heart Rhythm. 2004;1:129-38.
5. Cummings JE, Pacifico A, Drago JL, Kilicaslan F, Natale A. Alternative energy sources for the ablation of arrhythmias. Pacing Clin Electrophysiol. 2005;28:434-43.
6. Straube F, Dorwarth U, Vogt J, Kuniss M, Heinz Kuck K, Tebbenjohanns J, Garcia Alberola A, Chun KR, Souza JJ, Ouarrak T, Senges J, Brachmann J, Lewalter T, Hoffmann E. Differences of two cryoballoon generations: insights from the prospective multicentre, multinational FREEZE Cohort Substudy. Europace. 2014;16:1434-42.
7. Khairy P, Chauvet P, Lehmann J, Lambert J, Macle L, Tanguay JF, Sirois MG, Santoianni D, Dubuc M. Lower incidence of thrombus formation with cryoenergy versus radiofrequency catheter ablation.Circulation. 2003;107:2045-50.
8. Manasse E, Colombo P, Roncalli M, Gallotti R. Myocardial acute and chronic histological modifications induced by cryoablation. Eur J Cardiothorac Surg. 2000;17:339-40.
9. Su W, Kowal R, Kowalski M, Metzner A, Svinarich JT, Wheelan K, Wang P. Best Practice Guide for Cryoballoon Ablation in Atrial Fibrillation: The compilation experience of over 3000 Procedures. Heart Rhythm. 2015;12:1658-66.
10. Kimman GP, Theuns DA, Szili-Torok T, Scholten MF, Res JC, Jordaens LJ. CRAVT: a prospective, randomized study comparing transvenous cryothermal and radiofrequency ablation in atrioventricular nodal re-entrant tachycardia. Eur Heart J. 2004;25:2232-7.
11. Zrenner B, Dong J, Schreieck J, Deisenhofer I, Estner H, Luani B, Karch M, Schmitt C. Transvenous cryoablation versus radiofrequency ablation of the slow pathway for the treatment of atrioventricular nodal re-entrant tachycardia: a prospective randomized pilot study. Eur Heart J. 2004;25:2226-31.
12. Packer DL, Kowal RC, Wheelan KR, Irwin JM, Champagne J, Guerra PG, Dubuc M, Reddy V, Nelson L, Holcomb RG, Lehmann JW, Ruskin JN; STOP AF Cryoablation Investigators. Cryoballoon ablation of pulmonary veins for paroxysmal atrial fibrillation: first results of the North American Arctic Front (STOP AF) pivotal trial. J Am Coll Cardiol. 2013;61:1713-23.
13. Reddy VY, Sediva L, Petru J, Skoda J, Chovanec M, Chitovova Z, Di Stefano P, Rubin E, Dukkipati S, Neuzil P. Durability of Pulmonary Vein Isolation with Cryoballoon Ablation: Results from the SUstained PV Isolation with ARctic Front Advance (SUPIR) Study. J Cardiovasc Electrophysiol. 2015;26:493-500.
14. Andrade JG, Khairy P, Guerra PG, Deyell MW, Rivard L, Macle L, Thibault B, Talajic M, Roy D, Dubuc M. Efficacy and safety of cryoballoon ablation for atrial fibrillation: a systematic review of published studies. Heart Rhythm. 2011;8:1444-51.
15. Mugnai G, Chierchia GB, de Asmundis C, Sieira-Moret J, Conte G, Capulzini L, Wauters K, Rodriguez-Mañero M, Di Giovanni G, Baltogiannis G, Ciconte G, Saitoh Y, Juliá J, Brugada P. Comparison of pulmonary vein isolation using cryoballoon versus conventional radiofrequency for paroxysmal atrial fibrillation. Am J Cardiol. 2014;113:1509-13.
16. Fürnkranz A, Bordignon S, Schmidt B, Perrotta L, Dugo D, De Lazzari M,Schulte-Hahn B, Nowak B, Chun JK. Incidence and characteristics of phrenic nerve palsy following pulmonary vein isolation with the second-generation as compared with the first-generation cryoballoon in 360 consecutive patients. Europace. 2015;17:574-8.
17. Kowalski M, Ellenbogen KA, Koneru JN. Prevention of phrenic nerve injury during interventional electrophysiologic procedures. Heart Rhythm. 2014;11:1839-44.
18. Fürnkranz A, Bordignon S, Schmidt B, Böhmig M, Böhmer MC, Bode F, Schulte-Hahn B, Nowak B, Dignaß AU, Chun JK. Luminal esophageal temperature predicts esophageal lesions after second-generation cryoballoon pulmonary vein isolation. Heart Rhythm. 2013;10:789-93.
19. Metzner A, Burchard A, Wohlmuth P, Rausch P, Bardyszewski A, Gienapp C, Tilz RR, Rillig A, Mathew S, Deiss S, Makimoto H, Ouyang F, Kuck KH, Wissner E. Increased incidence of esophageal thermal lesions using the second-generation 28-mm cryoballoon. Circ Arrhythm Electrophysiol. 2013;6:769-75.
20. Calkins H, Kuck KH, Cappato R, Brugada J, Camm AJ, Chen SA, Crijns HJ, Damiano RJ Jr, Davies DW, DiMarco J, Edgerton J, Ellenbogen K, Ezekowitz MD, Haines DE, Haissaguerre M, Hindricks G, Iesaka Y, Jackman W, Jalife J, Jais P, Kalman J, Keane D, Kim YH, Kirchhof P, Klein G, Kottkamp H, Kumagai K, Lindsay BD, Mansour M, Marchlinski FE, McCarthy PM, Mont JL, Morady F, Nademanee K, Nakagawa H, Natale A, Nattel S, Packer DL, Pappone C, Prystowsky E, Raviele A, Reddy V, Ruskin JN, Shemin RJ, Tsao HM, Wilber D; Heart Rhythm Society Task Force on Catheter and Surgical Ablation of Atrial Fibrillation. 2012 HRS/EHRA/ECAS expert consensus statement on catheter and surgical ablation of atrial fibrillation: recommendations for patient selection, procedural techniques, patient management and follow-up, definitions, endpoints, and research trial design: a report of the Heart Rhythm Society (HRS) Task Force on Catheter and Surgical Ablation of Atrial Fibrillation. Developed in partnership with the European Heart Rhythm Association (EHRA), a registered branch of the European Society of Cardiology (ESC) and the European Cardiac Arrhythmia Society (ECAS); and in collaboration with the American College of Cardiology (ACC), American Heart Association (AHA), the Asia Pacific Heart Rhythm Society (APHRS), and the Society of Thoracic Surgeons (STS). Endorsed by the

governing bodies of the American College of Cardiology Foundation, the American Heart Association, the European Cardiac Arrhythmia Society, the European Heart Rhythm Association, the Society of Thoracic Surgeons, the Asia Pacific Heart Rhythm Society, and the Heart Rhythm Society. Heart Rhythm. 2012;9:632-696.e21.

21. Meininger GR, Calkins H, Lickfett L, Lopath P, Fjield T, Pacheco R, Harhen P, Rodriguez ER, Berger R, Halperin H, Solomon SB. Initial experience with a novel focused ultrasound ablation system for ring ablation outside the pulmonary vein. J Interv Card Electrophysiol. 2003;8:141-8.
22. Laughner JI, Sulkin MS, Wu Z, Deng CX, Efimov IR. Three potential mechanisms for failure of high intensity focused ultrasound ablation in cardiac tissue. Circ Arrhythm Electrophysiol. 2012;5:409-16.
23. Nakagawa H, Antz M, Wong T, Schmidt B, Ernst S, Ouyang F, Vogtmann T, Wu R, Yokoyama K, Lockwood D, Po SS, Beckman KJ, Davies DW, Kuck KH, Jackman WM. Initial experience using a forward directed, high-intensity focused ultrasound balloon catheter for pulmonary vein antrum isolation in patients with atrial fibrillation. J Cardiovasc Electrophysiol. 2007;18: 136-44.
24. Neven K, Schmidt B, Metzner A, Otomo K, Nuyens D, De Potter T, Chun KR, Ouyang F, Kuck KH. Fatal end of a safety algorithm for pulmonary vein isolation with use of high-intensity focused ultrasound.Circ Arrhythm Electrophysiol. 2010;3:260-5.
25. Metzner A, Chun KR, Neven K, Fuernkranz A, Ouyang F, Antz M, Tilz R, Zerm T, Koektuerk B, Wissner E, Koester I, Ernst S, Boczor S, Kuck KH, Schmidt B. Long-term clinical outcome following pulmonary vein isolation with high-intensity focused ultrasound balloon catheters in patients with paroxysmal atrial fibrillation. Europace. 2010;12:188-93.
26. Schmidt B, Chun KR, Metzner A, Fuernkranz A, Ouyang F, Kuck KH. Pulmonary vein isolation with high-intensity focused ultrasound: results from the HIFU 12F study. Europace 2009;11:1281-8.
27. Garcia R, Sacher F, Oses P, Derval N, Barandon L, Denis A, Hocini M, Roques X, Haïssaguerre M, Labrousse L, Jaïs P. Electrophysiological study 6 months after Epicor high-intensity focused ultrasound atrial fibrillation ablation. J Interv Card Electrophysiol. 2014;41:245-51.
28. Neven K, Metzner A, Schmidt B, Ouyang F, Kuck KH. Two-year clinical follow-up after pulmonary vein isolation using high-intensity focused ultrasound (HIFU) and an esophageal temperature-guided safety algorithm. Heart Rhythm. 2012;9: 407-13.
29. Reddy VY, Neuzil P, Themistoclakis S, Danik SB, Bonso A, Rossillo A, Raviele A, Schweikert R, Ernst S, Kuck KH, Natale A. Visually-guided balloon catheter ablation of atrial fibrillation: experimental feasibility and first-in-human multicenter clinical outcome. Circulation. 2009;120:12-20.
30. Dukkipati SR, Neuzil P, Kautzner J, Petru J, Wichterle D, Skoda J, Cihak R, Peichl P, Dello Russo A, Pelargonio G, Tondo C, Natale A, Reddy VY. The durability of pulmonary vein isolation using the visually guided laser balloon catheter: multicenter results of pulmonary vein remapping studies. Heart Rhythm. 2012;9:919-25.
31. Dukkipati SR, Kuck KH, Neuzil P, Woollett I, Kautzner J, McElderry HT, Schmidt B, Gerstenfeld EP, Doshi SK, Horton R, Metzner A, d'Avila A, Ruskin JN, Natale A, Reddy VY. Pulmonary vein isolation using a visually guided laser balloon catheter: the first 200-patient multicenter clinical experience. Circ Arrhythm Electrophysiol. 2013;6:467-72.
32. Sediva L, Petrů J, Škoda J, Janotka M, Chovanec M, Reddy V, Neužil P. Visually guided laser ablation: a single-centre long-term experience. Europace. 2014;16:1746-51.
33. Bordignon S, Chun KR, Gunawardene M, Fuernkranz A, Urban V, Schulte-Hahn B, Nowak B, Schmidt B. Comparison of balloon catheter ablation technologies for pulmonary vein isolation: the laser versus cryo study. J Cardiovasc Electrophysiol. 2013;24:987-94.
34. Gal P, Smit JJ, Adiyaman A, Ramdat Misier AR, Delnoy PP, Elvan A. First Dutch experience with the endoscopic laser balloon ablation system for the treatment of atrial fibrillation. Neth Heart J. 2015;23:96-9.
35. Keane D, Ruskin J, Norris N, Chapelon PA, Bérubé D. In vitro and in vivo evaluation of the thermal patterns and lesions of catheter ablation with a microwave monopole antenna. J Interv Card Electrophysiol. 2004;10:111-9.
36. Wonnell TL, Stauffer PR, Langberg JJ. Evaluation of microwave and radiofrequency catheter ablation in a myocardium-equivalent phantom model. IEEE Trans Biomed Eng. 1992; 39:1086-95.
37. Vander Brink BA, Gilbride C, Aronovitz MJ, Lenihan T, Schorn G, Taylor K, Regan JF, Carr K, Schoen FJ, Link MS, Homoud MK, Estes NA 3rd, Wang PJ. Safety and efficacy of a steerable temperature monitoring microwave catheter system for ventricular myocardial ablation. J Cardiovasc Electrophysiol. 2000;11:305-10.
38. Wisser W, Khazen C, Deviatko E, Stix G, Binder T, Seitelberger R, Schmidinger H, Wolner E. Microwave and radiofrequency ablation yield similar success rates for treatment of chronic atrial fibrillation. Eur J Cardiothorac Surg. 2004;25:1011-7.
39. Schuetz A, Schulze CJ, Sarvanakis KK, Mair H, Plazer H, Kilger E, Reichart B, Wildhirt SM. Surgical treatment of permanent atrial fibrillation using microwave energy ablation: a prospective randomized clinical trial. Eur J Cardiothorac Surg. 2003;24:475-80.
40. Vicol C, Kellerer D, Petrakopoulou P, Kaczmarek I, Lamm P, Reichart B. Long-term results after ablation for long-standing atrial fibrillation concomitant to surgery for organic heart disease: is microwave energy reliable? J Thorac Cardiovasc Surg. 2008;136:1156-9.
41. Lin Z, Shan ZG, Liao CX, Chen LW. The effect of microwave and bipolar radiofrequency ablation in the surgical treatment of permanent atrial fibrillation during valve surgery. Thorac Cardiovasc Surg. 2011;59:460-4.
42. Tanaka K, Satake S, Saito S, Takahashi S, Hiroe Y, Miyashita Y, Tanaka S, Tanaka M, Watanabe Y. A new radiofrequency thermal balloon catheter for pulmonary vein isolation. J Am Coll Cardiol 2001;38:2079-86.
43. Satake S, Tanaka K, Saito S, Tanaka S, Sohara H, Hiroe Y, Miyashita Y, Takahashi S, Murakami M, Watanabe Y. Usefulness of a new radiofrequency thermal balloon catheter for pulmonary vein isolation: a new device for treatment of atrial fibrillation. J Cardiovasc Electrophysiol. 2003; 14:609-15.
44. Sohara H, Takeda H, Ueno H, Oda T, Satake S. Feasibility of the radiofrequency hot balloon catheter for isolation of the posterior left atrium and pulmonary veins for the treatment of atrial fibrillation. Circ Arrhythm Electrophysiol. 2009;2: 225-32.

45. Sohara H, Satake S, Takeda H, Yamaguchi Y, Nagasu N. Prevalence of esophageal ulceration after atrial fibrillation ablation with the hot balloon ablation catheter: what is the value of esophageal cooling? J Cardiovasc Electrophysiol. 2014; 25:686-92.
46. Avitall B, Reddy V, McElderry T, Kouth J, Schneider. New and novel low intensity collimated ultrasound for the creation of continuous linear lesions. Heart Rhythm. 2013;10(Suppl):S129 (abstr).
47. Koruth JS, Schneider C, Avitall B, Ribeiro L, Dukkipati S, Walcott GP, Phillips P, McElderry HT, Reddy VY. Pre-clinical investigation of a Low-Intensity Collimated Ultrasound system for pulmonary vein isolation in a porcine model. JACC: Clinical Electrophysiology. 2015;1:306-14.

EDITORS' SUMMARY

Drs Gunda, Atoui, and Lakkireddy provide a practical summary of non-radiofrequency sources that are either being used or have been significantly investigated for ablation procedures. Of these sources, the most detailed discussion is on the most commonly used alternative to radiofrequency energy, i.e. cryoablation. The authors succinctly compare the risks, techniques, and efficacy of cryo energy use with radiofrequency ablation, particularly for paroxysmal atrial fibrillation.

There follows a summary of high-intensity focused ultrasound and the yet unsolved problems with this energy source related to collateral damage, especially related to the esophagus.

Newer and more recently investigated energy sources are described and a bottomline summary provided that will be useful for quick review by the reader. This chapter should ideally be read after the section on the biophysics of RF ablation and serves as a useful adjunct, essentially describing the alternatives available once the limitations of RF energy use have been learned.

Not covered in this chapter are newer non-thermal methods of ablation, particularly reversible and irreversible electroporation. As new data emerges with this initially promising energy source, future summaries of alternative ablation approaches will likely compare electroporation with thermal (heating and cooling) techniques for ablation.

SECTION C

Supraventricular Tachyarrhythmias: AV Node-dependent Tachycardias

CHAPTER 12

Vikas Kalra, Mithilesh K Das

Supraventricular Arrhythmias: Classification

LIST OF ABBREVIATIONS

AF	Atrial Fibrillation	AVRT	Atrioventricular Reciprocating Tachycardia
AFL	Atrial Flutter	LA	Left Atrium
AP	Accessory Pathway	MAT	Multifocal Atrial Tachycardia
APC	Atrial Premature Complex	PJRT	Permanent Junctional Reciprocating Tachycardia
AT	Atrial Tachycardia	RA	Right Atrium
AV	Atrioventricular	SVT	Supraventricular Tachycardia
AVNRT	Atrioventricular Nodal Reentrant Tachycardia	VPC	Ventricular Premature Complex

INTRODUCTION

Supraventricular tachycardia (SVT) is defined as any tachycardia with origin above the ventricle [atrium, atrioventricular (AV) node or His bundle]. There are multiple types of SVT as mentioned in **Table 12.1**. Atrial flutter (AFL) and atrial fibrillation (AF), though supraventricular arrhythmias, are typically not included in the classification of SVT.

Electrocardiographically, SVT can be broadly classified into short RP tachycardia and long RP tachycardia based on the timing of the P-wave in relation to the R-R interval. In short RP tachycardia, the RP interval is less than half of the RR interval and in long RP tachycardia, the RP interval is more than the half of RR interval **(Table 12.2 and Figure 12.1)**. The supraventricular arrhythmias can also be classified into AV node dependent [atrioventricular nodal reentrant tachycardia (AVNRT) and atrioventricular reciprocating tachycardia (AVRT)] and AV node independent [atrial tachycardia (AT), AFL and AF]. This classification has clinical implications in that any means like vagal maneuvers (carotid massage) or drugs that transiently block or slow the conduction in the AV node can terminate the AV node-dependent tachycardias but not the AV node independent arrhythmias. These measures may also help in reaching a diagnosis in a patient with supraventricular arrhythmia.

ATRIOVENTRICULAR NODAL REENTRANT TACHYCARDIA

Atrioventricular nodal reentrant tachycardia (AVNRT) is the most common form of paroxysmal SVT. The circuit of this tachycardia involves two pathways of the AV node (dual AV nodal physiology) with different conduction velocities and refractory periods. The common type of AVNRT (slow-fast) involves anterograde conduction down the slow AV nodal pathway and retrograde conduction via the fast AV nodal pathway. Typically, an atrial premature complex (APC) initiates AVNRT by blocking conduction

Table 12.1: Types of supraventricular arrhythmias

- Sinus tachycardia
- Atrial tachycardia (AT)
- Atrioventricular nodal reentrant tachycardia (AVNRT)
- Atrioventricular reciprocating tachycardia (AVRT)
- Permanent junctional reciprocating tachycardia (PJRT)
- Junctional tachycardia
- Atrial flutter
- Atrial fibrillation

Table 12.2: Classification of supraventricular tachycardia based on R-P interval

Short RP tachycardia	*Long RP tachycardia*
Typical AVNRT (slow-fast)	Sinus tachycardia
AVRT	AT
Junctional tachycardia with retrograde atrial conduction	Atypical AVNRT (fast-slow)
AT with a long PR interval	PJRT

Abbreviations: AVNRT, atrioventricular nodal reentrant tachycardia; AVRT, atrioventricular reciprocating tachycardia; AT, atrial tachycardia; PJRT, permanent junctional reciprocating tachycardia

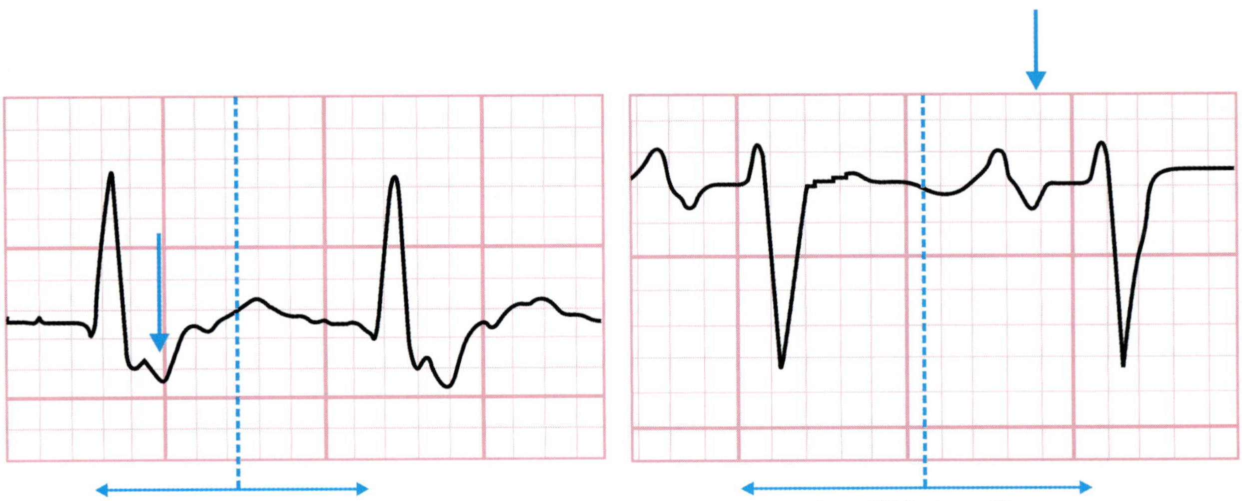

Figure 12.1: Classification of supraventricular tachycardia based on R-P interval

anterogradely via the fast pathway, but conducting down the slow pathway to the His bundle. The conduction also occurs from the AV node retrogradely via the fast pathway, which has recovered by this time, and excites the atria (retrograde P-wave). This retrograde P-wave is called the *echo beat.* If the impulse that reaches the atrium via the fast pathway can conduct down the slow pathway again, then the reentrant circuit of AVNRT gets completed and the tachycardia is initiated. It continues until an APC or a ventricular premature complex (VPC) enters the circuit to block the conduction **(Figures 12.2A to C)** in either limb resulting in its termination. Alternatively, a change in autonomic tone can alter the conduction or refractoriness of one of the pathways (usually the slow pathway) to terminate the tachycardia. The less common fast-slow type of AVNRT involves antegrade conduction down the fast pathway and retrogradely up the slow pathway. A slow-slow or slow-intermediate form of AVNRT with the retrograde P-wave occurring in the mid-cycle probably involves reentry by the way of a slow and an intermediate pathway.

ATRIOVENTRICULAR RECIPROCATING TACHYCARDIA

Atrioventricular reciprocating tachycardia (AVRT) is a form of a reentrant tachycardia involving the accessory pathway as at least one of the two limbs of the reentrant circuit. It can be further classified as orthodromic AVRT if AV node-His Purkinje system serves as the antegrade limb of the reentrant circuit **(Figures 12.3A and 12.4A)** and antidromic AVRT if the accessory pathway serves as the antegrade limb of the reentrant circuit **(Figures 12.3B and 12.4B)**.

ATRIAL TACHYCARDIA

Atrial tachycardia (AT) is defined as a regular rhythm originating from the atrium at a rate of 100 bpm to 240 bpm. The presence of an atrial rate above 100 bpm with at least three morphologically distinct P-waves signifies

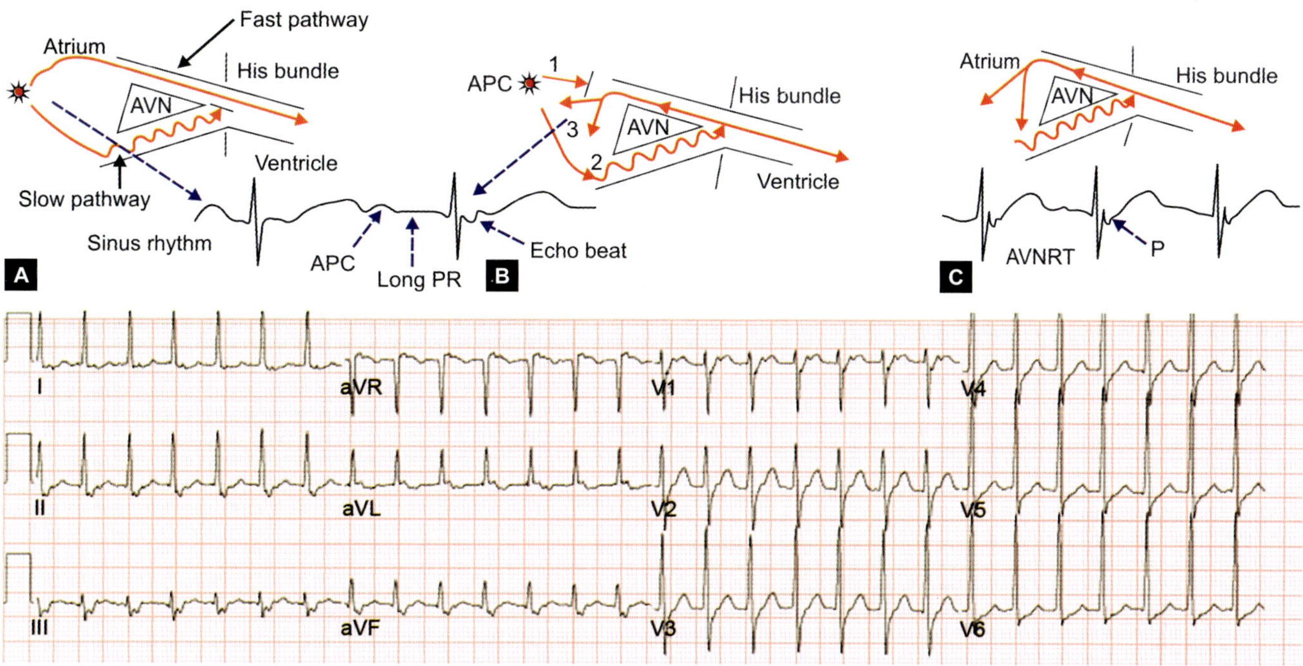

Figures 12.2A to C: AVNRT—Mechanism of initiation and its ECG
Abbreviations: APC, atrial premature complex; AVN, atrioventricular node; AVNRT, atrioventricular nodal reentrant tachycardia

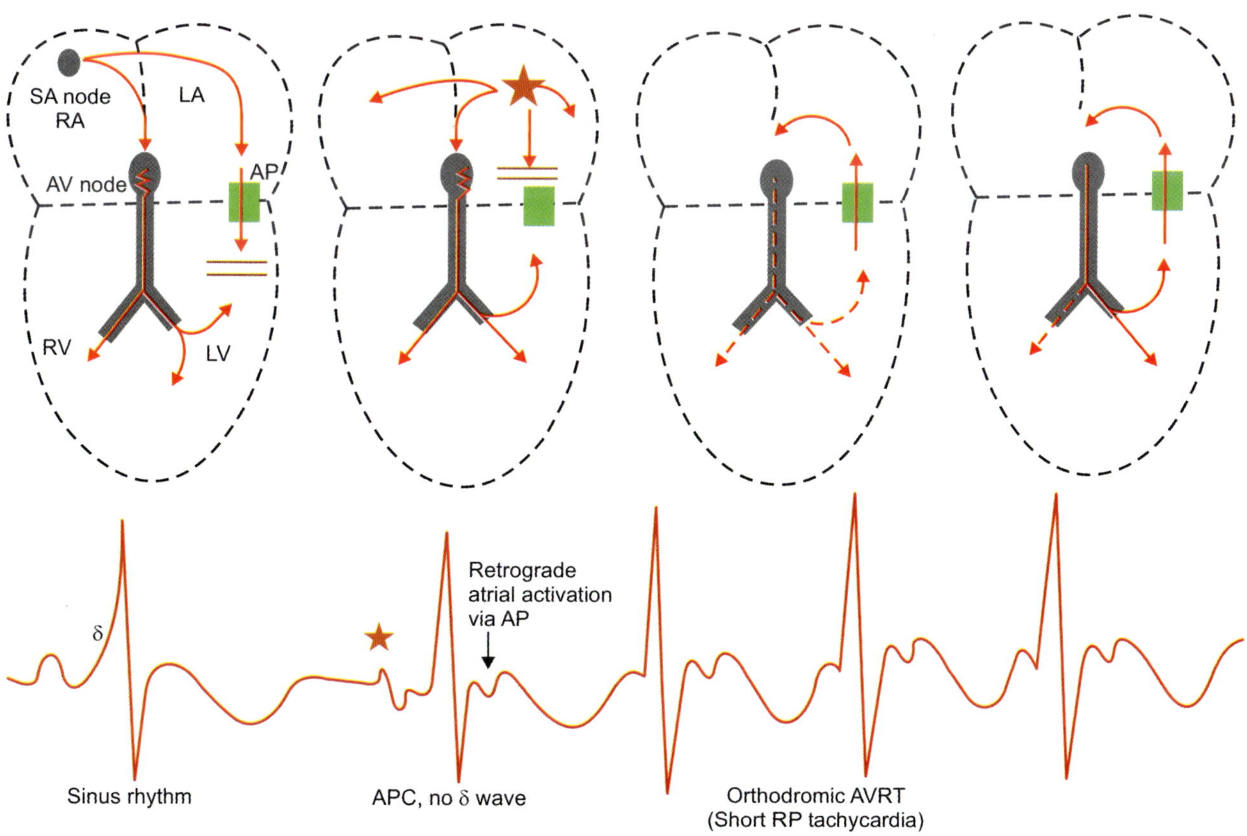

Figure 12.3A: Initiation of orthodromic AVRT with APC originating in the left atrium with antegrade block in the accessory pathway (AP) and conduction over the AV node and retrograde conduction over the left sided AP
Abbreviations: AP, accessory pathway; APC, atrial premature complex; AV, atrioventricular; AVRT, atrioventricular reciprocating tachycardia; LA, left atrium; LV, left ventricle; RA, right atrium; RV, right ventricle; SA, sinoatrial

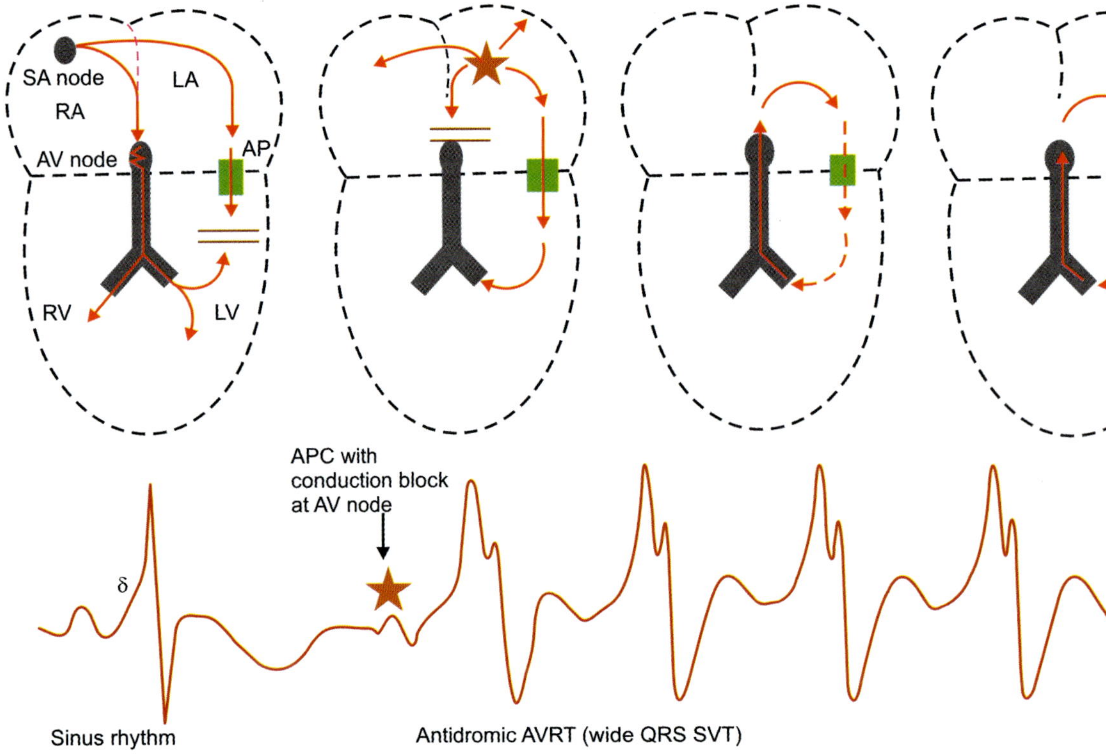

Figure 12.3B: Initiation of antidromic AVRT with APC originating in left atrium with antegrade block in the AV node and conduction over the accessory pathway and retrograde conduction over the AV node

Abbreviations: AP, accessory pathway; APC, atrial premature complex; AV, atrioventricular; AVRT, atrioventricular reciprocating tachycardia; LA, left atrium; LV, left ventricle; RA, right atrium; RV, right ventricle; SA, sinoatrial

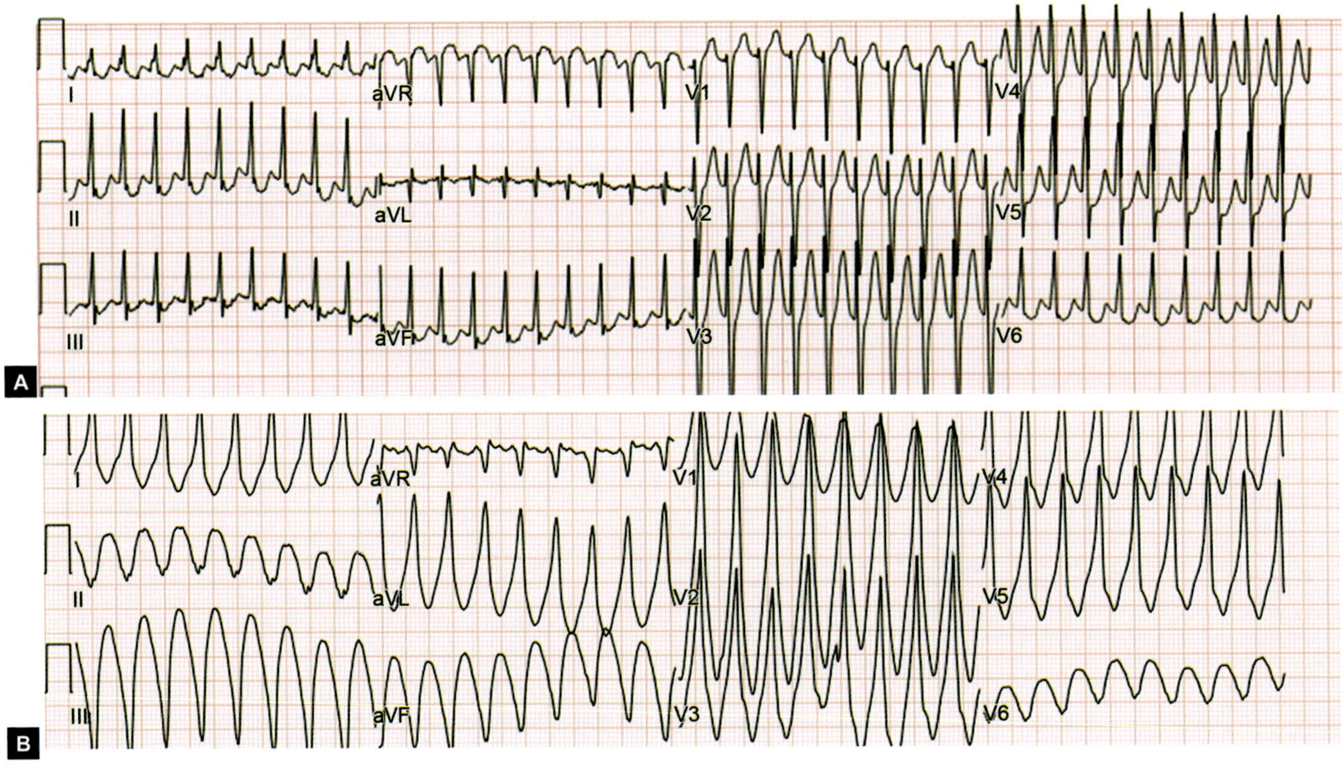

Figures 12.4A and B: AVRT. (A) ECG of orthodromic AVRT; (B) ECG of antidromic AVRT

different foci of atrial depolarization and is called a *multifocal atrial tachycardia (MAT)*. However, more commonly the P waves during AT are of same morphology. Underlying mechanism of atrial tachycardia could either be focal (automatic or triggered activity or microreentry) or macroreentrant. ECG is a useful tool to help localize the site of origin of focal atrial tachycardia. In general, lead V1 and inferior leads (II, III, aVF) of ECG determine the P-wave vector that can help in localization of focal atrial tachycardia. Since the left atrium (LA) is posterior, positive P-wave in lead V1 during a focal AT suggests origin in LA while a negative P-wave in lead V1 suggests origin in the right atrium (RA). A superior P-wave vector indicated by negative P-waves in inferior leads suggests origin in lower part of the atrium and inferior P-wave vector (positive P-waves in inferior leads) indicates origin in upper part of atrium **(Figures 12.5A and B)**. P-wave duration during tachycardia is also important to distinguish septal origin (narrow P-wave) versus origin from lateral wall (wider P-wave).

ATRIAL FLUTTER

Atrial flutter (AFL) is a macroreentrant arrhythmia with an electrocardiographic diagnosis based on regular atrial (flutter) waves usually without an underlying isoelectric line, at rates between 240 and 340 bpm. The ventricular rate varies depending on the AV conduction. AFL is classified into right atrial cavotricuspid isthmus dependent flutter (typical), that can be either counter-clockwise **(Figure 12.6A)** or clockwise **(Figure 12.6B)**, and noncavotricuspid isthmus dependent (atypical) flutter **(Figure 12.6C)** that can be left or right atrial or scar related. The most common flutter is the typical counter-clockwise right atrial flutter that shows regular saw-toothed flutter waves which are negative in the inferior leads and show a terminal positivity in lead V1 of the ECG **(Figure 12.6A)**.

ATRIAL FIBRILLATION

Atrial fibrillation (AF) is characterized by rapid (300–600 bpm), and irregular atrial fibrillatory waves (f waves) with an undulating baseline **(Figure 12.6D)**. It is the most common cardiac tachyarrhythmia and is classified as paroxysmal (self-terminating episodes that last <7 days), persistent (last 8 days to <1 year and may require electric versus pharmacologic cardioversion), and permanent (>1 year with no intention for further rhythm control). Patients with persistent AF existing for longer than 1 year who are considered for rhythm control have been referred to as having *longstanding persistent AF.* Underlying mechanism of atrial fibrillation is not clearly understood but is believed to be related to factors that trigger and

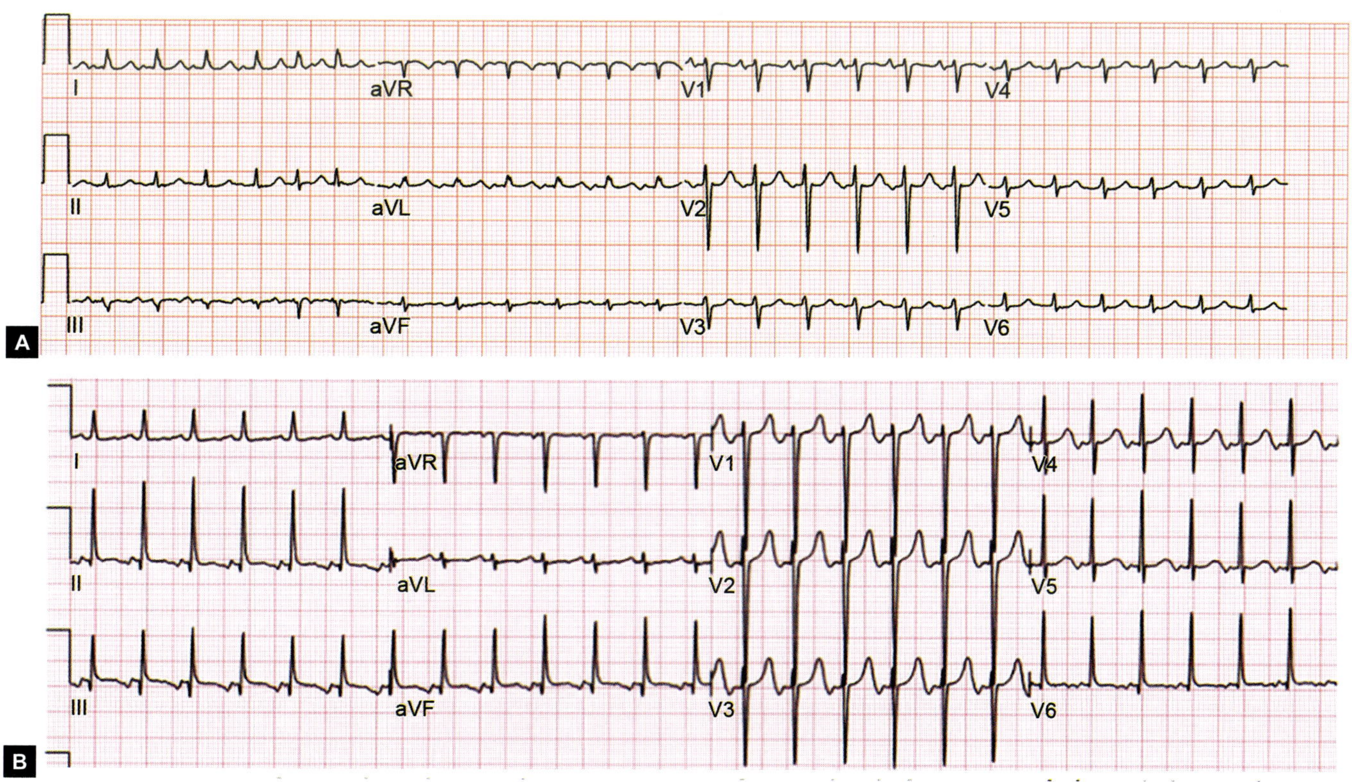

Figures 12.5A and B: ECG of atrial tachycardia originating from the left atrium (A) and the right atrium (B)

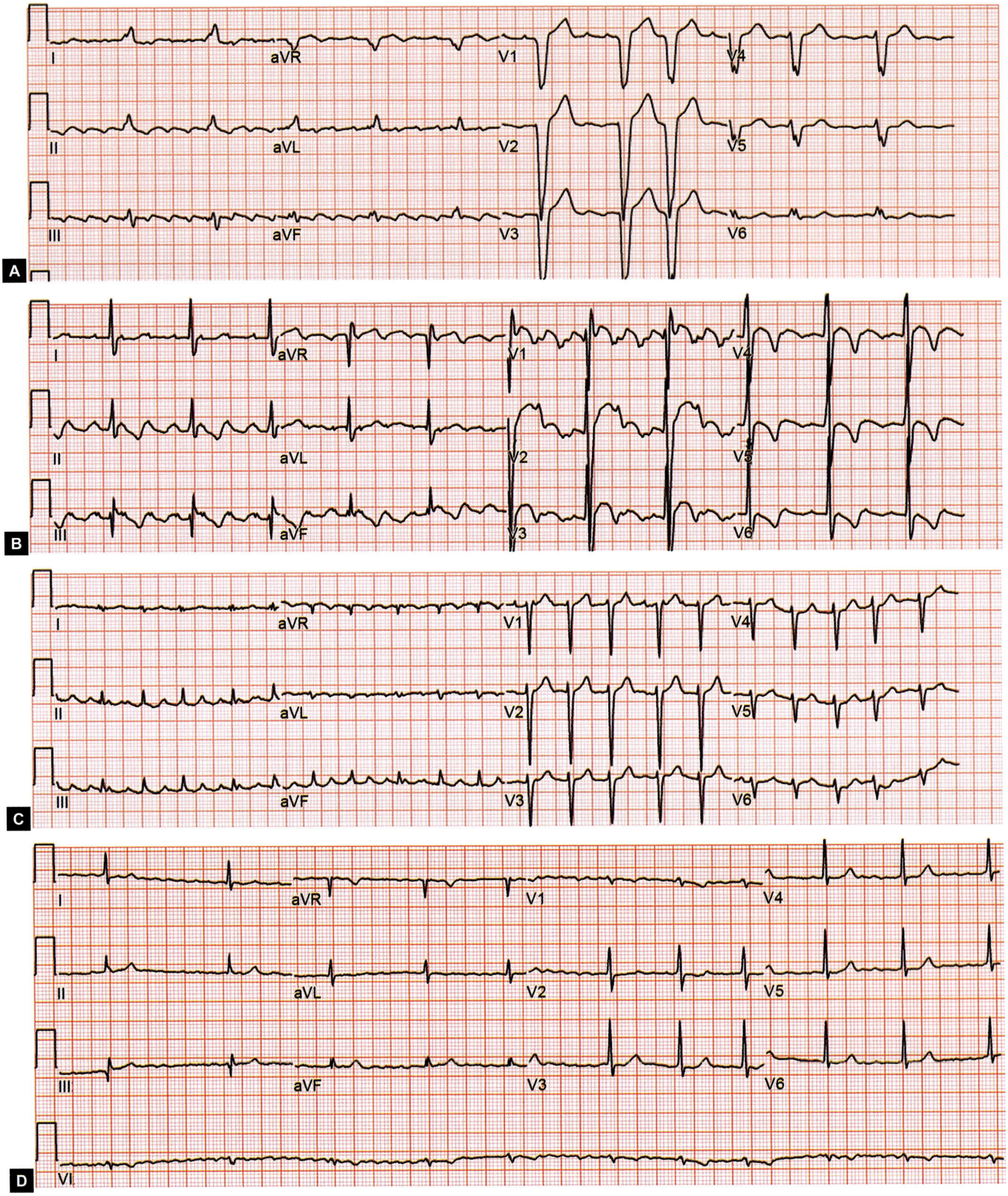

Figures 12.6A to D: Atrial flutter and atrial fibrillation: (A) Typical counter-clockwise atrial flutter; (B) Typical clockwise atrial flutter; (C) Atypical atrial flutter originating from left atrium; (D) Atrial fibrillation

factors that perpetuate the arrhythmia (substrate). Rapid electrical firing from the sleeves of atrial myocytes extending into the veins most commonly (90%) the pulmonary veins is known to trigger the initiation of AF. Other foci that can trigger AF include foci within the superior vena cava, small muscle bundles in the ligament of Marshall, and the musculature of the coronary sinus.

EDITORS' SUMMARY

In this chapter, Drs Kalra and Das provide a well-illustrated electrocardiogram-based review of supraventricular arrhythmias. The material represents platform novel for the invasive electrophysiologist to be well versed in prior to planning the course of a supraventricular tachycardia ablation procedure.

1. ***Accessory pathway-related tachycardias***: The best clear pathology and physiology correlation that we have to date established for the mechanism of arrhythmia are those related to an accessory pathway. Even the novice student understands the circuits for orthodromic and antidromic tachycardia, and the possibility that an accessory pathway may be a bystander and not directly participate in the tachycardia. Specific variants that require more detailed study and we do not as clearly understand the pathophysiology and anatomy for include slowly and decrementally conducting retrograde pathways that produce the syndrome of PJRT (permanent form of junctional reciprocating tachycardia), nodoventricular and nodofascicular tracts, and variants of antegradely conducting decremental pathways.
2. ***AV node reentry***: The authors use simple and clear circuit diagrams to help the student understand the basics of this very complex arrhythmia. The reader, however, must use this information in conjunction with those in other chapters in this book and other excellent writings such as by Jackman's group (Lockwood D, Nakagawa H, Jackman W. Electrophysiologic Characteristics of Atrioventricular Nodal Reentry Tachycardia: Implications for Reentrant Circuits. In: Zipes D, Jalife J (Eds). Cardiac Electrophysiology From Cell to Bedside. Philadelphia: Elsevier Saunders; 2009. pp. 615-46. [Book Chapter]). The exact circuits in AVNRT and indeed the nature of the AV node inputs (fast and slow pathways) remain inadequately described and require correlative anatomic, physiological and invasive EP studies.
3. ***Automatic and macroreentrant atrial tachycardias***: The electrocardiogram can be of immense value in planning an EP procedure for atrial tachycardias. In combination with the clinical nature of the arrhythmia, point source or focal tachycardias are relatively straightforward conceptually to map and ablate at the earliest site of origin when compared to reference electrocardiographic or intracardiac marker. On the other hand, reentrant arrhythmia can be very challenging to map and define the complete circuit. Of the multiple potential macroreentrant atrial tachycardias, cavotricuspid isthmus flutter, described excellently in this chapter, and its variants have to be anticipated and well understood as this pattern remains the only one in our field where the electrocardiogram predicts the circuit and an anatomic site for successful ablation (the cavotricuspid isthmus). The complete absence of an isoelectric interval in all ECG leads during an atrial tachycardia suggests a large circuit reentry. On the other hand, a significant isoelectric period with a smaller flutter wave may suggest a microreentrant circuit. Smaller circuit reentry like microreentry may be approached in the EP lab with methods similar to focal source tachycardia whereas macroreentry requires a careful mapping approach with combined activation and entrainment mapping.

CHAPTER 13

Peter Cheung, Taresh Taneja, Shoei K Stephen Huang

Supraventricular Tachycardias: Approach during Electrophysiology Study

LIST OF ABBREVIATIONS

AP	Accessory Pathway	HP	His-Purkinje
ART	Antidromic Reciprocating Tachycardia	ORT	Orthodromic Reciprocating Tachycardia
AT	Atrial Tachycardia	PAC	Premature Atrial Complex
AVN	Atrioventricular Node	PPI	Postpacing Interval
AVNRT	Atrioventricular Nodal Reentrant Tachycardia	PVC	Premature Ventricular Complex
AVRT	Atrioventricular Reciprocating Tachycardia	RV	Right Ventricle
CL	Cycle Length	SP	Slow Pathway
EP	Electrophysiology	SVT	Supraventricular Tachycardia
EPS	Electrophysiology Study	TCL	Tachycardia Cycle Length
FP	Fast Pathway		

INTRODUCTION

Diagnosis of supraventricular tachycardia (SVT) is a challenging and rewarding aspect of cardiac electrophysiology. In this chapter, we describe a systematic approach to diagnose SVT in the electrophysiology (EP) laboratory. Details of individual maneuvers should be found in subsequent chapters. For the sake of discussion, we define SVT loosely to include atrial tachycardia (AT), atrioventricular nodal reentrant tachycardia (AVNRT), and atrioventricular reciprocating tachycardia (AVRT), even though technically, this definition may be debated.

Before taking the patient to the EP laboratory, there should be clinical evidence of SVT such as ECG documentation, history of abrupt onset and termination, or termination with Valsalva maneuver or adenosine, etc. Such evidence is helpful in postulating a mechanism of SVT. For example, an ECG in which P-wave is clearly visible during SVT, so-called long RP tachycardia, has differential diagnosis of AT, AVRT, or atypical AVNRT. SVT with P-wave at the terminal portion of QRS can be either AVNRT, or less likely, AT. However, P-wave is not always discernable as it may be hidden in the QRS or T wave. Histories that are helpful, include sensation of neck pounding which indicates simultaneous contraction of atria and ventricles, suggesting AVNRT. Termination of tachycardia with Valsalva maneuver suggests a crucial role of the AV node (AVN) in the circuit, favoring AVNRT or AVRT. On the other hand, palpitation alone, without any additional descriptive feature, is nonspecific for SVT. Non-SVT etiologies of palpitation include sinus tachycardia, atrial or ventricular ectopics, atrial fibrillation, prominent heartbeat, or anxiety. EP study (EPS) under this ill-defined circumstance is of low yield. The purpose of EPS is not only to diagnose, but more importantly to treat SVT. It is not useful as a tool to rule out arrhythmia. Therefore, a careful history should be performed to assess whether EPS has an important therapeutic role prior to the undertaking.

EPS may be divided into 2 parts: baseline study and SVT study. Baseline study is an evaluation of electrophysiological properties of the electrical components in the heart. These components include atrial tissue, AVN, accessory pathway (AP), His-Purkinje system (HP), and ventricular tissue. Baseline study exposes potential substrate for SVT. Examples of potential substrates are dual AVN physiology and AP. However, presence of a substrate does not automatically render a diagnosis as it could be an innocent bystander. Uncommonly, multiple substrates are present. An example of an innocent bystander would be dual AVN physiology in a patient with AVRT, or an AP in a patient with AVNRT. Even less commonly, multiple tachycardia mechanisms are possible in an individual patient.

In contrast, SVT study consists of observations, induction, termination, and pacing maneuvers during SVT. Because of its actual interaction with tachycardia itself, SVT study is more diagnostic than a baseline study. Maneuvers to differentiate mechanisms of SVT will be briefly discussed. In-depth discussions are found in the subsequent chapters. Often, a combination of maneuvers and observations are required to make a diagnosis. Therefore, it is essential that a systematic and integrative approach be adopted. This chapter will provide a framework of such an approach.

BASELINE STUDY

During baseline EPS, the goal should be to assess AVN physiology and presence of AP. Simultaneous surface ECG may offer a clue. Preexcitation and a short or negative HV interval are seen with manifest AP. During sinus rhythm, a long PR interval and a long AH interval suggest anterograde conduction via AVN slow pathway (SP), which may be substrate for atypical AVNRT. Incremental pacing and programmed stimulation are essential to interrogate electrophysiological substrate. Parahisian and differential pacing in the right ventricle (RV) are helpful to detect concealed septal accessory pathway. **Table 13.1** lists baseline observations that are helpful in anticipating a mechanism for SVT.

Incremental Pacing

Incremental pacing is performed at a gradually increased rate until conduction block occurs.

Incremental atrial pacing assesses AV conduction through AVN fast pathway (FP), SP, and AP. AV conduction in normal physiology is through the FP. PR interval is normal at baseline. With incremental atrial pacing, there is gradual prolongation of AH; no sudden prolongation of AH interval should occur; and AV interval < VV interval **(Figure 13.1)**. In contrast, dual AVN physiology is seen when anterograde conduction shifts from FP to SP. With incremental pacing, there is lengthening of AH interval, whether gradual

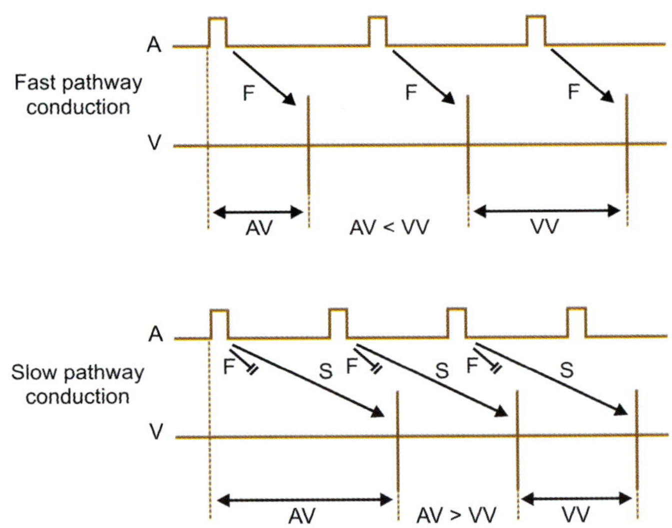

Figure 13.1: Fast and slow pathway conduction

Table 13.1: Baseline characteristics associated with a possible mechanism

Possible diagnosis	*Typical AVNRT*	*Atypical AVNRT*	*AVRT*	*AT*
Abrupt onset	+	+	+	+
Long RP	–	+	+	+
Neck pounding	+			+/–
Dual AV node physiology	+	+		
Preexcitation			+	
Extranodal response to parahisian pacing			+	
Differential pacing: $S\text{-}A^{*}_{\text{RV septum}} < S\text{-}A_{\text{RV apex}}$			+	
Eccentric atrial activation during VA conduction			+	

*S-A: stimulus to atrial signal.

or abrupt, such that AV interval is > VV interval. At this point, anterograde conduction is through the SP.

For manifest AP, preexcitation increases with incremental pacing due to delayed (decremental) conduction through the AVN, and hence preferential conduction through the AP. AP block may precede or follow AVN block. During incremental pacing, if preexcitation is lost and QRS becomes narrow, AP block has preceded AVN block. This favors orthodromic reciprocating tachycardia (ORT), an AVRT in which the AVN serves as the anterograde limb of the circuit. On the contrary, when the loss of preexcitation is associated with AV block, AP block has followed AVN block. Antidromic reciprocating tachycardia (ART) where AVN serves as the retrograde limb of the circuit is possible. Since ART is rare, ORT is still possible and more common; though in this situation, induction of ORT may require isoproterenol to "wake-up" the AVN.

Incremental ventricular pacing assesses VA conduction. Normal VA conduction through the AVN is decremental, increasing VA interval with incremental pacing. On the other hand, non-decremental conduction suggests retrograde AP conduction. During baseline study, when VA block occurs at a relatively long pacing interval, isoproterenol to facilitate VA conduction is usually required to induce AVNRT or AVRT. VA conduction with concentric (midline) atrial activation during ventricular pacing is consistent with AVN or septally located AP conduction. VA conduction with eccentric atrial activation is consistent with laterally located AP conduction. However, retrograde AVN conduction may appear eccentric with earliest atrial activation in the late proximal or early middle coronary sinus (CS).[1] In this case, comparison of atrial activation sequence to that recorded by the His catheter is helpful. Early retrograde atrial activation in the His catheter is evidence against a lateral AP.

Through meticulous study of AV or VA conduction properties, it is possible to unmask SVT substrates with incremental pacing technique.

Programmed Stimulation

In programmed stimulation, a train of stimulations at a fixed interval (S1) is followed by a premature extrastimulus (S2). This exploits the differential conduction properties of FP, SP, and AP. Dual AVN physiology may be unmasked by this maneuver with block in the FP because of its longer refractory period. An "AH jump" is described as lengthening of AH interval by ≥ 50 ms when S2 is shortened by 10 ms. When this occurs, conduction shifts from FP to SP. Dual AV nodal physiology is supportive but not diagnostic of AVNRT. It is only seen in 60% of patients with AVNRT.[2] Furthermore, it can be seen in patients without AVNRT.[1] In fact, elimination of dual AVN physiology is not a requirement for successful treatment of AVNRT. Therefore, dual AVN physiology is neither sensitive nor specific for AVNRT.

Programmed stimulation is also useful in studying AP. Because of its composition of cardiac myocytes, AP refractory period is increased by prolonging S1 interval, rendering AP more likely to block with S2. In contrast, AVN refractory period is decreased by a prolonged S1 interval, rendering it more likely to conduct with S2. Exploiting this difference by increasing S1 interval is useful to induce ORT.

Premature Atrial Complex

A PAC may be seen after incremental pacing or programmed stimulation. This atrial beat may be atrial in origin or it may be a result of retrograde VA conduction (AV echo). AV echo may be due to retrograde conduction through the AVN or AP. The activation sequence and morphology of electrogram is useful to distinguish atrial origin from AV echo **(Table 13.2)**. A high-to-low morphology may be from either atrial ectopy or AP with a high atrial or free wall connection. This excludes AVN echo which has a low-to-high morphology due to its low central location. Premature atrial activation before His activation supports atrial origin as it is not dependent on the AV node. Early atrial activation after the His deflection with VA < 80 ms excludes AP echo as it requires time to exit the HP fiber, traverse ventricular tissue and engage the AP **(Figure 13.2)**. Keep in mind that the analysis of PAC is helpful but not diagnostic of the clinical arrhythmia. However, when applying to a sustained clinical arrhythmia, this analysis is very useful.

Parahisian Pacing

Parahisian pacing is useful to detect the presence of a concealed septal AP. High output pacing is performed at the His catheter (20 mA) so as to capture the His-RBB axis in addition to the ventricle. The resultant QRS is narrow as a result of fusion between global ventricular activation by the HP system and local ventricular activation by the His catheter. Pacing output is then decreased to capture only local ventricular tissue and not the His bundle. This can be identified when QRS widens due to loss of His capture. If a septal AP is present, VA conduction is predominantly

Table 13.2: Origin of PAC after pacing

Origin	Fast pathway	Slow pathway	Accessory pathway	Atrium
Morphology—high-low	–	–	+	+
Morphology—low-high	+	+	+	+
Timing- pre-His	+/–	–	–	+
Septal VA < 80 ms	+	–	–	+/–
Septal VA > 80 ms	–	+	+	+

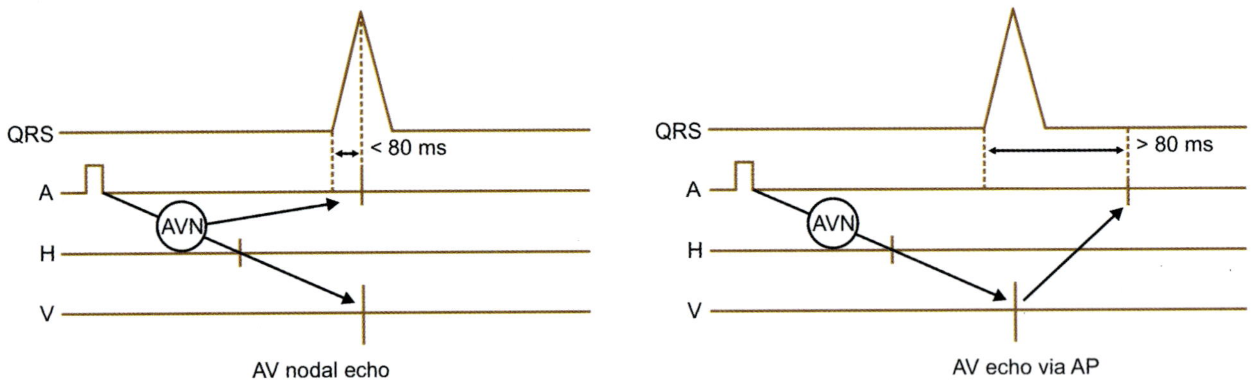

Figure 13.2: Timing of AV echo and mechanism

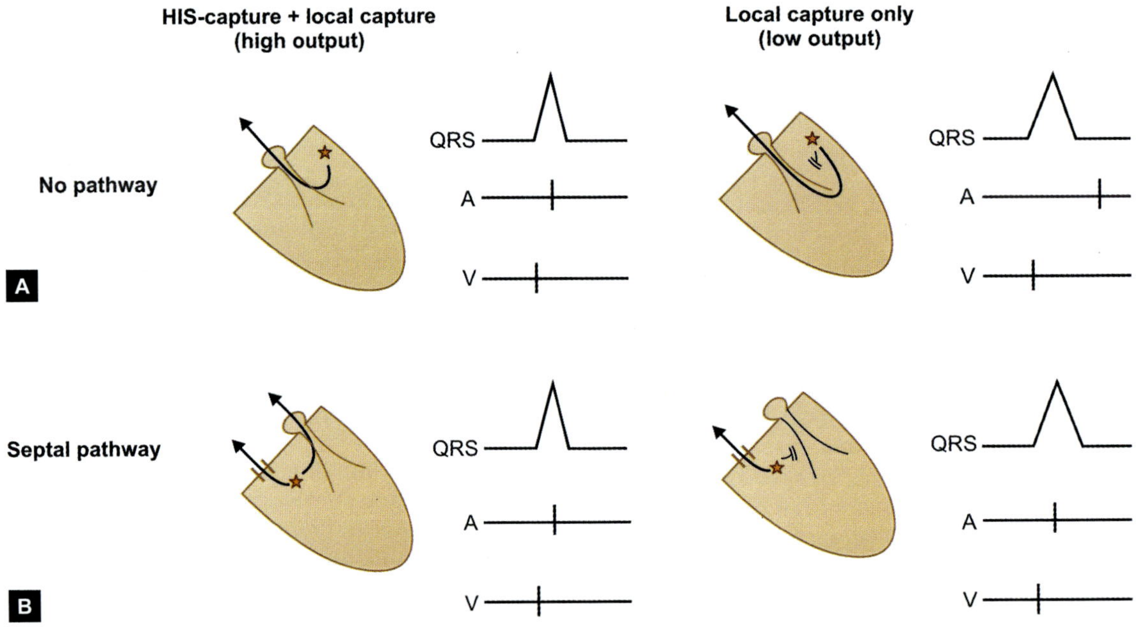

Figures 13.3A and B: Parahisian pacing

via AP due to decremental conduction in the AVN and faster retrograde conduction in the AP. In that case, whether His is captured or not, VA timing is unaffected **(Figure 13.3B)** and the response to parahisian pacing is termed an *"extranodal response."* In the absence of septal AP, VA conduction is via AV node. With His capture, VA conduction time is shorter because of the short distance between His and AVN. With loss of His capture, VA conduction time is longer because HP system is engaged at a more distal portion **(Figure 13.3A)**. This is termed a *"nodal response."* An extranodal response is diagnostic of an AP. A nodal response, however, does not exclude AP because VA conduction is competitive between the AVN and AP. Slow retrograde AP and non-septal AP conduction may yield a nodal response.

Differential Pacing

Differential pacing from the right ventricle (RV) is similar to parahisian pacing. Instead of alternating between His capture and loss of His capture, pacing alternates between RV septum and apex. In the presence of septal AP, VA time is shorter when pacing in the RV septum. In the absence of septal AP, VA time is longer in the RV septum as it takes time for impulse to reach and enter the distal portion of the HP fiber.

SUPRAVENTRICULAR TACHYCARDIA STUDY

SVT study comprises induction and analysis of SVT by studying initiation, perturbation, termination, and response to pacing maneuvers.

Induction of SVT

SVT may not be inducible at baseline. Baseline study and analysis should point to a possible mechanism. However, induction is a crucial part of SVT study. We will discuss baseline findings that one may expect with AVNRT and AVRT as well as some tips on inducing these SVTs.

In typical AVNRT, dual AVN physiology may be seen. With incremental atrial pacing, AV interval is longer than RR interval. AVN echo may be present. Multiple AVN echo beats are possible. With AVN echo, the site of block pinpoints location where SVT fails to propagate—antegrade (AV) block implicates SP, while retrograde (VA) block implicates FP. Isoproterenol can stimulate conduction in either pathway facilitating initiation of and sustaining AVNRT. On the other hand, isoproterenol may overstimulate the FP rendering AVNRT noninducible as SP may block first and become refractory **(Figure 13.4)**. In that case, washout of isoproterenol may allow AVNRT to be induced. Another technique is to decrease S1 interval, which stresses the FP and causes it to block; this may also delay slow pathway conduction, which allows time for FP to recover for retrograde conduction. Adding more than 1 extrastimulus (S3 or higher) has a similar effect.

In atypical AVNRT, first degree AV block may or may not be present; VA conduction time is usually long. AVN echo cannot be differentiated from that of septal AP. Parahisian or differential pacing may be helpful to exclude the presence of AP. Retrograde conduction is via the SP, and anterograde conduction may be via FP or another SP. Isoproterenol is helpful to stimulate both slow and fast pathways to initiate and sustain tachycardia.

In AVRT, AP may be manifest or concealed. In presence of a manifest AP, increase in preexcitation should be seen with incremental atrial pacing. If preexcitation morphology and HV remains fixed on incremental atrial pacing, then a fasciculoventricular pathway is present and this does not contribute to SVT. Concealed left lateral or right free wall AP may be detected by studying the atrial activation sequence during ventricular pacing. Septal AP may be detected by parahisian or differential ventricular pacing during sinus rhythm. Rarely, retrograde AVN conduction can be robust such that a concealed pathway may be masked. Isoproterenol may rarely be required to enhance AP conduction. Once a pathway is detected, pacing close to the pathway will preferentially conduct through the AP over the AVN.

Incremental pacing and programmed stimulation are useful to induce SVT. If block in a manifest AP precedes AVN and tachycardia is not initiated, this may be due to concealed anterograde conduction in the AP **(Figure 13.5A)**. Lengthening of S1 may enhance AVN conduction and anterograde AP block, facilitating induction of ORT. The same trick is useful, if manifest AP block follows AVN block. On the other hand, if AV echo is seen and does not conduct into the ventricle **(Figure 13.5B)**, use of isoproterenol may facilitate induction of ORT by enhancing

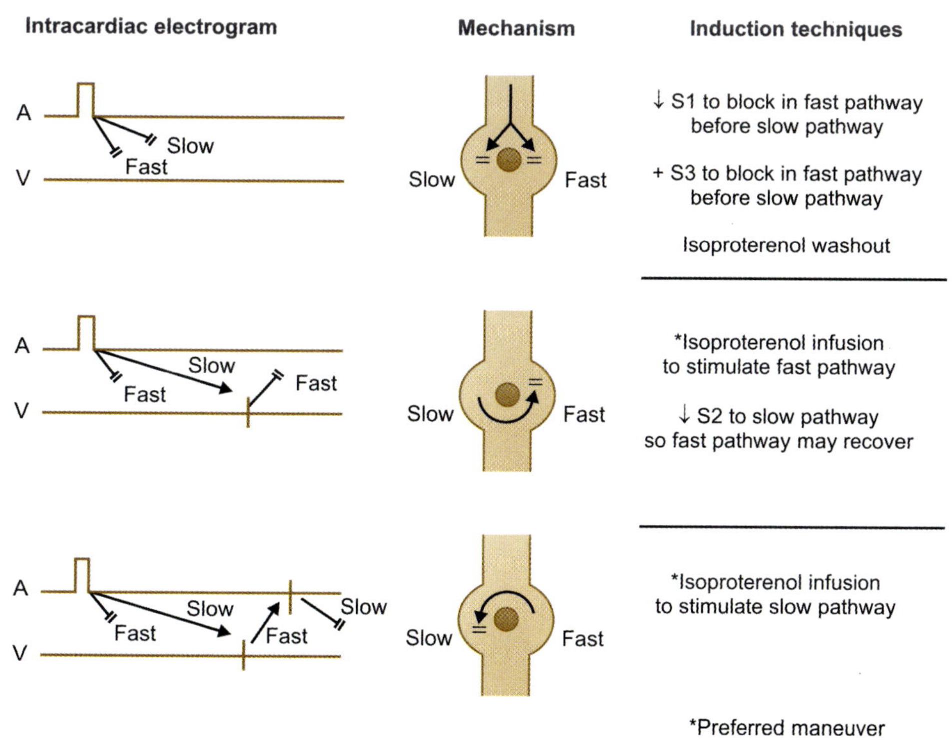

Figure 13.4: Sites of failure to propagate AVNRT

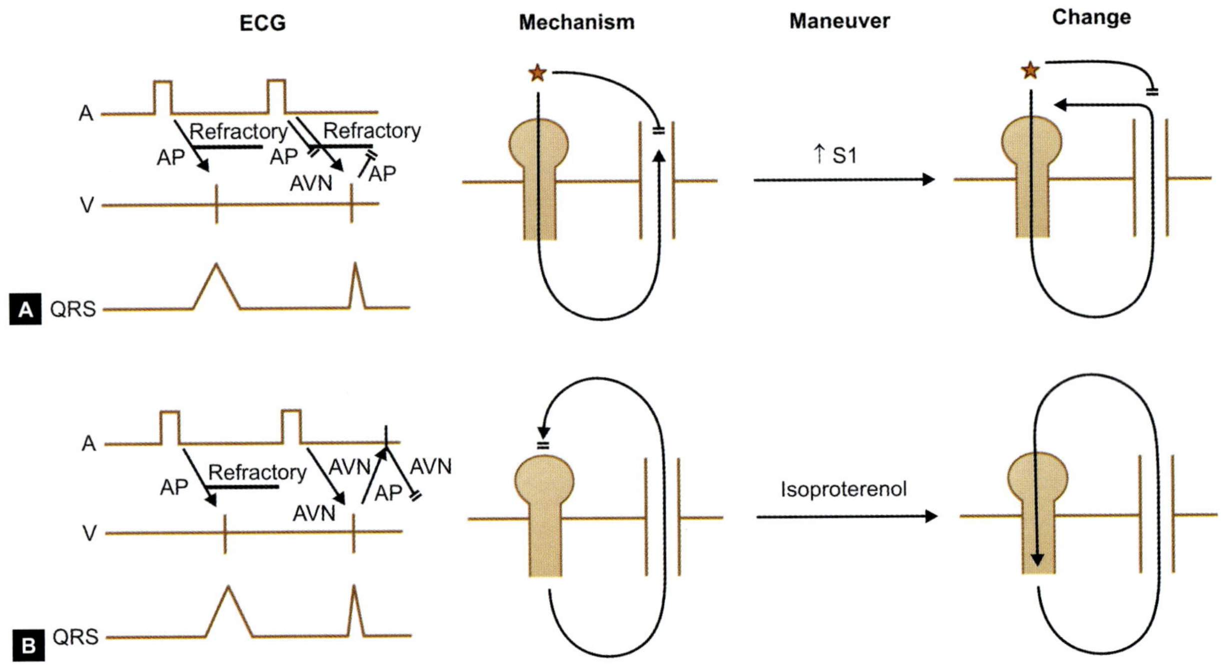

Figures 13.5A and B: Sites of failure to propagate ORT

Table 13.3: Observable characteristics during SVT that suggest a mechanism

Possible diagnosis	*AVNRT*	*Atypical AVNRT*	*AVRT*	*Atrial tachycardia*
Initiation dependent on long AH	+	+ (slow-slow variant)		
ΔAA precedes ΔHH or ΔVV	–	–	–	+
ΔHH or ΔVV precedes ΔAA	+	+	+	–
Termination with AV block	+	+	+	–
His deflection within QRS	–	–	– ORT + ART	bystander AP
AV block during SVT	+/–		–	+

AVN conduction. In ART, preexcitation is seen at baseline and on atrial pacing. The strategy to induce ART is opposite to that of ORT although induction of ART is usually difficult. S1 interval may be shortened to cause AVN block. This strategy may not work with AP that has decremental property.

Atriofascicular (Mahaim) fiber presents a unique challenge as its electrophysiological properties are distinct from that of the usual atrioventricular APs. It is a manifest accessory pathway with decremental conduction. Preexcitation may not be apparent during sinus rhythm due to slow AP conduction. With incremental pacing, QRS may have a typical left bundle-branch block morphology. It may not have any retrograde conduction even with isoproterenol.

If an SVT is not inducible with atrial pacing, similar techniques of programmed stimulation may be performed in the ventricle.

Analysis of SVT

Initiation of SVT offers a diagnostic clue to the mechanism. Initiation of SVT with a long AH interval suggests AVNRT **(Table 13.3)**. Spontaneous variation of cycle length (CL) offers another clue. Variation of CL is more likely with AT than AVNRT or AVRT. If CL variation in the atrium precedes that in the His or ventricle, then a diagnosis of AT is suggested. Conversely, if variation in His or ventricle (HH, or VV interval) precedes that in atrium (AA interval), then AT is excluded. Termination of tachycardia provides another diagnostic clue. Termination of the tachycardia with AV block demonstrates that AV conduction is crucial to the tachycardia, making AT highly unlikely. Be careful that this observation is not made with a PAC, as a non-conducted PAC can terminate atrial tachycardia with apparent AV block. His deflection within the QRS during tachycardia usually excludes ORT and AVNRT, which utilize His for anterograde conduction. AV block during tachycardia excludes AVRT (AVRT via an atrioventricular AP) as ventricular participation is essential for this SVT. Other characteristics, such as analysis of atrial electrogram morphology or VA time are also useful during SVT. It is important to bear in mind that a confounder does rarely exist and may lead to an erroneous diagnosis. An example of a confounder would be presence of 2 or more substrates with one acting as a bystander (e.g. any combination of dual AVN, > 1 SP, ≥ 1 AP).

Pacing Maneuvers during SVT

Two techniques are essential during an SVT study: ventricular overdrive pacing and His-synchronized premature ventricular complex (PVC) insertion during SVT.

Ventricular Overdrive Pacing

Ventricular overdrive pacing is a powerful diagnostic maneuver during SVT. A train of ventricular stimuli is delivered at a CL slightly below the tachycardia CL (TCL). Capture of atria by retrograde conduction should be confirmed. When pacing is terminated, atrial and ventricular events are analyzed **(Figure 13.6)**. VAAV sequence is diagnostic of AT whereas a VAV sequence rules out AT.[3]

Many powerful observations from ventricular overdrive pacing lead to diagnosis of a SVT.

1. For long RP tachycardia with concentric atrial activation, differential diagnosis of VAV response is atypical AVNRT or AVRT utilizing a septal AP. Postpacing interval (PPI), which is the interval between the last stimulus and the first returning complex recorded from the pacing electrode, offers important diagnostic information. PPI in the RV apex differentiates atypical AVNRT from AVRT via septal AP[4] **(Figure 13.7)**. A PPI-TCL < 115 ms suggests AVRT as the RV apex is in the vicinity of the circuit. Conversely, a PPI minus TCL difference that is greater than 115 ms (PPI-TCL >115 ms) shows that RV apex is far from the circuit and favors a diagnosis of AVNRT.
2. Refinement of the PPI approach by adjusting for difference in AH allows differentiation of atypical AVNRT from AVRT not limited to septal AP.[5] The rationale is that accelerated ventricular pacing perturbs AVN conduction and lengthens the returning AH interval comparing to that of tachycardia. Apparent PPI becomes exaggerated, and the diagnosis is biased towards AVNRT. Correction of this change ($\Delta AH = AH_{after\ pacing} - AH_{during\ tachycardia}$) increases the power of the PPI to diagnose AVRT via any pathway with a cut-off value of 110 ms (PPI-TCL-ΔAH < 110 ms).
3. During ventricular pacing, if tachycardia is terminated without affecting the atrium (i.e. atrial electrogram is not advanced), then AT is excluded. This demonstrates that a circuit outside of the atrium is critical to propagation of SVT. By definition, this rules out AT.
4. During ventricular pacing, if atrial signal is advanced while there is variable fusion of QRS, AVRT is diagnosed.[6] Variable fusion is due to different degrees of fusion in QRS between the paced wavefront and the tachycardia QRS. Fusion is variable because fusion or collision is occurring at a higher point with each subsequent stimulus until either AVN penetration (in AVRNT or AT) or manifested entrainment (in AVRT) occurs. During variable fusion, AVN-HP system is not available for retrograde conduction

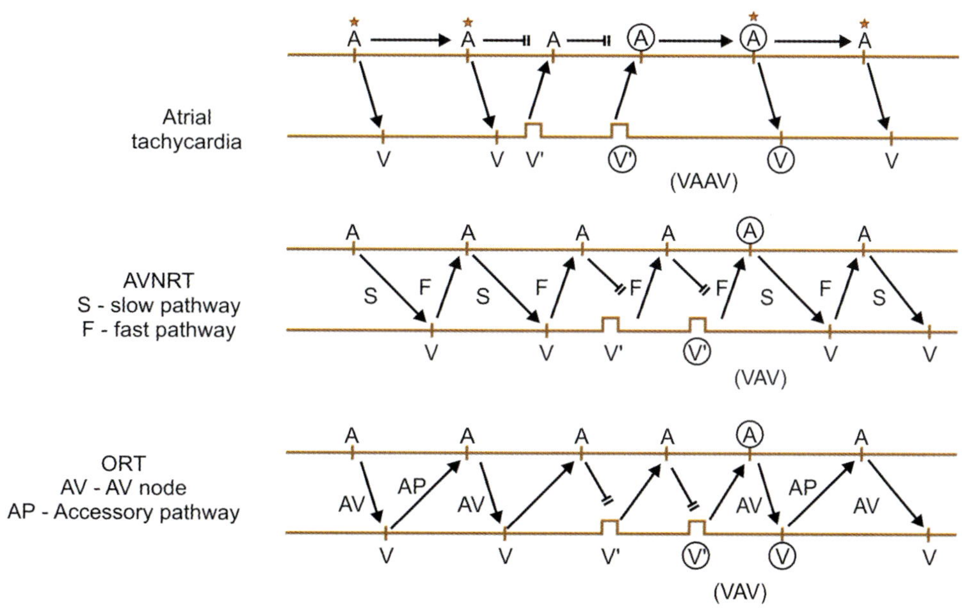

Figure 13.6: Ventricular overdrive pacing and response based on mechanism of SVT

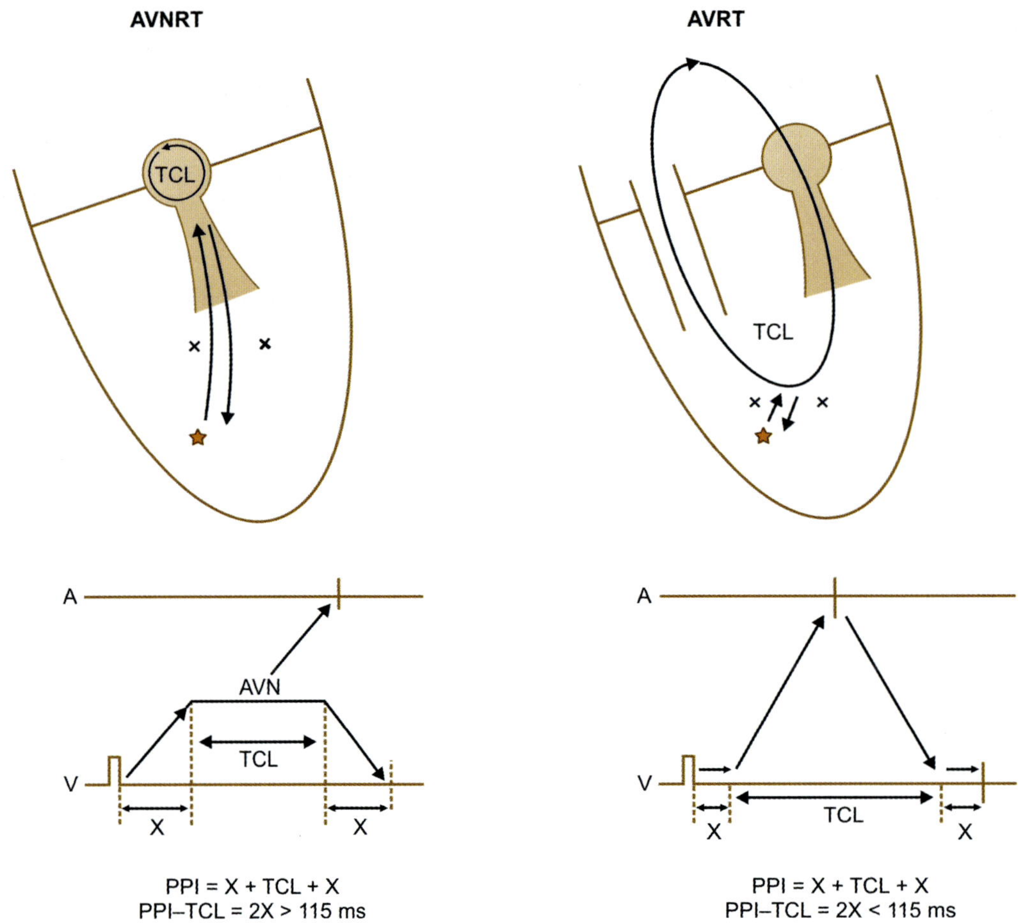

Figure 13.7: Difference of ventricular postpacing interval in AVNRT and AVRT

and the only mechanism by which the atrial signal can be advanced is by an AP **(Figure 13.8)**. To apply this analysis correctly, it is crucial to limit this to the transition zone where fusion is variable. Once the QRS has achieved a stable morphology (2 consecutively identical QRS complexes), VA conduction is no longer diagnostic of presence of AP. The limitation of this observation is that an innocent bystander pathway may confound the diagnosis.

5. Sometimes ventricular overdrive pacing fails to yield a diagnosis due to termination of tachycardia or failure to capture the atrium. In that case, atrial pacing maneuver is helpful. A train of atrial stimuli is delivered below TCL. After cessation of pacing, a fixed returning V-A interval (VA linking) that is consistent between trains suggests dependence of atrial event on VA conduction, favoring AVNRT and AVRT over AT.
6. If ventricular pacing below TCL dissociates ventricle from tachycardia (VA dissociation), AVRT is excluded.

Table 13.4 summarizes important diagnostic responses seen on pacing maneuvers.

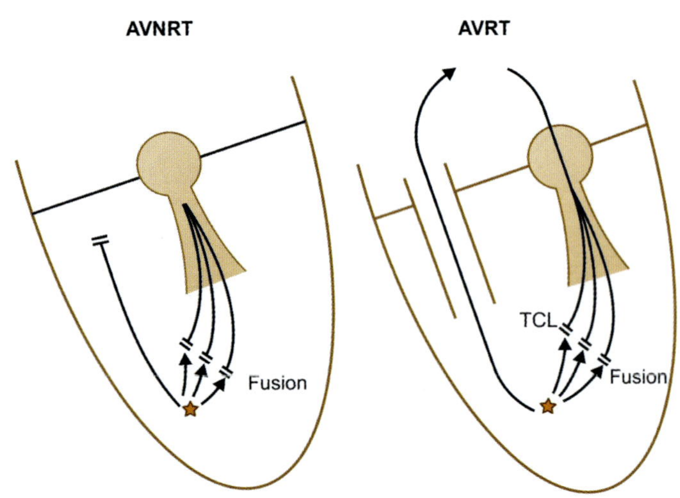

Figure 13.8: Variable fusion from anterograde conduction of SVT and retrograde wavefront from pacing. His is not available for retrograde conduction. Advancement of atrial activation proves the presence of accessory pathway

His Synchronized PVC

His synchronized PVC is another important technique wherein during tachycardia, PVC is introduced in the RV by a single stimulus near the time of His activation. Observable changes may differentiate AVRT from AVNRT. Observations include advancing the tachycardia or terminating the tachycardia. If tachycardia is terminated without conducting into the atrium, AVRT is the only possible diagnosis. AT is excluded because termination occurs without affecting the atrium. AVNRT is excluded because termination occurs without affecting the AVN (His refractory). Similarly, if the tachycardia is advanced and atrial morphology and activation sequence remains unchanged, an AVRT is diagnosed. In the unusual circumstance where a patient has an innocent bystander pathway that does not participate in the SVT, the atrial signal is advanced but with a different activation sequence. Finally, instead of advancing, PVC may delay the subsequent atrial event of the tachycardia (V_{stim}-A > V_{SVT}-A interval). In that case, AVRT with a decremental AP is diagnosed.

Incorporating various observations, **Flow chart 13.1** depicts one algorithm to diagnose SVT. In situations where ventricular overdrive pacing and His synchronous PVC insertion fail to differentiate AVRT and AVNRT due to lack of VA conduction, other observations are required to make

Table 13.4: Diagnostic responses to pacing maneuvers

	Typical AVNRT	*Atypical AVNRT*	*AVRT*	*Atrial tachycardia*
VAAV	–	–	–	+
VAV	+	+	+	–
PPI-TCL-ΔAH > 110 ms		+	–	N/A
PPI-TCL-ΔAH < 110 ms		–	+	N/A
PVC* advanced SVT	–	–	+	bystander AP
PVC* terminated SVT without affecting atrium	–	–	+	–

*His synchronized

Flow chart 13.1: Algorithm for diagnosing SVT

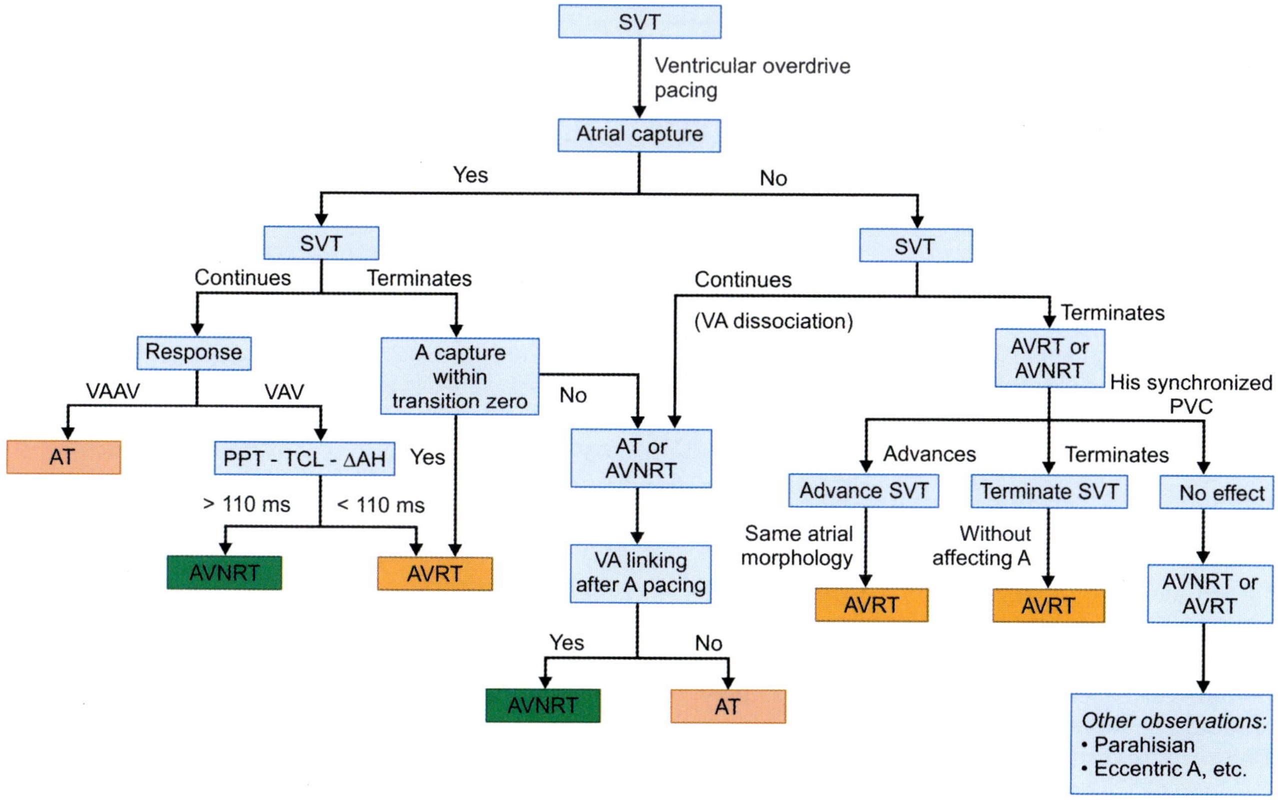

a diagnosis (**Flow chart 13.1**, right lower corner). During SVT, eccentric atrial activation (especially comparing to His catheter atrial activation) locates lateral and free wall AP. Once AP is identified, pacing the ventricle close to AP insertion site render pacing maneuver more successful; this will also confirm whether an AP is crucial to SVT or an innocent bystander. In SVT with concentric atrial activation, pacing at the septum can be helpful in detecting a septal AP. Unlike parahisian pacing, VA conduction during AVRT is noncompetitive as AVN is not available. In the event that none of these maneuvers was positive, AVRT should be unlikely. In AVNRT, it is not surprising that the AVN may prevent impulse from ventricular pacing to penetrate into the atrium. In AVRT, since ventricle is part of the circuit, it is less likely for paced impulse to fail to penetrate the atrium via an AP. Therefore, an SVT in which the atrium is unaffected by ventricular pacing close to earliest atrial activation is unlikely to be AVRT.

Familiarity with ventricular overdrive pacing and His synchronized PVC insertion is critical to accurate diagnosis of SVT.

CONCLUSION

For successful treatment of SVT, it is crucial that an accurate diagnosis be made with a systematic approach. Diagnosis starts with clinical history. Baseline EPS helps to detect arrhythmia substrates. Keen observation of electrophysiological events before and during SVT, combined with appropriately focused diagnostic maneuvers ensures success in accurate diagnosis of SVT mechanism.

REFERENCES

1. Lockwood, DJ, Nakagawa, H, Dyer, JW, et al. Electrophysiological Characteristics of Atrioventricular Nodal Reentrant Tachycardia: Implications for the Reentrant Circuits. In: Zipes DP, Jalife J (Eds). Cardiac Electrophysiology From Cell to Bedside, 6th edn. Philadelphia: WB Saunders. pp. 767-788.
2. McElderry, HT, Kay GN. Ablation of Atrioventricular Nodal Reentry by the Anatomic Approach. In: Huang SKS, Wood MA (Eds). Catheter Ablation of Cardiac Arrhythmias, 1st edn. WB Saunders. pp, 325-346.
3. Knight BP, Zivin A, Souza J, Flemming M, Pelosi F, Goyal R, Man C, Strickberger SA, Morady F. A technique for the rapid diagnosis of atrial tachycardia in the electrophysiology laboratory. J Am Coll Cardiol. 1999;33:775-81.
4. Michaud GF, Tada H, Chough S, Baker R, Wasmer K, Sticherling C, Oral H, Pelosi F, Jr, Knight BP, Strickberger SA, Morady F. Differentiation of atypical atrioventricular node re-entrant tachycardia from orthodromic reciprocating tachycardia using a septal accessory pathway by the response to ventricular pacing. J Am Coll Cardiol. 2001;38:1163-67.
5. González-Torrecilla E, Arenal A, Atienza F, Osca J, Garcia-Fernandez J, Puchol A, Sanchez A, Almendral J. First postpacing interval after tachycardia entrainment with correction for atrioventricular node delay: a simple maneuver for differential diagnosis of atrioventricular nodal reentrant tachycardias versus orthodromic reciprocating tachycardias. Heart Rhythm. 2006;3:674-79.
6. Al Mahameed ST, Buxton AE, Michaud GF. New criteria during right ventricular pacing to determine the mechanism of supraventricular tachycardia. Circ Arrhythm Electrophysiol. 2010;3:578-84.

EDITORS' SUMMARY

This chapter serves as an introduction to the fundamental principles, correct execution, and interpretation of the common maneuvers performed in the invasive EP laboratory to define the mechanism of supraventricular tachycardia. While the basics need to be completely understood, important exceptions and less common variant responses to the executed maneuvers also need to be mastered for the electrophysiologist.

AV node reentry is among the most complex arrhythmias that we deal with in our practice despite the fact that we are usually successful in curing this SVT. The present chapter should be used in conjunction with reference 1 (Lockwood DJ, Nakagawa H, Dyer JW, et al. Electrophysiological Characteristics of Atrioventricular Nodal Reentrant Tachycardia: Implications for the Reentrant Circuits. In: Zipes DP, Jalife J (Eds). Cardiac Electrophysiology From Cell to Bedside, 6th edn. Philadelphia: WB Saunders. pp. 767-688.) to fully appreciate the variations and the importance of anatomic definitions for this rhythm disorder. For example, although as a generalization, typical AVNRT has a short RP interval and atypical AVNRT does not, many exceptions abound. This is because the RP interval is defined by the relative time from a center portion of the AVNRT circuit to the ventricle and the atrium. In some patients with typical AVNRT, the limb to atrial activation may occur sooner than antegrade conduction to the ventricle producing a long RP tachycardia. On the other hand, when a long lower common pathway is present, near simultaneous ventriculoatrial activation and a short RP interval may be manifest. Both the definition for the variants of AVNRT and indeed the approach to ablation remains primarily anatomic and is well illustrated in the discussion by Cheung, et al.

The important technical details and the spectrum of responses to ventricular pacing maneuvers for SVT are excellently discussed and well-illustrated in the comprehensive flow chart that will be invaluable, particularly for the early student of interventional electrophysiology.

CHAPTER 14

John William Schleifer, Komandoor Srivathsan

Supraventricular Tachycardias: Baseline Features during Sinus Rhythm and Tachycardia

LIST OF ABBREVIATIONS

AT	Atrial Tachycardia	PJRT	Permanent Junctional Reciprocating Tachycardia
AVNRT	Atrioventricular Nodal Reentrant Tachycardia	PVC	Premature Ventricular Complex
AVRT	Atrioventricular Reciprocating Tachycardia	RBBB	Right Bundle Branch Block
CS	Coronary Sinus	SVT	Supraventricular Tachycardia
LBBB	Left Bundle Branch Block	WPW	Wolff-Parkinson-White
ORT	Orthodromic Reciprocating Tachycardia		

INTRODUCTION

Supraventricular tachycardia (SVT) is broadly defined as any arrhythmia originating above the bundle of His with rates higher than 100 beats per minute. This definition includes atrial fibrillation, atrial flutter, and multifocal atrial tachycardia. From the clinical perspective, however, these arrhythmias are addressed separately because of their distinct clinical presentation, mechanisms of origination, and management strategies.

The SVTs described below are similar because they occur in structurally normal hearts and in the absence of cardiopulmonary disease; as opposed to atrial fibrillation, atrial flutter, and multifocal atrial tachycardia which usually present in patients with underlying cardiopulmonary disease states.

Due to their similar clinical presentations and consequences, the SVTs are classified by mechanism of formation as atrioventricular nodal reentrant tachycardia (AVNRT), atrioventricular reciprocating tachycardia (AVRT), and atrial tachycardia (AT).

EPIDEMIOLOGY

The prevalence of SVT is approximately 2.3 per 1000 in the general population,[1] with atrioventricular nodal reentrant tachycardia (AVNRT) accounting for 60% of all cases, atrioventricular reciprocating tachycardia (AVRT) accounting for 30%, and atrial tachycardia (AT) accounting for 10%. This distribution of SVTs is evolving—with increase in the mean age of the population, the proportion of patients with AT is increasing.

MECHANISMS AND PATHOPHYSIOLOGY

The most common mechanism of SVT, reentry, is responsible for both AVNRT and AVRT. Macroreentrant atrial tachycardias that do not involve the AV node are classified as atrial flutters and will be covered separately. The basic requirement of a reentrant circuit is the presence of an anatomical or functional area of no conduction or of poor conduction around which a propagating impulse travels in two distinct paths. A reentrant circuit develops when these paths have different refractory periods and different velocities of propagation. An oncoming impulse when timed correctly while one path is refractory may propagate via only one path, and then it returns via the second path in a circuitous fashion. By the time, the impulse returns, the original path is ready to be activated and can therefore, transmit the impulse repeatedly, thereby setting up a continuous self-propagating circuit.

In AVNRT, the two limbs of the circuit are the fast and slow pathways that bring impulses to the AV node from the rest of the right atrium. The impulse usually travels antegrade down the slow pathway and returns retrograde via the fast pathway (slow-fast or typical AVNRT). Occasionally the impulse goes in the opposite direction around this circuit, giving rise to fast-slow or atypical AVNRT.

In AVRT, an accessory atrioventricular conduction pathway and either the AV node or another accessory pathway form the two limbs of the circuit. The impulse travels from the atrium down the accessory pathway and returns retrograde via the AV node (antidromic conduction) or may travel in the opposite direction (orthodromic conduction, antegrade through the AV node and retrograde via accessory pathway). If the accessory pathway responsible for AVRT conducts in the antegrade direction, a Wolff-Parkinson-White (WPW) pattern is seen during sinus rhythm in which the accessory pathway and AV node conduct concurrently causing fusion of QRS complex between two different activations. Depending on competitive conduction properties of the accessory pathway and AV node, the QRS complex may be variably preexcited. As the accessory pathway is not gated, it preexcites the ventricle resulting in initial part of the QRS; but once the impulse crosses AV node, conduction through fast His Purkinje system will form the latter part of the QRS complex (in effect PJ interval between preexcited and normal QRS complex is the same but PR may be shorter secondary to initial portion preexcited by accessory pathway). The degree to which a QRS is preexcited is determined by the location of the accessory pathway and the conduction properties of the intervening atrial tissue compared to the AV nodal conduction properties. Left lateral pathways tend to be minimally preexcited in contrast to the septal and right free wall pathways that are closer to the sinus node. Fixed preexcitation at various heart rates raises the possibility of preexcitation occurring beyond the AV node such as that occurs with a fasciculoventricular pathway.

Because accessory pathways often do not share the decremental conduction properties of the AV node, they can conduct at very fast rates with short refractory periods. Hence, in the presence of an accessory pathway with antegrade conduction, patients with atrial tachycardia or atrial fibrillation can conduct to the ventricle at excessively fast rates, potentially leading to ventricular fibrillation. Blocking AV node conduction in such situations may remove the influence of concealed conduction from the AV node, further enhancing conduction through the accessory pathway and accelerating ventricular rates.

In contrast to the reentrant mechanisms causing AVNRT and AVRT, atrial tachycardia is caused by increased automaticity or triggered activity in an ectopic atrial focus. Atrial tissue in the crista terminalis and myocytes extending into the pulmonary veins commonly develop increased automaticity causing atrial tachycardia. Reentrant atrial tachycardias, with all the components of the reentrant circuit located entirely within the atrium, do not involve the AV node or ventricular tissue and are classified as atrial flutters.

CLINICAL PRESENTATION

Clinically, the presentation of AVNRT, AVRT, or AT will be the sudden development of episodic (paroxysmal) rapid narrow QRS complex rhythm with rates reaching up to 250 beats per minute. Although some patients are asymptomatic during these episodes, most will experience symptoms ranging from palpitations to syncope. There are three common mechanisms for syncope in patients with SVT. Most commonly, syncope is a result of extremely fast ventricular rates leading to incomplete ventricular filling and ejection and reduction in blood pressure especially at the onset of the SVT. Secondly, a sinus pause following the termination of an SVT episode can also cause syncope. Least commonly, a vasovagal event may be triggered by tachycardia. Since most episodes are paroxysmal or transient and terminate spontaneously, there are usually no long-term adverse effects of this arrhythmia and tachycardia-induced cardiomyopathy in patients with AVNRT or AVRT is rare. One exception is a special form of AVRT, called permanent junctional reciprocating tachycardia (PJRT) which involves a slowly-conducting accessory pathway that conducts only retrogradely. The arrhythmia of PJRT may be sustained for long periods, which increases the propensity for tachycardia-induced cardiomyopathy. The slow conduction through the pathway, however, also limits the rate of the tachycardia.

ELECTROCARDIOGRAPHIC FINDINGS

Careful analysis of the 12-lead ECG prior to any electrophysiological study is critical.

Initiation and Onset

If the initiating P-wave is different from tachycardia P-wave and conducts with long PR interval prior to tachycardia initiation, the tachycardia is AV node dependent favoring slow/fast typical AV node reentry. If the initiating P-wave is similar to subsequent P-wave, then it favors atrial tachycardia.

Warm Up and Cool Down

Warm up (an increasing heart rate after initiation) or cool down (a decreasing heart rate before termination) is suggestive of automaticity and is most commonly seen in atrial tachycardia.

RP Relationship

A short RP tachycardia with RP duration of less than 60 ms favors typical slow/fast AVNRT. Because the conduction retrograde up the fast pathway to activate the atria occurs at the same time as the conduction down the His-Purkinje system to activate the ventricles, the RP is very short. If the RP duration is greater than 80 ms in a short RP tachycardia, it favors a pathway-mediated orthodromic reciprocating tachycardia. The ECG in **Figure 14.1A** shows very short RP interval (<60 ms) with inverted P-waves in leads III and aVF making slow/fast AVNRT likely. The ECG in tachycardia must be compared with the sinus rhythm ECG **(Figure 14.1B)** when available and examined for the location and morphology of P-wave. The "s" wave in leads III and aVF is confirmed to be a pseudo "s" in comparison to the sinus rhythm ECG, which does not have "s" waves in these leads, suggesting that they are rather "P" waves. In rare instances, either due to rapid retrograde conduction of the fast pathway (mostly in pediatric patients) or slow anterograde conduction through the lower common pathway and His-Purkinje system (mostly in elderly patients), typical AVNRT can be a long RP tachycardia.

On the other hand, in a short RP tachycardia with an RP interval >80 ms as shown in the **Figure 14.2**, an accessory pathway is likely. This patient had a left lateral accessory pathway that was ablated.

Long RP tachycardia typically favors atrial tachycardia. Atypical AVNRT and accessory pathways with long conduction times **(Figure 14.3)** are other potential causes of a long RP tachycardia which need to be considered. The patient with the ECG in **Figure 14.3** had a slow conducting decremental accessory pathway that was ablated in the posteroseptal region near the coronary sinus os.

P-wave Duration and Vector

Narrow P-waves with a P-wave duration 40 ms or less suggest an anterior interatrial septum source of atrial activation from either atrial tachycardia or typical AVNRT. P-waves wider than 80 ms suggest sequential activation of the atria. Very wide P-waves >120 ms are likely originating

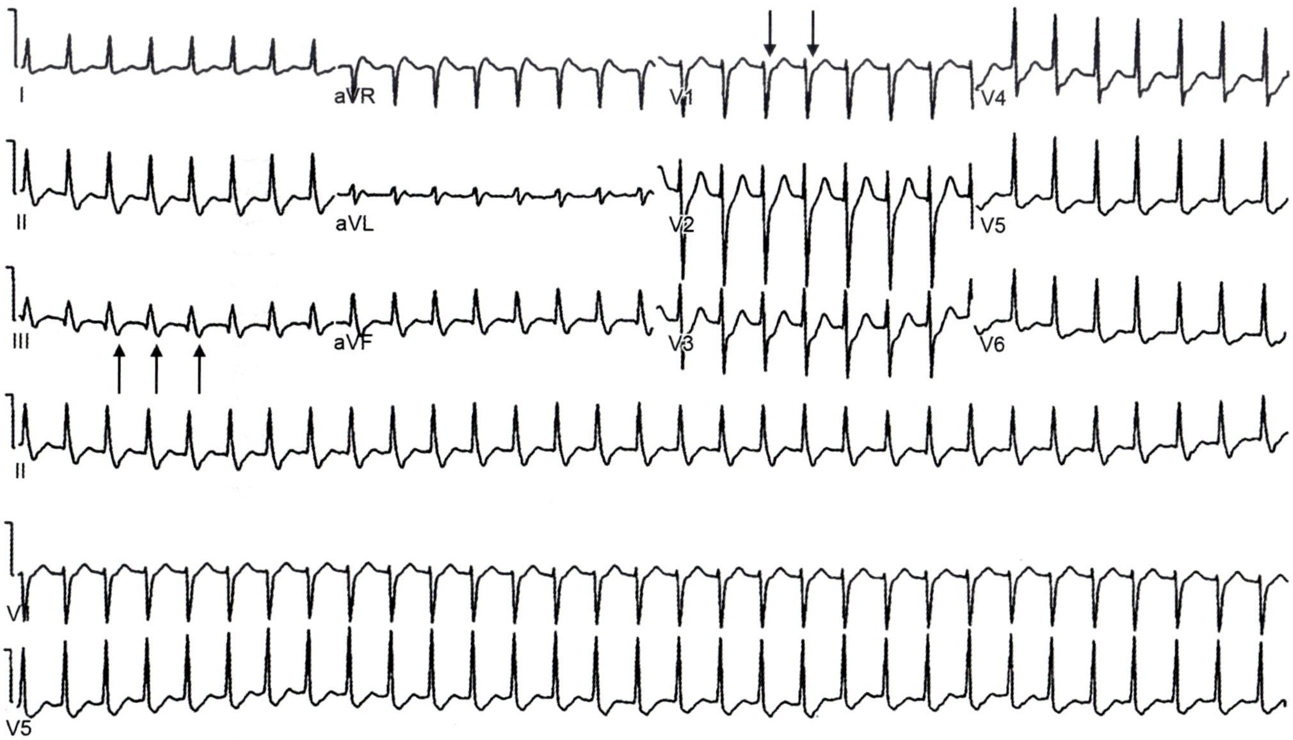

ECG during tachycardia

Figure 14.1A

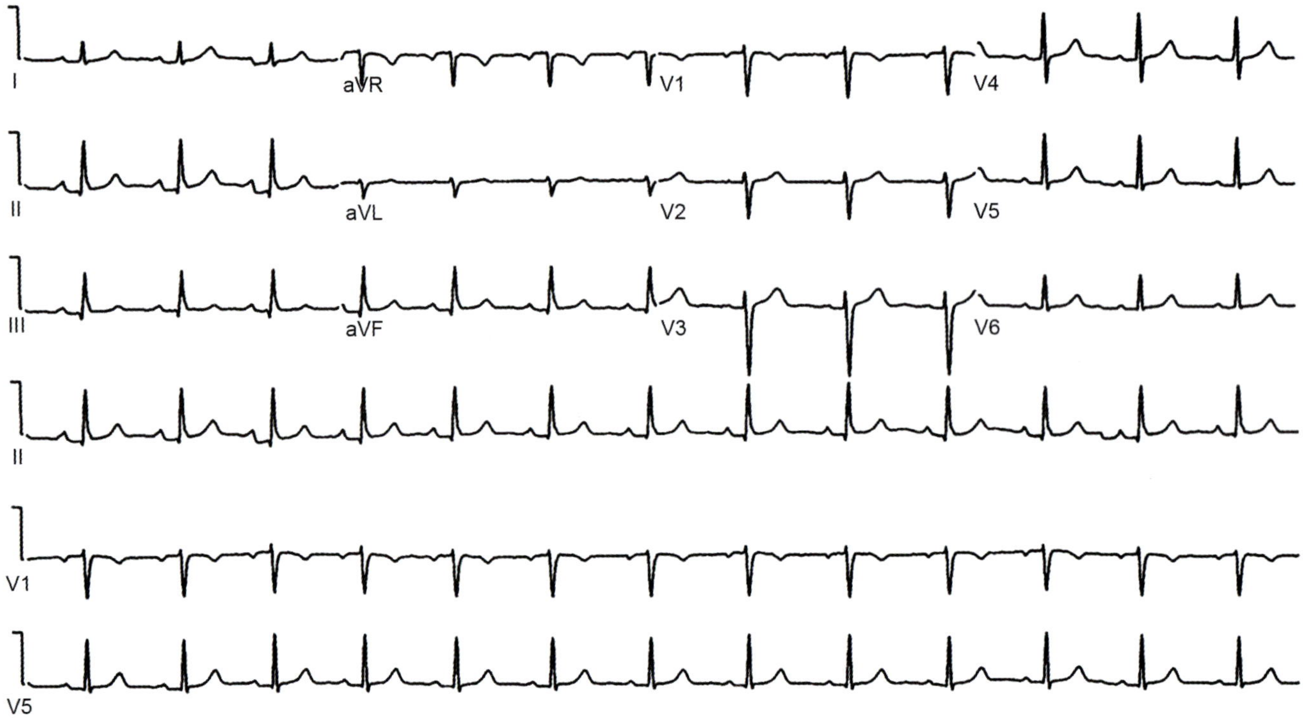

ECG during sinus rhythm

Figure 14.1B

Figures 14.1A and B: The P-wave during tachycardia (A) is at the end of the QRS complex with an RP interval less than 60 ms; the P-waves (arrows) form pseudo-S waves that are not present in sinus rhythm (B)

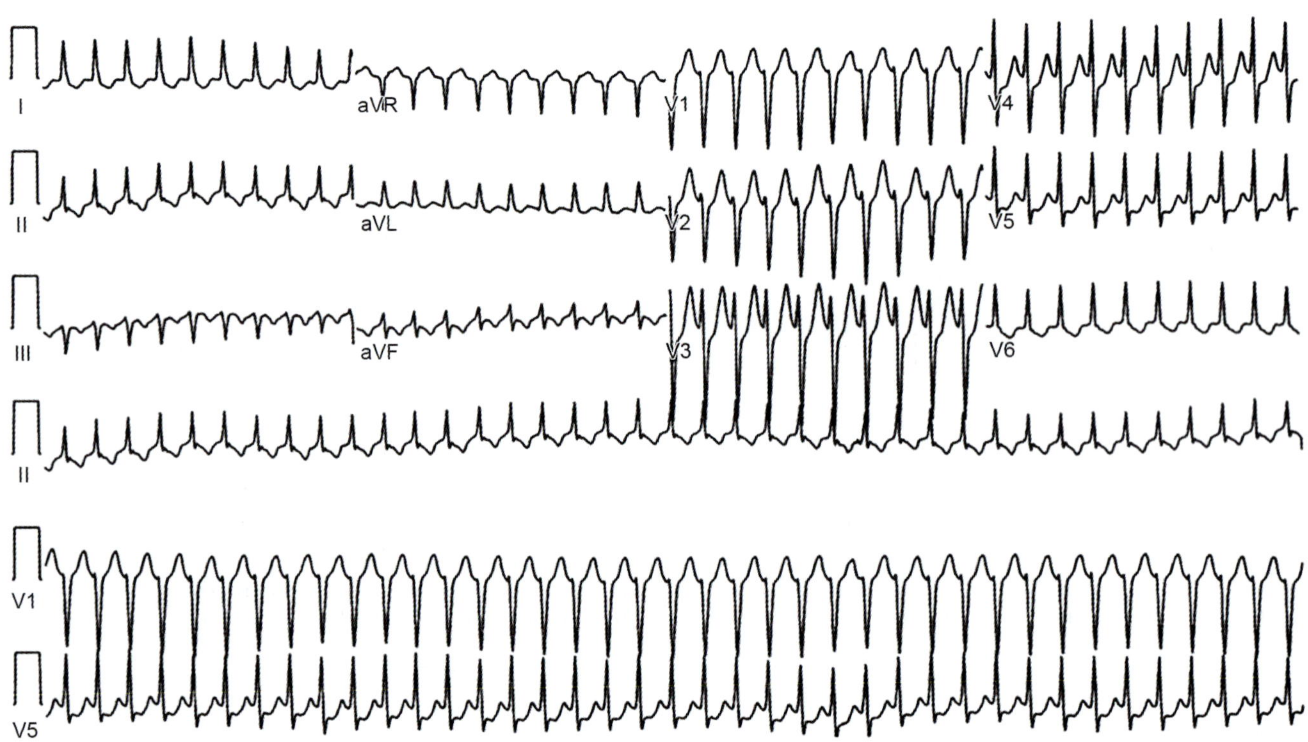

Figure 14.2: Short RP tachycardia with RP duration >80 ms, suggestive of an accessory pathway-mediated orthodromic reciprocating tachycardia

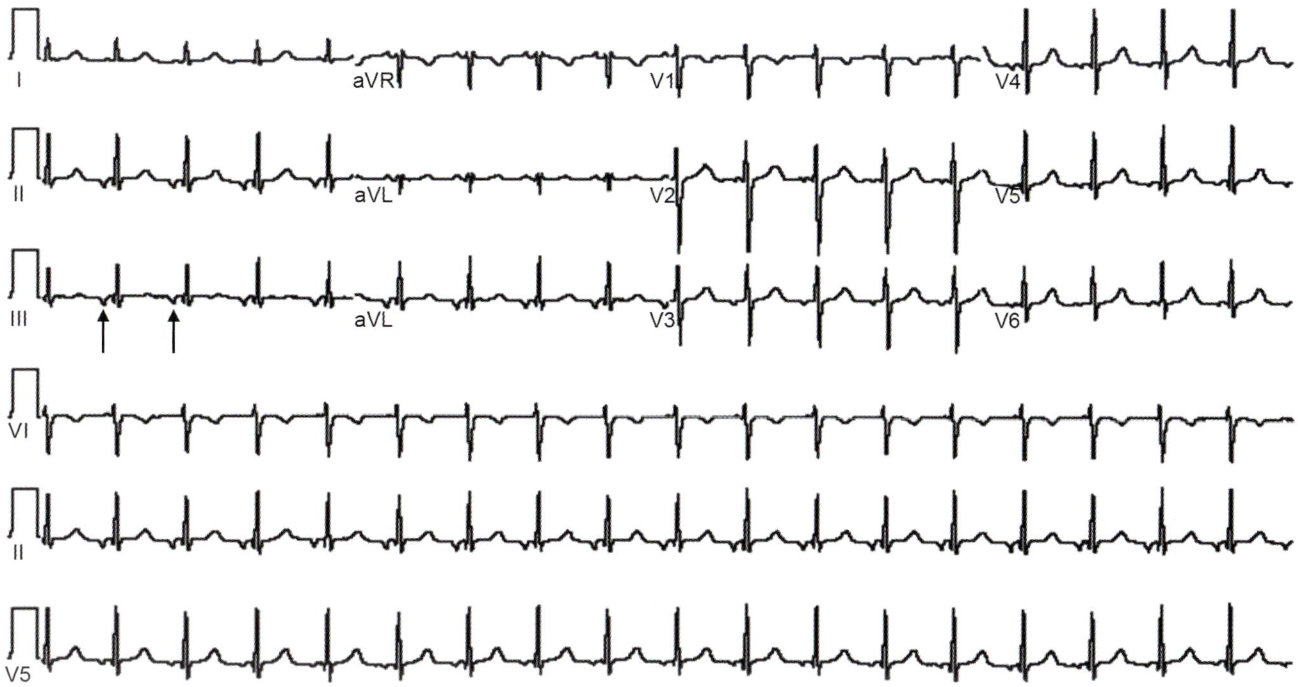

Figure 14.3: Long RP tachycardia secondary to accessory pathway with long conduction times because of decremental properties. P-waves are indicated by arrows

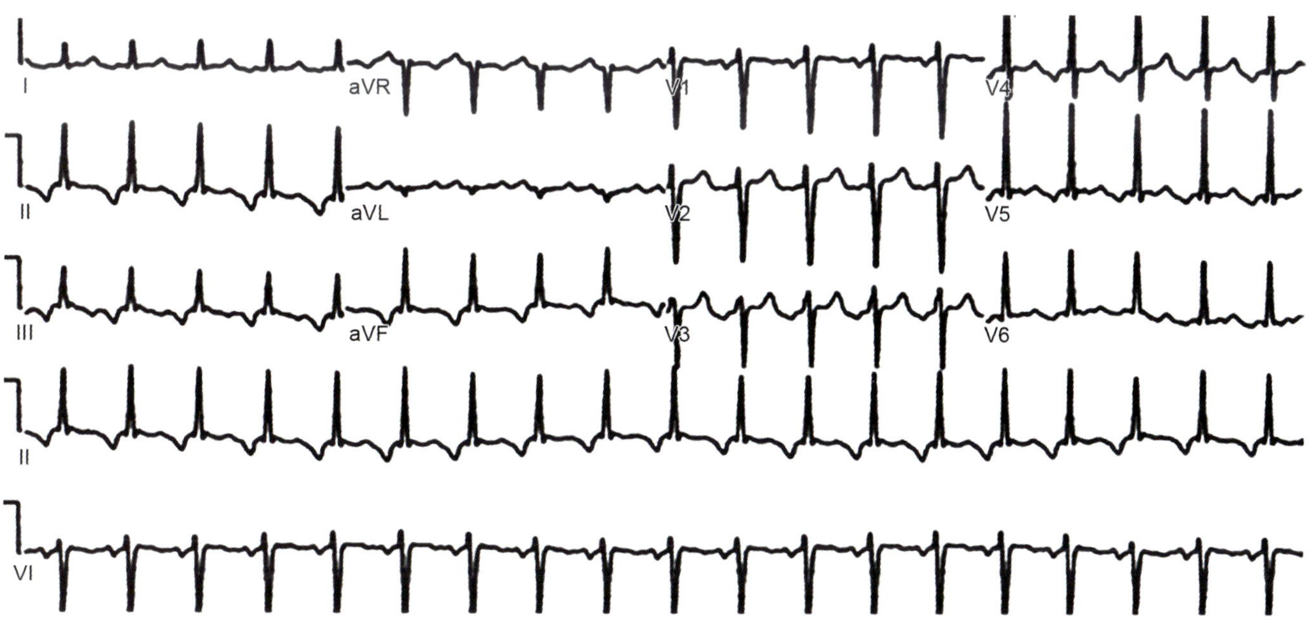

Figure 14.4: Note the long P-wave duration of 80 ms during an atrial tachycardia. This tachycardia was ablated at posterior tricuspid annulus (Unlike anterior interatrial septum, posterior interatrial septum is not contiguous between the right and left atria, leading to a wider P-wave)

near the atrial appendage, although previous surgery, ablation, scarring, and fibrosis may alter P-wave duration significantly. Negative P-waves in the inferior leads indicate most likely that the tricuspid annulus adjacent to coronary sinus is the source **(Figure 14.4)**. Inverted P-waves in aVL suggest a left atrial source either as a result of automatic AT or AVRT due to a left-sided accessory pathway. Positive P-waves in V1 indicate a posterior origin typically seen in left AT.

Termination

Termination with an A is suggestive of AV nodal dependence. Termination with a V is generally not specific of any type tachycardia mechanism. A spontaneous premature ventricular complex (PVC) that terminates a supraventricular tachycardia is in favor of accessory pathway-mediated tachycardia **(Figure 14.5)**, although AVNRT cannot be excluded.

Preexcitation

The presence of obvious preexcitation on the surface ECG in patients with narrow QRS SVT makes ORT (orthodromic reciprocating tachycardia) likely, but both AVNRT with a poorly-conducting bystander pathway and atrial tachycardia remain possibilities. Maximal preexcitation aids in localization of the pathway, whether it happens in sinus rhythm or during atrial fibrillation. Location of the pathway, AV nodal conduction, and intra-atrial conduction delay may influence the degree of preexcitation seen on an ECG. The ECGs in **Figures 14.6 and 14.7** are from two different patients with posteroseptal pathways, one in sinus rhythm and other during atrial fibrillation. Anterograde conduction properties of the accessory pathway are better assessed by measuring the shortest preexcited RR interval atrial fibrillation, with extremely short RR intervals <250 ms potentially increasing the risk of sudden death **(Figure 14.7)**.

Bundle Branch Block and Surface ECG

In the example shown in **Figure 14.8**, right bundle branch block (RBBB) does not prolong the cycle length of the tachycardia, which makes right sided accessory pathway-mediated ORT unlikely. In fact, a short RP interval with an RP duration less than 60 ms is in favor of slow/fast AVNRT. The spontaneous development of a bundle branch block that results in an increase in tachycardia cycle length is indicative of an ORT using an accessory pathway lying ipsilateral to the bundle branch block. For example, increase in tachycardia cycle length with left bundle branch block (LBBB) during an SVT indicates that the SVT in question is an ORT involving a left lateral accessory pathway.

BASELINE INTRACARDIAC ELECTROGRAM FINDINGS

Similar to surface ECG, findings on intracardiac electrograms of short RP versus long RP tachycardia are useful in the differential diagnosis of an SVT and are summarized in **Figure 14.9**.

Baseline observations of intracardiac electrograms have to be carefully analyzed for several features as outlined in **Figure 14.10**.

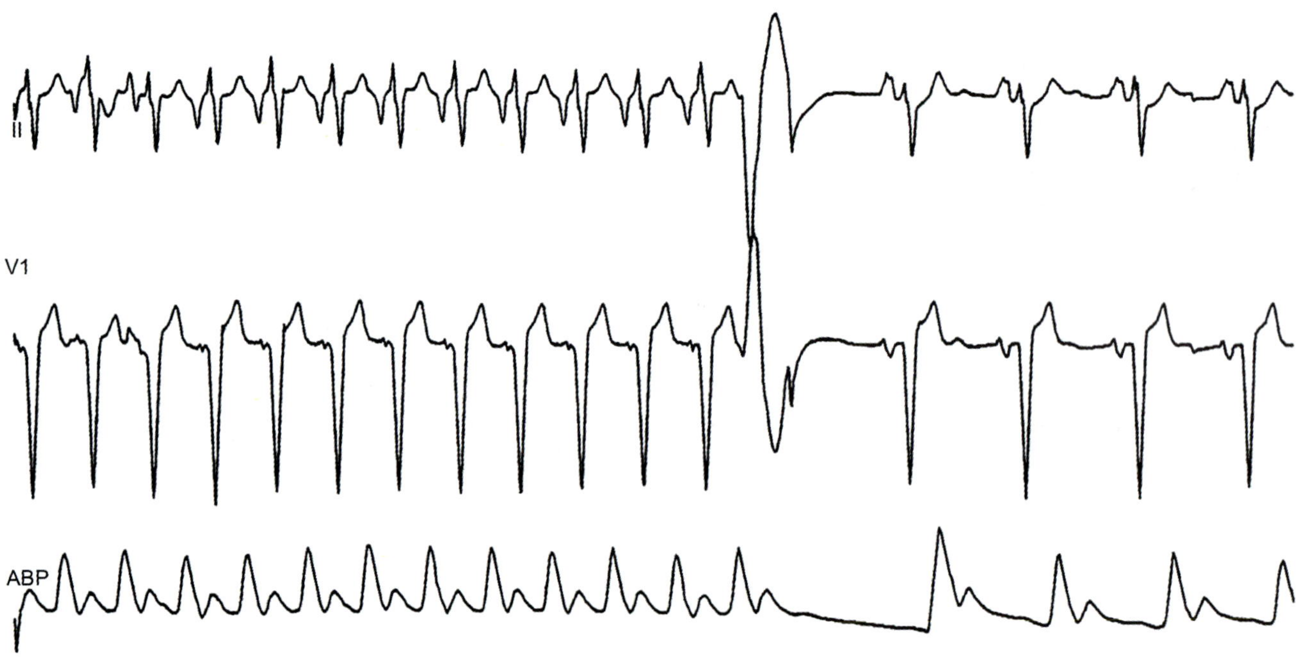

Figure 14.5: A long RP tachycardia terminated repeatedly by a PVC favors orthodromic reciprocating tachycardia in spite of being a long RP tachycardia

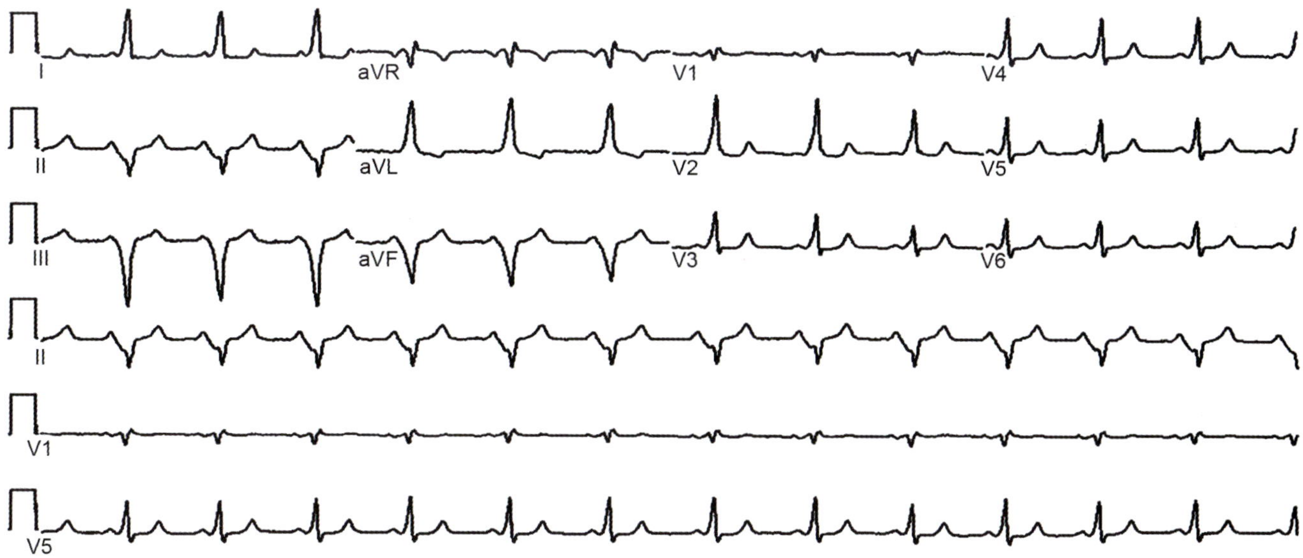

Figure 14.6: QRS morphology during sinus rhythm suggests preexcitation due to a posteroseptal accessory pathway that was confirmed to be in a coronary sinus diverticulum during ablation

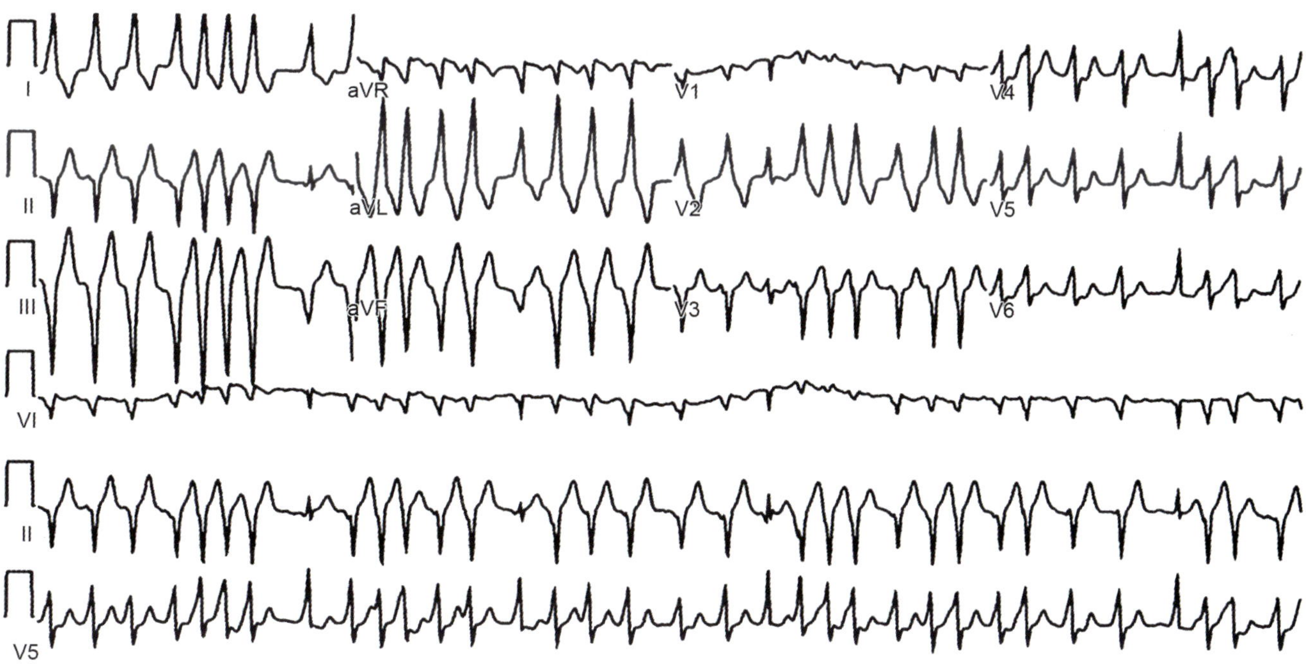

Figure 14.7: Preexcited atrial fibrillation with variable degrees of preexcitation via a right posteroseptal pathway. The shortest RR intervals being 240 ms predict an increased risk of sudden death

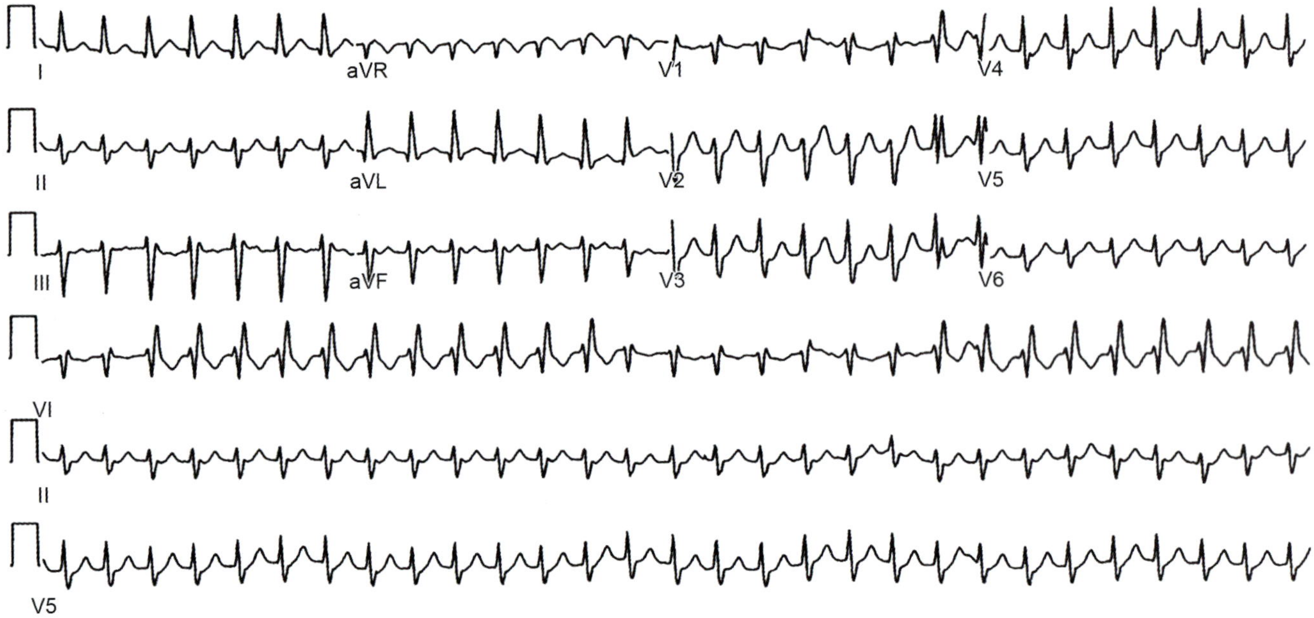

Figure 14.8: A RBBB does not alter the cycle length of the tachycardia, making right free wall accessory pathway-mediated ORT unlikely. In fact, because this is a short RP tachycardia with an RP duration of 40 ms, it is most likely typical slow/fast AVNRT with incidental RBBB

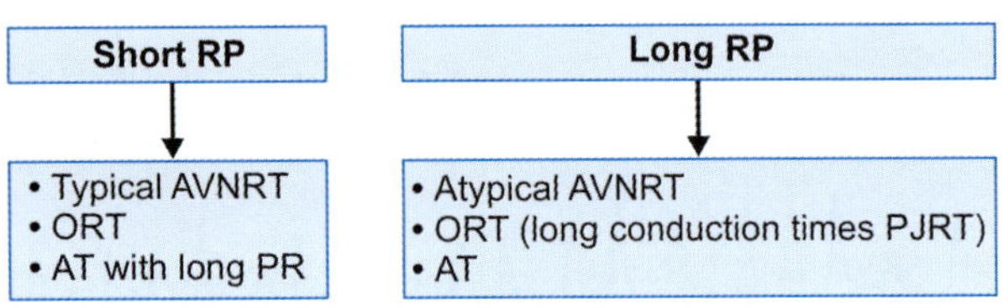

Typical AVNRT in children and elderly can be long RP

Figure 14.9: RP relationship in supraventricular tachycardia
Abbreviations: AT, atrial tachycardia; AVNRT, atrioventricular nodal reentrant tachycardia; ORT, orthodromic reciprocating tachycardia

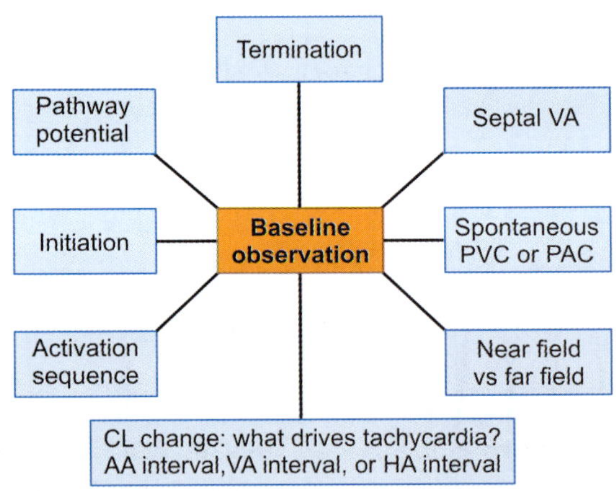

Figure 14.10: Analysis of baseline features on intracardiac electrograms during electrophysiologic study
Abbreviations: CL, cycle length; PAC, premature atrial complex; PVC, premature ventricular complex

Initiation

A 2:1 QRS response to a single atrial stimulus demonstrates the presence of two functionally distinct AV nodal pathways. If a 2:1 QRS response to a single atrial stimulus initiates a short RP tachycardia, this observation is very suggestive of typical slow-fast AVNRT **(Figure 14.11)**.

Atypical AVNRT (fast/slow type) is more commonly initiated while pacing the ventricle. The ventricular extrastimulus conducts through the slow pathway (with the earliest atrial electrogram near the CS os) as part of the retrograde limb of the tachycardia. The antegrade limb produces a very short AH interval, indicating the conduction occurs through the fast pathway. The reason that the AH interval is very short for the cycle length of the tachycardia is that the conduction to the His via fast pathway takes place concurrently while the impulse is still breaking out to the atrium **(Figure 14.12)**.

It is not uncommon to see intra-atrial reentry precipitating AVNRT as shown in **Figure 14.13**. The nonsustained reentry is unable to enter the fast pathway due to its longer repolarization time. However, the slow pathway area is eventually engaged, leading to slow/fast AV node reentry.

The most common way to initiate typical AVNRT is shown in **Figure 14.14**. A timed atrial extrastimulus finds the fast pathway refractory but conducts through the slow pathway.

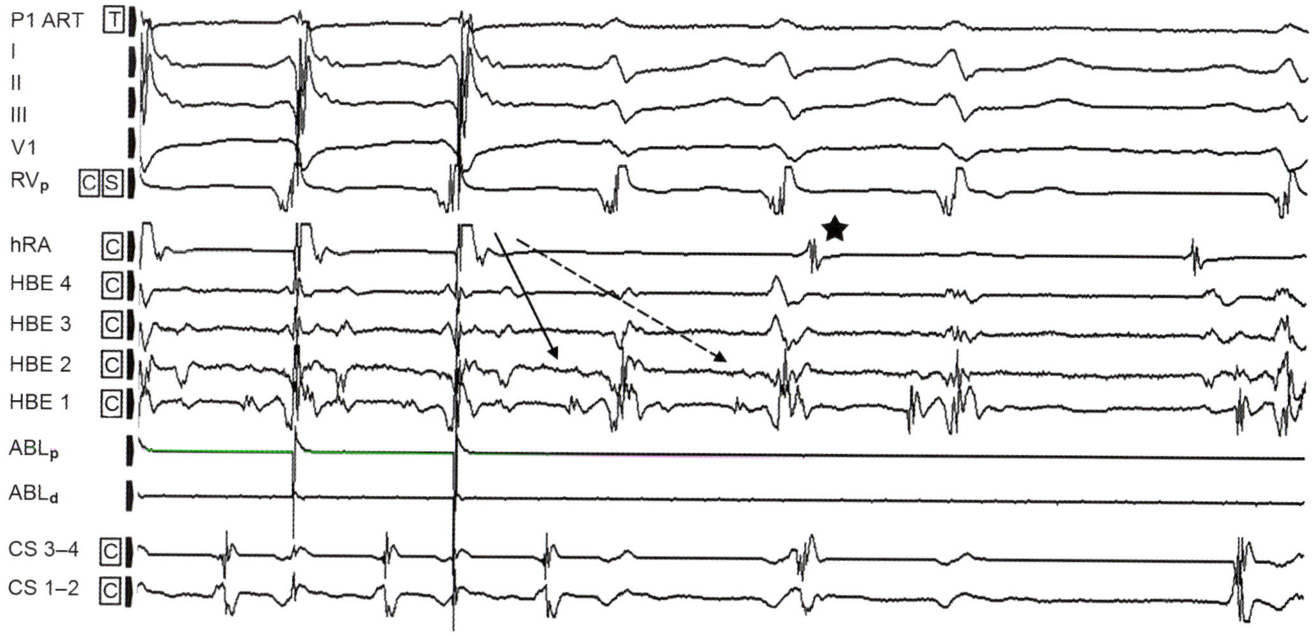

Figure 14.11: A single timed atrial extrastimulus causes the first QRS complex through the fast pathway (solid arrow) and the second QRS complex through the slow pathway (dash type arrow) with a return echo via the recovered fast pathway (star). The impulse then conducts through the atrium and slow pathway, resulting in an intermediary AH interval, before encountering the refractory fast pathway and terminating. Even if this is only observation in a patient with documented short RP SVT, AVNRT becomes the most likely diagnosis, and the slow pathway may be ablated

From top to bottom are—intra-arterial blood pressure (P1ART); surface ECG leads I, II, III and V1; right ventricular proximal electrogram (RV_p); high right atrium (hRA); His bundle proximal (HBE 4), mid (HBE 3 and 2) and distal (HBE 1); ablation proximal and distal (ABL_p and ABL_d); and coronary sinus mid (CS 3–4) and distal (CS 1–2)

It encounters the now-repolarized fast pathway to complete the reentry circuit. The earliest atrial electrogram is at anterior interatrial septum near the His bundle catheter.

Effect of a Spontaneous Bundle Branch Block

In **Figure 14.15**, both the paced ventricular extrastimulus and the nonsustained bundle branch reentry beat with a LBBB pattern have an eccentric atrial activation with longer VA interval in contrast to the SVT beats with a narrow QRS. The correlation of a different atrial activation pattern with a different ventricular site of activation suggests that the eccentric activation sequence is due to ventriculoatrial conduction via an accessory pathway, rather than an atrial extrasystole arising from left atrium. During a right bundle branch block, the VA interval is similar to the VA interval during a narrow QRS, providing additional evidence that the eccentric activation sequence is due to a left sided accessory pathway. The fact that the tachycardia cycle length shortens with a narrow QRS indicates that the accessory pathway participates in this tachycardia. The same principle mentioned above when discussing ECG features applies to intracardiac electrogram interpretation: an ipsilateral bundle branch block will lengthen the cycle length of an accessory pathway-mediated tachycardia. However, during contralateral bundle branch block, AH lengthening due to slowing of conduction in the AV node may result in a slower tachycardia cycle length.

SVT with AV Block

While any lack of 1:1 AV relationship excludes almost all ORT with atrioventricular accessory pathways, AVNRT is not ruled out completely. Since block at the His or infra-His level is outside of the AVNRT reentry circuit, the tachycardia can continue despite the existence of AV block. Whenever the P-wave is at mid-point between two successive QRS complexes, typical AVNRT with 2:1 atrioventricular conduction should be considered in the differential diagnosis (*see* **Figures 14.16A and B**). The site of block is usually at the infra-His level. In **Figure 14.16A**, 2:1 block may appear to be in the lower common pathway, however, closer inspection of the proximal His catheter electrogram reveals far-field His in intracardiac electrogram without QRS complexes (not an unusual finding), confirming that the block is at infra-His level. Later on in the

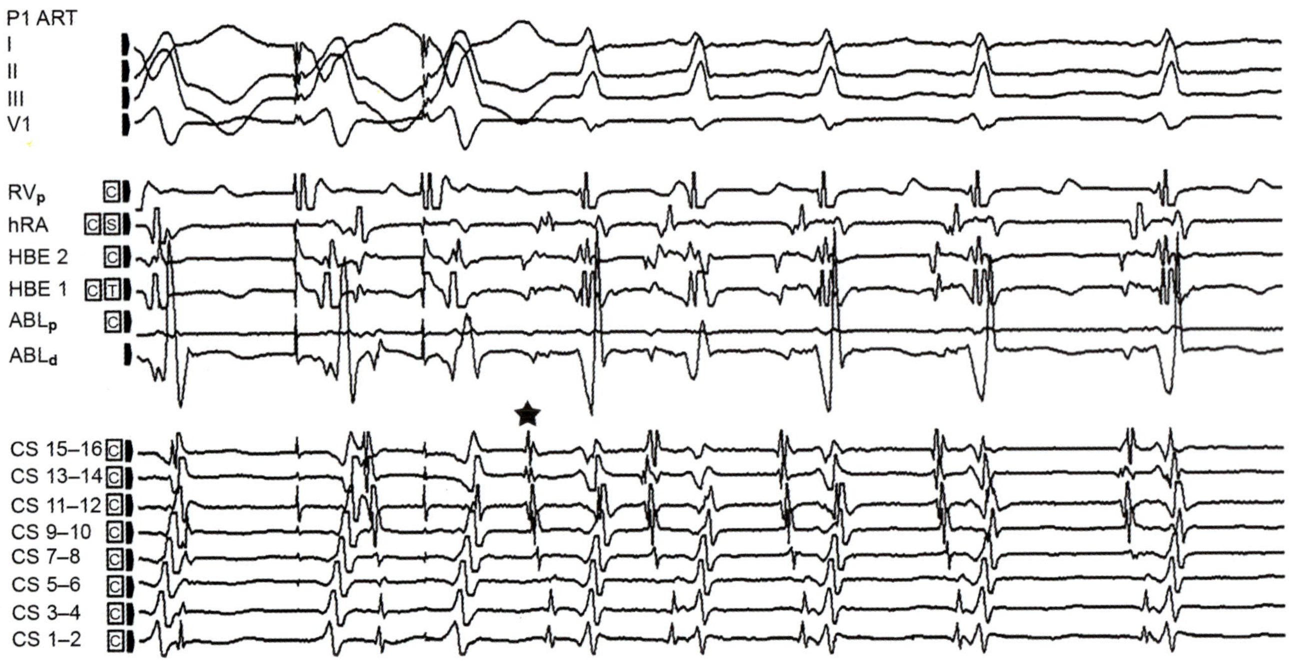

Figure 14.12: A timed ventricular extrastimulus conducts retrograde via the slow pathway (the earliest atrial electrogram occurs near the CS os, indicated by a star). The antegrade AH interval is very short because it is a pseudointerval; conduction via the fast pathway is already taking place while the impulse is still conducting through the slow pathway to reach the atrium. Although changes in the VA interval are largely determining the changes in tachycardia cycle length fluctuation, the AH interval is too short for sequential conduction that would be expected in an ORT
From top to bottom are—intra-arterial blood pressure (P1ART); surface ECG leads I, II, III and V1; right ventricular proximal electrogram (RV_p); high right atrium (hRA); His bundle proximal (HBE 4), mid (HBE 3 and 2) and distal (HBE 1); ablation proximal and distal (ABL_p and ABL_d); and coronary sinus proximal (CS 15–16) to distal (CS 1–2)

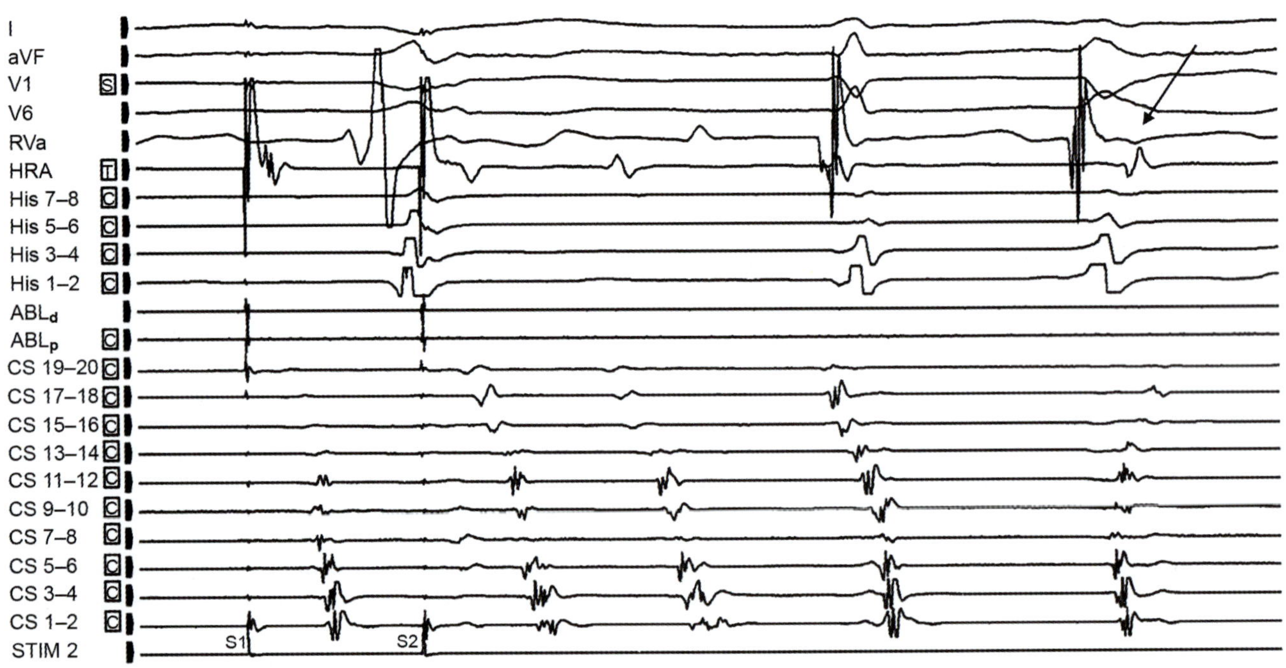

Figure 14.13: Intra-atrial reentry precipitates typical slow/fast AVNRT. The solid arrow points to the first beat of subsequent AVNRT
From top to bottom are—surface ECG leads I, aVF, V1 and V6; right ventricular electrogram (RVa); high right atrium (HRA); His bundle proximal (His 7–8), mid (His 5–6 and His 3–4) and distal (His 1–2); ablation distal and proximal (ABL_d and ABL_p); and coronary sinus proximal (CS 19–20) to distal (CS 1–2)

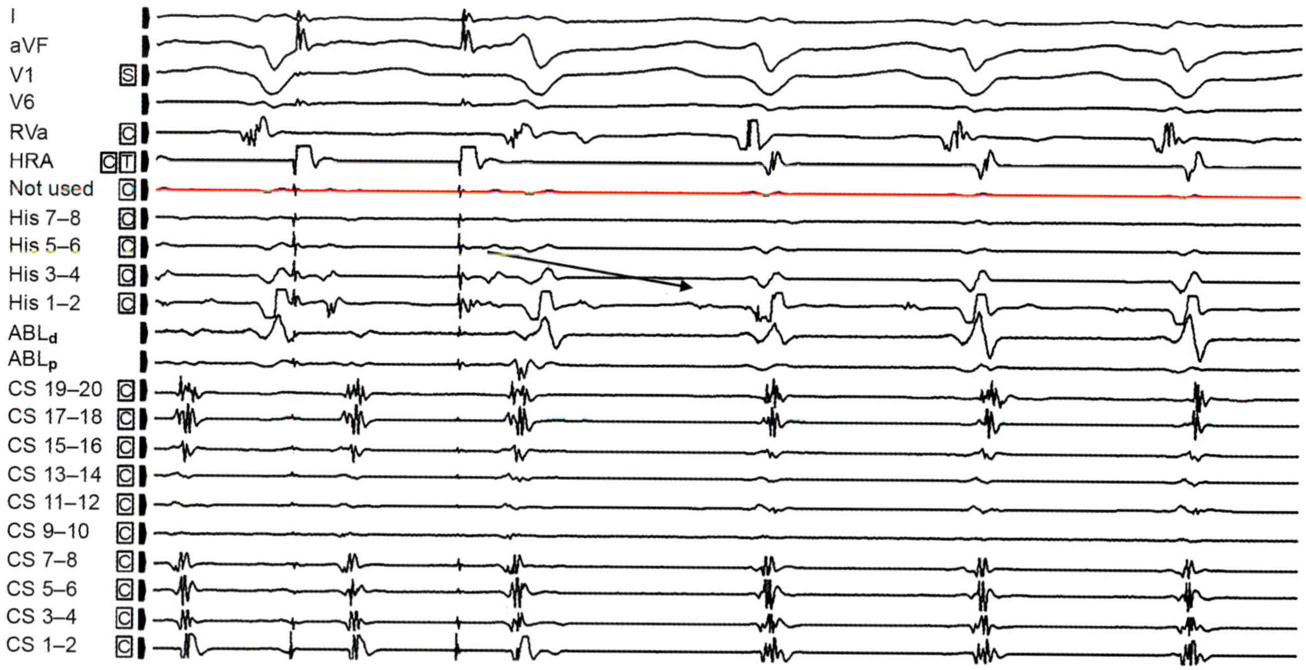

Figure 14.14: A timed atrial extrastimulus conducts through the slow pathway, initiating slow/fast AVNRT. The initiating AH interval is marked with a solid arrow. Note that the initial atrial electrogram is recorded by the His catheter and the VA interval during tachycardia is <70 ms
From top to bottom are—surface ECG leads I, aVF, V1 and V6; right ventricular electrogram (RVa); high right atrium (HRA); His bundle proximal (His 7–8), mid (His 5–6 and His 3–4) and distal (His 1–2); ablation distal and proximal (ABL_d and ABL_p); and coronary sinus proximal (CS 19–20) to distal (CS 1–2)

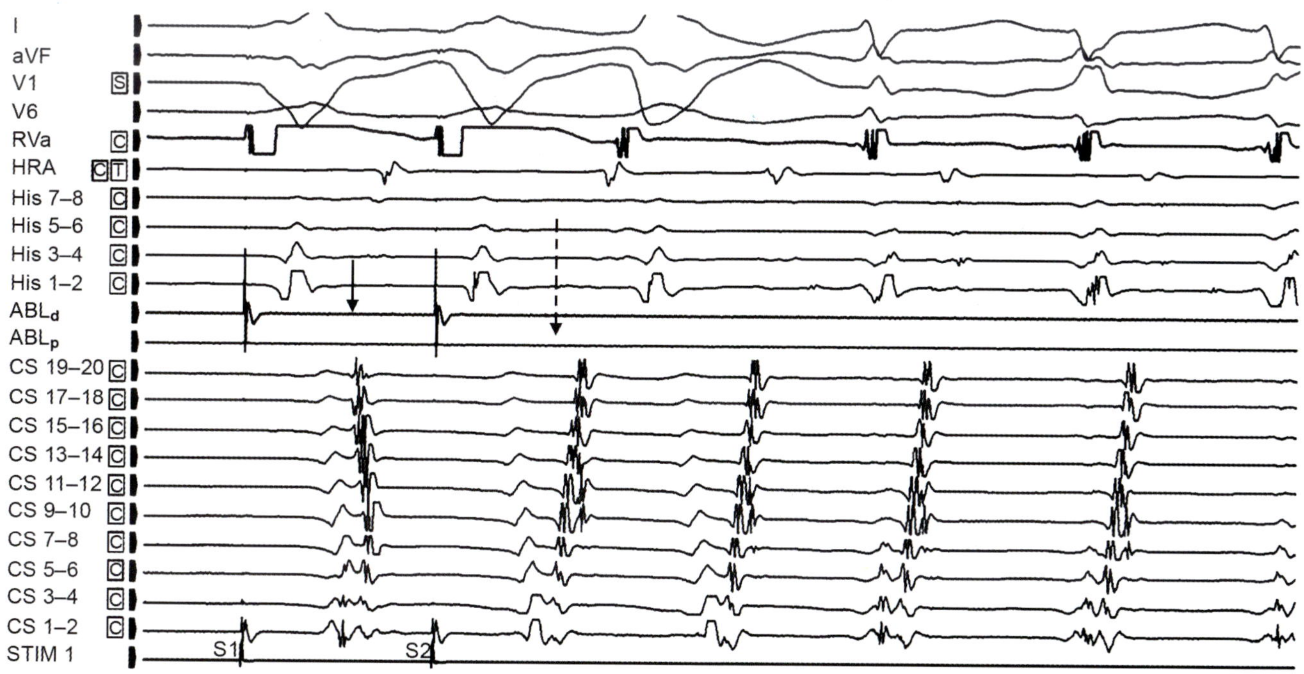

Figure 14.15: Ventricular drive train pacing conducts through both the AV node and an accessory pathway (first arrow). A ventricular extrastimulus conducts through the accessory pathway with eccentric activation (second arrow). See text for additional details
From top to bottom are—surface ECG leads I, aVF, V1 and V6; right ventricular electrogram (RVa); high right atrium (HRA); His bundle proximal (His 7–8), mid (His 5–6 and His 3–4) and distal (His 1–2); ablation distal and proximal (ABL_d and ABL_p); and coronary sinus proximal (CS 19–20) to distal (CS 1–2)

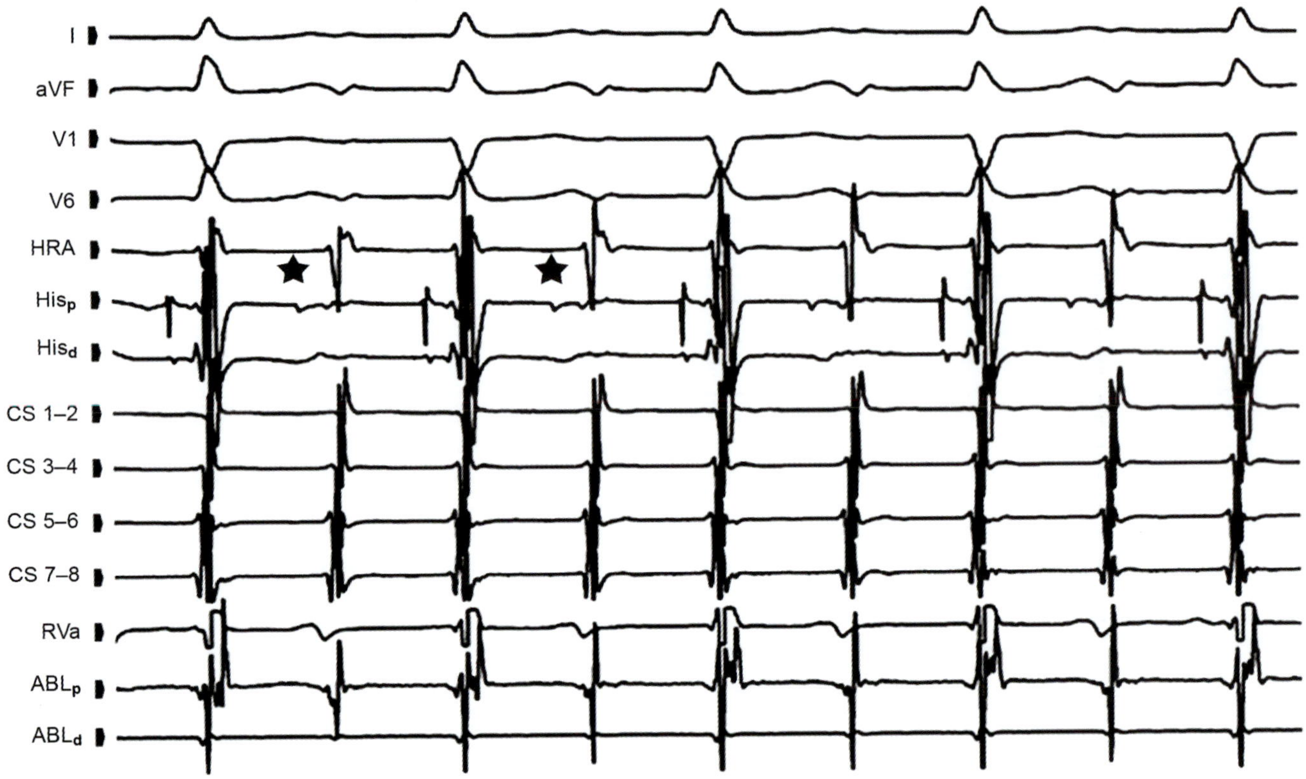

Figure 14.16A: Typical slow/fast AVNRT with 2:1 AV conduction. The stars point to far-field His electrograms consistent with typical AVNRT with 2:1 infra-His block. See text for details

From top to bottom are—surface ECG leads I, aVF, V1 and V6; high right atrium (HRA); His bundle proximal (His_p) and distal (His_d); coronary sinus distal (CS 1–2) to proximal (CS 7–8); right ventricular apex (RVa); and ablation proximal (ABL_p) and distal (ABL_d) signals

study, 1:1 conduction was consistent (*see* **Figure 14.16B**), and the activation pattern was consistent with typical slow/fast AVNRT with the earliest atrial electrogram at the anterior interatrial septum, seen on the His catheter.

A lack of 1:1 response more commonly favors atrial tachycardia. In **Figure 14.17**, even though the interval between the atrial (HRA) electrograms and the QRS complexes is increasing, the atrial cycle length is unaltered, suggesting that the atrial activation is independent from AV nodal conduction, making AVNRT unlikely. These findings, along with an eccentric activation sequence in the coronary sinus catheter, make it likely that this is an atrial tachycardia arising from the left atrium.

Septal VA Interval

Septal VA interval is an important observation that helps in rapid assessment of tachycardia. The septal VA interval is usually <70 ms at the truly contiguous anterior interatrial septum in AVNRT (note that the posterior interatrial septum near the coronary sinus is not contiguous, but separated by a triangular space). The short septal VA interval indicates that the retrograde depolarization of the fast pathway is taking place at the same time when the antegrade stimulation of the ventricle is occurring. This is not a true interval because the conduction is not from the ventricle to the atrium, but conduction is bidirectional to atrium and ventricle concurrently from a point where the slow pathway meets the fast pathway. A septal VA interval of <70 ms is used to differentiate AVNRT from accessory pathway-mediated ORT (*see* **Figure 14.18**). While this is not absolutely diagnostic (as it is possible that atrial electrogram may conduct to subsequent ventricular electrogram), it is more probable to be typical AVNRT. In ORT, the impulse must activate the ventricle and reach the base of the heart before conducting to the atrium through the accessory pathway. Thus, a septal VA interval even in an anteroseptal pathway is >80 ms because at least 80 ms is required for the ventricular activation to reach the base of the heart.

Even though the atrial electrogram is earliest at the His catheter in typical AVNRT, when high density electrodes are used on His catheter (2 mm spacing), it is not uncommon to see that the fast pathway breaks through at the proximal electrodes of His catheter and then spreads towards the annular atrial tissue as evidenced by the atrial electrogram on the distal His catheter (*see* **Figure 14.19**).

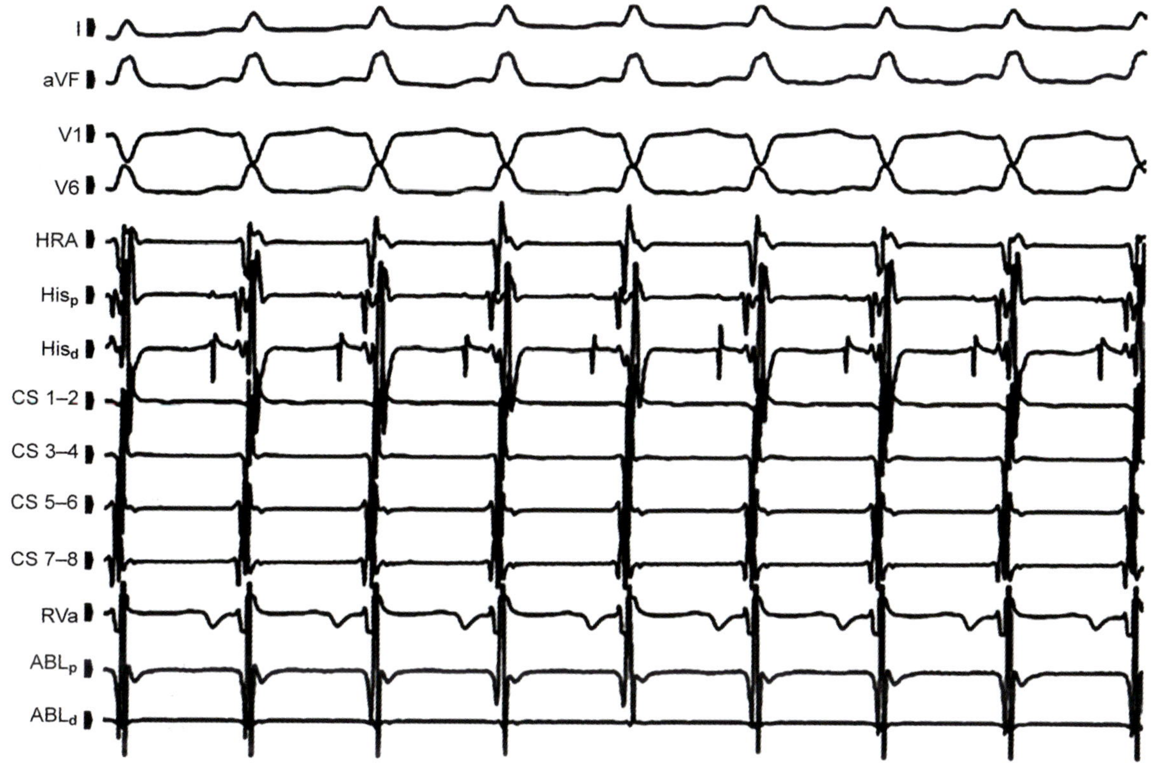

Figure 14.16B: Later in the study, the tachycardia conducts 1:1, consistent with typical slow/fast AVNRT
From top to bottom are—surface ECG leads I, aVF, V1 and V6; high right atrium (HRA); His bundle proximal (His_p) and distal (His_d); coronary sinus distal (CS 1–2) to proximal (CS 7–8); right ventricular apex (RVa); and ablation proximal (ABL_p) and distal (ABL_d) signals

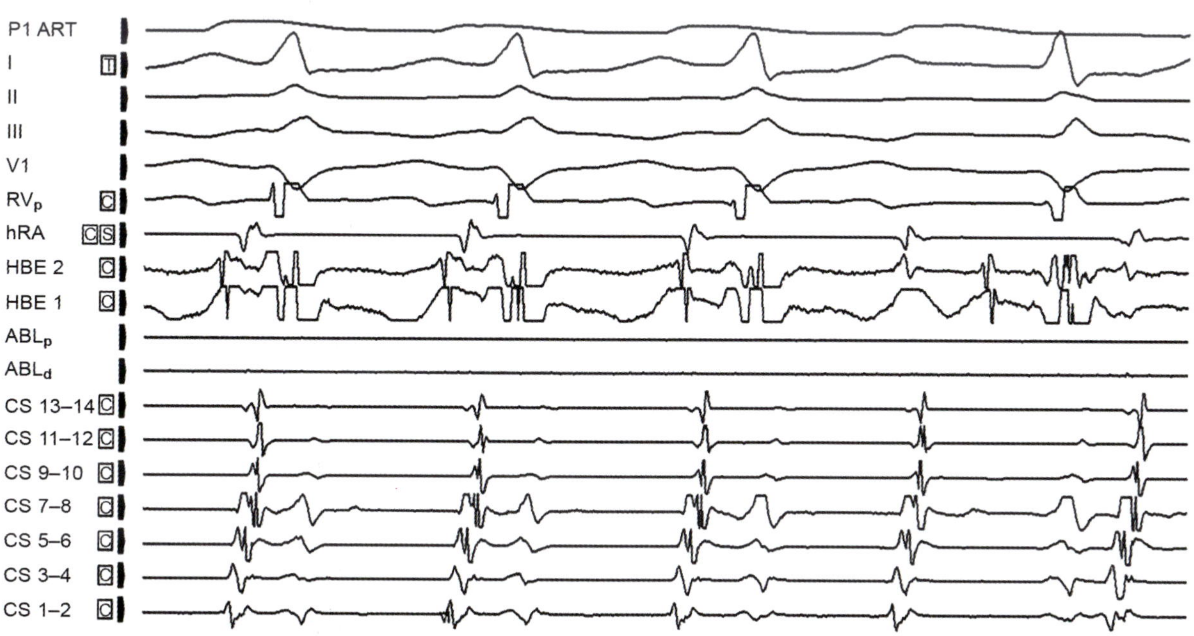

Figure 14.17: Ectopic left atrial tachycardia showing independence from AV node conduction and eccentric activation of the coronary sinus catheter. See text for details
From top to bottom are—intra-arterial blood pressure (P1ART); surface ECG leads I, II, III and V1; right ventricular proximal electrogram (RV_p); high right atrium (hRA); His bundle proximal (HBE 4), mid (HBE 3 and 2) and distal (HBE 1); ablation proximal and distal (ABL_p and ABL_d); and coronary sinus proximal (CS 13–14) to distal (CS 1–2)

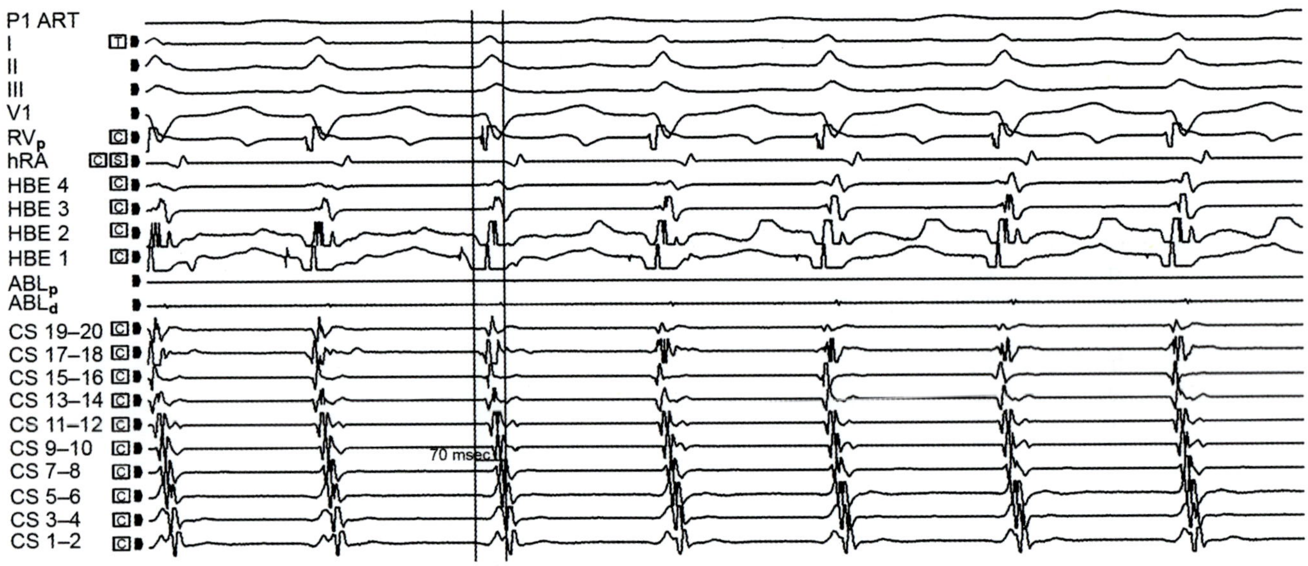

Figure 14.18: A septal VA interval of <70 ms favors typical AVNRT. See text for details
From top to bottom are—intra-arterial blood pressure (P1 ART); surface ECG leads I, II, III and V1; right ventricular proximal electrogram (RV_p); high right atrium (hRA); His bundle proximal (HBE 4), mid (HBE 3 and 2) and distal (HBE 1); ablation proximal and distal (ABL_p and ABL_d); and coronary sinus proximal (CS 15–16) to distal (CS 1–2)

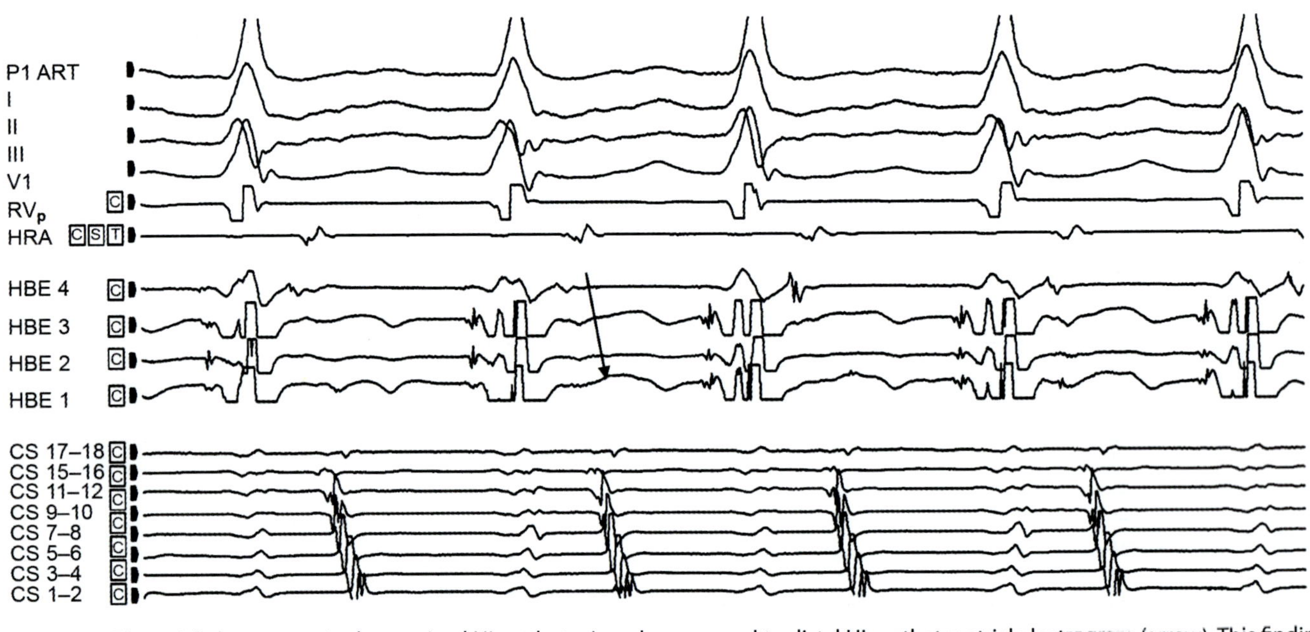

Figure 14.19: The atrial electrogram in the proximal His catheter is early compared to distal His catheter atrial electrogram (arrow). This finding is observed because of better atrial activation sequence resolution from 2 mm-spaced electrodes. The fast pathway breaks out away from the annulus, and activation spreads towards the annulus from the break out site. In accessory pathway-mediated ORT, the earliest electrogram occurs closer to the annulus. See text for further details
From top to bottom are—intra-arterial blood pressure (P1ART); surface ECG leads I, II, III and V1; right ventricular proximal electrogram (RV_p); high right atrium (hRA); His bundle proximal (HBE 4), mid (HBE 3 and 2) and distal (HBE 1); and coronary sinus proximal (CS 17–18) to distal (CS 1–2)

Baseline EP Study Findings before Tachycardia Induction

During ventricular extrastimuli, if the HRA electrogram precedes or coincides with the septal electrogram, then a right sided accessory pathway must be in the differential diagnosis **(Figure 14.20)**.

When there is a right-sided accessory pathway in the differential diagnosis, it is worthwhile placing a halo catheter around the tricuspid annulus to identify the region of interest by bracketing the annular electrogram **(Figures 14.21A and B)**.

In short RP tachycardia, when the P-waves are upright in the inferior leads or the high right atrial electrogram precedes the annular electrogram, atrial tachycardia is likely. **(Figure 14.22)**.

What Drives the Tachycardia?

Any fluctuation or wobble in the cycle length of the tachycardia needs to be carefully explored. This usually happens at the onset of tachycardia, but may occur anytime during the study. The tachycardia cycle length in reentry is dependent on the sum of multiple subintervals. For example, in typical AVNRT, the cycle length is a sum of the AH interval and the HA interval. In ORT, it is sum of the AV interval and the VA interval. In atrial tachycardia, a change of subintervals is of no consequence to the subsequent tachycardia cycle length, because the area of automaticity driving the tachycardia is not affected by the activation of distant structures.

Fixed AA Interval and AV Node Independence

The AA interval is the only interval of significance in atrial tachycardia. Subinterval changes such as AH interval change does not predictably influence the subsequent tachycardia, suggestive of independence from AV nodal conduction (*see* **Figures 14.22 and 14.23**).

VA Interval Change and the Influence of a Spontaneous Bundle Branch Block on the Tachycardia

VA interval change influencing tachycardia cycle length change is usually due to accessory pathway-mediated

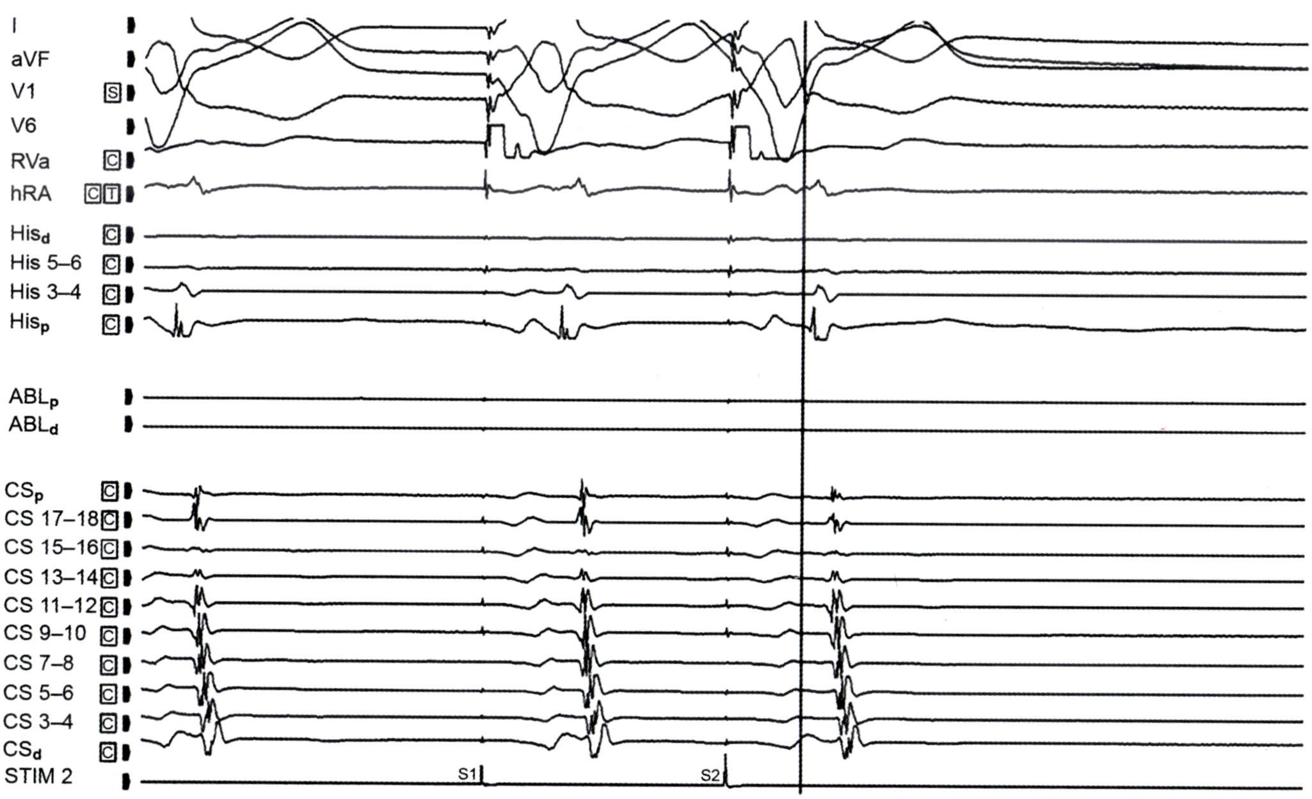

Figure 14.20: During baseline ventricular extrastimulus testing, the HRA electrogram precedes the annular septal electrogram, suggesting a right-sided accessory pathway

From top to bottom are—surface ECG leads I, aVF, V1 and V6; right ventricular apex (RVa); high right atrium (hRA); His bundle distal (His$_d$) mid (His 5–6 and His 3–4) and proximal (His$_p$); ablation proximal and distal (ABL$_p$ and ABL$_d$); and coronary sinus proximal (CS$_p$), mid (CS 17–18 to CS 3–4), and distal (CS$_d$)

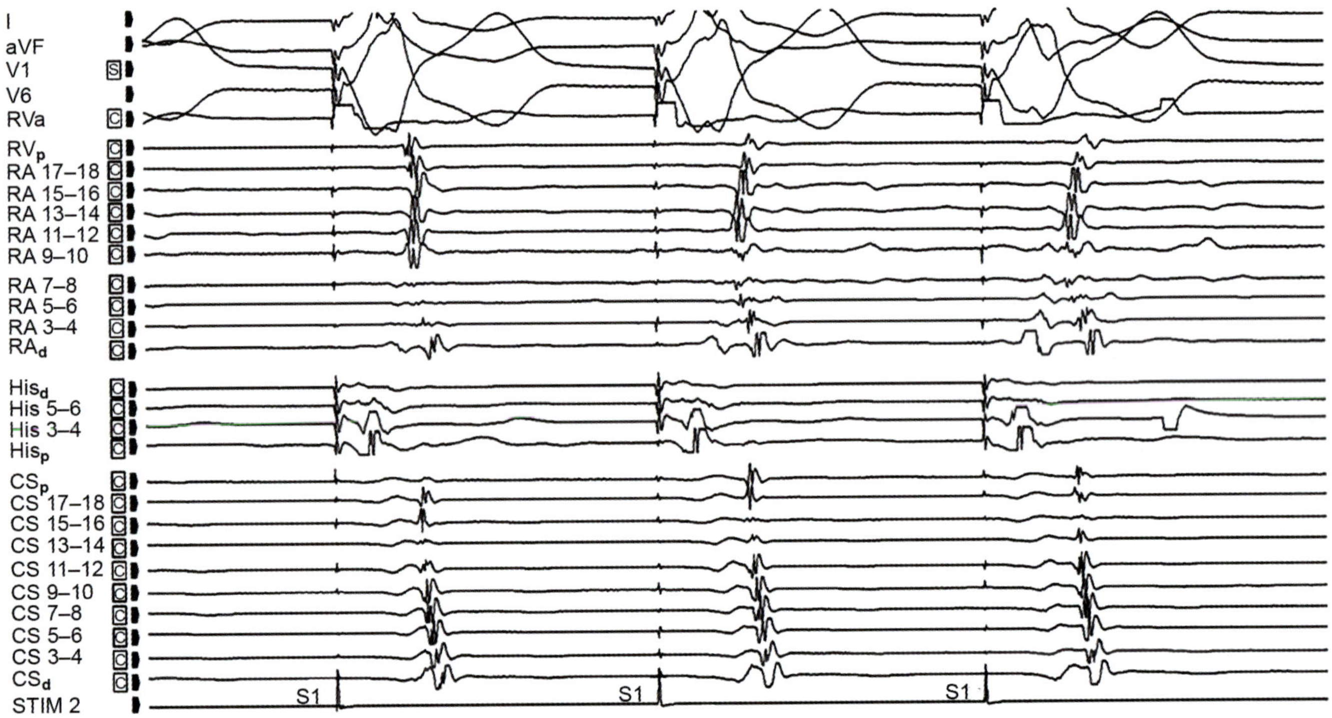

Figure 14.21A: Halo catheter electrograms bracket the right sided accessory pathway location
From top to bottom are—surface ECG leads I, aVF, V1 and V6; right ventricle distal (RVa) and proximal (RV_p); halo catheter proximal (RA 17–18) to proximal (RA_d); His bundle distal (His_d), mid (His 5–6 and His 3–4), and proximal (His_p); coronary sinus proximal (CS_p), mid (CS 17–18 to CS 3–4), and distal (CS_d); and stim channel

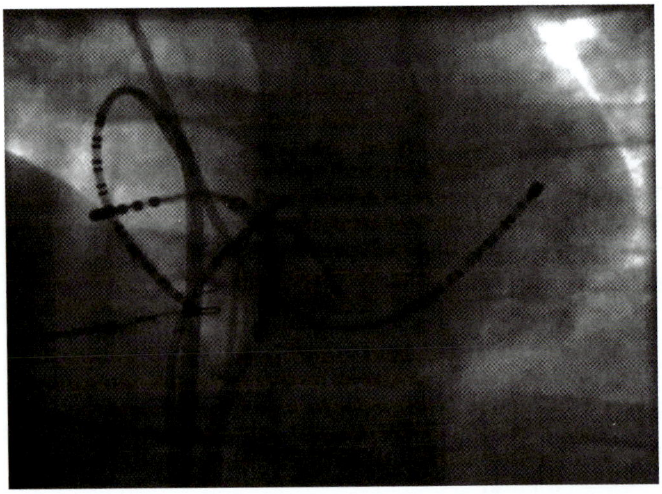

Figure 14.21B: The fluoroscopic image of the halo catheter bracketing the right sided-accessory pathway being used to guide the ablation catheter to the accessory pathway location

tachycardia although atypical AVNRT (fast/slow) may exhibit such a feature (*see* **Figure 14.12**). However, a spontaneous bundle branch block is particularly useful in evaluating the effect of a change in the VA interval, and, if it happens, it requires careful assessment. If the tachycardia cycle length is lengthened by the development of a bundle branch block, the presence of ipsilateral accessory pathway participating in tachycardia is confirmed (*see* **Figures 14.24 and 14.25**). Conversely, if there is no change in tachycardia cycle length with the spontaneous development of a bundle branch block,

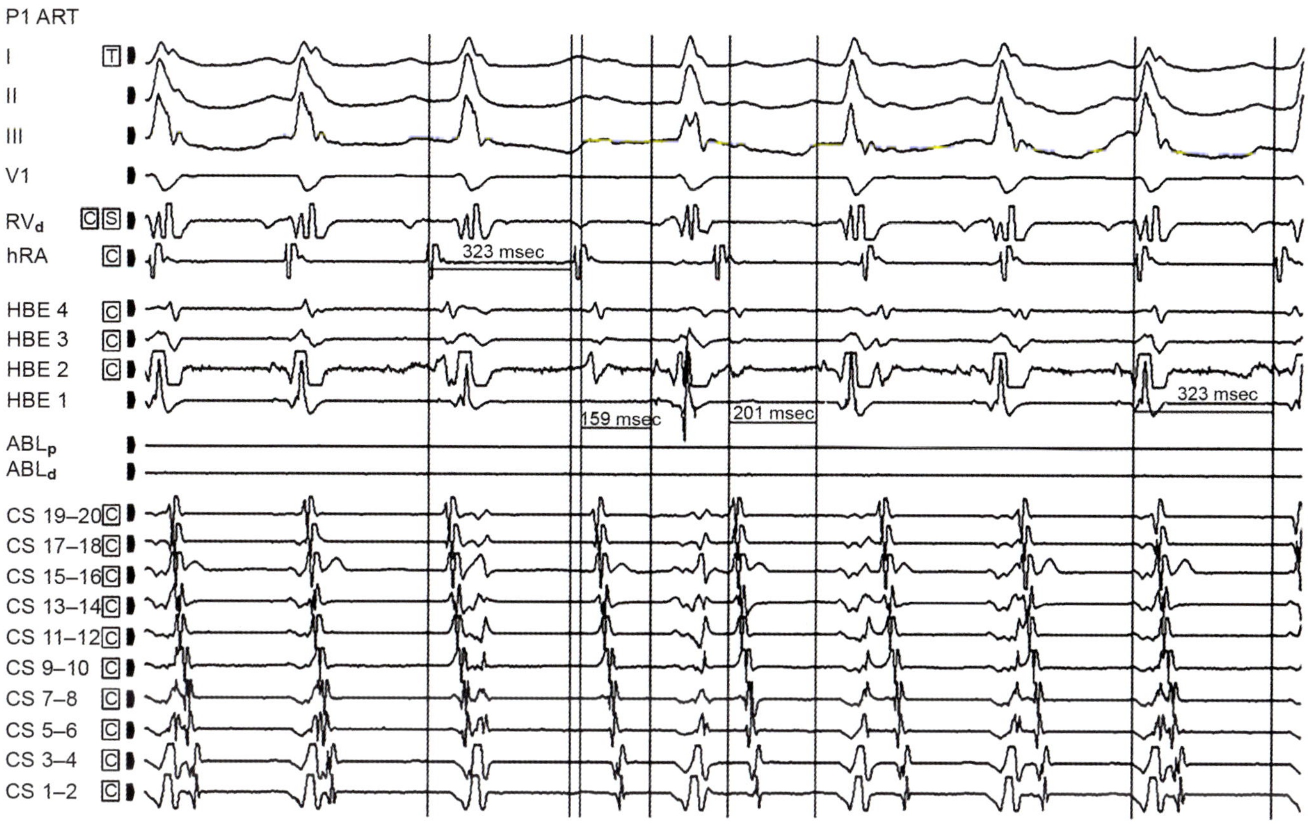

Figure 14.22: Atrial tachycardia shows independence from the AV nodal conduction, because the AH subinterval change has no effect on the AA interval

From top to bottom are—intra-arterial blood pressure (P1 ART); surface ECG leads I, II, III and V1; right ventricular distal electrogram (RV_d); high right atrium (hRA); His bundle proximal (HBE 4), mid (HBE 3 and 2) and distal (HBE 1); ablation proximal and distal (ABL_p and ABL_d); and coronary sinus proximal (CS 19–20) to distal (CS 1–2)

then a free wall accessory pathway on the same side as the bundle branch block is unlikely (*see* **Figure 14.26**).

HA Interval

The HA interval is a pseudointerval in typical AVNRT. Because the lower common pathway is very small in patients with typical AVNRT, an HA interval change that results in a change in the tachycardia cycle length is usually reflective of typical AVNRT. Conversely, an HA interval change that does not affect the tachycardia cycle length makes typical AVNRT unlikely (*see* **Figures 14.27 and 14.28**).

Spontaneous AV Block

If the tachycardia continues despite spontaneous AV block, in other words, without 1:1 AV relationship, not only is an accessory pathway-mediated tachycardia excluded, but an atrial tachycardia becomes much more likely (*see* **Figure 14.29**). However, 2:1 AV conduction can occur in AVNRT.

Tachycardia termination with a ventricular electrogram is not diagnostic, but it is common in atrial tachycardia (*see* **Figure 14.30**).

On the other hand, termination with an atrial electrogram is suggestive of AV node dependence, and indicates either AVNRT or an accessory pathway-mediated ORT (*see* **Figure 14.31**).

Pathway Potentials

Pathway potentials (sharp near-field electrograms occurring between ventricular and atrial activation, *see* **Figure 14.32**) indicate great locations for successful ablation, provided pathway participation is confirmed on further testing.

Spontaneous PVC during His Refractoriness

A spontaneous PVC falling while the His bundle is refractory is rare. If it fortuitously happens as in **Figure 14.33**, and the subsequent atrial signal is advanced, then presence

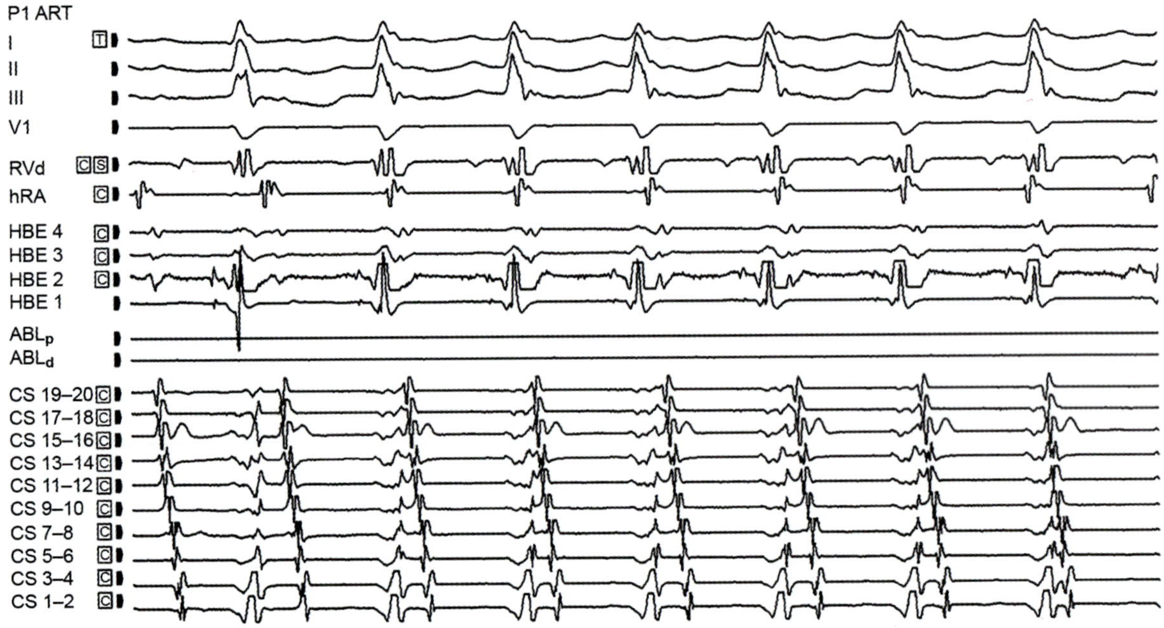

Figure 14.23: A short septal VA interval is seen, but the VA relationship is slowly changing without AA interval change, indicating that AA interval is independent of AV node conduction (AH interval) and VA interval. Additionally, positive P-wave in lead III also favors atrial tachycardia
From top to bottom are—intra-arterial blood pressure (P1 ART); surface ECG leads I, II, III and V1; right ventricular distal electrogram (RV_d); high right atrium (hRA); His bundle proximal (HBE 4), mid (HBE 3 and 2) and distal (HBE 1); ablation proximal and distal (ABL_p and ABL_d); and coronary sinus proximal (CS 19–20) to distal (CS 1–2)

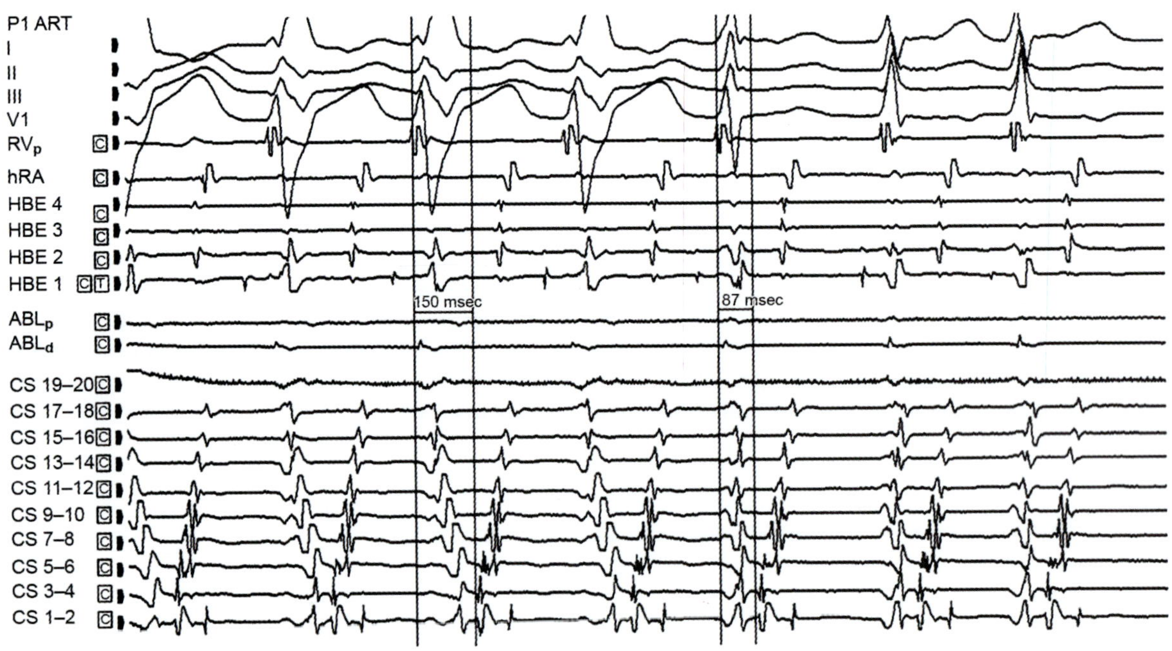

Figure 14.24: A spontaneous LBBB lengthens the tachycardia cycle length, corresponding to a VA interval change, confirming the participation of an accessory pathway in the left free wall. Additionally, on close inspection the CS 3,4 electrogram reveals the earliest near-field electrogram (CS origin) and far-field left atrial electrogram, suggesting that the pathway is inserted into the CS (coronary sinus) muscle coat. Ablation inside the CS was successful
From top to bottom are—intra-arterial blood pressure (P1 ART); surface ECG leads I, II, III and V1; right ventricular distal electrogram (RV_d); high right atrium (hRA); His bundle proximal (HBE 4), mid (HBE 3 and 2) and distal (HBE 1); ablation proximal and distal (ABL_p and ABL_d); and coronary sinus proximal (CS 19–20) to distal (CS 1–2)

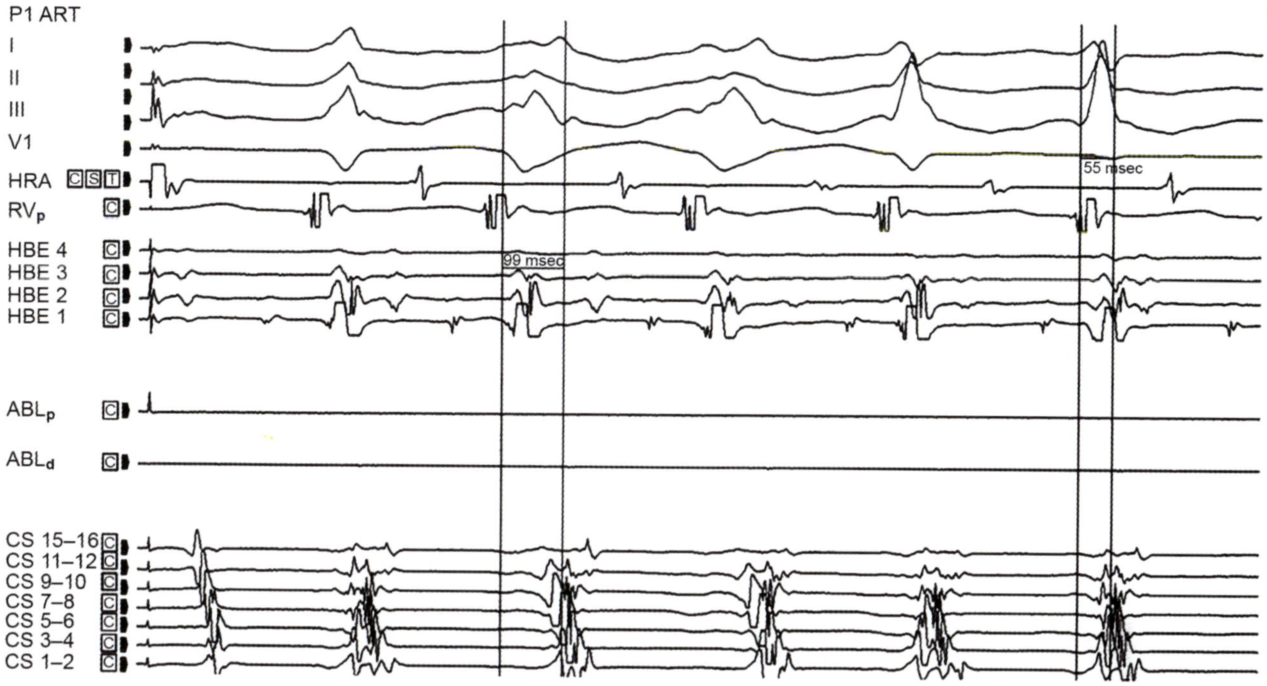

Figure 14.25: A spontaneous LBBB lengthens the VA interval and the tachycardia cycle length, indicating a left-sided accessory pathway participating in the tachycardia. See text for details

From top to bottom are—intra-arterial blood pressure (P1 ART); surface ECG leads I, II, III and V1; high right atrium (HRA); right ventricular proximal electrogram (RV_p); His bundle proximal (HBE 4), mid (HBE 3 and 2) and distal (HBE 1); ablation proximal and distal (ABL_p and ABL_d); and coronary sinus proximal (CS 15–16) to distal (CS 1–2)

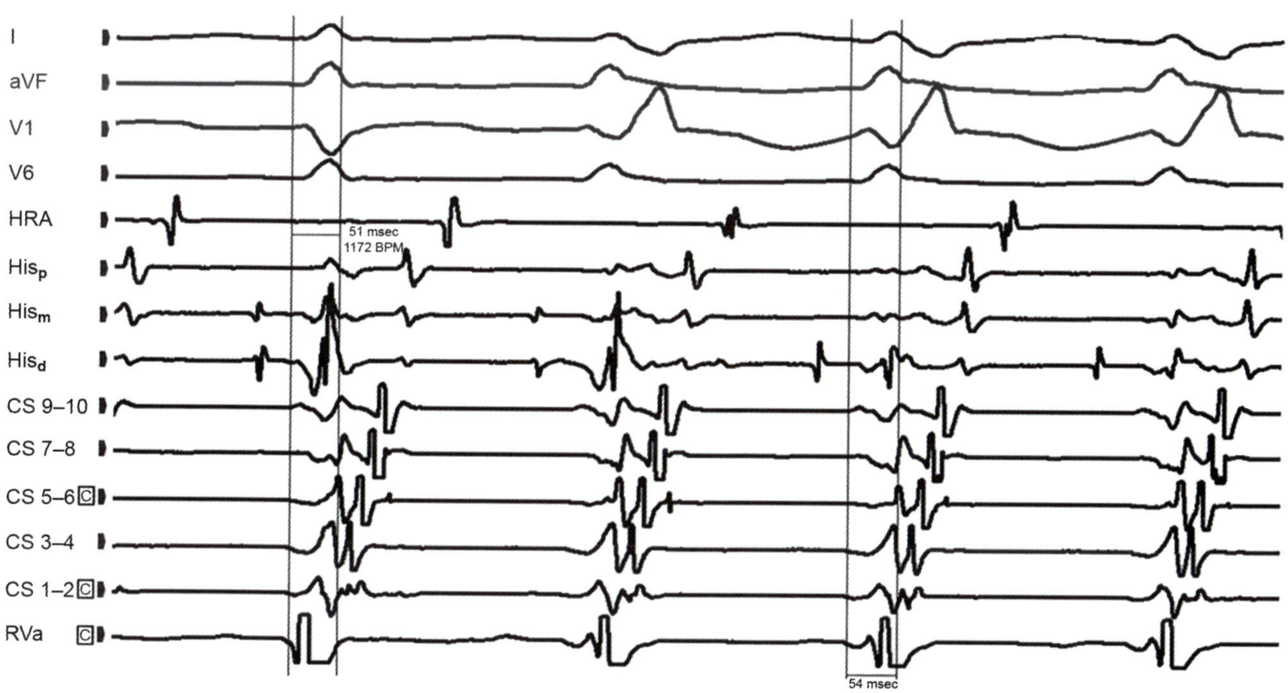

Figure 14.26: A spontaneous RBBB in a patient with a left-sided accessory pathway (contralateral bundle branch block) shows no VA interval or tachycardia cycle length change

From top to bottom are—surface ECG leads I, aVF, V1 and V6; high right atrium (HRA); His bundle proximal (His_p), mid (His_m), and distal (His_d); coronary sinus proximal (CS 9–10) to distal (CS 1–2) and right ventricle (RVa)

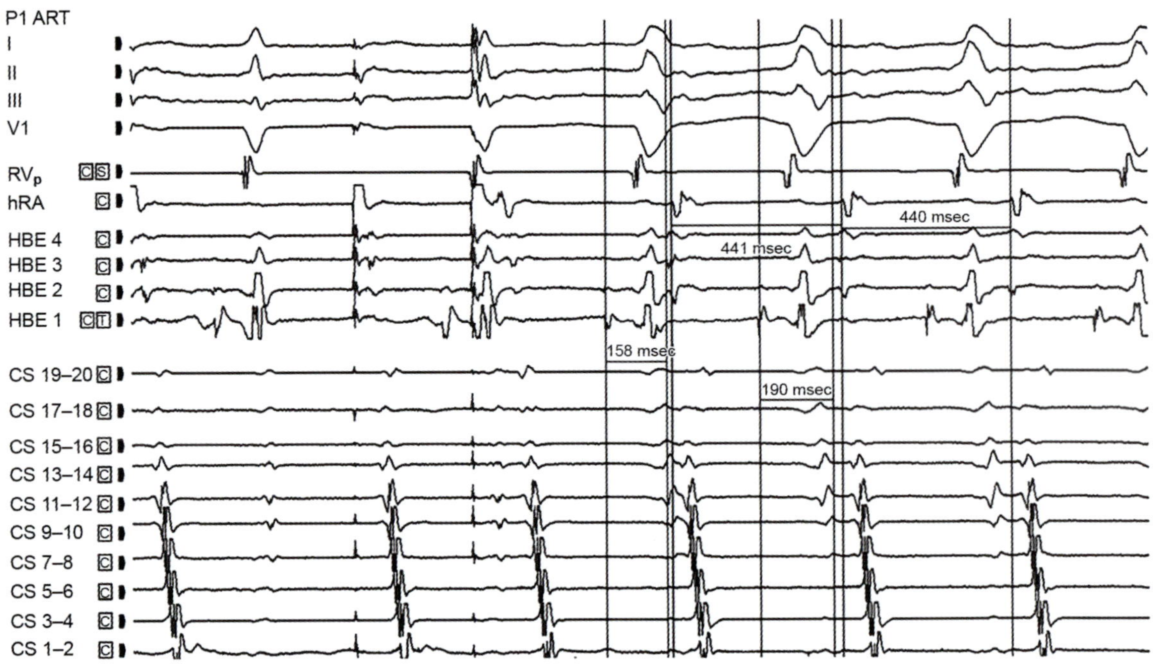

Figure 14.27: Changing HA interval does not change tachycardia cycle length, suggesting a diagnosis of atrial tachycardia, even though the initiation was with atrial extrastimuli

From top to bottom are—intra-arterial blood pressure (P1 ART); surface ECG leads I, II, III and V1; right ventricular electrogram (RV$_p$); high right atrium (hRA); His bundle proximal (HBE 4), mid (HBE 3 and 2) and distal (HBE 1); and coronary sinus proximal (CS 19–20) to distal (CS 1–2)

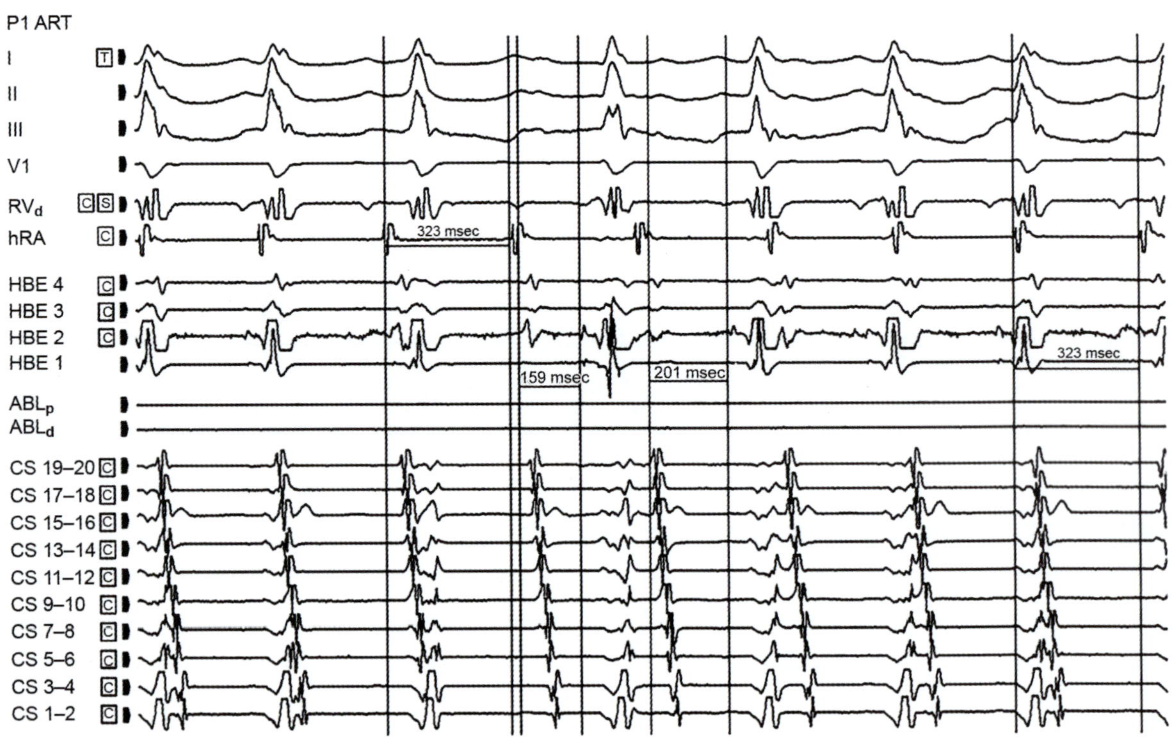

Figure 14.28: In this tracing, an AH interval change does not change the tachycardia cycle length, making the diagnosis of atrial tachycardia very likely

From top to bottom are—intra-arterial blood pressure (P1 ART); surface ECG leads I, II, III and V1; right ventricular distal electrogram (RV$_d$); high right atrium (hRA); His bundle proximal (HBE 4), mid (HBE 3 and 2) and distal (HBE 1); ablation proximal and distal (ABL$_p$ and ABL$_d$); and coronary sinus proximal (CS 19–20) to distal (CS 1–2)

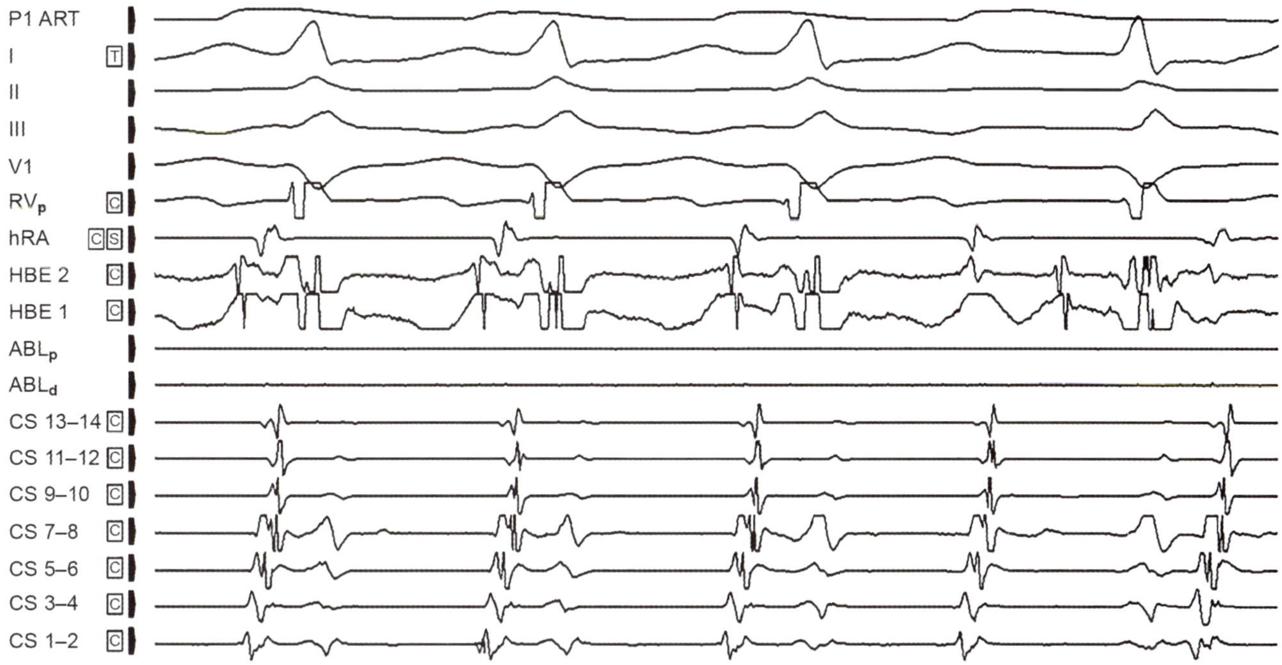

Figure 14.29: Spontaneous AV block leads to the likely diagnosis of atrial tachycardia and excludes ORT. Notice that changes in HA interval do not affect the atrial tachycardia cycle length, and that there is absence of both His and ventricular electrograms at time of AV block, making AVNRT unlikely

From top to bottom are—intra-arterial blood pressure (P1 ART); surface ECG leads I, II, III and V1; right ventricular electrogram (RV_p); high right atrium (hRA); His bundle proximal (HBE 2) and distal (HBE 1); ablation proximal and distal (ABL_p and ABL_d); and coronary sinus proximal (CS 13–14) to distal (CS 1–2)

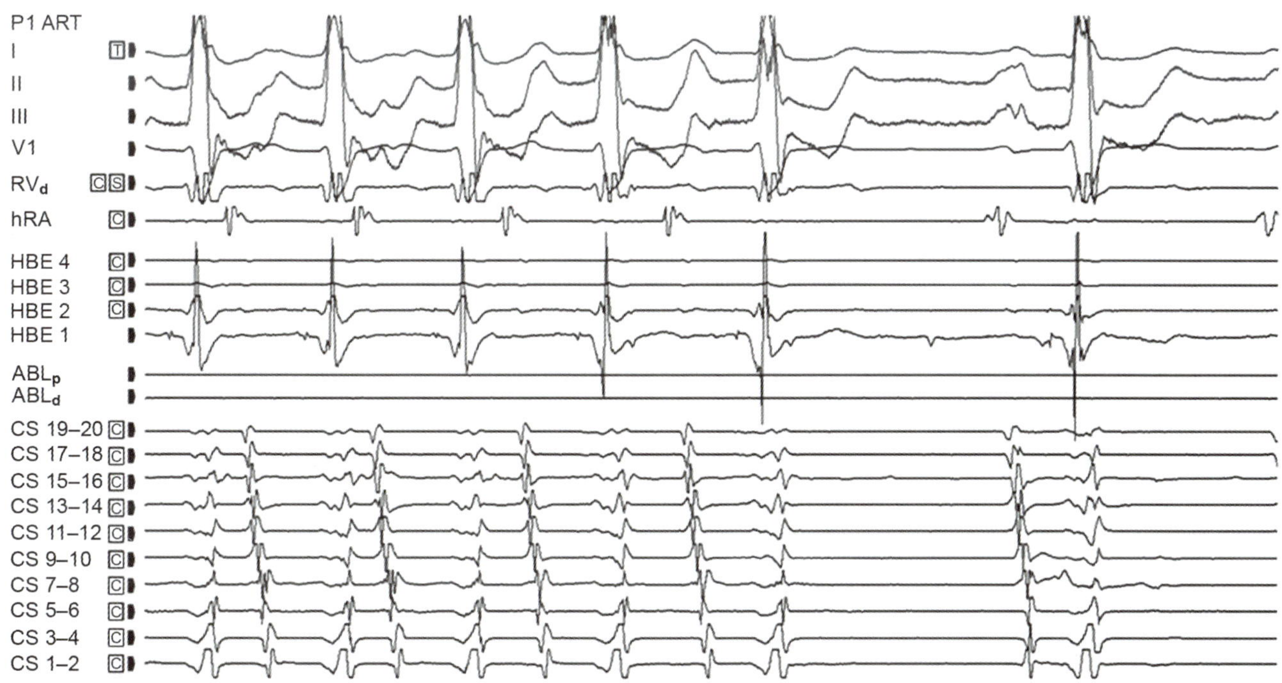

Figure 14.30: Tachycardia terminating with a ventricular electrogram preceded by a high-to-low atrial activation sequence is suggestive of atrial tachycardia

From top to bottom are—intra-arterial blood pressure (P1 ART); surface ECG leads I, II, III and V1; right ventricular distal electrogram (RV_d); high right atrium (hRA); His bundle proximal (HBE 4), mid (HBE 3 and 2) and distal (HBE 1); ablation proximal and distal (ABL_p and ABL_d); and coronary sinus proximal (CS 19–20) to distal (CS 1–2)

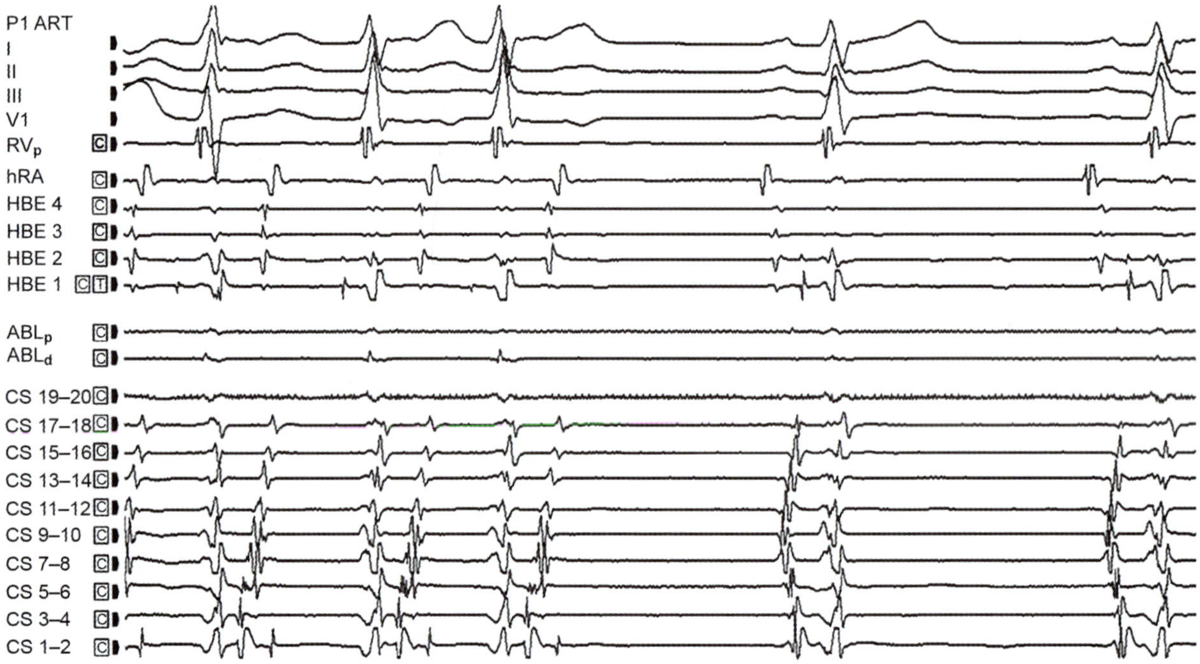

Figure 14.31: ORT terminating with an atrial electrogram confirms AV node dependence. See text for details
From top to bottom are—intra-arterial blood pressure (P1 ART); surface ECG leads I, II, III and V1; right ventricular electrogram (RV_p); high right atrium (hRA); His bundle proximal (HBE 4), mid (HBE 3 and 2) and distal (HBE 1); ablation proximal and distal (ABL_p and ABL_d); and coronary sinus proximal (CS 19–20) to distal (CS 1–2)

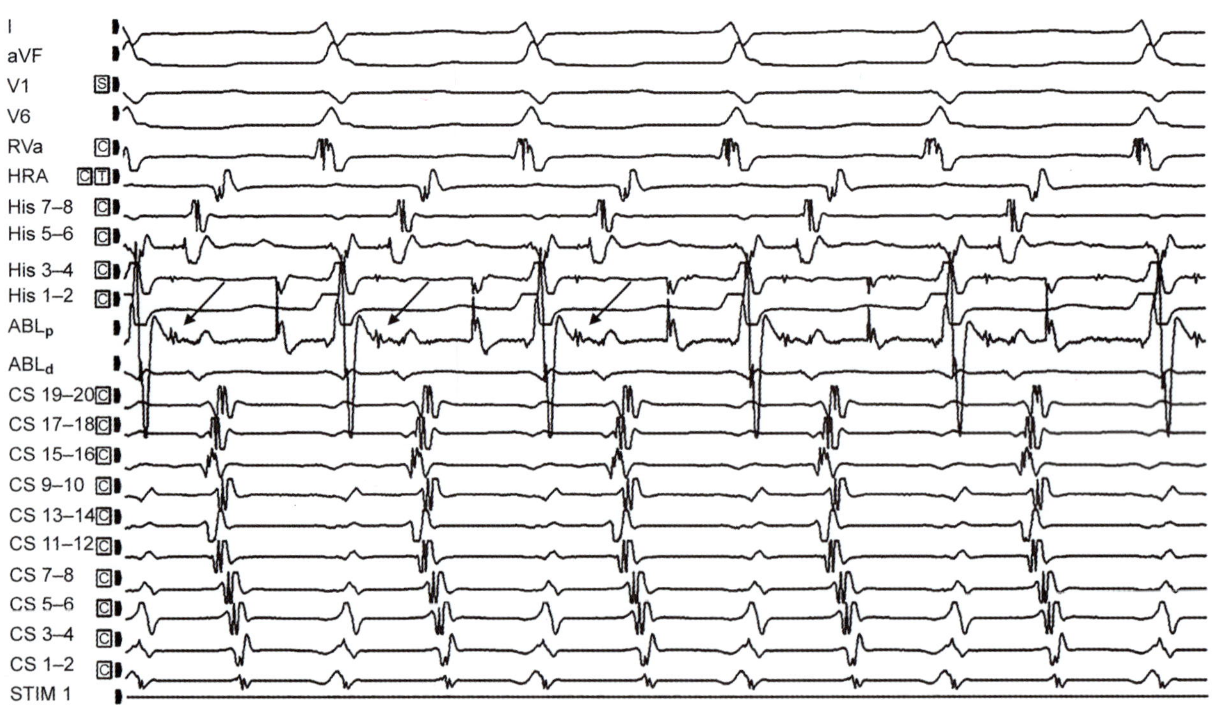

Figure 14.32: Pathway potentials (marked by arrows) are seen in the proximal ablation catheter. See text for details
From top to bottom are—surface ECG leads I, aVF, V1 and V6; right ventricular electrogram (RVa); high right atrium (HRA); His bundle proximal (His 7–8), mid (His 5–6 and His 3–4) and distal (His 1–2); ablation proximal and distal (ABL_p and ABL_d); and coronary sinus proximal (CS 19–20) to distal (CS 1–2)

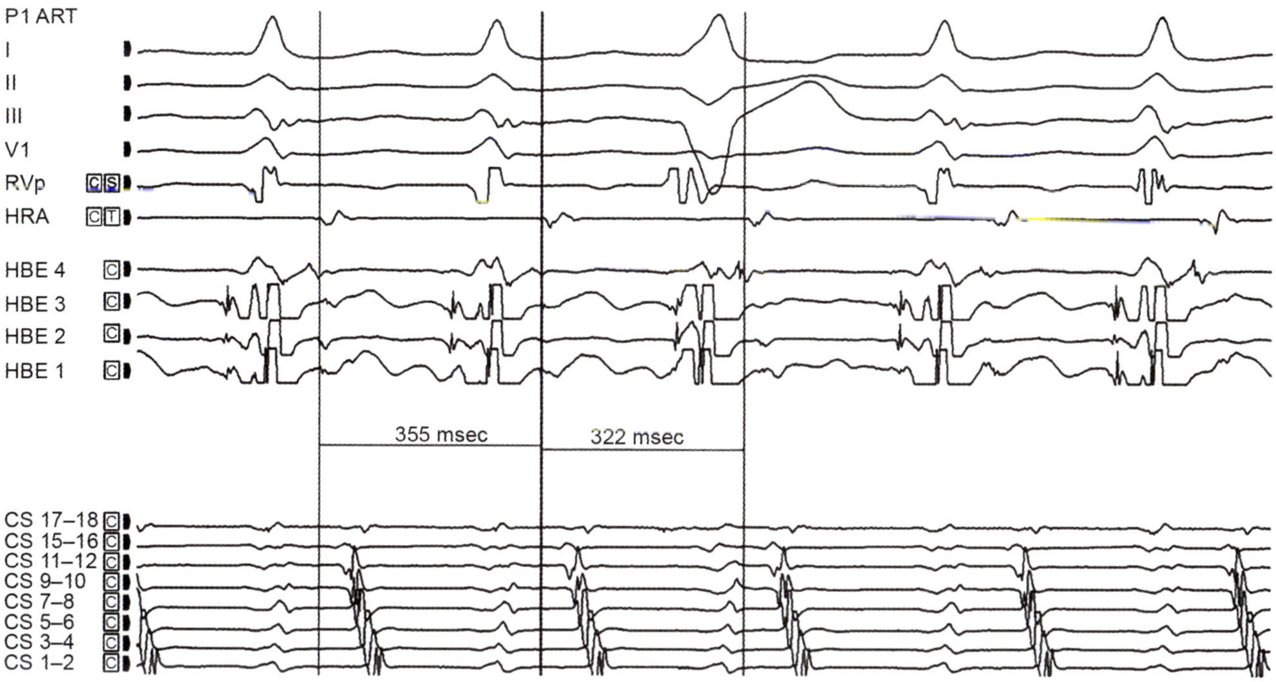

Figure 14.33: A spontaneous PVC concurrent with the antegrade His (thus occurring while the His bundle is refractory) advances the subsequent atrial electrogram, confirming the presence of an accessory pathway. However, the subsequent His electrogram was not advanced. Participation of an accessory pathway in this tachycardia cannot be confirmed with this finding alone. The right atrial electrogram (assuming the catheter is located in high right atrium) occurs ahead of the CS electrogram and simultaneously with the His electrogram; this also suggests the presence of a right-sided accessory pathway. However, AVNRT with a bystander pathway cannot be excluded based on this figure
From top to bottom are—intra-arterial blood pressure (P1 ART); surface ECG leads I, II, III and V1; right ventricular electrogram (RV_p); high right atrium (HRA); His bundle proximal (HBE 4), mid (HBE 3 and 2) and distal (HBE 1); and coronary sinus proximal (CS 17–18) to distal (CS 1–2)

of an accessory pathway is confirmed provided the feature is reproducible with pacing maneuvers. If the subsequent His is also advanced, resetting the tachycardia, then the accessory pathway is integral to the tachycardia.

CONCLUSION

Observing some of the baseline features as outlined above should enable one to reasonably assess the type of tachycardia before performing maneuvers that confirm the type of tachycardia and its mechanism.

REFERENCE

1. Orejarena LA, Vidaillet H, DeStefano F, Nordstrom DL, Vierkant RA, Smith PN, Hayes JJ. Paroxysmal supraventricular tachycardia in the general population. J Am Coll Cardiol. 1998;31:150-7.

EDITORS' SUMMARY

This contribution from Dr Srivathsan is a delightful blend of practicality and comprehensiveness. The author analyzes at multiple levels the most critically important determination in invasive electrophysiology—defining a mechanism of conduction from one site to another. Specifically, retrograde and antegrade conduction via the AV node and utilizing that information in a series of maneuvers meant to diagnose the mechanism of tachycardia.

1. ***Pseudointervals:*** The reader should be cognizant of the fact that in AV node reentry, there is no true ventriculoatrial conduction. As a result, the VA interval, HA interval, and the RP interval do not represent actual conduction time from the ventricle or His bundle to the atrium, but rather a relative conduction time between a common turnaround point in the AVNRT circuit concurrently conducting to both the ventricle and atrium. Thus, although a short RP interval favors typical AVNRT, because of the pseudointerval phenomenon, very fast retrograde fast pathway conduction or slow conduction to the ventricle distal to the His bundle may produce a P-wave or atrial activation before ventricular activation in typical AVNRT that would result in a long RP interval tachycardia. Similarly, the presence of a lower common pathway with certain atypical AVNRT such as slow-slow AVNRT (Lockwood D, Nakagawa H, Jackman W. Electrophysiologic Characteristics of Atrioventricular Nodal Reentry Tachycardia: Implications for Reentrant Circuits. In: Zipes D, Jalife J (Eds). Cardiac Electrophysiology From Cell to Bedside. Philadelphia: Elsevier Saunders; 2009. pp. 615-46. [Book Chapter]; and Asirvatham SJ, Friedman PA, Cha YM. Mayo Clinic Electrophysiology Manual; Rochester: Mayo Clinic Scientific Press; 2014. p. 711) can change the expected P and R relationship. The relatively longer conduction to the AV node and then to the ventricle will result in extremely short RP intervals despite the fact that this is an atypical AVNRT.
2. ***P-wave morphology and atrial activation sequence:*** The intracardiac equivalent to the P-wave morphology is the atrial activation sequence measured with multiple electrodes. The morphology of the P-wave in the various types of AV node reentry or retrograde accessory pathway locations is a direct consequence of the specific exit site to the atrium from where activation spreads during ventricular pacing or tachycardia. Anatomically, the fast pathway is located behind the tendon of Todaro on the true interatrial septum, whereas the slow pathway is related to the ostial coronary sinus myocardium and not far from the true interatrial septum. As a result, retrograde fast pathway activation (or anteroseptal accessory pathway conduction) results in a narrow negative P-wave in leads II, III, and aVF. On the other hand, retrograde slow pathway conduction (or posteroseptal accessory pathway) results in a wide (often wider than the sinus P-wave) negative P-wave in leads II, III, and aVF. Intracardiac equivalent is that the catheter placed behind and slightly inferior to the proximal His electrodes (behind the tendon of Todaro) will be the earliest site of atrial activation with typical AVNRT whereas the electrodes near the proximal coronary sinus will show the earliest atrial activation with atypical AVNRT and retrograde slow pathway conduction.
3. ***Wobble:*** The presence of wobble helps in determining which ventricular sequence corresponds to which atrial sequence. Dr Srivathsan emphasizes the importance of carefully analyzing what actually came first during wobble (spontaneously changing intervals during tachycardia) as well as analyzing retrograde conduction during ventricular pacing. With wobble, what was the first to change and then subsequently drives the next beat in tachycardia? Would ventricular pacing be responsible for this? Which was the first atrial activation that was advanced or in some cases delayed by ventricular pacing?

Dr Srivathsan has provided a truly instructional beginner's manual in this detailed chapter for students of electrophysiology, yet intermediate and experienced operators will still find well explained, new information for their continued learning as well.

CHAPTER 15

Supraventricular Tachycardias: Ventricular Pacing Maneuvers

Jeffrey Munro, Dan Sorajja, Win-Kuang Shen

LIST OF ABBREVIATIONS

AP	Accessory Pathway	PI	Preexcitation Index
ART	Antidromic Reciprocating Tachycardia	PPI	Postpacing Interval
AT	Atrial Tachycardia	PVC	Premature Ventricular Complex
AV	Atrioventricular	RBB	Right Bundle Branch
AVNRT	Atrioventricular Nodal Reentrant Tachycardia	RV	Right Ventricle
AVRT	Atrioventricular Reciprocating Tachycardia	SA	Stimulus to Atrial
ECG	Electrocardiogram	SVT	Supraventricular Tachycardia
JT	Junctional Tachycardia	TCL	Tachycardia Cycle Length
LV	Left Ventricle	VA	Ventriculoatrial
ORT	Orthodromic Reciprocating Tachycardia	VES	Ventricular Extrasystole

INTRODUCTION

The ability to distinguish causes of supraventricular tachycardia in the electrophysiology lab requires knowledge of multiple diagnostic maneuvers to come to an accurate diagnosis. Each of the maneuvers has specific applications depending on the rhythm and reproducibility of the maneuver, and certain caveats which may limit the conclusiveness of the maneuver. While many of the diagnostic maneuvers have attached "cut-off" values to favor one diagnosis over another, we feel it is just as important to understand the principles behind the maneuver. When presented with a supraventricular tachycardia (SVT), ventricular pacing maneuvers are the initial part of programmed electrical stimulation that we perform in our laboratory after obtaining baseline observations. In this section, we will cover these maneuvers and the rationale behind them.

SITE OF PACING: GENERAL CONSIDERATIONS

Ventricular pacing maneuvers are often performed from the right ventricular apex as this is usually a stable position for the catheter, but diagnostic limitations of this location could warrant positioning the catheter at the basal portion of the ventricle. Specifically, when identifying a retrograde His-bundle potential, pacing at the ventricular apex often results in a ventricular electrogram on the His catheter and a retrograde His-bundle potential that is concurrent with the ventricular portion of the electrogram, making its identification challenging. If the pacing catheter is repositioned at

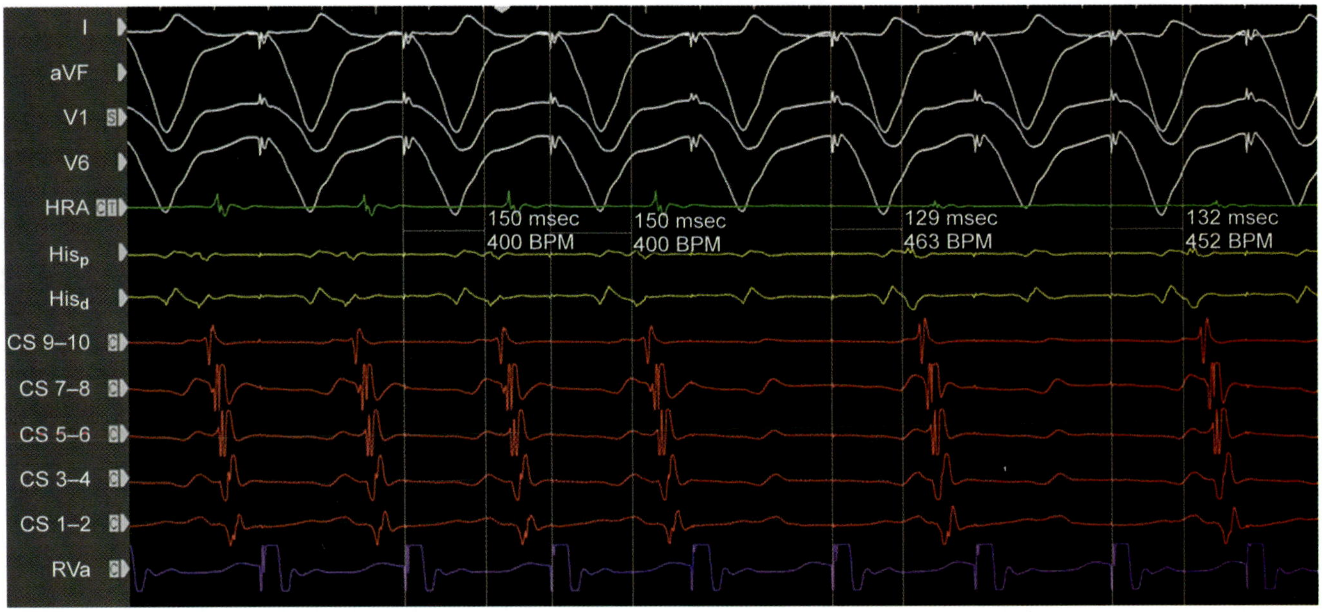

Figure 15.3: Pacing at the right ventricular apex shows concentric retrograde atrial activation with the earliest atrial electrogram on the His catheter

bypass tract, over a fusion of the AV node and bypass tract, or even fusion of multiple bypass tracts.

Concentric: In a patient with exclusively AV nodal retrograde conduction, the earliest site of atrial activation with VA conduction should occur in either the region of the His-bundle catheter, slightly posterior to the tendon of Todaro, when occurring over the fast pathway **(Figure 15.3)** or at the proximal coronary sinus when retrograde conduction is over the slow pathway. Some confusion may occur when there is earliest activation in the area of the mid-portion of the muscular coronary sinus, since this may represent either a left posterior extension of the AV node or a left posterior-septal or left posterior accessory pathway.[2,3] Certainly, additional information is required to differentiate one from the other including the characteristics of retrograde block and para-Hisian pacing as well as maneuvers during tachycardia. The presence of concentric retrograde atrial activation does not exclude retrogradely conducting accessory pathways, even septal ones.

Eccentric: When performing ventricular pacing, if the earliest retrograde atrial activation is clearly away from the septal structures, eccentric activation is present **(Figure 15.4)** and suggests the presence of an accessory pathway. However, there are a number of pitfalls when assessing the presence of eccentric atrial activation. Insufficient mapping around the tricuspid and mitral annulus could falsely give the impression that the earliest retrograde atrial activation is occurring at the septum. For example, when the accessory pathway is along the left free wall, pacing from the right ventricle can result in atrial activation via retrograde conduction over the AV node **(Figure 15.5)** before any evidence of conduction over the accessory pathway can manifest because of the greater distance of pacing site from the AP. This scenario is more likely in the presence of catecholamines that enhance AV nodal conduction. These limitations can be overcome with more extensive mapping along the mitral and tricuspid annuli, ventricular pacing at different cycle lengths, as well as differential pacing in the RV and LV.

Characteristics of VA Block

The AV node utilizes predominantly calcium current for depolarization, and therefore AV nodal block occurs with the Wenckebach phenomenon and decremental conduction. Accessory pathways have predominantly sodium channel-dependent depolarization and therefore, block in a 2:1 pattern with decremental ventricular pacing. While Wenckebach VA block is usually suggestive of retrograde conduction over the AV node, accessory pathways infrequently display decremental conduction properties. Non-decremental VA conduction with 2:1 retrograde block is very unlikely to occur in the AV node and likely signifies block in the His-bundle or possibly the presence of an accessory pathway.[4]

Para-Hisian Pacing

The diagnostic challenge of differentiating atypical atrioventricular nodal reentrant tachycardia (AVNRT) and ORT (using a septal AP) partly stems from the similar retrograde activation patterns seen, with both commonly having a

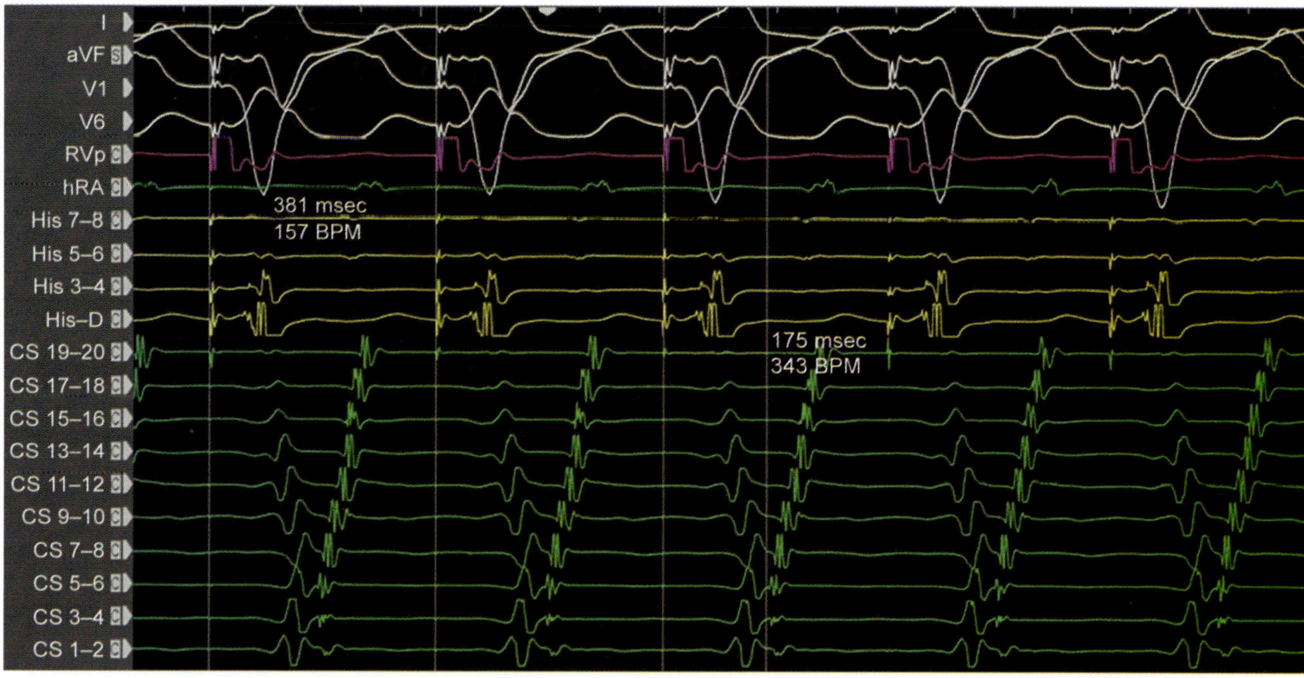

Figure 15.4: Right ventricular pacing demonstrating eccentric retrograde atrial activation in the presence of a left lateral accessory pathway. The distal coronary sinus poles 3,4 have the earliest atrial activation with bracketing seen

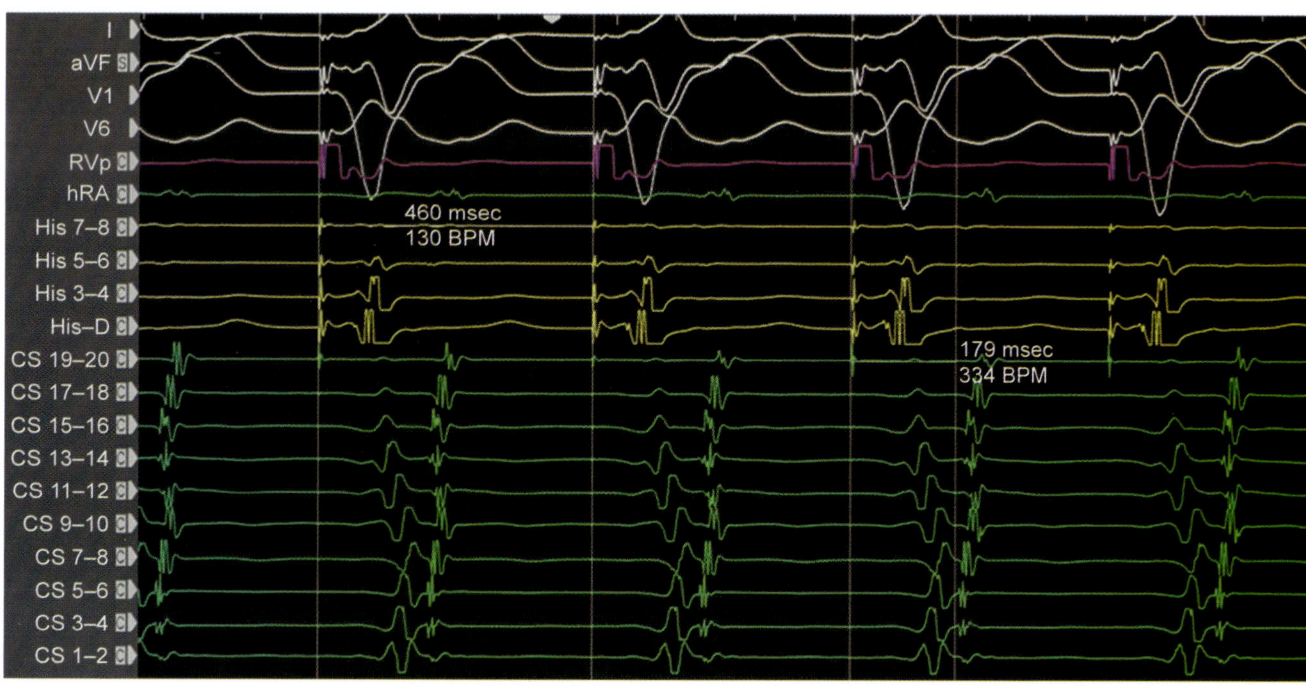

Figure 15.5: Retrograde atrial activation is a result of fusion of the activation wavefront over both the AV node and a left lateral accessory pathway

concentric pattern. Other difficulties with diagnosis may occur due to inability to induce sustained tachycardia to perform diagnostic maneuvers, or inconsistent retrograde conduction when pacing at short cycle lengths, similar to the tachycardia cycle length (TCL). When assessing retrograde atrial activation, retrograde conduction over the AV node or a septal accessory pathway may both produce a pattern that appears concentric with the earliest atrial depolarization along the septum.

In order to engage the AV node for retrograde conduction, the impulse must first conduct retrograde along the His-bundle or proximal right bundle branch (RBB), which are electrically insulated from the adjacent myocardium. Assuming there is no extranodal path for VA conduction, para-Hisian high output pacing will overcome the impedance of insulation of these structures resulting in His-RBB capture with retrograde conduction through the His-bundle and subsequently through the AV node. On the surface electrocardiogram (ECG), His-RBB capture will be noted by narrowing of the paced QRS complex. Unwanted local atrial activation may occur and is indicated by an atrial electrogram within 60 ms of the pacing stimulus, and the maneuver may require a more distal para-Hisian pacing site to prevent atrial capture. At low output pacing, a pacing stimulus will not be able to capture the His-RBB, and capture of only the local ventricular myocardium will result in a wide QRS complex. The impulse will travel via local myocardial capture along the septum to the apex then followed by engagement and depolarization of the Purkinje fibers with subsequent retrograde conduction along the right bundle branch, His bundle, and then AV node. With this longer course, the SA interval should be longer at low output pacing if there is no retrogradely conducting accessory pathway present **(Figure 15.6)**.

In the case of extranodal conduction through an accessory pathway, retrograde conduction continues through the same sequence at high output pacing or low output pacing. Pacing would result in local myocardial capture with conduction over the accessory pathway followed by retrograde atrial activation, and therefore no change in the SA interval is observed at various pacing outputs **(Figure 15.7)**. Depending on the retrograde conduction time over the His-Purkinje system and AV node, a fusion of nodal and extranodal retrograde atrial activation may be present. Seven patterns have been described and are summarized in **Table 15.1**. Of note, the SA interval should not change at high output pacing when an accessory pathway, specifically a rapidly conducting septal pathway, is present.

Limitations of para-Hisian pacing are primarily related to the distance of the pacing site to the accessory pathway as well as position of the pacing catheter to capture the right bundle at high output and local myocardium at low output for an interpretable response. Therefore, the maneuver may not exclude free wall AP or slowly conducting AP despite a difference the SA interval with high versus low output pacing. Occasionally with low output pacing not close to the accessory pathway insertion, the SA interval may be longer than at high output, but without any change in the atrial activation sequence.

Delta VA Interval

In AVNRT, there is simultaneous parallel activation of the His-bundle in an antegrade fashion during retrograde activation of the atria; therefore the VA interval represents

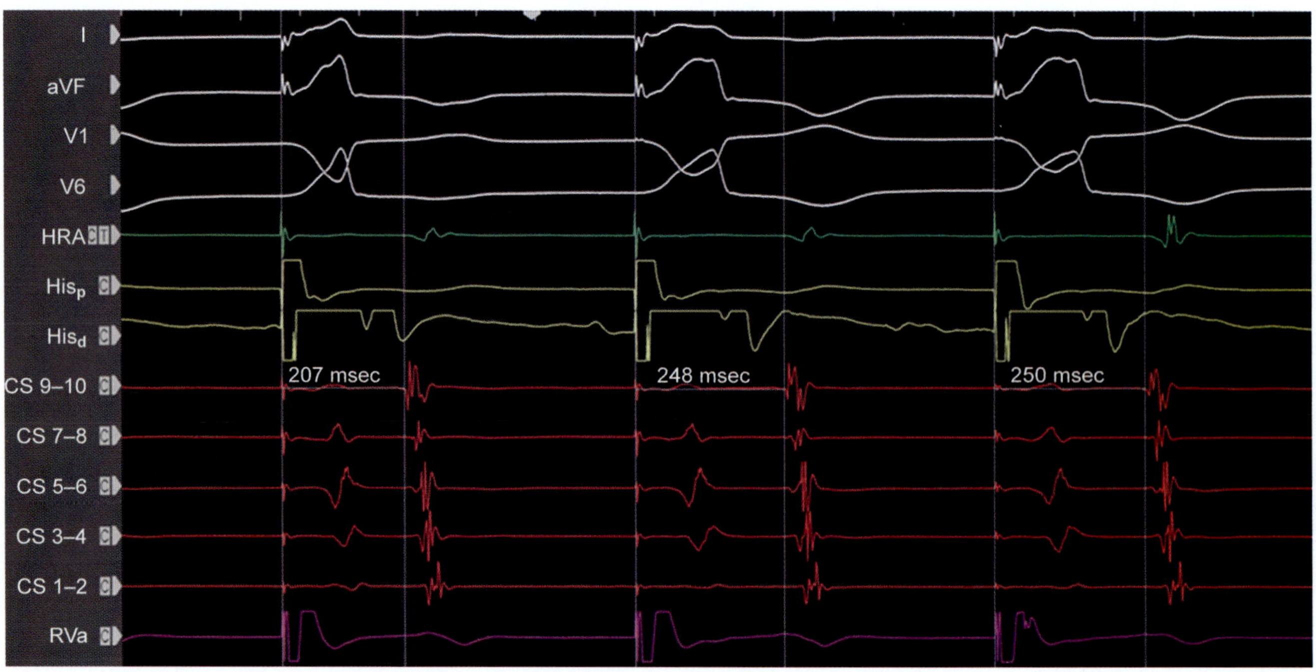

Figure 15.6: Para-Hisian pacing in a patient with atypical AVNRT demonstrates retrograde atrial activation exclusively over the AV node. During His/Right bundle capture with a narrow QRS complex, the SA interval is shorter than during capture of the local septal myocardium

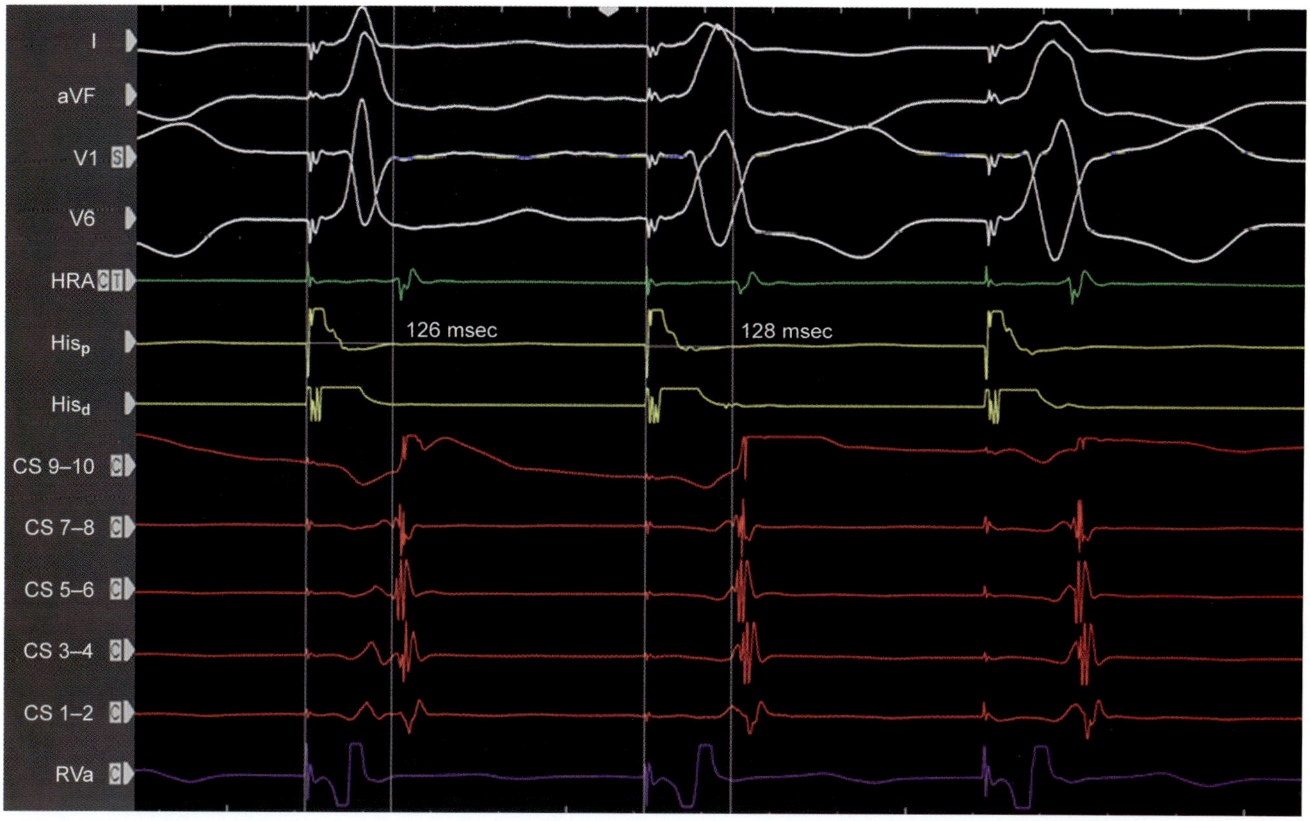

Figure 15.7: Para-Hisian pacing in a case with a left posteroseptal accessory pathway. The SA interval does not change with capture of the His/right bundle and local septal myocardium versus capture of the local septal myocardium only, and the atrial activation sequence remains unchanged

Table 15.1: Different responses to para-Hisian pacing

S.No.	*Retrograde VA conduction C versus NC*	*Atrial activation C versus NC*	*SA*	*HA*	*Local VA*
1.	AVN/AVN	Unchanged	$SA_C < SA_{NC}$	$HA_C = HA_{NC}$	–
2.	AP/AP	Unchanged	$SA_C = SA_{NC}$	–	–
3.	AP/AP_L	Unchanged	$SA_C < SA_{NC}$	–	$VA_C = VA_{NC}$
4.	AVN/AP	Different	–	$HA_C > HA_{NC}$	$VA_C < VA_{NC}$
5.	AVN/Fusion	Different	–	$HA_C = HA_{NC}$	$VA_C < VA_{NC}$
6.	Fusion/AP	Different	–	$HA_C > HA_{NC}$	$VA_C = VA_{NC}$
7.	Fusion/Fusion	Different	–	$HA_C = HA_{NC}$	$VA_C = VA_{NC}$

"C" notates capture of the right bundle branch or His-bundle by the pacing stimulus. "NC" notates capture of the local ventricular myocardium adjacent to the His-bundle without capture of the right bundle or His-bundle by the pacing stimulus. The SA, HA, and local VA intervals with the subscripts "C" and "NC" notate those intervals when there is either capture (C) of the right bundle/His-bundle and capture only of the local myocardium (NC) by the pacing stimulus respectively. AP_L notates a case when retrograde conduction occurs over an accessory pathway and the SA_{NC} interval is lengthened with little to no change in the local VA interval. Examples include a left lateral accessory pathway that may be activated from myocardium that is activated via the His-Purkinje system during right bundle/His-bundle capture or delay in ventricular myocardial capture with decreasing pacing output. Fusion notates retrograde atrial activation over both the AVN and AP. Adapted from Hirao K, et al., 1996.[5]

a pseudointerval. On the other hand, ventricular pacing results in a sequential activation of the local myocardium, His-Purkinje system, AV node and atria representing a true interval, (SA or VA_{pacing}). When comparing the VA interval during AVNRT to the SA interval during ventricular pacing at the tachycardia cycle length, the difference is due to parallel ventricular and atrial activation (during AVNRT) as opposed to the sequential activation (during ventricular pacing). Thus, the delta VA interval that is the difference between SA during pacing and VA during SVT in typical AVNRT is long **(Figures 15.8A and B)**. In contrast, during ORT, ventricular activation is followed by retrograde conduction over an accessory pathway followed by retrograde atrial activation, and therefore the VA interval represents a true interval. During ventricular pacing, the SA interval also represents sequential activation of the local ventricular myocardium followed retrograde atrial activation via the His and AV node with possible fusion from contribution of retrograde atrial activation by the accessory pathway. The VA interval during ORT and the SA interval

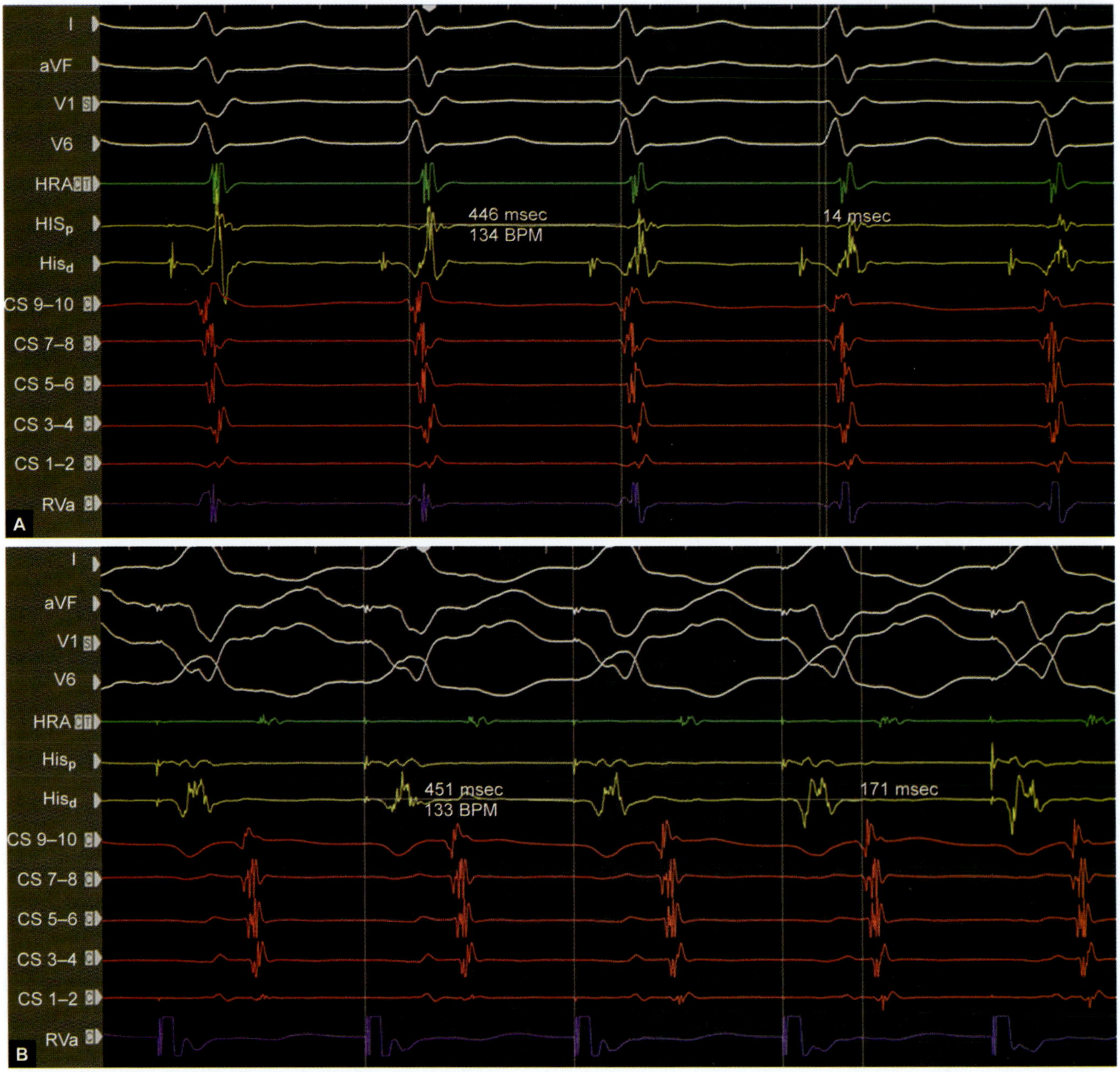

Figures 15.8A and B: (A) The VA interval during typical AVNRT is short (14 ms); (B) Pacing the ventricle in the same patient at the tachycardia cycle length results in a longer SA time of 171 ms and the difference (delta VA) is greater than 90 ms, consistent with AVNRT rather than ORT

while pacing at the tachycardia cycle length will be much closer in value since they are both measuring sequential activation.

In a study of 30 patients with ORT using a septal accessory pathway and 30 patients with slow-fast or slow-intermediate AVNRT, the delta VA was evaluated for its ability to differentiate ORT from AVNRT. With delta VA equal to $VA_{pacing} - VA_{SVT}$, there was a significant difference for AVNRT (138 +/– 26 ms) versus ORT (27 +/– 20 ms, P <0.001). When using a cut-off value of 90 ms, the sensitivity, specificity and positive predictive value are 100% for the delta VA to differentiate AVNRT from ORT.[6] Similar results were observed in a study using a cutoff of 85 ms for the delta VA, but with slightly less specificity and sensitivity.[7]

Delta HA Interval

Differentiating AVNRT from ORT utilizing a septal accessory pathway, both with concentric appearing retrograde atrial activation, can be a diagnostic challenge. Maneuvers can include ventricular overdrive pacing to determine the post-pacing interval. One can also introduce His-refractory premature ventricular complexes (PVCs) to determine if there is preexcitation, postexcitation or termination without terminal retrograde atrial activation. While these pacing maneuvers can help differentiate one mechanism of tachycardia from the other, not uncommonly these may terminate the tachycardia and render the postpacing interval unmeasurable or the tachycardia terminates with a His refractory PVC with terminal atrial activation which is non-diagnostic to differentiate AVNRT from ORT.

When the diagnosis remains uncertain, additional information must be gathered to determine the mechanism of the tachycardia. AVNRT activates the His bundle in an antegrade fashion followed by conduction over the retrograde limb of the circuit (usually the fast or slow pathway), and then depolarizes the atria with the HA interval representing a nearly linear interval. With pacing the ventricle at tachycardia cycle length, the SA and HA intervals will be truly linear, and they should both be longer than the VA and HA seen during tachycardia **(Figures 15.9A and B)**.

In ORT, the His bundle depolarization is sequentially followed by the Purkinje system, ventricles, the accessory pathway in a retrograde direction, and then the atria. The HA interval in ORT represents serial activation of the components involved. When pacing the ventricle at the tachycardia cycle length, in the absence of an accessory pathway, retrograde atrial activation occurs after depolarization of the His bundle and conduction over the AV node. When an accessory pathway is present, pacing the ventricle at the tachycardia cycle length would result in parallel conduction over the accessory pathway and His-Purkinje system and therefore can result in a pseudointerval of a shorter HA interval **(Figures 15.10A and B)**.

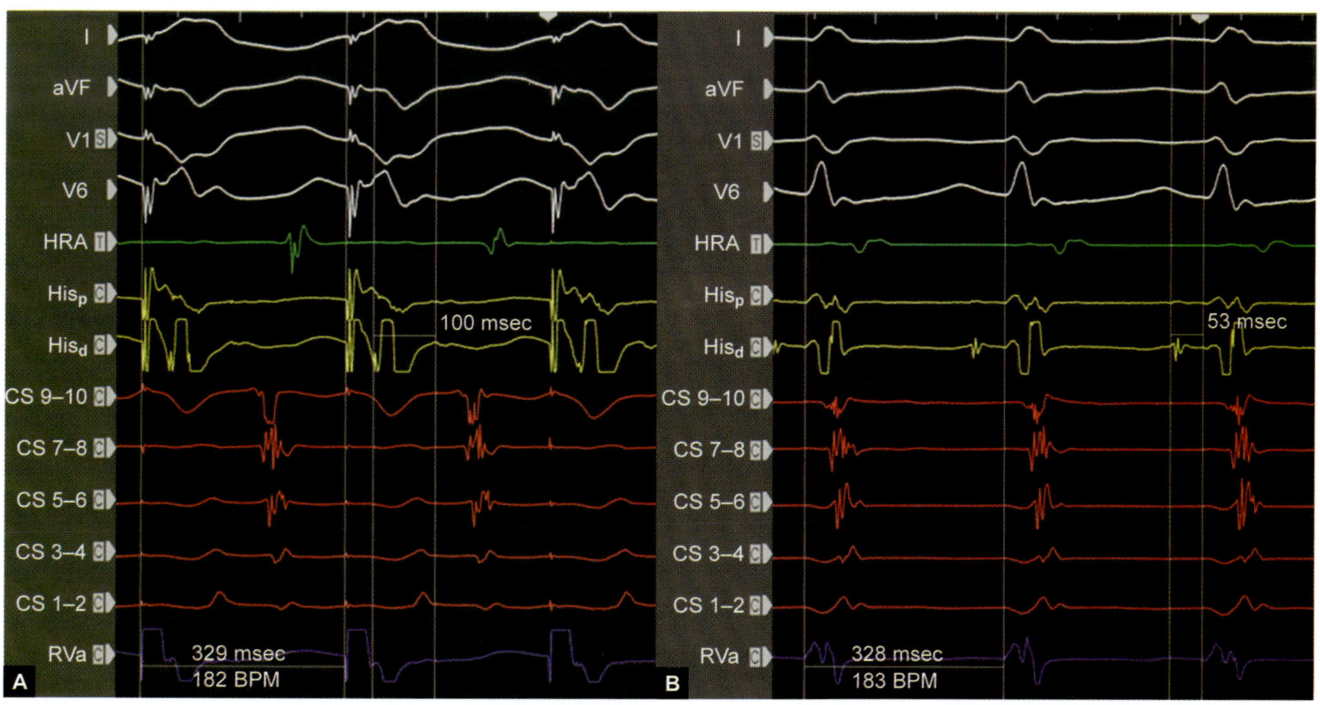

Figures 15.9A and B: Demonstration of Delta HA interval in a patient with AVNRT. (A) The right ventricle is being paced at the tachycardia cycle length with an HA interval of 100 ms; (B) The HA interval during tachycardia is 53 ms. The Delta HA interval is 47 ms, consistent with AVNRT

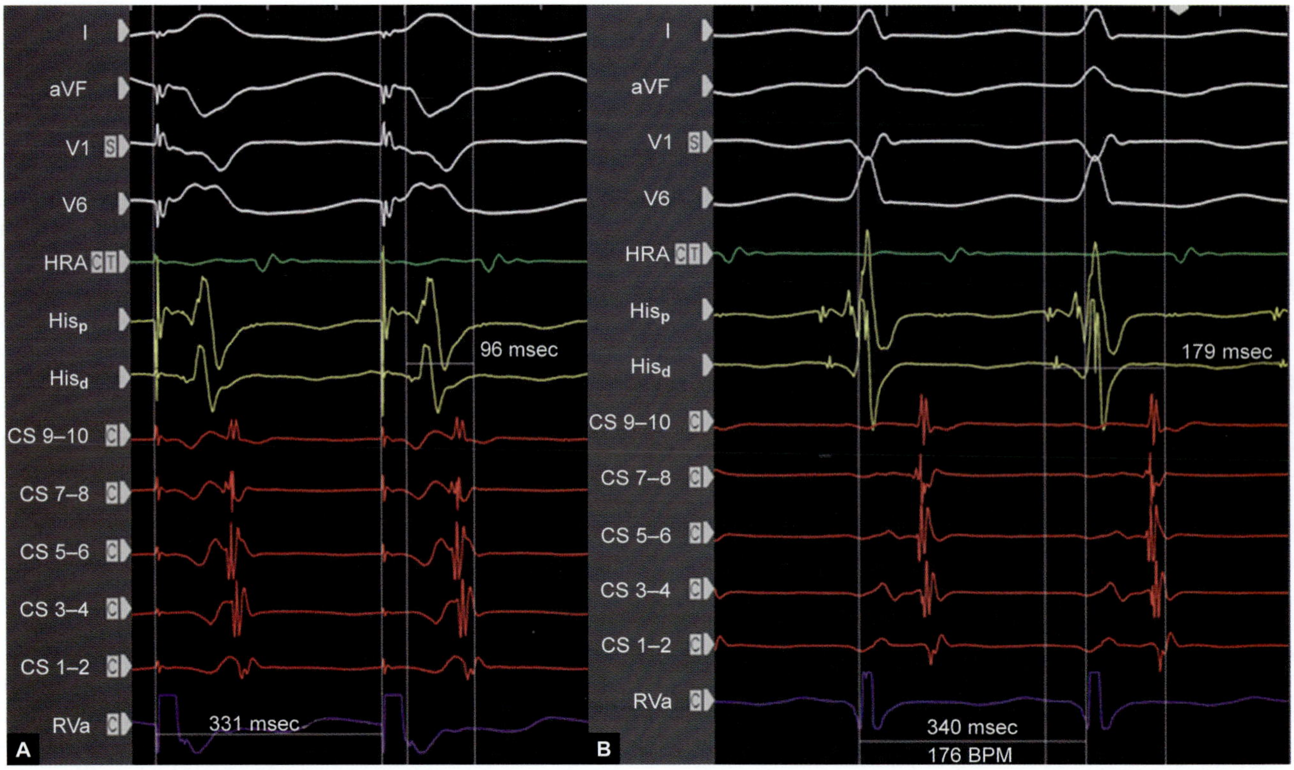

Figures 15.10A and B: In a patient with ORT involving a left posteroseptal accessory pathway, the HA interval during pacing the right ventricle at the tachycardia cycle length (A) is 96 ms, while the HA interval during tachycardia (B) is 179 ms. The Delta HA interval is therefore –83 ms and consistent with ORT

In one study with AVNRT (60 patients) and ORT (24 patients) utilizing a septal atrioventricular accessory pathway, the HA interval was able to differentiate between the two diagnoses. When comparing the HA during ventricular pacing at the tachycardia cycle-length (HA_{pacing}) to the HA during tachycardia (HA_{tachy}) they found that the delta HA defined as $HA_{pacing} - HA_{tachy}$ was significantly less in patients with ORT (less than –27 ms) versus those with AVNRT (greater than 0 ms). When the delta HA value is more positive than –10 ms, the sensitivity, specificity and predictive accuracy were 100% for the diagnosis of AVNRT.[8]

In another study looking at the HA interval in ORT versus AVNRT, the HA was evaluated in 61 patients during entrainment versus during tachycardia. A retrograde His bundle deflection was identified in 93% of their patients. A cutoff of delta HA > 0 ms identified AVNRT as opposed to ORT with a sensitivity, specificity and positive predictive value of 100%.[9]

Some potential limitations of the maneuver include the potential of having a bystander accessory pathway in a patient with AVNRT that conducts retrograde during ventricular pacing and therefore, produces a shorter HA interval than expected, or autonomic tone that differs at the time of tachycardia and pacing. Another limitation is the difficulty with visualizing the retrograde His electrogram during ventricular pacing. Conceptually, the pacing portion of this technique does not evaluate the mechanism and properties of the tachycardia itself but rather the electrophysiologic framework present.

In one series of patients with junctional tachycardia (JT) or AVNRT, the delta HA was used to differentiate the diagnoses. Using the delta HA interval with pacing from the basal RV there was a statistically significant difference between the group of patients with JT (delta HA = 9 ms) and those with AVNRT (delta HA = –10 ms) with $p < 0.00001$. Using a cutoff of delta HA ≥ 0 ms, there was a sensitivity of 89%, specificity of 83% positive predictive value of 84% and negative predictive value of 88% to diagnose junctional tachycardia. With a delta HA <0 ms, the sensitivity was 83% for diagnosing AVNRT.[10]

VENTRICULAR PACING MANEUVERS DURING TACHYCARDIA

Ventricular Overdrive Pacing during Tachycardia

AVNRT and atrioventricular reciprocating tachycardia (AVRT) use the AV node as an obligatory component of the tachycardia whereas atrial tachycardia (AT) does not need

AV node for its initiation or persistence. The response to ventricular burst pacing at cycle lengths shorter than the tachycardia, so called ventricular overdrive pacing, can be used to differentiate them. Of note, the general term of ventricular overdrive pacing is not necessarily entrainment since the overdrive pacing maneuver can also be performed with AT, which is often due to triggered or automatic mechanism.

Ventricular Overdrive Pacing: Entrainment and Fusion

Ventricular overdrive pacing during supraventricular tachycardia may result in entrainment of a reentrant tachycardia, with obligatory advancement of the atrial activation to the pacing cycle length and no change in the retrograde atrial activation sequence. To help differentiate AVNRT from ORT, a number of observations have been made regarding the response of a tachycardia to the first ventricular paced beats for attempted entrainment.

The number of ventricular paced beats that are delivered prior to entrainment of the tachycardia, and advancement of the atrial activation, is significantly different for AVNRT and ORT. The distance from the right ventricular pacing site to the reentrant tachycardia circuit is usually farther in AVNRT than in ORT, with the possible exception of a left free wall accessory pathway. When right ventricular overdrive pacing commences during AVNRT, progressive fusion will occur between the paced ventricular activation wavefront and the antegrade activation of the ventricles over the His bundle. When entrainment is achieved with retrograde conduction over the His bundle with subsequent retrograde advancement of atrial activation, ventricular fusion will no longer be present from lack of antegrade conduction over the His bundle. This situation is in contrast to ventricular overdrive pacing during ORT wherein pacing is performed within or proximal to the circuit with progressive fusion for very few beats prior to entrainment of the tachycardia **(Figure 15.11)**. Left lateral accessory pathways can limit the usefulness of these observations but pacing in the left ventricle, more proximal to or within the circuit, usually eliminates these exceptions. It is critical that the retrograde atrial activation does not change with ventricular overdrive pacing and attempted entrainment, as this may indicate a bystander accessory pathway.

A group of patients with either AVNRT or ORT were reviewed to determine if there was a significant difference in the number of fully RV paced (nonfused) beats observed prior to advancement of the tachycardia and entrainment with ventricular overdrive pacing. In the group of patients with AVNRT compared to those with ORT, 3.7 ± 1.1 versus 1 ± 0 ($p < 0.0001$) fully RV paced beats were observed prior to advancement of the tachycardia. A cutoff of > 1 beat had a positive and negative predictive value of 100% for predicting

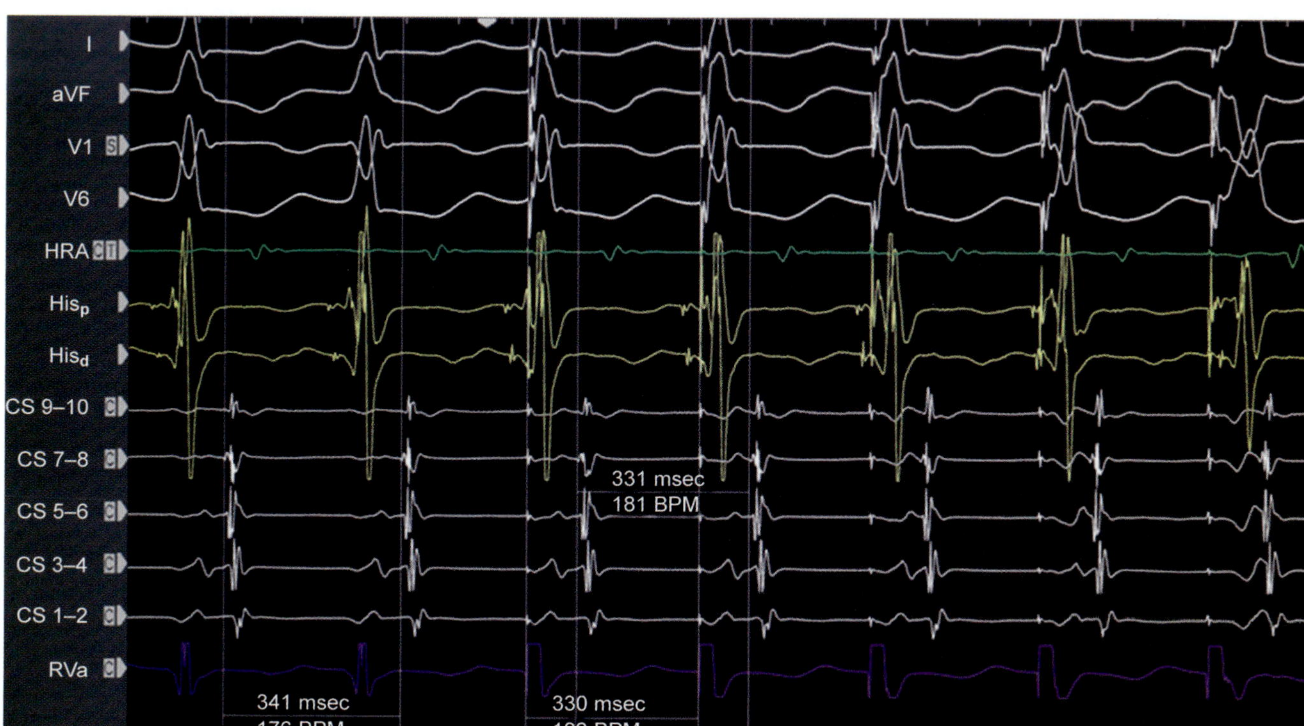

Figure 15.11: Right ventricular overdrive pacing with advancement of the atrial activation to the pacing cycle length after the second paced beat and entrainment, with manifest fusion of the surface QRS which is diagnostic of ORT

AVNRT. Of note a significant proportion (21%) of the patients in this study had ORT utilizing a left lateral accessory pathway.[11]

If entrainment is achieved with ventricular overdrive pacing, it is important to identify when in the pacing train atrial activation was first advanced, and if ventricular fusion was present at the time of advancement of the atrial activation. During AVNRT, ventricular fusion indicates that there is still antegrade conduction over the His bundle and therefore, advancement of the atrial activation to the pacing cycle length cannot occur unless there is a bystander accessory pathway and likely a change in the atrial activation sequence. Ventricular fusion of the wavefront from ventricular pacing and antegrade activation over the His bundle can occur with entrainment during ORT since retrograde atrial activation and advancement of the tachycardia will occur over an accessory pathway. Initially fusion was not observed with entrainment during ORT, but these cases involved left lateral pathways and overdrive pacing in the right ventricle. The anatomical distance of the left lateral pathway would be great enough that retrograde capture of the His bundle occurs before advancement of the tachycardia over a distant left lateral accessory pathway. Pacing in the left ventricle would provide a means to overcome this limitation.[12]

Ventricular Overdrive Pacing: Response on Cessation of Pacing

V-A-A-V response: When ventricular overdrive pacing is performed during atrial tachycardia, retrograde activation of the AV node is usually achieved with capture and acceleration of the atrial depolarization rate. When 1:1 VA conduction while pacing during tachycardia is lacking, the application of the maneuver is limited. With intact VA conduction at the pacing rate, the result is a ventricular electrogram driving an atrial electrogram (the 'V-A' portion of the V-A-A-V). Cessation of burst pacing results in the last retrograde depolarization of the atria, which is unable to conduct through the AV node at that point due to AV node refractoriness. The resumption of the atrial tachycardia results in an atrial depolarization, with subsequent antegrade conduction over the AV node, His-Purkinje system and depolarization of the ventricle (resulting in the 'A-V' portion of V-A-A-V) **(Figure 15.12)**. In one study evaluating the usefulness of this maneuver in 163 patients with atrial tachycardia, ORT, and AVNRT, atrial tachycardia was identified by a "V-A-A-V" response with high sensitivity and specificity.[13]

V-A-V response: During typical AVNRT, ventricular overdrive pacing will advance the atrial depolarization via retrograde fast pathway conduction to the atria, with antidromic collision of wavefronts in the slow pathway. When ventricular burst pacing is stopped, the last impulse that conducted retrograde over the fast pathway will then conduct down the slow pathway without encountering an antidromic wavefront, with subsequent antegrade His-Purkinje depolarization and continuation of the tachycardia. This response to ventricular overdrive pacing is a "V-A-V" response **(Figure 15.13)**.

A similar response is observed with ORT. When ventricular burst pacing is performed, retrograde conduction over

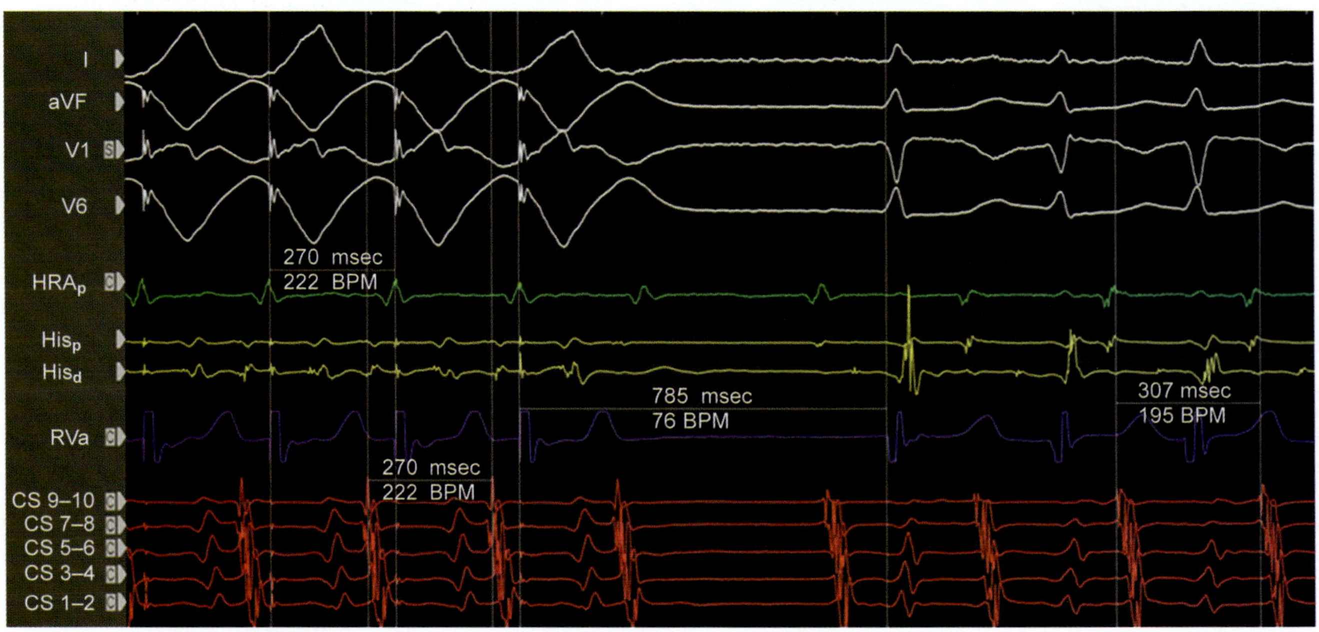

Figure 15.12: Ventricular overdrive pacing from the right ventricular apex results in advancement of the atrial rate to the pacing rate. The response after cessation of pacing is a "V-A-A-V" response consistent with atrial tachycardia

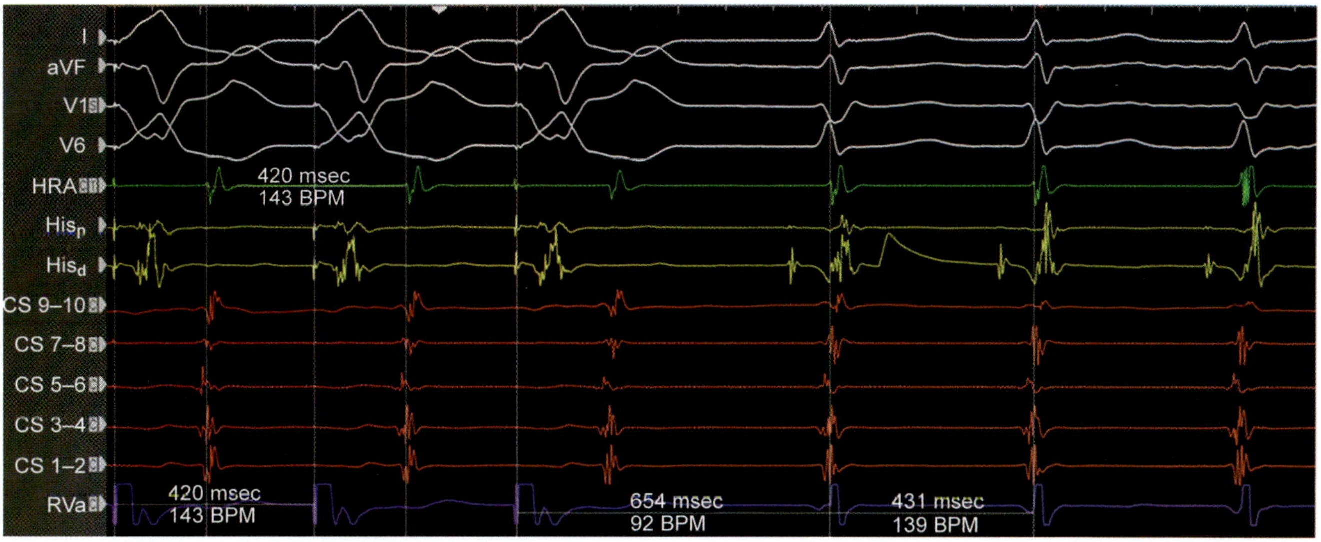

Figure 15.13: Ventricular overdrive pacing from the right ventricle during typical (slow-fast) AVNRT has a VAHV response. The PPI-TCL is 223 ms, consistent with AVNRT

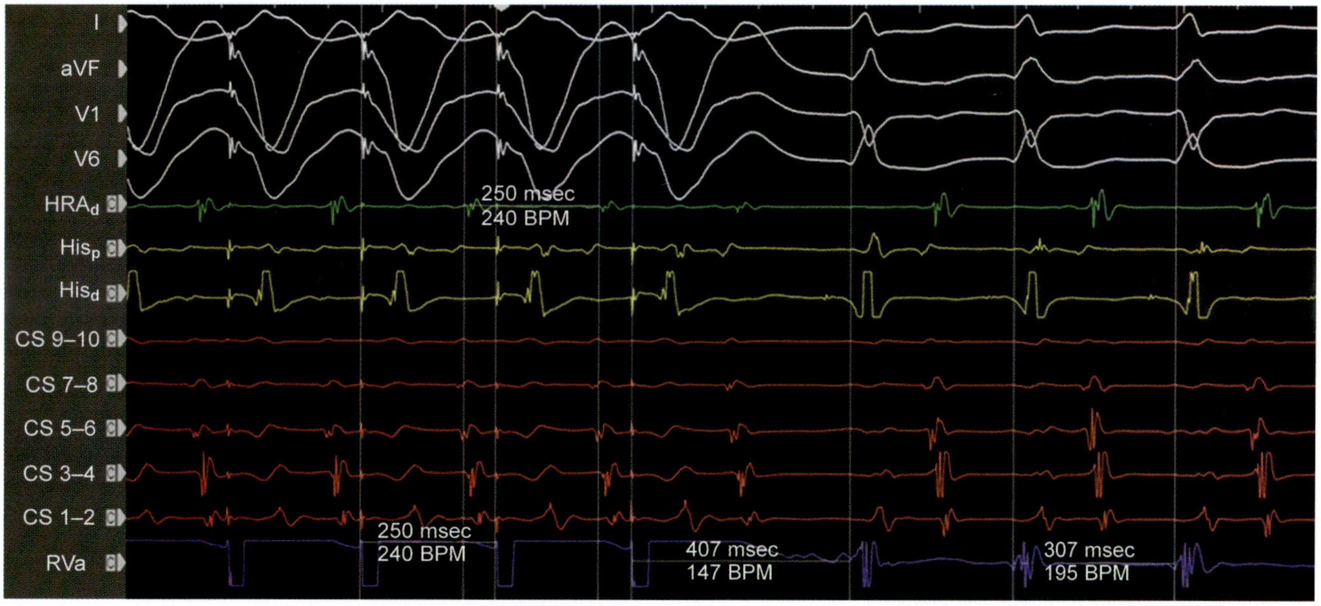

Figure 15.14: An example of ventricular overdrive pacing during ORT with an anteroseptal accessory pathway resulting in a VAHV response. Additionally, the PPI-TCL is 100 ms, consistent with ORT rather than AVNRT

the accessory pathway is followed by atrial depolarization advanced to the pacing rate. Cessation of ventricular overdrive pacing will allow the last paced ventricular beat to conduct over the accessory pathway to the atrium (the 'V-A' portion of V-A-V), and then conduct antegrade over the AV node and His-Purkinje system with subsequent ventricular depolarization resulting in the "V-A-V" response **(Figure 15.14)**. Of note, antidromic reciprocating tachycardia has a similar response but with the retrograde limb of the tachycardia being the AV node and the antegrade limb the accessory pathway.

Pseudoresponses: A number of situations may cause difficulty in interpretation of the response to ventricular overdrive pacing. It is important to verify that the rate of atrial depolarization is advanced to the cycle length of the ventricular overdrive pacing, otherwise one has not affected the atrium and the response after pacing is not a reliable indicator of the mechanism of the tachycardia. Also, accurate determination of the last atrial electrogram resulting from ventricular pacing is critical in order to determine which components of the maneuver should be evaluated in the response. In addition, the relationship of the His to the ventricular electrogram should be evaluated closely.[13,14]

Fast-slow and slow-slow atypical AVNRT as well as AVRT with a slow conducting septal AP can result in a pseudo "V-A-A-V" response, but careful inspection reveals a "V-A-H-A-V" response rather than "V-A-A-H-V" response as would be expected in atrial tachycardia **(Figure 15.15)**. Lack of 1:1 VA conduction during overdrive pacing may also result in a pseudo V-A-A-V response. Also, a pseudo "V-A-V" response may result with atrial tachycardia if a junctional beat occurs after cessation of pacing that does not conduct retrogradely to the atria, especially during catecholamine infusion such as isoproterenol.

Postpacing Interval with Entrainment of SVT during Ventricular Pacing

Entrainment is a powerful tool to identify whether the site of pacing is involved in a tachycardia circuit. Michaud et al. used entrainment to differentiate atypical AVNRT from ORT using a septal accessory pathway. They studied 30 patients with atypical AVNRT and 44 patients with ORT using a septal accessory pathway and found that every patient within the study group with atypical AVNRT had a postpacing interval (PPI) and TCL difference of greater than 115 ms and SA-VA interval > 85 ms as opposed to none of those with ORT.[7]

The PPI is the time from the last paced beat to the return of the first local electrogram at the site of pacing. In the case of ORT, the ventricle is an obligatory component of the circuit and therefore, entrainment of the tachycardia with ventricular pacing is such that one is pacing "in the circuit." Anatomically, the PPI (of the last paced beat during entrainment) represents the sum of the time of conduction from the site of pacing to the reentry circuit, the time of conduction through the entire reentry circuit, and the time of conduction from the reentry circuit back to the site of pacing. Because the ventricular site of pacing in ORT is in close proximity to the circuit, the PPI is close to the tachycardia cycle length **(*see* Figure 15.14)**.

For AVNRT, entrainment of the tachycardia with ventricular pacing results in a longer PPI than seen with ORT because conduction of the last paced beat must conduct along the ventricular myocardium and then retrogradely conduct over the His-Purkinje system, right bundle branch,

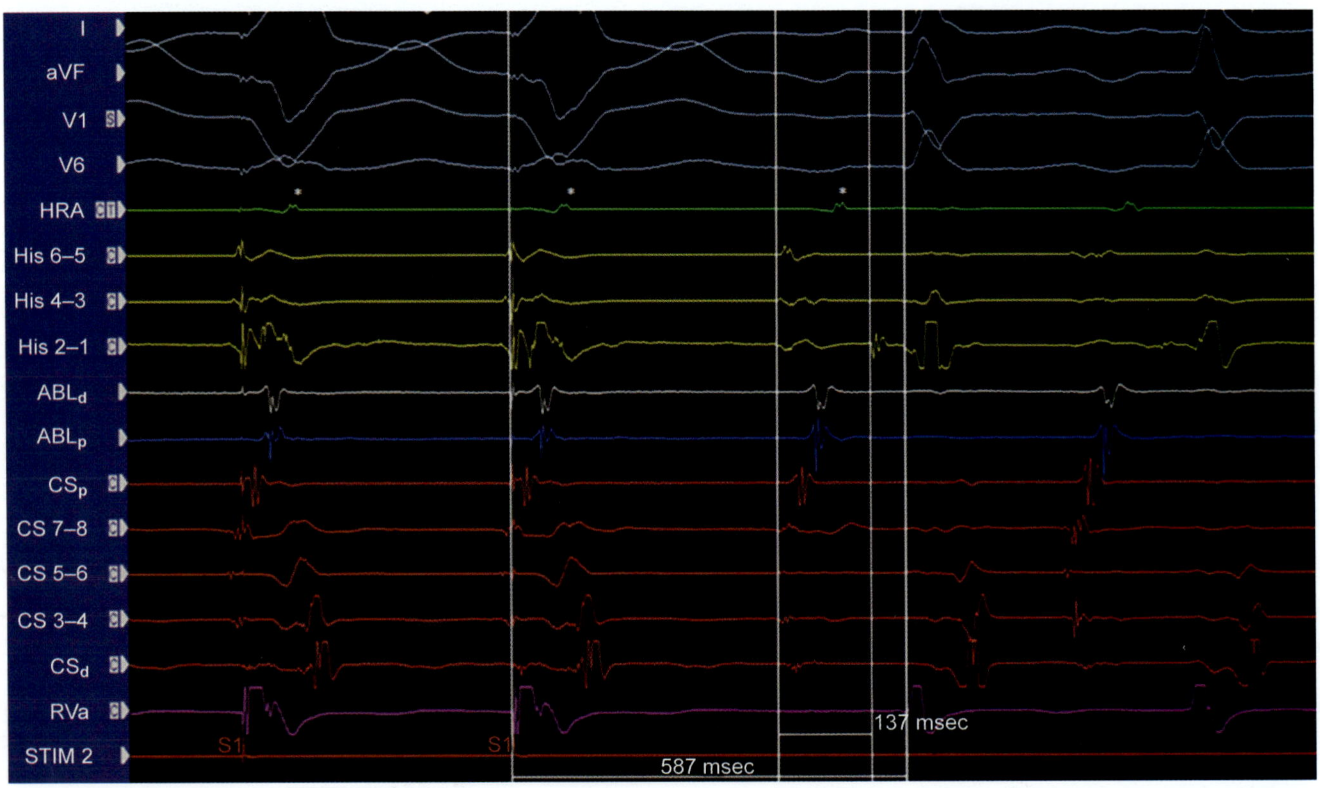

Figure 15.15: An example of a pseudo "VAAV" response in a patient with atypical AVNRT. The asterisk (*) denote retrograde atrial activation at the HRA catheter. The third atrial signal is the result of the last entrained beat and therefore this is a "VAV" response
Image courtesy: Luis Scott MD

and His-bundle before it reaches the reentry circuit. After conduction around the reentry circuit, the conduction has to proceed antegrade over the His-bundle, right bundle branch, and the ventricular myocardium to return to the pacing catheter site. The conduction time to and from the reentry circuit in AVNRT is significantly longer resulting in a PPI markedly longer than the tachycardia cycle length (*see* **Figure 15.13**). To further increase the PPI in AVNRT, the ventricular pacing can be performed from the base (at lower output) rather than the apex, as the base is farther from the circuit due to insulation around the AV node and His bundle.

Ventricular Extrasystoles Introduced during Supraventricular Tachycardia

During tachycardia, introduction of a ventricular extrasystole (VES) can produce a number of responses depending on the coupling interval of the VES as well as the available routes of retrograde VA conduction. Most commonly, a VES is introduced when the His-bundle is refractory, and therefore retrograde conduction to the atria can only occur if there is an accessory pathway. Furthermore, information can be ascertained as to whether the accessory pathway is participating in the tachycardia or if it is only a bystander (with the tachycardia having antegrade and retrograde limbs other than the accessory pathway).

His-Refractory Ventricular Extrasystole

When a VES is placed while the His-bundle is refractory (within 60 ms of the His electrogram), an advancement in the timing of atrial activation (preexcitation) documents an extranodal path of VA conduction (i.e. accessory pathway with retrograde conduction). In order to determine whether or not the accessory pathway is participating in the tachycardia, the PVC must reset the timing of the tachycardia, either by advancement **(Figure 15.16)** or delay of the subsequent His-bundle activation or QRS complex. Delay of the subsequent atrial activation, or postexcitation, is suggestive of a decremental conducting accessory pathway but advancement of the subsequent atrial activation with delay in the next His-bundle activation represents decremental conduction in the AV node. When either of these responses is observed with a His-refractory VES, the accessory pathway is integral to the tachycardia circuit. Of note, the atrial activation sequence during advancement or delay should be the same atrial activation sequence seen during SVT. The observation that a His-refractory VES reproducibly terminates the tachycardia without conducting to the atria is also diagnostic of ORT, since the tachycardia terminates due to the VES causing retrograde block in the accessory pathway. When there is termination of the SVT with conduction to the atrium (with similar atrial activation to the SVT), atrial tachycardia is practically excluded except for

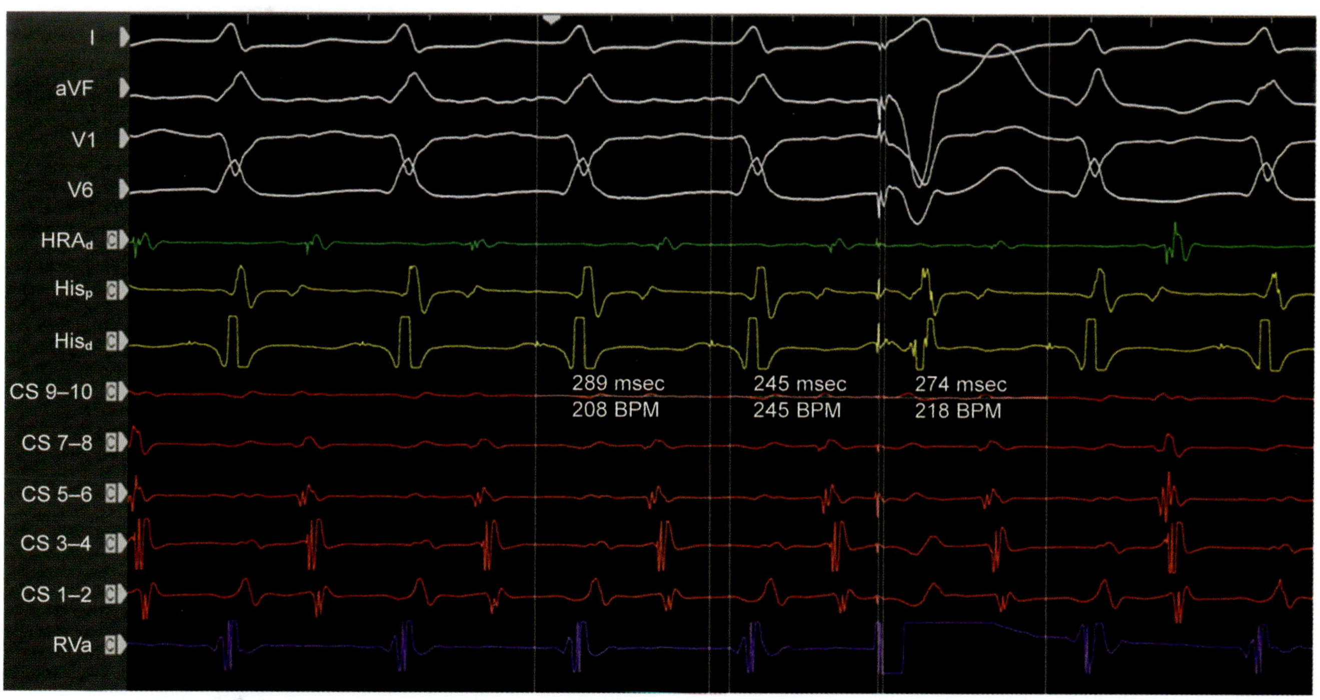

Figure 15.16: A VES is introduced at the time of His-bundle refractoriness in a patient with ORT involving an anteroseptal accessory pathway, with subsequent advancement of the next His-bundle potential and therefore advancement and reset of the tachycardia. Also, the preexcitation index in this case is 43 ms, consistent with ORT rather than AVNRT

the rare construct of an atrial tachycardia focus originating close to the atrial insertion of a bystander pathway.

Ventricular Extrasystole with a Short Coupling Interval

A VES placed earlier during tachycardia (prior to the His-bundle being refractory) could result in retrograde conduction over the His-bundle and AV node with advancement of the subsequent atrial activation. As a result, the tachycardia could also advance with retrograde conduction over an accessory pathway, and with advancement of the subsequent atrial activation. If there is advancement of the subsequent His-bundle activation and ventricular activation, there has been preexcitation of the tachycardia. The difference between the TCL and coupling interval of the VES (that has advanced the tachycardia) has been termed the *preexcitation index* which can yield diagnostically useful information as described in the section below.

The response to the shorter-coupled VES is similar diagnostically as the ventricular overdrive pacing maneuver. If the VES is followed by an advanced atrial activation and then an advanced His-bundle depolarization and ventricular activation, the response is similar to the "V-A-H-V" response as described in the ventricular overdrive pacing section, and therefore, inconsistent with atrial tachycardia. Similarly, if the VES advances the subsequent atrial activation followed by an additional atrial activation and then a His-bundle activation and ventricular depolarization, a so called "V-A-A-H-V" response, ORT and AVNRT are excluded.

Retrograde Right Bundle Branch Block

A VES introduced at a short enough coupling interval could encounter a RBB that is refractory from the previous depolarization. The extrasystole would then conduct transseptally with retrograde conduction over the left bundle branch. The retrograde His-bundle deflection would be delayed, representing the transseptal activation time and conduction over the left bundle branch, but the HA interval would remain unchanged if retrograde conduction is exclusively over the AV node. If the HA interval is shorter, then extranodal retrograde conduction exists since the retrograde conduction over the accessory pathway is not dependent on retrograde conduction over the right bundle branch.

Preexcitation Index

If a VES introduced during the His-bundle refractory period advances the subsequent atrial activation, then there is extranodal retrograde activation. Furthermore, if it advances the tachycardia, an accessory pathway is not only present but also participating in the tachycardia mechanism. As progressively more premature VES are introduced, especially before the His-bundle is activated, there is the potential for retrograde activation of the His-bundle, AV node, and atrium. In the case of an AVNRT, a VES introduced prior to His-bundle activation will be able to conduct to the AV node and through the retrograde limb of the tachycardia circuit (fast pathway in typical slow-fast or slow pathway in atypical fast-slow or slow-slow AVNRT) to advance the atrial activation. Subsequent to this, activation would proceed down the antegrade limb of the circuit (if it is no longer refractory) with advancement of the tachycardia.

This concept was studied by Miles, et al. who looked at 55 patients with ORT and 22 patients with AVNRT.[15] They defined the preexcitation index (PI) as the TCL minus the longest coupling interval of the VES that advanced the atrial activation. Introduction of VES achieved atrial preexcitation in 89% of patients with ORT and 14% of patients with AVNRT. The PI was > 100 ms in all patients with AVNRT, and among patients with ORT, all of those with a septal pathway participating in tachycardia had a PI < 45 ms and only left lateral pathways had a PI > 75 ms **(Table 15.2)**. A significant limitation of the study is that the group of patients with AVNRT was very small, and there was significant overlap of PI values for the groups with AVNRT and ORT with a left free wall pathway. A potential approach to overcome this limitation is introduction of VES using differential pacing; when the PI using a right VES is longer than the PI using a left VES, a left lateral pathway participating in ORT is probable.

Introduction of Ventricular Extrasystoles to Identify Accessory Pathway Potential

When mapping an accessory pathway, differentiating the ventricular component from the atrial component and identification of an accessory pathway potential can be challenging as these signals often are immediately adjacent to each other on the bipolar recording. Identification of an accessory pathway potential during mapping and ablation

Table 15.2: The mean preexcitation index and derived cutoff values from a group of 55 patients

	Mean Preexcitation Index (ms)	*Preexcitation Index Cutoff (ms)*
Location of Pathway		
Left Free Wall	88	> 75
Posterior Septal	38	< 45
Anterior Septal	17	< 45
AVNRT	108	> 100

Significant overlap occurred in the preexcitation index between the group with a left free wall accessory pathway and AVNRT. Adapted from Miles et al., 1986.[15]

at that site has been associated with higher success rates of ablation with fewer radiofrequency ablation lesions.[16] By introduction of extrasystoles—either ventricular or atrial, the components of the electrogram can be separated from each other. If an atrial extrasystole is introduced, effectively advancing the atrial activation and electrogram, the resultant residual of the electrogram under question would be the ventricular electrogram and possibly the accessory pathway potential. If a ventricular extrasystole is similarly introduced, then the residual of the electrogram being evaluated would be the atrial electrogram and pathway potential. Using these two maneuvers, the component of the electrogram representing the accessory pathway potential can be identified.[17]

REFERENCES

1. Martinez-Alday JD, Almendral J, Arenal A, Ormaetxe JM, Pastor A, Villacastin JP, Medina O, Peinado R, Delcan JL. Identification of concealed posteroseptal Kent pathways by comparison of ventriculoatrial intervals from apical and posterobasal right ventricular sites. Circulation. 1994;89: 1060-7.
2. Otomo K, Okamura H, Noda T, Satomi K, Shimizu W, Suyama K, Kurita T, Aihara N, Kamakura S. J Left-Variant atypical atrioventricular nodal reentrant tachycardia: Electrophysiological characteristics and effect of slow pathway ablation within the coronary sinus. J Cardiovasc Electrophysiol. 2006;17:1177-83.
3. Katritsis DG, Becker AE, Ellenbogen KA, Karabinos I, Giazitzoglou E, Korovesis S, Camm AJ. Right and left inferior extensions of the atrioventricular node may represent the anatomic substrate of the slow pathway in humans. Heart Rhythm. 2004;1:582-6.
4. Issa ZF, Miller JM, Zipes DP. Atrioventricular Reentrant Tachycardia. In: Clinical Arrhythmology and Electrophysiology: A Companion to Brunwald's Heart Disease, 2nd ed. Philadelphia, PA: Saunders; 2012. pp. 411-67.
5. Hirao K, Otomo K, Wang X, Beckman KJ, McClelland JH, Widman L, Gonzalez MD, Arruda M, Nakagawa H, Lazzara R, Jackman WM. Para-Hisian Pacing. A New method for differentiating retrograde conduction over and accessory AV pathway from conduction over the AV node. Circulation. 1996;94:1027-35.
6. Tai C, Chen S, Chiang C, Chang M. Characteristics and Radiofrequency Catheter Ablation of Septal Accessory Atrioventricular Pathways. Pacing Clin Electrophysiol. 1999; 22:500-11.
7. Michaud GF, Tada HT, Chough, S, Baker R, Wasmer K, Sticherling C, Oral H, Pelosi F Jr, Knight BP, Strickberger SA, Morady F. Differentiation of atypical atrioventricular node re-entrant tachycardia from orthodromic reciprocating tachycardia using a septal accessory pathway by the response to ventricular pacing. J Am Coll Cardiol. 2001;38:1163-7.
8. Miller JM, Rosenthal ME, Gottlieb CD, Vassallo JA, Josephson ME. Usefulness of the delta HA interval to accurately distinguish atrioventricular nodal reentry from orthodromic septal bypass tract tachycardias. Am J Cardiol. 1991;68:1037-44.
9. Ho R, Mark GE, Rhim ES, Pavri BB, Greenspon AJ. Differentiating atrioventricular nodal reentrant tachycardia from atrioventricular reentrant tachycardia by delta HA values during entrainment from the ventricle. Heart Rhythm. 2008;5:83-8.
10. Srivathsan K, Gami AS, Barrett R, Monahan K, Packer D, Asirvathsam S. Differentiating Atrioventricular Nodal Reentrant Tachycardia from Junctional Tachycardia: Novel Application of the Delta H-A Interval. J Cardiovasc Electrophysiol. 2008;19:1-6.
11. Dandimudi G, Mokabberi R, Assal C, Das MK, Oren J, Storm R, Vijayaraman P, Miller JM. A novel approach to differentiating orthodromic reciprocating tachycardia from atrioventricular nodal reentrant tachycardia. Heart Rhythm. 2010;7: 1326-9.
12. Ormaetxe JM, Almendral J, Arenal A, Martinez-Alday JD, Pastor A, Villacastin JP, Delcan JL. Ventricular Fusion During Resetting and Entrainment of Orthodromic Supraventricular Tachycardia Involving Septal Accessory Pathways: Implications for the Differential Diagnosis With Atrioventricular Nodal Reentry. Circulation. 1993;88:2623-31.
13. Knight BP, Zivin A, Souza J, Flemming M, Pelosi F, Goyal R, Man C, Strickberger SA, Morady F. A technique for the rapid diagnosis of atrial tachycardia in the electrophysiology laboratory. J Am Coll Cardiol. 1999;33:775-81.
14. Knight BP, Ebinger M, Oral H, Kim MH, Sticherling C, Pelosi F, Michaud GF, Strickberger SA, Morady F. Diagnostic value of tachycardia features and pacing maneuvers during paroxysmal supraventricular tachycardia. J Am Coll Cardiol. 2000;36: 574-82.
15. Miles W, Yee R, Klein GJ, Zipes DP, Prystowsky EN. The preexcitation index: an aid in determining the mechanism of supraventricular tachycardia and localizing accessory pathways. Circulation. 1986;74:493-500.
16. Otomo K, Gonzakez MD, Beckman KJ, Nakagawa H, Becker AE, Shah N, Matsudaira K, Wang Z, Lazzara R, Jackman WM. Reversing the direction of paced ventricular and atrial wavefronts reveals an oblique course in accessory AV pathways and improves localization for catheter ablation. Circulation. 2001;104:550-6.
17. Jackman WM, Friday KJ, Scherlag BJ, Dehning MM, Schechter E, Reynolds DW, Olson EG, Berbari EJ, Harrison LA, Lazzara R. Direct endocardial recording from an accessory atrioventricular pathway: localization of the site of block, effect of antiarrhythmic drugs, and attempt at nonsurgical ablation. Circulation. 1983;68:906-16.

EDITORS' SUMMARY

Munro et al. provide for us an incredibly comprehensive, lucid review of one of the cornerstone maneuvers of invasive electrophysiology—ventricular pacing to diagnose the mechanism of SVT. The classic, common, and some relatively obscure but pertinent maneuvers are all covered in a practical manner with outstanding illustrations.

The authors describe the importance of the pacing site, the relative spatiotemporal relationship to pacing site and the entrant site to the conduction system versus the accessory pathway, and the importance of pacing rate and pacing output. A well-summarized discussion of para-Hisian pacing follows, and when used along with the provided reference will be a complete theoretic basis for student operator to execute this important maneuver. The authors also explain for us physiologically well-defined but less commonly executed maneuvers such as the comparative timing from His-bundle to atrial activation in tachycardia and with ventricular pacing. Their final summary providing their insights from experience on the hierarchical importance of each of these myriad maneuvers and a systematic approach to defining the mechanism of supraventricular tachycardia will be found greatly valuable for all electrophysiologists.

CHAPTER 16

Nishant Verma, Bradley P Knight

Supraventricular Tachycardias: Atrial Pacing Maneuvers

LIST OF ABBREVIATIONS

AT	Atrial Tachycardia	PAC	Premature Atrial Contraction
AV	Atrioventricular	SVT	Supraventricular Tachycardia
AVNRT	Atrioventricular Nodal Reentrant Tachycardia	VA	Ventriculoatrial
AVRT	Atrioventricular Reciprocating Tachycardia	VT	Ventricular Tachycardia
JT	Junctional Tachycardia		

INTRODUCTION

The introduction of atrial extrastimuli and atrial overdrive pacing are often overlooked maneuvers to help establish the diagnosis of a supraventricular tachycardia (SVT). Tachycardias can be reset and entrained with atrial pacing in the same manner as with ventricular pacing. In routine clinical practice, atrial resetting and entrainment are of most benefit in a few, specific situations. These include the distinction of a focal atrial tachycardia (AT) from atrioventricular nodal reentrant tachycardia (AVNRT) and atrioventricular reciprocating tachycardia using an accessory pathway (AVRT), to help differentiate typical AVNRT from junctional tachycardia (JT), and to distinguish a preexcited SVT from ventricular tachycardia (VT). The tachycardia response to both atrial extrastimulus pacing and atrial overdrive pacing has diagnostic utility in each of these situations. This chapter will serve to look at both maneuvers and help guide the reader in their use for SVT diagnosis.

ATRIAL EXTRASTIMULUS PACING

Scanning diastole with atrial extrastimuli can be a useful maneuver to aid in the diagnosis of a narrow complex tachycardia **(Figure 16.1)**. While tachycardia resetting with premature atrial extrastimuli can help to establish the diagnosis of a reentrant rhythm, it is of limited value in helping to differentiate between AVNRT, AVRT and even a microreentrant atrial tachycardia. However, if resetting with manifest fusion can be demonstrated, it would establish the diagnosis of AVRT or a macroreentrant atrial tachycardia rather than AVNRT or a focal atrial tachycardia.[1,2] Manifest fusion in the P-wave with atrial pacing is much more difficult to visualize than QRS fusion with ventricular pacing; therefore, this is most often seen in the intracardiac electrograms.

The introduction of atrial extrastimuli, or premature atrial contractions (PACs), during tachycardia can also be useful to help distinguish typical AVNRT from junctional tachycardia **(Figures 16.2A and B)**. In this situation, both early PACs and His-refractory PACs can be diagnostically useful.

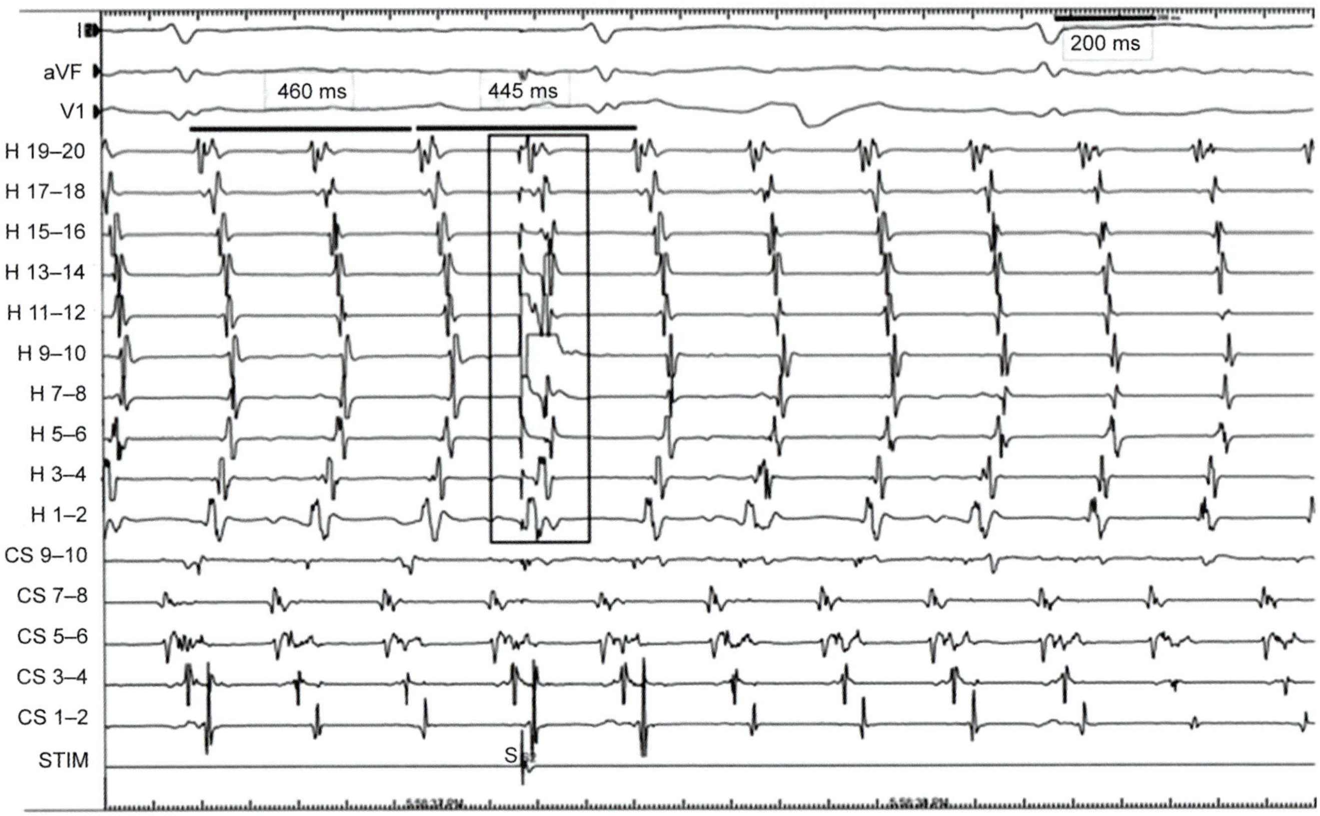

Figure 16.1: Atrial resetting with manifest intracardiac fusion during atypical atrial flutter. In a narrow-complex tachycardia with 1:1 AV conduction, this finding would rule out AVNRT or a focal AT

Abbreviations: H, halo; CS, coronary sinus; S, stimulus

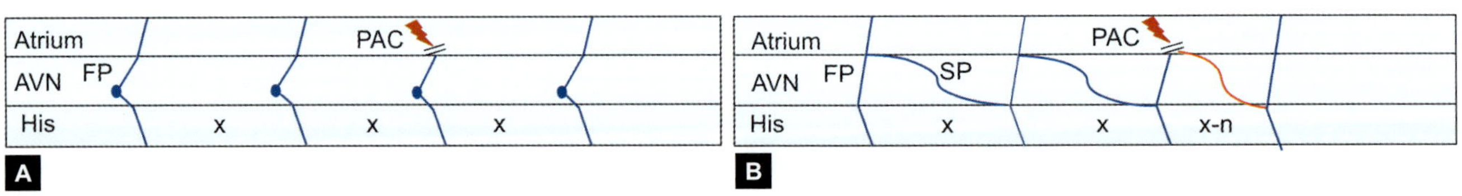

Figures 16.2A and B: The response to a His-refractory atrial extrastimulus during junctional tachycardia (A) and typical AVNRT (B) is demonstrated via a ladder diagram. During junctional tachycardia, the AV node cannot be penetrated by a His-refractory PAC because the fast pathway is refractory; however, during AVNRT, the slow pathway is available for antegrade conduction and the His signal is advanced

Abbreviations: PAC, premature atrial complex; FP, fast pathway; SP, slow pathway. [Adapted from reference (3)]

During junctional tachycardia, a His-refractory PAC will not be able to conduct through the AV node as the junction has already been depolarized and the node is refractory. However, during typical AVNRT, the retrograde limb of the tachycardia is the fast pathway and the antegrade limb is the slow pathway. Therefore, a His-refractory PAC could still affect the next beat of tachycardia with antegrade conduction down the slow pathway. Any perturbation of the next beat (advancement, delay or termination) by a His-refractory PAC is consistent with AVNRT and not junctional tachycardia.[3]

With earlier PACs, the antegrade fast pathway is available in both junctional tachycardia and typical AVNRT **(Figures 16.3A and B)**. Therefore, advancement of the next, immediate His can occur in both situations. However, in AVNRT, after the antegrade fast pathway is engaged by the atrial extrastimulus, the tachycardia will terminate, as there is no viable retrograde limb to perpetuate tachycardia. In junctional tachycardia, the PAC will advance the His timing; however, tachycardia will continue. Therefore, termination of tachycardia with an early-coupled PAC that advances the next, immediate His is diagnostic for typical AVNRT and not consistent with junctional tachycardia.[3]

Another clinical situation where atrial extrastimulus pacing has utility is to help distinguish a wide complex supraventricular tachycardia from ventricular tachycardia

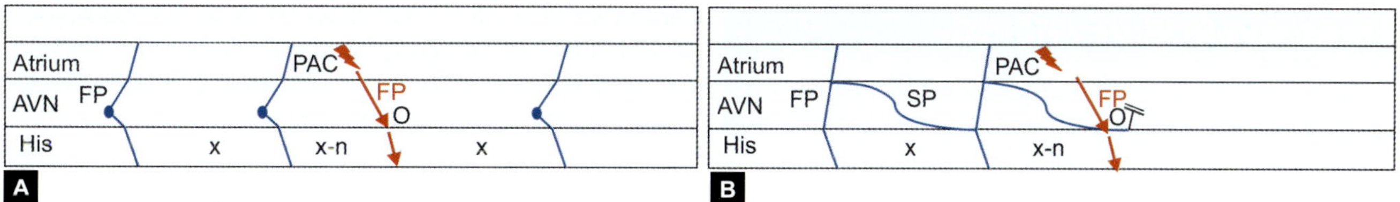

Figures 16.3A and B: The response to an early-coupled atrial extrastimulus during junctional tachycardia (A) and typical AVNRT (B) is demonstrated via a ladder diagram. An early atrial extrastimulus or PAC can engage the fast pathway (FP) for both JT and AVNRT and advance the His recording; however, in AVNRT, the antegrade conduction down the fast pathway terminates the rhythm, as there is no retrograde limb available for the tachycardia to perpetuate

Abbreviations: PAC, premature atrial complex; FP, fast pathway; SP, slow pathway; AVN, atrioventricular node. [Adapted from reference (3)]

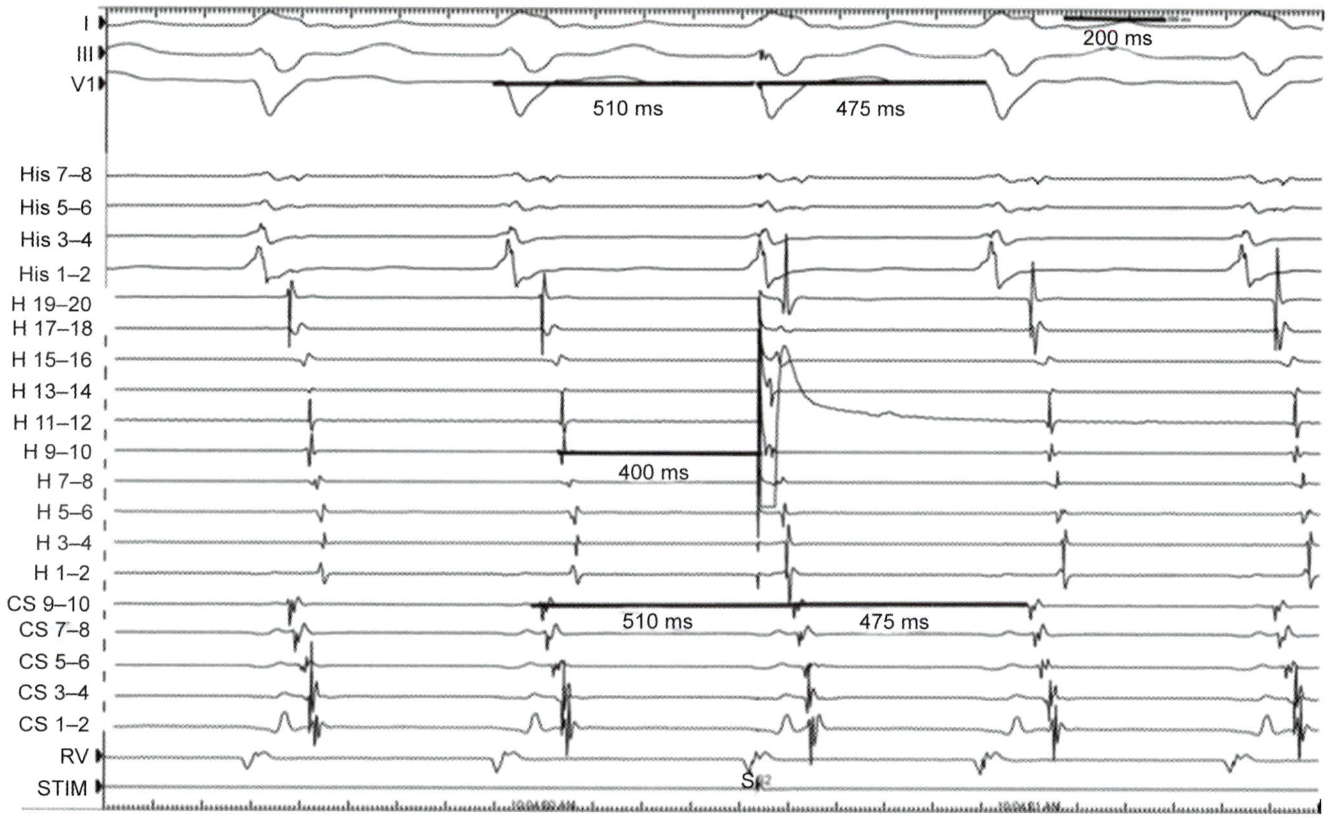

Figure 16.4: A lateral atrial extrastimulus with a coupling interval of 400 ms is introduced during antidromic tachycardia via an atriofascicular pathway. The septal atrial signal (CS 9–10) is not advanced, indicating that this atrial extrastimulus is His-refractory. The ventricular signal is advanced, ruling out VT, and the QRS morphology remains constant, proving a preexcited SVT. The subsequent atrial electrogram is also advanced confirming the diagnosis of antidromic tachycardia

Abbreviations: H, halo; CS, coronary sinus; RV, right ventricle; S, stimulus

(Figure 16.4). Any atrial stimulus that is able to advance or delay the next ventricular activation and generate the same QRS complex without fusion excludes myocardial VT. If a His-refractory atrial extrastimulus is able to advance the next ventricular activation, it proves the existence of an antegradely conducting accessory pathway but does not prove pathway participation in the tachycardia. If the QRS morphology remains constant while the ventricle is advanced, the diagnosis of a preexcited SVT can be made; however, it does not distinguish the type of SVT. If both the ventricular and subsequent atrial timings are advanced with a His-refractory PAC, then a diagnosis of antidromic AVRT can be made. Delay of the ventricular signal with a His-refractory PAC is also diagnostic for antidromic AVRT.[1,2]

ATRIAL OVERDRIVE PACING

Just as ventricular overdrive pacing can be used to aid in SVT diagnosis, atrial overdrive pacing can provide a similar diagnostic benefit. Reentrant rhythms can be continuously reset, or entrained, by atrial overdrive pacing. In fact, Waldo describes an early breakthrough in the understanding of entrainment during a case of slow VT with 1:1 ventriculoatrial (VA) conduction. Tachycardia entrainment was accomplished with atrial pacing and lead to a better understanding of the first two entrainment criteria.[4] Atrial overdrive pacing has utility in one common scenario, trying to distinguish an atrial tachycardia from AVNRT and AVRT; however, it can also be useful to distinguish AVNRT from junctional tachycardia and to distinguish AVRT from myocardial VT in the setting of a wide complex tachycardia.

VA linking is a concept that describes when atrial activation is dependent on ventricular activation and the VA times are fixed during tachycardia **(Figure 16.5)**. During both AVNRT and AVRT, atrial activation is dependent on ventricular activation and fixed VA intervals are expected. During atrial tachycardia, atrial activation is not dependent on ventricular activation and VA times are often variable. This can be observed at the onset of tachycardia as well as during atrial overdrive pacing. To perform this maneuver, the atrium is paced, during tachycardia, at a cycle length just below the tachycardia cycle length. If the tachycardia is accelerated to the pacing rate and continues after pacing is terminated, then the VA interval of the first return beat can be compared to the VA interval during tachycardia. If these VA intervals vary by 10 msec or less, VA linking is demonstrated. Showing this consistently at various pacing cycle lengths and various pacing locations is strong evidence against an atrial tachycardia.[2,5,6]

Examination of the AH intervals during atrial overdrive pacing can also be used to distinguish atrial tachycardia from AVNRT and AVRT **(Figure 16.6)**. During AVNRT and AVRT, there is generally a critical AH interval required to allow tachycardia to perpetuate. However, atrial tachycardia continuation is not dependent on the AH interval. During tachycardia, if the atrium is paced near the atrioventricular

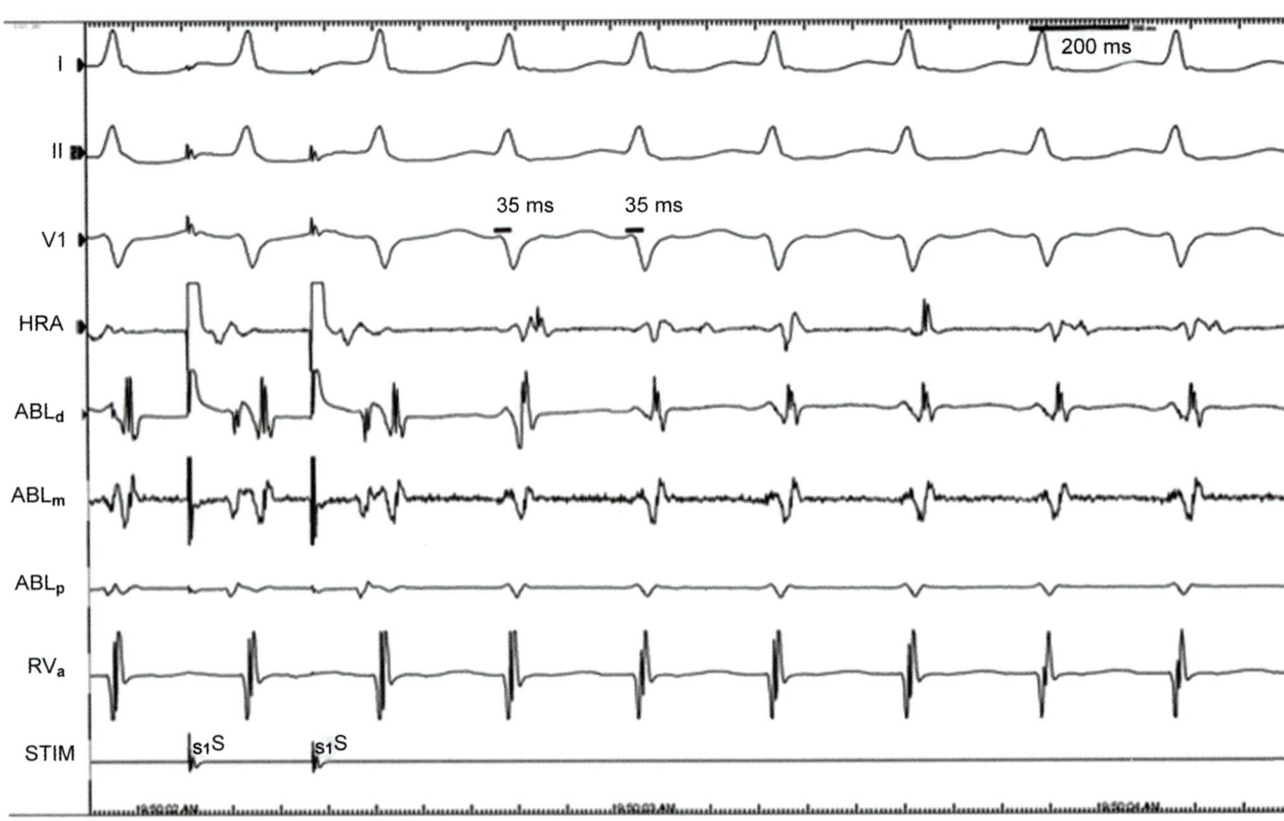

Figure 16.5: VA linking is shown during induction of typical AVNRT with right atrial pacing. The first beat of tachycardia has the same VA interval as the subsequent beats. This finding can also be demonstrated with entrainment of the tachycardia by atrial pacing and examination of the first return beat after pacing. This is not a consistent finding during atrial tachycardia
Abbreviations: HRA, high right atrium; ABL, ablation; RVa, RV apex; S, stimulus

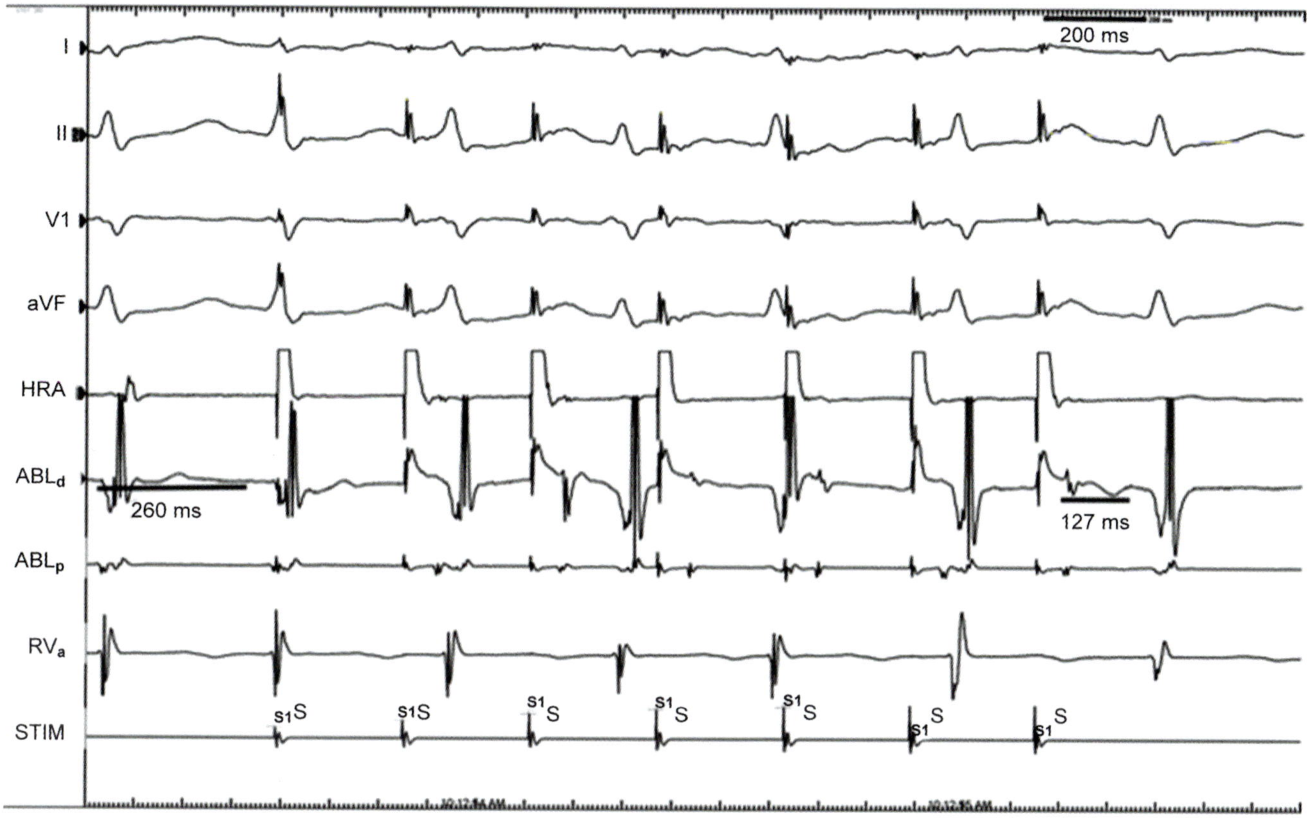

Figure 16.6: Typical AVNRT terminates with atrial pacing. The last AH interval after pacing is much shorter when the tachycardia terminates compared to the AH interval during tachycardia, and to the last AH interval when the tachycardia continues after atrial pacing. Therefore, tachycardia termination is thought to be dependent on a short AH interval. This finding is not consistent with atrial tachycardia
Abbreviations: HRA, high right atrium; ABL, ablation; RVa, RV apex; S, stimulus

(AV) block cycle length until tachycardia termination, the AH interval of the last paced beat can be examined. If the AH interval seen after tachycardia termination is shorter than the AH interval during tachycardia, or is shorter than the last AH interval at the end of other pacing attempts when the tachycardia continues, then the termination of tachycardia is said to be dependent on a short AH interval. An atrial tachycardia is not expected to be dependent on any AH interval.[5,6]

Atrial overdrive pacing has diagnostic utility to help distinguish junctional tachycardia from typical AVNRT as well **(Figures 16.7A and B)**. For this maneuver, the atrium is paced at a cycle length just below the tachycardia cycle length during tachycardia. After the tachycardia is accelerated to the pacing rate, atrial pacing is stopped with the anticipation that the tachycardia will continue. If the tachycardia terminates, then it can be reinitiated and the maneuver can be repeated. In the setting of AVNRT, the tachycardia is entrained while with junctional tachycardia, the tachycardia is overdrive suppressed. Conceptually similar to ventricular overdrive pacing, the response at cessation of pacing is examined. If the tachycardia continues with an "A-H-H-A" response after atrial pacing, then the diagnosis of a junctional tachycardia can be made. However, if there is an "A-H-A" response to atrial overdrive pacing, a diagnosis of typical AVNRT can be made.[7]

In the setting of a wide complex tachycardia, atrial overdrive pacing can help distinguish VT from a preexcited tachycardia **(Figures 16.8A and B)**. The ability to entrain a wide complex tachycardia from the atrium with concealed QRS fusion excludes the diagnosis of myocardial VT. However, it does not exclude bundle branch re-entry as a possible tachycardia mechanism. The converse of this concept, that atrial overdrive pacing results in manifest QRS fusion, is not diagnostic for myocardial VT as there could be more than one antegradely conducting accessory pathways and hence fusion may be seen with both VT and antidromic AVRT. Rapid atrial pacing that dissociates the atrium from the ventricle without a change in the ventricular cycle length and QRS morphology rules out preexcited SVT, AVRT and AT with aberrancy and strongly favors VT.[1,2,8]

In an analogous fashion to the use of ventricular overdrive pacing to distinguish atrial tachycardia from AVNRT and AVRT, the response to atrial overdrive pacing during a

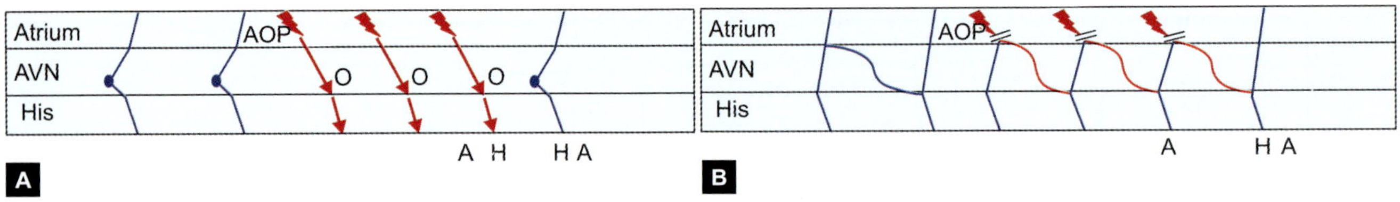

Figures 16.7A and B: The response to atrial overdrive pacing in junctional tachycardia (A) and typical AVNRT (B) is demonstrated via a ladder diagram. Overdrive suppression of the junctional tachycardia results in an "AHHA" response with tachycardia resumption while entrainment of AVNRT results in an "AHA" response

Abbreviations: AOP, atrial overdrive pacing; AVN, atrioventricular node. [Adapted from reference (7)]

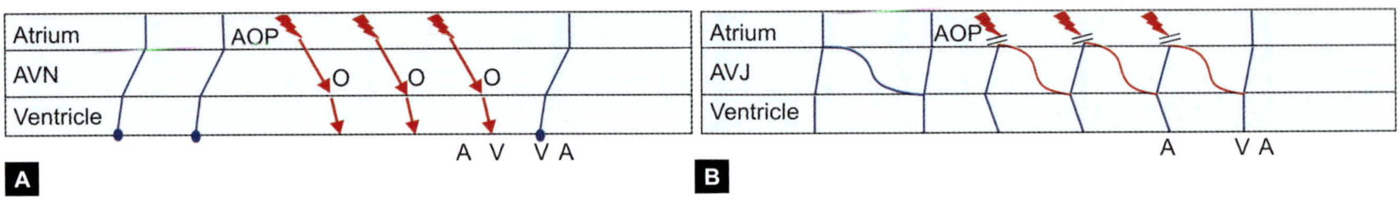

Figures 16.8A and B: The response to atrial overdrive pacing in ventricular tachycardia (A) and during antidromic AVRT or AVNRT with aberrant intraventricular conduction; (B) is demonstrated via a ladder diagram. Overdrive suppression of the VT results in an "AVVA" response with tachycardia resumption while entrainment of antidromic AVRT or AVNRT results in an "AVA" response

Abbreviations: AOP, atrial overdrive pacing; AVN, atrioventricular node; AVJ, atrioventricular junction. [Adapted from reference (8)]

wide complex tachycardia with 1:1 VA conduction can be examined. After the tachycardia cycle length is accelerated to that of the pacing rate, pacing is ceased with the goal of tachycardia continuing. During ventricular tachycardia, two useful findings can be observed. The first is that there is a change in the QRS morphology with either a narrowing or fusion, which is different from the tachycardia QRS morphology. In addition, after the last entrained ventricular complex, the response to atrial pacing is an "A-V-V-A" response. However, in the setting of a wide complex SVT, the ventricular response to atrial entrainment will be an "A-V-A".[8]

CONCLUSION

Atrial pacing maneuvers have tremendous utility to help diagnose SVT; however, they are most helpful in particular clinical scenarios. The most commonly encountered situation is during a supraventricular tachycardia with a short septal VA time (<70 ms). In this setting, an atrial tachycardia with a long AH time can be effectively ruled out with the reproducible demonstration of VA linking at multiple sites with multiple pacing rates. This maneuver would also be helpful for tachycardias with septal VA times >70 ms; however, other diagnostic maneuvers would need to be performed to distinguish between AVNRT and orthodromic AVRT.

A second increasingly important, albeit less common, scenario is when dealing with junctional tachycardia. Junctional tachycardia is a rare entity with unique clinical characteristics; however, it shares many of the same electrophysiologic characteristics of typical AVNRT. Ablation of junctional tachycardia is much more likely to result in AV block; therefore, a clear diagnosis is necessary prior to ablation. Both early and His-refractory extrastimulus pacing can help distinguish these two tachycardias as can atrial overdrive pacing during tachycardia.

The most clinically necessary use of atrial pacing maneuvers is in the setting of a wide complex tachycardia where SVT is being considered. Since the differential includes VT, preexcited SVTs and aberrant SVTs, these maneuvers are critical to help establish a diagnosis. Both extrastimulus pacing as well as overdrive pacing should routinely be used in this scenario to help clarify the diagnosis and guide the ablation strategy. A common adage is that when the tachycardia has a wide QRS, pace the atrium, and when it has a narrow QRS, pace the ventricle.

REFERENCES

1. Josephson ME. Clinical Cardiac Electrophysiology, 4th edn. Philadelphia, PA: Lippincott Williams and Wilkins; 2008. pp. 175-284, 339-445.
2. Issa ZF, Miller JM, Zipes DP. Clinical Arrhythmology and Electrophysiology, 2nd edn. Philadelphia, PA: Elsevier Inc; 2012. pp. 488-9, 509-10.
3. Padanilam BJ, Manfredi JA, Steinberg LA, Olson JA, Fogel RI, Prystowsky EN. Differentiating junctional tachycardia and atrioventricular node re-entry tachycardia based on response

to atrial extrastimulus pacing. J Am Coll Cardiol. 2008;52: 1711-7.
4. Waldo AL. From bedside to bench: entrainment and other stories. Heart Rhythm. 2004;1:94-106.
5. Kadish AH, Morady F. The response of paroxysmal supraventricular tachycardia to overdrive atrial and ventricular pacing: can it help determine the tachycardia mechanism? J Cardiovasc Electrophysiol. 1993;4:239-52.
6. Knight BP, Ebinger M, Oral H, Kim MH, Sticherling C, Pelosi F, Michaud GF, Strickberger SA, Morady F. Diagnostic value of tachycardia features and pacing maneuvers during paroxysmal supraventricular tachycardia. J Am Coll Cardiol. 2000;36:574-82.
7. Fan R, Tardos JG, Almasry I, Barbera S, Rashba EJ, Iwai S. Novel use of atrial overdrive pacing to rapidly differentiate junctional tachycardia from atrioventricular nodal reentrant tachycardia. Heart Rhythm. 2011;8:840-4.
8. Abdelwahab A, Gardner MJ, Basta MN, Parkash R, Khan A, Sapp JL. A technique for the rapid diagnosis of wide complex tachycardia with 1:1 AV relationship in the electrophysiology laboratory. Pacing Clin Electrophysiol. 2009;32: 475-83.

EDITORS' SUMMARY

The principle role for atrial pacing maneuvers is in the context of an undefined wide complex tachycardia. The rationale and nuances of using atrial extrastimuli and atrial pacing when confronted with a wide QRS tachycardia in the EP laboratory is also covered elsewhere in this book (Chapter 44) and in an another book (Asirvatham SJ, Friedman PA, Cha YM. Mayo Clinic Electrophysiology Manual Rochester: Mayo Clinic Scientific Press; 2014. p. 711). In essence, pacing in the atrium can help define whether the atrium is necessary for the maintenance of a wide QRS tachycardia as with antidromic tachycardia or AV node reentry with bundle-branch block, etc. or if the tachycardia can continue without atrial involvement as in all ventricular tachycardias and rare variants of AV node reentry.

In the present chapter, Drs. Verma and Knight describe the role of atrial pacing in SVT regardless of whether the QRS is narrow or wide. The most important utility as they comprehensively and clearly explain is distinguishing between AV node reentry and a rapid junctional tachycardia. Their description should form the foundation for any student of electrophysiology to begin understanding this often unclear distinction.

This differential diagnostic problem is made more complex by the fact that neither AV node reentry nor junctional tachycardia represents single uniform entities. AV node reentry may involve block of an upper common pathway resulting in more ventricular events than atrial events or intermittent antegrade atrioventricular block potentially at multiple levels. Similarly, junctional tachycardia may be from an automatic focus within the compact AV node or in the region of the His bundle and potentially in the slow or fast pathway inputs to the AV node. The heterogeneous nature of these entities provides ample opportunity for confusing overlap in specific variants, for example, slow pathway automatic tachycardia with retrograde block versus typical AVNRT. Using the principles outlined in this chapter, a foundation for excluding possible mechanisms of an unusual SVT can usually quickly be made, and then the operator needs to decide whether the arrhythmia can be solved without direct ablation on the compact AV node itself.

CHAPTER 17

Demosthenes G Katritsis, Mark E Josephson

Atrioventricular Nodal Reentrant Tachycardia: Classification, Electrophysiological Features, and Ablation

LIST OF ABBREVIATIONS

AV	Atrioventricular	VA	Ventriculoatrial
AVNRT	Atrioventricular Nodal Reentrant Tachycardia		

CLASSIFICATION

Atrioventricular nodal reentrant tachycardia (AVNRT) denotes reentry in the area of the atrioventricular (AV) node, and although several models have been proposed to explain the mechanism of the arrhythmia in the context of the complex anatomy of the AV node and its atrial extensions,[1] the actual circuit of the arrhythmia remains elusive.[2] Classification schemes have been mainly based on the conventional concept of longitudinally dissociated dual AV nodal pathways that conduct around a central obstacle **(Table 17.1)**.

In typical, *slow-fast* AVNRT the onset of atrial activation appears prior, at the onset, or just after the QRS complex, thus maintaining an atrial-His/His-atrial ratio, AH/HA >1. The HA interval is usually <70 ms, measured from earliest deflection of the His bundle activation to the earliest rapid deflection of the atrial activation in the His bundle electrogram, and the VA interval, measured from the onset of

Table 17.1: Conventional classification of AVNRT types

	AH/HA	*VA (His)*	*Usual ERAA*
Typical AVNRT			
Slow-fast	>1	<60 ms	RHis, CS os, LHis
Atypical AVNRT			
Fast-slow	<1	>60 ms	CS os, LRAS, dCS
Slow-slow	>1	>60 ms	CS os, dCS

Variable earliest retrograde atrial activation has been described for all types

Abbreviations: AH, atrial to His interval; HA, His to atrium interval; VA, interval measured from the onset of ventricular activation on surface ECG to the earliest deflection of the atrial activation in the His bundle electrogram; ERAA, earliest retrograde atrial activation; RHis, His bundle electrogram recorded from the right septum; LHis, His bundle electrogram recorded from the left septum; LRAS, low right atrial septum; CS os, ostium of the coronary sinus; dCS, distal coronary sinus

From: Katritsis DG, Camm AJ. Atrioventricular nodal reentrant tachycardia. Circulation. 2010;122:831-40

ventricular activation on surface ECG to the earliest rapid deflection of the atrial activation on the His bundle electrogram, is <60 ms.[2-4] In atypical, *fast-slow form* of atypical AVNRT, the retrograde atrial electrogram begins after ventricular activation with an AH/HA ratio <1. The HA interval is prolonged, ≥ 70 ms, and the VA interval is ≥60 ms.[2-4] The atypical, *slow-slow form*, represents, by definition, an arrhythmia utilizing two slow pathways. The AH/HA ratio is ≥ 1 but the HA interval is ≥70 ms, and the AH interval exceeds 200 ms.[5-7]

There are several inherent limitations of this classification. The distinction between fast-slow and slow-slow atypical AVNRT is often arbitrary in view of the lack of a unanimously accepted definition. In order to establish the diagnosis of a truly fast-slow form, it has been proposed that the AH interval should be less than 185 ms[8] or 200 ms.[4] This criterion, however, has not been adopted by other investigators.[9-11] Thus, tachycardias with a relatively prolonged AH interval but an AH/HA ratio <1 cannot be reliably classified as either fast-slow or slow-slow **(Figure 17.1)**. Furthermore, the term "fast-slow" implies that the fast component of slow-fast AVNRT is the same as the fast in the fast-slow type. There is now evidence that this is not the case in patients who present with both types of tachycardia.[12,13] Typical slow-fast and atypical fast-slow AVNRT appear to utilize different anatomical pathways for fast conduction. In addition, electrophysiological behavior compatible with multiple pathways may also be seen, and in some patients, several forms of AVNRT may be inducible at electrophysiology study.

We have therefore, proposed a different classification scheme **(Table 17.2)** that takes into account the short-

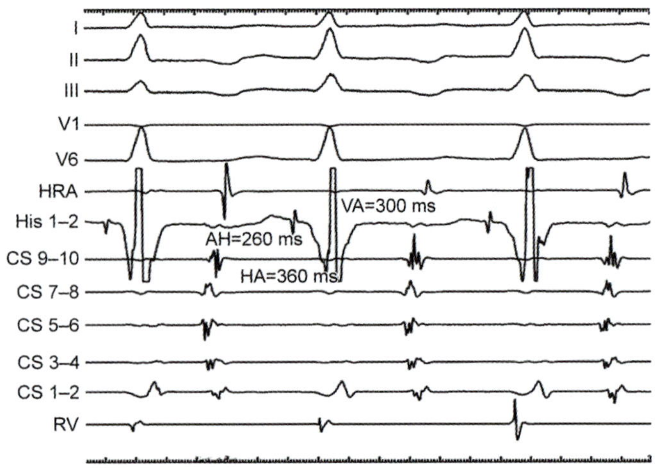

Figure 17.1: Atypical AVNRT. The form is fast-slow according to the AH<HA definition, but slow-slow according to the AH>200 ms criterion From top to bottom are—surface ECG leads I, II, III, V1 and V6; high right atrium (HRA); His bundle distal (His 1–2); coronary sinus proximal (CS 9–10) to distal (CS 1–2); and right ventricle (RV)

From: Katritsis DG, Josephson ME. Classification of electrophysiological types of atrioventricular nodal re-entrant tachycardia: a reappraisal. Europace. 2013;15:1231-40

Table 17.2: Novel proposed classification of AVNRT types

	HA	*VA (His)*	*AH/HA*
Typical AVNRT	≤70 ms	≤60 ms	>1
Atypical AVNRT	>70 ms	>60 ms	Variable

The distinction is for categorization only, and not relevant for mechanism or therapy. Atypical AVNRT has been traditionally classified as fast-slow (HA>70 ms, VA>60, AH/HA<1, and AH<200 ms) or slow-slow (HA>70 ms, VA>60 ms, AH/HA>1, and AH>200 ms). Not all of these criteria are always met and atypical AVNRT may not be subclassified accordingly

Abbreviations: AH, atrial to His interval; HA, His to atrium interval; VA, interval measured from the onset of ventricular activation on surface ECG to the earliest deflection of the atrial activation on the His bundle electrogram

From: Katritsis DG, Josephson ME. Classification of electrophysiological types of atrioventricular nodal re-entrant tachycardia: a reappraisal. Europace. 2013;15:1231-40.

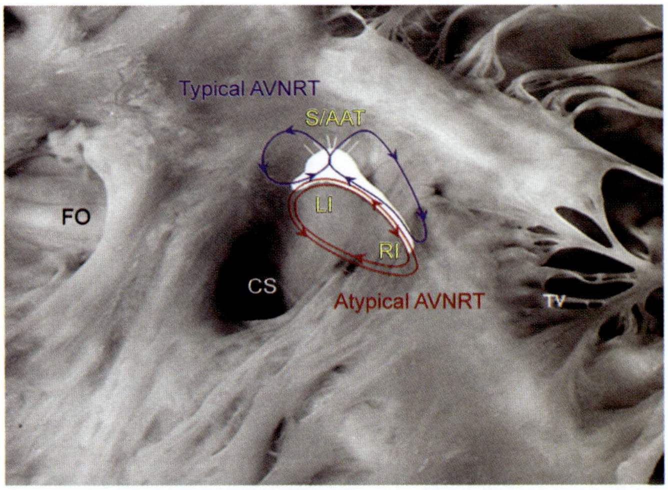

Figure 17.2: Proposed circuit of AVNRT. During typical AVNRT (slow-fast), right- or left-sided circuits may occur with antegrade conduction through the inferior inputs and retrograde conduction through the superior inputs (S) or the anisotropic atrionodal transitional area (AAT). In atypical AVNRT conduction occurs anterogradely through one of the inferior inputs, left (LI) or right (RI) and retrogradely through the other one. Depending on the orientation of the circuit we may record the so-called "fast-slow" or "slow-slow" types

Abbreviations: AAT, anisotropic atrionodal transitional area; AVNRT, atrioventricular nodal reentrant tachycardia; CS, coronary sinus; FO, fossa ovalis; LI, left inferior input; RI, right inferior input; S, superior input; TV, tricuspid valve

From: Katritsis DG, Josephson ME. Classification of electrophysiological types of atrioventricular nodal re-entrant tachycardia: a reappraisal. Europace. 2013;15:1231-40

comings of conventional classification, and reflects evolving concepts regarding the nature of the AVNRT circuit in various forms of the arrhythmia **(Figure 17.2)**.[3]

AVNRT should be classified either as typical or atypical. In addition, only the AH/HA and absolute HA intervals should be used as criteria for diagnosis of typical AVNRT.[8] The VA interval is also a practical and easily obtainable criterion, when the His bundle potential cannot be reproducibly and reliably recorded during tachycardia **(Table 17.2)**. As discussed later, retrograde atrial activation sequence or demonstration of a lower common pathway, should not be necessarily considered as reliable criteria for classification of AVNRT types.

ELECTROPHYSIOLOGICAL FEATURES

Earliest Atrial Retrograde Activation

Heterogeneity of both fast and slow conduction patterns has been well described, and all forms of AVNRT may display anterior, posterior and middle retrograde activation patterns. In typical, slow-fast AVNRT, posterior or even left atrial fast pathways may occur in up to 8% of patients.[10,11,14,15] There has also been evidence that were left septal His recordings routinely performed in patients with AVNRT, the proportion of left-sided retrograde fast pathways might be considerably higher than previously reported.[16] **Figures 17.3 and 17.4** present typical AVNRT (slow-fast) with variable earliest retrograde atrial activation.

In atypical AVNRT, the earliest retrograde atrial activation is traditionally reported at the base of the triangle of Koch, near the coronary sinus ostium. Detailed mapping of retrograde atrial activation in large series of patients, however, has produced variable results. Earliest atrial activation can be well recorded at the coronary sinus ostium, the low right atrial septum, or the His bundle area.[9-11,15] In certain cases of atypical AVNRT, retrograde atrial activation is even suggestive of a left lateral accessory pathway.[6,7]

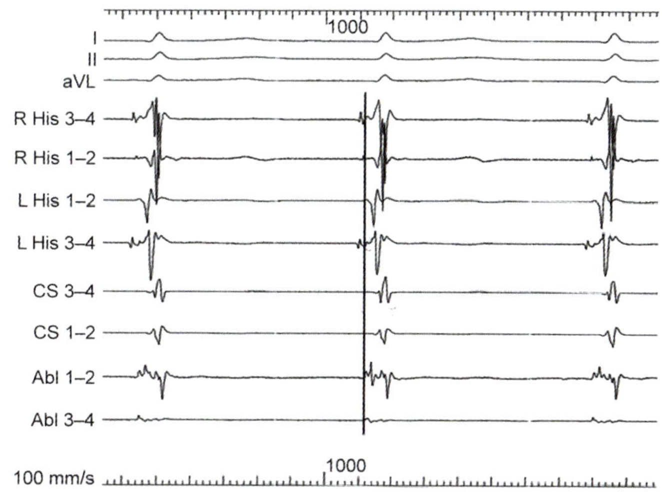

Figure 17.4: Typical slow-fast AVNRT. Simultaneous mapping of the right septum (R His), left septum (L His), and the anatomic area of the slow pathway is undertaken. Earliest retrograde atrial activation is recorded on the left septum

From top to bottom are—surface ECG leads I, II, and aVL; His bundle proximal recorded at the right septum (R His 3–4); His bundle recorded at left septum distal (L His 1–2) and proximal (L His 3–4); coronary sinus mid (CS 3–4) and distal (CS 1–2); and ablation catheter proximal (Abl 3–4) and distal (Abl 1–2) recordings from the anatomical area of the slow pathway

From: Katritsis DG, Josephson ME. Classification of electrophysiological types of atrioventricular nodal re-entrant tachycardia: a reappraisal. Europace. 2013;15:1231-40

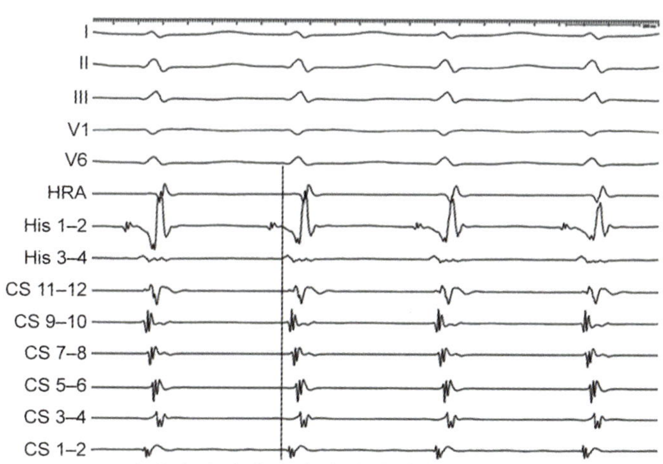

Figure 17.3: Typical slow-fast AVNRT. Earliest retrograde atrial activation is simultaneously recorded at distal CS (CS 1–2) and proximal His (His 3–4)

From top to bottom are—surface ECG leads I, II, III, V1 and V6; high right atrium (HRA); His bundle distal (His 1–2) and proximal (His 3–4); coronary sinus proximal (CS 11–12) to distal (CS 1–2)

From: Katritsis DG, Josephson ME. Classification of electrophysiological types of atrioventricular nodal re-entrant tachycardia: a reappraisal. Europace. 2013;15:1231-40

It is obvious, therefore, that classification based on earliest atrial retrograde activation is inappropriate. **Figures 17.5 and 17.6** depict fast-slow and slow-slow AVNRT, respectively, with earliest retrograde atrial activation at the His bundle electrode.

Upper and Lower Common Pathways

Early studies have considered the possibility of additional AV nodal tissue extrinsic to the tachycardia circuit in order to explain various electrophysiologic phenomena observed during AVNRT,[17] and the concepts of upper and lower common pathways have been long-standing controversies of AVNRT. The existence of an upper common pathway can now be rather easily refuted by subsequent evidence indicating that multiple atrial breakthroughs are extremely common, and retrograde activation often changes in timing and/or activation without significant alteration in tachycardia cycle, thus negating the notion of a simplistic focal atrial exit

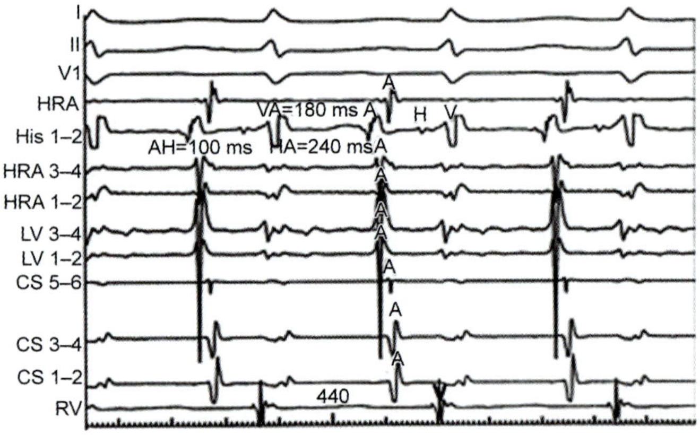

Figure 17.5: Atypical AVNRT. The form is conventionally fast-slow (AH<HA, HA>70 ms, AH<200 ms), and earliest retrograde atrial activation recorded at the His bundle electrode

From top to bottom are—surface ECG leads I, II, and V1; high right atrium (HRA); His bundle distal (His 1–2) and proximal (His 3–4); high right atrium distal (HRA 1–2) and proximal (HRA 3–4); left septum proximal (LV 3–4 and distal (LV 1–2); coronary sinus mid (CS 5–6) to distal (CS 1–2); and right ventricle (RV)

From: Katritsis DG, Josephson ME. Classification of electrophysiological types of atrioventricular nodal re-entrant tachycardia: a reappraisal. Europace. 2013;15:1231-40

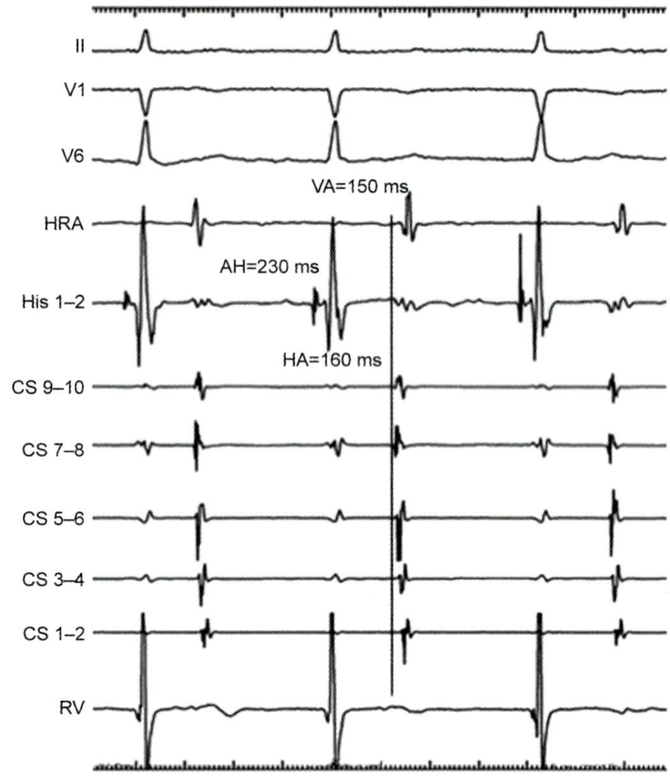

Figure 17.6: Atypical AVNRT. The form is conventionally slow-slow (AH>HA, HA>60 ms, AH>200 ms), and earliest retrograde atrial activation is recorded at the His bundle

From top to bottom are—surface ECG leads II, V1 and V6; high right atrium (HRA); His bundle distal (His 1–2); coronary sinus proximal (CS 9–10) to distal (CS 1–2); and right ventricle (RV)

From: Katritsis DG, Josephson ME. Classification of electrophysiological types of atrioventricular nodal re-entrant tachycardia: a reappraisal. Europace. 2013;15:1231-40

site.[18-20] The perinodal transitional tissue is the route to the atrium, and in this context it may be considered as a common pathway of tissue but not a discrete site. The breakthrough is whatever leads to atrial activation via transitional tissue; thus there are many possibilities **(Figures 17.3 and 17.6)**.

The lower common pathway, as initially considered by Mendez and Moe,[21] has been more reluctant to die. There is also evidence, however, that if anything, it represents a concept the mechanism and relevance of which remain speculative.[22] The notion of a lower common pathway has been utilized in order to explain phenomena of AV block without recording of a His electrogram as well as retrograde Wenckebach periodicity during AVNRT.[22-25] The lower common pathway is defined as the conduction path between the distal turnaround point of the AVNRT circuit and the His bundle. The conduction time over the lower common pathway has been usually estimated by subtracting the His to atrium interval during tachycardia (measured from the onset of the His electrogram to the onset of the atrial electrogram) from that during ventricular pacing (measured from the end of the His electrogram to the onset of the atrial electrogram) at the same cycle length and considered a measurable interval in the majority of typical AVNRT cases. Initially, a lower common pathway was demonstrated in up to 75% of 28 patients with AVNRT who were studied,[17] whereas in subsequent studies with the use of para-Hisian pacing, the presence of a lower common pathway was identified in 78% of 23 patients studied.[24] No evidence of a lower common pathway has been detected in typical slow-fast AVNRT.[26]

However, AV block during AVNRT without recording activation of the His bundle can also be explained by proximal intra-Hisian block.[27] In up to one-third of patients with AVNRT the lower turnaround point of the circuit is within the His bundle, thus arguing against an intranodal circuit as a universal feature of AVNRT.[28] Differences in the location of the lower turnaround sites of AV nodal reentry relatively to the His bundle have also been shown in experimental studies.[29] Thus, block during AVNRT does not necessarily define a "lower common pathway"; it just defines longer refractory period below the circuit. This is often seen at the onset of very fast AVNRT, which may expose the His-Purkinje tissue to long-short periods and can lead to functional phase 3 block, having nothing to do with the reentrant circuit.

The electrophysiologic proof of the existence of a lower common pathway depends on several assumptions that may not be valid. These necessary conditions are: retrograde fast pathway conduction is the same during pacing and tachycardia, the recording of the proximal His bundle potential corresponds to the proximal end of the His bundle, the beginning of the antegrade His bundle potential during tachycardia and the end of the retrograde His bundle potential during ventricular pacing represent activation at the same site, and autonomic tone remains the same during tachycardia and ventricular pacing. These assumptions are far from proven. Detailed mapping of both sides of the septum has revealed that earliest retrograde atrial activation may well be on the left side for both fast and slow pathways,[16,30] and that the breakthrough of atrial activation is discordant from that observed during ventricular pacing in up to 43% of patients with slow-fast AVNRT.[16] Even if a lower common pathway exists, therefore, applied methodologies are unable to detect and measure it. Thus, electrophysiologic findings suggesting the presence of a lower common pathway can be interpreted in various ways outside the context of a common pathway in most cases. Recent studies suggest a three-dimensional AV node with greater variability in the space constant of tissue and poor gap junction connectivity due to differential expression of connexin isoforms, that provide an explanation of dual conduction and nodal reentrant arrhythmogenesis.[31,32] It is very difficult to conceive the presence of "common" pathways in this environment.

Furthermore, the practical applicability of the method is questionable. There are certain cases in the electrophysiology laboratory where an antegrade, let alone a retrograde, His bundle electrogram may not be reproducibly and reliably recorded.[17,33]

Relative AH/HA Intervals

The AH time and the relative AH/HA intervals have been proposed as a criterion for distinction between fast-slow and slow-slow AVNRT. However, both absolute and relative values may be meaningless in certain occasions. They depend on autonomic status, age, use of isoprenaline and sedatives, and conduction properties of pathways involved, and may change during a single electrophysiology study. We have often noticed different AH/HA times in the same patient at similar or different tachycardia cycle lengths. Furthermore, when a His bundle electrogram cannot be recorded during tachycardia, a diagnosis-based exclusively on them is impossible.[34]

ABLATION

Chronic administration of antiarrhythmic drugs (such as beta blockers, nondihydropyridine calcium channel blockers, flecainide or propafenone) may be ineffective in up to 50% of cases.[2] Thus, catheter ablation is the current treatment of choice.

Slow pathway ablation or modification is effective in both typical and atypical AVNRT. Usually, a combined anatomical and mapping approach is employed with ablation lesions delivered at the inferior or mid part of the triangle of Koch.[35,36] Multicomponent atrial electrograms or low amplitude potentials, although not specific for identification of slow pathway conduction, are successfully used to guide ablation at these areas. Ablation should be only directed towards the anatomic position of the slow pathway. If right septal attempts are unsuccessful, the left septal side should be tried.[36] This approach offers a success rate of 95%, is associated with a risk of 0.5–1% AV block and has an approximately 4% recurrence rate. Although a <0.6% mortality has been reported in earlier studies,[37] no deaths are seen in recent trials.[38] Advanced age is not a contraindication for slow pathway ablation.[39] The pre-existence of first-degree heart block may carry a higher risk for late AV block and slow pathway modification, as opposed to complete elimination, is probably preferable in this setting.[40] Cryoablation may carry a lower risk of AV block, but it is rather negligible and this mode of therapy is associated with a significantly higher recurrence rate.[41]

CONCLUSION

1. AVNRT should be classified as typical or atypical. The term "fast-slow AVNRT" is rather misleading.
2. Retrograde atrial activation during tachycardia should not be relied upon as a diagnostic criterion. Both typical and atypical AVNRT are compatible with varying retrograde atrial activation patterns.
3. Attempts at establishing the presence of a "lower common pathway" are scientifically unjustified and of no practical significance.
4. When the diagnosis of AVNRT is established, ablation should be only directed towards the anatomic position of the slow pathway. If right septal attempts are unsuccessful, the left septal side should be tried.
5. Ablation targeting earliest atrial activation sites during typical AVNRT or the fast pathway in general for any kind of typical or atypical AVNRT, are not justified.

REFERENCES

1. Katritsis DG, Becker A. The atrioventricular nodal reentrant tachycardia circuit: A proposal. Heart Rhythm. 2007;4: 1354-60.
2. Katritsis DG, Camm AJ. Atrioventricular nodal reentrant tachycardia. Circulation. 2010;122:831-40.
3. Katritsis DG, Josephson ME. Classification of electrophysiological types of atrioventricular nodal re-entrant tachycardia: a reappraisal. Europace. 2013;15:1231-40.
4. Heidbüchel H, Jackman WM. Characterization of subforms of AV nodal reentrant tachycardia. Europace. 2004;6:316-2.
5. Goldberger J, Brooks R, Kadish A. Physiology of "atypical" atrioventricular junctional reentrant tachycardia occurring

following radiofrequency catheter modification of the atrioventricular node. Pacing Clin Electrophysiol. 1992;15: 2270-82.
6. Sakabe K, Wakatsuki T, Fujinaga H, Oishi Y, Ikata J, Toyoshima T, Hiura N, Nishikado A, Oki T, Ito S. Patient with atrioventricular node reentrant tachycardia with eccentric retrograde left-sided activation: treatment with radiofrequency catheter ablation. Jpn Heart J. 2000;41:227-34.
7. Vijayaraman P, Kok LC, Rhee B, Ellenbogen KA. Unusual variant of atrioventricular nodal reentrant tachycardia. Heart Rhythm. 2004;2:100-102.
8. Lockwood D, Nakagawa H, Jackman WM. Electrophysiologic characteristics of atrioventricular nodal reentrant tachycardia: implications for reentrant circuits. In: Zipes DP, Jalife J (Eds). Cardiac electrophysiology: from cell to bedside, 5th edn. Saunders. 2009. pp. 615-45.
9. Nawata H, Yamamoto N, Hirao K, Miyasaka N, Kawara T, Hiejima K, Harada T, Suzuki F. Heterogeneity of anterograde fast-pathway and retrograde slow-pathway conduction patterns in patients with the fast-slow form of atrioventricular nodal re-entrant tachycardia: electrophysiologic and electrocardiographic considerations. J Am Coll Cardiol. 1998;32: 1731-40.
10. Nam, G-B, Rhee K-S, Kim J, Choi K-J, Kim Y-H. Left atrionodal connections in typical and atypical atrioventricular nodal re-entrant tachycardias: activation sequence in the coronary sinus and results of radiofrequency catheter ablation. J Cardiovasc Electrophysiol. 2006;17:1-7.
11. Hwang C, Martin DJ, Goodman JS, Gang ES, Mandel WJ, Swerdlow CD, Peter CT, Chen PS. Atypical atrioventricular node reciprocating tachycardia masquerading as tachycardia using a left-sided accessory pathway. J Am Coll Cardiol. 1997;30:218-25.
12. Katritsis DG, Sepahpour A, Marine JE, Katritsis GD, Tanawuttiwat T, Calkins H, Rowland E, Josephson ME. Atypical atrioventricular nodal reentrant tachycardia: prevalence, electrophysiologic characteristics, and tachycardia circuit. Europace. 2015;17:1099-106.
13. Katritsis DG, Marine JE, Latchamsetty R, Zografos T, Tanawuttiwat T, Sheldon SH, Buxton AE, Calkins H, Morady F, Josephson ME. Coexistent Types of Atrioventricular Nodal Reentrant Tachycardia: Implications for the Tachycardia Circuit. Circ Arrhythm Electrophysiol. 2015;8:1189-93.
14. Engelstein ED, Stein KM, Markowitz SM, Lerman BB. Posterior fast atrioventricular node pathways: implications for radiofrequency catheter ablation of atrioventricular node reentrant tachycardia. J Am Coll Cardiol. 1996;27:1098-105.
15. Chen J, Anselme F, Smith TW, Zimetbaum P, Epstein LM, Papageorgiou P, Josephson ME. Standard right atrial ablation is effective for atrioventricular nodal reentry with earliest activation in the coronary sinus. J Cardiovasc Electrophysiol. 2004;15:2-7.
16. Katritsis DG, Ellenbogen KA, Becker AE. Atrial activation during atrioventricular nodal reentrant tachycardia: studies on retrograde fast pathway conduction. Heart Rhythm. 2006;3:993-1000.
17. Miller JM, Rosenthal ME, Vassalo JA, Josephson ME. Atrioventricular nodal reentrant tachycardia: Studies on upper and lower "common pathways". Circulation. 1987;75: 930-40.
18. McGuire MA, Lau KC, Johnson DC, Richards DA, Uther JB, Ross DL. Patients with two types of atrioventricular junctional (AV nodal) reentrant tachycardia. Evidence that a common pathway of nodal tissue is not present above the reentrant circuit. Circulation. 1991;83:1232-46.
19. Anselme F, Hook B, Monahan K, Frederiks J, Callans D, Zardini M, Epstein LM, Zebede J, Josephson ME. Heterogeneity of retrograde fast-pathway conduction pattern in patients with atrioventricular nodal reentry tachycardia: observations by simultaneous multisite catheter mapping of Koch's triangle. Circulation. 1996;93:960-8.
20. Katritsis DG. Upper and lower common pathways in atrioventricular nodal reentrant tachycardia: refutation of a legend? Pacing Clin Electrophysiol. 2007;30:1305-8.
21. Mendez C, Moe GK. Demonstration of a dual A-V nodal conduction system in the isolated rabbit heart. Circ Res. 1966;19:378-93.
22. Otomo K, Okamura H, Noda T, Satomi K, Shimizu W, Suyama K, Epstein LM, Zebede J, Josephson ME. Unique electrophysiologic characteristics of atrioventricular nodal re-entrant tachycardia with different ventriculoatrial block patterns: effects of slow pathway ablation and insights into the location of the reentrant circuit. Heart Rhythm. 2006;3:544-54.
23. Otomo K, Nagata Y, Uno K, Fujiwara H, Iesaka Y. Atypical atrioventricular nodal reentrant tachycardia with eccentric coronary sinus activation: Electrophysiological characteristics and essential effects of left-sided ablation inside the coronary sinus. Heart Rhythm. 2007;4:421-32.
24. Anselme F, Poty H, Cribier A, Josephson ME, Saoudi N. Entrainment of typical AV nodal reentrant tachycardia using para-Hisian pacing: evidence for a lower common pathway within the AV node. J Cardiovasc Electrophysiol. 1999;10: 655-61.
25. Kazemi B, Haghjoo M, Arya A, Sadr-Ameli MA. Spontaneous high degree atrioventricular block during AV nodal re-entrant tachycardia. Europace. 2006;8:421-2.
26. Heidbuchel H, Ector H, Van de Werf F. Prospective evaluation of the length of the lower common pathway in the differential diagnosis of various forms of AV nodal reentrant tachycardia. Pacing Clin Electrophysiol. 1998;21:209-16.
27. Man KC, Brinkman K, Bogun F, Knight B, Bahu M, Weiss R, Goyal R, Harvey M, Daoud EG, Strickberger SA, Morady F. 2:1 atrioventricular block during atrioventricular node reentrant tachycardia. J Am Coll Cardiol. 1996;28:1770-4.
28. Li YG, Bender B, Bogun F, Gronefeld G, Hohnloser SH. Location of the lower turnaround point in typical AV nodal reentrant tachycardia: a quantitative model. J Cardiovasc Electrophysiol. 2000;11:34-40.
29. Patterson E, Scherlag BJ. Slow:fast and slow:slow AV nodal reentry in the rabbit resulting from longitudinal dissociation within the posterior AV nodal input. J Interv Card Electrophysiol. 2003;8:93-102.
30. Katritsis DG, Ellenbogen KA, Becker AE, Camm AJ. Retrograde slow pathway conduction in patients with atrioventricular nodal re-entrant tachycardia. Europace. 2007;9:458-65.
31. Hucker WJ, McCain ML, Laughner JI, Iaizzo PA, Efimov IR. Connexin 43 expression delineates two discrete pathways in the human atrioventricular junction. Anat Rec (Hoboken). 2008;291:204-15.
32. Nikolaidou T, Aslanidi OV, Zhang H, Efimov IR. Structure-function relationship in the sinus and atrioventricular nodes. Pediatr Cardiol. 2012;33:890-9.
33. Kapa S, Henz BD, Dib C, Friedman PA, Munger TM, Ladewig DJ, Hammill SC, Packer DL, Asirvatham SJ. Utilization

of retrograde right bundle branch block to differentiate atrioventricular nodal from accessory pathway conduction. J Cardiovasc Electrophysiol. 2009;20:751-8.
34. Katritsis DG, Josephson ME. Differential diagnosis of regular, narrow-QRS tachycardias. Heart Rhythm. 2015;12: 1667-76.
35. Kalbfleisch SJ, Strickberger SA, Williamson B, Vorperian VR, Man C, Hummel JD, Langberg JJ, Morady F. Randomized comparison of anatomic and electrogram mapping approaches to ablation of the slow pathway of atrioventricular node reentrant tachycardia. J Am Coll Cardiol. 1994;23: 716-23.
36. Katritsis DG, Giazitzoglou E, Zografos T, Ellenbogen KA, Camm AJ. An approach to left septal slow pathway ablation. J Interv Card Electrophysiol. 2011;30:73-9.
37. Spector P, Reynolds MR, Calkins H, Sondhi M, Xu Y, Martin A, Williams CJ, Sledge I. Meta-analysis of ablation of atrial flutter and supraventricular tachycardia. Am J Cardiol. 2009;104: 671-7.
38. Bohnen M, Stevenson WG, Tedrow UB, Michaud GF, John RM, Epstein LM, Albert CM, Koplan BA. Incidence and predictors of major complications from contemporary catheter ablation to treat cardiac arrhythmias. Heart Rhythm. 2011;8: 1661-6.
39. Rostock T, Risius T, Ventura R, Klemm HU, Weiss C, Keitel A, Meinertz T, Willems S. Efficacy and safety of radiofrequency catheter ablation of atrioventricular nodal reentrant tachycardia in the elderly. J Cardiovasc Electrophysiol. 2005;16: 608-10.
40. Li YG, Gronefeld G, Bender B, Machura C, Hohnloser SH. Risk of development of delayed atrioventricular block after slow pathway modification in patients with atrioventricular nodal reentrant tachycardia and a pre-existing prolonged pr interval. Eur Heart J. 2001;22:89-95.
41. Deisenhofer I ZB, Yin YH, Pitschner HF, Kuniss M, Grossmann G, Stiller, S LA, Veltmann C, Frank J, Linner J, Estner HL, Pflaumer A, Wu J, von Bary, C UE, Reents T, Tzeis S, Fichtner S, Kathan S, Karch MR, Jilek C, Ammar S, Kolb C LZ, Haller B, Schmitt C, Hessling G. Cryoablation versus radiofrequency energy for the ablation of atrioventricular nodal reentrant tachycardia (the cyrano study): Results from a large multicenter prospective randomized trial. Circulation. 2010;122:2239-45.

EDITORS' SUMMARY

Despite the years of intensive study, AV node reentry remains a poorly understood arrhythmia both in terms of its anatomy and primary electrophysiological circuit. Even more complex are the many variants of this arrhythmia that in essence, usually involve a portion of the atrium and a portion of the AV node and its primary extensions. Drs Katritsis and Josephson–leaders in the electrophysiological characterization of this arrhythmia–provide an excellent framework classifying the arrhythmias describing the electrophysiological features and provide a rationale for how we approach ablation for AVNRT. When used in conjunction with references 4 and 8, the student will have a simultaneously practical and clear review from the present chapter and a detailed theoretical as well as case-based analysis of the multiple variants of AVNRT.

CHAPTER 18

Rahul Jain, John M Miller

Wolff-Parkinson-White Syndrome and Atrioventricular Accessory Pathway-related Arrhythmias: Localization, Mapping and Ablation

LIST OF ABBREVIATIONS

AF	Atrial Fibrillation	HRA	High Right Atrium
AP	Accessory Pathway	ORT	Orthodromic Reciprocating Tachycardia
APD	Atrial Premature Depolarization	PCL	Pacing Cycle Length
AV	Atrioventricular	PPI	Postpacing Interval
AVN	Atrioventricular Node	RA	Right Atrium
AVNRT	Atrioventricular Nodal Reentrant Tachycardia	RBB	Right Bundle Branch
AVRT	Atrioventricular Reentrant Tachycardia	RF	Radiofrequency
BT	Bypass Tract	RV	Right Ventricle
CL	Cycle Length	SA	Stimulus-Atrial
CS	Coronary Sinus	SR	Sinus Rhythm
ECG	Electrocardiogram	SVT	Supraventricular Tachycardia
EP	Electrophysiology	TCL	Tachycardia Cycle Length
HA	His Bundle-Atrial	VA	Ventriculoatrial
HB	His Bundle	VES	Ventricular Extrastimulus
HOP	His Overdrive Pacing	WPW	Wolff-Parkinson-White
HPS	His-Purkinje System		

INTRODUCTION

Accessory pathways (APs), also called bypass tracts (BTs), are anomalous muscular tracts that result from incomplete embryological development of the atrioventricular (AV) annuli and failure of complete fibrous separation between the atria and the ventricles. Free wall locations are the most common for APs in clinical practice; right and left free-wall APs account for 10 to 20% and 50 to 60% respectively, of all APs.[1] The posteroseptal region (anatomically posterior-paraseptal) is the second most common location for these connections and accounts for 25 to 30% of APs in most series.[2-5] Midseptal (true septal) APs account for 5% or less of all APs and superoparaseptal APs (previously called "anteroseptal" pathways) comprise 6 to 7% of all APs in most large series.[6]

The anatomy of the tricuspid annulus is different from that of the mitral annulus.[7-9] In contrast to the mitral annulus, the tricuspid valve annulus is less well formed and discontinuous in many individuals.[7-9] Right free-wall APs may cross discontinuities in the less distinct fibrous annulus or skirt the epicardial aspect of the annulus (as do left free-wall APs). Because these pathways might represent developmental abnormalities, they may be associated with congenital cardiac abnormalities and multiple pathways may be present in the same individual.

While anterogradely conducting APs produce the classic electrocardiogram (ECG) of Wolff-Parkinson-White (WPW) pattern, the actual importance of APs derives from their role in tachyarrhythmias. APs may have an integral role in tachycardias (that is, participating) or a bystander role (anomalous activation of the ventricles during a separate tachycardia process). These will be explored later in this chapter.

ELECTROCARDIOGRAPHIC CHARACTERISTICS AND LOCALIZATION

Several algorithms have been developed to regionalize anterogradely-conducting (manifest) APs to a relatively specific anatomic location, using the delta wave polarity **(Figure 18.1)**.

However, surface ECG localization of manifest free-wall APs is imperfect, especially if minimal preexcitation is present (QRS duration < 120 ms; **Figures 18.2 and 18.3**), or if multiple anterogradely-conducting pathways are present.

ECG algorithms for AP localization are most accurate for the diagnosis of left free-wall APs compared with all other locations, achieving at least 90% sensitivity and almost 100% specificity. If significant preexcitation is present, all left free wall APs should demonstrate a positive delta wave in V1, with the R wave greater than S wave (R > S) in lead V1 or V2. A negative delta wave in lead I, aVL, or V6 is pathognomonic of a left lateral pathway. As the pathway location moves from posterior to lateral to anterior, the delta waves in the

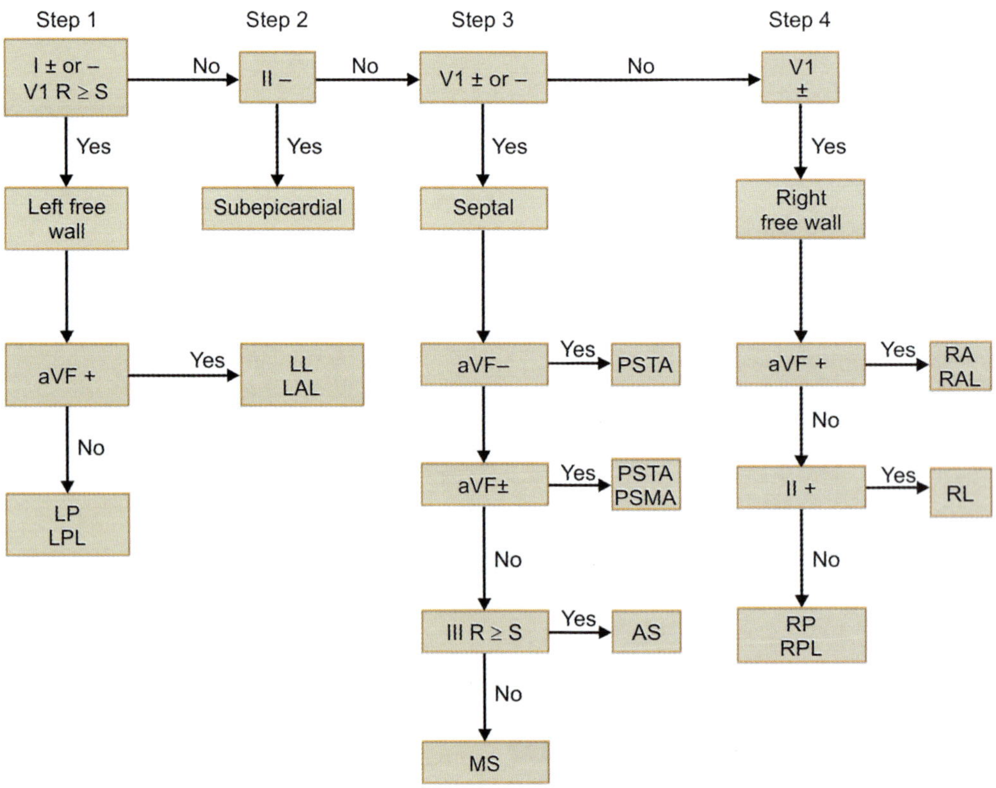

Figure 18.1: Algorithm for accessory pathway localization by surface electrogram (ECG) based on the first 20 ms of the delta wave
Abbreviations: ±, isoelectric delta wave; –, negative isoelectric wave; +, positive delta wave; LP, left posterior; LPL, left posterolateral; LL, left lateral; LAL, left anterolateral; PSTA, posteroseptal tricuspid annulus; PSMA, posteroseptal mitral annulus; AS, anteroseptal; RA, right anterior; RAL, right anterolateral; RL, right lateral.

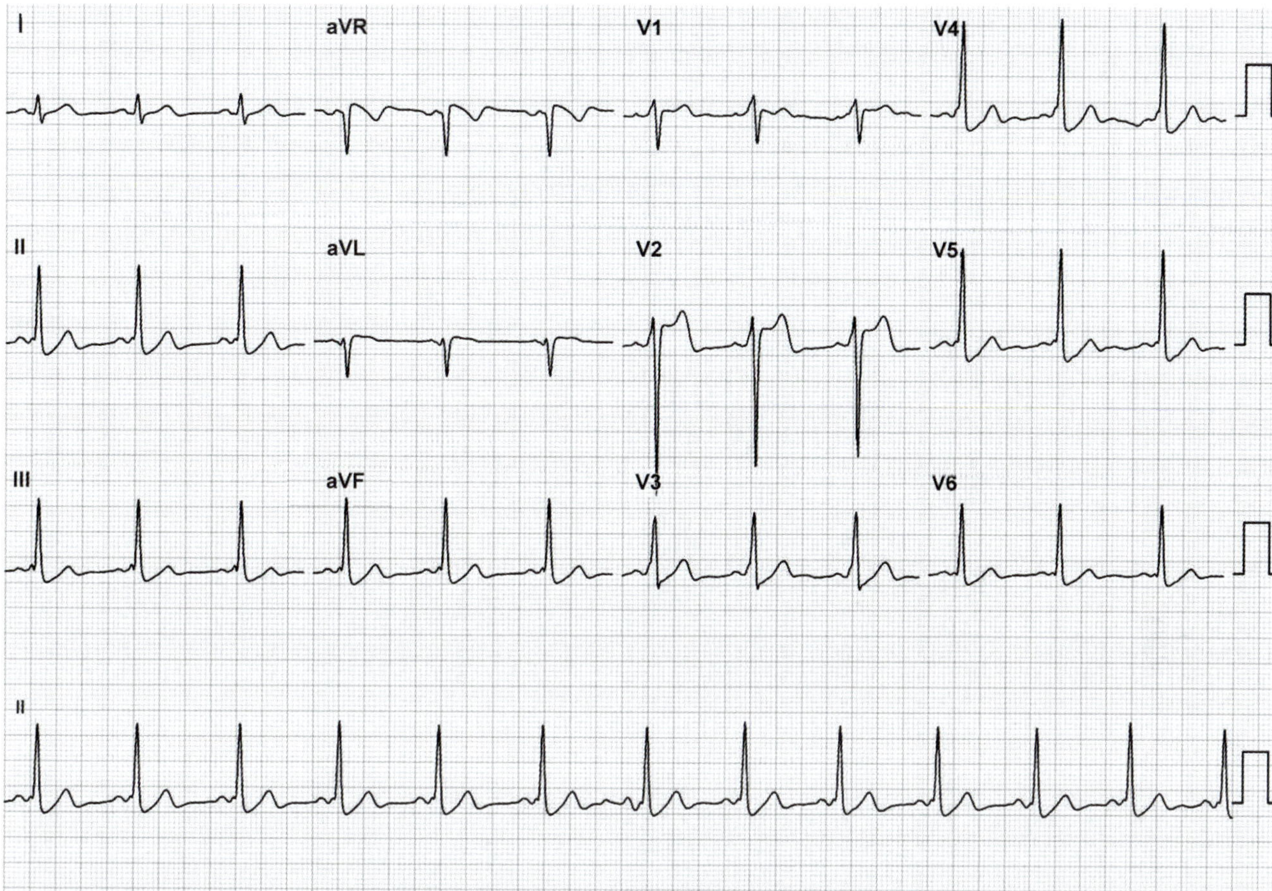

Figure 18.2: Surface electrogram of a patient with left lateral accessory pathway. Because of good AVN conduction the pathway is not fully manifest and therefore R/S ratio in lead V1 is not more than 1. Similarly, Lead I does not show a negative or isoelectric delta wave. The figure shows why sometimes the ECG algorithm fails to accurately localize an accessory pathway

inferior leads, especially aVF and III, change from negative to isoelectric to positive in polarity.

A positive delta wave with R < S in V1 is consistent with a right free wall AP or a minimally preexcited left free wall AP **(Figure 18.2)**. Most algorithms identify right free-wall APs by a positive initial delta wave in V1 but a late transition to R > S in the precordial leads at V3 or later, coupled with leftward orientation of the initial delta wave (delta wave positivity in lead I or aVL).[10-12] As the pathway location moves from the right superior free wall to the right middle and right inferior wall, the delta wave in inferior leads (aVF and II) changes from positive to isoelectric to negative.[10-12]

The location of the AP can also be inferred from the surface ECG by the polarity of the retrograde P wave during orthodromic atrioventricular reciprocating (AVRT).[13,14] Analysis of P waves in leads I and V1 and in the inferior leads is most helpful. A negative P wave in I is highly suggestive of a left free wall AP (95% positive predictive value). A positive P wave in lead I and/or in V1 is highly suggestive of right free wall AP. P wave polarity in the inferior leads, positive or negative, suggests superior or inferior location of the AP, respectively. In orthodromic SVT involving superoparaseptal APs, the P wave is typically situated in the early portion of the ST segment, and it is usually positive in the inferior leads whereas retrograde P waves related to posteroseptal pathways are usually inverted in the inferior leads.[6]

ATRIOVENTRICULAR ACCESSORY PATHWAYS AND RELATED ARRHYTHMIAS

Atrioventricular Reciprocating Tachycardia

Atrioventricular reentry is a macroreentrant tachycardia with an anatomically defined circuit that consists of two distinct pathways, the normal AV conduction system and an AV AP, linked by common proximal (atrial) and distal

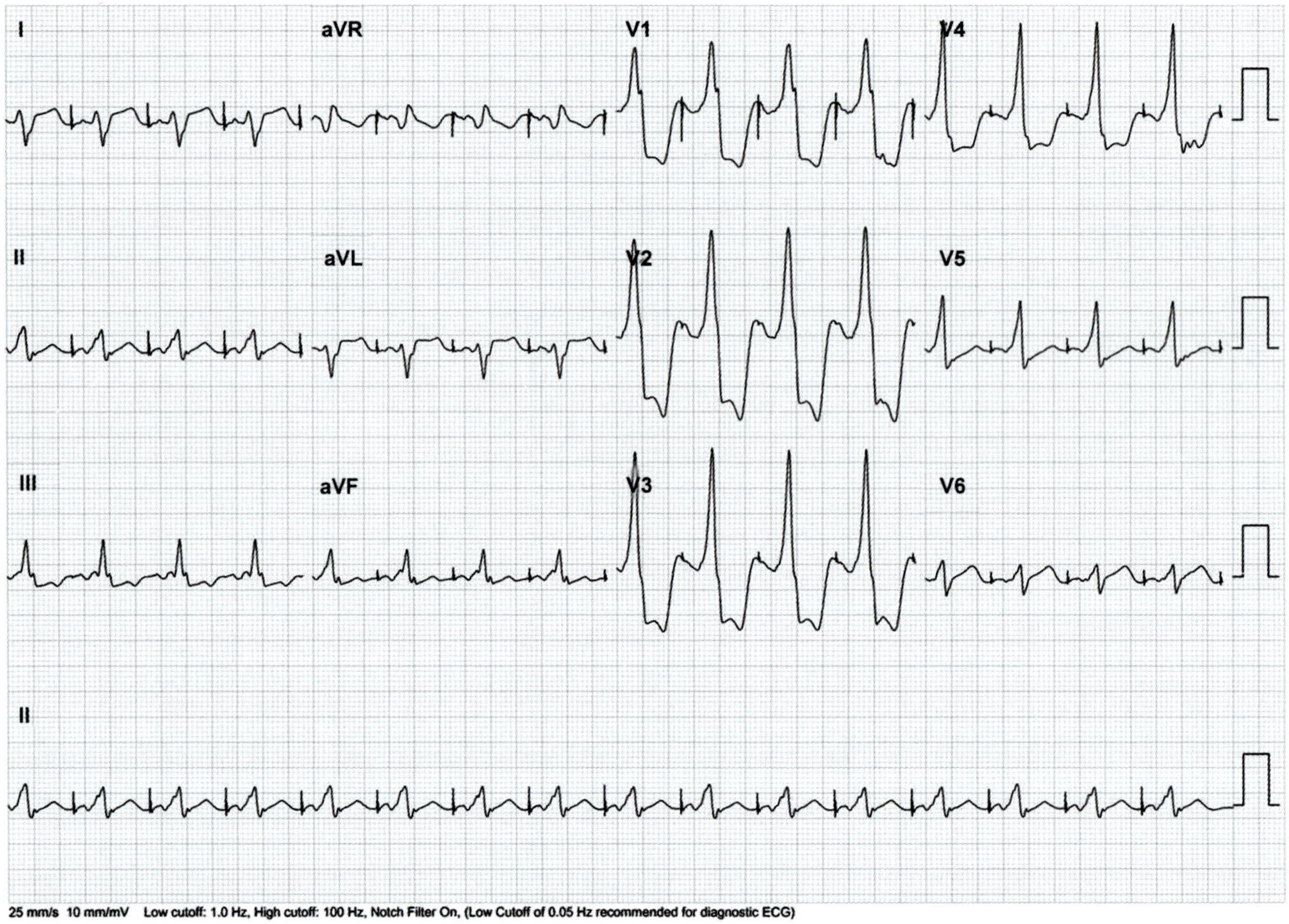

Figure 18.3: Surface electrogram of the same patient with left lateral accessory pathway but during pacing from the lateral coronary sinus at 600 ms. The pathway is fully manifest with R/S ratio being greater than 1 in lead V1

(ventricular) tissues. AVRTs are the most common (80%) tachycardias associated with WPW syndrome. AVRT is divided into orthodromic and antidromic according to direction of propagation in the normal conduction system (atrioventricular node, His-Purkinje system [AVN-HPS]).

Orthodromic Atrioventricular Reciprocating Tachycardia

In orthodromic AVRT, the AVN-HPS serves as the anterograde limb of the reentrant circuit and AV AP serves as the retrograde limb. Approximately, 50% of the APs that participate in orthodromic AVRT by conducting retrogradely are manifest (also able to conduct anterogradely) whereas 50% are "concealed" (able to conduct retrogradely only). In the latter case, preexcitation is absent on the surface ECG during sinus rhythm (SR). The QRS complex during orthodromic AVRT is either normal or shows a typical bundle branch block pattern. Orthodromic AVRT accounts for approximately 95% of AVRTs and 35% of all paroxysmal supraventricular tachycardias (SVTs).

The heart rate during AVRT ranges from 100 to 250/min; symptoms related to AVRT range from almost none to palpitations, lightheadedness, syncope, dyspnea and chest tightness. Because the AP is present even before birth, SVTs that use it may occur at any time during life (even during gestation). At whatever age an individual begins having episodes, they tend to become more frequent as time passes.

Antidromic Atrioventricular Reciprocating Tachycardia

In antidromic AVRT, the anterograde limb of the reentrant circuit is the AP. Consequently, the QRS complex during antidromic AVRT is fully preexcited. During classic antidromic AVRT, retrograde (ventriculoatrial [VA]) conduction occurs over the AVN-HPS. In other less common, non-classic forms of antidromic AVRT, the retrograde limb consists of another AP, or both another AP and the AVN-HPS. Antidromic AVRT occurs in 5 to 10% of patients with WPW syndrome. From 50 to 75% of patients with spontaneous antidromic AVRT have multiple APs (manifest or concealed), which may or may not be used as the retrograde limb during the tachycardia. Interestingly, susceptibility to antidromic AVRT appears to be facilitated by a distance of several centimeters between the AP and the normal AV conduction system. Consequently, most antidromic AVRTs use a lateral AP as the anterograde limb.

Wolff-Parkinson-White Pattern

The incidence of AV accessory pathways detected electrocardiographically has been variously reported as 0.1 to 3.1/1000 in the general population, and it has been noted in people of all ages, although its incidence decreases with increasing age.[15,16] The WPW pattern on the ECG can be intermittent and can even permanently disappear (in up to 40% of cases) over time. In a longitudinal study of patients with symptomatic WPW, Chen et al.[17] noted a loss of anterograde preexcitation in 22.5% over a 10-year follow-up. There is an increased familial incidence of the disorder; Vidaillet et al.[18] demonstrated a 3.4% incidence of accessory pathway in first-degree relatives of patients with preexcitation, an incidence significantly higher than that of the general population ($p < 0.001$). In isolated situations, the incidence among family members is much higher.

WPW pattern refers to the constellation of ECG abnormalities related to the presence of an AV AP (short PR interval, delta wave) in asymptomatic patients whereas *WPW syndrome* refers to a WPW ECG pattern associated with tachyarrhythmia.

Functioning AV APs are associated with certain congenital abnormalities, particularly Ebstein's anomaly of the tricuspid valve (in which up to 10% of patients are affected). Patients with Ebstein's anomaly and preexcitation invariably have right-sided connections.[19-21] Among patients with WPW syndrome presenting with SVT early in childhood, only 5% have Ebstein's anomaly, despite the fact that it is the most common form of congenital heart disease associated with WPW.

Atrial Fibrillation and Accessory Pathways

Atrial fibrillation (AF) is seen in up to 50% of patients with WPW syndrome, and in approximately 20% it is the presenting arrhythmia **(Figure 18.4)**.

It is the most common preexcited arrhythmia, and is of the so-called bystander category (that is, the AP is not necessary for continuation of the arrhythmia but is merely a means for ventricular activation during a separate process). It is clinically important since extremely rapid rates can occur during anterograde conduction over the AP leading to ventricular fibrillation and sudden death. Fortunately, not all individuals with AP and atrial fibrillation conduct rapidly enough to pose a risk of ventricular fibrillation. There are no known clinical features or AP locations that distinguish patients with preexcitation who are likely to have atrial fibrillation from those who are not. Induction of atrial fibrillation with ventricular pacing or during AVRT episodes may be related to intra-atrial pressure changes. In >90% of patients in most series, successful ablation of the AP cures atrial fibrillation (especially those <30 years of age). However, Haïssaguerre et al.[22] have reported persistent vulnerability to atrial fibrillation in 56% of patients.

Other Preexcited Tachycardias

Other forms of preexcited tachycardia are much less common (1 to 3% of WPW patients), and include atrial tachycardia and flutter and atrioventricular nodal reentry. These are important in that successful ablation of the AP by itself will have no effect on the basic rhythm disturbance, which must be addressed separately.

NONINVASIVE EVALUATION

In patients with newly diagnosed preexcitation, a minimal evaluation consists of history, physical examination and ECG. Relevant items of the patient's history include symptoms (type and severity) and age of onset of symptoms, as well as frequency of episodes of tachycardia if present. Family history is relevant in some individuals, in whom there is an increased familial prevalence of the disorder. Physical examination is usually unaffected by the presence of preexcitation, although some individuals with substantial right-sided preexcitation may have a paradoxically split second heart sound, as with left bundle branch block. The ECG is obviously relevant for determining the presence of preexcitation and ventricular insertion of the AP. ECGs during tachycardia episodes can also be used to infer the AP's atrial insertion site as noted above. Patients should be counseled as to the potential importance of the AP in the genesis of symptomatic episodes, as well as treatment options (no treatment, medical therapy or catheter ablation). In some cases, further diagnostic tests such as echocardiography (if Ebstein's anomaly is suspected) or stress test (to ascertain whether pre-excitation suddenly disappears at a relatively low heart rate, indicating a pathway that has very low risk for rapidly conducted atrial fibrillation) are used. Since stress testing rarely has this outcome, and provides no information as to how rapidly the AP can conduct during orthodromic AVRT, the study is not usually performed as part of the evaluation of these patients.

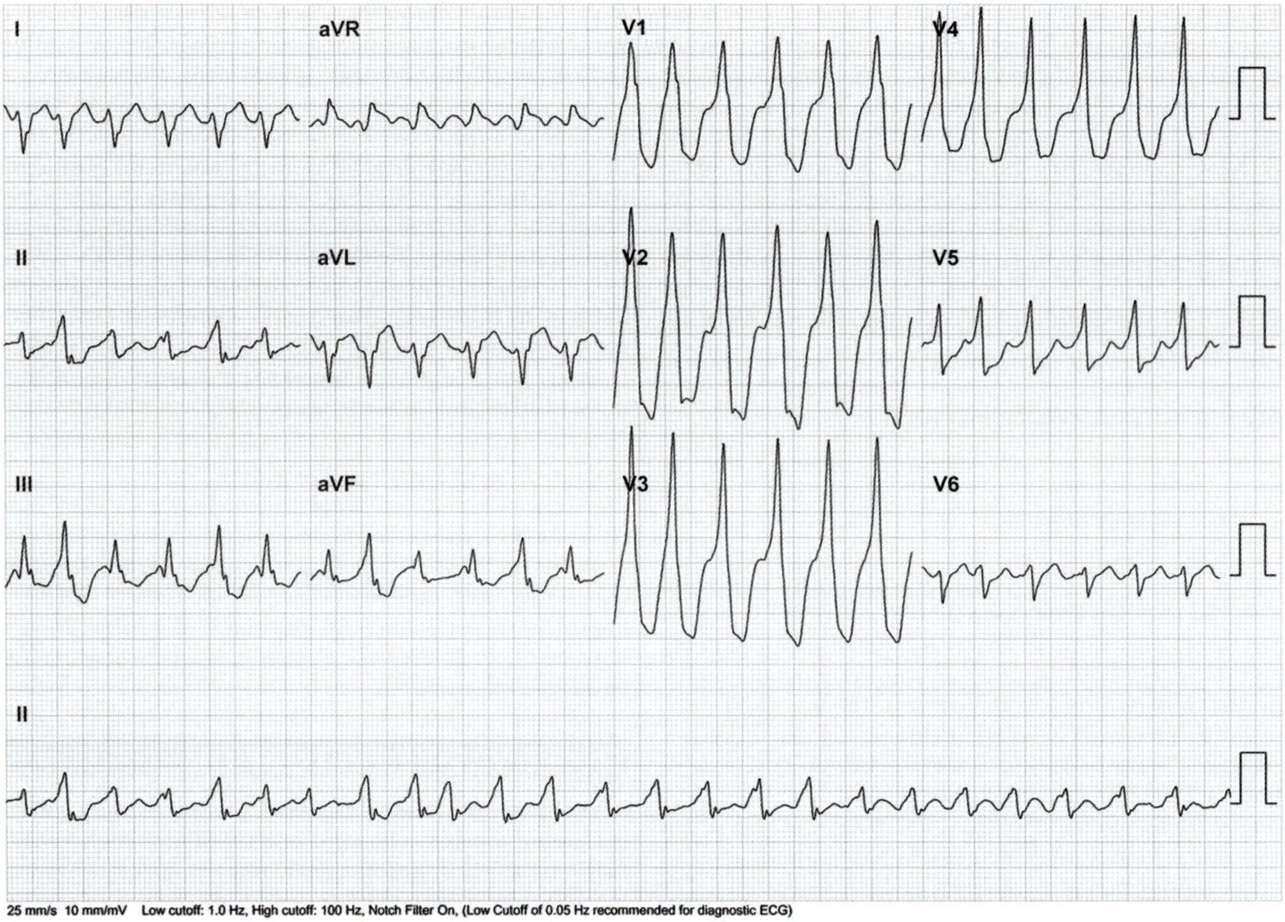

Figure 18.4: Preexcited atrial fibrillation in the same patient as in Figures 18.2 and 18.3

ELECTROPHYSIOLOGICAL EVALUATION

Indications for EP Study

The role of EP study in asymptomatic patients with preexcitation is controversial.

In one study, one third of asymptomatic individuals younger than 40 years of age when preexcitation was identified eventually developed symptoms, whereas no patients in whom preexcitation was first uncovered after the age of 40 years developed symptoms. Studies have shown that approximately 20% of asymptomatic patients will demonstrate a rapid ventricular rate during atrial fibrillation during electrophysiological testing. During follow-up, however, very few patients developed symptomatic arrhythmias, and none of these individuals experienced a cardiac arrest. Based on the above reasons and the fact that the positive predictive value of invasive electrophysiology testing is so low, it is difficult to justify routine use of EP study in asymptomatic patients.[4] Therefore, catheter ablation in asymptomatic preexcitation was classified as Class IIA indication with B level of evidence.[23] American College of Cardiology and European Society of Cardiology guidelines on the management of patients with asymptomatic WPW pattern suggest catheter ablation of AP in individuals in high-risk occupations such as school bus drivers, pilots, police and in scuba divers.[4,23]

However, studies from Pappone et al.[24-26] have questioned the above-mentioned approach. In their studies they have shown that asymptomatic WPW, with a negative EP study (i.e. no AVRT or AF inducible) identifies a subset of subjects with a very low risk profile. On the other hand, inducibility of sustained preexcited AF with a rapid ventricular response, particularly in the presence of multiple APs, may help select individuals at definite high-risk of dying suddenly, and catheter ablation of APs is warranted. This approach can be justified since noninvasive markers of lower risk such as intermittent preexcitation, sudden loss of AP conduction on exercise testing and loss of AP conduction after treatment with antiarrhythmic drugs are limited by poor sensitivity and specificity.

The potential value of electrophysiological testing in identifying high-risk patients who may benefit from catheter ablation must be balanced against the 1 to 2% risk of major complications associated with catheter ablation.

Patient Preparation for EP Study

Once it is determined that a patient is a candidate for EP study for further management of his/her arrhythmias a detailed description of the procedural details along with possible complications should be explained. If the pathway is manifest it will help to determine if left sided access is needed (retrograde aortic or transseptal approach). A realistic estimate of procedural success and complication rates should be provided.

Vascular Access and Catheters Used

The purposes of the EP study are to confirm the presence and number of APs, determine its conduction properties and location, and define its role in the patient's clinical arrhythmia. Typically, three quadripolar catheters are positioned in the high RA, right ventricle (RV) apex or septum, His bundle (HB) region and a decapolar catheter is positioned in the coronary sinus (CS). These catheters are introduced through femoral access sites. If a right-sided AP is suspected, a multipolar catheter along the tricuspid annulus can be helpful. When ablation is to be performed, catheter stability can be enhanced by the use of preformed long sheaths and catheters with sufficient curvature or reach to access the ablation target site. Ablation is usually performed during sinus rhythm or atrial or ventricular pacing. If ablation has to be performed during tachycardia, sudden displacement of the ablation catheter during ablation (if tachycardia suddenly terminates) can be avoided by atrial or ventricular pacing 5 to 10 ms faster than tachycardia cycle length. For difficult right-sided pathway ablation, some operators prefer to ablate with a catheter introduced from the internal jugular vein approach, either positioning the catheter tip on the atrial aspect or advancing across the tricuspid annulus to ablate from the ventricular aspect.

In case of left free wall APs there are two approaches: trans-septal and transaortic. The transaortic (retrograde) approach is directed at sites below the mitral annulus with the ablation catheter perpendicular to the site, whereas the trans-septal approach is directed to sites on or above the annulus with the electrodes more parallel to the annulus. However, many factors play into selecting the approach. These include physician's preference, presence of peripheral vascular disease, aortic valve disease or prosthesis, small ventricular chambers, presence of congenital heart disease, dilated aorta, and the location of the AP.

Baseline Measurements

In a person without an AP, a normal sinus P wave is conducted to the ventricles over the AV node where the impulse encounters an obligatory delay, resulting in an isoelectric interval between the end of the P-wave and onset of the normal QRS complex. In the presence of an anterogradely conducting AV AP (composed of normal myocardial tissue with rapid transmission), activation of some part of the ventricles begins earlier than it would occur with normal AV conduction, resulting in a short PR interval and delta wave (slurred upstroke of the QRS due to early activation of ventricular muscle at the AP insertion site that is remote from the HPS). The HV interval is shorter than normal since, while the His bundle is activated normally after AV nodal conduction, the early ventricular activation over the AP brings the QRS onset earlier. This can be observed readily on intracardiac recordings in the CS in patients with a manifest left lateral AP, in which case CS ventricular electrograms occur earlier than anticipated, often even before the onset of the QRS complex. Since the QRS complex is a fusion of conduction over a typically rapidly conducting AP as well as the AVN-HPS, accentuation of the inherent slowing of conduction in the AV node results in a greater degree of preexcitation (*see* **Figure 18.3**). This can be achieved by carotid sinus massage, atrial stimulation (*see* **Figure 18.3**) or pharmacologically.

Ventricular Pacing during Sinus Rhythm

Ventricular pacing during sinus rhythm is useful for determining the presence of retrograde conduction over an AP and/or AVN, as well as the AP's atrial insertion site. Pacing is typically performed at slow cycle lengths, gradually shortening the cycle length of pacing until block occurs. Presence of an AP may be manifested by a change in atrial activation pattern as one or more pathways ceases to conduct, or sudden cessation of retrograde conduction (if only the AP conducts retrogradely). Typically, while AV nodal conduction shows progressive delay in retrograde conduction times, APs show very little change in retrograde conduction time over the entire range of paced cycle lengths tested.

Atrial Pacing during Sinus Rhythm

Atrial pacing during sinus rhythm is performed to determine the paced cycle length at which AP conduction blocks, compared to that of the AV node and His bundle. As with ventricular pacing during sinus rhythm, atrial pacing starts at long cycle lengths, evaluating the degree of preexcitation. As the cycle length of pacing is progressively shortened, AV nodal conduction is delayed whereas AP conduction stays relatively constant, yielding greater degrees of preexcitation. The timing of the His bundle becomes progressively delayed ("moving in" to the QRS complex) until AV nodal block occurs and the His bundle is activated retrogradely, assuming a fixed relationship to the beginning of the preexcited QRS complex despite further shortening of paced cycle length (which would ordinarily further prolong the AH interval).

Atrial pacing should be performed from several sites (right atrium, coronary sinus) to assess for the presence of multiple anterogradely-conducting pathways, having multiple preexcitation patterns.

Initiation of Arrhythmias

Conduction and refractoriness of the accessory pathways in most cases behave like working muscle; therefore accessory pathways demonstrate rapid conduction, and have refractory periods that tend to shorten at decreasing paced cycle lengths. The reentrant arrhythmias involving APs allow one to see all the requirements of reentrant rhythms: (a) two anatomically or functionally determined pathways of conduction; (b) unidirectional block in one of the pathways (in this instance, either in the accessory pathway or in the AVN-His pathway); (c) sufficient slowing in the other part of the circuit (most commonly in AV node) to overcome refractoriness ahead of the circulating impulse; and (d) conduction time must exceed the longest effective refractory period of any component in the circuit.

The only difference between orthodromic tachycardias in patients with concealed AP and those with overt preexcitation is that unidirectional block is already present in patients with concealed AP.

Coupling intervals of atrial premature depolarizations (APDs) required to produce block in the AP are usually short, simultaneously producing enough AV nodal delay, so that the tachycardia is initiated at the onset of AP block. This is particularly true in cases with dual AV nodal pathways but no AV nodal reentry. Early coupled APDs conduct over the "slow" pathway, providing enough delay to initiate the tachycardia. Similar delay is provided by bundle branch block ipsilateral to the pathway's ventricular insertion.

The site of atrial stimulation may also be important, particularly if the limiting factor for initiation of the tachycardia is atrial refractoriness. The differentiation is for two reasons: (a) generally speaking, the closer the stimulation site to the AP, the easier it is for a premature wavefront to encroach on its refractory period; and (b) the earlier the atrium (or the AP) is activated, the earlier it will recover, thereby facilitating reentry. Occasionally single atrial extrastimuli cannot induce block and/or enough delay to initiate tachycardia. Rapid atrial pacing or multiple atrial extrastimuli can produce sudden block in those circumstances and initiate SVT. Sometimes, AV nodal echoes or intra-atrial reentry beats can induce tachycardia by either blocking the AP and/or producing enough delay in the normal AV nodal/His-Purkinje system to reenter the atria via the AP.

Initiation of orthodromic tachycardia by ventricular stimulation is possible in 80% of patients. Several patterns of VA conduction can be seen during ventricular pacing and ventricular extrastimuli; (a) conduction over the AP alone, commonly seen at short pacing CLs and short coupling intervals; VA conduction time is the same over a wide range of VPD coupling intervals and paced CLs in the absence of intraventricular conduction delay, (b) conduction over the AP and AV node, (c) conduction over the AV node only and (d) no conduction over either the AV node or AP. Because retrograde conduction over the AP is typically an all-or-none phenomenon, the prime determinant of initiating orthodromic SVT in response to ventricular stimulation is the extent of retrograde conduction and/or concealment in the normal pathway. Exclusive retrograde atrial activation over the AP is necessary to initiate SVT, while three potential responses can occur in a normal AV conduction system: (a) block in the His-Purkinje system; (b) block with or without concealment in the AV node; or (c) block in the AP with retrograde conduction over the normal conduction system to the His bundle resulting in a bundle branch reentrant complex. Whenever the tachycardia is initiated by development of block in the His-Purkinje system, the first AH interval of the tachycardia may be shorter than subsequent AH intervals because no concealment occurred in the AV node during the initiating impulse.

At shorter paced cycle lengths, with or without ventricular extrastimuli, penetration into the AV node usually occurs. In such cases the first AH interval of SVT will be longer than subsequent AH intervals due to concealment into the AV node on the first cycle. SVT initiation by a bundle branch reentrant complex can be seen in up to one third of patients. However, multiple modes of initiation may be seen in many patients.

Para-Hisian Pacing

Para-Hisian pacing is a useful maneuver to differentiate retrograde conduction over an accessory pathway (particularly septal pathways) and retrograde conduction over the fast or slow atrioventricular nodal pathway. This pacing maneuver uses RV pacing close to the His bundle or proximal right bundle branch (RBB). With slight changes in pacing output, the pacing stimulus changes capture among (1) basal anteroseptal RV plus His bundle or proximal RBB capture, (2) capture of the basal anteroseptal RV alone, and (3) His bundle-RBB capture alone. The differences among which tissue is directly captured produces differences in the timing of His activation relative to the timing of the ventricular activation. The presence or absence of a change in atrial activation sequence, stimulus-atrial (SA) intervals, and His bundle-atrial (HA) interval identifies whether retrograde conduction is dependent on ventricular activation, His bundle activation, or both (AP and AVN). The loss of His bundle-RBB (HB-RB) capture is usually identified by the widening of the QRS complex, whereas a narrower QRS results when some of the ventricular myocardium (farthest from the RV basal septum pacing site) is activated by the His-Purkinje system during both RV and His bundle-RBB capture (**Figure 18.5**).

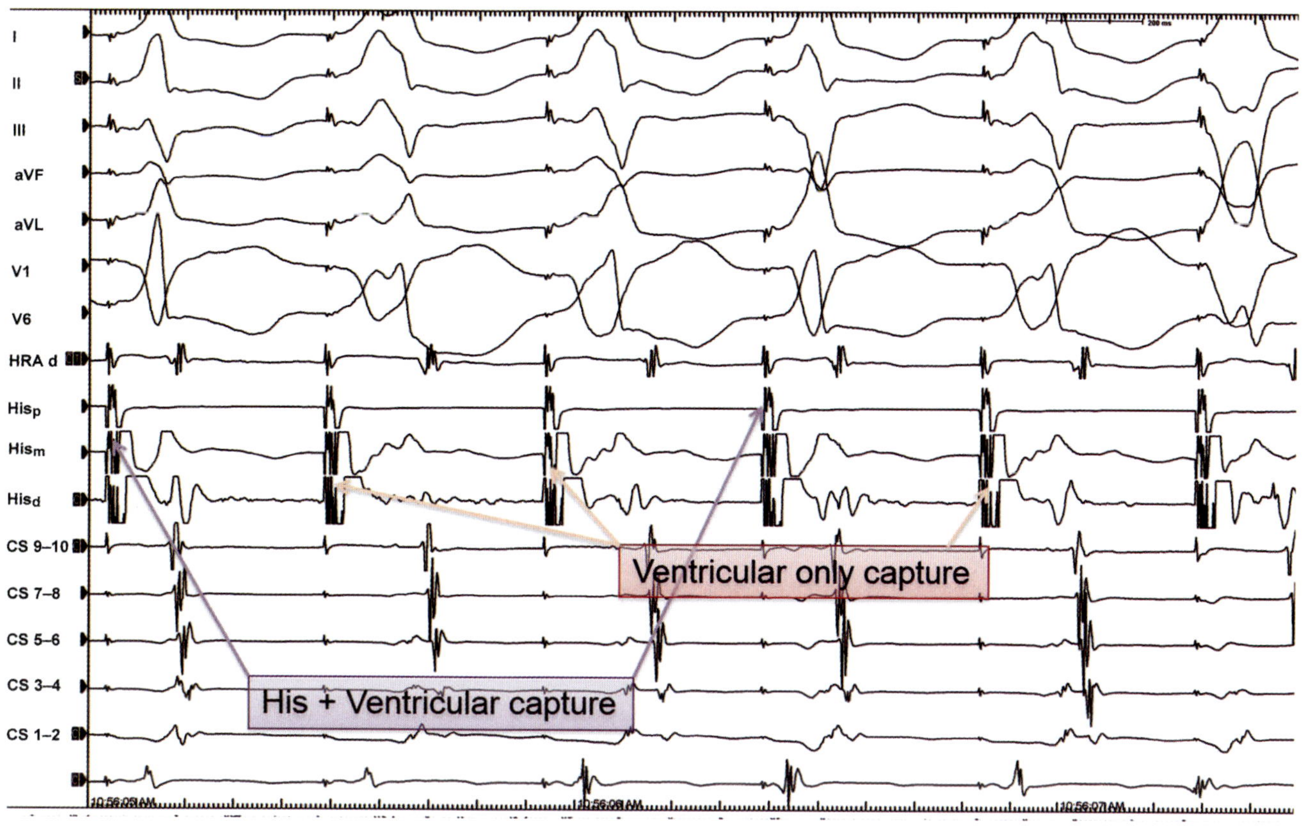

Figure 18.5: Para-Hisian pacing showing "Nodal Response". 1st and 4th para-Hisian paced beat has His and ventricular capture with stim-HRA interval of 146 ms. 2nd, 3rd and 5th paced beat is V-only capture with stim-HRA of 208 ms

Seven different patterns of Para-Hisian pacing response have been described.[27] **Figure 18.5** shows a nodal response or Pattern 1. Retrograde conduction occurs exclusively over the AVN regardless of whether the HB-RB is captured. Loss of His bundle capture results in a wide QRS with a long SA interval, and a shorter SA with HB-RB capture. **Figure 18.6** shows Pattern 3 para-Hisian pacing response.

Retrograde conduction is exclusively over the AP. In pattern 3, loss of HB-RB capture is associated with a delay in the timing of ventricular activation close to the AP. This results in an increase in SA interval in all electrograms with no change in atrial activation.

Singh et al.[28] recently reported a new maneuver to help differentiate AVRT from AV nodal reentrant tachycardia (AVNRT) using His overdrive pacing (HOP) during tachycardia. Once SVT is induced, HOP was performed by pacing the His bundle 10 to 30 ms faster than the SVT cycle length. The maneuver was determined to have entered the tachycardia circuit when a non-fused His capture beat advanced or delayed subsequent atrial electrogram by 10 ms or when the tachycardia was terminated. Entry into the circuit within one beat had a sensitivity of 92% and specificity of 92%. Contrariwise, a cut off ≥3 beats to enter the circuit had a sensitivity of 90% and specificity of 92% to confirm the diagnosis.

Ventricular Pacing and Ventricular Extrastimuli

Ventricular pacing and ventricular extrastimuli (VES) during SVT help in diagnosis and localization of the accessory pathways. VES or ventricular pacing with eccentric atrial activation is highly suggestive of accessory pathway. A VES delivered when the HB is refractory (i.e. when the His potential is already manifest or within 35 to 55 ms before the time of the expected His potential) can result in three responses that are helpful in diagnosis:

1. Advancement in timing of next atrial activation. This is diagnostic of the presence of an AP but does not prove that it is necessarily participating in the SVT. This excludes AVNRT, but does not exclude concomitant AT. However, if the VES advances atrial activation with an activation sequence identical to that during the SVT and resets the

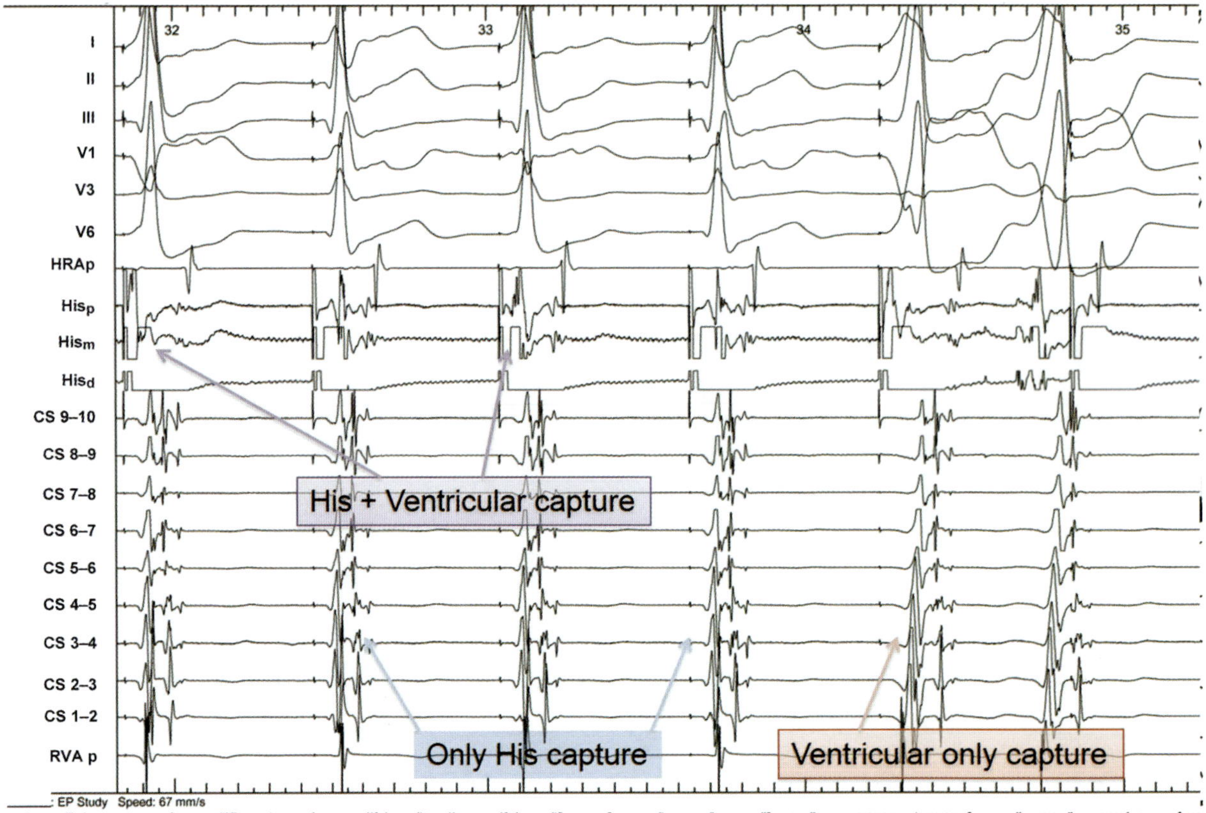

Figure 18.6: Para-Hisian pacing in a patient with a left lateral accessory pathway. RF application at the lateral mitral annulus resulted in successful ablation of the pathway. Para-Hisian pacing shows His-only capture on 2nd and 4th complexes with stim-HRA interval of 204 ms, ventricular-only capture in the 5th complex with stim-HRA of 240 ms and His + ventricular capture on the 1st and 3rd complexes (stim-HRA 204 ms). The activation pattern remains same and is eccentric. This is an example of Pattern 3 of Para-Hisian response ($AP\text{-}AP_L$)

tachycardia such that the VA relationship on the next SVT complex is identical to the rest, this strongly suggests that the SVT is orthodromic AVRT and the AP is participating in the SVT **(Figure 18.7)**.

2. Termination of SVT without atrial activation is diagnostic of AVRT (this should be a reproducible finding) **(Figure 18.8)**.
3. Delay in the next atrial activation. This proves that AP is participating in the SVT, denoting orthodromic AVRT as the mechanism.

As mentioned, VES can also be used to regionalize the accessory pathway. This is through the calculation of the preexcitation index.[29] This index is based on the coupling interval of the VES delivered from right ventricle that resets orthodromic AVRT as a percentage of the tachycardia cycle length (TCL). A relative preexcitation index of more than 90% of a VES that advances atrial activation during orthodromic AVRT suggests that the AP is close to the site of ventricular stimulation (i.e. it is septal AP). An absolute preexcitation index (TCL- VES coupling interval) of at least 75 ms suggests a left free wall AP, an index of < 45 msec suggests a septal AP and an index of 40 to 75 msec is indeterminate.

Entrainment by right ventricular apical pacing is an effective way to differentiate orthodromic AVRT using a right lateral or septal AP from AVNRT. The two numerical values that are important are stimulus-A (SA)-VA interval and post-pacing interval (PPI)–tachycardia cycle length (TCL).

It is important to understand the concept behind this maneuver. The VA interval during ventricular pacing is compared with that during SVT. The ventricle and atrium are activated in series during orthodromic AVRT and while ventricular pacing during AVRT, but in parallel during AVNRT. Also, the ventricular pacing site is physically and electrically closer to an AVRT circuit than it is to the AVNRT circuit. Therefore, the SA interval approximates VA interval during AVRT but is more than 85 ms longer than the VA interval during AVNRT.[30]

In addition, evaluation of PPI versus TCL is of value. In typical or atypical AVNRT, PPI reflects time it takes from the RV pacing site, through the RV muscle and HPS, once around the reentry circuit and back. Since the circuit is remote from the pacing site, the PPI-TCL difference is relatively long. During orthodromic AVRT using a septal AP, the PPI reflects the conduction time through the RV to the

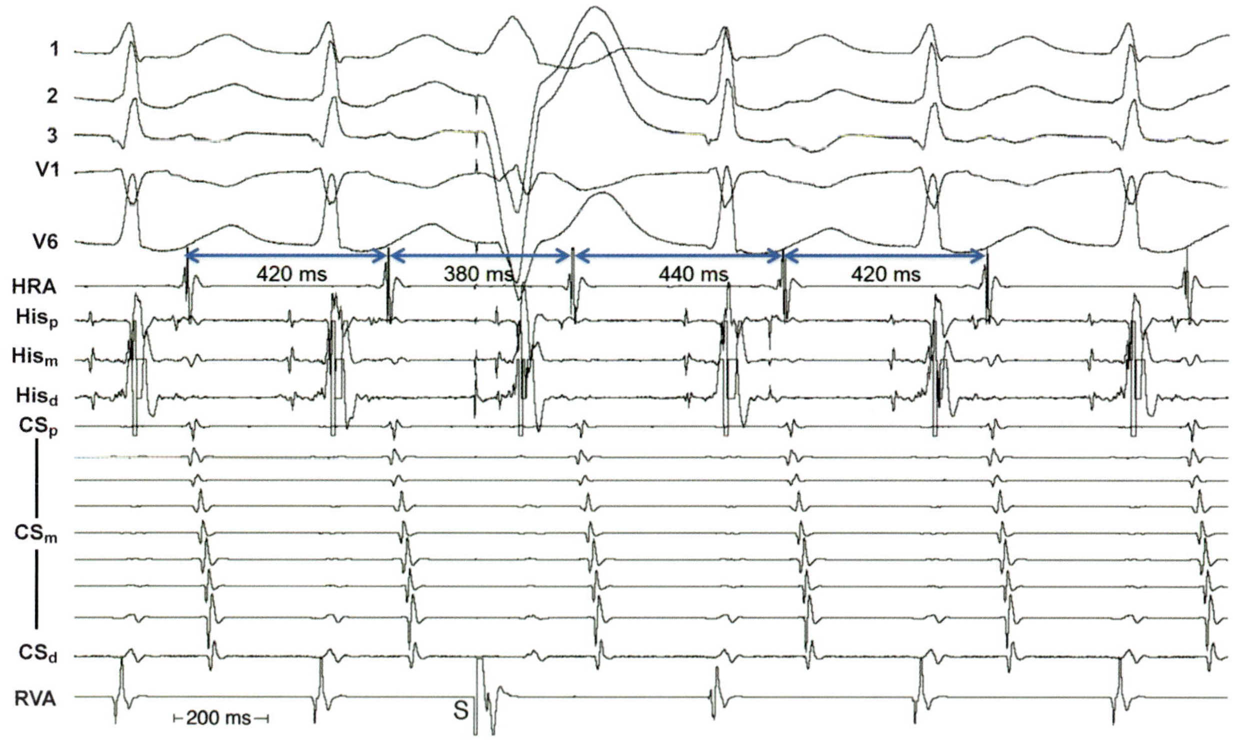

Figure 18.7: His refractory PVC advances the next atrial electrocardiogram followed by resetting of the tachycardia

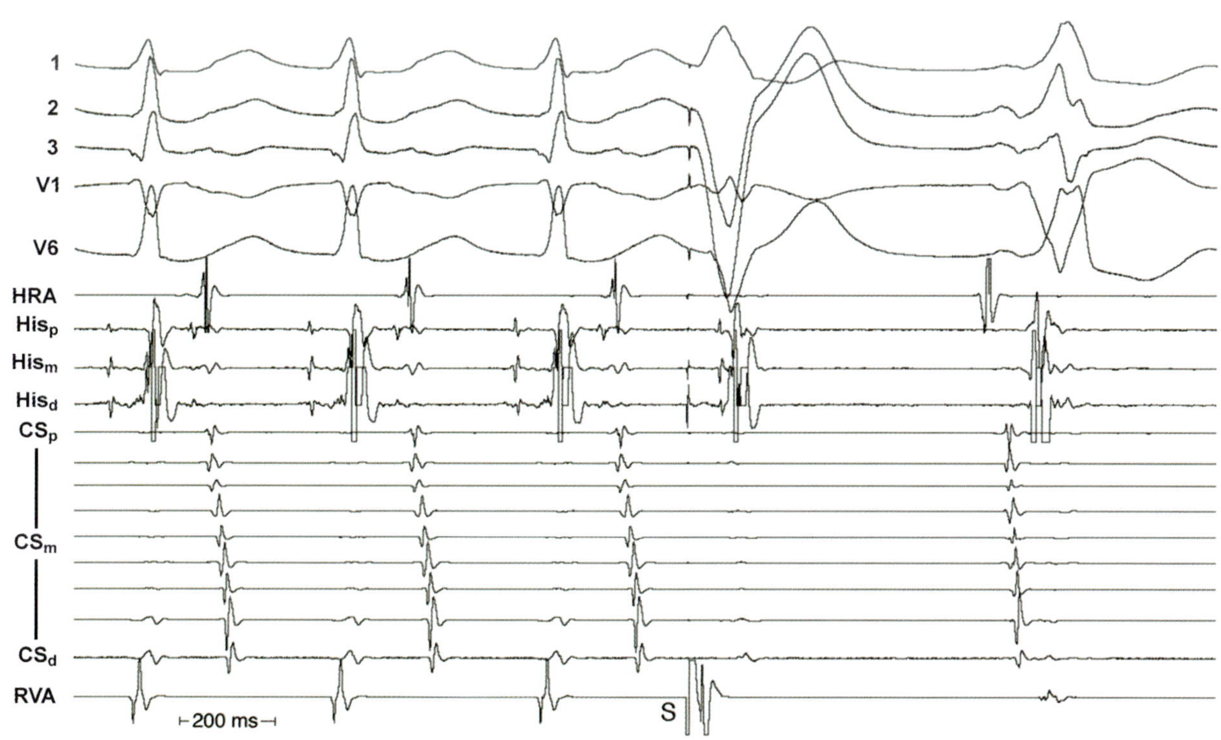

Figure 18.8: Termination of tachycardia with a His refractory PVC; the on-time, anterograde His potential (H) is evident

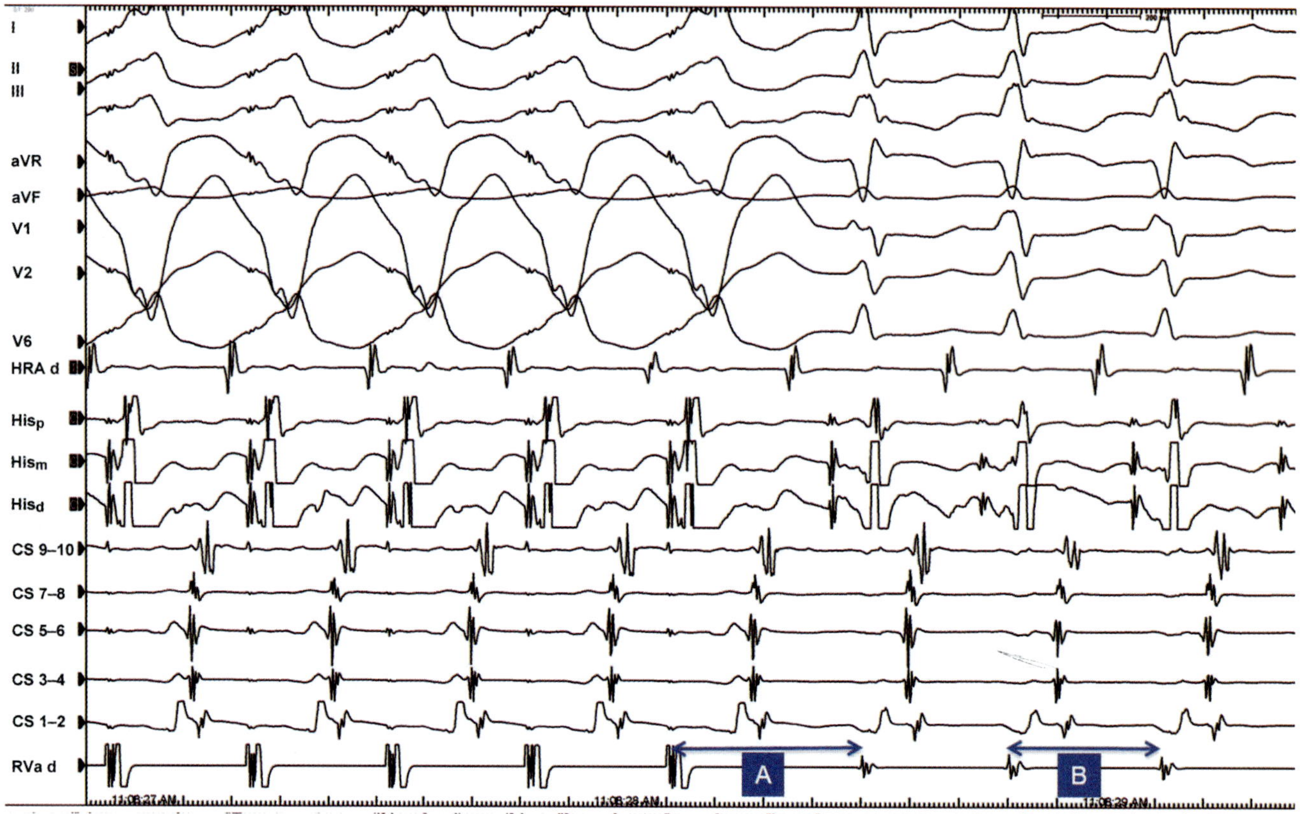

Figure 18.9: End of overdrive pacing (ODP) with entrainment in a patient with a left sided pathway. PPI (A) – TCL (B) of 401 ms – 304 ms = 97 ms. When corrected for AH immediately following ODP (129 ms) to the AH during tachycardia (119 ms) the corrected PPI-TCL was 87 ms. We can also deduce that this is a left sided pathway since right ventricular pacing is in effect a left bundle branch block and surface VA interval during RV pacing was 153 ms compared to the VA of 118 ms interval during tachycardia

septum, once around the reentry circuit and back. Since the RV pacing site is near or within the SVT circuit, in this case, the PPI more closely approximates the TCL. Thus, PPI-TCL of less than 115 ms is consistent with orthodromic AVRT.[30] Since rapid input to the AV node from the last paced complex may prolong the AH interval on that cycle and confound the PPI-TCL measurement, one should correct for any AVN delay (AH prolongation) using this index. A corrected PPI-TCL difference <110 ms is consistent with orthodromic AVRT **(Figure 18.9)**.[31]

These two criteria were initially reported to differentiate atypical AVNRT from orthodromic AVRT using a septal accessory pathway. However, in our experience this also holds true for typical AVNRT and right lateral pathways, but not for slowly conducting or decrementally conducting APs or far left lateral pathways. If the VA interval is greater than 40% of TCL with eccentric atrial activation one should always consider a decremental septal AP and should be very careful in making a diagnosis based on PPI-TCL alone. If there is oscillation in TCL and VA intervals of more than 30 ms then also one should be careful in interpreting results of overdrive pacing or extrastimuli.

Ventricular pacing during sinus rhythm at TCL results in an HA interval that is shorter than that during orthodromic AVRT, because the HB and atrium are activated in series during orthodromic AVRT and in parallel when ventricular pacing during sinus rhythm. In the setting of orthodromic AVRT the ΔHA (HA pacing – HA SVT) is typically less than –10 ms. In contrast, if AVNRT is present the ΔHA interval is more than –10 ms. This criterion has 100% specificity and sensitivity and positive predictive accuracy for differentiation between AVNRT and orthodromic AVRT. The main limitation of this criterion is identification of His potential during ventricular pacing. The HA during SVT is usually measured from the beginning of the His potential to the atrial electrogram in the high RA recording, and during ventricular pacing, from the end of the His potential to the same atrial recording.[32]

Differential right ventricular pacing during sinus rhythm is another useful maneuver to help in diagnosis of septal APs. The VA interval while pacing from the apex is compared to that while pacing from the base at the same CL. The VA intervals from apex pacing is same or longer than that from the base in the presence of an AP whereas the VA interval from apex

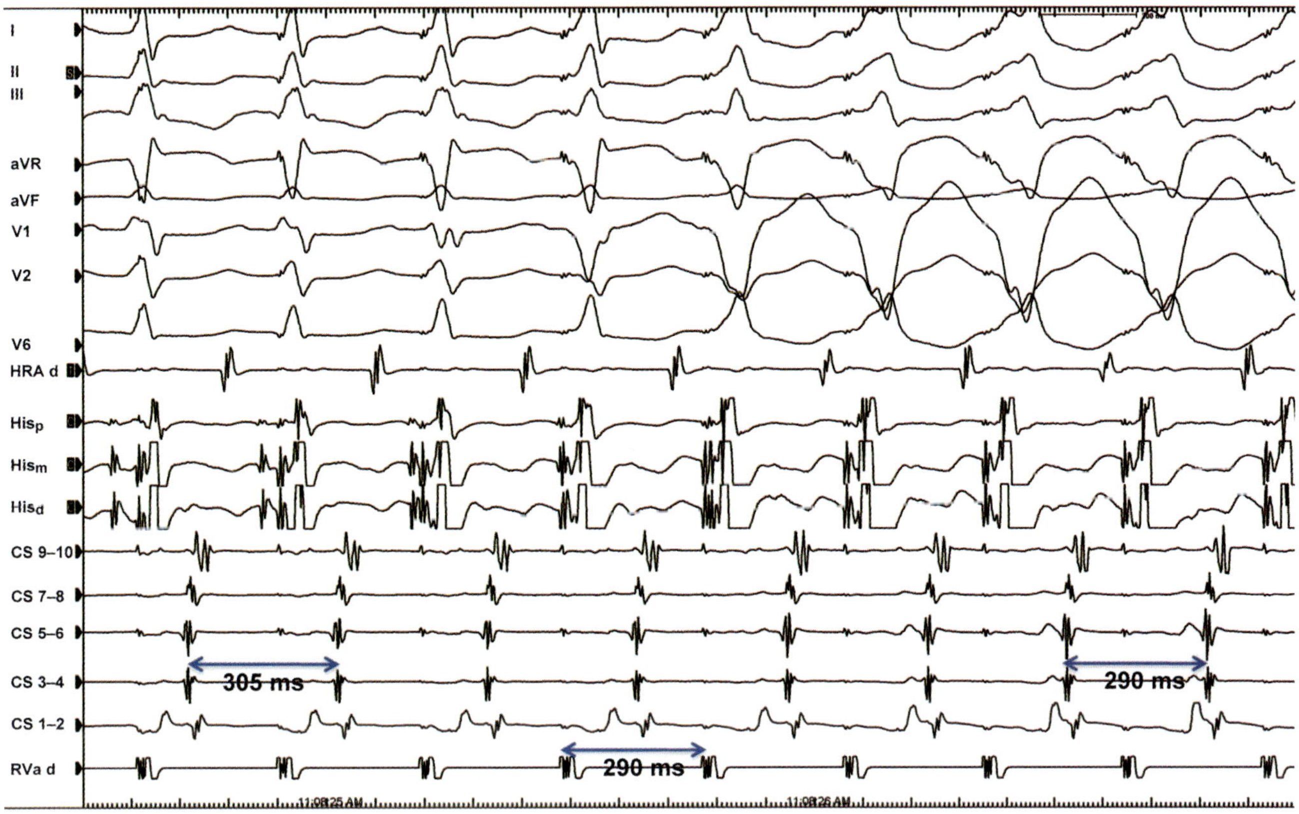

Figure 18.10: Start of overdrive pacing in a patient with left sided pathway. Within one beat of fully paced QRS the atrial electrograms are at pacing cycle length indicating ORT as the mechanism of the tachycardia

pacing is shorter than that from base in the absence of AP.[33] A similar maneuver can be performed during SVT (differential entrainment) to differentiate orthodromic AVRT using septal AP from AVNRT. This is conceptually based on the fact that in orthodromic AVRT, the ventricle is part of the circuit. A basal pacing site is closer to the circuit relative to the apex in septal accessory pathways but equidistant in case of free wall accessory pathways. A paced wave front from base or apex has equal access to the circuit and therefore the PPI tends to be similar in case of orthodromic AVRT.

In AVNRT pacing from the base of the RV is electrically more distant than the RV apex to the tachycardia circuit, given that the His-Purkinje network is close to the RV apex.[33,34] However, this requires consistent placement of the catheter at the apical site relatively near the right bundle terminus. Derval et al.[35] proposed differential sequential septal pacing as a simple maneuver to differentiate nodal versus extranodal VA conduction to circumvent this difficulty. The septal pacing site is progressively moved from the basal region towards the apex, near the entrance of the His-Purkinje system, and this shortens the VA time for nodal but not for the AP conduction.[35] The stimulus-atrial (SA) interval at the high midventricular site minus SA interval at the base (site 1) ≤ 0 ms for nodal and > 0 ms for extranodal conduction had optimal sensitivity and specificity (nodal: sensitivity = 97% and specificity = 85.3%; extranodal: sensitivity = 85.3% and specificity = 97.0%).

It is as important to evaluate the onset of overdrive pacing as it is to look at the end of the pacing train, since attempts at overdrive pacing during SVT results in termination of tachycardia in about half of AVNRT cases and 65% of AVRT cases.[35] Dandamudi et al.[36] showed that once completely RV paced complexes are present during SVT, a cut off ≤1 beat to accelerate TCL to pacing cycle length (PCL) could identify all orthodromic reciprocating tachycardia (ORT) cases as opposed to AVNRT **(Figure 18.10)**.

If ≥ 2 complexes are required to accelerate SVT to the PCL once a fixed morphology RV pacing is achieved, AVNRT is diagnosed with high confidence.

An absolute value of the VA interval of 70 ms during SVT separates septal AP from AVNRT. Benditt et al.[37] have demonstrated that using the electrogram at the high right atrium, the VA interval recorded during orthodromic AVRT with septal or left lateral APs exceeds 95 ms.

Effect of Bundle Branch Block

Patients with left free wall accessory pathways show prolongation of the surface VA interval (≥ 35 ms) with the

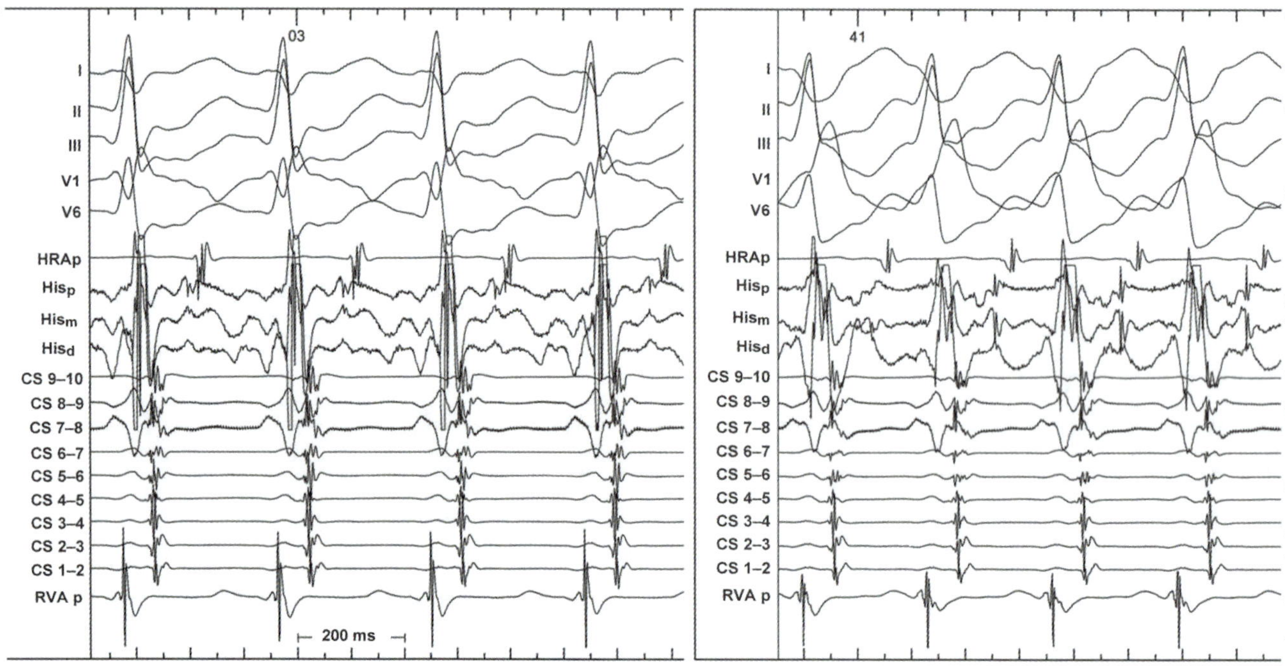

Figure 18.11: Effect of right bundle branch block in the same patient with a left sided pathway. The surface VA interval measured to earliest atrial electrogram with (right panel) and without RBBB (left panel) remains the same (85 ms)

development of left bundle branch block compared to that with a normal QRS complex or right bundle branch block, and those with right-sided APs show a VA prolongation (≥ 35 ms) with right bundle branch block compared to normal QRS or left bundle branch block **(Figures 18.9 and 18.11)**. In patients with superoparaseptal and posteroparaseptal APs, the development of bundle branch block produces either no increase in the VA interval or an increase ≤25 ms.[38,39] In patients with orthodromic tachycardia using a posterior paraseptal AP, left bundle branch block may produce a small increase in the VA interval (13 ± 8 msec), while in those using a superoparaseptal AP, right bundle branch block may be associated with a small increase in VA interval (16 ± 9 msec).[38] Jazayeri et al.[40] demonstrated a 15–35 msec increase in the VA interval with the development of left anterior fascicular block in patients with left free wall APs.

Atrial Pacing and Atrial Extrastimulation

Atrial stimulation close to or at the AV accessory pathway insertion site during sinus rhythm results in maximal preexcitation and the shortest P-delta interval. During preexcited SVT, if a late-coupled atrial extrastimulus delivered when the AV junctional portion of the atrium is refractory advances the next ventricular activation, it proves the presence of an anterogradely conducting AV accessory pathway (a concept similar to giving His refractory PVC). If it not only advances the next ventricular activation but the QRS morphology is similar to that of the wide complex tachycardia, it proves that the accessory pathway is responsible for the ventricular activation during the wide complex tachycardia. An atrial extrastimulus can also result in termination of the tachycardia **(Figure 18.12)**.

MAPPING AND ABLATION

Kenichiro Otomo et al.[41] very elegantly showed that the APs do not typically cross the AV groove perpendicularly, but have a slant. A wavefront propagating during ventricular pacing from the direction of the ventricular end ("concurrent" with AP activation) produced a short local apparent VA, because activation along the AP proceeds to the site of earliest atrial activation concomitant with the ventricular wavefront. A ventricular wavefront propagating in the opposite (countercurrent) direction would produce a longer local VA because the ventricular wavefront must pass the site of earliest atrial activation before reaching the ventricular end of the AP **(Figures 18.13A to D)**.

This has important implications, the most significant of which was further disproving the erroneous concept that the site with the shortest local VA interval signified the AP insertion site. For example, if the velocity of the ventricular wavefront along the annulus is slower than the AP and atrial wavefront, the shortest local VA interval would be shifted

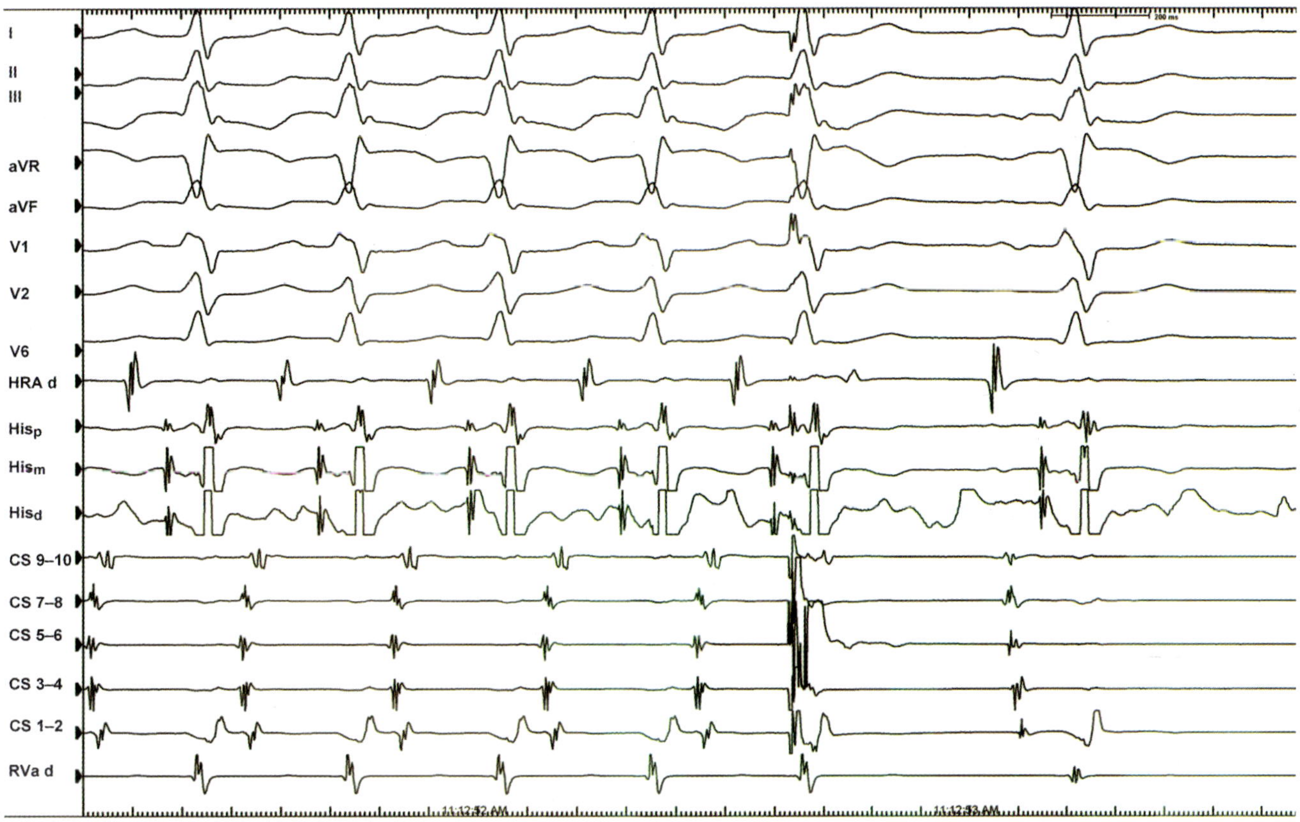

Figure 18.12: Atrial extrastimuli given during tachycardia from the CS in a patient with left lateral accessory pathway. The atrial stimulus results in termination of the tachycardia

away from the AP, with the shortest VA interval giving a false indicator of AP location (CS_d in **Figure 18.13, A2**).[41] Another important issue that can be resolved by knowing the concept of pacing from different sites is the fact that ventricular potential may overlap and mask the AP potential and site of earliest atrial activation during pacing from one direction and not the other.

During atrial pacing **(Figures 18.13C and D)**, a concurrent atrial wavefront would shorten the local AV interval at the site of earliest ventricular activation (local AV) and may mask the AP potential and site of earliest ventricular activation **(Figure 18.13 C2)**. A countercurrent wavefront lengthens the local AV interval and exposes the AP potential and ventricular activation sequence **(Figure 18.13 D1)**.[41]

The most widely used approaches to mapping of accessory pathways rely on the identification of the earliest ventricular activation during anterograde AP conduction and earliest retrograde atrial activation during ORT. Mapping can be performed either transaortically or trans-septally for left-sided APs. The transaortic approach is well-suited for mapping sites below the mitral valve (that is, when the ventricular insertion is being mapped) and transseptal when the atrial insertion is being mapped. In general terms, when using the transaortic approach the mapping/ablation catheter is perpendicular to the annulus whereas in the transseptal approach it is parallel. This point is helpful when there is a question about catheter stability and its impact on the success of the procedure. Posterior/inferior annular sites are more readily approached using transseptal access; whereas APs at other sites may be accessed equally well with either transseptal or retrograde aortic approaches.

The effect of bundle branch block and preexcitation index have already been described, both of which help in regionalizing the AP. AP potentials are seen in 35 to 94% of successful ablation sites but it can be difficult to differentiate AP potentials from other signals.[2,42,43] AP potentials are defined as discrete, high-frequency potentials of 0.5 to 1 mV in amplitude recorded 10 to 30 ms before the delta wave during anterograde preexcitation or between ventricular and atrial electrogram during orthodromic AVRT or ventricular pacing. A sharp QS deflection with maximum negative dV/dt is usually seen on the unipolar recording at successful ventricular insertion ablation sites (especially right-sided). The local VA interval at these sites is 25 to 50 ms but, as noted

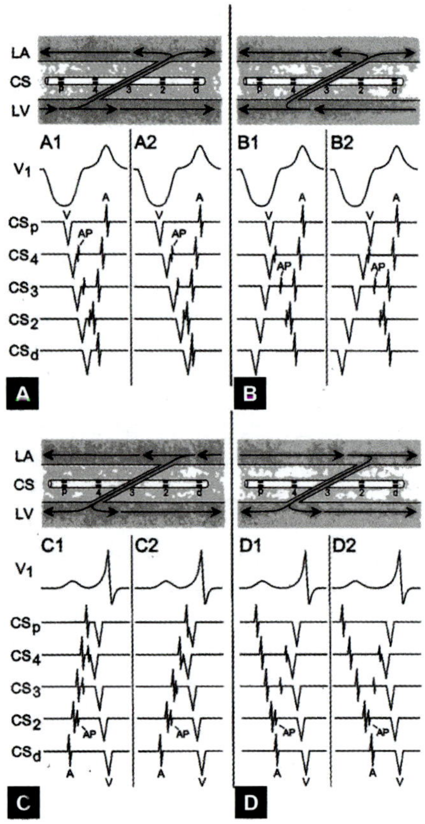

Figures 18.13A to D: Activation of slant accessory pathways from opposing directions. A and B show retrograde activation of a left free wall accessory pathway from the basal-posteroseptal RV producing a counterclockwise wavefront (A) and from the right ventricular outflow tract (B) producing a clockwise wavefront. (C and D) Activation of the atrial insertion from the distal-to-proximal direction and proximal-to-distal directions, respectively

From: Kenichiro O, Gonzalez M, Beckman K, et al. Reversing the direction of paced ventricular and atrial wavefronts reveals an oblique course in accessory AV pathways and improves localization for catheter ablation. Circulation 2001;104:550-6. With permission

above, basing choice of ablation sites primarily on the shortest local VA interval is incorrect.[41,44,45] In practice, sites with the shortest local VA interval are at or near sites with the earliest atrial electrogram during ventricular pacing or ORT, but it is not always true; a better guide is to target the AP potential or the site of earliest atrial activation during retrograde AP conduction or site of earliest ventricular activation during preexcitation. In a subannular position the atrial to ventricular electrogram ratio should be greater than 0.1. In supra-annular approach, an atrial to ventricular electrogram amplitude ratio <1 is sought. In cases of posterior paraseptal AP, fragmentation or double potentials are commonly seen at the site of earliest retrograde AP conduction in the CS.[46,47]

Atrial, ventricular electrograms and AP potentials can be differentiated by atrial extrastimuli, ventricular extrastimuli, or burst pacing to block in the AP **(Figures 18.14A to C)**. This differentiation is especially important when ablating a superoparaseptal and true septal pathways where AP has to be differentiated from the His potential. Spending extra time in carefully defining the area with best timing and configuration of unipolar and bipolar electrograms is helpful in achieving optimal results, using the least amount of radiofrequency (RF) energy and avoiding complications like AV block in case of superoparaseptal and midseptal pathways.

Rare pathways have been reported in which the atrial or ventricular insertion, or both, are relatively far from the AV groove. Atrial insertions are typically in either left or right atrial appendage while ventricular insertions are more variable. In such cases, sites at the annulus are not suitable for ablation and other sites such as in an atrial appendage must be explored.

Once the optimal ablation site has been identified and catheter stability is ensured, RF energy is given with a standard 4 mm-tip ablation catheter using a power setting of 50 W and targeting a temperature of 60°C. For superoparaseptal and midseptal pathway ablation a low power (30 W) and low temperature settings (50°C) to start may be used. If there is no evidence of pathway ablation in 15 seconds, RF application should be stopped and reasons for failed ablation should be evaluated. These are generally related to catheter instability or mapping error. It is important to assess AV nodal conduction after failed RF applications during superoparaseptal and midseptal pathways ablation to ensure normal AV conduction has not been inadvertently injured. At the end of the procedure it is important that tachycardia is not inducible and there is no evidence of any AP conduction in either antero- or retrograde directions.

CRYOABLATION FOR SEPTAL PATHWAYS: ADVANTAGES AND DISADVANTAGES

Cryoablation is an excellent option for septal pathways because of 3 properties. First, a transient and reversible loss of function can be created (cryomapping) before additional deep cooling results in an irreversible effect (cryoablation); second, the catheter tip adheres to the endocardial tissue, thus avoiding the risk of dislodgement during the procedure; and third, if normal AV conduction begins to be affected during ablation, cessation of freezing almost always leads to normalization of conduction. However, it is less successful on long-term follow-up than RF ablation (up to 20% recurrence after hospital discharge) and the larger ablation electrode is less desirable if precise mapping is needed; thus, it is generally reserved for cases in which there is a high perceived risk of AV block (midseptal, superoparaseptal APs).

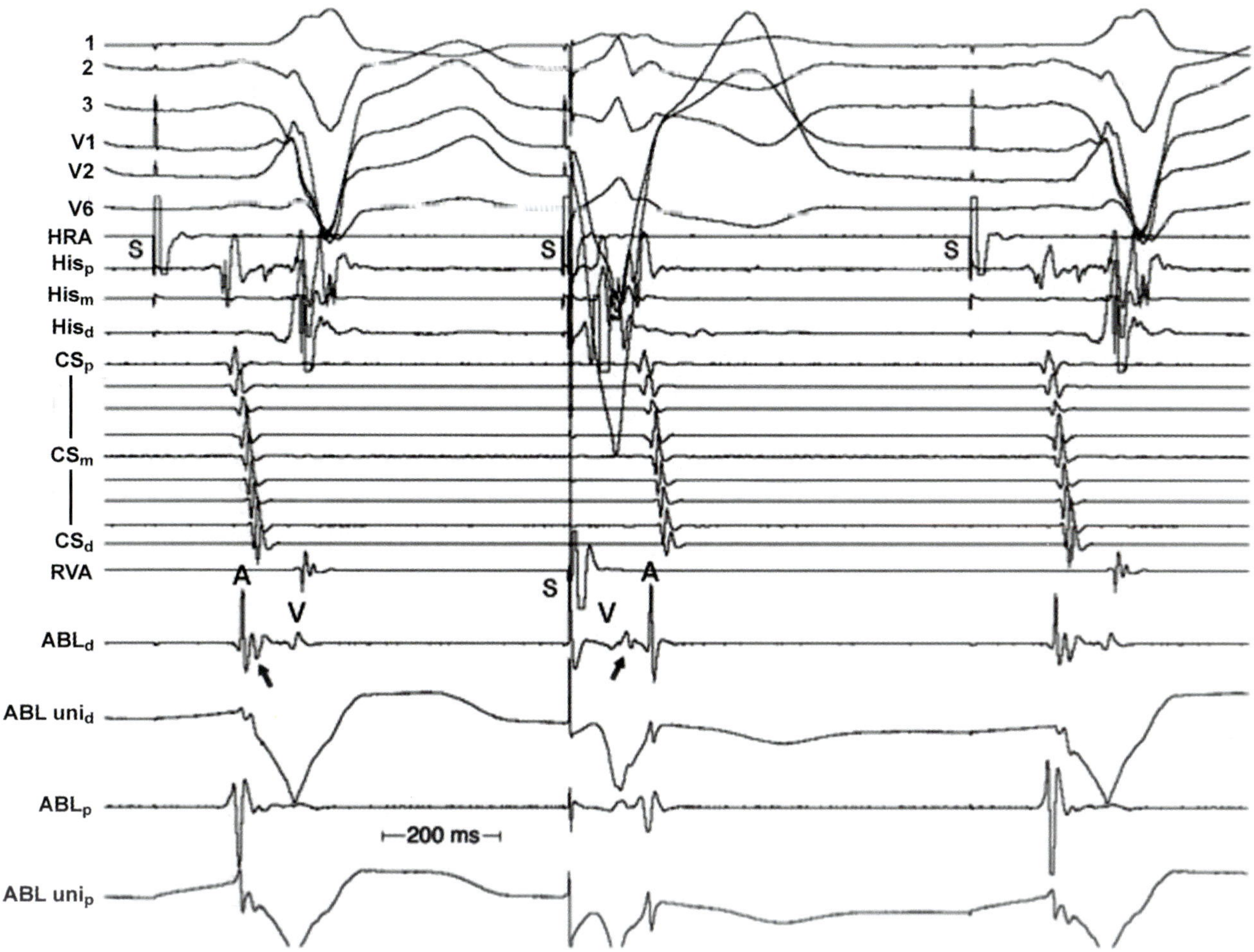

Figure 18.14A: Determination of bypass tract potential. Atrial pacing (S) with preexcitation is ongoing throughout with a single ventricular extrastimulus introduced at a time that will not advance the timing of atrial activation. The small arrow indicates a possible bypass tract potential between atrial (A) and ventricular (V) electrograms during anterograde conduction; with the ventricular extrastimulus, the atrial signal is exactly on time from atrial pacing, but the signal indicated by the arrow is advanced. Thus, it is not part of the atrial electrogram

RESULTS: SUCCESS RATE BY SITE; COMPLICATION RATE, RECURRENCE RATE

Success rates for ablation of left free wall APs is the highest of any AP location, ranging from 92 to 100%.[48,49] The recurrence rate (after apparent successful ablation) for left free wall AP is the lowest of any location, at 2 to 5%. The success rate does not vary depending on transaortic or transseptal approach.[48,49] The complication rates for transaortic approach of left sided APs range from 0% to 8%.[48-50] They include myocardial perforation with cardiac tamponade, access site hematomas, dissections, pseudoaneurysms, AV fistulas, damage to aortic or mitral valve, dissection or thrombosis of the left main coronary artery, and thromboembolic events. The incidence of complications with the transseptal approach ranges from 0% to 6% in adults and 0% to 25% in pediatric series.[48-50] The vascular complications are less with this approach but complications related to atrial septal puncture may be seen.

The success rate for right-free wall AP ablation varies from 66% to 100%, being the lowest of any AP location.[4,50] The lower success rate is attributed to catheter instability during ablation and an AP insertion away from the annulus. Likewise, the recurrence rate for right-free wall APs ranges from 9% to 16.7% and is higher than of any location.[4,50] Complications from right-free wall AP ablation are less common than for other AP location.[4,50] Cardiac perforation and pulmonary embolism may rarely occur.

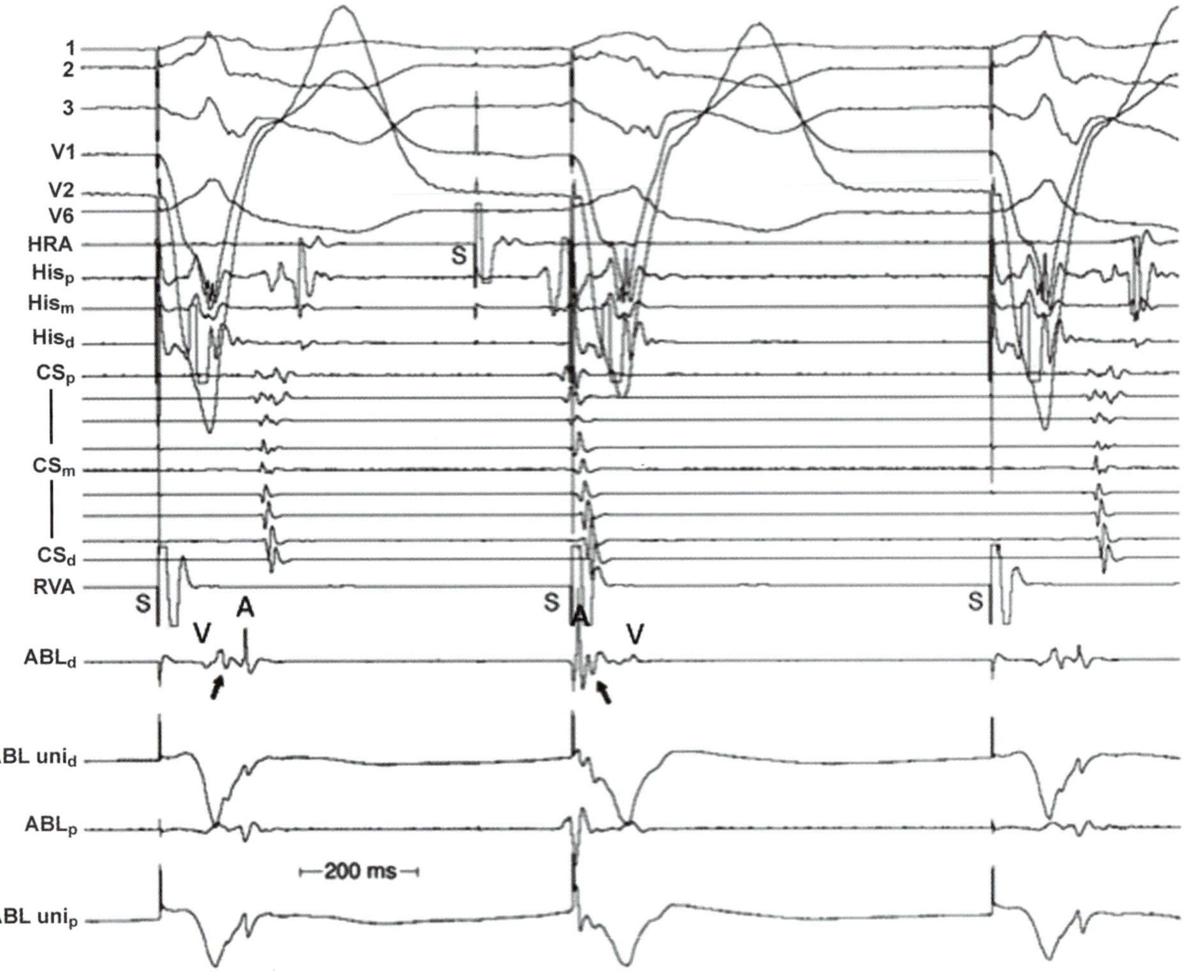

Figure 18.14B: Determination of bypass tract potential. Ventricular pacing (S) with retrograde conduction is ongoing throughout with a single atrial extrastimulus introduced at a time that will not advance the timing of ventricular activation. The small arrow indicates a possible bypass tract potential between ventricular (V) and atrial (A) electrograms during retrograde conduction on the 1st complex; with the atrial extrastimulus, the ventricular signal is exactly on time from ventricular pacing, but the atrial electrogram and signal indicated by the arrow are advanced. Thus, the small potential is not part of the ventricular electrogram. This information, taken with the prior figure, indicates that the signal is neither atrial nor ventricular but must instead be the bypass tract recording. Ablation here quickly eliminated pathway conduction both antero- and retrogradely

The success rate for posterior paraseptal AP ablation varies from 88% to 100%.[3,4,50] and recurrence rates vary from 12% to 0%. Complications are comparable to ablation of APs at other locations. Ablation within the CS or its branches (necessary in some cases with left posterior APs) carries the risk of perforation, tamponade, venous occlusion or damage to the right coronary artery (acute thrombosis or spasm, or chronic stenosis).

The success rate for ablation of superoparaseptal APs is more than 95% and that for midseptal APs is 98%. There is a 1% risk of complete AV block when ablating superoparaseptal and midseptal APs. An overall 1.5% risk of cardiac perforation with tamponade, tamponade, stroke, pericardial effusion or valve damage is reported for ablations at all locations.

CONCLUSION

Ablation of accessory pathways is a technical and physio logical challenge to an electrophysiologist. A thorou understanding of physiology, detailed and accurate mappi gives success rate that varies from 62% to 100% depending the site of AP (epicardial versus left-free wall pathway). Th highly favorable risk-benefit ratio justifies ablation as a first line therapy for patients with AP-dependent tachycardia.

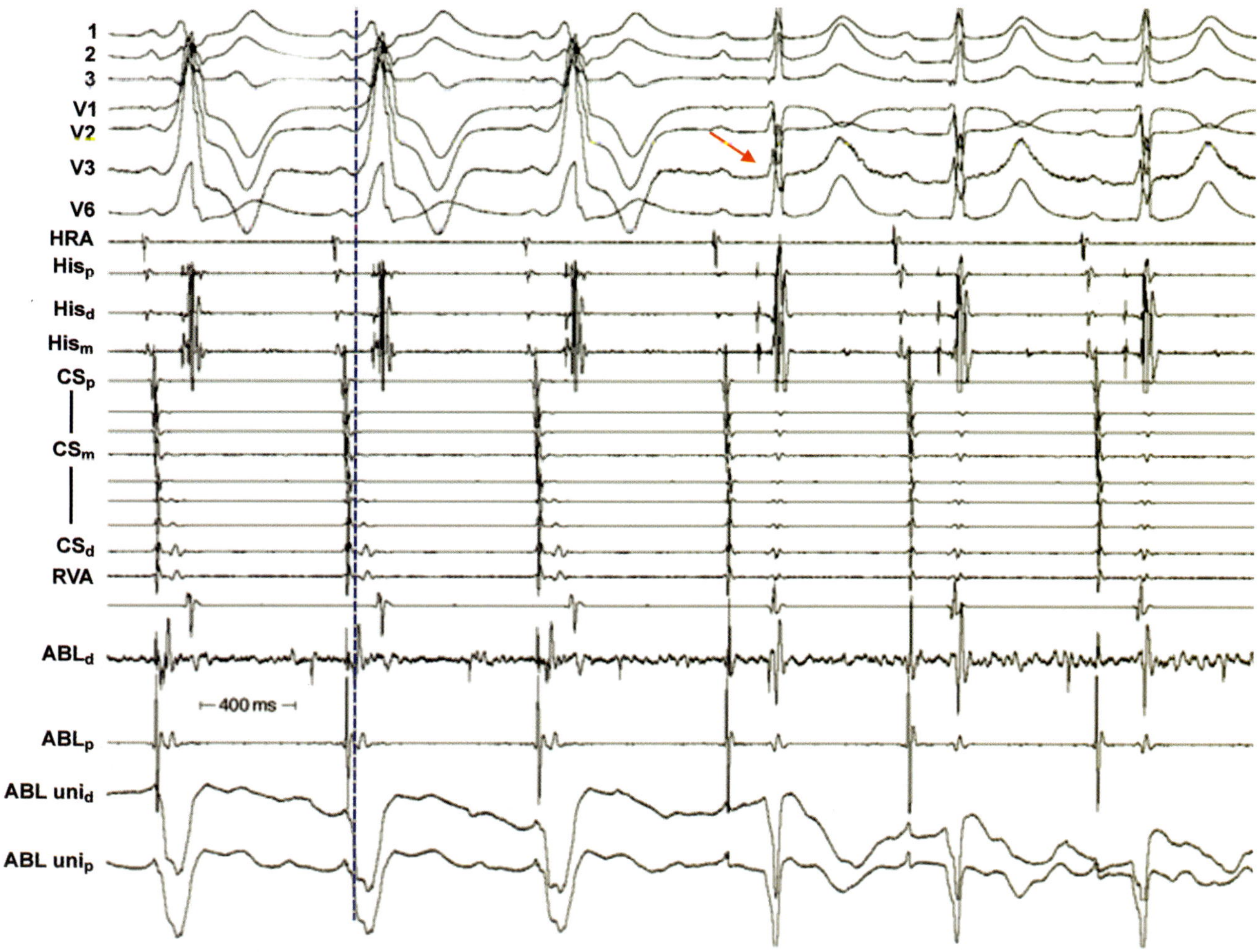

Figure 18.14C: Onset of RF application at inferolateral mitral annulus. Approximately 1 sec after beginning RF energy delivery at a site with a QS configuration in the distal unipolar recording (ABL uni$_d$), with the distal bipolar recording having a ventricular electrogram just before the delta wave onset (blue dashed line), the delta wave disappears (red arrow). At this time, a marked separation occurs between atrial and ventricular electrograms in the CS and ablation recordings

REFERENCES

1. Yee RK, GJ, Prystowsky, EN. The Wolff-Parkinson-White syndrome and related variants. In: Zipes DP (Ed). Philadelphia: WB Saunders; 2000. pp. 845-61.
2. Calkins H, Kim YN, Schmaltz S, Sousa J, el-Atassi R, Leon A, Kadish A, Langberg JJ, Morady F. Electrogram criteria for identification of appropriate target sites for radiofrequency catheter ablation of accessory atrioventricular connections. Circulation. 1992;85:565-73.
3. Calkins H, Yong P, Miller JM, Olshansky B, Carlson M, Saul JP, Huang SK, Liem LB, Klein LS, Moser SA, Bloch DA, Gillette P, Prystowsky E. Catheter ablation of accessory pathways, atrioventricular nodal reentrant tachycardia, and the atrioventricular junction: final results of a prospective, multicenter clinical trial. The Atakr Multicenter Investigators Group. Circulation. 1999;99:262-70.
4. Jackman WM, Wang XZ, Friday KJ, Roman CA, Moulton KP, Beckman KJ, McClelland JH, Twidale N, Hazlitt HA, Prior MI, et al. Catheter ablation of accessory atrioventricular pathways (Wolff-Parkinson-White syndrome) by radiofrequency current. N Engl J Med. 1991;324:1605-11.
5. Jazayeri MR, Deshpande S, Dhala A, Blanck Z, Sra J, Akhtar M. Transcatheter mapping and radiofrequency ablation of cardiac arrhythmias. Curr Probl Cardiol. 1994;19:287-395.
6. Miller JM DK, Jain R, et al. Ablation of supraparaseptal (anteroseptal) and mid septal accessory pathways, 3rd edn. In: Huang SK (Ed). Elsevier; 2015.
7. Anderson RH, Ho SY. Anatomy of the atrioventricular junctions with regard to ventricular preexcitation. Pacing Clin Electrophysiol. 1997;20:2072-6.
8. Becker AE, Anderson RH. The Wolff-Parkinson-White syndrome and its anatomical substrates. Anat Rec. 1981; 201:169-77.

9. Becker AE, Anderson RH, Durrer D, Wellens HJ. The anatomical substrates of Wolff-Parkinson-White syndrome. A clinicopathologic correlation in seven patients. Circulation. 1978;57:870-9.
10. Arruda MS, McClelland JH, Wang X, Beckman KJ, Widman LE, Gonzalez MD, Nakagawa H, Lazzara R, Jackman WM. Development and validation of an ECG algorithm for identifying accessory pathway ablation site in Wolff-Parkinson-White syndrome. J Cardiovasc Electrophysiol. 1998;9:2-12.
11. Boersma L, Garcia-Moran E, Mont L, Brugada J. Accessory pathway localization by QRS polarity in children with Wolff-Parkinson-White syndrome. J Cardiovasc Electrophysiol. 2002;13:1222-6.
12. Chiang CE, Chen SA, Teo WS, Tsai DS, Wu TJ, Cheng CC, Chiou CW, Tai CT, Lee SH, Chen CY, et al. An accurate stepwise electrocardiographic algorithm for localization of accessory pathways in patients with Wolff-Parkinson-White syndrome from a comprehensive analysis of delta waves and R/S ratio during sinus rhythm. Am J Cardiol. 1995;76:40-6.
13. Chen SA, Tai CT. Ablation of atrioventricular accessory pathways: current technique-state of the art. Pacing Clin Electrophysiol. 2001;24:1795-809.
14. Fitzgerald DM, Hawthorne HR, Crossley GH, Simmons TW, Haisty WK, Jr. P wave morphology during atrial pacing along the atrioventricular ring. ECG localization of the site of origin of retrograde atrial activation. J Electrocardiol. 1996;29:1-10.
15. Chung KY, Walsh TJ, Massie E. Wolff-Parkinson-White Syndrome. Am Heart J. 1965;69:116-33.
16. Garson A, Jr., Gillette PC, McNamara DG. Supraventricular tachycardia in children: clinical features, response to treatment, and long-term follow-up in 217 patients. J Pediatr. 1981;98: 875-82.
17. Chen SA, Chiang CE, Tai CT, Lee SH, Chiou CW, Ueng KC, Wen ZC, Cheng CC, Chang MS. Longitudinal clinical and electrophysiological assessment of patients with symptomatic Wolff-Parkinson-White syndrome and atrioventricular node reentrant tachycardia. Circulation. 1996;93:2023-32.
18. Vidaillet HJ, Jr., Pressley JC, Henke E, Harrell FE, Jr., German LD. Familial occurrence of accessory atrioventricular pathways (preexcitation syndrome). N Engl J Med. 1987;317:65-9.
19. Deal BJ, Keane JF, Gillette PC, Garson A, Jr. Wolff-Parkinson-White syndrome and supraventricular tachycardia during infancy: management and follow-up. J Am Coll Cardiol. 1985;5:130-5.
20. Giardina AC, Ehlers KH, Engle MA. Wolff-Parkinson-White syndrome in infants and children. A long-term follow-up study. Br Heart J. 1972;34:839-46.
21. Lev M, Gibson S, Miller RA. Ebstein's disease with Wolff-Parkinson-White syndrome; report of a case with a histopathologic study of possible conduction pathways. Am Heart J. 1955;49:724-41.
22. Haissaguerre M, Fischer B, Labbe T, Lemetayer P, Montserrat P, d'Ivernois C, Dartigues JF, Warin JF. Frequency of recurrent atrial fibrillation after catheter ablation of overt accessory pathways. Am J Cardiol. 1992;69:493-7.
23. Blomstrom-Lundqvist C, Scheinman MM, Aliot EM, Alpert JS, Calkins H, Camm AJ, Campbell WB, Haines DE, Kuck KH, Lerman BB, Miller DD, Shaeffer CW, Stevenson WG, Tomaselli GF, Antman EM, Smith SC, Jr., Faxon DP, Fuster V, Gibbons RJ, Gregoratos G, Hiratzka LF, Hunt SA, Jacobs AK, Russell RO, Jr., Priori SG, Blanc JJ, Budaj A, Burgos EF, Cowie M, Deckers JW, Garcia MA, Klein WW, Lekakis J, Lindahl B, Mazzotta G, Morais JC, Oto A, Smiseth O, Trappe HJ. ACC/AHA/ESC guidelines for the management of patients with supraventricular arrhythmias—executive summary. A report of the American college of cardiology/American heart association task force on practice guidelines and the European society of cardiology committee for practice guidelines (writing committee to develop guidelines for the management of patients with supraventricular arrhythmias) developed in collaboration with NASPE-Heart Rhythm Society. J Am Coll Cardiol. 2003;42:1493-531.
24. Pappone C, Santinelli V. Should catheter ablation be performed in asymptomatic patients with Wolff-Parkinson-White syndrome? Catheter ablation should be performed in asymptomatic patients with Wolff-Parkinson-White syndrome. Circulation. 2005;112:2207-15; discussion 16.
25. Pappone C, Santinelli V, Manguso F, Augello G, Santinelli O, Vicedomini G, Gulletta S, Mazzone P, Tortoriello V, Pappone A, Dicandia C, Rosanio S. A randomized study of prophylactic catheter ablation in asymptomatic patients with the Wolff-Parkinson-White syndrome. N Engl J Med. 2003;349: 1803-11.
26. Pappone C, Santinelli V, Rosanio S, Vicedomini G, Nardi S, Pappone A, Tortoriello V, Manguso F, Mazzone P, Gulletta S, Oreto G, Alfieri O. Usefulness of invasive electrophysiologic testing to stratify the risk of arrhythmic events in asymptomatic patients with Wolff-Parkinson-White pattern: results from a large prospective long-term follow-up study. J Am Coll Cardiol. 2003;41:239-44.
27. Hirao K, Otomo K, Wang X, Beckman KJ, McClelland JH, Widman L, Gonzalez MD, Arruda M, Nakagawa H, Lazzara R, Jackman WM. Para-Hisian pacing. A new method for differentiating retrograde conduction over an accessory AV pathway from conduction over the AV node. Circulation. 1996;94:1027-35.
28. Singh DK, Viswanathan MN, Tanel RE, Lee RJ, Lee BK, Marcus GM, Olgin JE, Han F, Vedantham V, Tseng ZH, Pellegrini C, Kawamura M, Gerstenfeld EP, Badhwar N, Scheinman M. His overdrive pacing during supraventricular tachycardia: a novel maneuver for distinguishing atrioventricular nodal reentrant tachycardia from atrioventricular reciprocating tachycardia. Heart Rhythm. 2014;11:1327-35.
29. Miles WM, Yee R, Klein GJ, Zipes DP, Prystowsky EN. The preexcitation index: an aid in determining the mechanism of supraventricular tachycardia and localizing accessory pathways. Circulation. 1986;74:493-500.
30. Michaud GF, Tada H, Chough S, Baker R, Wasmer K, Sticherling C, Oral H, Pelosi F, Jr., Knight BP, Strickberger SA, Morady F. Differentiation of atypical atrioventricular node re-entrant tachycardia from orthodromic reciprocating tachycardia using a septal accessory pathway by the response to ventricular pacing. J Am Coll Cardiol. 2001;38:1163-7.
31. Gonzalez-Torrecilla E, Arenal A, Atienza F, Osca J, Garcia-Fernandez J, Puchol A, Sanchez A, Almendral J. First postpacing interval after tachycardia entrainment with correction for atrioventricular node delay: a simple maneuver for differential diagnosis of atrioventricular nodal reentrant tachycardias versus orthodromic reciprocating tachycardias. Heart Rhythm. 2006;3:674-9.
32. Miller JM, Rosenthal ME, Gottlieb CD, Vassallo JA, Josephson ME. Usefulness of the delta HA interval to accurately distinguish

atrioventricular nodal reentry from orthodromic septal bypass tract tachycardias. Am J Cardiol. 1991;68:1037-44.

33. Martinez-Alday JD, Almendral J, Arenal A, Ormaetxe JM, Pastor A, Villacastin JP, Medina O, Peinado R, Delcan JL. Identification of concealed posteroseptal Kent pathways by comparison of ventriculoatrial intervals from apical and posterobasal right ventricular sites. Circulation. 1994;89:1060-7.
34. Segal OR, Gula LJ, Skanes AC, Krahn AD, Yee R, Klein GJ. Differential ventricular entrainment: a maneuver to differentiate AV node reentrant tachycardia from orthodromic reciprocating tachycardia. Heart Rhythm. 2009;6:493-500.
35. Derval N, Skanes AC, Gula LJ, Gray C, Denis A, Lim HS, Krahn AD, Yee R, Sacher F, Haissaguerre M, Klein GJ. Differential sequential septal pacing: a simple maneuver to differentiate nodal versus extranodal ventriculoatrial conduction. Heart Rhythm. 2013;10:1785-91.
36. Dandamudi G, Mokabberi R, Assal C, Das MK, Oren J, Storm R, Vijayaraman P, Miller JM. A novel approach to differentiating orthodromic reciprocating tachycardia from atrioventricular nodal reentrant tachycardia. Heart Rhythm. 2010;7:1326-9.
37. Benditt DG, Pritchett EL, Smith WM, Gallagher JJ. Ventriculoatrial intervals: diagnostic use in paroxysmal supra-ventricular tachycardia. Ann Intern Med. 1979;91:161-6.
38. Kerr CR, Gallagher JJ, German LD. Changes in ventriculoatrial intervals with bundle branch block aberration during reciprocating tachycardia in patients with accessory atrioventricular pathways. Circulation. 1982;66:196-201.
39. Pritchett EL, Tonkin AM, Dugan FA, Wallace AG, Gallagher JJ. Ventriculo-atrial conduction time during reciprocating tachycardia with intermittent bundle-branch block in Wolff-Parkinson-White syndrome. Br Heart J. 1976;38: 1058-64.
40. Jazayeri MR, Caceres J, Tchou P, Mahmud R, Denker S, Akhtar M. Electrophysiologic characteristics of sudden QRS axis deviation during orthodromic tachycardia. Role of functional fascicular block in localization of accessory pathway. J Clin Invest. 1989;83:952-9.
41. Otomo K, Gonzalez MD, Beckman KJ, Nakagawa H, Becker AE, Shah N, Matsudaira K, Wang Z, Lazzara R, Jackman WM. Reversing the direction of paced ventricular and atrial wavefronts reveals an oblique course in accessory AV pathways and improves localization for catheter ablation. Circulation. 2001;104:550-6.
42. Cappato R, Schluter M, Mont L, Kuck KH. Anatomic, electrical, and mechanical factors affecting bipolar endocardial electrograms. Impact on catheter ablation of manifest left free-wall accessory pathways. Circulation. 1994;90:884-94.
43. Jackman WM, Friday KJ, Fitzgerald DM, Bowman AJ, Yeung-Lai-Wai JA, Lazzara R. Localization of left-free wall and posteroseptal accessory atrioventricular pathways by direct recording of accessory pathway activation. Pacing Clin Electrophysiol. 1989;12:204-14.
44. Chen X, Borggrefe M, Shenasa M, Haverkamp W, Hindricks G, Breithardt G. Characteristics of local electrogram predicting successful transcatheter radiofrequency ablation of left-sided accessory pathways. J Am Coll Cardiol. 1992;20:656-65.
45. Xie B, Heald SC, Camm AJ, Rowland E, Ward DE. Successful radiofrequency ablation of accessory pathways with the first energy delivery: the anatomic and electrical characteristics. Eur Heart J. 1996;17:1072-9.
46. Pap R, Traykov VB, Makai A, Bencsik G, Forster T, Saghy L. Ablaon of posteroseptal and left posterior accessory pathways guided by left atrium-coronary sinus musculature activation sequence. J Cardiovasc Electrophysiol. 2008;19:653-8.
47. Takahashi A, Shah DC, Jais P, Hocini M, Clementy J, Haissaguerre M. Specific electrocardiographic features of manifest coronary vein posteroseptal accessory pathways. J Cardiovasc Electrophysiol. 1998;9:1015-25.
48. De Ponti R, Zardini M, Storti C, Longobardi M, Salerno-Uriarte JA. Trans-septal catheterization for radiofrequency catheter ablation of cardiac arrhythmias. Results and safety of a simplified method. Eur Heart J. 1998;19:943-50.
49. Yip AS, Chow WH, Yung TC, Chau EM, Chan TF. Radiofrequency catheter ablation of left-sided accessory pathways using a transseptal technique and specialized long intravascular sheaths. Efficacy, recurrence rate and complications. Jpn Heart J. 1997;38:643-50.
50. Swartz JF, Tracy CM, Fletcher RD. Radiofrequency endocardial catheter ablation of accessory atrioventricular pathway atrial insertion sites. Circulation. 1993;87:487-99.

EDITORS' SUMMARY

The cornerstone arrhythmogenic substrate for learning the principal skills of electrophysiology is the accessory pathway. In this chapter, Drs Miller and Jain provide a classic and comprehensive review of exactly what needs to be understood when we try to define arrhythmia mechanism and utilize our background in anatomy, fluoroscopy, and biophysics to effectively cure the arrhythmia. The principles and tenets of rhythm diagnosis so lucidly explained by Dr Miller will be useful for electrophysiology students when invasively diagnosing or treating any arrhythmia.

Arrhythmia mechanism: Following the principles of defining the arrhythmia mechanism with accessory pathway-related arrhythmias, for example orthodromic reciprocating tachycardia, we first define that a reentrant process is present, and then sequentially determine what all are the components of the circuit, then conclusively identify that the accessory pathway is a part of that circuit.

Similar reasoning is essential in complex ventricular tachycardia and post-AF ablation, reentrant, atypical flutter ablation. For the early entrant to invasive electrophysiology, multiple teaching points made in this chapter, and extending that reasoning along with a mastery of entrainment techniques and the unique regional anatomy of the specific sites being targeted, the student would be well on his or her way to mastery in this field.

Identifying appropriate targets: With pathway-related reentrant tachycardia, we may identify earliest atrial activation sites during ORT or ventricular pacing; earliest ventricular sites, when antegrade preexcitation or antidromic tachycardia is present; and when pacing close to the pathway where we identify atrial and ventricular electrograms occurring nearly simultaneously. As explained in this chapter, however, each has their own pitfalls. For example, even when a pathway is not present, pacing the right atrium in someone with left bundle branch block may show atrioventricular fusion in the lateral mitral annulus because of simultaneous atrial and ventricular activation occurring at that site. Pacing close to the suspected site of abnormal atrioventricular conduction will eliminate this pitfall. When we wish to ablate an accessory pathway, the principal signal of interest is the conduction signal from pathway activation—pathway potential. Drs Miller and Jain explain important tips to maximize identifying these sites and using all available evidence to find the best location to target energy delivery.

Biophysics: With both radiofrequency and cryoablation, no success can be anticipated if contact is not present. Knowledge of various catheters, sheaths, details of regional anatomy, and methods to assess contact are all essential skills for the electrophysiologist and is germane to any arrhythmia ablation. However, the skills are best learned with pathway ablation since we get immediate, real-time feedback on success. Unlike for example with atrial fibrillation ablation, we may not know whether we are successful until the line or perivenous circular ablation is complete, or in many instances success may be unknown for several months after the ablation. However, with pathway ablation, we usually know immediately, and this immediate feedback is a powerful learning tool to know whether our assumptions of contact and anatomy, as well as the biophysics of energy delivery, have been learned and executed correctly.

CHAPTER 19

Shomu Bohora

Mahaim Fiber Accessory Pathways and Other Variants of Preexcitation

LIST OF ABBREVIATIONS

AP	Accessory Pathway	LBBB	Left Bundle Branch Block
ARVC	Arrhythmogenic Right Ventricular Cardiomyopathy	RBB	Right Bundle Branch
AV	Atrioventricular	RBBB	Right Bundle Branch Block
AVNRT	Atrioventricular Nodal Reentrant Tachycardia	RF	Radiofrequency
AVRT	Atrioventricular Reciprocating Tachycardia	RV	Right Ventricle
EP	Electrophysiology	SVT	Supraventricular Tachycardia

INTRODUCTION

Mahaim and Winston were the first to describe Mahaim fiber, as a tract, which connects the atrioventricular (AV) node to the ventricular myocardium.[1] It was initially believed that Mahaim accessory pathways represent nodofascicular or nodoventricular connections. In 1978, Becker et al.[2] found specialized fibers present at the lateral tricuspid annulus and coursing through the right ventricle mimicking a second AV node. Mahaim fiber conducts slowly and only antegradely and has decremental conduction properties, and these features represent the Mahaim physiology. Later, electrophysiology (EP) studies, catheter and surgical ablation established the fact that the so called Mahaim fiber tachycardia are caused usually by atriofascicular fibers connecting the atrium near the lateral tricuspid annulus to the right bundle branch.[3-12]

ETIOPATHOGENESIS

Less than 3% of patients with ventricular preexcitation have decrementally conducting accessory pathway. About 6% of patients presenting with a wide QRS supraventricular tachycardia (SVT) with left bundle branch block (LBBB) morphology have a Mahaim bypass tract. Mahaim fibers are better described by the structures connected by it proximally (atrium or AV node) and distally (fascicle or ventricle). Accordingly, the accessory pathways are termed as atriofascicular, atrioventricular, nodofascicular, nodoventricular and fasciculoventricular accessory pathways. The pathway from the atrium can connect and insert basally into the ventricular myocardium close to the tricuspid annulus (short atrioventricular tract) or in the apical ventricular myocardium (long atrioventricular tract) or can travel along the right ventricular endocardial surface to insert into the right bundle branch (RBB), usually in its distal third (atriofascicular tract).[7] The long pathways have a wide distal insertion, which can be up to 0.5 to 2 cm in diameter.[13] Nodofascicular/ventricular pathways, similarly connect from the AV node to the fascicles/ventricle. Fasciculoventricular connections have also been described that connect from the His bundle or right bundle branch to the right ventricle; however, clinical arrhythmias mediated by these pathways have not been seen. The proximal component of the pathway is thought to have node-like features and is largely responsible for the decremental conduction properties of the pathway.[2,7,8] Atriofascicular pathways represent the majority of these slow conducting accessory pathways (APs) with decremental conduction properties. The atrial insertion site is predominantly situated on the right side along the tricuspid annulus generally at the 5–10 o'clock position with the ventricular insertion site being the distal right bundle branch **(Figure 19.1)**. Atrial insertion site can rarely be present at the superior or medial region of the tricuspid annulus necessitating careful mapping. Very rare reports of a left sided pathway have also been described.[14,15] Mahaim fibers are likely AV node like tissues which have failed to involute at other sites or appear due to duplication of AV conduction tissue at site other than the normal sites.

MAHAIM PHYSIOLOGY

Mahaim physiology refers to the following specific features of these tracts making them unique among all the accessory pathways:

- Antegrade conduction only
- Long conduction time at baseline

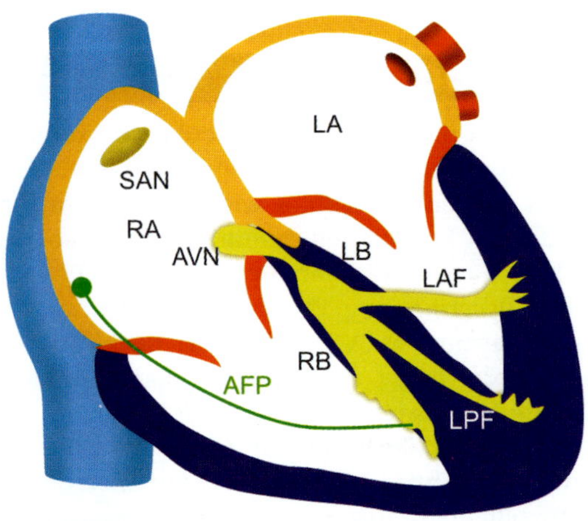

Figure 19.1: Schematic diagram showing the connection of the atriofascicular bypass tract

Abbreviations: AFP, atriofascicular pathway; AVN, atrioventricular node; LA, left atrium; LAF, left anterior fascicle; LB, left bundle branch; LPF, left posterior fascicle; RA, right atrium; RB, right bundle branch; SAN, sinoatrial node

- Decremental conduction on atrial pacing
- Wenckebach on atrial pacing and
- Conduction block in response to adenosine.

Mahaim fiber tachycardia, therefore, has to be an antidromic tachycardia, with antegrade conduction via the accessory pathway and retrograde conduction via the AV node or another accessory pathway. Since a right sided atriofascicular bypass tract constitutes the majority of the Mahaim fiber-related tachycardia, an atriofascicular tract-related tachycardia is described further in detail.

ATRIOFASCICULAR BYPASS TRACT

Atriofascicular bypass tract is the most common of the Mahaim physiology pathways and as the name suggests the fiber connects the atrium to the ventricle at the fascicle which is nearly always right sided.

Though, most commonly seen in patients without structural heart disease, it is not uncommon to see it in patients with Ebstein's anomaly.[10,11,13,16-21] Palpitation is the most common presentation and is related to either an antidromic atrioventricular reciprocating tachycardia (AVRT) or other supraventricular tachycardias, wherein the atriofascicular bypass tract acts as an innocent bystander. Associated atrioventricular nodal reentrant tachycardia (AVNRT) is not uncommon. The tachycardia generally manifests in the age group of 20–50 years. As almost all the atriofascicular bypass tracts are situated on the right side, further description is for a right sided atriofascicular bypass tract.

ECG Features

During the typical antidromic AVRT, ECG shows typical LBBB morphology with a QRS interval of ≤150 msec. Left axis deviation of the QRS in the frontal plane is common with an axis between 0 and –75° and a late R > S transition at V4 or V5. QRS complex in V1 shows an initial sharp r deflection and is an important differentiating point from other non-decremental AP-mediated antidromic tachycardias or ventricular tachycardia **(Figure 19.2)**.

During sinus rhythm, there generally is no evidence of preexcitation due to slow conduction in the AP. Subtle signs of atriofascicular tract activation during a sinus rhythm ECG can be absent q in leads I, aVL, V5 and V6, late precordial transition in V4-5 or even in V6 and rS complex in lead III **(Figure 19.3)**. Occasionally, there may be presence of LBBB like pattern during sinus rhythm due to preferential conduction over the atriofascicular bypass tract. However, the PR interval is not short as the pathway conducts with a delay. The QRS complex is not very wide as the distal insertion is over the right bundle branch **(Figure 19.4)**. Occasionally evidence of automatic beats arising from the atriofascicular tract can be seen on ECG with a same LBBB morphology and left axis deviation in the frontal plane **(Figure 19.5)**.

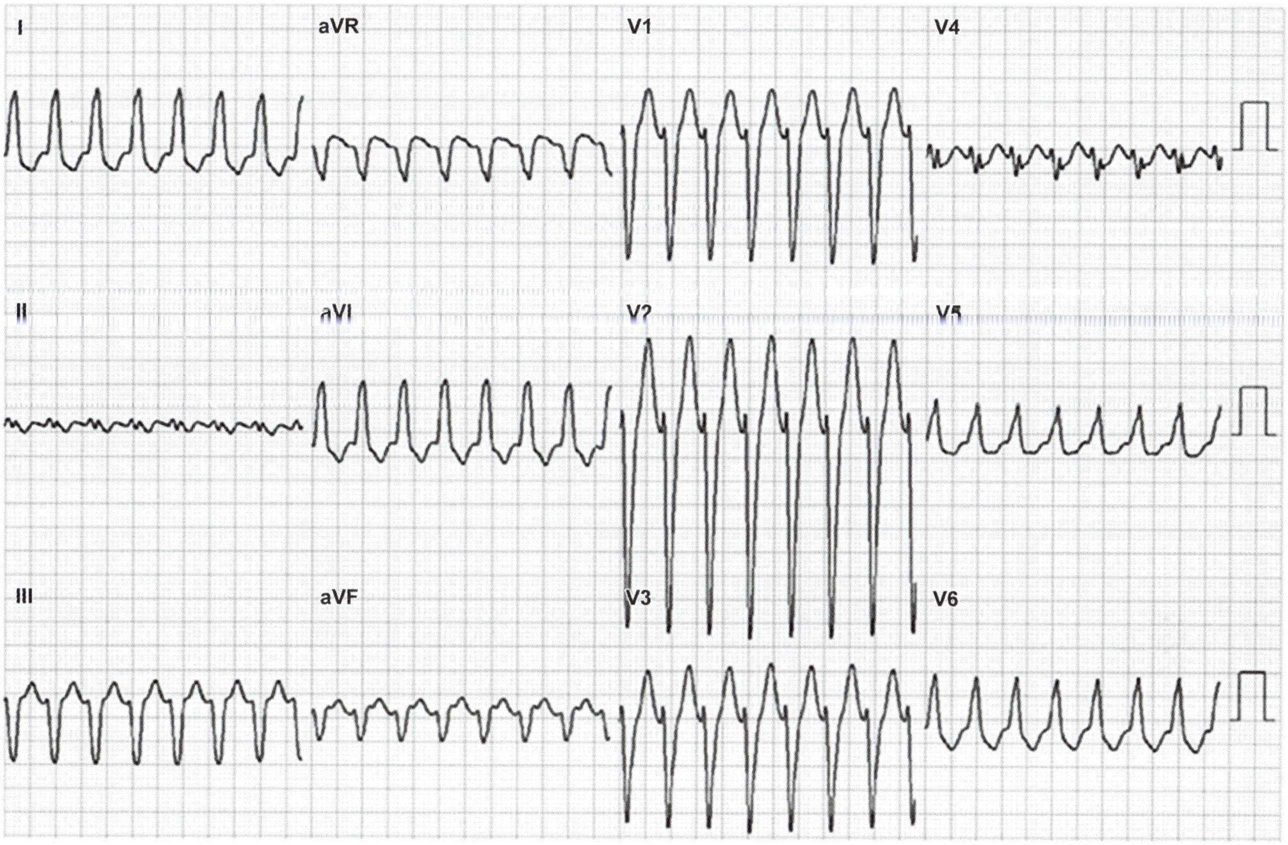

Figure 19.2: Twelve-lead ECG of a broad QRS tachycardia with LBBB morphology and left axis deviation in a patient with no structural heart disease. Likelihood of atriofascicular bypass tract-mediated antidromic tachycardia should be considered in this patient in view of initial sharp r in V1 with late precordial transition in V4-5

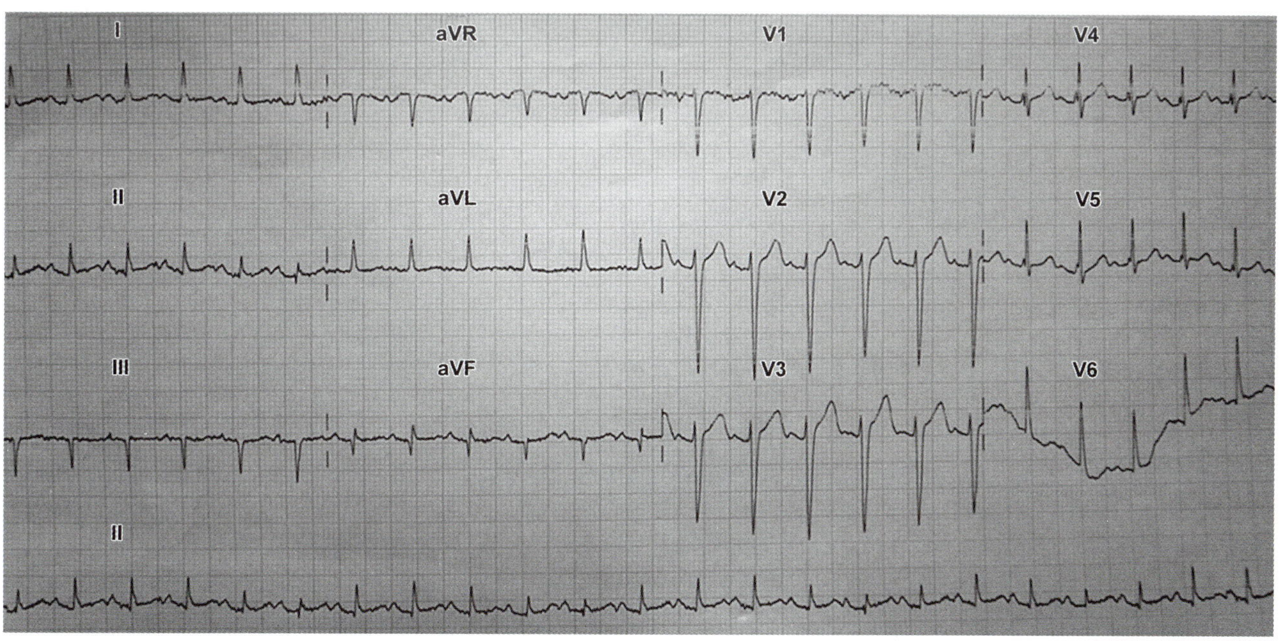

Figure 19.3: Twelve-lead ECG of the patient having atriofascicular bypass tract during sinus rhythm. Features suggesting subtle preexcitation due to atriofascicular bypass tract include absence of q in leads I, aVL, V5 and V6 with normal PR interval in this example. Also, note the rS pattern in lead III

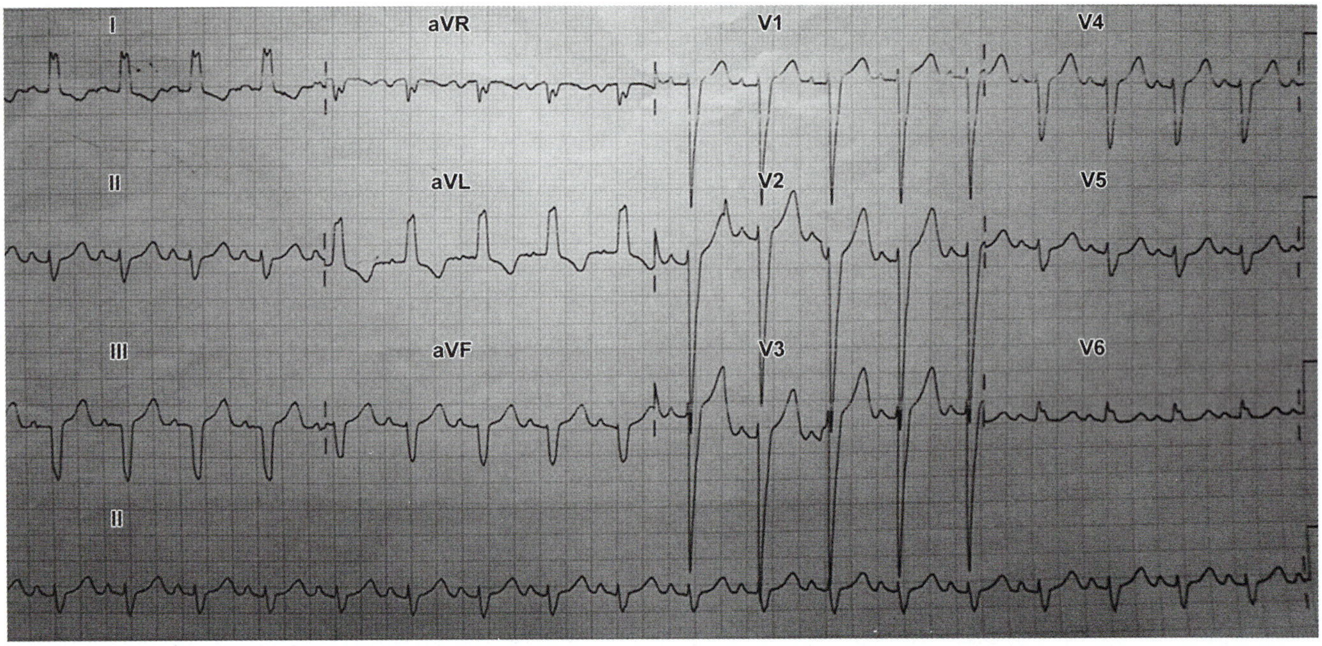

Figure 19.4: Twelve-lead ECG of the same patient as in Figure 19.3 at another time. A broad QRS with LBBB pattern, left axis deviation and a late transition in V5-6 during sinus rhythm with normal PR interval, very likely suggests preferential conduction over the atriofascicular bypass tract. It is very uncommon to see preexcitation during sinus rhythm

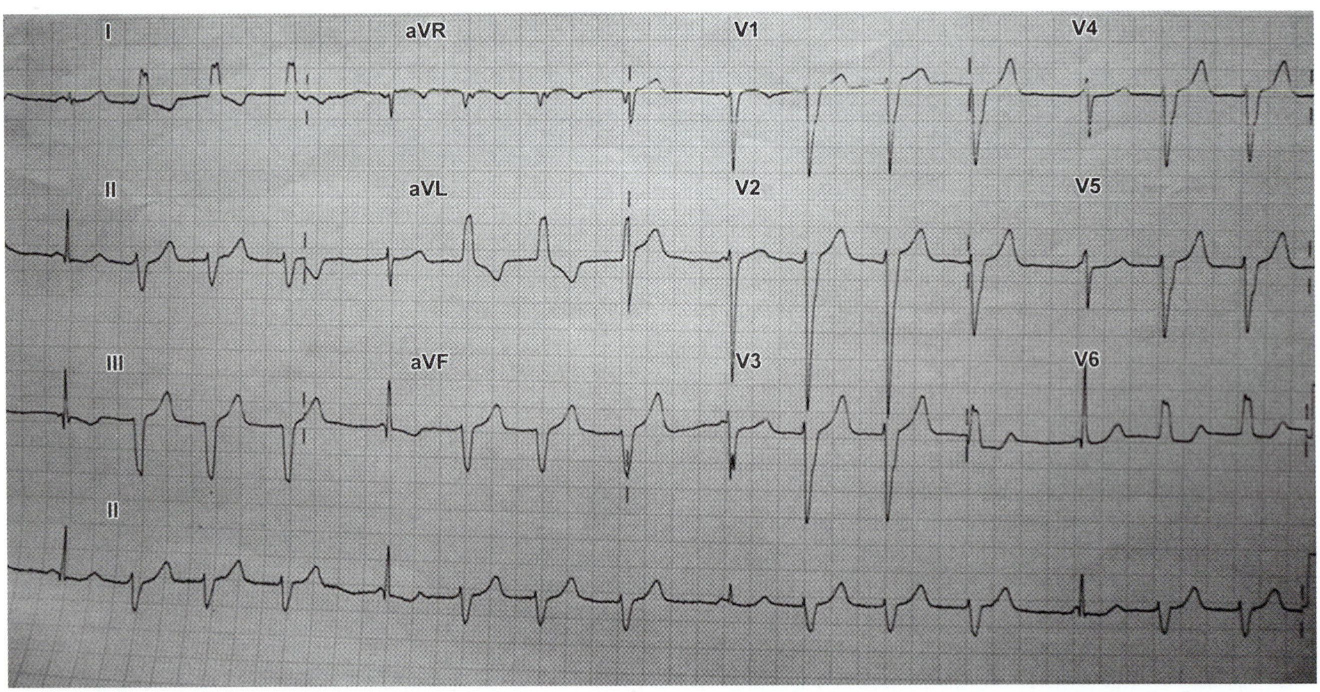

Figure 19.5: Twelve-lead ECG of the same patient, post-tachycardia termination, shows intermittent broad QRS beats with LBBB morphology and left axis deviation similar to the preexcited beats, however with no preceding P-waves, suggesting an atriofascicular bypass tract automatic rhythm. The beats with narrower QRS demonstrate a short PR interval and are likely to be junctional escape beats. This phenomenon is likely due to sinus node suppression post-tachycardia termination

Electrophysiology Study

Catheter Placement

The preexcitation due to right sided atriofascicular pathways becomes manifest during pacing from the right atrium. Pacing the right atrial free wall is more likely to reveal these pathways than pacing the coronary sinus. Hence, the site of catheter placement especially in a study with limited catheters is important. The author prefers to place a decapolar catheter along the tricuspid annulus similar to that when doing an atrial flutter ablation for need of pacing from different sites along the tricuspid annulus. A traditionally placed decapolar catheter in the coronary sinus **(Figures 19.6A and B)** is repositioned to the tricuspid annular site once there is evidence of an atriofascicular bypass tract on basal protocols if an additional access site is to be avoided **(Figures 19.6C and D)**. A quadripolar catheter records His potentials and ablation catheter initially can be placed in the right ventricle near the RBB. These pathways are occasionally very sensitive to mechanical trauma and conduction through the pathway may get blocked for minutes to hours. Hence, catheter manipulation should be gentle and performed with care especially near the lateral tricuspid annular region.

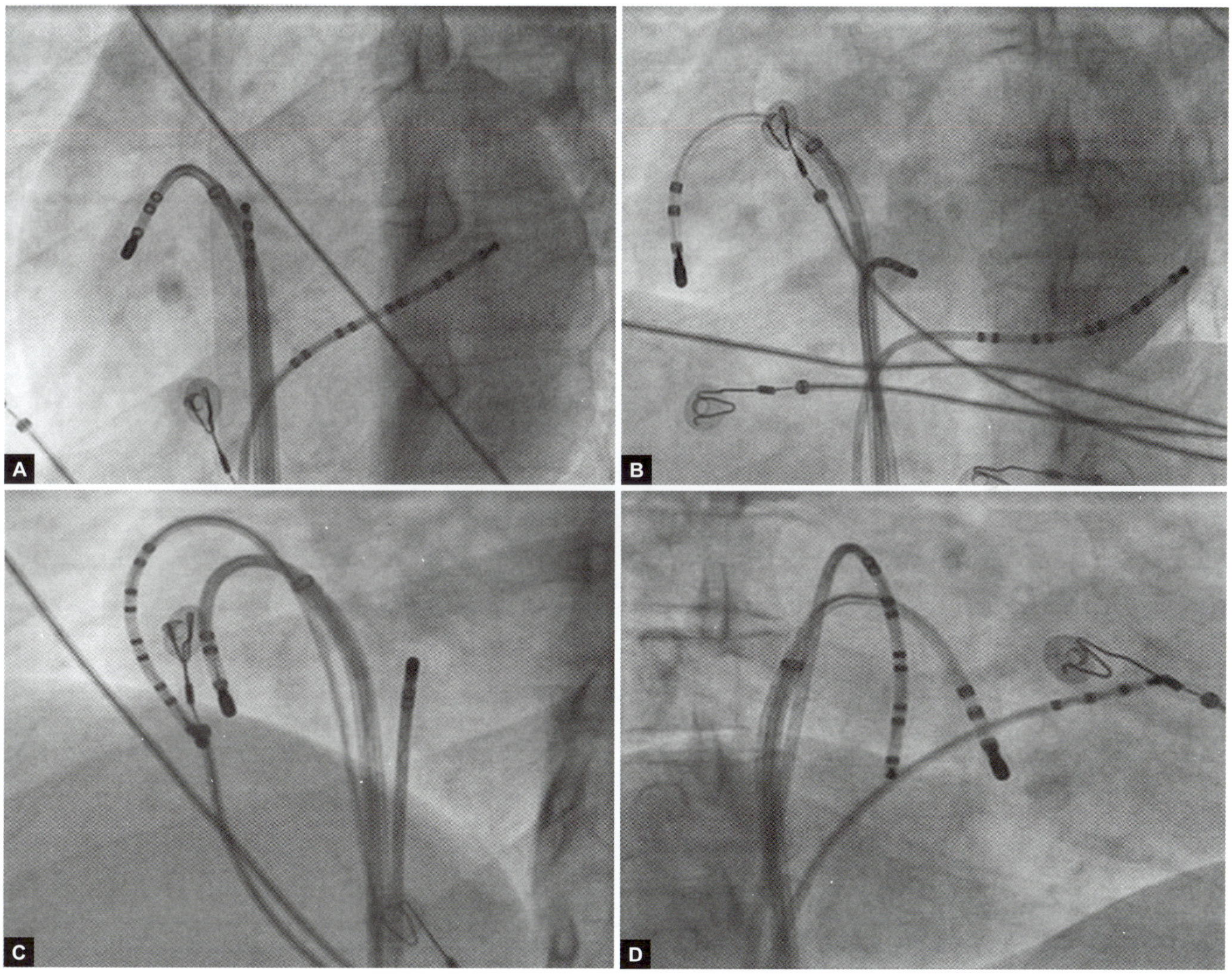

Figures 19.6A to D: Standard placement of catheters when three catheters are used. Mapping along the tricuspid annulus is done with the ablation catheter introduced in a long sheath in this example. The sites of ablation in left anterior oblique (LAO) view at 9 o'clock in (A) and 8 o'clock in (B) are generally the most common. (C and D) are LAO and right anterior oblique (RAO) views respectively showing an alternative way to place the catheters wherein the decapolar catheter from the CS is repositioned at the tricuspid annulus. Pacing and mapping the tricuspid annulus becomes much easier with this approach. The decapolar catheter also provides a useful anatomical reference in a procedure without 3D mapping. Use of a long sheath for ablation catheter helps to minimize sudden movements of the catheter and makes it more stable. Keeping the sheath high up helps to map the tricuspid annulus in a vertical direction easily as catheter movement along the annulus is parallel and smooth

Electrophysiologic Findings

During sinus rhythm, in absence of preexcitation, the AH and HV interval appear normal. Subtle preexcitation, when present may lead to a shortened HV interval. Ventricular pacing shows central and decremental conduction, and may occasionally induce tachycardia. There is no evidence of retrograde conduction over the accessory pathway. Atrial pacing, when done from the coronary sinus catheter may show no evidence of preexcitation initially due to earlier engagement of the nearby AV node. However, right atrial free wall pacing easily and promptly brings out antegrade conduction through a right sided atriofascicular bypass tract. A gradual increase in the AV interval, simultaneous with the development of LBBB and shortening of the His-ventricular (HV) interval in response to atrial pacing is characteristic and is due to long conduction time through the atriofascicular bypass tract.[3,4] A decreasing HV interval to finally a negative value during maximal preexcitation and then a fixed value after maximal preexcitation has been achieved is characteristic **(Figure 19.7A)**. HV interval, better described as VH interval when HV is negative, is related to the insertion site of the bypass tract. More distal the insertion of the bypass tract in the RBB, longer is the VH interval. VH interval is generally less than 20 ms and always <50 ms in an atriofascicular bypass tract. During maximal preexcitation right bundle branch (RBB) activation is seen earlier than the His bundle activation. The activation pattern is reversed to a RBB → His Distal → His proximal activation during maximal preexcitation **(Figure 19.7B)** and is schematically shown in **Figure 19.7C**. Atrial extrastimulus demonstrates decremental conduction through the atriofascicular bypass tract **(Figure 19.8A)**. The antegrade refractory period of the bypass tract is similar to that of the AV node and ranges commonly from 250 to 400 ms **(Figure 19.8B)**.

Tachycardia can be induced on atrial pacing **(Figure 19.9A)** as well as ventricular pacing. Atriofascicular bypass tract tachycardia is an antidromic tachycardia, with antegrade conduction over the atriofascicular bypass tract and retrograde conduction via the AV node or another accessory pathway. Antidromic tachycardia through the atriofascicular bypass tract demonstrates a negative HV interval (VH interval < 50 ms) with an activation pattern earliest in the RV at the mid septum near the presumed insertion of the bypass tract and thereafter RB-> His D-> His P activation sequence as seen during maximal preexcitation **(Figure 19.9B)** and is demonstrated in the schematic diagram **(Figure 19.9C)**. VA interval is generally >70 ms and atrial activation is concentric if the retrograde limb of the tachycardia is AVN-His Purkinje system. Differential RV pacing (entrainment) during tachycardia results in a shorter postpacing interval with apical pacing compared to basal pacing.

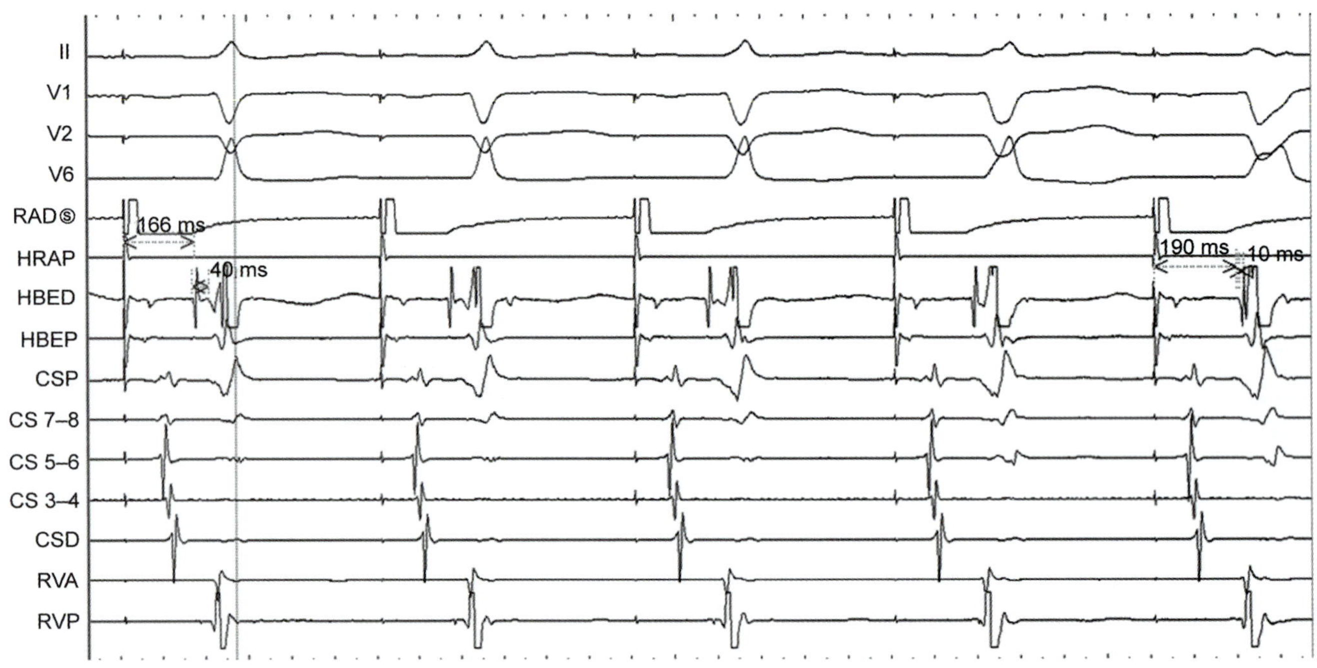

Figure 19.7A: Atrial pacing shows progressive HV shortening with increase in the AV interval. Note that the QRS also widens progressively. Finally the VH interval is 10 ms at maximum preexcitation. This feature is classically seen with Mahaim physiology, i.e. long conduction time and decremental conduction

Abbreviations: CSP, coronary sinus proximal; CSD, coronary sinus distal; CS 7–8 to CS 3–4, coronary sinus mid; HRAP, high right atrium proximal; RAD, right atrium distal; RVA, right ventricular apex distal; RVP, right ventricular proximal

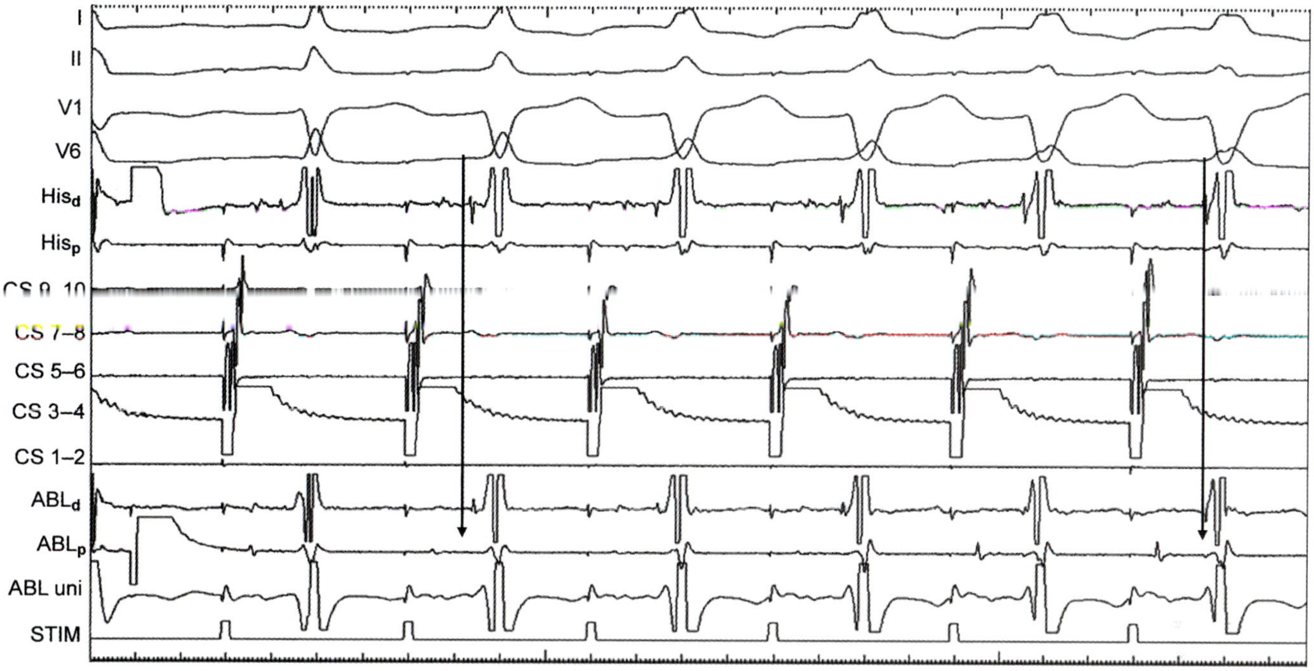

Figure 19.7B: EP tracing during atrial pacing. The ablation catheter (ABL_d and ABL_p) is positioned to record the right bundle branch electrogram. With lesser preexcitation in the initial part, RB activation occurs after the His bundle. However, with more preexcitation (right half), RB activation is seen as early as the surface QRS and His activation suggesting reversal of HB-RBB activation pattern

Abbreviations: ABL_d, ablation distal; ABL_p, ablation proximal; ABL uni, ablation unipolar; CS 9–10 to CS 1–2, coronary sinus proximal to distal; His_p and His_d, His bundle proximal and distal; STIM, stimulation

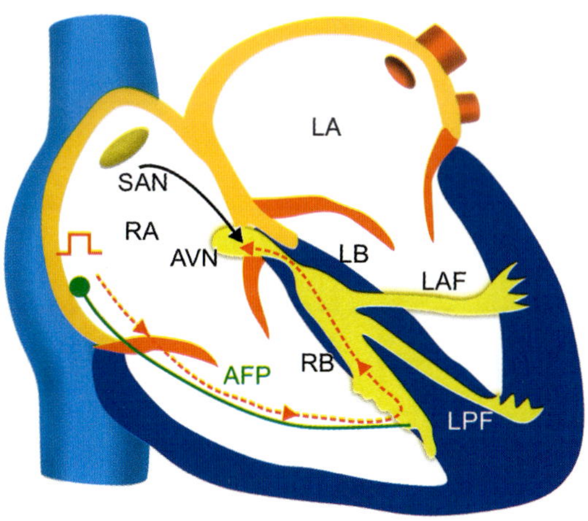

Figure 19.7C: Schematic diagram showing preexcitation on atrial pacing. Preferential conduction to the ventricle occurs via the atriofascicular tract, which causes right bundle activation earlier/at same time as the His activation during maximal preexcitation. (Red interrupted line showing the activation path from the atriofascicular pathway, while the black arrow shows normal antegrade atrial and AV nodal activation)

Abbreviations: AFP, atriofascicular pathway; AVN, atrioventricular node; LA, left atrium; LAF, left anterior fascicle; LB, left bundle branch; LPF, left posterior fascicle; RA, right atrium; RB, right bundle branch; SAN, sinoatrial node

Recognition of this pattern of activation sequence which mimics an atrial paced maximally preexcited rhythm does not however, confirm active participation of the atriofascicular bypass tract and needs to be differentiated from an innocent bystander activation of the atriofascicular pathway during another SVT like an AVNRT. That this is a true antidromic AVRT can be confirmed by delivering a late atrial extrastimulus, when the His bundle is refractory, and demonstrating advancement of the next V as well as the following A (resetting). Advancement of only the V with a late atrial extrastimulus without an advancement in timing of the next A can occur during bystander activation **(Figures 19.10A and B)**.

Increase in VA and VH intervals and slowing of the tachycardia with mechanical retrograde RBBB without change in QRS morphology; VH in SVT< VH with RV pacing

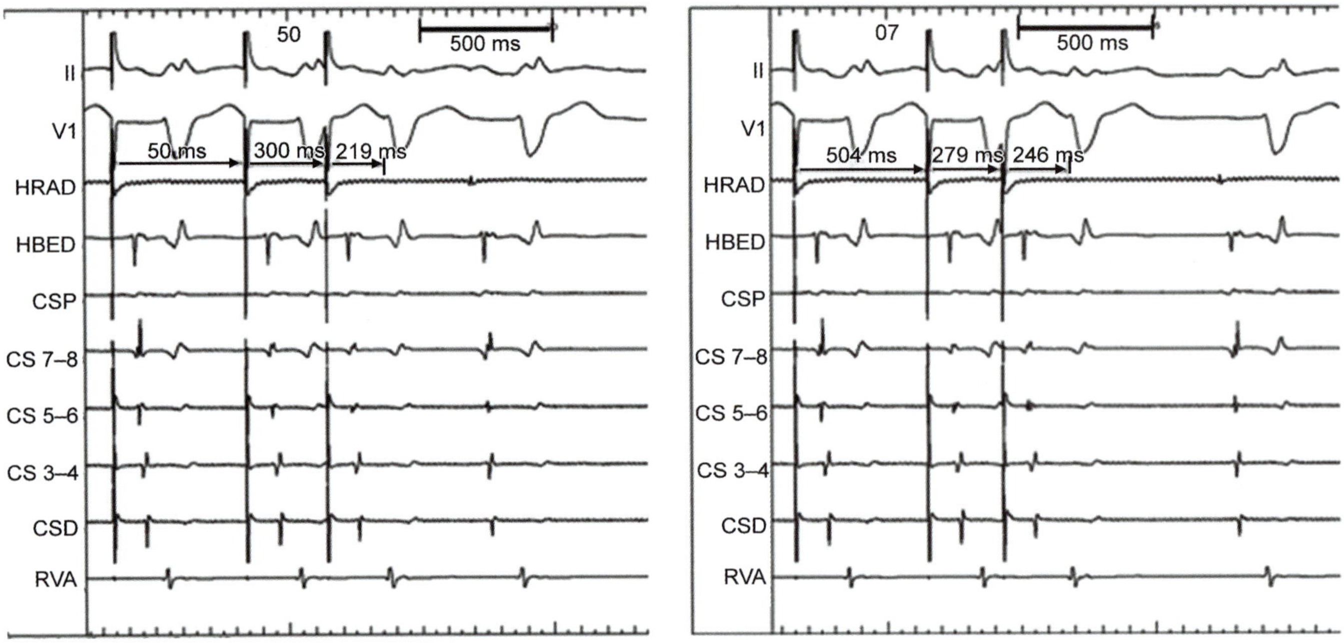

Figure 19.8A: Decremental conduction characteristics on atrial extrastimuli. An atrial extra at a shorter coupling interval leads to increase in the AV interval with maximal preexcitation evident

Abbreviations: CSD, coronary sinus distal; CSP, coronary sinus proximal; CS 3–4 to CS 7–8, coronary sinus mid; HBED, His bundle electrogram distal; HRAD, high right atrium distal; RVA, right ventricular apex

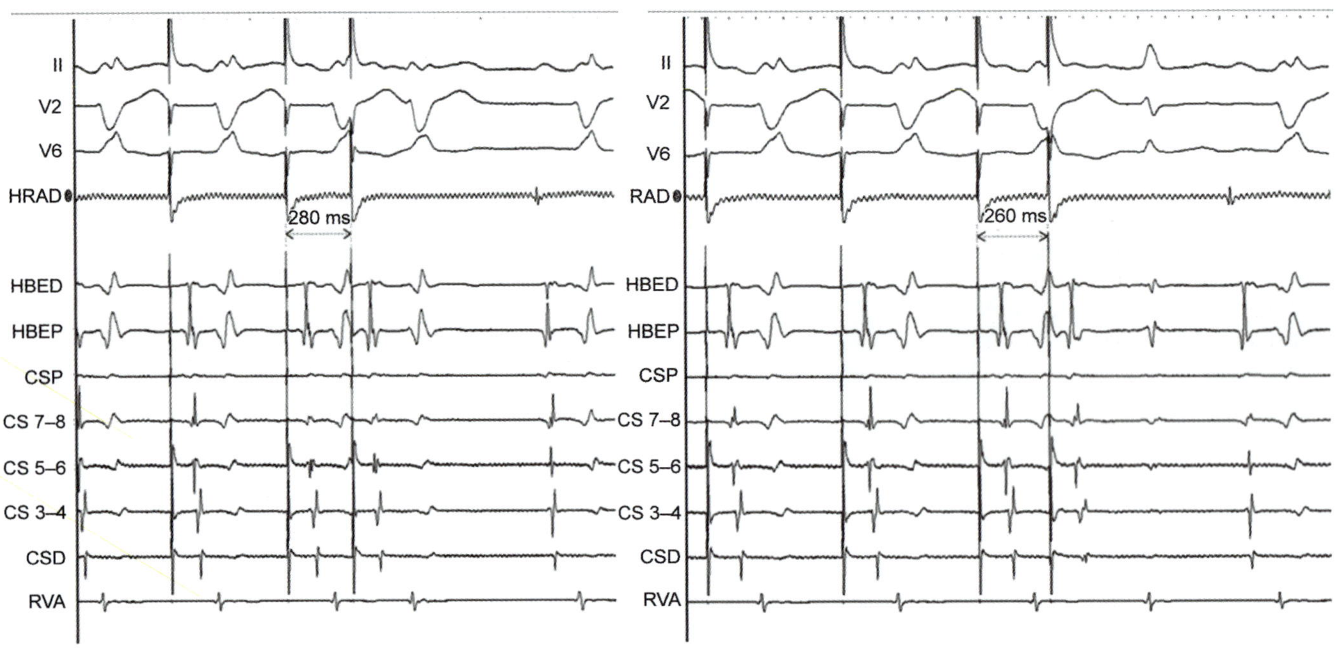

Figure 19.8B: Refractory period of atriofascicular bypass tract is long and generally competes with the AV nodal refractory period. An atrial extrastimulus at a shorter coupling interval causes conduction via the AV node as shown by a narrow QRS as the refractory period of the atriofascicular tract is reached

Abbreviations: CSD, coronary sinus distal; CSP, coronary sinus proximal; CS 3-4 to CS 7-8, coronary sinus mid; HBED, His bundle electrogram distal; HBEP, His bundle electrogram proximal; HRAD, high right atrium distal; RVA, right ventricular apex

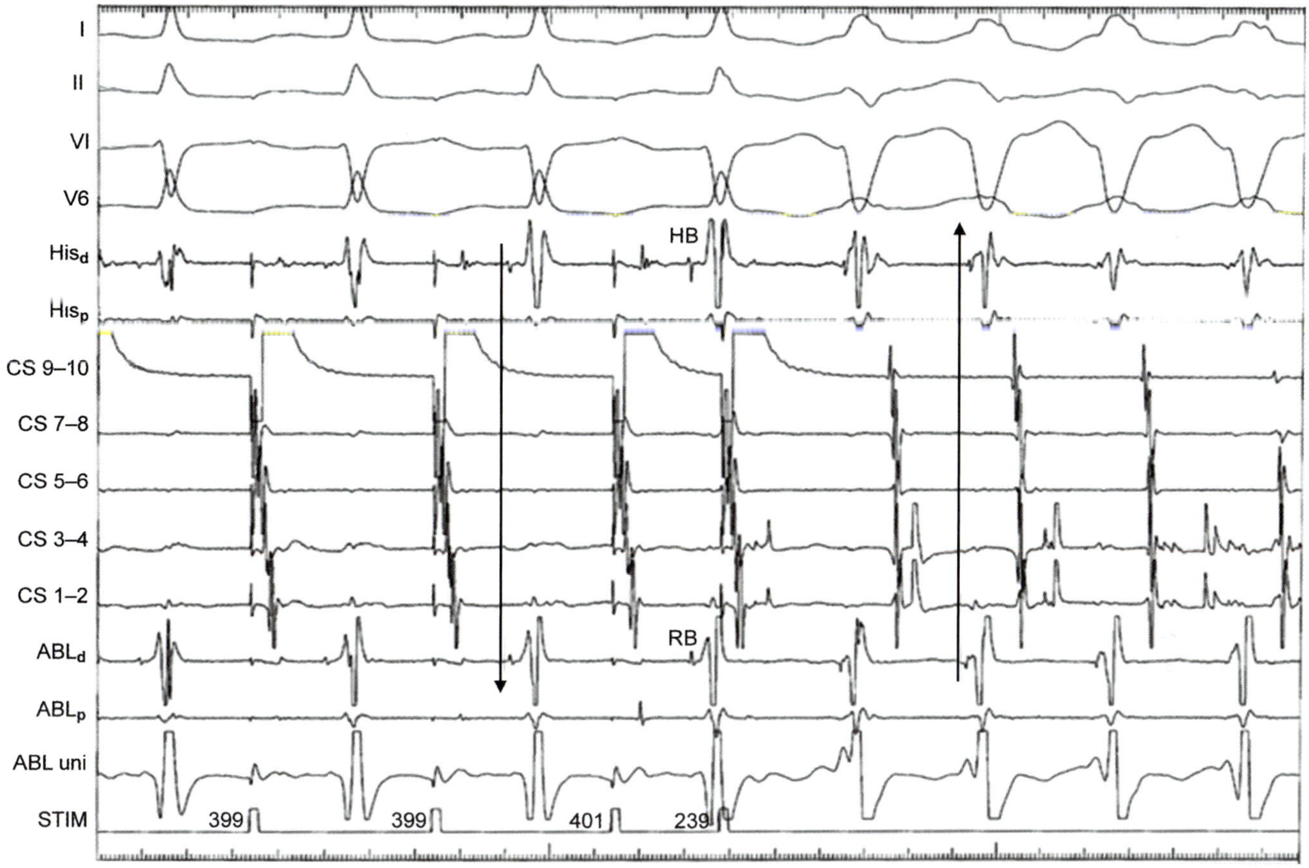

Figure 19.9A: Induction of tachycardia during atrial extrastimulus. The HB->RB activation sequence gets reversed with the onset of tachycardia. This suggests an antidromic atriofascicular bypass tract tachycardia supported also by a negative HV interval during the tachycardia

Abbreviations: ABL uni, ablation unipolar; ABLp, ablation proximal; ABL$_d$, ablation distal; CS 9–10 to CS 1–2, coronary sinus proximal to distal; HB, His bundle; His$_p$ and His$_d$, His bundle proximal and distal; STIM, stimulation; RB, right bundle branch

at same cycle length and HA in SVT = HA during RV pacing also help to recognize an antidromic atriofascicular bypass tract tachycardia. The electrophysiological properties are well elucidated by many previous studies.[4,5,7,8]

Innocent Bystander Activation of the Atriofascicular Bypass Tract

Bystander activation of atriofascicular bypass tract during other SVTs like AVNRT, orthodromic AVRT mediated by another accessory pathway or atrial tachycardia can occur creating confusion in the diagnosis. Continuation of broad complex tachycardia with conduction over the bypass tract at the same cycle length (CL) as the narrow complex tachycardia **(Figure 19.11A)**, varying fusion of QRS complex with varying HV (VH) interval **(Figures 19.11A and B)**, HA during tachycardia < HA during RV pacing, His activation before or on time with RBB in absence of RBBB, VH during tachycardia equal to VH during RV pacing and late atrial extra when septal A refractory advances V and but not the next A, help to differentiate the same.

Other rarely seen features of atriofascicular bypass tract as seen by the author are:

- Incessant tachycardia.
- Tachycardia being induced by spontaneous automatic beats arising from the atriofascicular bypass tract.
- A change in the cycle length during tachycardia with a constant VA interval can be due to changing AV interval due to change in the antegrade conduction characteristics.
- A change in the QRS width and QRS complex morphology in an ongoing antidromic tachycardia, due to change in the exit site, due possibly to a broad-based insertion of the AP in the ventricular myocardium.
- Accelerated automatic rhythm from the atriofascicular bypass tract on isoprenaline.

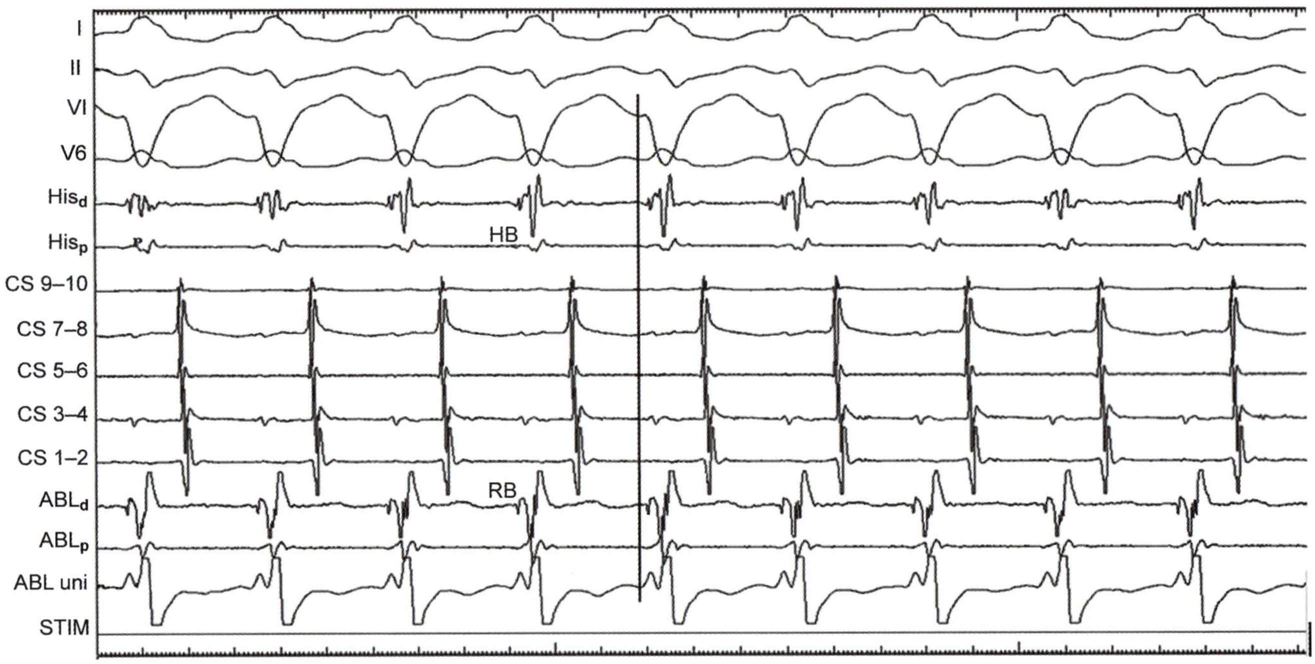

Figure 19.9B: During tachycardia, RB activation is seen earlier than the His activation with a negative HV interval
Abbreviations: ABL uni, ablation unipolar; ABL$_p$, ablation proximal; ABL$_d$, ablation distal; CS 9–10 to CS 1–2, coronary sinus proximal to distal; HB, His bundle; His$_p$ and His$_d$, His bundle proximal and distal; STIM, stimulation; RB, right bundle branch

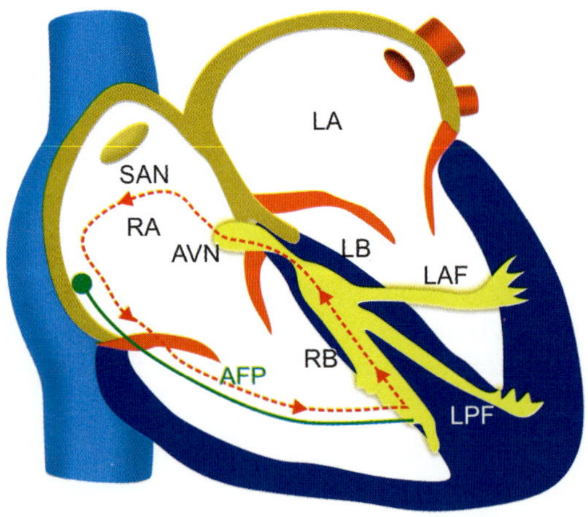

Figure 19.9C: Schematic diagram of an antidromic atriofascicular bypass tachycardia
Abbreviations: AFP, atriofascicular pathway; AVN, atrioventricular node; LA, left atrium; LAF, left anterior fascicle; LB, left bundle branch; LPF, left posterior fascicle; RA, right atrium; RB, right bundle branch; SAN, sinoatrial node

Differential Diagnosis of Antidromic AVRT due to Atriofascicular AP

- *SVT with aberrancy:* HV interval is normal or mildly prolonged with activation of the His antegradely further to the RB. Presence of narrow complex tachycardia of the same cycle length reinforces the diagnosis.
- *Bundle branch reentrant tachycardia:* HV interval at baseline is generally prolonged and further increases during the tachycardia. The activation sequence in the more common LBBB type of bundle branch reentry shows His activation is before RB activation. VA 1:1 relationship is not necessary and hence when absent is easy to recognize.
- *Ventricular tachycardia:* The QRS morphology does not resemble the typical LBBB morphology. VA association is not necessary. Absence of preexcitation on atrial pacing or ability of tachycardia to reset during atrial pacing when His bundle is refractory, or with a random atrial extrastimulus usually makes the diagnosis apparent.

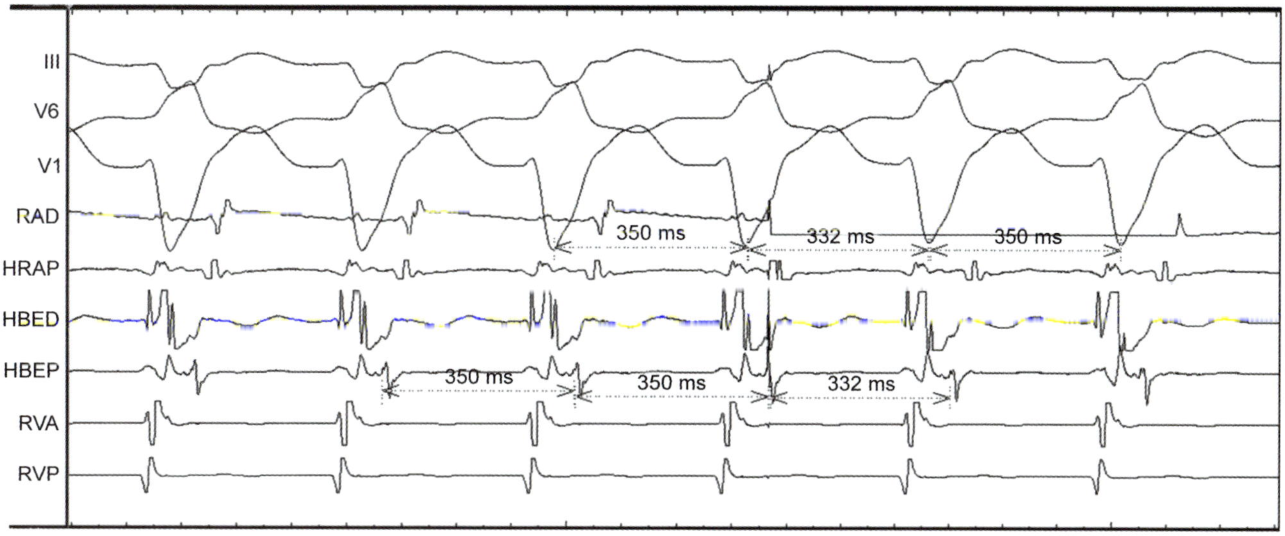

Figure 19.10A: Right atrial free wall late extrastimulus advanced V and the next A at the septum which confirms the ongoing tachycardia to be an antidromic atriofascicular bypass tract tachycardia

Abbreviations: HBED, His bundle electrogram distal; HBEP, His bundle electrogram proximal; HRAP, high right atrium proximal; RAD, right atrium distal; RVA, right ventricular apex distal; RVP, right ventricle proximal

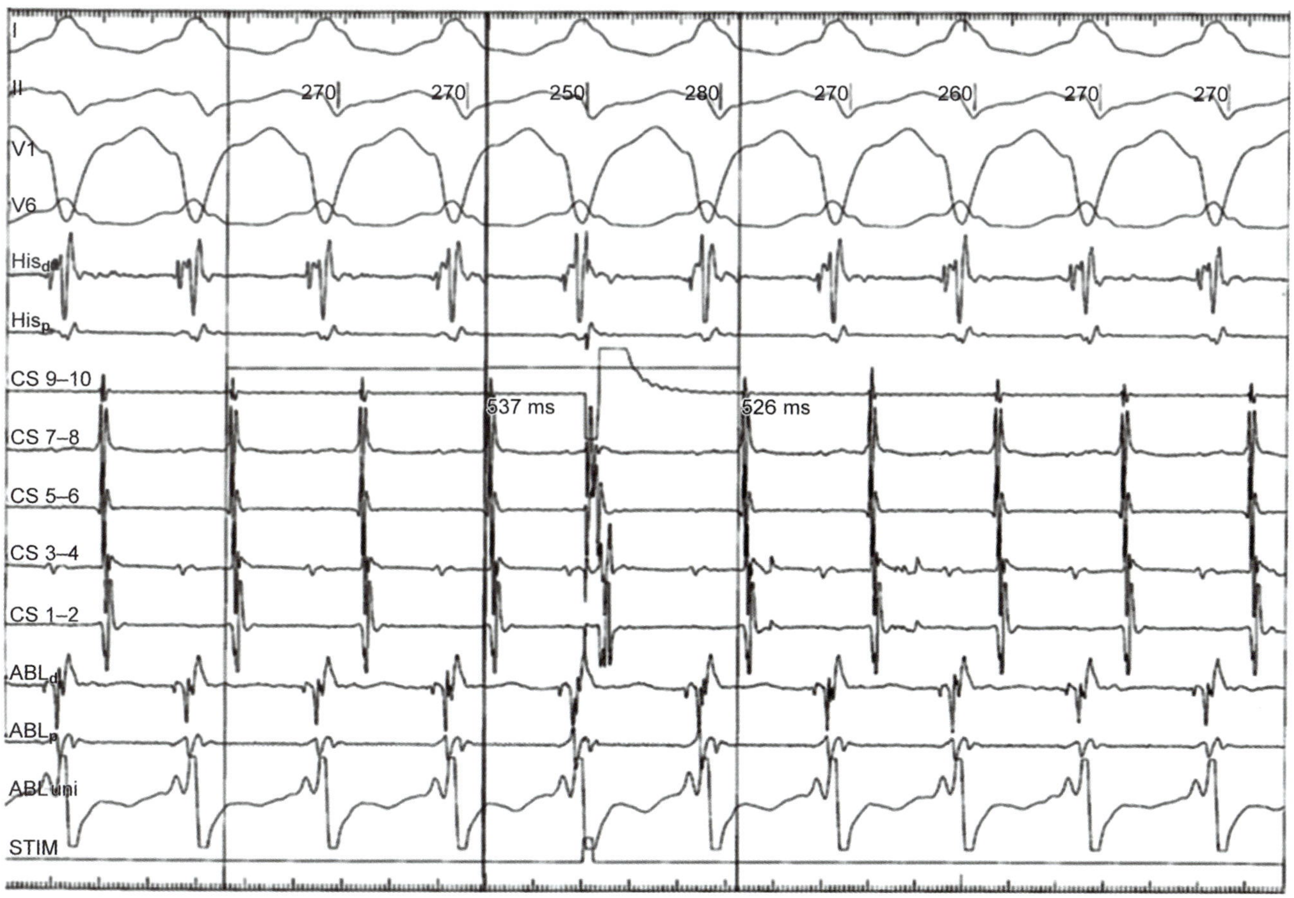

Figure 19.10B: Advancement and resetting of atrial activation by a right atrial free wall late extrastimulus is demonstrated by measuring twice the cycle length, which sometimes is easier and faster

Abbreviations: ABL uni, ablation unipolar; ABL_p, ablation proximal; ABL_d, ablation distal; CS 9–10 to CS 1–2, coronary sinus proximal to distal; His_p and His_d, His bundle proximal and distal; STIM, stimulation

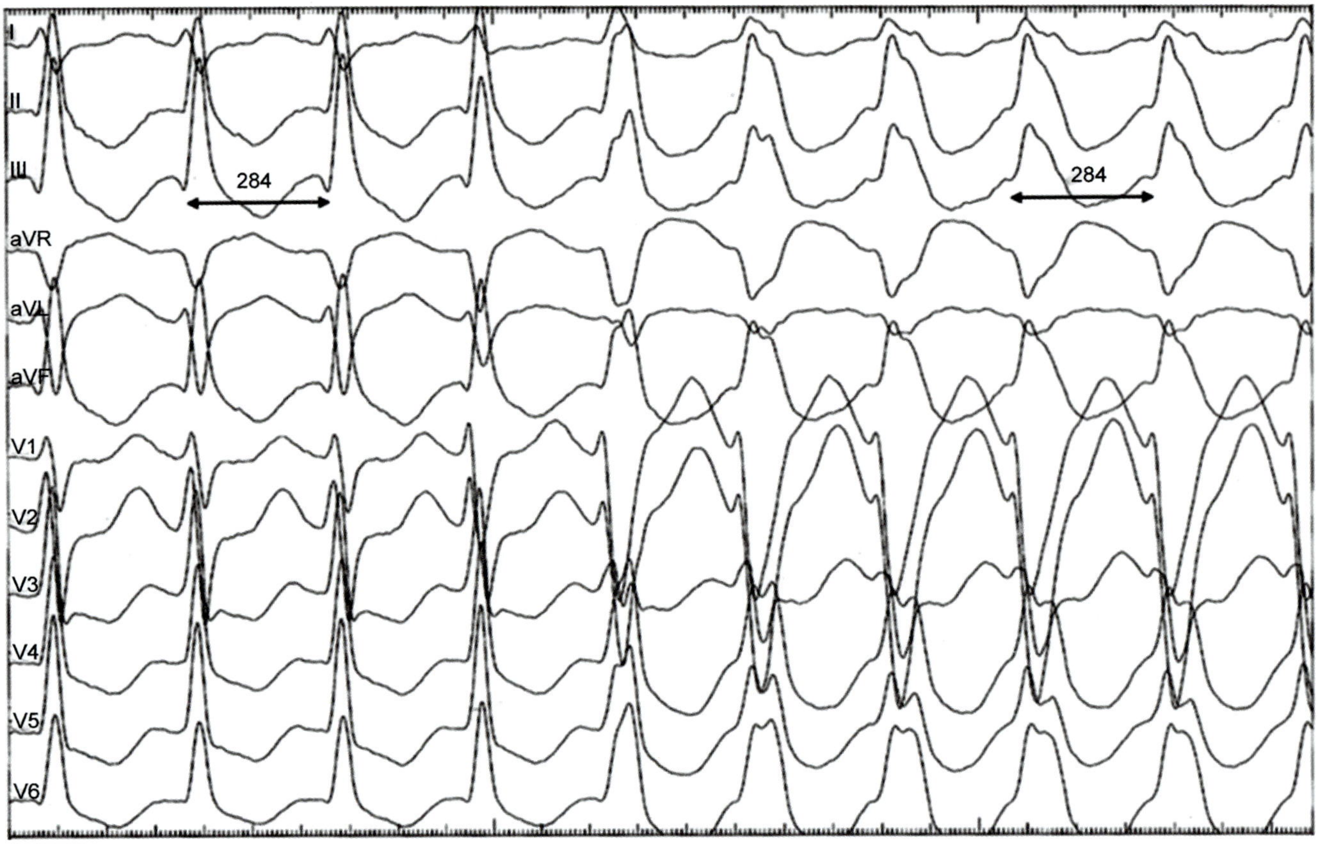

Figure 19.11A: Twelve-lead ECG shows a narrow complex tachycardia transiting into a broad complex tachycardia with the same CL. There is gradually increasing fusion in the mid part with maximal preexcitation in the later part. Here an atriofascicular bypass tract was an innocent bystander during an orthodromic AVRT using another AP

A capture beat of different QRS morphology may be seen. VH interval is generally prolonged and is generally associated with structural heart disease. Arrhythmogenic right ventricular cardiomyopathy (ARVC), cardiac sarcoidosis and idiopathic ventricular tachycardia arising from the RV are common differentials of myocardial VT of LBBB morphology.

- *Antidromic AVRT using a right sided Kent (typical atrioventricular) bypass tract:* Not uncommon in patients with Ebsteins anomaly, this can be demonstrated by absence of decremental conduction characteristics and commonly present retrograde conduction through the bypass tract. The QRS is wider during preexcitation and VH interval during the tachycardia is longer than 20 ms. The QRS morphology during maximal preexcitation and antidromic AVRT usually does not resemble typical LBBB morphology.

Mapping and Radiofrequency Ablation

Unlike routine bypass tracts, a 12-lead ECG is not of great importance in predicting the site of ablation at the annulus as the site of distal insertion determines the QRS morphology. Because of their conduction properties and anatomic location, it is difficult to map both the proximal (atrial) and distal (ventricular) insertion of atriofascicular bypass tract. Atriofascicular bypass tract do not conduct retrogradely, so the proximal insertion cannot be identified by ventricular pacing. There are several reports on ablation of atriofascicular bypass tract with a very high success rate.[7,10,11,13,16-22] Different strategies can be adapted for successful localization of the pathway for ablation[23] and include:

- Atriofascicular bypass tract potential ("M" potential) based mapping and ablation.
- Activation mapping of earliest ventricular activation and ablation in the ventricle.
- Shortest interval from atrial stimulus to ventricular activation technique.
- Atrial extrastimulus mapping during antidromic tachycardia.
- Mechanical trauma mapping.
- Electroanatomic mapping.

The most common and successful strategy is atriofascicular bypass tract potential ("M potential") based mapping

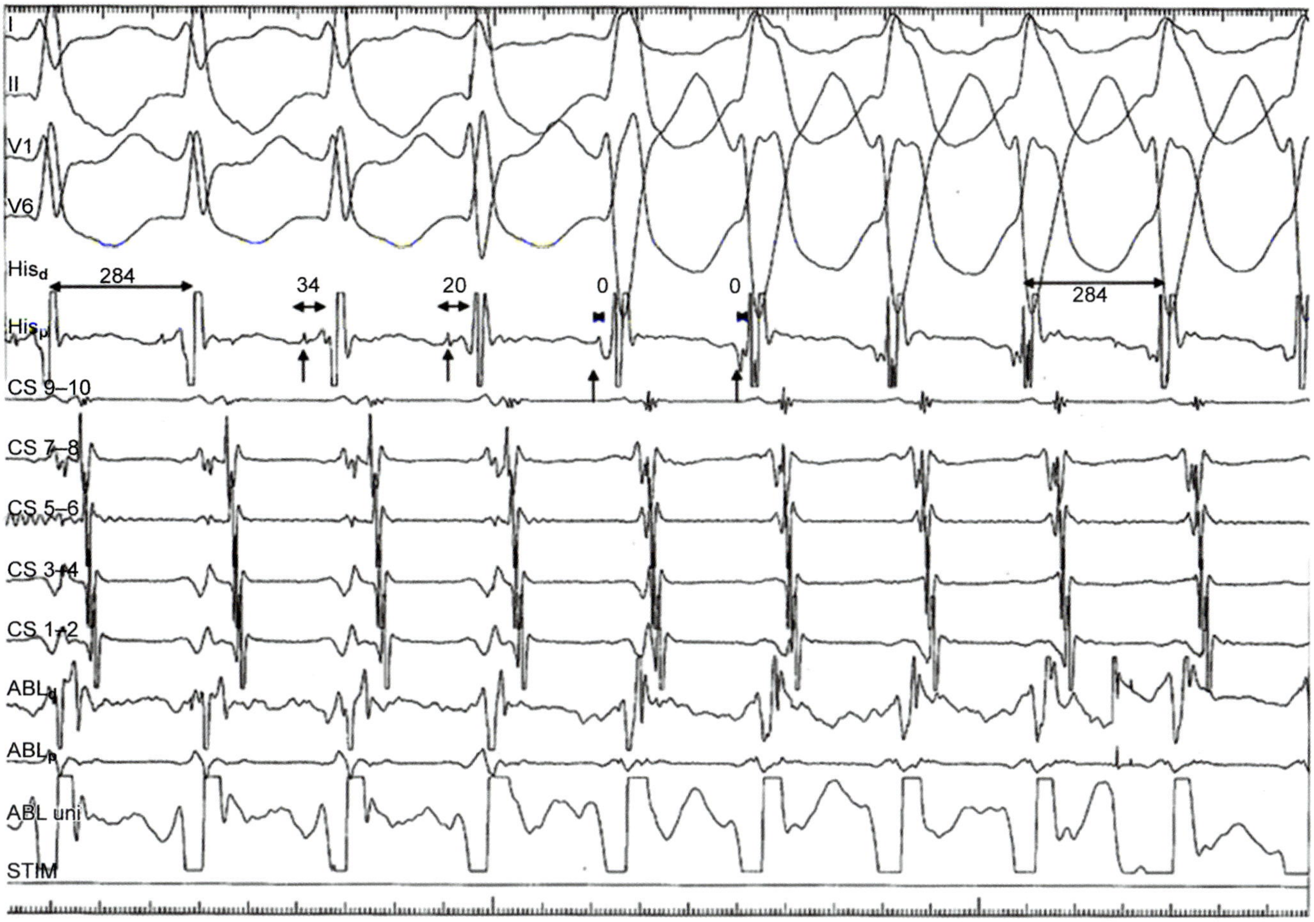

Figure 19.11B: Intracardiac recordings of the tracing of Figure 19.11A shows that, with an increasing QRS width, a decrease in the HV interval is seen progressively suggesting increasing preexcitation, with no change in CL of the tachycardia. H is marked with arrows and HV intervals are mentioned in ms. Differentiation from SVT with aberrancy is evident, where HV interval will be normal

Abbreviations: ABL uni, ablation unipolar; ABL_p, ablation proximal; ABL_d, ablation distal; CS 9–10 to CS 1–2, coronary sinus proximal to distal; His_p and His_d, His bundle proximal and distal; STIM, stimulation

and ablation at the tricuspid annulus. However, other strategies may sometimes be useful for ablation in cases where "M" potential is not obtained, which are described further. Target temperature during radiofrequency (RF) energy delivery should be 60 to 70°C. The energy delivery should be stopped if 10 to 12 seconds of application does not abolish the accessory pathway conduction, and further mapping to look for alternative ablation sites should be performed.

Atriofascicular Bypass Tract Potential ("M" Potential)-based Mapping and Ablation

"M" potentials commonly appear as a discrete sharp potential lying between the atrial and ventricular electrogram recorded at the tricuspid annulus **(Figure 19.12A)**. The interval between the M potential and V remains constant during atrial pacing at different cycle lengths. The potential may be as large as the His bundle potential **(Figure 19.12B)** or small and sharp **(Figure 19.12C)** or small and wide **(Figure 19.12D)**. M potential will be recorded only in very close proximity to the atrial insertion of the accessory pathway and, therefore, is likely to be a good predictor of a successful ablation site as described by various studies.[7,11,13,17-20] Mapping is done using the ablation catheter starting commonly from the 10 o'clock position on the tricuspid annulus and down. Catheter movement should be gentle to avoid mechanical trauma. A long sheath may provide stability during mapping. Most commonly, the M potential is located between tricuspid annular 6 o'clock to 10 o'clock region,[7,11,13,16-19] and hence this region should be thoroughly mapped during sinus rhythm. Once an M potential is obtained, RF energy is delivered during sinus rhythm, during which Mahaim automatic rhythm is seen in

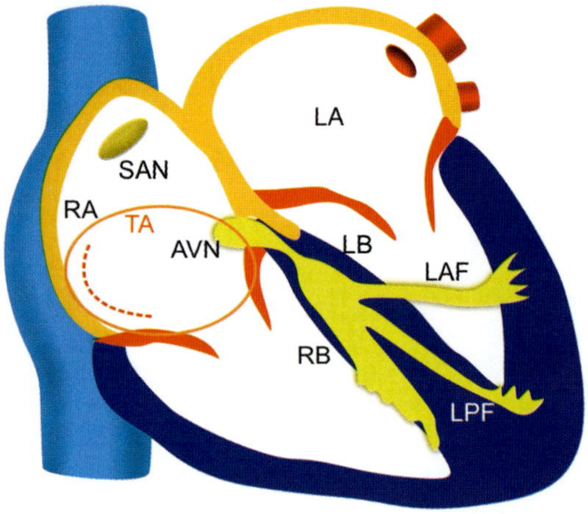

Figure 19.12A: Schematic diagram showing common site of M potential at the annulus. Red interrupted line from tricuspid annulus (TA) 6 o'clock to 10 o'clock position shows the most common sites of presence of M potential

Abbreviations: AVN, atrioventricular node; LA, left atrium; LAF, left anterior fascicle; LB, left bundle branch; LPF, left posterior fascicle; RA, right atrium; RB, right bundle branch; SAN, sinoatrial node; TA, tricuspid annulus

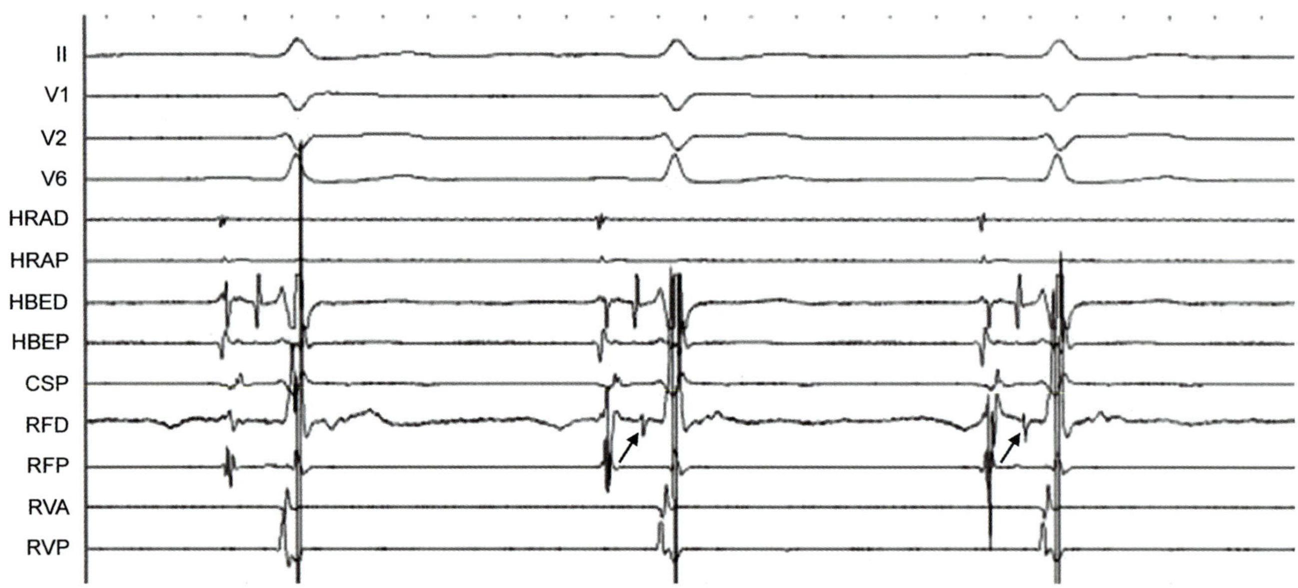

Figure 19.12B: Atriofascicular bypass tract potential as marked with arrow in the RF distal (RFD) channel shows a sharp and large potential similar to a His bundle recording

Abbreviations: CSP, coronary sinus proximal; HBED and HBEP, His bundle electrogram distal and proximal; HRAD and HRAP, high right atrium distal and proximal; RFD and RFP, radiofrequency (ablation) distal and proximal; RVA and RVP, right ventricular apex distal and proximal

most instances. This is similar and analogous to the junctional accelerated rhythm seen during slow pathway ablation in patients with AVNRT. To improve catheter stability, ablation is preferably done during continuous atrial pacing that also enables easy recognition of loss of preexcitation. Successful ablation site generally has an equal A-V ratio. Occasionally, a site that is more ventricular results in successful ablation. Recurrence has rarely been reported once successful ablation has been done by this method.[19,21]

Activation Mapping of Earliest Ventricular Activation and Ablation in the Ventricle

This is the only technique where ablation of atriofascicular AP is targeted at the ventricular insertion site **(Figure 19.13A)**. Activation mapping is done either during tachycardia or during atrial pacing with maximum preexcitation. Most commonly the insertion site is at the distal aspect of the RBB, though there may be a lot of variations.[13] The right

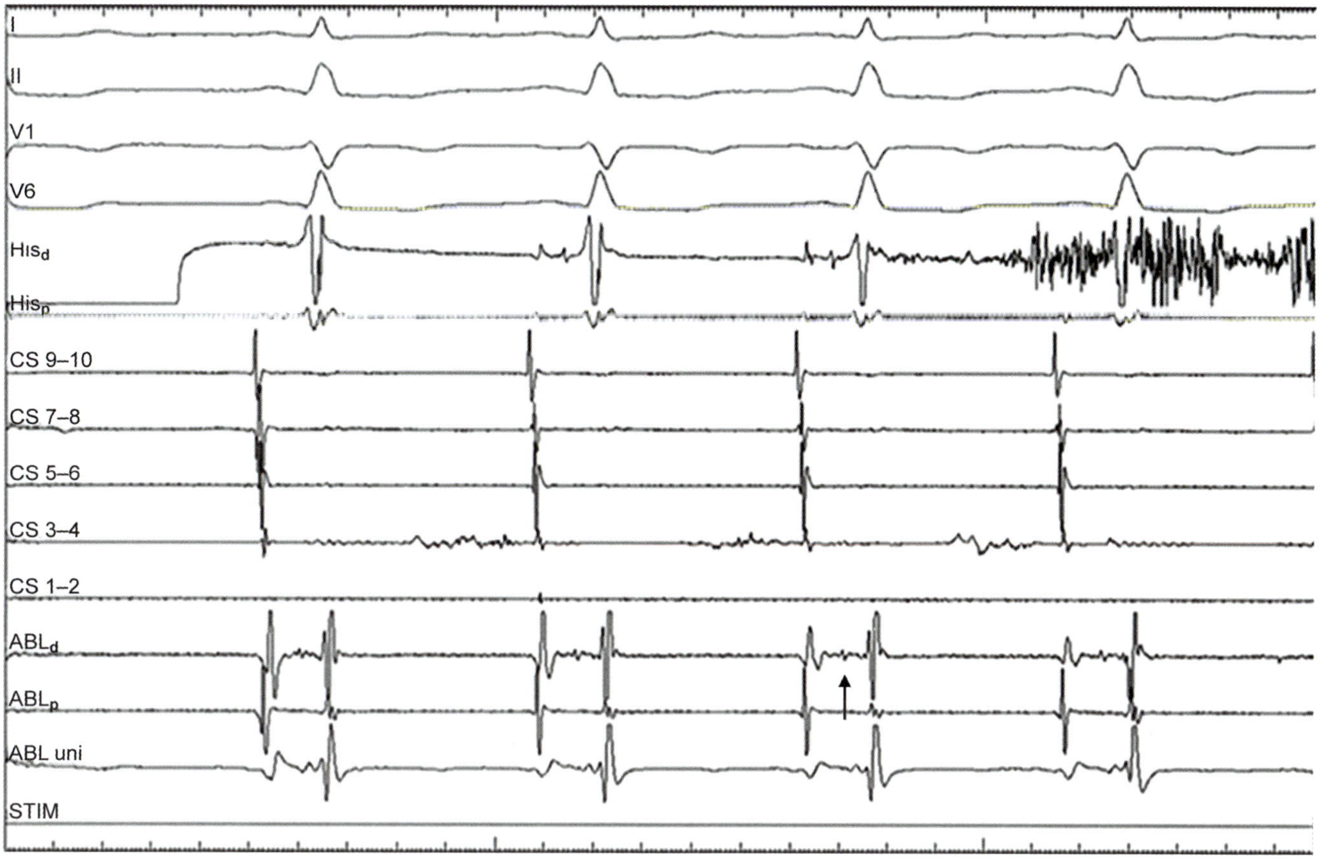

Figure 19.12C: Atriofascicular bypass tract potential as marked with arrow in the RF distal (ABL_d) channel shows a sharp but small potential
Abbreviations: ABL_d, ABL_p and ABL uni, ablation distal, proximal and unipolar; CS 9–10 to CS 1–2, coronary sinus proximal to distal; His_d and His_p, His bundle electrogram distal and proximal; STIM, stimulation

bundle branch is identified till its distal aspect by the presence of a right bundle potential. Thereafter with a slight counterclockwise torque the site with the earliest ventricular activation is mapped **(Figure 19.13B)**. There is occasionally a distinct sharp potential preceding the earliest ventricular electrogram with a small intervening isoelectric baseline, which possibly signifies the insertion site of the atriofascicular bypass tract and which is a good site for ablation. Activation mapping of the earliest local ventricular potential targeting distal branches is sometimes a time consuming task. Atriofascicular or atrioventricular pathways tend to have generally a long course and often show extensive arborization over a wide area of ventricular muscle making ablation at the ventricular insertion site difficult.[13] Though, it is possible to ablate using this technique but a complete elimination is very unlikely. Some patients with atriofascicular bypass tract who undergo ablation at the distal insertion can develop a pro-arrhythmic response with facilitation of antidromic tachycardia occurrence due to slow conduction induced by radiofrequency ablation.[7,10] Also, ablation of the right bundle branch within the ventricle can result in lengthening of the tachycardia circuit and possibly a more incessant tachycardia. Because of these problems, ablation is usually aimed at the proximal (atrial) insertion of the pathway. In some cases, however, mapping and subsequent ablation of the ventricular insertion has been achieved leading to successful clinical outcome.[24]

Shortest Interval from Atrial Stimulus to Ventricular Activation Technique

Shortest interval from stimulus to ventricular activation is a method to identify a right atrial site on the tricuspid annulus, pacing from where has the shortest interval from the stimulus to the earliest preexcited QRS. Right atrium is paced at the tricuspid annulus at a constant rate at which maximum preexcitation is noted, during which the interval from the stimulus/local activation at atrium to the ventricular activation is measured. Thereafter, the catheter is moved along the annulus and similar intervals noted at other pacing sites. Stimulation sites remote from the atrial insertion of the accessory pathway result in long stimulus-QRS interval due

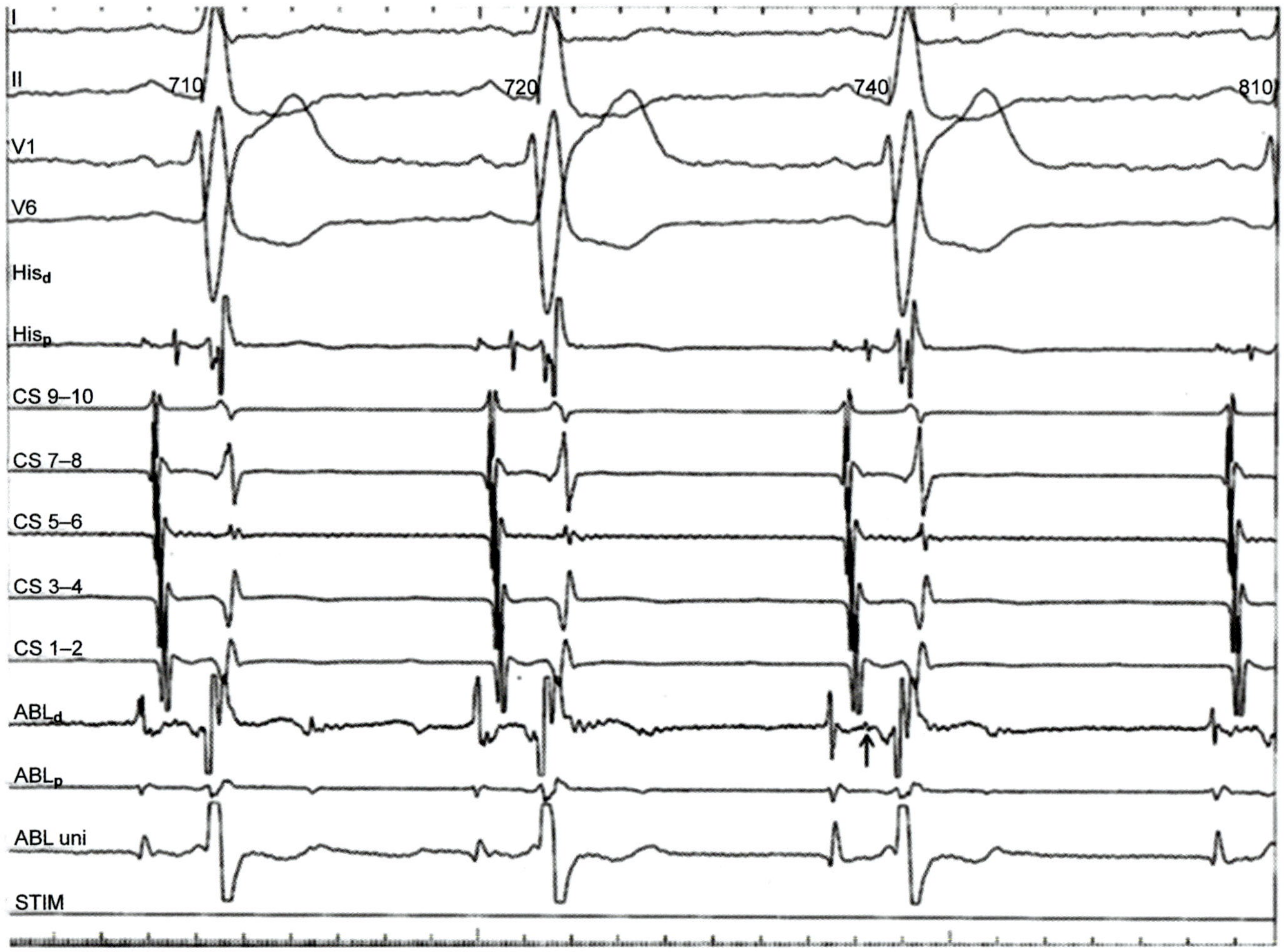

Figure 19.12D: Atriofascicular bypass tract potential as marked with arrow in the RF distal (ABL$_d$) channel shows a small and wider potential
Abbreviations: ABL$_d$, ABL$_p$ and ABL uni, ablation distal, proximal and unipolar; CS 9-10 to CS 1-2, coronary sinus proximal to distal; His$_d$ and His$_p$, His bundle electrogram distal and proximal; STIM, stimulation

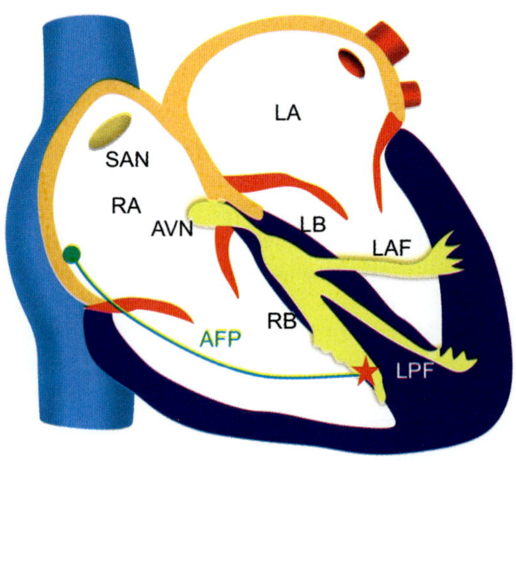

Figure 19.13A: Schematic diagram showing target site (red star) of ablation by earliest ventricular activation method
Abbreviations: AFP, atriofascicular pathway; AVN, atrioventricular node; LA, left atrium; LAF, left anterior fascicle; LB, left bundle branch; LPF, left posterior fascicle; RA, right atrium; RB, right bundle branch; SAN, sinoatrial node

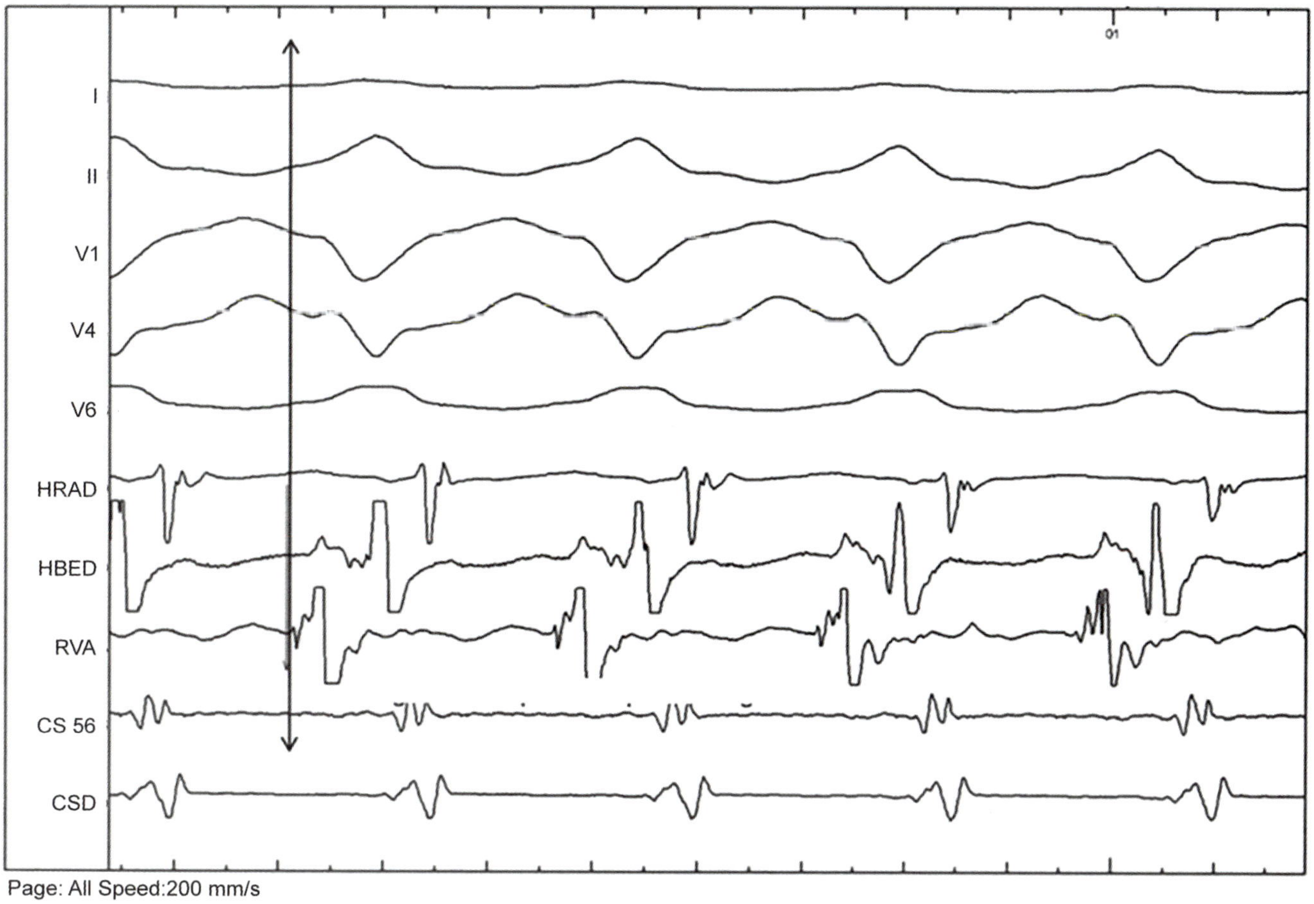

Figure 19.13B: Activation mapping during tachycardia shows earliest ventricular activation signals in the RVA channel which may be an appropriate site for ablation

Abbreviations: HBED, His bundle electrogram distal; HRAD, high right atrium distal; CSD, coronary sinus distal; CS 56, coronary sinus mid; RVA, right ventricle apex distal

to the amount of interposed atrial tissue. Ablation is done at the site of shortest atrial stimulus to ventricular activation as it represents the atrial insertion site of the atriofascicular bypass tract **(Figure 19.14)**. The result of RF ablation at the site of the shortest interval has remained inconsistent as seen in various studies and varies from 0 to 100%.[10,18-21] This method is time and labor intensive and very inaccurate because it is difficult to stimulate from many sites at the same distance from the annulus. However, in the absence of a proper M potential, this method is helpful in localization of the atriofascicular bypass tract.

Atrial Extrastimulus Mapping during Antidromic Tachycardia

Atrial extrastimulus mapping during antidromic tachycardia is a method for finding the atrial insertion site for ablation. During tachycardia a late atrial extrastimulus is delivered at sites along the tricuspid annulus. Advancement of the following ventricular beat is noted. The site in the tricuspid annulus where the longest coupled atrial stimulus causes resetting with the least interposing tissue separating it from the accessory pathway proximal insertion is obtained, which is a suitable site for attempting ablation **(Figure 19.15)**. However, it is an inaccurate and tedious method.

Mechanical Trauma Mapping

Atriofascicular bypass tract is located very close to the endocardium and thus catheter movement-related mechanical trauma may result in transient loss of conduction. Unintentional mechanical trauma during catheter positioning sometimes results in transient abolition of conduction through the pathway for minutes to hours,[10,18] which may hamper successful localization and ablation thereafter and may be responsible for unsuccessful procedure outcome.

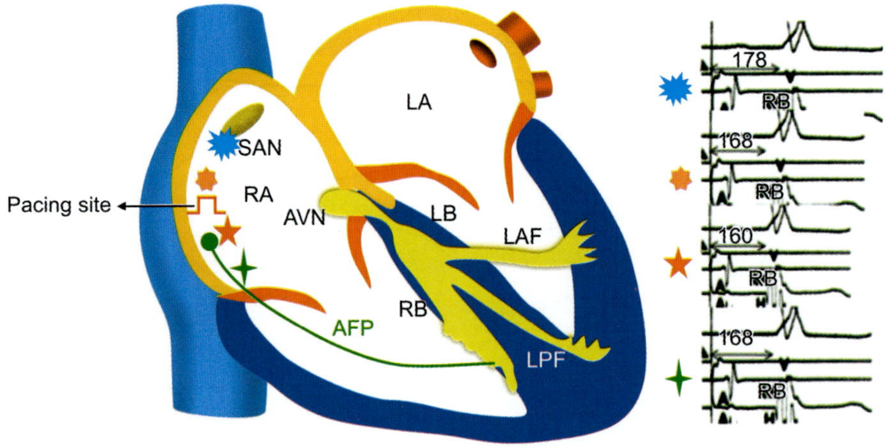

Figure 19.14: Schematic diagram showing as to how the target site is determined. The shortest stimulus to V interval represents the least amount of interposed atrial tissue and possibly the atrial insertion site as represented by site marked by red star in the diagram. Ablation at the site should be successful

Abbreviations: AFP, atriofascicular pathway; AVN, atrioventricular node; LA, left atrium; LAF, left anterior fascicle; LB, left bundle branch; LPF, left posterior fascicle; RA, right atrium; RB, right bundle branch; SAN, sinoatrial node

Judicious use of mechanical trauma in a controlled way during antidromic tachycardia or atrial pacing and causing transient AP conduction block locates the AP insertion at the atrial insertion site and then ablation is done at the site where conduction block occurred. However, when conduction block occurs, the catheter may move away from the target site and relocate leading to false sense of successful ablation. Mapping and RF ablation guided by this method has been useful to an extent.[21,22] Studies have shown a very high immediate success rate with this method, but predictably there were high recurrences at follow-up.[22]

Electroanatomic Mapping

Electroanatomic mapping[20,25] can be helpful in cases where accessory pathway potential cannot be found and/or there has been a failed attempt with above conventional techniques. The earliest annular or ventricular activation can be known and the sites can be tagged as the probable sites for ablation. This technique allows the operator to reach the tagged sites and further ablations can be attempted in and around the area. It is also useful when mechanical trauma precludes adequate mapping. In case of transient conduction block, the catheter can be manipulated back to the tagged location for ablation. However, success rates have not been encouraging.[20]

Important Practical Points with Regard to Ablation

- Ablation catheter should be moved slowly and carefully along the annulus, avoiding bumps on the tissue so as to avoid mechanical trauma and accidental loss of preexcitation, for which long sheaths can be used for improving stability. The sheath can be positioned high, so that movement of the catheter occurs in a vertical direction by giving a push to the catheter from the sheath.
- Ablation, if possible, should be done during atrial pacing. Stability is improved during atrial pacing as compared with ablation during antidromic tachycardia when catheter is likely to "jump" with tachycardia termination. Mahaim accelerated rhythm that occurs commonly during ablation can also cause catheter displacement and therefore atrial pacing during ablation is beneficial. Also, atrial pacing increases preexcitation and hence make it easier to assess conduction block with ablation.
- Ablation at a site with a larger ventricular signal at the annulus occasionally can lead to success.
- In case of difficulty in finding the appropriate site at the tricuspid annulus, a presumptive ablation carried out in a line from the tricuspid annular 7 o'clock to 9 o'clock region can be helpful in possibly localizing and treating in difficult cases, rather than mapping and treating at the ventricular insertion site. This has helped the author in occasional cases.
- In occasional patients in spite of all attempts to localize the pathway, ablation may not be successful.[20,21] This may be due to presence of accessory pathway at uncommon sites including an epicardial location.
- Coexistence of other tachycardia, especially atrioventricular nodal reentrant tachycardia (association of up to 10–40%) and WPW syndrome due to Kent bundle has been described in literature.[7,16-20] Coexisting atrial flutter

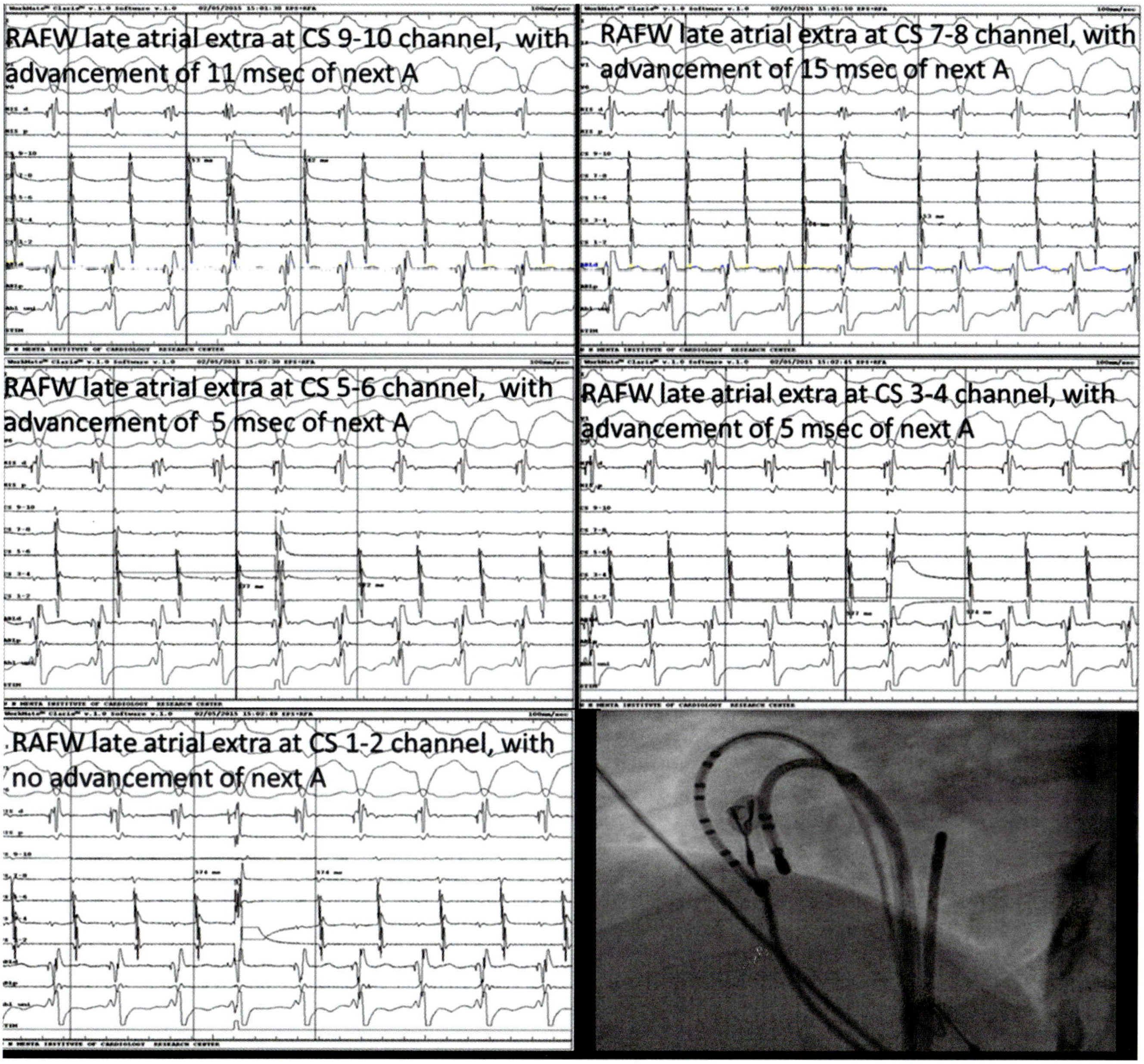

Figure 19.15: Method of atrial extrastimulus. The decapolar catheter when positioned in the right atrial free wall (RAFW) helps in performing the maneuver easily. Stimulus is given at the RAFW during the tachycardia at the same coupled interval from the five paired electrodes. The site which shows the maximum advancement of V and the next A is the site most nearby to the site of atrial insertion of the atriofascicular bypass tract and should be the target site of mapping and ablation. In this figure the maximum advancement is seen best in the CS 7–8 channel and hence mapping should be done nearby the same site

Abbreviations: RAFW, right atrial free wall; CS, coronary sinus has also been described.[21] Therefore after successful ablation, programmed electrical stimulation to exclude the presence of other arrhythmias is a must.

Atriofascicular Bypass Tract (Mahaim) Automatic Tachycardia

Atriofascicular bypass tract automatic rhythm is generally brought about during radiofrequency current delivery **(Figure 19.16A)**, and is probably due to heat-related automaticity of nodal-like tissue (in a similar fashion to junctional rhythm that arises during slow AV nodal pathway ablation). Accelerated automatic beats during RF ablation have been considered as a marker of successful result.[7,16,19-21] The morphology is similar to the preexcited beats/tachycardia **(Figure 19.16B)** and disappears immediately after successful ablation. Occasionally, few automatic beats with LBBB morphology and left axis deviation in the frontal plane occur spontaneously or on isoprenaline, even after successful ablation and possibly is likely due to automaticity arising from lower down along the bypass tract.

OTHER VARIANTS OF PREEXCITATION WITH MAHAIM PHYSIOLOGY

Atrioventricular Bypass Tract

The features of atrioventricular bypass tract with Mahaim physiology are similar to the atriofascicular connection. Differences are few and are as follows:

- The connection occurs from the atrium to the ventricle instead of the fascicle. The AV bypass tracts can be short or long depending on the sites of insertion **(Figure 19.17)**.
- Wider QRS during maximal preexcitation and tachycardia with notching/fragmentation suggesting a slow conduction of the activation wavefront **(Figure 19.18)**.
- A longer VH interval during tachycardia of 50–80 msec **(Figure 19.18)** and VH during tachycardia is generally more than VH during RV apical pacing as it takes a

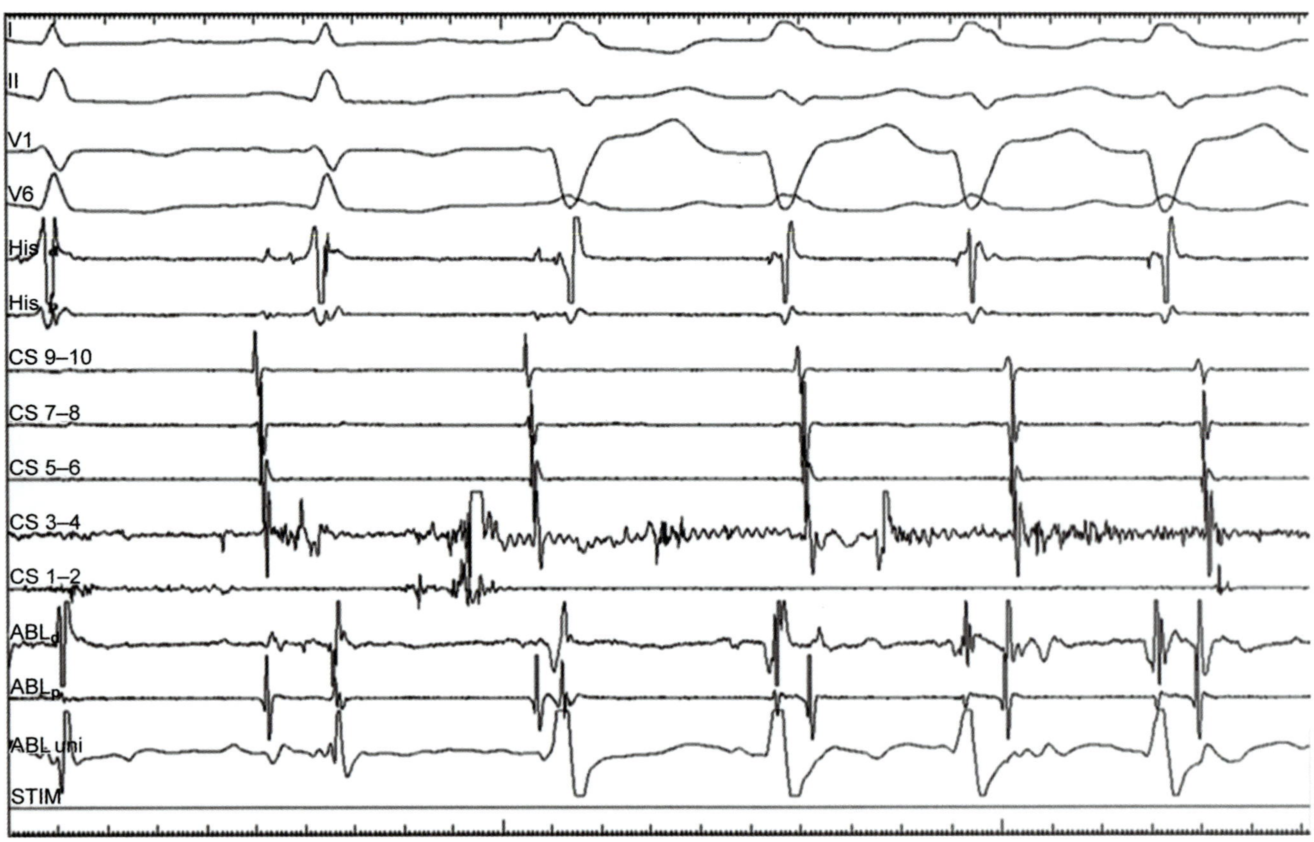

Figure 19.16A: Radiofrequency ablation at the site of M potential (seen in ABL_d channel) causes an immediate atriofascicular bypass tract automatic rhythm

Abbreviations: ABL_d, ABL_p and ABL uni, ablation distal, proximal and unipolar; CS 9–10 to CS 1–2, coronary sinus proximal to distal; His_d and His_p, His bundle electrogram distal and proximal; STIM, stimulation

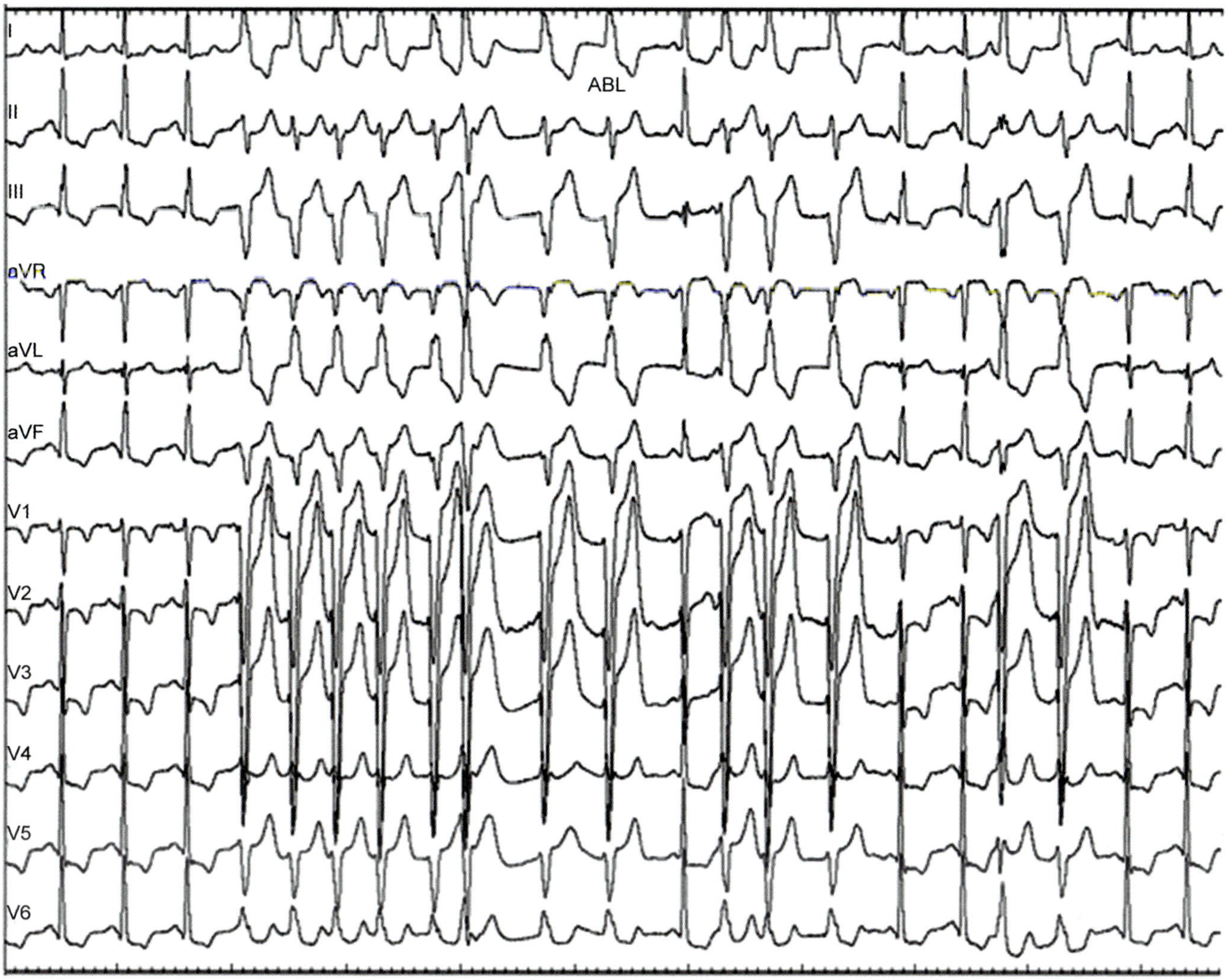

Figure 19.16B: During ablation of the atriofascicular bypass tract, automatic rhythm with QRS morphology similar to preexcited/tachycardia QRS beat occurs and generally disappears once ablation has been successfully done

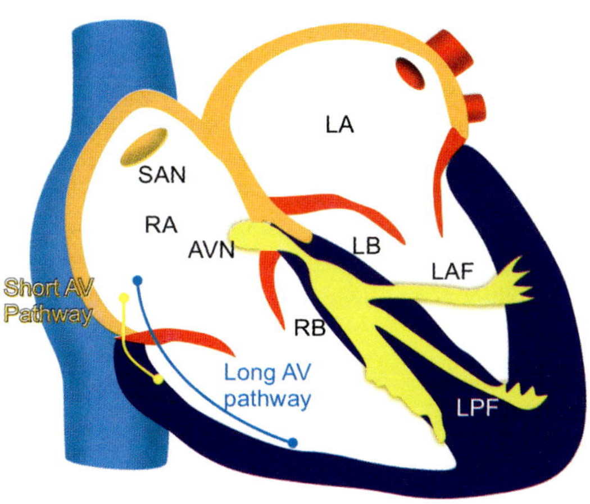

Figure 19.17: Schematic diagram demonstrating long and short atrioventricular bypass tracts. The distal insertion site is the ventricular myocardium and is near the annulus in a short pathway, while in a long atrioventricular bypass tract is away from the annulus at varying distances

Abbreviations: AVN, atrioventricular node; LA, left atrium; LAF, left anterior fascicle; LB, left bundle branch; LPF, left posterior fascicle; RA, right atrium; RB, right bundle branch; SAN, sinoatrial node

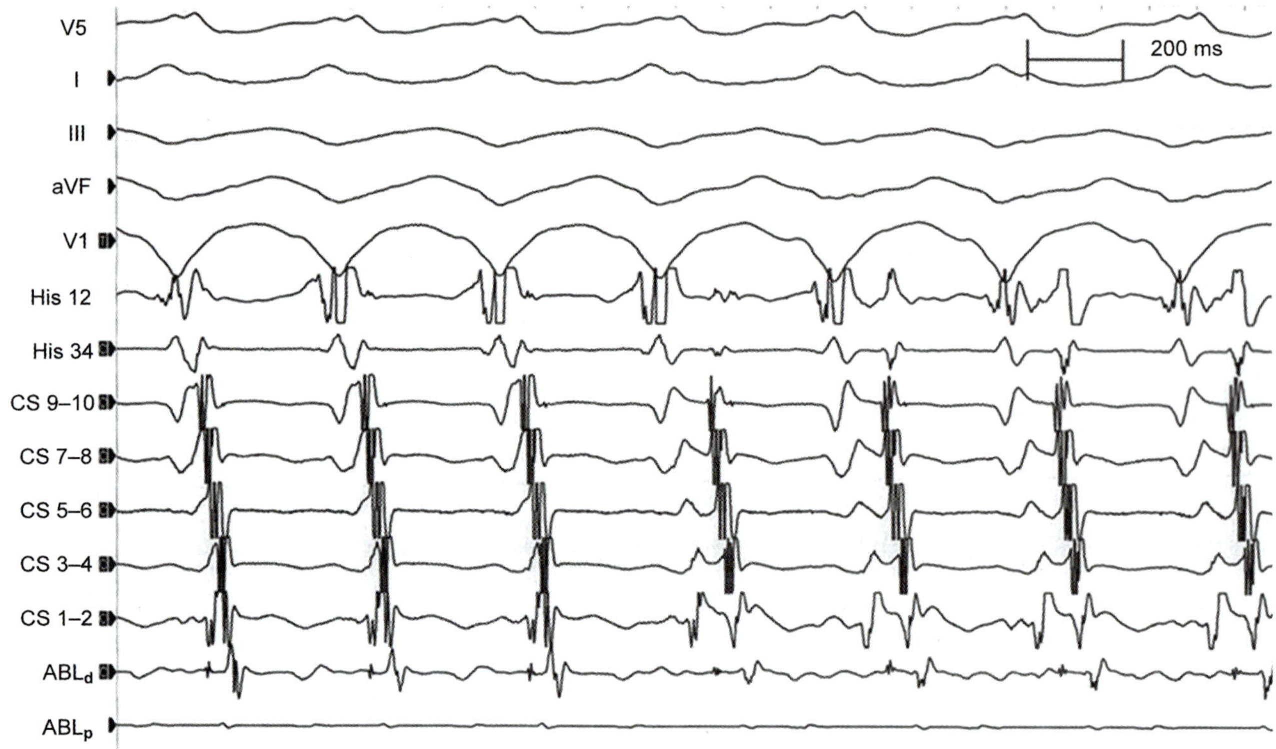

Figure 19.18: Antidromic tachycardia in a patient with atrioventricular bypass tract, showing a wider QRS of 178 ms. The VH interval was 62 ms

Abbreviations: ABL_d and ABL_p, ablation distal and proximal; CS 9–10 to CS 1–2, coronary sinus proximal to distal; His 12 and His 34, His bundle distal and proximal

longer time for the ventricular activation from the base to activate the bundles and reach the His.

- The site of earliest activation is near the tricuspid annulus in a short AV connection, while may be towards the apex in a long AV connection.
- Methods of ablation are similar as the atriofascicular bypass tract.

Nodofascicular/Nodoventricular Bypass Tract

Nodofascicular fibers were the originally described Mahaim fiber connections histologically. As the name suggests in nodofascicular and nodoventricular bypass tracts, the proximal insertion site is at the AV node, while the distal insertion site is at the conduction system (His bundle, Right bundle, or rarely other fascicles) or the septal region of the ventricle respectively **(Figure 19.19)**. These pathways may demonstrate only antegrade conductions as in atriofascicular tracts but rarely may demonstrate only retrograde or bidirectional conduction. The retrogradely conducting pathway can result in an orthodromic AVRT that appears as a narrow QRS tachycardia. These are not described here in this chapter.

In an antegradely conducting pathway, tachycardia occurs with similar characteristics as an atriofascicular/atrioventricular bypass tract **(Figure 19.20A)** except with the following differences:

- AV dissociation is possible during tachycardia and may be brought out by advancement of the ventricular activation **(Figure 19.20B)**.
- Advancement of V occurs only if septal A is advanced by an atrial extrastimulus during tachycardia.
- Ablation needs to be done at the distal insertion site **(Figure 19.20C)**. Ablation at the proximal insertion site has chances of causing complete heart block. Mostly the successful site of ablation exists in the mid right ventricular septum **(Figure 19.20D)**.
- Commonly it is associated with AVNRT and hence may exist as innocent bystander and a differentiation between true antidromic tachycardia should always be made.

Fasciculoventricular Bypass Tract

As the name suggests the bypass tract connects the His bundle or bundle branch to the ventricle at the septum on either the right or the left side **(Figure 19.21)**. The HV interval remains fixed and less than 35 ms during atrial pacing at various rates indicating no change in the degree of preexcitation **(Figure 19.22)**. The preexcitation is seen not only during sinus rhythm and atrial pacing but also during AV nodal rhythm and even during His bundle pacing. The presence of preexcited beats during junctional rhythm or His bundle pacing is diagnostic of the presence of this pathway. Fasciculoventricular pathways may present confusion in diagnosis as they may act as innocent bystander during other SVTs. There is no evidence to suggest involvement of these pathways in genesis of any arrhythmia and hence they do not require ablation.

CONCLUSION

Atriofascicular bypass tracts are the most common Mahaim fibers and are responsible for antidromic tachycardia that presents with LBBB morphology and left axis deviation of

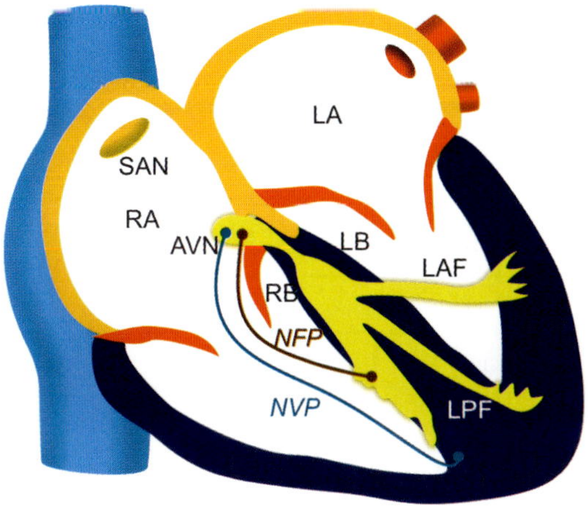

Figure 19.19: Schematic diagram demonstrating nodofascicular and nodoventricular bypass tract. The distal insertion site is the His bundle, right bundle, or rarely other fascicles in a nodofascicular pathway (NFP). The distal insertion site is the ventricular myocardium at the septum in a nodoventricular pathway (NVP)

Abbreviations: AVN, atrioventricular node; LA, left atrium; LAF, left anterior fascicle; LB, left bundle branch; LPF, left posterior fascicle; NFP, nodo-fascicular pathway; NVP, nodo-ventricular pathway; RA, right atrium; RB, right bundle branch; SAN, sinoatrial node

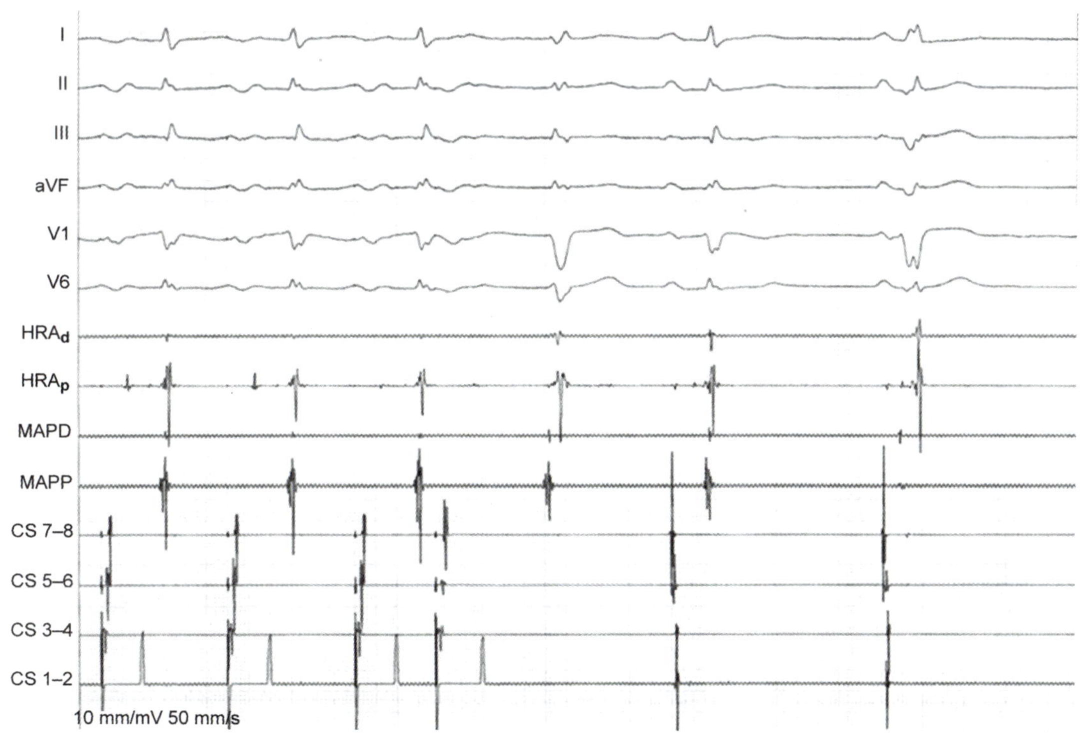

Figure 19.20A: Atrial pacing in a patient with Ebstein's anomaly and recurrent palpitations shows preexcitation with QRS morphology similar to that during tachycardia. The accessory pathway had decremental conduction characteristics and an antidromic bypass tract tachycardia was induced easily on atrial pacing

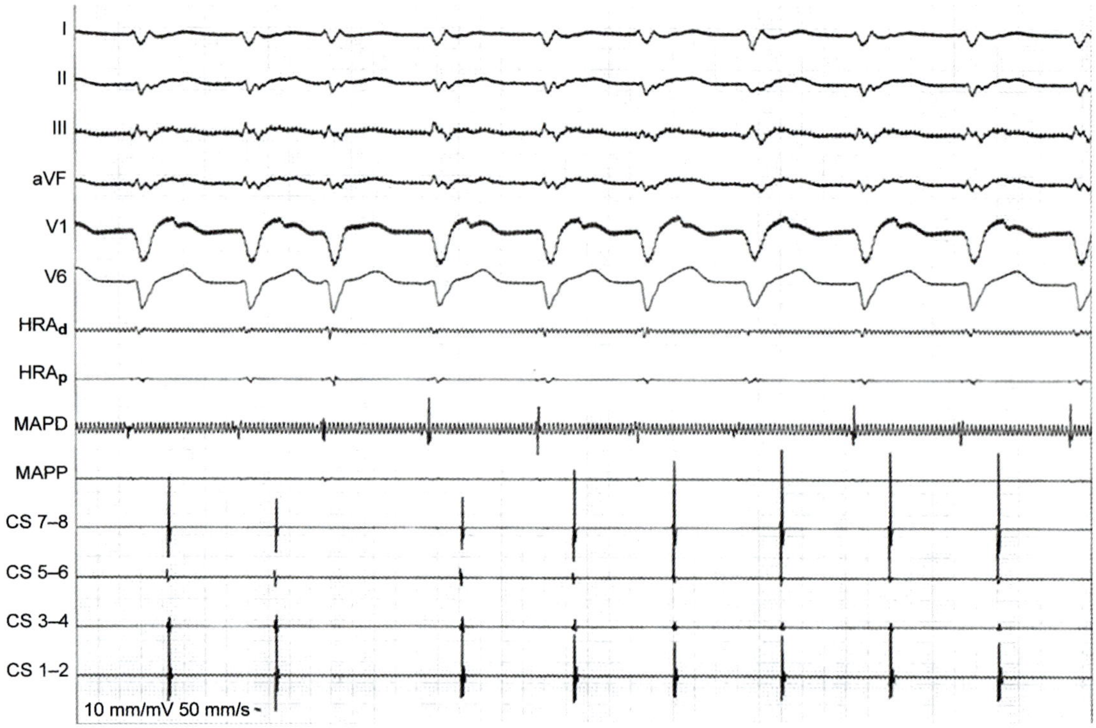

Figure 19.20B: Transient episode of VA dissociation during antidromic AVRT brought out by a spontaneous premature ventricular beat with QRS morphology identical to that during the tachycardia indicates that A is not necessarily a part of the circuit. Hence, the antidromic AVRT had to be mediated by a nodofascicular bypass tract

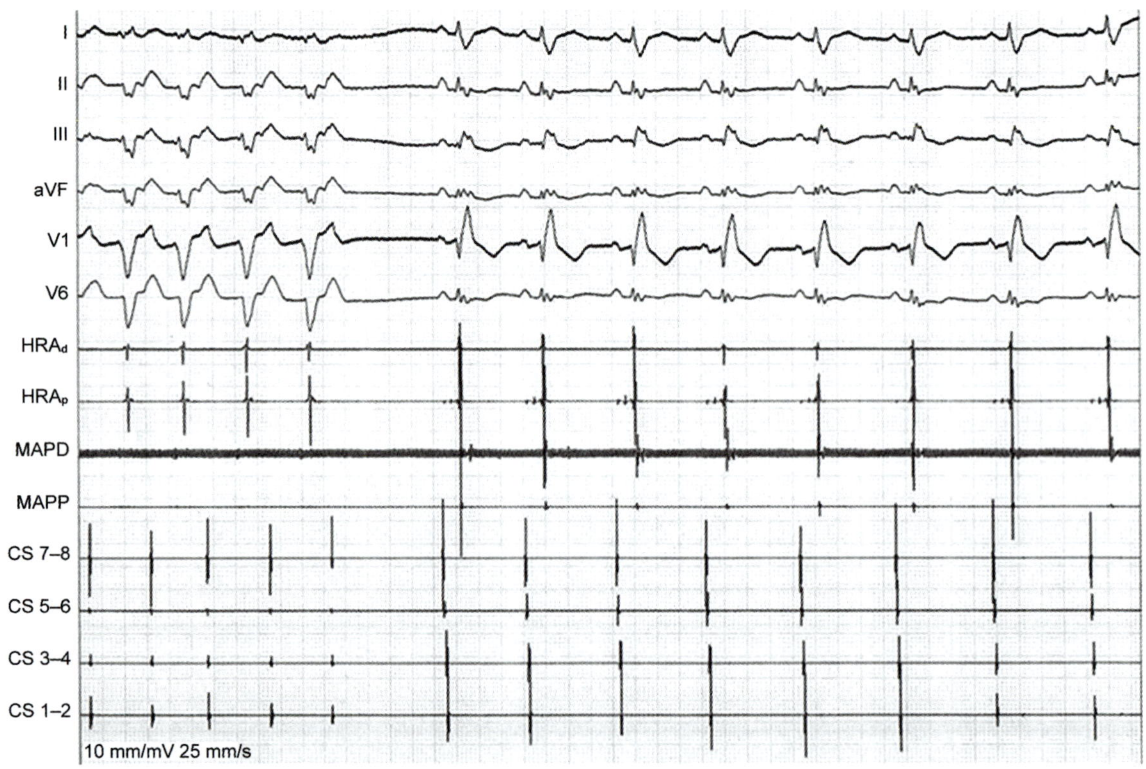

Figure 19.20C: Ablation in the right ventricle at the distal RBB caused automaticity followed by loss of preexcitation and appearance of RBBB that is expected in Ebstein's anomaly. No tachycardia was inducible following ablation

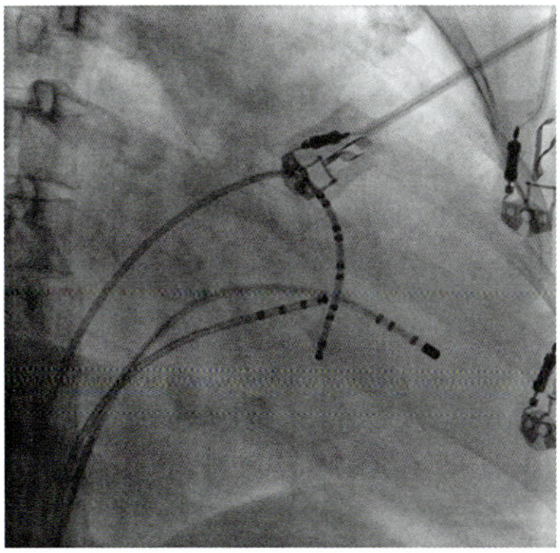

Figure 19.20D: Site of ablation in the right ventricle at the distal insertion site in RAO view. The site is typically described to be in the mid RV septum

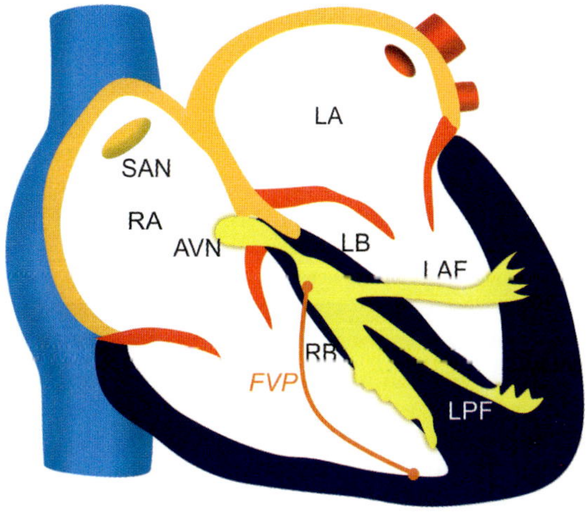

Figure 19.21: Schematic diagram depicting a fasciculoventricular bypass tract connecting the right bundle branch to the right ventricle
Abbreviations: AVN, atrioventricular node; FVP, fasciculo-ventricular pathway; LA, left atrium; LAF, left anterior fascicle; LB, left bundle branch; LPF, left posterior fascicle; RA, right atrium; RB, right bundle branch; SAN, sinoatrial node

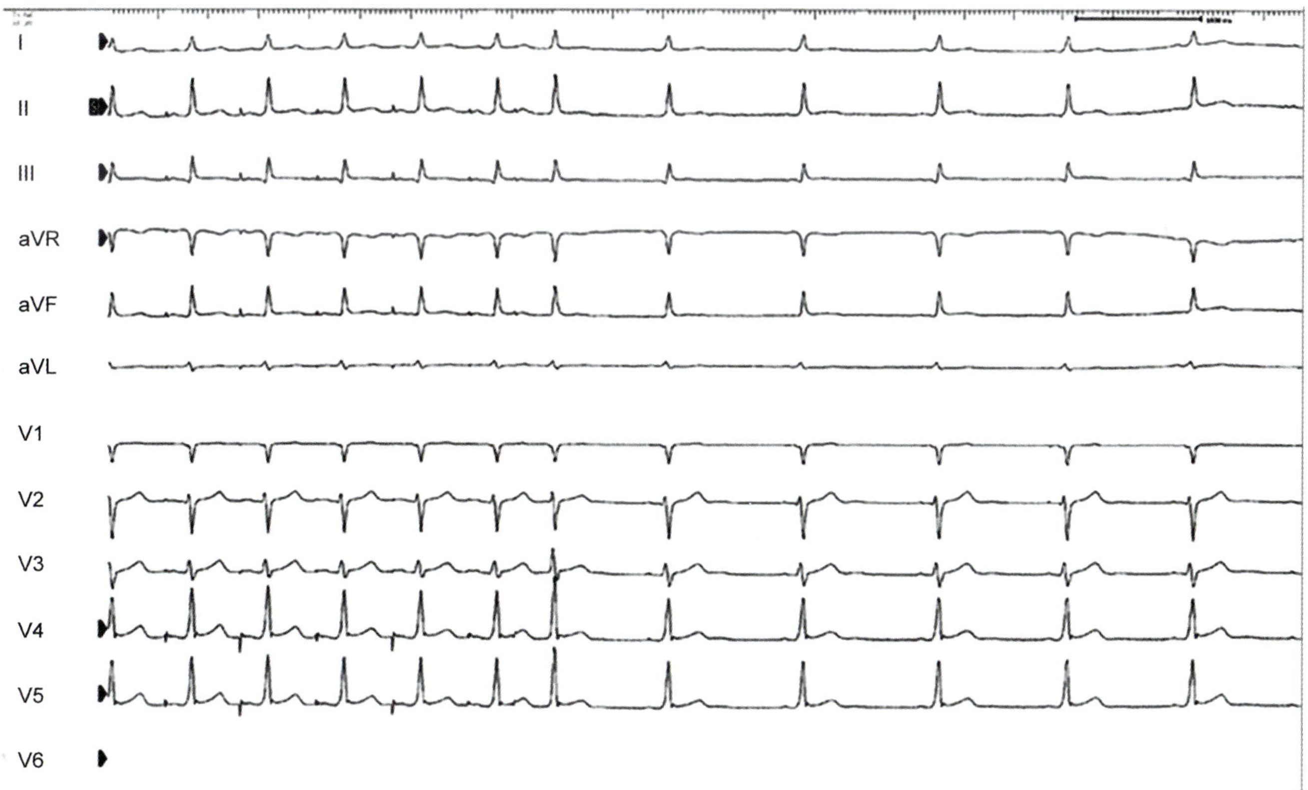

Figure 19.22: ECG of a patient with fasciculoventricular bypass tract during atrial pacing (initial half) and sinus rhythm (latter half). There is fixed degree of preexcitation at all rates. No tachycardia was inducible in this patient with recurrent syncope that were likely vasovagal

the QRS in the frontal plane. These pathways exhibit AV node like properties and generally are localized at the lateral aspect of the tricuspid annulus. High success rate of radiofrequency ablation of the accessory pathway is achieved using varying methods, the most successful being the site of the "M" Potential. Mahaim automatic rhythm is generally obtained during application of RF energy and predicts successful ablation.

REFERENCES

1. Mahaim I, Winston MR. Recherches d'lanatomic comparee et du pathologic experimentale sur les connexions hautes du faisceau de His-Tawara. Cardiologia. 1941;5:189-260.
2. Becker AE, Anderson RH, Path MRC, Durrer D, Wellens HJJ. The anatomical substrates of Wolff-Parkinson-White syndrome: a clinic-pathologic correlation in seven patients. Circulation. 1978;57:870-9.
3. Gallagher JJ, Smith WM, Kasell JH, Benson DW Jr, Sterba R, Grant AO. Role of Mahaim fibers in cardiac arrhythmias in man. Circulation. 1981;64:176-89.
4. Gillette PC, Garson A Jr, Cooley DA, McNamara DG. Prolonged and decremental antegrade conduction properties in right anterior accessory connections: wide QRS antidromic tachycardia of left bundle branch block pattern without Wolff-Parkinson-White configuration in sinus rhythm. Am Heart J. 1982;103:66-74.
5. Tchou P, Lehmann MH, Jazayeri M, Akhtar M. Atriofascicular connection or a nodoventricular Mahaim fiber? Electrophysiologic elucidation of the pathway and associated reentrant circuit. Circulation. 1988;77:837-48.
6. Bhandari A, Morady F, Shen EN, Schwartz AB, Botvinick E, Scheinman MM. Catheter-induced His bundle ablation in a patient with reentrant tachycardia associated with a nodoventricular tract. J Am Coll Cardiol. 1984;4:611-6.
7. McClelland JH, Wang X, Beckman KJ, Hazlitt HA, Prior MI, Nakagawa H, Lazzara R, Jackman WM. Radiofrequency catheter ablation of right atriofascicular (Mahaim) accessory pathways guided by accessory pathway activation potentials. Circulation. 1994;89:2655-66.
8. Tchou PJ, Keim SG, Kinn RM, Rist KE, Setter SF, Adhar G. Electrophysiologic evidence for an ectopic node-His like atrioventricular conduction system in an atriofascicular pathway (Abstract). Pacing Clin Electrophysiol. 1992;15:51.
9. Haissaguerre M, Warin JF, Le Metayer P, Maraud L, De Roy L, Montserrat P, Massiere JP. Catheter ablation of Mahaim fibers with preservation of atrioventricular nodal conduction. Circulation. 1990;82:418-27.
10. Klein L, Hackett FK, Zipes DP, Miles WM. Radiofrequency catheter ablation of Mahaim fibers at the tricuspid annulus. Circulation. 1993;87:738-47.
11. Brugada J, Martinez-Sanchez J, Kuzmicic B, Figueiredo MO, Matas M, Pava LF, Navarro-Lopez F. Radiofrequency catheter ablation of atriofascicular pathways guided by discrete electrical potentials recorded at the tricuspid annulus. Pacing Clin Electrophysiol. 1995;18:1388-94.
12. Klein GJ, Guiraudon GM, Kerr CR, Sharma AD, Yee R, Szabo T, Wah JA. "Nodoventricular" accessory pathway: evidence for a distinct accessory atrioventricular pathway with atrioventricular node-like properties. J Am Coll Cardiol. 1988;11:1035-40.
13. Haissaguerre M, Cauchemez B, Marcus F, Le Metayer P, Lauribe P, Poquet F, Gencel L, Clémenty J. Characteristics of the ventricular insertion sites of accessory pathways with anterograde decremental conduction properties. Circulation. 1995;91:1077-85.
14. Johnson CT, Brooks C, Jaramillo J, Mickelsen S, Kusumoto FM. A left free-wall, decrementally conducting, atrioventricular (Mahaim) fiber: diagnosis at electrophysiological study and radiofrequency catheter ablation guided by direct recording of a Mahaim potential. Pacing Clin Electrophysiol. 1997;20: 2486-8.
15. Faizel Osman, Peter J Stafford, G Andre Ng. Looks Like VT But Isn't - Successful Ablation Of A Left Free Wall Accessory Pathway With Mahaim-like Properties. Indian Pacing Electrophysiol J. 2009;9:112-8.
16. Grogin HR, Randall JL, Kwasman M, Epstein LM, Schamp DJ, Lesh MD, Scheinmann MM. Radiofrequency catheter ablation of atriofascicular and nodoventricular Mahaim tracts. Circulation. 1994;90:272-81.
17. Heal SC, Davies DW, Ward DE, Garrat CJ, Rowland E. Radiofrequency catheter ablation of Mahaim tachycardia by targeting Mahaim potentials at the tricuspid annulus. Br Heart J. 1995;73:250-7.
18. Kottkamp H, Hindricks G, Shenasa H, Chen X, Wichter T, Borggrefe M, Breithardt G. Variants of preexcitation-specialized atriofascicular pathways, nodofascicular pathways, and fasciculoventricular pathways: electrophysiologic findings and target sites for radiofrequency catheter ablation. J Cardiovasc Electrophysiol. 1996;7:916-30.
19. Sternick EB, Gerken LM, Vrandecic MO. Appraisal of "Mahaim" automatic tachycardia. J Cardiovasc Electrophysiol. 2002;13:244-9.
20. Singh B, Gupta RK, Dhall A, Ghose T, Trehan R, Kaul U. Mahaim Automatic Accelerated Rhythm: A Marker of Successful Radiofrequency Ablation. Indian Heart J. 2004;56: 215-9.
21. Bohora S, Dora SK, Namboodiri N, Valaparambil A, Tharakan J. Electrophysiology study and radiofrequency catheter ablation of atriofascicular tracts with decremental properties (Mahaim fibre) at the tricuspid annulus. Europace. 2008;10:1428-33.
22. Cappato R, Schluter M, Weiss C, Siebels J, Hebe J, Duckeck W, Mletzko R, Kuck KH. Catheter-induced mechanical conduction block of right-sided accessory fibers with Mahaim-type preexcitation to guide radiofrequency ablation. Circulation. 1994;90:282-90.
23. Bohora S, Tharakan J. "Ablation Techniques for Mahaim Fiber Tachycardia." Indian Pacing Electrophysiol. 2009;9: 75-80.
24. Valentino Ducceschi, Raffaele Vitale, Ewa Anna Sokola, Luca Ottaviano, Raffaele Sangiuolo, Giovanni Gregorio. Ablating The Ventricular Insertion Of Atrio-fascicular Mahaim Fiber: Could Be Performed Safely? Indian Pacing Electrophysiol J. 2009;9: 119-24.
25. Fung JWH, Chan HCK, Chan WWL, Sanderson JE. Ablation of the Mahaim pathway guided by noncontact mapping. J Cardiovasc Electrophysiol. 2002;13:1064.

EDITORS' SUMMARY

Dr Bohora provides in this chapter a practical yet detailed review of one of the most fascinating and often difficult to ablate arrhythmia substrate—an atriofascicular accessory bypass tract or fiber ("Mahaim fiber"). As explained in the text, the pathways that Mahaim described initially were completely different from what we today use his name in connection with (atriofascicular tracts). The terminology used in this chapter and book reflects contemporary usage of "Mahaim pathways". In fact however, atriofascicular and atrioventricular accessory pathways that do not demonstrate retrograde conduction and do exhibit antegrade decremental conduction were not described by Mahaim, yet since the usage has stuck we have kept with this inaccuracy. What makes this arrhythmia so interesting and difficult to treat?

1. ***Defining the target***: For accessory pathway ablation, we may target the earliest retrograde A, earliest antegrade V during pathway conduction, or a site where there is near-simultaneous atrioventricular activation during pathway conduction. None of these methods are of any value whatsoever with Mahaim fiber ablation. First, there is no retrograde conduction through these tracts. Thus, the early A has no value. Second, the earliest ventricular site is often the exit site of the normal conduction system to which the atriofascicular tract inserts. Thus, mapping and ablating the earliest ventricular activation with these pathways is nothing more than mapping the normal conduction system exit and unlikely to yield a successful result. Finally, there is no site for atrioventricular fusion with the common type of Mahaim fiber because the pathway does not insert into the annulus and has a decremental AV node like structure between the atrial input point and ventricular exit. In this sense, looking for AV fusion with Mahaim ablation would be as pointless a task as identifying the AV node or His bundle by trying to find AV fusion along the annulus!

   What then is an appropriate target? The only one is identifying the accessory pathway potential itself similar to a His bundle recording on the tricuspid annulus. Fortunately, however, the pathway potential with Mahaim fibers is among the clearest that we see in electrophysiology because of the lack of AV fusion.
2. ***Mechanical trauma and transient pathway loss***: Similar to the ease with which the right bundle may be mechanically "bumped," we often transiently lose conduction and it becomes impossible to find an appropriate target necessitating at times a repeat procedure.
3. ***Catheter contact***: Since Mahaim fibers most commonly occur from the free wall of the tricuspid annulus—a notoriously difficult site to maintain catheter contact—the ablationist will be challenged to use all available skills and imaging technique to optimize contact, particularly with the use of guiding sheaths and sometimes the internal jugular or subclavian vein access routes to place the catheter under the tricuspid leaflet for stability.
4. ***Difficulty with identifying the annulus***: Unlike mitral annular pathways where the coronary sinus serves as an excellent fixed reference proximating the annulus and stable activation patterns that can be used for point-to-point mapping and ablation, no such structure is present beyond the tricuspid valve epicardially. The use of multielectrode recordings mentioned and illustrated by Dr Bohora can be very helpful in facilitating success for these cases.

CHAPTER 20

Leonard A Steinberg, Benzy J Padanilam

Junctional Tachycardia

LIST OF ABBREVIATIONS

AV	Atrioventricular	PSVT	Paroxysmal Supraventricular Tachycardia
AVNRT	Atrioventricular Nodal Reentrant Tachycardia	RF	Radiofrequency
AVRT	Atrioventricular Reciprocating Tachycardia	SVT	Supraventricular Tachycardia
ECMO	Extracorporeal Membrane Oxygenation	VA	Ventriculoatrial
JET	Junctional Ectopic Tachycardia	VSD	Ventricular Septal Defect
JT	Junctional Tachycardia	VT	Ventricular Tachycardia
PAC	Premature Atrial Contraction		

INTRODUCTION

Non-reentrant or focal junctional tachycardia is an uncommon arrhythmia that originates in the AV node or the proximal aspect of the His bundle. Often referred to as junctional ectopic tachycardia, or JET, the word “ectopic” is superfluous, but has persisted in the medical literature. Junctional tachycardia is recognized in three distinct clinical scenarios: as an incessant infantile arrhythmia (congenital JET); as a transient arrhythmia following repair of congenital heart disease (postoperative JET); and as a sporadic, often paroxysmal arrhythmia in adolescents and adults [Junctional tachycardia (JT)]. It may also manifest secondary to drug toxicities (e.g. digoxin, theophylline) and inflammatory conditions (e.g. rheumatic carditis).

GENERAL CONSIDERATIONS

The AV Junction

The atrioventricular (AV) junction consists of the atrial approaches to the AV node, the compact AV node and the penetrating portion of the His bundle **(Figure 20.1)**. Automaticity is a normal characteristic of AV junctional tissues. Early studies in rabbits suggested that junctional escape rhythms arise from automaticity at the atrionodal and nodal-His regions, not the compact node.[1] Recent human optical mapping studies place the leading AV junctional escape pacemaker in the compact node and suggest that the focus shifts to the rightward AV nodal extensions (slow pathway region) during autonomic stimulation.[2-4]

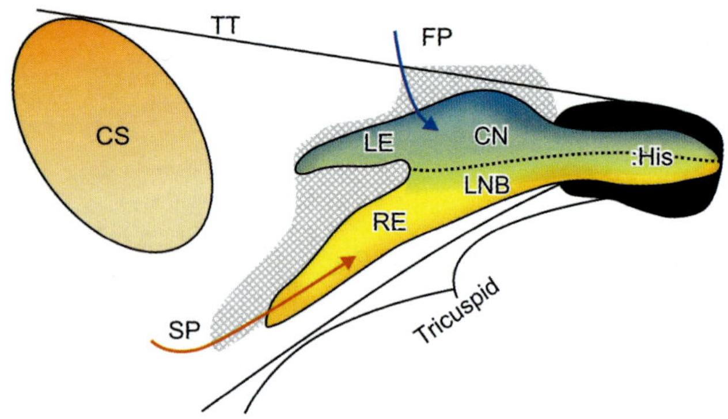

Figure 20.1: Proposed functional anatomy of the AV junction: AV node is located in the triangle of Koch bounded by coronary sinus (CS), tendon of Todaro (TT) and septal leaflet of tricuspid valve. The lower nodal bundle (LNB) leads into rightward extension (RE) forming the slow pathway (SP) area. The compact node (CN) forms the fast pathway (FP) area and leads into a smaller leftward extension (LE). The directional arrows illustrate the functional inputs—FP in blue and SP in red. Adapted from reference 4

The precise origin of pathologic focal junctional rhythms is less well defined. Structural abnormalities of the AV node have been reported in patients with congenital JET,[5,6] but a link connecting these abnormalities to the site of origin and mechanism of JT remains undiscovered. Ablation of the JT focus has commonly been successful in the slow pathway region, without compromising AV nodal conduction. Thus, most JT foci are presumably located in the AV nodal extensions rather than the compact node.

Rhythm Characterization and Differential Diagnosis

Focal junctional tachycardia is most often characterized by a narrow QRS complex, often irregular tachycardia, with or without a constant ventriculoatrial (VA) relationship. Warm up and cool down phenomena are commonly seen. When retrograde conduction occurs, P-waves commonly fall just after the QRS complex, though they can fall just before or within the QRS. Longer VA intervals or VA block may occur depending on a variety of factors, including the junctional rate, the proximity of the focus to the atrium (proximal AV nodal tissue vs His origin), and the conduction properties of the AV junction. Retrograde atrial activation is concentric, resulting in P-waves that are negative in the inferior leads, isoelectric to slightly positive in lead I, and positive in the anterior precordial leads. Because of the electrical proximity of the junctional focus to the atrium, retrograde conduction over an accessory pathway would be expected only when retrograde AV nodal conduction is slow or absent. Thus, 1:1 conduction with non-concentric P-waves should raise suspicion for other arrhythmias. Likewise, the proximity of the junctional focus to the His-Purkinje system generally precludes the possibility of ventricular preexcitation from an atrioventricular accessory pathway. Preexcited JT could rarely occur in the presence of a fasciculoventricular, nodoventricular, or nodofascicular connection. When VA block is present, sinus or atrial beats may occasionally penetrate the AV junction leading to capture beats, but termination is rare.[6]

Focal JT must be differentiated from other supraventricular arrhythmias. The common presentation with rate variability and VA dissociation is highly suggestive of junctional tachycardia, particularly in infants and in patients following surgical repair of congenital heart disease. When irregular, the rhythm may be mistaken for multifocal atrial tachycardia or, in adult patients, for atrial fibrillation. When P waves are clearly visible on ECG, the presence of VA dissociation with more QRS complexes than P waves excludes most other forms of supraventricular tachycardia (SVT). In particular, the vast majority of accessory pathway mediated SVTs require a 1:1 AV relationship. Tachycardias mediated by nodofascicular and nodoventricular accessory pathways constitute rare exceptions, and could potentially mimic junctional tachycardia with VA dissociation.[7] Atrioventricular nodal reentrant tachycardia (AVNRT) can occasionally present with VA dissociation as well.[8] When JT occurs with a 1:1 VA relationship and very short VA intervals, the rhythm can be mistaken for AVNRT or atrial tachycardias conducted over an AV nodal slow pathway. When the VA interval is longer, atrioventricular reciprocating tachycardia (AVRT) should be considered.

Additional evaluation may be required to establish the diagnosis. Adenosine often terminates AVNRT and AVRT, and it may terminate or transiently expose atrial tachycardias. In contrast, congenital and postoperative JET rarely slow with adenosine, though VA dissociation may be observed, suggesting a focal junctional mechanism. At electrophysiology study, the rhythm originates from the AV junction with a normal HV interval.[9] Overdrive atrial pacing leads to 1:1 atrioventricular conduction, but neither atrial nor ventricular pacing will suppress congenital and postoperative JET. The response to ventricular overdrive pacing should be similar to that seen with AVNRT: a V-A-V pattern is expected on termination of pacing, and this response largely excludes atrial tachycardia. Observance of a V-A-A-V pattern excludes the possibility of junctional tachycardia and suggests an atrial tachycardia.[10] Accessory pathway mediated tachycardias, including nodofascicular and nodoventricular, are diagnosed (and JT excluded) when ventricular extrastimuli timed to His depolarization perturb the tachycardia, or when bundle branch block increases the tachycardia cycle length.

Differentiating junctional tachycardia from typical AVNRT during electrophysiology study can be difficult. Proposed diagnostic maneuvers have attempted to leverage differences between focal and reentrant arrhythmias. In our laboratory, we have evaluated the response of the two tachycardias to atrial extrastimuli [premature atrial contractions (PACs)]. A response to this maneuver, when present, demonstrated a 100% specificity for differentiating the arrhythmias, though AVNRT could not always be perturbed using this protocol. A PAC timed to His bundle depolarization that perturbs the timing of the next His indicates antegrade conduction through AV nodal slow pathway and favors the diagnosis of AVNRT. An earlier PAC that advances the immediate His without terminating the tachycardia suggests JT.[11] Tachycardia response to atrial overdrive pacing has also been used to differentiate between JT and AVNRT. Fan et al identified an A-H-H-A response on termination of pacing in 8 of 8 patients with JT. Atrial overdrive pacing during AVNRT resulted in an A-H-A response in 19 of 21 patients and terminated tachycardia in the other two.[12]

CLINICAL SYNDROMES

Congenital Junctional Ectopic Tachycardia

This rare arrhythmia of increased junctional automaticity usually presents in infancy or early childhood. Congenital JET was first described by Coumel in 1976[13] as an incessant, refractory arrhythmia in 7 infants. Additional sporadic reports on increasing numbers of patients[6,14] have culminated in a recent description of 99 infants and children with congenital JET.[15] The heart rate is commonly greater than 200 bpm,[6,9,14,15] and may occasionally exceed 300 bpm. Heart failure symptoms and left ventricular systolic dysfunction are common, occurring in ~50% and ~75%, respectively, at presentation.[6,14] The impairment in cardiac function is proportional to the extent of elevated heart rate, but not the age of the patient at presentation.[6,14]

Partly because of the young age at presentation, the diagnosis is most frequently established by non-invasive means. Electrocardiograms usually demonstrate a rapid narrow QRS rhythm with warm up, cool down, and rate variability.[9] Ventriculo-atrial (VA) dissociation is present in two-thirds or more of patients.[6,14,15] When a 1:1 VA relation is initially present, prolonged monitoring may reveal intermittent VA dissociation **(Figures 20.2A and B)**. Rarely, congenital JET presents as a wide QRS complex rhythm. JET with aberrant conduction can be confirmed when other supraventricular complexes conduct with an identical QRS morphology. When the diagnosis is not evident, invasive electrophysiology studies may be required for differentiation from ventricular tachycardia.

The incidence and etiology of congenital JET remain ill defined. The condition is assumed to be rare, though less severe presentations with only mild increase in heart rate may go undiagnosed: most asymptomatic newborns and infants do not undergo routine ECG evaluation. The pathophysiology of this condition is equally enigmatic. Associated congenital heart disease is uncommon.[15] However, postmortem evaluations of congenital JET cases have revealed structural abnormalities of the AV junction.[5,6,13] A case report of pathology findings in 3 such patients revealed left sided extension of the AV node and His bundle, engulfment of the AV node within the central fibrous body, and a cranial displacement of the coronary sinus os.[5] On histologic examination, the summit of the ventricular septum demonstrated inflammation and fibrosis in one and necrosis in another. In Villian et al's case series of 26 patients with congenital JET, all 3 autopsied patients demonstrated one or more abnormalities, including degeneration of the His bundle, a left sided His bundle, and the presence ventricular fibroelastosis.[6]

In the largest and most recent study of congenital JET, a family history of JET was reported in 20% of patients.[15] Two previous case series have reported a familial association in 50% of congenital JET cases,[6,14] signifying the likelihood of a genetic contribution to this uncommon arrhythmia. Recent data suggests that at least some cases may result from fetal exposure to anti-Ro or anti-La antibodies,[16] suggesting JT may—in some cases—be a forme fruste of neonatal lupus. Fetal magnetocardiography has identified intermittent episodes JET in a significant proportion of fetuses known to have congenital complete heart block.[17] Postnatal progression from JET to complete heart block has been documented in rare instances,[15,18] and may be one mechanism for sudden death in this condition. Other sudden deaths have been attributed to ventricular fibrillation, possibly precipitated by electrolyte imbalances and use of antiarrhythmic mediations.[6]

Multiple antiarrhythmic agents have been used in the treatment of congenital JET with variable success. Because of the rare nature of this arrhythmia, no controlled trials are available. Therapy is guided by case reports and retrospective reviews of relatively small patient cohorts, as well as by trial and error. In a report of 4 infants diagnosed with JET before 2 months of age, propafenone reduced the rate to <150 bpm in 2 infants and completely suppressed the arrhythmia in 2 others.[19] However, in a 20 year experience with congenital JET, Sarubbi et al reported propafenone provided successful rate control in only 3 of 9 subjects.[14] Fenrich reported successful treatment of congenital JET with the combination of flecainide and amiodarone in 3 of 3 patients.[20] Ivabradine was successfully used in one patient who had not responded to combination therapy with flecainide and sotalol.[21] The largest retrospective review to date[15] followed 99 patients with congenital JET for a median 4.5 years, and included many patients described in previous case reports. Amiodarone, alone or in combination with other antiarrhythmic medications was most commonly reported to control or completely suppress the rhythm.

Historically, atrioventricular junction ablation and permanent pacing were used to control congenital JET. Ablation therapy has now evolved to target the JET focus

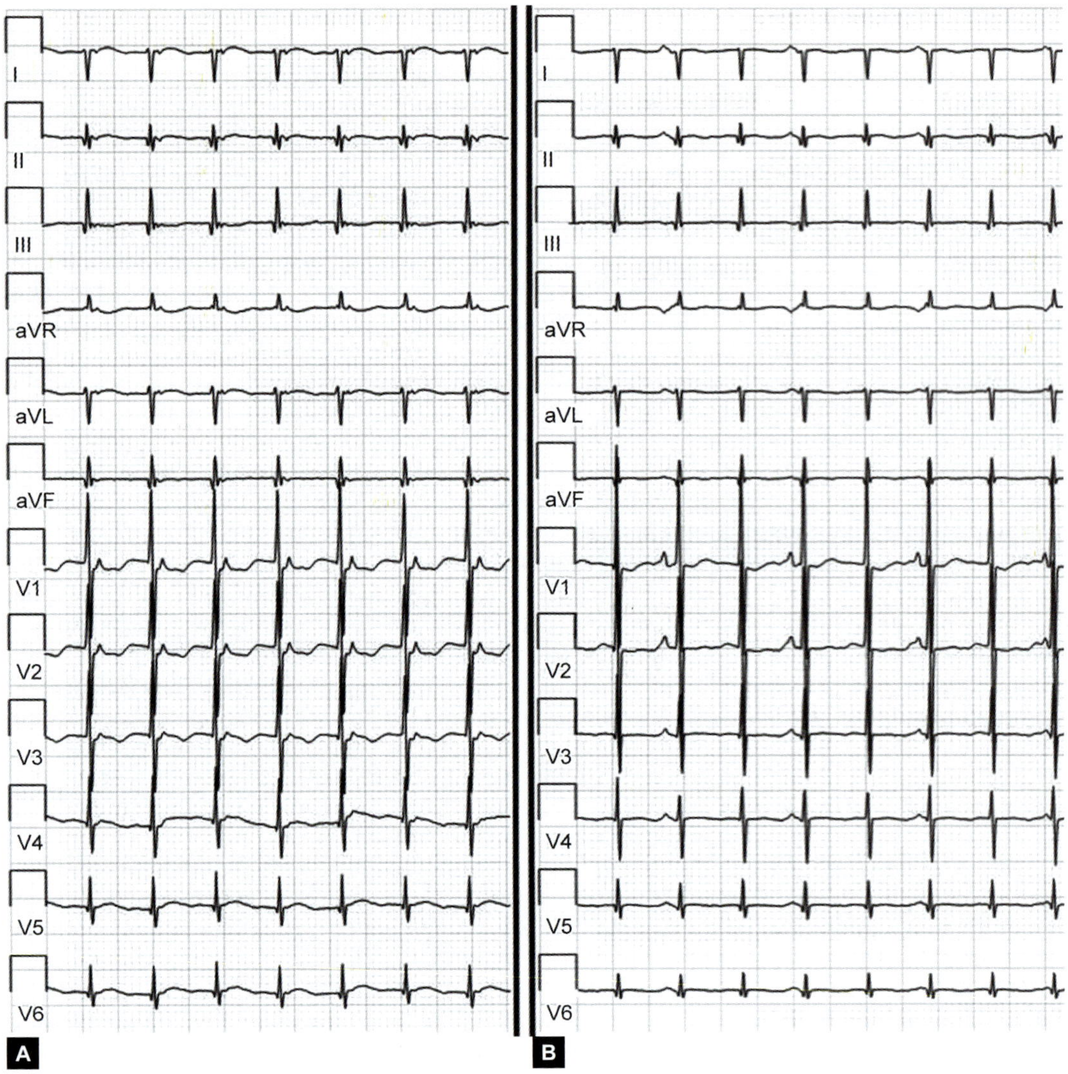

Figures 20.2A and B: Neonatal congenital junctional ectopic tachycardia. Twelve lead ECG recording of a newborn infant in junctional tachycardia. The recordings are obtained at 25 mm/s and 5 mm/mV. (A) Obtained shortly after birth, the heart rate is 175 bpm. There is 1:1 retrograde conduction to the atrium with a constant VA interval. P-waves are typical of concentric retrograde conduction; (B) This recording was obtained several hours later. The junctional rate has slowed slightly. There is dissociated sinus rhythm

without intentionally causing AV block. Radiofrequency (RF) catheter ablation of the junctional focus has been successfully employed with preservation of AV conduction.[22-25] Successful sites have targeted earliest atrial activation and have ranged from the posterior septum, near the slow pathway inputs to the anterior septum, close to His bundle potentials. Despite success, RF ablations are still associated with considerable risk of complete AV block. Cryoablation, with its minimal risk of heart block, has become the preferred ablation modality for congenital JET. In the largest reported series, Collins et al reported inadvertent heart block in 3 of 17 patients (18%) undergoing RF ablation, whereas there was no permanent heart block in 26 patients undergoing cryoablation.[15] Acute success rates (~84%) and recurrence rates (~14%) were similar between the two modalities.

The prognosis for patients with congenital JET is guarded. They have traditionally been considered a high-risk population. In Villain et al's[6] review of 26 patients presenting between 1970 and 1987, left ventricular dysfunction was present in 80% of the entire cohort and in all 16 patients with symptoms of congestive heart failure. The mortality rate was 35%. Sudden deaths accounted for more than half the mortality, including 2 witnessed ventricular fibrillation events and one witnessed asystole. Other deaths were largely complications of diagnostic or therapeutic procedures. In contrast, Collins et al recent review of 96[15] patients revealed a mortality rate of just 4%. These patients presented between 1969 and 2008, but cases were heavily weighted towards the modern era. Advancements in ablation and pacing technology, availability of amiodarone, and widespread accessibility of noninvasive imaging may have played a significant role in the improved outcomes. However, the more recent cohort also presented at an older age, exhibited a lower mean ventricular rate, and incurred a lower incidence of both heart failure symptoms and left ventricular dysfunction. These variances suggest that innate differences in patient populations may have played some role in the divergent outcomes.

For patients who survive the early course without significant sequelae, the long-term outlook appears favorable. Junctional tachycardia spontaneously resolves in a great many or slows to the point where medical therapy is no longer indicated.[6,15] A minority may require permanent pacing as a result of AV junction ablation, a complication of junctional tachycardia ablation, or a natural progression of the disease to complete heart block.[15] A small minority will continue to require antiarrhythmic therapy. Because of the reported propensity to develop heart block and limited available long-term outcome data, periodic follow-up for the development of conduction abnormalities may be warranted.

Postoperative Junctional Ectopic Tachycardia

The most frequently encountered setting for junctional tachycardia is in the cardiac intensive care unit following surgical correction of congenital heart disease. The arrhythmia can occur after any cardiovascular surgery.[26-29] JET has been estimated to occur in 5 to 14% of all pediatric congenital cardiac surgeries[26,28,30,31] and may occur in 21% of high-risk procedures.[32] Surgeries associated with highest risk of JET include surgical repair of a ventricular septal defect, either as an isolated defect or a component of complex congenital heart disease; tetralogy of Fallot repair especially when the surgical repair involves extensive resection of muscle bundles or relief of right ventricular outflow tract obstruction repair of an atrioventricular canal defect; the Norwood procedure; and the arterial switch operation.[26,27,29,31] Other potential factors include younger age at repair,[28,29] higher bypass temperature,[27] longer ischemic time,[26,30] elevation of CKMB,[30] and postoperative use of dopamine for hemodynamic support.[28]

The arrhythmia is often seen within the first 24 hours following surgery and usually resolves within the first week.[27] Some patients may present with a mildly accelerated junctional rhythm. This can be an early sign of impending rapid JT or an accelerated 'escape' rhythm associated with sinus node dysfunction in the postoperative patient. The emergence and the rate of the tachycardia often wax and wane with variations in the autonomic state. Increased catecholamine levels and fever may exacerbate the condition. Despite the short-lived nature of this arrhythmia, it can cause significant hemodynamic sequelae. Postoperative JET has been associated with increased mortality, prolonged mechanical ventilation, higher risk of extracorporeal membrane oxygenation (ECMO) support, and longer ICU and hospital admissions.[30,31]

Postoperative JET may compromise the hemodynamic state by the synergistic effect of a variety of mechanisms. The rapid ventricular rate—coupled with the loss of AV synchrony—diminish ventricular filling in the already noncompliant, postoperative myocardium. The resulting low cardiac output state leads to higher endogenous (or exogenous) catecholamine levels. A faster junctional rate ensues, inciting worsening heart failure, and leading to a spiraling cycle of decline. In severe cases, heart failure results in shunting of blood away from the skin and an inability to dissipate heat. Fever may further accelerate the junctional rate. These concerns have led to the use of an axiom borrowed from another, more common arrhythmia: JET begets JET. Indeed, the phrase may be more apropos of postoperative JET than of atrial fibrillation.

Although the exact mechanism underlying postoperative JET is unknown, clinical characteristics of the tachycardia suggest increased automaticity of the AV junction. Seghaye et al reported elevated histamine levels in patients with postoperative arrhythmias, including JET, when compared to postoperative patients without arrhythmias.[33] Infiltrative hemorrhage and direct trauma to the conduction system have been observed on postmortem evaluation of patients with postoperative JET.[34] Transient injury to the atrioventricular junction may increase junctional automaticity.[27] In support of this theory, JET is associated with postoperative complete heart block.[29] Heart block may occur transiently, or it may be a permanent complication of the surgical repair. Recently, an insertion/deletion polymorphism in the angiotensin converting enzyme predicted an almost 2 fold risk of postoperative JET. Thirty one percent of patients homozygous for the deletion polymorphism developed JET following high-risk surgical procedures, whereas JET occurred in only 16% of heterozygotes or those with the insertion polymorphism.[32] Modulation of the renin-angiotensin-aldosterone system via increased levels of angiotensin converting enzyme and angiotensin II is the proposed mechanism.[35]

Similar to the congenital form, the typical ECG of postoperative JET consists of a rapid tachycardia with the "usual" QRS complex. Retrograde P waves may rarely precede the QRS complex in this rhythm, but more commonly they are buried within the QRS, fall within the ST segment, or are dissociated. Ventricular septal defect (VSD) repairs often result in right bundle branch block. The presence of a typical right bundle branch block pattern tachycardia with no visible P waves or with AV dissociation following VSD repair suggests junctional tachycardia, but ventricular tachycardia (VT) must also be considered. P waves seen conducting with an identical QRS morphology at other times makes VT unlikely **(Figure 20.3)**.

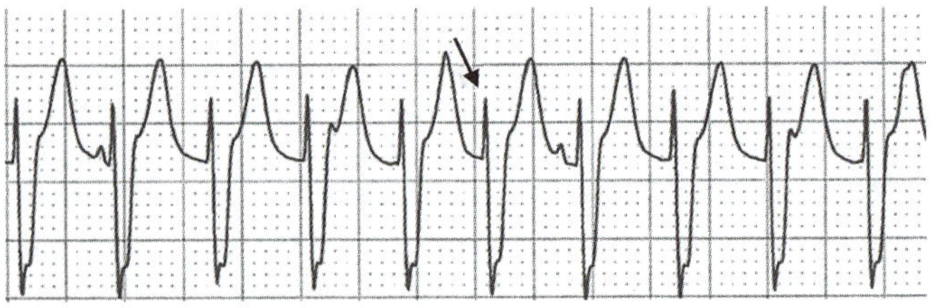

Figure 20.3: Postoperative Junctional ectopic tachycardia (JET) in a 4-month-old infant following VSD repair. The heart rate is ~ 180 bpm. ECG lead I is shown at 25 mm/s. The QRS complex has a sharp upstroke and a slurred S wave, and the QRS duration of 100 ms is wide for this age group, consistent with right bundle branch block or delay. Dissociated sinus rhythm at 150 bpm is also noted. P-waves falling at the peak of the T-wave reproducibly advanced the subsequent QRS (arrow) without change in the QRS morphology. In the setting of VSD repair, this tracing is diagnostic of postoperative JET

Therapy focuses on restoring AV synchrony and minimizing the junctional rate. A reduction of catecholamine levels and maintenance of normal body temperature are the first steps in treatment.[29] Endogenous catecholamine levels can be partially controlled with sedation. Reduction of exogenous catecholamines should be attempted when the patient's overall hemodynamic state will allow. When fever is present, establishing a euthermic state with use of a cooling blanket has been shown to be effective.[29] These measures may be of marginal benefit in difficult to control patients, but have minimal toxicity and can be rapidly employed, even while other therapies are in preparation or in process.

Further cooling with induced hypothermia has been used. Cooling to a goal temperature of 32 to 34°C (moderate hypothermia) was shown in one report to rapidly decrease the JET rate by an average of more than 50 bpm in 6 patients.[36] In another report of three patients with rapid postoperative JET, moderate hypothermia slowed the rate to less than 180 bpm in all three.[37] However, moderate hypothermia requires deep sedation and often paralysis. These measures may have had an independent influence on the JET rate in the reports suggesting effectiveness. In a prospective evaluation of therapies for postoperative JET using a staged approach, hypothermia (33–35°C) was effective only when used in combination with Procainamide.[29] Hypothermia may also trigger multiple undesirable effects in the postoperative patient, including immunosuppression, coagulopathy, electrolyte disturbances and decreased drug clearance.[38] For these reasons, and with the availability of other effective therapies, cooling below normal body temperature (or mild hypothermia) is only rarely employed at our institution.

Atrial pacing or AV sequential pacing therapy is a mainstay of treatment. Both forms of pacing may be performed via temporary epicardial pacing wires or atrial pacing may be accomplished with an esophageal lead. When the tachycardia rate is relatively slow, pacing slightly faster than the native rate may be sufficient to prevent further junctional acceleration and palliate the hemodynamic state until the rhythm spontaneously resolves.[29] The rate of pacing should be just fast enough to reestablish AV synchrony, with titration of the pacing rate based on frequent reassessment of the underlying rhythm. Ventricular synchronous atrial pacing has also been used to establish AV synchrony without increasing the ventricular rate.[39,40] At faster junctional rates, or when atrial pacing is not available, attempts are made to slow the junctional rate. Successful therapy may involve complete suppression of the rhythm or a decrease in the rate to allow for atrial pacing.

Amiodarone has become the drug treatment of choice for JET. It safely and effectively reduces the junctional rate in most patients.[41-44] Polymorphic ventricular tachycardia has been reported as a rare complication of amiodarone therapy for postoperative JET,[45] but proarrhythmia is rare. Hypotension, a common side effect of intravenous amiodarone in pediatric patients, occurs partially secondary to a preservative in the IV formulation,[46] rather than the drug itself. Administration of fluids and calcium can usually correct hypotension when secondary to amiodarone.

Some centers have found success with prophylactic therapy. Imamura et al evaluated the effect of amiodarone on the incidence of JET following tetralogy of Fallot repair. A dose of 2 mg/kg/day, started while rewarming after cardiac bypass and continued for 48 hours, decreased the incidence of JET from 37% to 10%, but did not demonstrate a significant effect on the length of ICU or hospital admission.[47] Manrique et al. demonstrated a dose-related decrease in the incidence of postoperative JET by administering magnesium during rewarming,[48] though as with amiodarone, ICU length of stay was not affected.

Other therapies have been employed with variable success. Limited data is available for most. Early reported therapy for junctional tachycardia employed ventricular paired pacing to limit the effective mechanical rate.[49] This technique saw continued use as recently as 1999.[50,51] Walsh et al's evaluation of a staged approach to therapy found no therapeutic benefit to digoxin, propranolol, phenytoin, or verapamil.[29] The only effective agent in this relatively large study was the combination of procainamide and hypothermia, which was 'clearly effective' in 80% of attempted therapies and 'possibly effective' in up to 97%. Procainamide, however, requires frequent monitoring of drug levels and titration of dose. It may cause hypotension, negative inotropy, and proarrhythmia. Garson reported control of postoperative JET with intravenous propafenone in 100% of 7 patients.[52] Intravenous flecainide was successfully employed in 7 patients with postoperative JET.[53] The IV formulations of both flecainide and propafenone have been associated with significant hypotension,[52,54,55] and neither is universally available.

There is no single standard approach to the treatment of postoperative JET, though treatment protocols across institutions have become similar. Our initial approach to postoperative JET involves minimizing catecholamine levels and eliminating fever. When the JET rate exceeds 160 bpm, or there is evidence of hemodynamic compromise, atrial overdrive pacing or AV sequential pacing is initiated. Mild hypothermia (35–37°C) is occasionally employed. Failing an adequate response, amiodarone is usually administered in 3–5 mg/kg boluses until the tachycardia is controlled. Initial doses in excess of 25 mg/kg have, rarely, been used to suppress rapid JET rates. Continuous amiodarone infusions are then variably employed at rates up to 20 mg/kg/day (~15 mcg/kg/min) depending on the perceived severity of the arrhythmia and the amount of amiodarone needed for initial control. Combination therapy with other medications is rarely required. When amiodarone fails to control JET, extracorporeal membrane oxygenation (ECMO) has been employed to sustain cardiac output until the arrhythmia resolves.[56] It is critical to continue amiodarone therapy during ECMO in order to reduce time on the circuit and to ensure adequate rhythm control following ECMO decannulation.

The long-term prognosis for patients with postoperative JET is excellent. Though some patients may have permanent heart block, the presence of JET does not appear to predict the likelihood of conduction system recovery. Rarely, we have seen patients with a persistent, mildly accelerated junctional rhythm lasting weeks after surgery, but these mildly elevated heart rates are generally well tolerated in otherwise stable patients, no longer in the immediate postoperative state. In the absence of sinus node dysfunction, long-term persistence of a postoperative junctional rhythm generally does not occur.

Junctional Tachycardia in Adults

Junctional tachycardia is relatively rare in adults and descriptions are limited to case reports and case series. The adult form has previously been referred to as nonparoxysmal JT to differentiate it from paroxysmal supraventricular tachycardias (PSVTs), or as automatic JT to denote the mechanism. These terminologies are no longer used because the adult form is clinically paroxysmal and its mechanism can be automatic or triggered.

Adult onset JT was initially described as a secondary disorder in the setting of acute myocardial ischemia, digoxin toxicity, chronic lung disease, rheumatic carditis, and metabolic derangements.[57] These JTs are slower (70–120/min) and usually regular. Wenckebach pattern may be present in digoxin toxicity associated JT.[58] JT may also manifest during catheter ablation of AVNRT. In addition to the junctional rhythms induced during application of radiofrequency current, persistent JT may occur post-ablation. These rhythms resolve spontaneously after minutes or hours, but can be mistaken for recurrent AVNRT leading to additional, unnecessary ablations.

Primary JT in adults was described by Ruder et al in a report of 5 adult patients.[59] The age at onset of tachycardia ranged from 13 to 23 years, and the tachycardia rates ranged from 110 to 180 bpm. The episodes are paroxysmal rather than incessant, lasting seconds to hours. In some patients, the tachycardia demonstrates inducibility with pacing and adenosine sensitivity, consistent with a triggered mechanism. In others, lack of inducibility or adenosine response suggests abnormal automaticity, as is seen with the pediatric forms of the arrhythmia.[60] Beta blockers effectively control rhythm in most adult patients. The lower heart rate, response to beta blockade, and the benign clinical course of adult JT are important distinctions from congenital JET. Catheter ablation may be considered in patients not responding to medical therapy although the risk of complete heart block during ablation is relatively high.[61] The use of cryoablation has been associated with reduction of complete heart block risk in the pediatric population.[15,62] The site of origin of the tachycardia can be the AV nodal slow pathway region, AV nodal fast pathway region or the His bundle. A distal to proximal His bundle activation suggest His origin of the tachycardia. The earliest atrial activation during JT may give clues to the region of AV nodal origin of the tachycardia although such sites may not be the sites of successful ablation. Hamdan et al proposed targeting the earliest retrograde atrial activation site when VA conduction is present. When AV dissociation predominates, they recommended and an empiric approach with of sequential ablations progressing from the slow pathway area to mid and anterior septum.[63] Others have proposed targeting sites of tachycardia termination during catheter manipulations.[22] Atrial overdrive pacing during ablation allows for observation of AV conduction, and may minimize the risk of AV block.[64]

CONCLUSION

Nonreentrant JTs are uncommon arrhythmias. The congenital and postoperative forms of JET may carry a poor prognosis unless promptly treated. Amiodarone is often required. Conversely, the adult forms of JT generally carry a benign prognosis and often respond to beta-blockers. When medical management is ineffective, ablation of the JT focus may be considered.

REFERENCES

1. Watanabe Y, Dreifus LS. Sites of impulse formation within the atrioventricular junction of the rabbit. Circ Res. 1968;22: 717-27.
2. Efimov IR, Mazgalev TN. High-resolution, three-dimensional fluorescent imaging reveals multilayer conduction pattern in the atrioventricular node. Circulation. 1998;98:54-7.
3. Fedorov VV, Ambrosi CM, Kostecki G, Hucker WJ, Glukhov AV, Wuskell JP, Loew LM, Moazami N, Efimov IR. Anatomic localization and autonomic modulation of atrioventricular

junctional rhythm in failing human hearts. Circ Arrhythm Electrophysiol. 2011;4:515-25.
4. Kurian T, Ambrosi C, Hucker W, Fedorov VV, Efimov IR. Anatomy and electrophysiology of the human AV node. Pacing Clin Electrophysiol. 2010;33:754-62.
5. Bharati S, Moskowitz WB, Scheinman M, Estes NA, 3rd, Lev M. Junctional tachycardias: anatomic substrate and its significance in ablative procedures. J Am Coll Cardiol. 1991;18:179-86.
6. Villain E, Vetter VL, Garcia JM, Herre J, Cifarelli A, Garson A, Jr. Evolving concepts in the management of congenital junctional ectopic tachycardia. A multicenter study. Circulation. 1990;81:1544-9.
7. Hamdan MH, Kalman JM, Lesh MD, Lee RJ, Saxon LA, Dorostkar P, Scheinman MM. Narrow complex tachycardia with VA block: diagnostic and therapeutic implications. Pacing Clin Electrophysiol. 1998;21:1196-206.
8. Otomo K, Okamura H, Noda T, Satomi K, Shimizu W, Suyama K, Kurita T, Aihara N, Kamakura S. Unique electrophysiologic characteristics of atrioventricular nodal reentrant tachycardia with different ventriculoatrial block patterns: effects of slow pathway ablation and insights into the location of the reentrant circuit. Heart Rhythm. 2006;3:544-54.
9. Garson A, Jr., Gillette PC. Junctional ectopic tachycardia in children: electrocardiography, electrophysiology and pharmacologic response. Am J Cardiol. 1979;44:298-302.
10. Knight BP, Ebinger M, Oral H, Kim MH, Sticherling C, Pelosi F, Michaud GF, Strickberger SA, Morady F. Diagnostic value of tachycardia features and pacing maneuvers during paroxysmal supraventricular tachycardia. J Am Coll Cardiol. 2000;36:574-82.
11. Padanilam BJ, Manfredi JA, Steinberg LA, Olson JA, Fogel RI, Prystowsky EN. Differentiating junctional tachycardia and atrioventricular node re-entry tachycardia based on response to atrial extrastimulus pacing. J Am Coll Cardiol. 2008;52: 1711-7.
12. Fan R, Tardos JG, Almasry I, Barbera S, Rashba EJ, Iwai S. Novel use of atrial overdrive pacing to rapidly differentiate junctional tachycardia from atrioventricular nodal reentrant tachycardia. Heart Rhythm. 2011;8:840-4.
13. Coumel P, Fidelle JE, Attuel P, Brechenmacher C, Batisse A, Bretagne J, Clementy J, Gerard R, Grolleau R, Huault G, Mouy A, Nouaille J, Kachaner J, Ribiere M, Toumieux MC. [Congenital bundle-of-his focal tachycardias. Cooperative study of 7 cases]. Arch Mal Coeur Vaiss. 1976;69:899-909.
14. Sarubbi B, Musto B, Ducceschi V, D'Onofrio A, Cavallaro C, Vecchione F, Musto C, Calabro R. Congenital junctional ectopic tachycardia in children and adolescents: a 20 year experience based study. Heart. 2002;88:188-90.
15. Collins KK, Van Hare GF, Kertesz NJ, Law IH, Bar-Cohen Y, Dubin AM, Etheridge SP, Berul CI, Avari JN, Tuzcu V, Sreeram N, Schaffer MS, Fournier A, Sanatani S, Snyder CS, Smith RT, Jr., Arabia L, Hamilton R, Chun T, Liberman L, Kakavand B, Paul T, Tanel RE. Pediatric nonpost-operative junctional ectopic tachycardia medical management and interventional therapies. J Am Coll Cardiol. 2009;53: 690-7.
16. Dubin AM, Cuneo BF, Strasburger JF, Wakai RT, Van Hare GF, Rosenthal DN. Congenital junctional ectopic tachycardia and congenital complete atrioventricular block: a shared etiology? Heart Rhythm. 2005;2:313-5.
17. Zhou T, Shen XQ, Zhou SH, Fang ZF, Hu XQ, Zhao YS, Qi SS, Zhou Z, Li J, Lv XL. Atrioventricular block: a serious complication in and after transcatheter closure of perimembranous ventricular septal defects. Clin Cardiol. 2008;31:368-71.
18. Henneveld H, Hutter P, Bink-Boelkens M, Sreeram N. Junctional ectopic tachycardia evolving into complete heart block. Heart. 1998;80:627-8.
19. Paul T, Reimer A, Janousek J, Kallfelz HC. Efficacy and safety of propafenone in congenital junctional ectopic tachycardia. J Am Coll Cardiol. 1992;20:911-4.
20. Fenrich AL, Jr., Perry JC, Friedman RA. Flecainide and amiodarone: combined therapy for refractory tachyarrhythmias in infancy. J Am Coll Cardiol. 1995;25:1195-8.
21. Al-Ghamdi S, Al-Fayyadh MI, Hamilton RM. Potential new indication for ivabradine: treatment of a patient with congenital junctional ectopic tachycardia. J Cardiovasc Electrophysiol. 2013;24:822-4.
22. Ehlert FA, Goldberger JJ, Deal BJ, Benson DW, Kadish AH. Successful radiofrequency energy ablation of automatic junctional tachycardia preserving normal atrioventricular nodal conduction. Pacing Clin Electrophysiol. 1993;16:54-61.
23. Emmel M, Sreeram N, Brockmeier K. Catheter ablation of junctional ectopic tachycardia in children, with preservation of atrioventricular conduction. Z Kardiol. 2005;94:280-6.
24. Fishberger SB, Rossi AF, Messina JJ, Saul JP. Successful radiofrequency catheter ablation of congenital junctional ectopic tachycardia with preservation of atrioventricular conduction in a 9-month-old infant. Pacing Clin Electrophysiol. 1998;21:2132-5.
25. Simmers TA, Sreeram N, Wittkampf FH, Derksen R. Radiofrequency catheter ablation of junctional ectopic tachycardia with preservation of atrioventricular conduction. Pacing Clin Electrophysiol. 2003;26:1284-8.
26. Batra AS, Chun DS, Johnson TR, Maldonado EM, Kashyap BA, Maiers J, Lindblade CL, Rodefeld M, Brown JW, Hubbard JE. A prospective analysis of the incidence and risk factors associated with junctional ectopic tachycardia following surgery for congenital heart disease. Pediatr Cardiol. 2006;27:51-5.
27. Dodge-Khatami A, Miller OI, Anderson RH, Goldman AP, Gil-Jaurena JM, Elliott MJ, Tsang VT, De Leval MR. Surgical substrates of postoperative junctional ectopic tachycardia in congenital heart defects. J Thorac Cardiovasc Surg. 2002;123:624-30.
28. Hoffman TM, Bush DM, Wernovsky G, Cohen MI, Wieand TS, Gaynor JW, Spray TL, Rhodes LA. Postoperative junctional ectopic tachycardia in children: incidence, risk factors, and treatment. Ann Thorac Surg. 2002;74:1607-11.
29. Walsh EP, Saul JP, Sholler GF, Triedman JK, Jonas RA, Mayer JE, Wessel DL. Evaluation of a staged treatment protocol for rapid automatic junctional tachycardia after operation for congenital heart disease. J Am Coll Cardiol. 1997;29:1046-53.
30. Andreasen JB, Johnsen SP, Ravn HB. Junctional ectopic tachycardia after surgery for congenital heart disease in children. Intensive Care Med. 2008;34:895-902.
31. Zampi JD, Hirsch JC, Gurney JG, Donohue JE, Yu S, LaPage MJ, Hanauer DA, Charpie JR. Junctional ectopic tachycardia after infant heart surgery: incidence and outcomes. Pediatr Cardiol. 2012;33:1362-9.
32. Borgman KY, Smith AH, Owen JP, Fish FA, Kannankeril PJ. A genetic contribution to risk for postoperative junctional

ectopic tachycardia in children undergoing surgery for congenital heart disease. Heart Rhythm. 2011;8:1900-4.

33. Seghaye MC, Duchateau J, Grabitz RG, Mertes J, Marcus C, Buro K, Messmer BJ, von Bernuth G. Histamine liberation related to cardiopulmonary bypass in children: possible relation to transient postoperative arrhythmias. J Thorac Cardiovasc Surg. 1996;111:971-81.
34. Till JA, Ho SY, Rowland E. Histopathological findings in three children with His bundle tachycardia occurring subsequent to cardiac surgery. Eur Heart J. 1992;13:709-12.
35. Smith AH, Flack EC, Borgman KY, Owen JP, Fish FA, Bichell DP, Kannankeril PJ. A common angiotensin-converting enzyme polymorphism and preoperative angiotensin-converting enzyme inhibition modify risk of tachyarrhythmias after congenital heart surgery. Heart Rhythm. 2014;11:637-43.
36. Pfammatter JP, Paul T, Ziemer G, Kallfelz HC. Successful management of junctional tachycardia by hypothermia after cardiac operations in infants. Ann Thorac Surg. 1995;60: 556-60.
37. Bash SE, Shah JJ, Albers WH, Geiss DM. Hypothermia for the treatment of postsurgical greatly accelerated junctional ectopic tachycardia. J Am Coll Cardiol. 1987;10:1095-9.
38. Polderman KH. Mechanisms of action, physiological effects, and complications of hypothermia. Crit Care Med. 2009;37:S186-202.
39. Janousek J, Vojtovic P, Chaloupecky V, Hucin B, Tlaskal T, Kostelka M, Reich O. Hemodynamically optimized temporary cardiac pacing after surgery for congenital heart defects. Pacing Clin Electrophysiol. 2000;23:1250-9.
40. Janousek J, Vojtovic P, Gebauer RA. Use of a modified, commercially available temporary pacemaker for R wave synchronized atrial pacing in postoperative junctional ectopic tachycardia. Pacing Clin Electrophysiol. 2003;26:579-86.
41. Laird WP, Snyder CS, Kertesz NJ, Friedman RA, Miller D, Fenrich AL. Use of intravenous amiodarone for postoperative junctional ectopic tachycardia in children. Pediatr Cardiol. 2003;24:133-7.
42. Perry JC, Fenrich AL, Hulse JE, Triedman JK, Friedman RA, Lamberti JJ. Pediatric use of intravenous amiodarone: efficacy and safety in critically ill patients from a multicenter protocol. J Am Coll Cardiol. 1996;27:1246-50.
43. Plumpton K, Justo R, Haas N. Amiodarone for post-operative junctional ectopic tachycardia. Cardiol Young. 2005;15:13-8.
44. Raja P, Hawker RE, Chaikitpinyo A, Cooper SG, Lau KC, Nunn GR, Cartmill TB, Sholler GF. Amiodarone management of junctional ectopic tachycardia after cardiac surgery in children. Br Heart J. 1994;72:261-5.
45. Yap SC, Hoomtje T, Sreeram N. Polymorphic ventricular tachycardia after use of intravenous amiodarone for post-operative junctional ectopic tachycardia. Int J Cardiol. 2000; 76:245-7.
46. Alade SL, Brown RE, Paquet A, Jr. Polysorbate 80 and E-Ferol toxicity. Pediatrics. 1986;77:593-7.
47. Imamura M, Dossey AM, Garcia X, Shinkawa T, Jaquiss RD. Prophylactic amiodarone reduces junctional ectopic tachycardia after tetralogy of Fallot repair. J Thorac Cardiovasc Surg. 2012;143:152-6.
48. Manrique AM, Arroyo M, Lin Y, El Khoudary SR, Colvin E, Lichtenstein S, Chrysostomou C, Orr R, Jooste E, Davis P, Wearden P, Morell V, Munoz R. Magnesium supplementation during cardiopulmonary bypass to prevent junctional ectopic tachycardia after pediatric cardiac surgery: a randomized controlled study. J Thorac Cardiovasc Surg. 2010;139: 162-9 e2.
49. Waldo AL, Krongrad E, Kupersmith J, Levine OR, Bowman FO, Jr., Hoffman BF. Ventricular paired pacing to control rapid ventricular heart rate following open heart surgery. Observations on ectopic automaticity. Report of a case in a four-month-old patient. Circulation. 1976;53:176-81.
50. Kohli V, Young ML, Perryman RA, Wolff GS. Paired ventricular pacing: an alternative therapy for postoperative junctional ectopic tachycardia in congenital heart disease. Pacing Clin Electrophysiol. 1999;22:706-10.
51. Sluysmans T, Moulin D, Jaumin P, Rubay J, Vliers A, DeJonghe D. Ventricular paired pacing to control intractable junctional tachycardia following open heart surgery in a child. Intensive Care Med. 1989;15:203-5.
52. Garson A, Jr., Moak JP, Smith RT, Jr., Norton JB, Jr. Usefulness of intravenous propafenone for control of postoperative junctional ectopic tachycardia. Am J Cardiol. 1987;59:1422-4.
53. Bronzetti G, Formigari R, Giardini A, Frascaroli G, Gargiulo G, Picchio FM. Intravenous flecainide for the treatment of junctional ectopic tachycardia after surgery for congenital heart disease. Ann Thorac Surg. 2003;76:148-51; discussion 51.
54. Till JA, Shinebourne EA, Rowland E, Ward DE, Bhamra R, Haga P, Johnston A, Holt DW. Paediatric use of flecainide in supraventricular tachycardia: clinical efficacy and pharmacokinetics. Br Heart J. 1989;62:133-9.
55. Wren C, Campbell RW. The response of paediatric arrhythmias to intravenous and oral flecainide. Br Heart J. 1987;57:171-5.
56. Azzam FJ, Fiore AC. Postoperative junctional ectopic tachycardia. Can J Anaesth. 1998;45:898-902.
57. Pick A, Dominguez P. Nonparoxysmal A-V nodal tachycardia. Circulation. 1957;16:1022-32.
58. Pick A, Langendorf R, Katz LN. A-V nodal tachycardia with block. Circulation. 1961;24:12-22.
59. Davis J, Scheinman MM, Ruder MA, Griffin JC, Herre JM, Finkebeiner WE, Chin MC, Eldar M. Ablation of cardiac tissues by an electrode catheter technique for treatment of ectopic supraventricular tachycardia in adults. Circulation. 1986;74:1044-53.
60. Shukla A, Curtis AB, Mehra MR, Albert NM, Gheorghiade M, Heywood JT, Liu Y, O'Connor CM, Reynolds D, Walsh MN, Yancy CW, Fonarow GC. Factors associated with improvement in utilization of cardiac resynchronization therapy in eligible heart failure patients: findings from IMPROVE HF. Pacing Clin Electrophysiol. 2013;36:433-43.
61. Hamdan M, Van Hare GF, Fisher W, Gonzalez R, Dorostkar P, Lee R, Lesh M, Saxon L, Kalman J, Scheinman M. Selective catheter ablation of the tachycardia focus in patients with nonreentrant junctional tachycardia. Am J Cardiol. 1996;78:1292-7.
62. Law IH, Von Bergen NH, Gingerich JC, Saarel EV, Fischbach PS, Dick M, 2nd. Transcatheter cryothermal ablation of junctional ectopic tachycardia in the normal heart. Heart Rhythm. 2006;3:903-7.
63. Hamdan MH, Badhwar N, Scheinman MM. Role of invasive electrophysiologic testing in the evaluation and management of adult patients with focal junctional tachycardia. Card Electrophysiol Rev. 2002;6:431-5.
64. Fukuhara H, Nakamura Y, Ohnishi T. Atrial pacing during radiofrequency ablation of junctional ectopic tachycardia--a useful technique for avoiding atrioventricular bloc. Jpn Circ J. 2001;65:242-4.

EDITORS' SUMMARY

Although an uncommon rhythm malady that confronts invasive electrophysiologists, junctional tachycardia and its difficult distinction from AV node reentry represents an outstanding training ground for a student to appreciate the elegance and logic of the diagnostic maneuvers we employ. In this chapter, one of the innovators of the most practical of these maneuvers used presently provides a balanced and usable description of the arrhythmia, its differential diagnosis, and invasive diagnostic and treatment options.

The most common scenarios where we need to be thorough with this background is when after anatomic slow pathway ablation has been completed, a slower short VA interval tachycardia remains, and we need to decide whether this represents an ablation-related accelerated junctional rhythm of no clinical consequence or recurrent slower AV node reentry that requires ablation.

The approach can be exceedingly complex given that junctional tachycardia itself is a heterogenous group of disorders ranging from His bundle automatic tachycardia, compact AV junctional tachycardia, slow pathway region tachycardia with retrograde block, and reentrant varieties sometimes related to abnormal His bundle conduction. In addition, the retrograde atrial sequence both with junctional tachycardias as well as AV node reentry can vary along with intermittent or absent retrograde conduction all leading to several layers of enhanced complexity. Nevertheless, the electrophysiologist who carefully studies Dr Padanilam's chapter and explanation to understand the arrhythmia and the diagnostic maneuvers in their simplest state should be able to vary these principles when confronted with more complex scenarios.

SECTION D

Supraventricular Tachyarrhythmias: Atrial Tachycardia, Flutter and Fibrillation

CHAPTER 21

Chrishan J Nalliah, Jonathan M Kalman

Focal Atrial Tachycardia and its Differentiation from Macroreentrant Atrial Tachycardia

LIST OF ABBREVIATIONS

AF	Atrial Fibrillation	PPI	Postpacing Interval
ANS	Autonomic Nervous System	PV	Pulmonary Vein
AT	Atrial Tachycardia	RA	Right Atrium
AV	Atrioventricular	RSPV	Right Superior Pulmonary Vein
CL	Cycle Length	SHD	Structural Heart Disease
CT	Crista Terminalis	SVT	Supraventricular Tachycardia
LSPV	Left Superior Pulmonary Vein	TCL	Tachycardia Cycle Length

INTRODUCTION

Atrial tachycardia (AT) can be broadly categorized based on its mechanism as focal or reentrant. Focal AT is characterized as a fast rhythm from a discrete origin, discharging at a rate that is generally regular, and conducting in a centrifugal manner throughout the atria.[1] Mechanisms that underlie focal AT include automaticity, triggered activity and microreentry.

Reentry refers to the presence of a circuit in the atria capable of sustaining repetitive circuitous atrial activation. Onset requires unidirectional conduction block and a region of slowed conduction is frequently present, such that the depolarizing wave-front does not encounter nonrefractory tissue. **(Figures 21.1A and B)**.

Reentry phenomena can be further classified as micro- or macroreentrant in character. By definition, macroreentry refers to circuits that are subtended by myocardium that spans > 2 cm.

The mechanism of focal tachycardias is not always readily determined by electrophysiologic techniques and it may be difficult to distinguish microreentry from automaticity or triggered activity.[2] From a practical standpoint attempts at distinguishing the underlying mechanism of focal AT is of relatively limited value. Diagnosis of focal versus macro reentrant AT has greater clinical and prognostic relevance. Thus, we will focus on this distinction in the present chapter.

Focal AT can present at any age and can occur in both normal (idiopathic) and diseased hearts (structural heart disease). It represents 3–17% of supraventricular tachycardia (SVT) cases referred for ablation.[1] Macroreentrant ATs are frequently associated with regions of atrial scar and are often noted in the context of structural heart disease, prior cardiac surgery and increasingly after catheter ablation of atrial fibrillation (AF).

Focal AT usually has a benign prognosis. However, 8–10% of patients with focal AT may develop a tachycardia-mediated cardiomyopathy.[3,4] Medi et al.[4] noted that focal AT leading to cardiomyopathy was more commonly associated with younger age, male gender and tended to be slower. Focal AT arising from the appendage has a high tendency to be incessant and thus, is more frequently associated with development of cardiomyopathy.

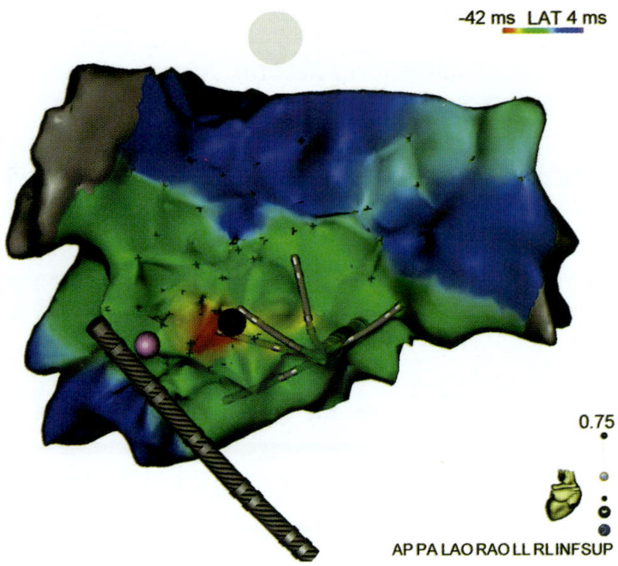

Figure 21.1A: Electroanatomic map of focal atrial tachycardia (AT) in a 24-year-old woman with recurrent palpitations. Characteristic of focal AT, activation spreads centrifugally from a single point. Red denotes earliest activation and blue/purple latest activation on a continuous color scale

AT mechanism is related to the atrial substrate maintaining the tachycardia which determines the mapping and ablation strategy. Thus, the first step when approaching AT from an electrophysiologic perspective is to clearly establish its mechanism. In this chapter, we will outline an approach to differentiate atrial tachycardia mechanism; specifically focal from macroreentrant AT.

FOCAL VERSUS MACROREENTRANT AT

At the outset it should be appreciated that AT mechanism is rarely distinguished utilizing any single criteria. All aspects of clinical and electrophysiologic evaluation should be considered to establish the mechanism. This includes:

- Clinical evaluation
- Surface ECG characteristics
- Electrophysiologic study
- Ablation strategy.

Clinical Evaluation

Clinical History

Determination of AT mechanism begins with careful consideration of the clinical context. As previously mentioned, focal AT classically occurs in patients without structural heart disease (SHD) but it can also occur when SHD

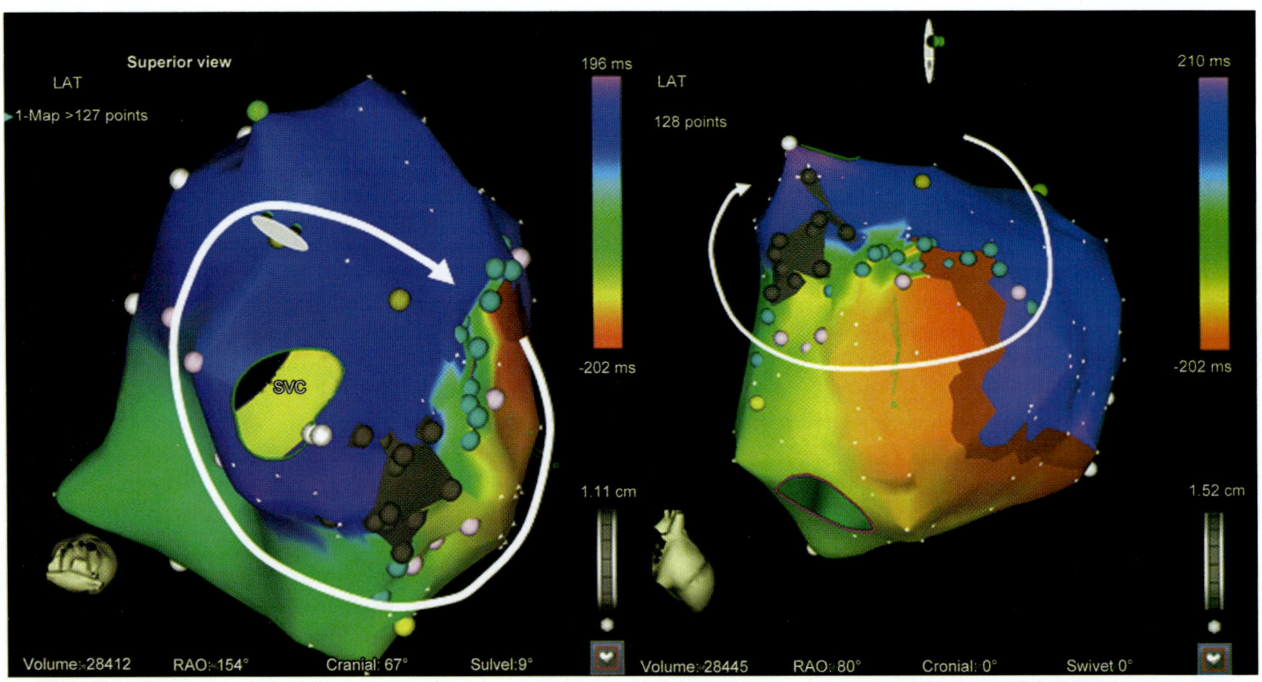

Figure 21.1B: Electroanatomic map of reentrant atrial tachycardia (AT) in a 52-year-old male patient with past history of atrial septal defect repair. Red denotes earliest activation and purple latest activation on a continuous color scale. Reentry is characterized by progressively later areas around the reentry circuit until the head meets tail (i.e. early meets late). The location around the SVC is diagnostic of upper loop reentry.

is present. Macroreentry typically occurs in the presence of atrial scar either related to prior surgery, atrial remodeling (e.g. in atrial stretch and heart failure) or occasionally spontaneously without obvious cause. Scar provides the appropriate milieu to stabilize reentrant circuits. Therefore, in the setting of a normal atrium, focal AT is the more likely mechanism for AT, while both mechanisms remain possibilities in a diseased atrium. Reentry has classically been described in the context of previous cardiac surgery, structural heart disease and more recently following catheter ablation for AF.

Tachycardia Profile

Clinical tachycardia behavior also provides insight into its mechanism. Focal AT is usually characterized by bursts of tachycardia, while reentrant AT tends to be sustained and protracted. Secondly, response to adenosine may provide some indications of tachycardia mechanism. Focal AT can be influenced by autonomic tone. Therefore, some cases of focal AT are susceptible to termination by adenosine. In contrast, adenosine administration during macroreentrant AT usually results in transient AV block without tachycardia termination.[5]

ECG Evaluation

Classically, atrial macroreentry causes the appearance of continuous undulation of the P-wave or flutter wave. In contrast, focal tachycardia more frequently demonstrates discrete P-waves separated by an isoelectric interval. It has been suggested that P-wave duration <160 ms and P-wave to atrial cycle length ratio of <45% indicates focal versus reentrant atrial activation.[6] However, there are many exceptions and one must be very circumspect about using the P-wave appearance to determine atrial tachycardia mechanism.

The P-wave can be utilized to approximately localize focal atrial tachycardia when the morphology is clearly discernible **(Flow chart 21.1)**. However, vector analysis is possible only when normal atrial conduction can be assumed. Thus, the surface ECG is of minimal utility for localizing ectopic AT in the diseased atrium.[7]

Secondly, during tachycardia the P-wave is often completely obscured by the QRS-complex or fused in varying degrees with the T-wave or sinus focus, making it difficult to interpret.[8]

Electrophysiologic Study

The approach to AT in the EP lab comprises three main steps: determination of AT mechanism, localization and ablation.

Atrial Cycle Length Stability

Stability of atrial cycle length (CL) provides a clue to the tachycardia mechanism. The atrial cycle length of macro-reentrant tachycardia is typically stable because the reentry circuit is not influenced by other factors. However, the focus in focal AT is often under the influence of the autonomic nervous system (ANS), which can result in a variable atrial cycle length.

Entrainment

Macroreentrant circuits can be readily entrained. When 2 sites >2 cm apart can be entrained and are within the circuit [based on postpacing interval (PPI) criteria], then macroreentry is defined. Some focal reentrant tachycardias can also be entrained but the PPI-TCL in this case will only

Flow chart 21.1: A P-wave algorithm that determines the origin of focal atrial tachycardia in normal hearts

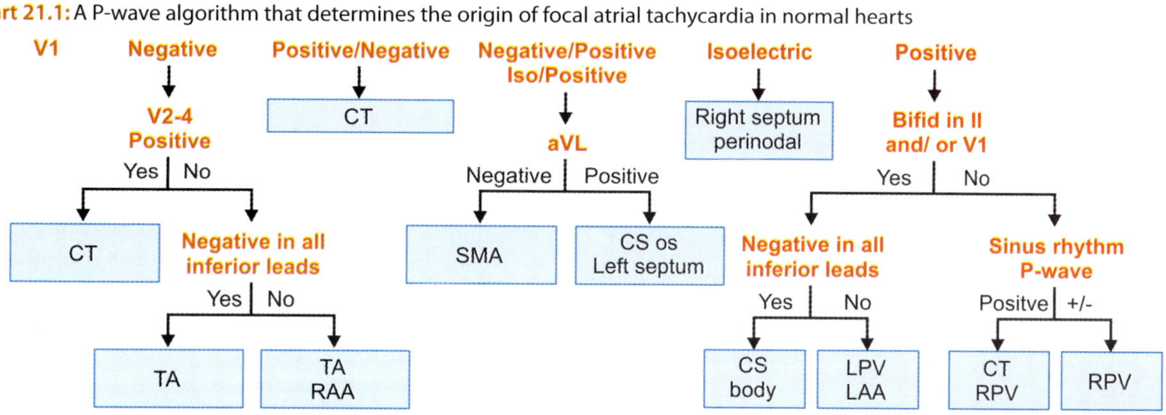

Abbreviations: CS, coronary sinus; CT, crista terminalis; LAA, left atrial appendage; LPV, left pulmonary veins; RAA, right atrial appendage; RPV, right pulmonary veins; SMA, superior mitral annulus; TA, tricuspid annulus

From: Kistler PM et al. P-wave morphology in focal atrial tachycardia: development of an algorithm to predict the anatomic site of origin. J Am Coll Cardiol. 2006;48:1010-7

be "in the circuit" at or immediately adjacent to the site of focal origin. Entrainment is thus, a very useful electrophysiologic maneuver for establishing the mechanism of AT. Waldo's traditional criteria for entrainment also include constant and progressive fusion. Thus, macroreentry can be reset with fusion. In contrast, pacing during a focal tachycardia may reset the tachycardia but reset with fusion is impossible.

The difference between the AT CL and postpacing interval (PPI-TCL) indicates the proximity of the pacing site to the circuit; a shorter PPI-TCL indicates greater proximity to the circuit. We use entrainment pacing with cycle length 10–20 ms less than the TCL in order to avoid introducing decrement by pacing at shorter cycle lengths. If the entraining cycle length is too short, it is possible to introduce decrement into the circuit, which will prolong the PPI and produce an erroneous result. It is also important to initiate entrainment with synchronization to the entraining electrode in order to avoid initial introduction of a tight-coupled stimulus, which may terminate or change the circuit. When entrainment is "in" at two sites more than 2 cm apart, the presence of macroreentry is confirmed.

Where the macroreentrant circuits location is suspected, such as in typical atrial flutter, entrainment should be performed at multiple locations within the purported circuit to demonstrate that all points do coincide with circuit route.[9] Entrainment maneuvers performed within a circuit will result in a PPI-TCL of 0.

A left versus right atrial circuit can be predicted following entrainment from the right atrium (RA). PPI-TCL ≤ 50 ms predicts a right atrial circuit and conversely > 50 ms implies a left atrial circuit. Entrainment from multiple atrial locations can facilitate circuit localization.[10]

Overdrive Pacing

Regardless of the mechanism of AT, focal AT can be overridden by atrial over-drive pacing. The PPI-TCL after atrial overdrive pacing of focal AT has a direct relationship to proximity of the pacing site to the focus, and may be clinically useful in finding a successful ablation site.[11]

Activation Mapping

Atrial activation mapping in its purest form refers to denotation of activation times to various points within the atrium to demonstrate directionality of wave-front propagation during tachycardia. This can be performed with point-by-point mapping using a single catheter or by deployment of multipolar catheters within the region of interest. Reentry is demonstrated by sequential circuitous electrode activation covering the entire cycle length.

Centrifugal activation emanating from a focal point versus sequential circuitous activation demonstrating reentry can be differentiated. Focal activation is represented by a localized region of earliest activation. Activation becomes progressively later distal to this point **(Figure 21.1A)**.

High density, three-dimensional (3D) electroanatomic mapping (contact or noncontact mapping) can delineate the reentrant circuit with the use of activation maps represented as a continuous progression of colors. A key point with activation mapping using electroanatomic mapping systems in macroreentrant circuits is that early activation is not applicable to any specific point in the circuit as activation is continuous and the origin of activation is always arbitrary with respect to the particular reference chosen for illustration. Thus, color coding will be represented in red or white at the site with earliest activation with respect to the arbitrarily defined zero point and will progress through a spectrum of colors to purple representing latest activation again with respect to the arbitrarily chosen point. Activation timing should span the entire cycle length of a macro-reentrant circuit. Where "earliest" meets "latest" activation in a continuous circuit is the point where "head meets tail" which is again an arbitrary anatomic point determined by choice of the zero point **(Figure 21.1B)**.

Dependence on circuit reentry is characterized by a region where early meets late activation. The most common example of this, which will be discussed in greater detail in subsequent chapters, is the use of a multipole catheter around the tricuspid annulus to map typical atrial flutter. Wave front propagation around the tricuspid annulus is represented by sequential activation of adjacent electrodes in an anticlockwise direction around the tricuspid annulus. Smaller circuits require more densely spaced electrodes to demonstrate sequential activation. Activation mapping of microreentry results in a map that is similar to focal AT. Relatively broad spacing of mapping electrodes results in poor spatial resolution that may not capture or delineate differences in timing of activation within a small region of atrial tissue. More recently, high-density catheters have been developed to enable mapping in higher resolution to facilitate delineation of critical components of smaller circuits.[12,13]

Additionally, electrophysiological mapping of the atrium allows characterization of the substrate maintaining AT and may provide some mechanistic cues. As previously discussed, macroreentry is often associated with diseased atrial tissue characterized by low voltage (e.g. scar) that provides a non-conducting obstacle capable of sustaining reentry. The raw signals utilized to perform activation mapping can also be used to generate a voltage map. Regions of scar often sustain reentry and can be targeted for further electrophysiologic interrogation. Although substrate characterization can be a useful adjunct to other electrophysiologic maneuvers, low voltage regions alone do not provide sufficient evidence for AT mechanism diagnosis. Focal mechanisms can exist in a scarred atrium **(Figure 21.2)** or alternatively both AT mechanisms can co-exist in the same atria.

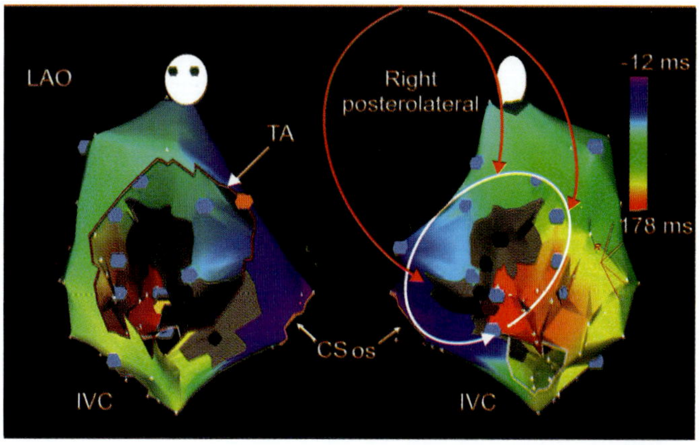

Figure 21.2: Electroanatomical map of an AT in a patient with prior atrial septal defect repair and cavotricuspid isthmus (CTI) ablation. A history of past atrial surgery does not automatically indicate macroreentrant tachycardia. The AT could not be successfully entrained at various sites around the tricuspid annulus. Consistent with this, the electroanatomic map clearly demonstrated focal AT with an early location lateral to the atriotomy site

Abbreviations: CS, coronary sinus; LAO, left anterior oblique; TA, tricuspid annulus; IVC, inferior vena cava

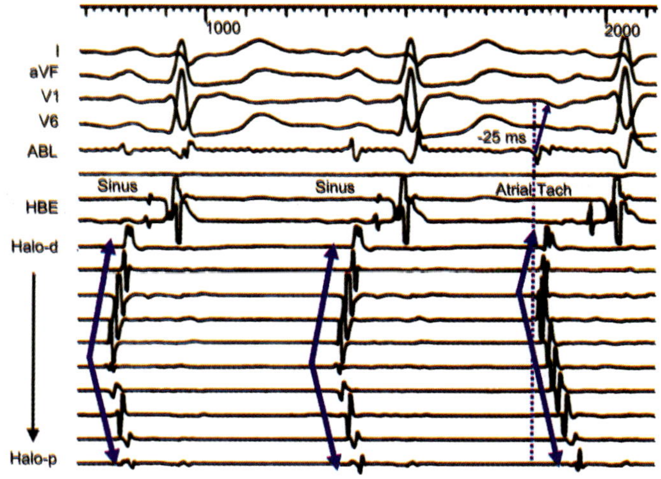

Figure 21.3: Activation mapping of the tricuspid annulus using a multipolar catheter. The activation sequence of a beat of AT is significantly different to the sinus beat. The site of successful ablation is on time with earliest activation of the multipolar catheter and −25 ms earlier than the surface P-wave and has both atrial and ventricular electrograms indicating tricuspid annular location. Note the abnormal morphology of the surface compared with the sinus P-wave

Abbreviations: d, distal; p, proximal; ABL, ablation catheter; Halo, multipolar catheter; HBE, His bundle electrogram

There are a number of limitations to mapping AT that must be borne in mind:

1. Acquisition of high fidelity electrograms to generate reliable activation maps require reproducible and preferably stable AT. However, ectopic AT often occurs in short bursts and become quiescent. Catheter trauma, anesthetic agents or changes of autonomic tone, can render a focal site quiescent making it challenging to map.
2. Catheters often cover only a limited portion of myocardium. A limited field of view may provide an erroneous impression of reentry or alternatively fail to capture reentry phenomena that occur beyond the field of view of the mapping catheters. A careful and methodical approach to activation mapping should be adopted.

Ablation Strategy

The tachycardia mechanism determines the curative ablation strategy. In focal AT, the critical focus that forms the target of ablation is assumed to arise at or near the earliest site of endocardial atrial activation **(Figure 21.3)**. The true focus may lie within the mid or epicardial layers of the atrial wall and break through the endocardial surface at the mapped position. While sometimes a single lesion or even catheter pressure can suppress focal AT, multiple lesions may be required to impact a concealed focal site. In contrast, successful ablation of macroreentry requires formation of a line of block within the reentry circuit that sustains AT. AT isthmus can be up to several centimeters in width (e.g. cavo tricuspid isthmus or the mitral isthmus) while at other times the critical isthmus can be very narrow and amenable to single point ablation. Tachycardia suppression with catheter pressure is less frequently a feature of macroreentry when the isthmus is wide but may occur at the site of a narrow isthmus. At these sites, subthreshold stimulation may terminate the tachycardia. The usual strategy for inducing conduction block within a circuit is to perform a line of ablation anchored to two nonconducting atrial regions such as an anatomic structure (like a valve annulus) or a region of scarring.

The site of successful AT ablation may in some circumstances harbor a fractionated electrogram that represents a region of slowed conduction critical for arrhythmia maintenance. However, it should be noted that similar signals can be located remote to regions of importance, and conversely regions of importance may be devoid of such signals. Therefore, fractionated atrial signals should only be considered of mechanistic importance where its location coincides with other electrophysiological markers indicating that the region is within the circuit. For example, regions of fractionation are often located at the crista terminalis (CT) which may not necessarily have pathophysiologic significance.

Recent data demonstrate that catheter contact force is a critical determinant for successful ablation. Developments in ablation catheter technology enable real time evaluation of tissue contact force.[14,15] Kumar et al.[15] observed that contact force in the context of typical atrial flutter ablation was highly variable even when other physiological and electrophysiological parameters indicated satisfactory contact. Adequate tissue contact correlated with better acute success rates.

COMMON SITES OF FOCAL ATRIAL TACHYCARDIA

Use of P-wave morphology to determine the anatomic location of focal tachycardia is limited by the spatial resolution of the surface ECG.[8] P-wave morphology in V1 can be utilized to broadly differentiate right from left sided ATs. Right ATs are characterized by a negative or a biphasic (+/–) P-wave in V1, while left ATs are characterized by a positive or biphasic (–/+) P-wave. However, as the anatomic location approaches the septum, the accuracy of this approach breaks down. Differentiation of left septal from right septal AT and superior CT from right superior pulmonary vein (RSPV) AT can be challenging due to anatomic proximity **(Figure 21.3)**.

- *Crista terminalis:* The CT is a common site for right AT comprising up to two-thirds of RA tachycardias. The distribution of RA tachycardia frequency in the CT appears to follow a gradation, with greatest frequency located superiorly and the lowest inferiorly. The CT is a complex structure consisting of marked anisotropy and poor transverse cell-to-cell coupling, making it well-suited for arrhythmia-genesis. Superiorly orientated sites of ectopy demonstrate upright P-waves in the inferior leads (II, III and aVF) while inferiorly situated sites demonstrate inverted P-waves inferiorly. Precordial lead V1 demonstrates a biphasic P-wave (positive-negative) due to initial right followed by left atrial activation. Right to left activation results in a negative P-wave in aVR and positive P-wave in aVL. The site of successful ablation of CT right AT often harbors fractionated signals.[16]
- *Coronary sinus:* The coronary sinus is a complex structure consisting of interwoven fibers and marked anisotropy particularly at the ostium. Ectopy can arise in any aspect of the coronary sinus, but the os contains the vast majority of foci. Atrial activation is directed superiorly due to the os' inferior-septal location. The P-wave is, therefore, negative in the inferior leads and positive in aVL. Atrial tachycardias, originating several centimeters inside the coronary sinus have also been described.
- *Tricuspid annulus:* The tricuspid annulus is also a common site of origin for focal atrial tachycardias. Various investigators have noted cells with 'nodal-like' properties distributed across the tricuspid annulus, leading to speculation that these may form the substrate for focal AT.[17,18] P-wave morphology is largely determined by the anatomic site of the focus around the tricuspid ring. The P-wave is usually inverted in V1, inverted in lead III, and upright in aVL. The P-wave is also inverted or biphasic across the precordium from V2 to V5.[19]
- *Pulmonary veins:* Once localized to the left atrium, the potential sources of ectopy include the pulmonary veins (PVs), left atrial appendage and coronary sinus body. The most common sites of left atrial tachycardias are the PVs. Right-sided PVs have positive P-waves in V1-V6 and are positive in lead I. Left sided PVs have bifid-positive P-waves in V1/II and isoelectric/negative in lead I. Differentiation of RSPV from superior CT and LSPV from appendage AT can be difficult due to anatomic proximity.
- *Venous structures:* Venous structures within the atria can harbor focal ectopy that drive AT. These structures include the superior vena cava, inferior vena cava, pulmonary veins and the vein of Marshall. Focal activity within structures can be at a higher rate than atrial activation, due to exit block into the atria. Venous structures within proximity of the site of earliest atrial activation should be explored to determine whether it is responsible for driving tachycardia **(Figure 21.4)**.

CONCLUSION

We have outlined an approach to diagnosis and treatment of focal AT, and importantly its differentiation from macroreentrant AT. Correct differentiation of tachycardia mechanism remains critical for successful treatment. Despite technological evolutions, fundamental principles of clinical electrophysiology including clinical history, ECG interpretation and basic laboratory maneuvers (e.g. entrainment, activation mapping) remain central to successful diagnosis and treatment. However, advancements such as high-density mapping and contact force sensing catheters are poised to enhance the efficacy and speed of these complex procedures.

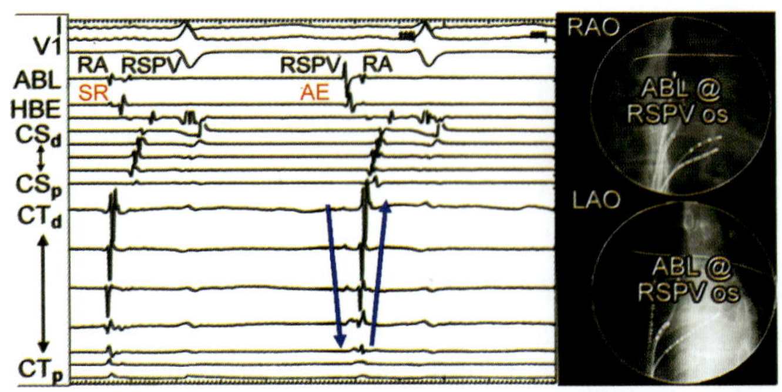

Figure 21.4: Focal atrial tachycardia (AT) arising from the right superior pulmonary vein (RSPV). Multipolar linear catheter deployed superior-inferiorly at the crista terminalis (CT) demonstrates earliest activation at the superior CT. However, probing of the RSPV demonstrated that the tachycardia focus was within the RSPV. Activation of the CT represented far field activation

Abbreviations: AE, atrial ectopic; RA, right atrium; SR, sinus rhythm, other abbreviations as in previous figures

REFERENCES

1. Page RL, Joglar JA, Caldwell MA, Calkins H, Conti JB, Deal BJ, Estes NA, 3rd, Field ME, Goldberger ZD, Hammill SC, Indik JH, Lindsay BD, Olshansky B, Russo AM, Shen WK, Tracy CM, Al-Khatib SM. 2015 ACC/AHA/HRS Guideline for the Management of Adult Patients With Supraventricular Tachycardia: A Report of the American College of Cardiology/ American Heart Association Task Force on Clinical Practice Guidelines and the Heart Rhythm Society. J Am Coll Cardiol, 2015.
2. Sanders P, Hocini M, Jais P, Hsu LF, Takahashi Y, Rotter M, Scavee C, Pasquie JL, Sacher F, Rostock T, Nalliah CJ, Clementy J, Haissaguerre M. Characterization of focal atrial tachycardia using high-density mapping. J Am Coll Cardiol. 2005;46: 2088-99.
3. Ju W, Yang B, Li M, Zhang F, Chen H, Gu K, Yu J, Cao K, Chen M. Tachycardiomyopathy complicated by focal atrial tachycardia: incidence, risk factors, and long-term outcome. J Cardiovasc Electrophysiol. 2014;25:953-7.
4. Medi C, Kalman JM, Haqqani H, Vohra JK, Morton JB, Sparks PB, Kistler PM. Tachycardia-mediated cardiomyopathy secondary to focal atrial tachycardia: long-term outcome after catheter ablation. J Am Coll Cardiol. 2009;53:1791-7.
5. Higa S, Tai CT, Lin YJ, Liu TY, Lee PC, Huang JL, Yuniadi Y, Huang BH, Hsieh MH, Lee SH, Kuo JY, Lee KT, Chen SA. Mechanism of adenosine-induced termination of focal atrial tachycardia. J Cardiovasc Electrophysiol. 2004;15:1387-93.
6. Brown JP, Krummen DE, Feld GK, Narayan SM. Using electrocardiographic activation time and diastolic intervals to separate focal from macro-re-entrant atrial tachycardias. J Am Coll Cardiol. 2007;49:1965-73.
7. Chugh A, Latchamsetty R, Oral H, Elmouchi D, Tschopp D, Reich S, Igic P, Lemerand T, Good E, Bogun F, Pelosi F, Jr., Morady F. Characteristics of cavotricuspid isthmus-dependent atrial flutter after left atrial ablation of atrial fibrillation. Circulation. 2006;113:609-15.
8. Kistler PM, Roberts-Thomson KC, Haqqani HM, Fynn SP, Singarayar S, Vohra JK, Morton JB, Sparks PB, Kalman JM. P-wave morphology in focal atrial tachycardia: development of an algorithm to predict the anatomic site of origin. J Am Coll Cardiol. 2006;48:1010-7.
9. Kalman JM, Olgin JE, Saxon LA, Lee RJ, Scheinman MM, Lesh MD. Electrocardiographic and electrophysiologic characterization of atypical atrial flutter in man: use of activation and entrainment mapping and implications for catheter ablation. J Cardiovasc Electrophysiol. 1997;8:121-44.
10. Miyazaki H, Stevenson WG, Stephenson K, Soejima K, Epstein LM. Entrainment mapping for rapid distinction of left and right atrial tachycardias. Heart Rhythm. 2006;3: 516-23.
11. Mohamed U, Skanes AC, Gula LJ, Leong-Sit P, Krahn AD, Yee R, Subbiah R, Klein GJ. A novel pacing maneuver to localize focal atrial tachycardia. J Cardiovasc Electrophysiol. 2007;18: 1-6.
12. Anter E, Tschabrunn CM, Contreras-Valdes FM, Li J, Josephson ME. Pulmonary vein isolation using the Rhythmia mapping system: Verification of intracardiac signals using the Orion mini-basket catheter. Heart Rhythm. 2015;12:1927-34.
13. Nakagawa H, Ikeda A, Sharma T, Lazzara R, Jackman WM. Rapid high resolution electroanatomical mapping: evaluation of a new system in a canine atrial linear lesion model. Circ Arrhythm Electrophysiol. 2012;5:417-24.
14. Kumar S, Chan M, Lee J, Wong MC, Yudi M, Morton JB, Spence SJ, Halloran K, Kistler PM, Kalman JM. Catheter-tissue contact force determines atrial electrogram characteristics before and lesion efficacy after antral pulmonary vein isolation in humans. J Cardiovasc Electrophysiol. 2014;25:122-9.
15. Kumar S, Morton JB, Lee G, Halloran K, Kistler PM, Kalman JM. High Incidence of Low Catheter-Tissue Contact Force at the Cavotricuspid Isthmus During Catheter Ablation of Atrial Flutter: Implications for Achieving Isthmus Block. J Cardiovasc Electrophysiol. 2015;26:826-31.
16. Kalman JM, Olgin JE, Karch MR, Hamdan M, Lee RJ, Lesh MD. "Cristal tachycardias": origin of right atrial tachycardias from the crista terminalis identified by intracardiac echocardiography. J Am Coll Cardiol, 1998;31:451-9.
17. McGuire MA, de Bakker JM, Vermeulen JT, Moorman AF, Loh P, Thibault B, Vermeulen JL, Becker AE, Janse MJ. Atrioventricular junctional tissue. Discrepancy between histological and electrophysiological characteristics. Circulation. 1996;94: 571-7.
18. Wit AL, Fenoglio JJ, Jr. Hordof AJ, Reemtsma K. Ultrastructure and transmembrane potentials of cardiac muscle in the human anterior mitral valve leaflet. Circulation. 1979;59: 1284-92.
19. Morton JB, Sanders P, Das A, Vohra JK, Sparks PB, Kalman JM. Focal atrial tachycardia arising from the tricuspid annulus: electrophysiologic and electrocardiographic characteristics. J Cardiovasc Electrophysiol. 2001;12:653-9.

EDITORS' SUMMARY

In this chapter, one of the pioneers who describe the mechanisms, physiology, and anatomy of atrial tachycardias targeted for ablation (Professor Kalman) and colleagues provide an updated guide to atrial tachycardia in the contemporary ablation era. The relationship between the mechanism for tachycardia (automaticity versus reentry) and the approach for mapping and ablation is carefully described. The student of electrophysiology will benefit from a detailed study of this chapter in conjunction with the chapters on mapping techniques (Chapter 8), three-dimensional mapping (Chapter 9), entrainment (Chapter 43), and anatomy (Chapter 6). The figures themselves are extraordinarily clear and instructive, and after carefully reading through the chapter, the electrophysiologist will benefit from using the figures as a review or test to refamiliarize ourselves with the concepts outlined prior to performing what can be complex procedures.

CHAPTER 22

Yanfei Yang, Melvin Scheinman

Atrial Flutter: Classification, Mechanisms and Management

LIST OF ABBREVIATIONS

AF	Atrial Fibrillation	LA	Left Atrium
AFL	Atrial Flutter	LAO	Left Anterior Oblique
AV	Atrioventricular	LLR	Lower Loop Reentry
CCW	Counter-clockwise	MA	Mitral Annulus
CS	Coronary Sinus	PPI	Postpacing Interval
CT	Crista Terminalis	PV	Pulmonary Vein
CTI	Cavotricuspid Isthmus	RA	Right Atrium
CW	Clockwise	RF	Radiofrequency
DWR	Double-wave Reentry	SVC	Superior Vena Cava
FO	Fossa Ovalis	TA	Tricuspid Annulus
IIR	Intraisthmus Reentry	TCL	Tachycardia Cycle Length
IVC	Inferior Vena Cava	ULR	Upper Loop Reentry

INTRODUCTION

Atrial flutter (AFL) was first described as a rapid, regular excitation of the atrium by MacWilliam and was subsequently differentiated from atrial fibrillation (AF) by Jolly and Ritchie,[1,2] of which the ECGs inscribed by these authors are compatible with a counter-clockwise cavotricuspid isthmus (CTI) dependent flutter.

With induction of sustained flutter in dogs, Sir Thomas Lewis and associates mapped the arrhythmia by direct recordings from the atrial epicardial surface together with surface ECG recordings.[3] They showed that the atrial activation was in an orderly manner involving both vena cava, and there was an absence of a true diastole which explained the surface pattern. The circulating wave front was inscribed either in a caudocranial or cranial-caudal fashion in the right atrium (RA). In their experiments, they also suspected a rotation around the atrioventricular (AV) valves. However, their observations were not universally accepted. Others favored enhanced automaticity as a mechanism of AFL.[4]

It is uncommon to induce stable AFL in normal canines. But by introducing a crush lesion between the cavae, Rosenblueth and Garcia Ramos successfully created a canine model of sustained AFL and found that the flutter wave front rotated around the crush lesion using epicardial mapping.[5] Of interest, they also noted that in some animals, an additional lesion that "was made starting at the lower edge of the orifice of the inferior vena cava (IVC) and extending the limit... toward the AV groove" could stop the flutter without reinducibility. The lesion is identical to the lesion currently used to ablate CTI-dependent AFL.

HISTORY OF NONPHARMACOLOGIC TREATMENT IN PATIENTS WITH ATRIAL FLUTTER

In the late 1970s, Waldo and his colleagues studied patients with postoperative flutter using fixed atrial electrodes.[6,7] They confirmed that the AFL cycle length was remarkably consistent with mean variations of less than 4 ms. Moreover in their study, they used entrainment for detecting the reentrant circuit as well as for discerning where the critical region is for tachycardia maintenance.[7] Another interesting finding from their studies is the relationship between AF and AFL in those patients in whom the onset of AFL was recorded, that the transition to AFL was preceded by short episodes of rapid transitional rhythm (or AF).[8]

Using a canine model with the intercaval lesion extended into the right atrial free wall, the studies by Frame et al. not only revealed evidence of electrical activation around the tricuspid orifice, but also proved the reentrant circuit around the annulus by entrainment pacing and showed the presence of an excitable gap.[9,10] These studies established the need of barriers for tachycardia initiation and perpetuation. The reentrant nature of AFL was further demonstrated in other studies.[11-15]

In a notable work by Klein and Guiraudon, who mapped two patients with AFL in the operating room, the evidence of a large right atrial reentrant circuit with its narrowest part of the circuit between the tricuspid valve and the IVC was revealed; and the flutter was successfully treated by cryoablation around the coronary sinus (CS) and surrounding atrium.[15]

Following the report of Klein et al., several studies used high energy shocks in an attempt to cure AFL (Saoudi,[16] Chauvin and Breckenmacher[17]).

In the early 1990s, both Drs Feld and Cosio reported treating patients with AFL by applying radiofrequency (RF) energy to the CTI region for disruption of AFL circuit.[18,19] In an elegant study Feld et al. used endocardial mapping techniques and entrainment pacing to prove that the area posterior or inferior to the CS was a critical portion of the AFL circuit and application of RF energy to this region could terminate AFL.[18] Cosio et al. used similar techniques but ablated the area more laterally, between the tricuspid annulus (TA) and IVC.[19] The latter approach becomes the basis for current ablation of CTI-dependent flutter.

TYPES OF ATRIAL FLUTTER AND THEIR CLINICAL IMPLICATIONS

Atrial flutter is rapid regular single macroreentrant atrial arrhythmia with little or no isoelectric interval, and was historically defined as typical, reverse typical or atypical AFLs. However, with increasing knowledge of its circuits and mechanisms, a new terminology appears to be appropriate.

Cavotricuspid Isthmus Dependent Atrial Flutter

In the majority of RA flutters, the CTI is a critical part of the reentrant circuit, and is also the target for AFL ablation.

Counterclockwise (CCW) or Clockwise (CW) AFL

These are macroreentrant circuits around the TA, with the flutter wave front activation in a CCW or CW fashion in the left anterior oblique (LAO) projection.[20-25] Counterclockwise AFL is the most common and the surface ECG shows continuous sawtooth-like flutter wave dominantly negative in the inferior leads (II, III and aVF) and positive in V1; whereas CW flutter shows positive waves in the inferior leads and negative waves in V1 **(Figures 22.1A and B)**. Both CCW and CW AFL can be seen in patients with or without structural heart disease or prior cardiac surgery. CTI-dependent flutter is readily diagnosed with entrainment mapping in the isthmus. The characteristic finding is concealed entrainment with a postpacing interval <30 ms compared with the tachycardia cycle length **(Figures 22.2 and 22.3)**. Ablation is usually begun from the inferior tricuspid valve region (anterior) with an ablation line drawn posteriorly to the inferior vena cava.

Double-wave Reentry

The flutter circuits have an excitable gap. If a critical timed premature beat is able to invade the circuit with only antidromic block, i.e. it is able to propagate orthodromically, then 2 wave fronts may travel within the circuit simultaneously.[26] Thus, the arrhythmia is manifest by acceleration of the tachycardia rate but with identical surface and intracardiac electrogram morphology. Double-wave reentry is usually produced by extrastimuli and is usually short-lived, but may serve as a trigger for AF.[27]

Lower Loop Reentry

Lower loop reentry is a type of CTI-dependent flutter that is confined to the lower part of the RA with a reentrant circuit around the IVC.[28-30] It often co-exists with typical CCW or CW flutter and involves posterior breakthrough(s) across the crista terminalis (CT). Since the CTI is still a critical part of the circuit, LLR is curable by CTI ablation **(Figure 22.4)**. The surface morphology of LLR usually is similar to that of CCW or CW flutter.[31] In patients with LLR physiology, proof of bidirectional isthmus block after CTI ablation may be problematic. For example, pacing from the coronary sinus

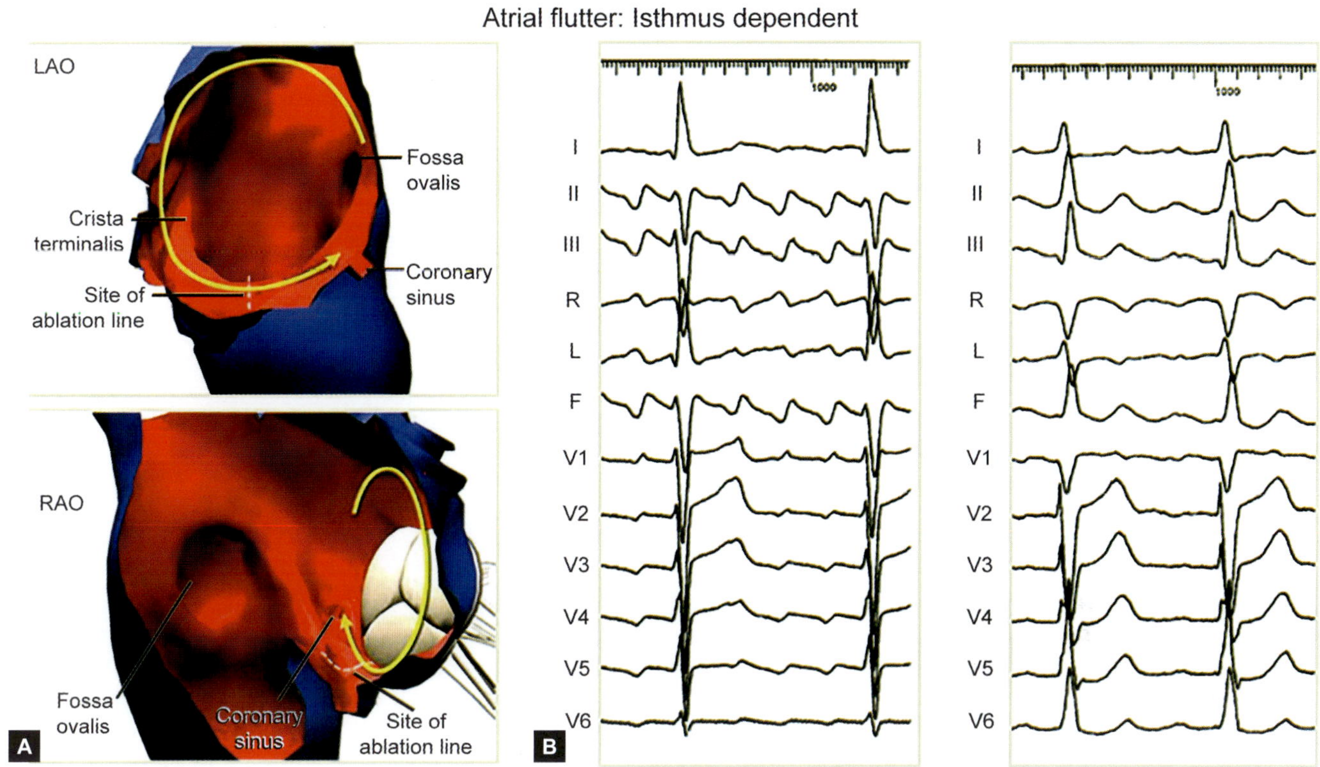

Figures 22.1A and B: Left anterior oblique (LAO) and right anterior oblique (RAO) projections of cavotricuspid isthmus dependent flutter (A) and typical ECG findings of counterclockwise (CCW) and clockwise (CW) flutter circuits (B)
Source: Adapted from the Mayo Foundation for Medical Education and Research

may produce a pattern on the duo-decapolar catheter identical to that of an isthmus leak despite complete CTI block. This problem can be obviated by insertion of a multipolar catheter across the isthmus into the coronary sinus. In this instance, pacing from the CS will clearly show block within the isthmus.

Intraisthmus Reentry

Intraisthmus reentry (IIR) is a novel reentrant circuit within the region of septal (medial) CTI and CS ostium.[32,33] In this flutter form, entrainment pacing from the anteroinferior (lateral) CTI shows PPI > TCL, indicating the lateral CTI is out of the reentrant circuit; whereas, pacing from the region of septal isthmus or CS ostium shows concealed entrainment with PPI = TCL. Fractionated or double potentials usually can be recorded in this area and can be entrained **(Figure 22.5)**. Applying RF energy at the site of maximal fractionated potentials can always abolish the tachycardia. IIR often occurs in patients who have undergone prior CTI ablation and may mimic recurrence of CTI flutter. Differentiation is readily made by entrainment of the lateral versus septal CTI. It is important to emphasize that IIR may occur even with complete bidirectional isthmus block. In this instance, flutter or pacing from the CS will produce block in the CTI and usually gives rise to a counter-clockwise pattern. If a leak in the isthmus is present then the activation pattern will change (simultaneous pattern).[33]

Non-Cavotricuspid Isthmus Dependent Atrial Flutter

Right Atrial Flutter Circuits

Scar-related RA macroreentrant Tachycardia

Previous studies have shown that macroreentrant tachycardia can occur in patients with or without atriotomy or congenital heart disease.[29,34,35] In the patients with such macroreentrant circuits, electroanatomic voltage maps from the RA often show "scar" or low-voltage area(s) which serves as the central obstacle or channel(s) for these reentrant circuits. The morphology of surface ECG may vary depending on where the scar(s) and low-voltage area(s) are and how the wave fronts exit the circuits. Frequently RA scar flutter occurs over lateral wall incisional scars which are present

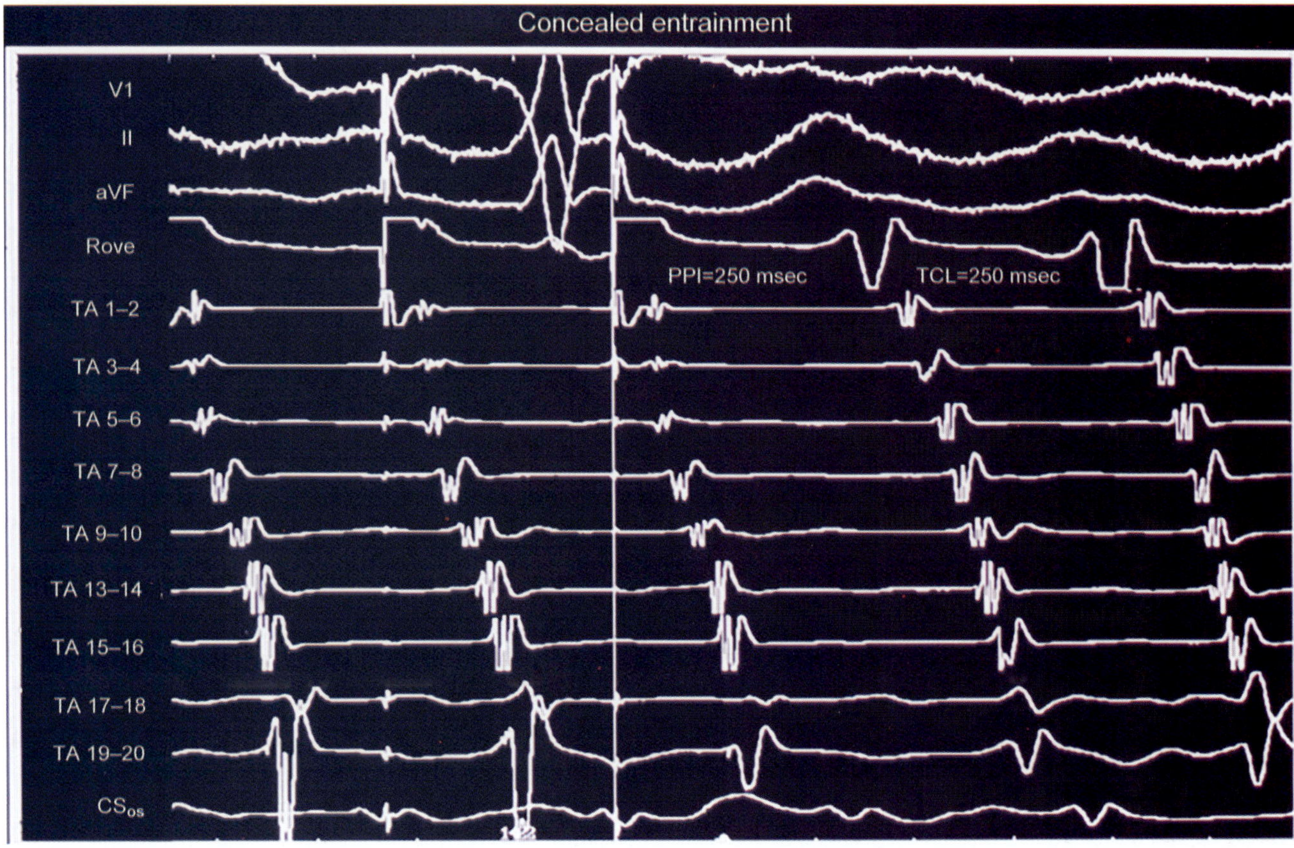

Figure 22.2: Entrainment pacing with duodecapolar catheter positioned across the tricuspid valve with TA 1–2 at the lateral isthmus. Note evidence of concealed entrainment (identical surface and intracardiac electrograms) with PPI (postpacing interval) equal to the tachycardia cycle length (TCL)

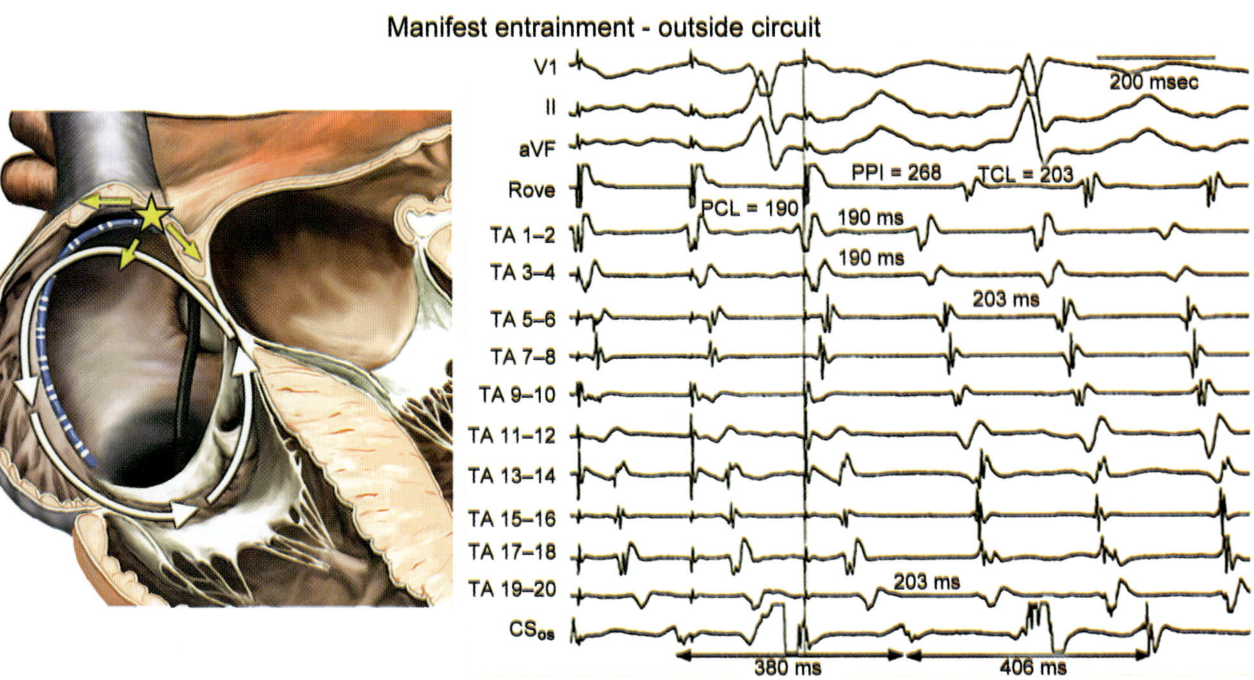

Figure 22.3: Pacing outside the flutter circuit shows manifest entrainment with PPI > TCL

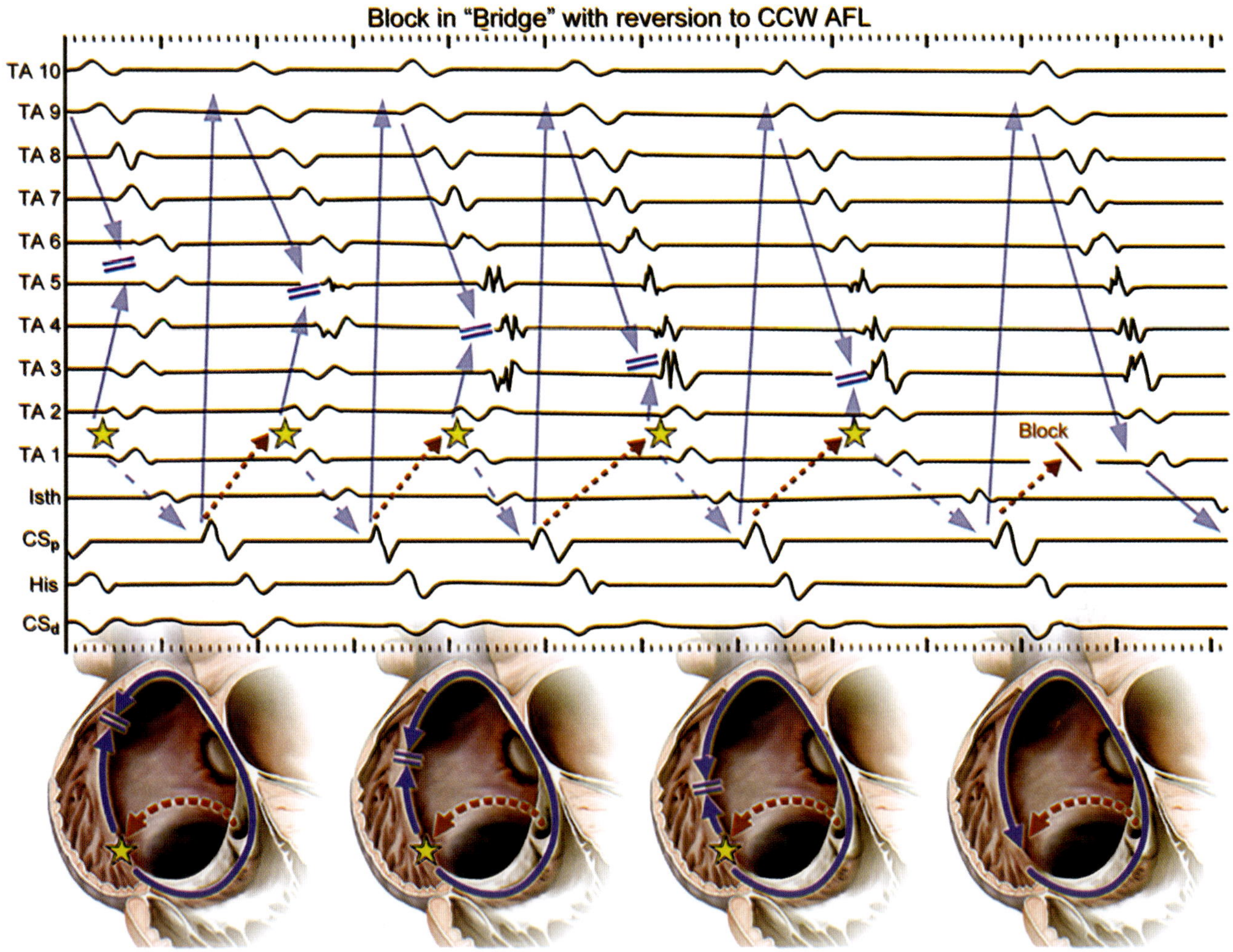

Figure 22.4: The schema at the bottom shows two potential flutter circuits with solid line showing typical CTI flutter while the dashed line shows the pattern of lower loop reentry (LLR). The first five beats show evidence of LLR with early break at TA 1 and collision at TA 5. The last complex shows reversion to typical CTI flutter

Source: Reprinted with permission from American Heart Association

after surgical correction of various congenital cardiac defects. The flutter circuit will rotate around the scar and is ablated by carrying the ablation from the center of the scar to the inferior vena cava. Of note is the possibility of double loop reentry involving a common isthmus between a CTI and lateral scar flutter circuits.

Upper Loop Reentry (ULR)

This is an atypical AFL involving the upper portion of RA with transverse conduction over the CT and wave front collision occurring at lower part of RA or within the CTI.[29,36] During this tachycardia, entrainment pacing in the region of CTI shows that the CTI is not part of the circuit, therefore, it is a non-CTI-dependent flutter. Upper loop reentry was initially felt to involve a reentrant circuit using the channel between the superior vena cava (SVC), fossa ovalis (FO) and CT.[29] A study by Tai et al. using non-contact mapping technique showed that this form of AFL was a macroreentrant tachycardia in the RA free wall with the CT as its functional central obstacle.[36] They successfully abolished ULR by linear ablation of the gap in the CT. Similar to LLR, ULR also can occur in conjunction with typical CW and/or CCW flutter, as well as LLR.

Left Atrial Flutter Circuits

Left AFL circuits are often related to AF ablation procedures. In recent years, these circuits have been better defined by use of electroanatomic or noncontact mapping techniques.[37]

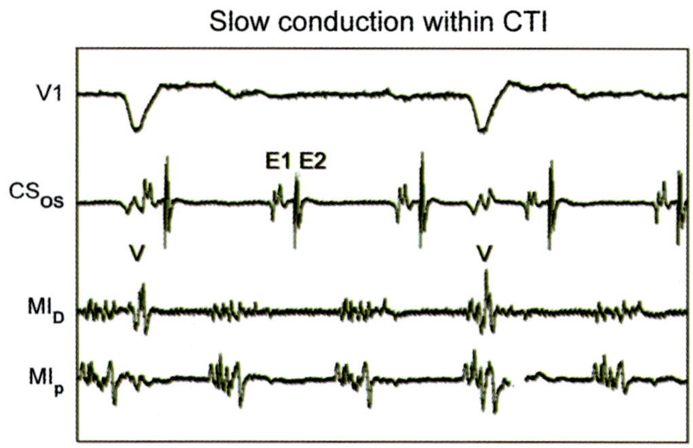

Figure 22.5: Characteristic intracardiac recording from a patient with intraisthmus reentry wherein Ml_P and Ml_D are recorded from the anterior-inferior cavotricuspid isthmus (CTI) adjacent to the coronary sinus (CS). Note the long-duration pan-diastolic potentials as well as the split potentials from the CS region

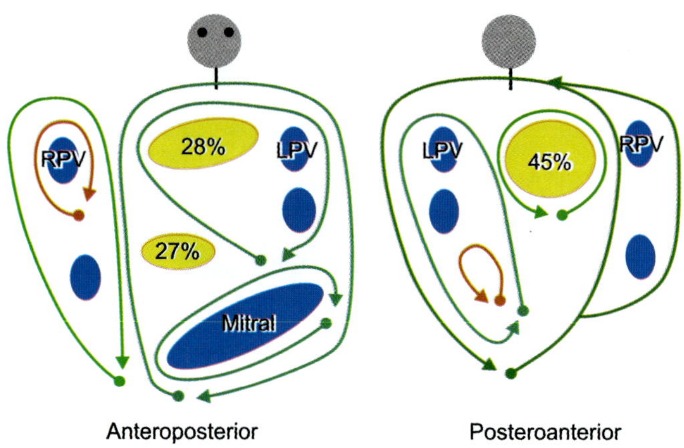

Figure 22.6: Major types of left atrial flutter patterns after AF ablation. These patterns may involve an isolated pulmonary vein, may be perimitral or due to a leak in the roof line

Abbreviations: LPV, left pulmonary veins; RPV, right pulmonary veins

Source: Jais P et al. Mapping and ablation of left atrial flutters. Circulation. 2000;101:2928-34. Reprinted with permission from American Heart Association

Cardiac surgery involving the left atrium (LA) or atrial septum or ablation of AF can produce different left flutter circuits **(Figure 22.6)**. But, left AFL circuits also can be found in patients without a history of atriotomy or prior ablation. Electroanatomic maps in these patients often show low-voltage or scar areas in the LA, which act as either a central obstacle or barrier in the circuit. The surface ECG of left AFLs are variable due to different reentrant circuits. Below are several common left flutter circuits.

Mitral Annular AFL

This AFL has a reentrant circuit around the mitral annulus (MA) either in a CCW or CW fashion. It is more common in patients with structural heart disease, but it has also been shown in patients without obvious structural heart disease.[31,37] The electroanatomic voltage map often shows scar or low-voltage area(s) on the posterior wall of LA as a posterior boundary of this circuit. The surface ECG of MA flutter can mimic CTI-dependent CCW or CW flutter, but usually shows low amplitude flutter waves in most of the 12 leads.[31] Mitral annular flutter is diagnosed when in circuit entrainment is found in response to both proximal and distal coronary sinus pacing or for pacing the proximal and distal left atrial annular sites. Ablation is usually performed by creating an ablation line from the left inferior pulmonary vein to the coronary sinus. This approach may prove difficult because of the coronary sinus musculature and often requires ablative lesions within the coronary sinus. If this approach fails a more anterior approach may be necessary.

Pulmonary Vein(s) with or without LA Scar Circuits

Various left AFL circuits involve the pulmonary veins (PVs), especially in patients with AF or mitral valve disease. Reentry can circle around one or more PVs and/or posterior scar or low-voltage area(s).[31,37] In order to cure these complex circuits, electroanatomic mapping is required to reveal the circuit and guide ablation **(Figure 22.7)**. Since these circuits are related to low-voltage or scar area(s), the surface ECG usually has low amplitude or flat flutter waves.

Atrial Flutter Related to Breaks in a Roof Line

A common procedure used for ablation of patients with persistent AF is construction of an ablation line between the upper left pulmonary venous orifices[38] known commonly as a roof line. One common source of atrial flutter after ablation is residual conduction through the roof line.[39] Three dimensional mapping and entrainment pacing is used to diagnoses this type of flutter. Ablative lesions are placed to seal the site of block and then pacing is utilized to prove bidirectional block across the roof line.

Left Atrial Flutter due to Septal Reentrant Circuits

An uncommon site of left atrial flutter relates to left septal circuits that rotate around the septum primum **(Figures 22.8A and B)**.[40] These circuits show entrainment in the region of the fossae on either the left or right atrium. Successful ablation involves creation of a flutter line from the septum primum to either the inferior pulmonary vein or mitral annulus to serve as a barrier to the flutter circuit.

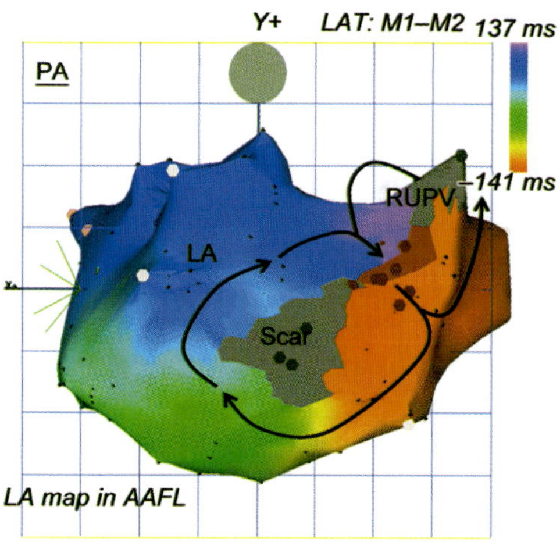

Figure 22.7: Electroanatomic activation map in a patient with left atrial (LA) flutter in the posterior-anterior (PA) project view. The activation map demonstrates a reentrant circuit (figure-of-8) around the right upper pulmonary vein (RUPV) and scar on the LA posterior wall, as shown by the arrows

Abbreviation: AAFL, atypical atrial flutter

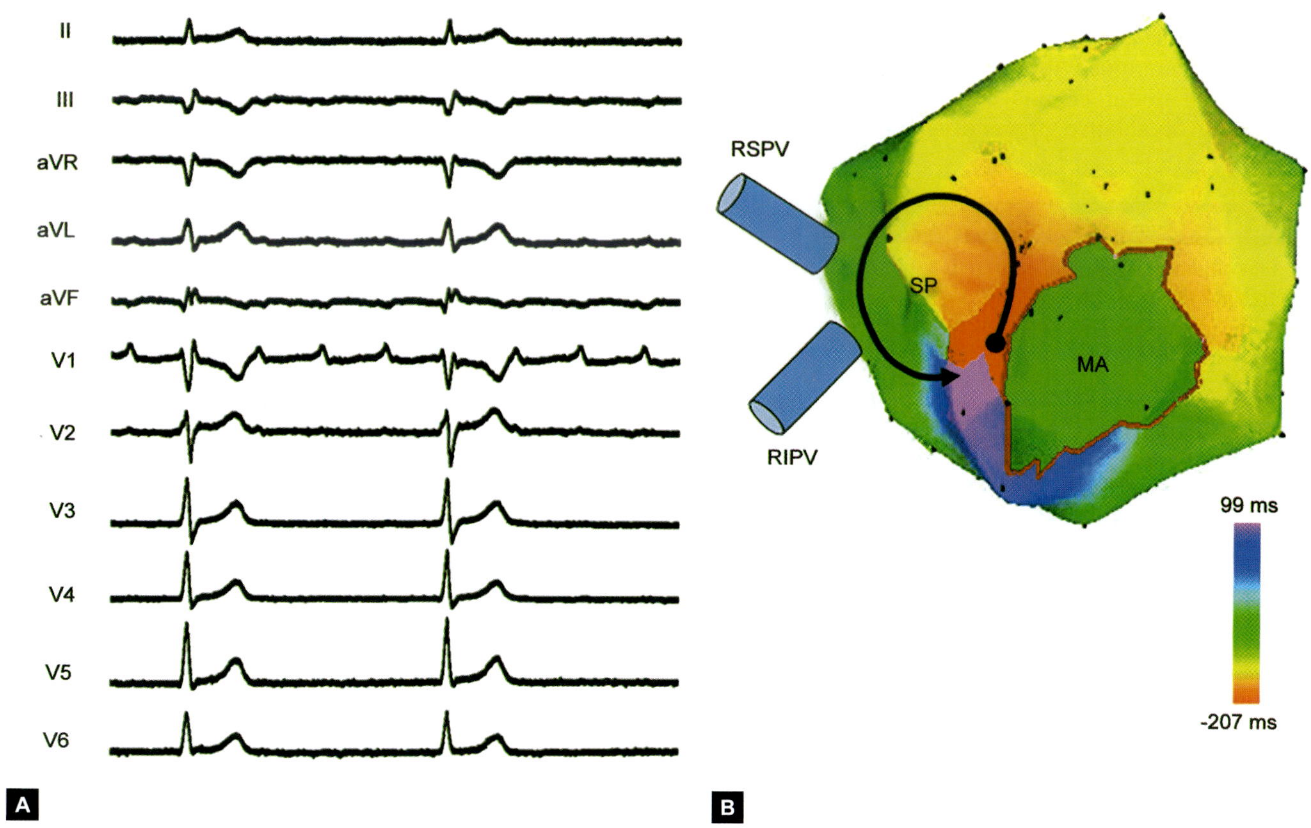

Figures 22.8A and B: Typical ECG pattern (A) and 3D anatomic map (B) from a patient with left septal atrial flutter. The flutter circuit rotates around the septum primum (SP) and a successful ablation line extends from the SP to either the right inferior pulmonary vein (RIPV) or the mitral annulus (MA)

Abbreviations: MA, mitral annulus; RIPV, right inferior pulmonary vein; RSPV, right superior pulmonary vein; SP, septum primum

Flow chart 22.1: This figure summarizes the newer designations of the various flutter circuits. Not shown are circuits that are figures of eight configurations involving one or more of the designated circuits or scarred areas

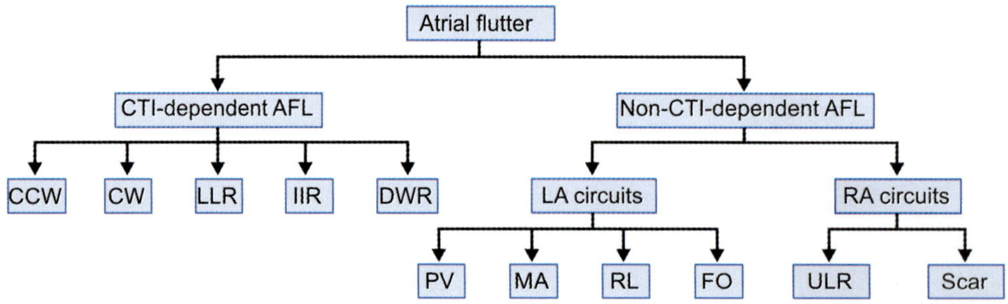

Abbreviations: AFl, atrial flutter; CCW, counter-clockwise; CTI, cavotricuspid isthmus; CW, clockwise; DWR, double-wave reentry; FO, fossa ovalis; IIR, intraisthmus reentry; LA, left atrial; LLR, lower loop reentry; MA, mitral annulus; PV, pulmonary vein; RA, right atrial; RL, roof line; Scar, scar based reentry (i.e., lateral wall incision site); ULR, upper loop reentry

CONCLUSION

The past two decades have produced an explosion of information related to the pathogenesis and variety of both right and left atrial flutter circuits **(Flow chart 22.1)**. We now appreciate that atrial flutter is much more than simple clockwise and counter-clockwise rotation around the tricuspid annulus. Appreciation of the diversity and complexity of flutter circuits has led to the introduction of a variety of ablative procedures that are most often curative.

REFERENCES

1. McWilliam JA. Fibrillar contraction of the heart. J Physiol. 1886;8:296.
2. Jolly WA, Ritchie TW. Auricular flutter and fibrillation. Heart. 1911;3:177-221.
3. Lewis T, Feil HS and Stroud WD. Observations upon flutter and fibrillation: Part II: the nature of auricular flutter and Part III: some effects of rhythmic stimulation of the auricle. Heart. 1920;7:191-292.
4. Scherf D, Schott A. Extrasystoles and allied arrhythmias. Chicago: Year Book Medical Publishers; 1973. pp. 402-20.
5. Rosenblueth A and Garcia Ramos J. Studies on flutter and fibrillation II. The Influence of artificial obstacles on experimental auricular flutter. Am Heart J. 1947;33:677-84.
6. Wells JL, MacLean WA, James TN, Waldo AL. Characterization of atrial flutter. Studies in man after open heart surgery using fixed atrial electrodes. Circulation. 1979;60:665-73.
7. Waldo AL, MacLean WAH, Karp RB, Kouchoukos NT, James TN. Entrainment and interruption of atrial flutter with atrial pacing. Studies in man following open heart surgery. Circulation. 1977;56:737-45.
8. Waldo AL, Cooper TB. Spontaneous onset of type I atrial flutter in patients. J Am Coll Cardiol. 1996;28:707-12.
9. Frame LH, Page RL, Hoffman BF. Atrial reentry around an anatomic barrier with a partially refractory excitable gap. A canine model for atrial flutter. Circ Res. 1986;58: 495-511.
10. Frame LH, Page RL, Boyden PA, Fenoglio JJ, Jr., Hoffman BF. Circus movement in the canine atrium around the tricuspid ring during experimental atrial flutter and during reentry in vitro. Circulation. 1987;76:1155-75.
11. Boineau JP, Mooney CR, Hudson RD, et al. Observations on re-entrant excitation pathways and refractory period distributions in spontaneous and experimental atrial flutter in the dog. In Re-entrant Arrhythmias—Mechanisms and Treatment. Kulbertus HE, Baltimore (Eds), University Park Press; 1977. p. 72.
12. Hayden WG, Hurley EJ, Rytand DA. The mechanism of canine atrial flutter. Circ Res. 1967;20:496-505.
13. Kimura E, Kato K, Murao S, Ajisaka H, Koyama S, Omiya Z. Experimental studies on the mechanism of the auricular flutter. Tohoku J Exp Med. 1954;60:197-207.
14. Kato K, Sato M, Harumi K, Sakamoto T, Koyama S, Murao S. Studies on auricular flutter. Observations upon F-wave. Resp Circ. (Tokyo) 1957;5:837-42.
15. Klein GJ, Guiraudon GM, Sharma AD, Milstein S. Demonstration of macroreentry and feasibility of operative therapy in the common type of atrial flutter. Am J Cardiol. 1986;57:587-91.
16. Saoudi N, Atallah G, Kirkorian G, Touboul P. Catheter ablation of the atrial myocardium in human type I atrial flutter. Circulation. 1990;81:762-71.
17. Chauvin M, Brechenmacher C. A clinical study of the application of endocardial fulguration in the treatment of recurrent atrial flutter. Pacing Clin Electrophysiol. 1989;12: 219-24.
18. Feld GK, Fleck RP, Chen PS, Boyce K, Bahnson TD, Stein JB, Calisi CM, Ibarra M. Radiofrequency catheter ablation for the treatment of human type 1 atrial flutter. Identification of a critical zone in the reentrant circuit by endocardial mapping techniques. Circulation. 1992;86:1233-40.
19. Cosio FG, Lopez-Gil M, Goicolea A, Arribas F, Barroso JL. Radiofrequency ablation of the inferior vena cava-tricuspid valve isthmus in common atrial flutter. Am J Cardiol. 1993; 71:705-9.
20. Cosio FG, Arribas F, Barbero JM, Kallmeyer C, Goicolea A. Validation of double-spike electrograms as markers of conduction delay or block in atrial flutter. Am J Cardiol. 1988;61:775-80.

21. Olshansky B, Okumura K, Hess PG, Waldo AL. Demonstration of an area of slow conduction in human atrial flutter. J Am Coll Cardiol. 1990;16:1639-48.
22. Olgin JE, Kalman JM, Fitzpatrick AP, Lesh MD. Role of right atrial endocardial structures as barriers to conduction during human type I atrial flutter. Activation and entrainment mapping guided by intracardiac echocardiography. Circulation. 1995; 92:1839-48.
23. Nakagawa H, Lazzara R, Khastgir T, Beckman KJ, McClelland JH, Imai S, Pitha JV, Becker AE, Arruda M, Gonzalez MD, Widman LE, Rome M, Neuhauser J, Wang X, Calame JD, Goudeau MD, Jackman WM. Role of the tricuspid annulus and the eustachian valve/ridge on atrial flutter. Relevance to catheter ablation of the septal isthmus and a new technique for rapid identification of ablation success. Circulation. 1996; 94:407-24.
24. Kalman J, Olgin J, Saxon L, Fisher WG, Lee RJ, Lesh MD. Activation and entrainment mapping defines the tricuspid annulus as the anterior barrier in typical atrial flutter. Circulation. 1996;94:398-406.
25. Friedman PA, Luria D, Fenton AM, Munger TM, Jahangir A, Shen WK, Rea RF, Stanton MS, Hammill SC, Packer DL. Global right atrial mapping of human atrial flutter: the presence of posteromedial (sinus venosa region) functional block and double potentials: a study in biplane fluoroscopy and intracardiac echocardiography. Circulation. 2000;101:1568-77.
26. Cheng J, Scheinman MM. Acceleration of typical atrial flutter due to double-wave reentry induced by programmed electrical stimulation. Circulation. 1998;97:1589-96.
27. Yang Y, Mangat I, Glatter KA, Cheng J, Scheinman MM. Mechanism of conversion of atypical right atrial flutter to atrial fibrillation. Am J Cardiol. 2003;91:46-52.
28. Cheng J, Cabeen WR, Scheinman MM. Right atrial flutter due to lower loop reentry; mechanism and anatomic substrates. Circulation. 1999;99:1700-5.
29. Yang Y, Cheng J, Bochoeyer A, Hamdan MH, Kowal RC, Page R, Lee RJ, Steiner PR, Saxon LA, Lesh MD, Modin GW, Scheinman MM. Atypical right atrial flutter patterns. Circulation. 2001; 103:3092-8.
30. Zhang S, Younis G, Hariharan R, Ho J, Yang Y, Ip J, Thakur RK, Seger J, Scheinman MM, Cheng J. Lower loop reentry as a mechanism of clockwise right atrial flutter. Circulation. 2004;109:1630-5.
31. Bochoeyer A, Yang Y, Cheng J, Lee RJ, Keung EC, Marrouche NF, Natale A, Scheinman MM. Surface electrocardiographic characteristics of right and left atrial flutter. Circulation. 2003;108:60-6.
32. Yang Y, Varma N, Scheinman MM. Reentry within the cavotricuspid isthmus: a novel isthmus dependent circuit. (abstract) J Am Coll Cardiol. 2003;41:119A.
33. Yang Y, Varma N, Keung EC, Scheinman MM. Reentry within the cavotricuspid isthmus: an isthmus dependent circuit. Pacing Clin Electrophysiol. 2005;28:808-18.
34. Kall JG, Rubenstein DS, Kopp DE, Burke MC, Verdino RJ, Lin AC, Johnson CT, Cooke PA, Wang ZG, Fumo M, Wilber DJ. Atypical atrial flutter originating in the right atrial free wall. Circulation. 2000;101:270-9.
35. Nakagawa H, Shah N, Matsudaira K, Overholt E, Chandrasekaran K, Beckman KJ, Spector P, Calame JD, Rao A, Hasdemir C, Otomo K, Wang Z, Lazzara R, Jackman WM. Characterization of reentrant circuit in macroreentrant right atrial tachycardia after surgical repair of congenital heart disease: isolated channels between scars allow "focal" ablation. Circulation. 2001;103:699-709.
36. Tai CT, Huang JL, Lin YK, Hsieh MH, Lee PC, Ding YA, Chang MS, Chen SA. Noncontact three-dimensional mapping and ablation of upper loop re-entry originating in the right atrium. J Am Coll Cardiol. 2002;40:746-53.
37. Jais P, Shah DC, Haissaguerre M, Hocini M, Peng JT, Takahashi A, Garrigue S, Le Metayer P, Clementy J. Mapping and ablation of left atrial flutters. Circulation. 2000;101: 2928-34.
38. Hocini M, Jais P, Sanders P, Takahashi Y, Rotter M, Rostock T, Hsu LF, Sacher F, Reuter S, Clementy J, Haissaguerre M. Techniques, evaluation, and consequences of linear block at the left atrial roof in paroxysmal atrial fibrillation: a prospective randomized study. Circulation. 2005;112:3688-96.
39. Calkins H, Kuck KH, Cappato R, Brugada J, Camm AJ, Chen SA, Crijns HJ, Damiano RJ, Jr., Davies DW, DiMarco J, Edgerton J, Ellenbogen K, Ezekowitz MD, Haines DE, Haissaguerre M, Hindricks G, Iesaka Y, Jackman W, Jalife J, Jais P, Kalman J, Keane D, Kim YH, Kirchhof P, Klein G, Kottkamp H, Kumagai K, Lindsay BD, Mansour M, Marchlinski FE, McCarthy PM, Mont JL, Morady F, Nademanee K, Nakagawa H, Natale A, Nattel S, Packer DL, Pappone C, Prystowsky E, Raviele A, Reddy V, Ruskin JN, Shemin RJ, Tsao HM, Wilber D. 2012 HRS/EHRA/ECAS expert consensus statement on catheter and surgical ablation of atrial fibrillation: recommendations for patient selection, procedural techniques, patient management and follow-up, definitions, endpoints, and research trial design: a report of the Heart Rhythm Society (HRS) Task Force on Catheter and Surgical Ablation of Atrial Fibrillation. Developed in partnership with the European Heart Rhythm Association (EHRA), a registered branch of the European Society of Cardiology (ESC) and the European Cardiac Arrhythmia Society (ECAS); and in collaboration with the American College of Cardiology (ACC), American Heart Association (AHA), the Asia Pacific Heart Rhythm Society (APHRS), and the Society of Thoracic Surgeons (STS). Endorsed by the governing bodies of the American College of Cardiology Foundation, the American Heart Association, the European Cardiac Arrhythmia Society, the European Heart Rhythm Association, the Society of Thoracic Surgeons, the Asia Pacific Heart Rhythm Society, and the Heart Rhythm Society. Heart Rhythm. 2012;9:632-96 e21.
40. Marrouche NF, Natale A, Wazni OM, Cheng J, Yang Y, Pollack H, Verma A, Ursell P, Scheinman MM. Left septal atrial flutter: electrophysiology, anatomy, and results of ablation. Circulation. 2004;109:2440-7.

EDITORS' SUMMARY

Professor Scheinman, one of the founders of modern cardiac electrophysiology, has provided a chapter for this textbook that gives us a detailed overview of reentrant atrial arrhythmias in a remarkably precise and summarized form. Cavotricuspid isthmus-dependent flutter along with its closely allied variants of double-wave reentry, lower loop reentry, etc. is introduced and explained. Professor Scheinman then teaches us how the same principles of approaching what creates the propensity for a reentrant circuit can be applied to the left atrium where most electrophysiologists now are presented with challenges, particularly in post-AF ablation reentrant tachycardia ablation.

CHAPTER 23

Ashok Shah, Nicolas Derval, Thomas Pambrun, Sana Amraoui, Seigo Yamashita, Benjamin Berte, Noora Al-Jefairi, Antonio Frontera, Darren Hooks, Arnaud Denis, Frédéric Sacher, Mélèze Hocini, Pierre Jais, Michel Haissaguerre

Atrial Fibrillation: Classification and Mechanisms of Initiation and Maintenance

LIST OF ABBREVIATIONS

AF	Atrial Fibrillation	PV	Pulmonary Vein
ECG	Electrocardiogram		

DEFINITION

Atrial fibrillation (AF) is the most common cardiac arrhythmia and is defined[1] by the following electrocardiographic characteristics:

- Absolutely irregular RR intervals, i.e. RR intervals that do not follow a repetitive pattern on 12-lead surface electrocardiogram (ECG).
- No distinct P waves on the ECG, although some apparently regular atrial electrical activity may be seen in some ECG leads, most often in lead V1.
- The atrial cycle length (when visible), i.e. the interval between two atrial activations, is usually variable and < 200 ms (> 300 beats per minute).

While an irregular pulse should always raise the suspicion of AF, an ECG recording is necessary to diagnose AF. Any arrhythmia that has the above ECG characteristics of AF and lasts sufficiently long for a 12-lead ECG to be recorded, or at least 30s on a rhythm strip, should be considered as *an episode of AF*.

CLASSIFICATION

There are several types and classifications of AF as mentioned below:

- Primary vs. secondary
- Nonvalvular vs. valvular
- Symptomatic vs. silent
- Lone vs. in structurally diseased heart
- First diagnosed (index episode) vs. recurrent

In the current cardiac electrophysiology practice, the most commonly used clinical classification of AF divides it into two broad categories as explained in **Table 23.1**.[2]

Paroxysmal and Persistent AF

Every patient who is diagnosed with AF for the first time is considered a patient with *first diagnosed AF*, irrespective of the duration of the arrhythmia or the presence and severity of AF-related symptoms. So, if a patient has been experiencing AF-related symptoms intermittently since short or

Table 23.1: Types and classification of atrial fibrillation**

AF Episode	An atrial fibrillation episode is defined as AF that is documented by ECG monitoring and has a duration of at least 30 seconds, or if less than 30 seconds, is present continuously throughout the ECG monitoring tracing. The presence of subsequent episodes of AF requires that sinus rhythm be documented by ECG monitoring between AF episodes.
Paroxysmal AF*	Paroxysmal AF is defined as recurrent AF (≥2 episodes) that terminates spontaneously within 7 days. Episodes of AF of ≤48 hours duration that are terminated with electrical or pharmacologic cardioversion should also be classified as paroxysmal AF episodes.
Persistent AF*	Persistent AF is defined as continuous AF that is sustained beyond seven days. Episodes of AF in which a decision is made to electrically or pharmacologically cardiovert the patient after ≥ 48 hours of AF, but prior to 7 days, should also be classified as persistent AF episodes.
Longstanding persistent AF	Longstanding persistent AF is defined as continous AF of greater than 12 months' duration.
Permanent AF	The term permanent AF is not appropriate in the context of patients undergoing catheter or surgical ablation of AF, as it refers to a group of patients for which a decision has been made not to restore or maintain sinus rhythm by any means, including catheter or surgical ablation. If a patient previously classified as having permanent AF is to undergo catheter or surgical ablation, the AF should be reclassified.

*It is recognized that patients may have both paroxysmal and persistent AF. A patient's AF type should be defined as the most frequent type of AF experienced within six months of an ablation procedure. Continuous AF is AF that is documented to be present on all ECG monitoring performed during a defined period of time

**We recommend that the term "chronic AF" not be used in the context of patients undergoing ablation of AF as it is ambiguous, and there is no standardized definition of this term.

Source: Permission to reproduce the table obtained from Heart Rhythm 2012;9:632-696.e21

long period in the past but never underwent an ECG-documentation to establish the diagnosis of AF, that past period will not be counted into the duration of arrhythmia. The arrhythmia duration will begin getting counted forwards from the first diagnosed episode of AF. All arrhythmia episodes occurring after the index episode are called *recurrent AF* (≥ 2 episodes). When recurrent AF terminates spontaneously within 7 days it is called *Paroxysmal AF*. When it is sustained for > 7 days, it is defined as *Persistent AF*. In addition to these simplified classification of two types of clinical AF, the expert guidelines[1,2] also recommend that the patients with continuous (sustained) AF who undergo cardioversion within 7 days be classified as having *paroxysmal AF* if the cardioversion is performed within 48 hours of AF-onset, and *persistent AF* if the cardioversion is performed more than 48 hours after AF-onset. Based on the clinical experience which evolved from advanced techniques enabling continuous monitoring (recording) of AF over long periods, the recently recommended definitions are more clinically relevant than the mutually exclusive simple definitions of persistent and paroxysmal AF. Moreover, in the context of current practice and AF-related clinical trials, the simple definitions did not take into account conversion of AF by different therapeutic means. Also, in an attempt to make the description of AF internationally uniform, the term *chronic AF*, which has been in use since very long to mean nonparoxysmal AF, has not been defined in the new guidelines.[1-3] Instead, persistent AF is specified as "*longstanding persistent AF*", when it remains sustained for greater than one-year's duration.

Permanent AF

The term "permanent AF" was meaningfully in vogue in the preablation era. AF was classified into *permanent* category when the patient accepted being in continuous AF after getting subjected to therapeutic attempts for reversal of the rhythm and despite which there was failure to maintain sinus rhythm. Within the context of any rhythm control strategy, including catheter ablation, the term permanent AF can be considered as historical. The term permanent AF represents a joint decision by the patient and a physician to cease further attempts to restore and/or maintain sinus rhythm at a particular point in time. It is important, therefore, to recognize that the term "permanent AF" represents a therapeutic attitude on the part of a patient and the physician rather than any inherent pathophysiological attribute of the AF.[1,2] Such decisions may change as symptoms, the efficacy of therapeutic interventions, and patient and physician preferences evolve. If after reevaluation, a rhythm control strategy is recommended, the permanent AF should be redesignated as paroxysmal, persistent, or longstanding persistent AF, as appropriate.[2]

Other Types of AF

The several other types and classifications of AF as mentioned above are defined here.

Silent AF is defined as asymptomatic AF often diagnosed by an opportune ECG or rhythm strip. Paroxysmal and persistent AF types may be symptomatic or silent (i.e. asymptomatic).

Nonvalvular AF is defined as AF occurring in the absence of rheumatic mitral stenosis, a mechanical or bioprosthetic heart valve, or mitral valve repair.[3]

Lone AF is defined as AF in patients with minimal or no heart disease (structurally normal heart).[1] There are a variety of cardiovascular and noncardiac disorders which predispose to AF.[1] They include but are not limited to valvular, congenital, ischemic and pericardial heart diseases, primary cardiomyopathy, endocrine, metabolic, renal and pulmonary disorders and dyselectrolytemia.

Primary AF is defined as AF occurring independent of or in the absence of any disorder (as mentioned above) known to predispose to AF. AF which occurs as a consequence of a predisposing condition and resolves upon reversal of the primary disorder is called *Secondary AF*.

It is recognized that a particular patient may have AF episodes that fall into one or more of these categories. So, it is recommended that patients be categorized by their most frequent pattern of AF during the last six months.[2]

MECHANISMS OF AF INITIATION AND MAINTENANCE

Atrial fibrillation is the clinical manifestation of a chain of subclinical events (happening at the cellular and intercellular-interstitial level) which lead to alterations in the structure (pathophysiology) and electrical properties (electrophysiology) of the atrial myocardium.[4] **Flow chart 23.1** displays the role and involvement of multiple factor-systems in the electropathophysiology of AF.[3] It is beyond the scope of this chapter in *Practical Cardiac Electrophysiology* to get into the cellular-level details of AF-conducive changes. The focus has been on the experimental and clinical aspects of AF mapping to describe the mechanisms of the initiation and maintenance of AF.

Flow chart 23.1: Mechanisms of atrial fibrillation

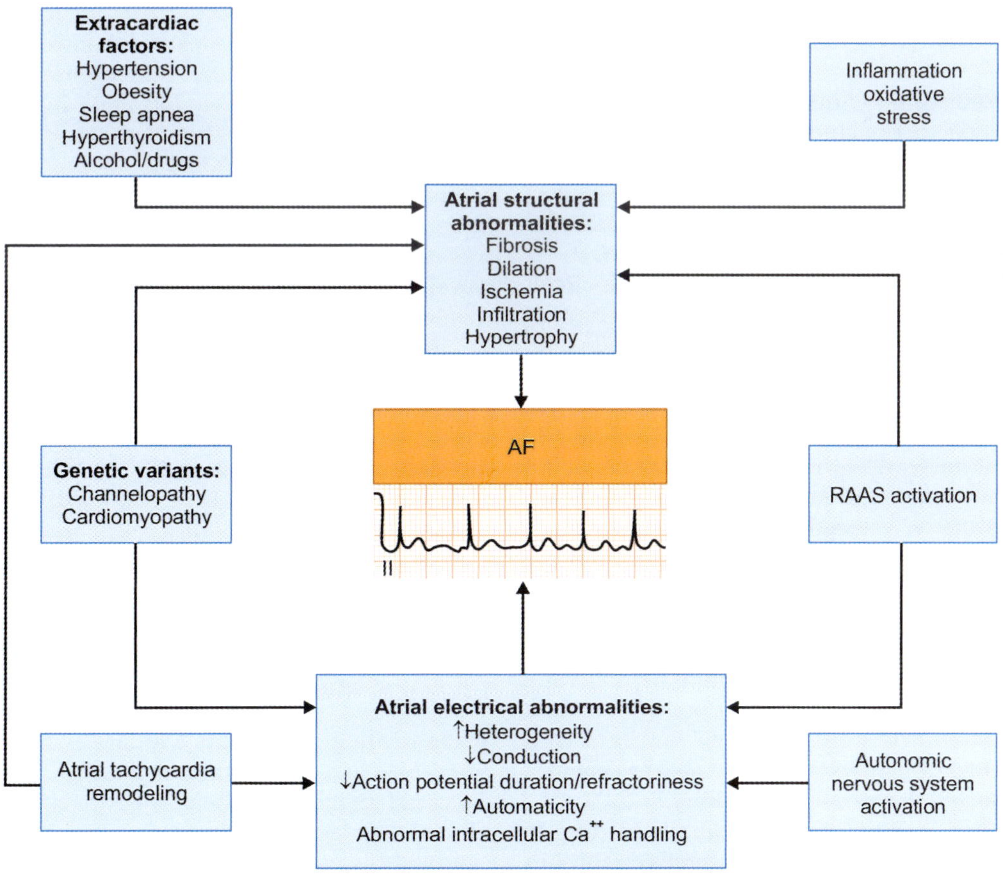

Abbreviations: AF, atrial fibrillation; Ca^{++}, ionized calcium; RAAS, renin-angiotensin-aldosterone system

Source: Permission to reproduce the figure obtained from J Am Coll Cardiol. 2014;64:2246-80.

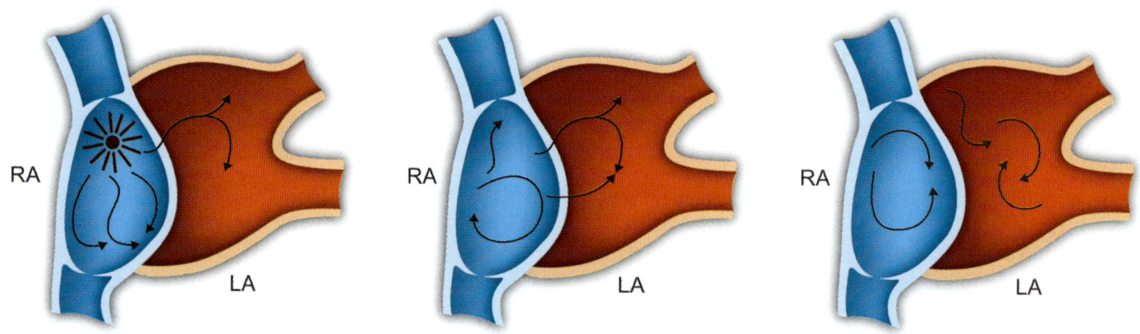

Figures 23.1A to C: Conceptual models of atrial fibrillation in the early twentieth century, along with therapeutic implications. Ectopic foci (A) and single reentrant circuits (B) generating atrial fibrillation can be located in either atrium, but are shown here as arising in the right atrium. In (C), atrial fibrillation is maintained by multiple reentry circuits with spatial and temporal variability
Abbreviations: LA, left atrium; RA, right atrium; RP, refractory period
Source: Permission to reproduce the figure obtained from Nattel S. Nature. 2002;415:219-26.

Classical Mechanisms of AF

Beginning early 20th century, many theories and concepts have been proposed to explain the mechanistic behavior of AF.[5] The principal of them were that AF is caused by rapidly discharging, spontaneously active, atrial ectopic foci **(Figure 23.1A)**, by a single reentry circuit **(Figure 23.1B)**, or by multiple functional reentrant circuits **(Figure 23.1C)**.

The rapidly discharging ectopic focus and single-circuit concepts lost the ground until the last decade of 20th century in favor of multiple-circuit reentry model which, therefore, dominated our mechanistic understanding of AF for the most part of the last century. Particularly influential was the work of Moe and co-workers,[6] who emphasized the role of multiple reentrant wavelets in the perpetuation of AF **(Figure 23.1C)**. An important component of Moe's theory is the concept of the 'wavelength of reentry' proposed by Allessie et al.[7] The wavelength is the distance traveled by the electrical impulse in one refractory period. It is the product of the refractory period and the conduction velocity. If the length of the electrical circuit is smaller than the wavelength, the impulse will traverse the circuit and return to its starting point in a time shorter than the refractory period, forcing it to impinge on still-refractory tissue and die out. In such a situation, arrhythmia cannot sustain. Thus, the wavelength is the shortest pathlength that can sustain reentry.

According to the 'leading circle' hypothesis of Allessie et al.[7] **(Figure 23.2A)**, functional reentry naturally establishes itself in a pathlength the size of the wavelength. The number of reexcitation waves that can be accommodated is then a simple function of atrial size and the wavelength: decreased wavelength decreases the minimum circuit size, which increases the number of circuits that can be accommodated, which in turn favors multiple-circuit reentry and tends to perpetuate AF **(Figure 23.2B)**.

This mechanistic concept significantly impacted the initial AF rhythm management, where the primary approach was to increase the refractory period (and thereby the wavelength), which limits the number of functional circuits that can be maintained so that AF cannot sustain itself. In addition to drugs that increase the refractory period to stop AF and disallow its maintenance, it was thought that multiple-circuit reentry should be amenable to interventions which reduce the electrically active atrial mass below the critical limit necessary for the reentering circuits to perpetuate themselves. In accordance with this school of thought, Cox pioneered surgical division of the atria into electrically isolated compartments, as exemplified by the 'Maze' procedure.[8]

Focal Initiation of AF Challenging the Classical Mechanism

While treating AF patients with antiarrhythmic drugs and/or with linear lesions to mimic surgical Maze procedure using percutaneous catheter-based technique, new clinical observations were made in the last decade of the 20th century.[9-11]

AF was spontaneously triggered by sustained monomorphic atrial tachycardias or repetitive atrial ectopic beats.

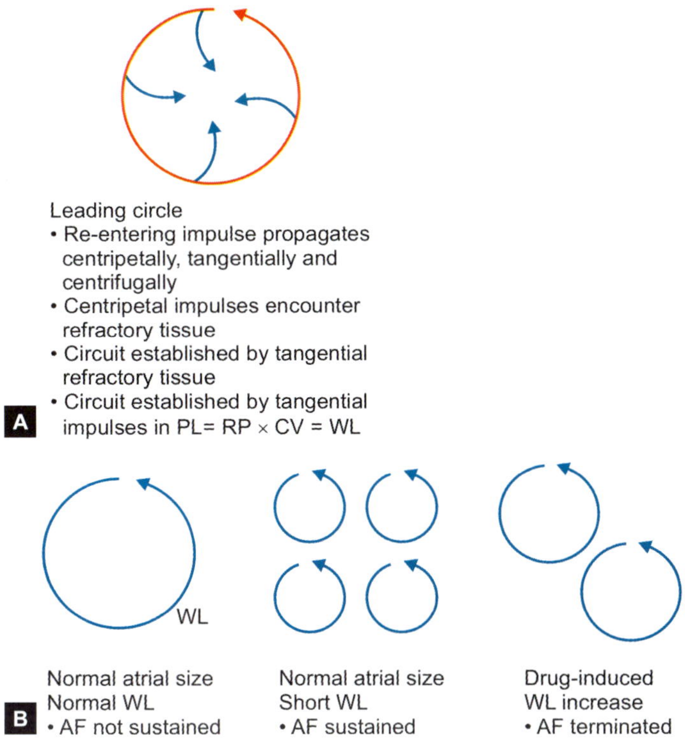

Figures 23.2A and B: Models of reentry and implications for atrial fibrillation. (A) Mechanism of functional reentry in the leading circle model; (B) Role of wavelength in the stability of atrial fibrillation according to the leading circle model. The size of functional reentry circuits depends on the wavelength. Short wavelengths allow several simultaneous circuits to be maintained, favoring continuation of atrial fibrillation. Drugs that increase the wavelength reduce the number of circuits that can be accommodated, favoring termination of atrial fibrillation

Abbreviations: CV, conduction velocity; PL, pathlength; RP, refractory period; WL, wavelength

Source: Permission to reproduce the figure obtained from Nattel S. Nature. 2002;415:219-26.

The latter were spontaneous, intermittent, isolated or occurred in bursts of irregular atrial tachycardia with episodes lasting for minutes or hours and ending spontaneously. All the atrial arrhythmias were due to the same focus firing irregularly and exhibiting a consistent and centrifugal pattern of activation **(Figures 23.3A to E)**. These observations challenged the previously prevailing notion that all AF is caused by multiple-circuit reentry especially when focal-source mechanism of AF was validated by discrete radiofrequency ablation of the source leading to acute termination of AF, its hypo/noninducibility and its sustained remission.[9-11]

In addition to shift in the mechanistic concept, the predominant fibrillogenic role of the right atrium was challenged by the observation that the majority of the focal sources were located in the pulmonary veins and in the contiguous posterior left atrium. These structures seemed to play a highly significant role in the focal mechanism **(Figures 23.4A and B)**.[10,11] The clinical observation was also substantiated by experimental AF mapping in sheep and dogs.[12,13]

Several clinical centers worldwide, subsequently, confirmed the preliminary observations made by Haissaguerre, Jais et al.[14,15] According to the new concept, paroxysms of AF are initiated by discharges from one or only a few focal sources **(Figure 23.5)**. The vast majority of atrial premature beats that suddenly and spontaneously initiate frequent bursts of AF originate in the pulmonary veins. This seminal observation has been made not only in the patients who underwent linear ablation in the right and left atria for AF but also in drug-refractory AF patients who did not have any ablation previously.[14] Although rarer than the pulmonary veins, focal sources spontaneously triggering AF are also found to be located in the ostia of the great veins and coronary sinus, appendages, septum, crista terminalis, etc.[16]

The electrophysiological mechanism underlying the focal theory of AF is not proven. The irregularly repetitive, rapid discharges from the focal source which are silenced by discrete radiofrequency application favor triggered activity or automaticity as the most likely electrophysiological mechanism of the initiation of AF. [14] Again, the AF-initiating first ectopic spike is closely coupled (linked) to the previous sinus beat without there being any intervening activity. This suggests triggered activity as a possible mechanism of AF initiation **(Figure 23.5)**. The abrupt burst of focal activity without gradual warm up and lack of gradual slow down before abrupt termination typically observed in automatic arrhythmias go against abnormal automaticity as the mechanism of AF initiation. Similarly, deep pulmonary venous origin contrasts with the juxtaostial origin of automatic focal left atrial tachycardias. On the other hand, the occurrence of dissociated pulmonary vein potentials after ablation favors automaticity.[14]

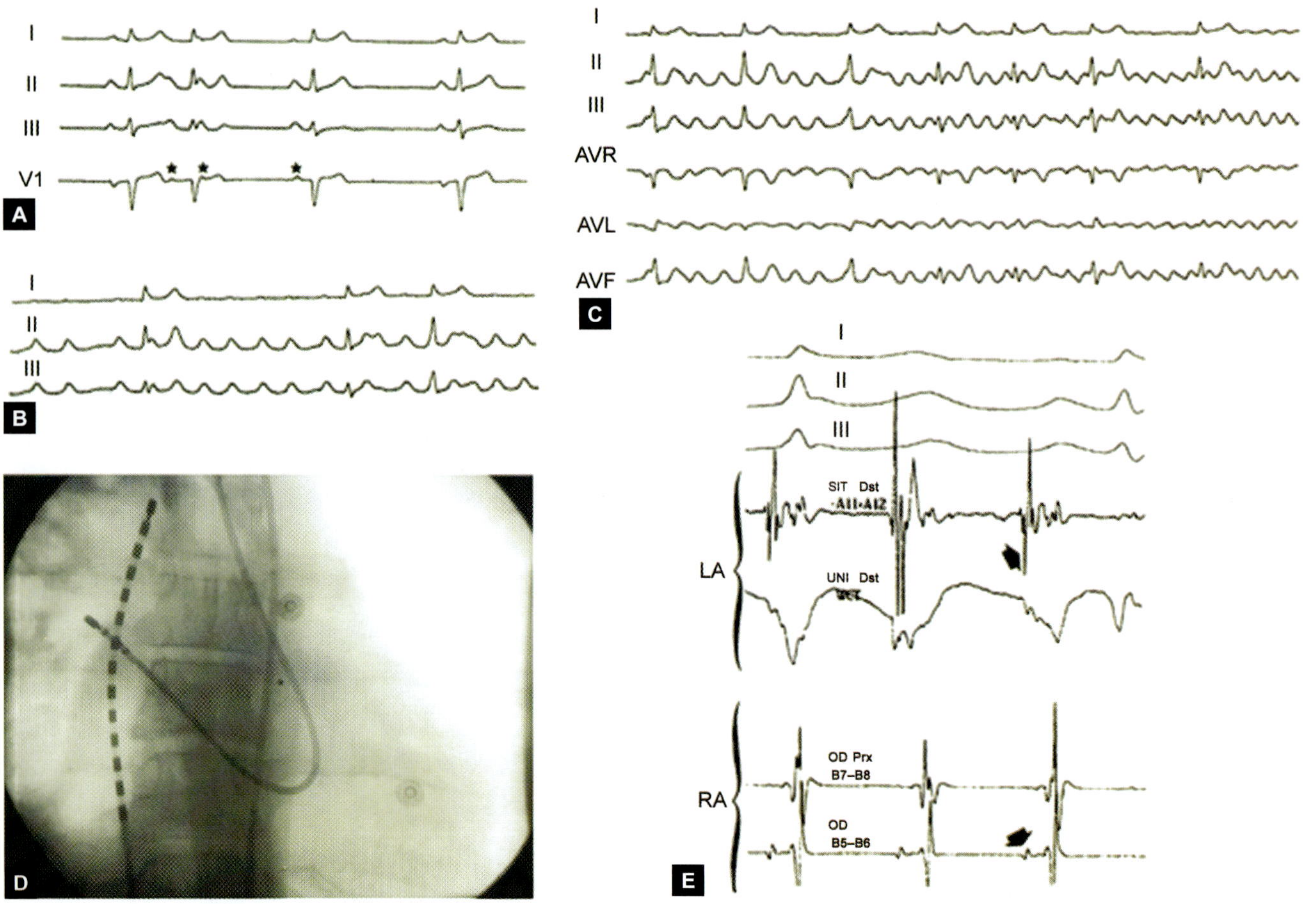

Figures 23.3A to E: Ablation of sources of paroxysmal AF (1997–98). (A to C) Different atrial arrhythmias observed in the same patient: three monomorphic extrasystoles with short and very long (third star) coupling intervals (A), a monomorphic and a very irregular atrial tachycardia with well discernible P waves of similar morphology (B), and the same monomorphic and irregular atrial tachycardia shown in the beginning of this tracing (C). At the end of the recording, the intrinsic rate of the focus is high enough to give an ECG pattern of a coarse AF. Mapping of the RA was performed first, and earliest bipolar activity was recorded in the posterior high RA by use of a multielectrode catheter positioned vertically along the border of the right side of the heart as shown in the radiograph (D). After six unsuccessful RF attempts in this area, LA mapping was performed. Earlier bipolar activity was found just behind the previous RA region, in the right superior pulmonary vein area. This is the position of the quadripolar ablation catheter shown in D, placed just inside the right superior pulmonary vein via the retrograde aortic approach. (E) Analysis of RA and LA activity. The timing of the earliest (arrows) component of each electrogram is the same, but the RA activity is slow and small in amplitude (far-field activity), whereas the LA activity is sharp and of higher amplitude, representing local activity. The first RF pulse delivered at this site successfully ablated all the atrial arrhythmias for this patient

Abbreviations: RA, right atrium; LA, left atrium; SIT Dst, indicates distal bipole of the ablation catheter; UNI Dst, unfiltered unipolar electrogram from the tip of the ablation catheter; OD Prx B7-B8 and OD B5-B6, two adjacent bipoles from the multielectrode catheter in the RA

Source: Permission to reproduce the figure obtained from Jais P et al. Circulation. 1997;95:572-6.

Maintenance of AF

The evolving evidence has thrown us back to the debates of the early 20th century, suggesting that spontaneous ectopic activity, single-circuit reentry and multiple circuit reentry may all be involved in the maintenance of AF.[17] It is important to note that the mechanisms involved in the maintenance of AF differ between paroxysmal and persistent/long-standing persistent varieties. While limited number of discretely localized sources are responsible for the maintenance of paroxysmal AF, the extent of sources gets wider with increasing duration of AF such that the sources spread over wide atrial substrate are involved in the maintenance of chronically persistent or permanent AF.[18] In addition to more widely spread sources, nonfocal mechanisms also play a dominant role in nonparoxysmal AF.

Maintenance of AF by Localized Sources

In the experimental studies, AF was produced by either rapid atrial pacing and vagal stimulation[19,20] or local application

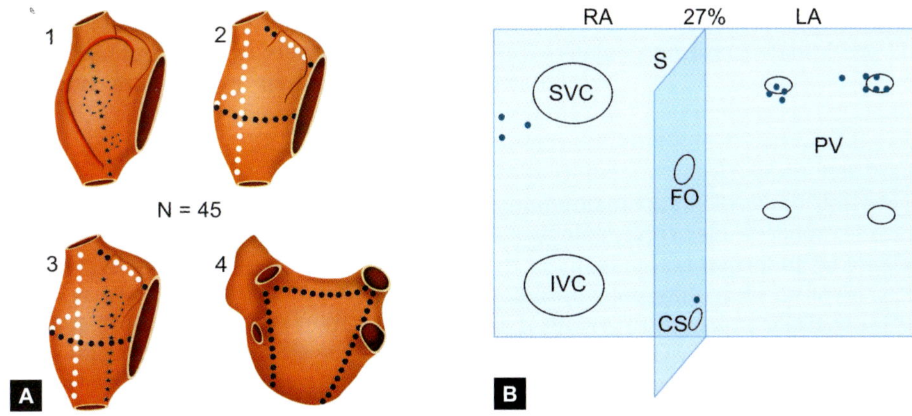

Figures 23.4A and B: Catheter ablation of AF initially involved linear ablation of the RA and LA and not pulmonary vein isolation (A). In a study by Haissaguerre et al. (J Cardiovasc Electrophysiol. 1996;7(12):1132-44), 27% patients showed evidence of focal triggers initiating AF from the pulmonary veins (PVs) and around the superior or inferior vena cava (SVC/IVC) after linear ablation was undertaken (B)

Abbreviations: CS, coronary sinus; FO, foramen ovale; IVC, inferior vena cava; LA, left atrium; PV, pulmonary vein; RA, right atrium; SVC, superior vena cava

Source: Permission to reproduce the figure obtained from Haissaguerre, et al. J Cardiovasc Electrophysiol. 1996;7(12):1132-44.

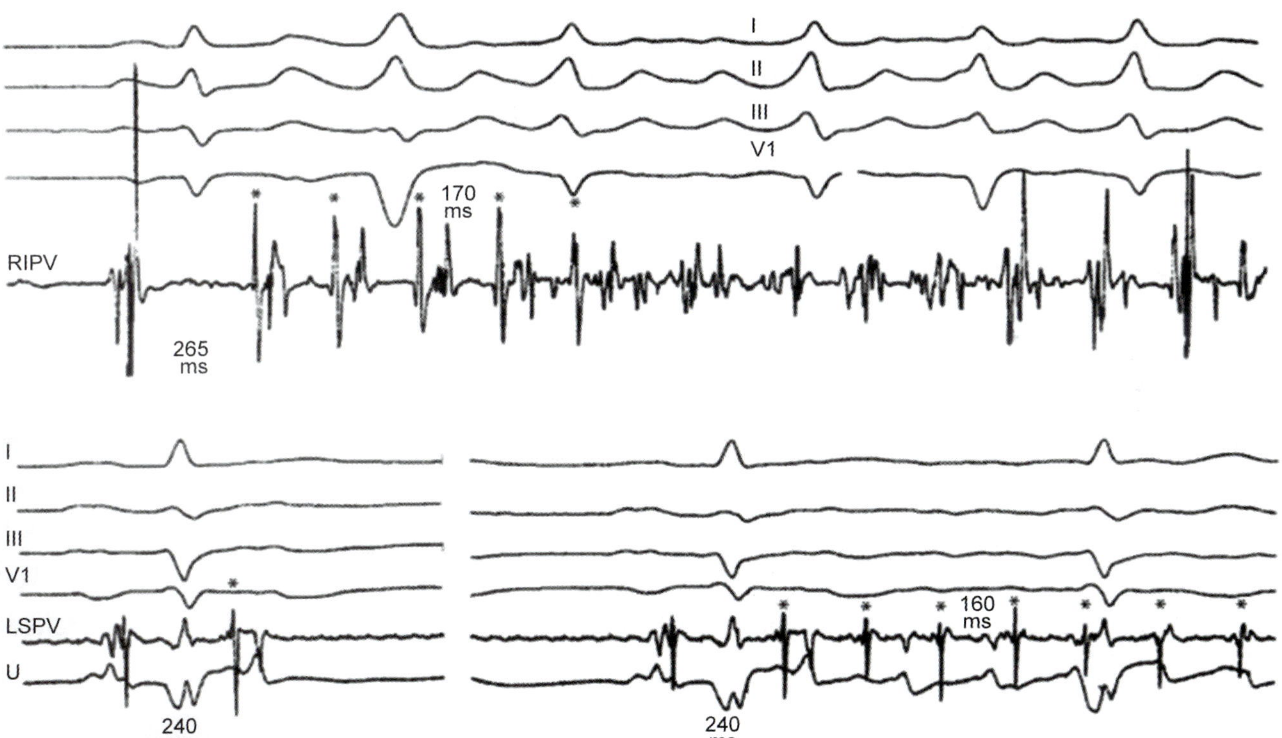

Figure 23.5: Two examples of the onset of atrial fibrillation from foci in a right inferior pulmonary vein (RIPV) and a left superior pulmonary vein (LSPV). The electrogram with the pulmonary vein spike is the terminal part of a two-component electrogram obtained during sinus rhythm. In the upper panel, a burst of five spikes (asterisks) with a mean cycle length of 170 ms induced continuous electrical activity in the RIPV, with coarse atrial fibrillation on the surface electrocardiogram. The coupling interval of the first spike was 265 ms. In the bottom panel on the left, a sinus beat (with a terminal spike) was followed by an isolated atrial ectopic beat (asterisk) at a coupling interval of 240 ms. The electrogram of the ectopic beat characteristically shows temporal reversal, with the rapid deflection spike preceding the lower-amplitude, slower far-field atrial activity. On the right, in the same patient, a train of spike discharges (asterisks) at a cycle length of 160 ms sets off atrial fibrillation. The spike discharges are also characterized by temporal reversal but exhibit a progressively prolonged conduction time to the atria. The coupling interval of the first spike on the right (240 ms) is identical to that of the isolated ectopic beat on the left. LSPV denotes left superior pulmonary vein, and U unipolar left atrial activity

Source: Permission to reproduce the figure obtained from Haïssaguerre M, et al. N Engl J Med. 1998;339:659-66.

of aconitine.[21] Both models resulted in a similar pattern of AF. Aconitine-induced AF was initiated and perpetuated from the same focus, whereas cholinergic AF was perpetuated as long as vagal stimulation was maintained but remained independent of the event that started it. Similarly, in a clinical setting, when pulmonary vein firing triggers initiation of AF, the same focal source possibly has a role in the maintenance of its paroxysmal episode, too.[11,14] Electrophysiologically, while the triggered activity or abnormal automaticity of the focus is the mechanism involved in spontaneous initiation of AF, reentry is the most likely mechanism involved in maintaining focal AF. While focus' automaticity cannot be denied to have a role in AF maintenance as evidenced by bursts of activity, the reentry in the region of focus (localized) is suggested by continuous activity between all subsequent local electrogram spikes **(Figure 23.5)**. Foci located distally in the pulmonary veins were found to have the least (shortest) effective refractory period in the atria in a study involving AF and control patients. Also, substantial gradients in refractoriness were recorded in their vicinity, thereby imparting the region the arrhythmogenic characteristic favoring reentry.[15] The long conduction time between pulmonary vein and left atrium indicates either discontinuous conduction or a tissue several centimetres long, since the sharp morphologic feature of the spike **(Figure 23.5)** indicate that focus is a rapidly conducting structure.

Haïssaguerre et al.[22] demonstrated that patients with AF organized by prior pulmonary vein and linear ablation show two types of sources maintaining AF, called AF-drivers: Focal triggers and localized reentry. A site or region centrifugally activating the remaining atrial tissue is defined as a source. AF was considered organized if mapping showed irregular but discrete atrial complexes exhibiting consistent activation sequences for >75% of the time-window using a 20-pole catheter with 5 radiating spines covering 3.5-cm diameter or sequential conventional mapping. Such AF was maintained by 1 to 3 sources predominantly in the left atrium. Electrograms at the earliest area varied from discrete centrifugal activation to an activity spanning 75% to 100% of the cycle length, the latter indicating complex local conduction or a reentrant circuit **(Figures 23.6A and B)**. The role in maintaining AF was confirmed by prolongation of the AF cycle length and a change in atrial activation sequence or AF termination during radiofrequency delivery at the source.

Focal Triggers

Focal triggers are rapidly discharging discrete sources which spread fibrillatory activation centrifugally into the atrial sink. Such sources were observed to generate impulses continuously or in bursts and demonstrate varying cycle lengths with gradient of cycle length (>20 ms) to the surrounding atrium **(Figure 23.7)**. Local radiofrequency ablation prolonged AF cycle length and either terminated AF or changed activation sequence to another organized rhythm. Their intrinsic properties were strikingly evidenced independently of external influence in patients with islands of permanent or intermittent fibrillatory activity isolated by ablation and surrounded by the atrium in sinus rhythm **(Figure 23.8)**.

Localized Reentry

Localized reentry is suggested by prolonged duration of fractionated local electrograms which is accounted for by the activation wavefront slowly moving in the region and covering the entire AF cycle length or a large portion of it or by alternating activation of the adjacent sites **(Figure 23.6)**. The latter observation is considered to be indicative of sequential activation from a rotating wave. A rotating wave concept is also in agreement with the observation of rotors during experimental AF in sheep, the wavelength of which was reported as 10 ± 3 mm.[12] Such sizeable regional rotor is identifiable with the spatial resolution of the presently used electrode spacing in ablation **(Figure 23.6B)** and mapping **(Figure 23.6A)** catheters.

Progression of Clinical AF

Temporally, AF is a progressive disorder and basic research has led to the hypothesis that 'AF begets AF', meaning that the changes in the atrial substrate caused by AF lead to persistence of AF.[23,24] Whether paroxysmal AF progresses to permanent AF in all patients has not been proven, and the frequency and rapidity of AF progression are unknown. Some studies have, however, reported that the progression of paroxysmal AF to persistent AF occurs at a rate of 5–15% annually,[25-28] and is marked by structural alterations in the atrial tissue associated with comorbidities, including aging, diabetes, hypertension, and heart failure.[28] These studies also showed that patients with paroxysmal AF who develop one or more comorbid conditions progress to persistent AF more frequently than those who have no comorbidities.

Maintenance of AF by Wider Atrial Substrate (Self-perpetuation)

Repetitive discharges from localized, discrete AF drivers can produce progressive pathologic changes in the atrial substrate that may lead to the self-perpetuation of atrial fibrillation. Thus, with the progression of AF to the persistent variety, the mechanisms involved in its maintenance do not remain limited to a small number of focal sources. Multiple reentrant wavelets (stable and unstable) and coexisting foci spread over wider atrial substrate have been implicated in the maintenance of such AF.

Several epicardial mapping studies in patients with persistent AF and structural heart disease have found evidence for multiple unstable wavefronts within the left atrium[29,30] while another observed regional regular short-cycle length

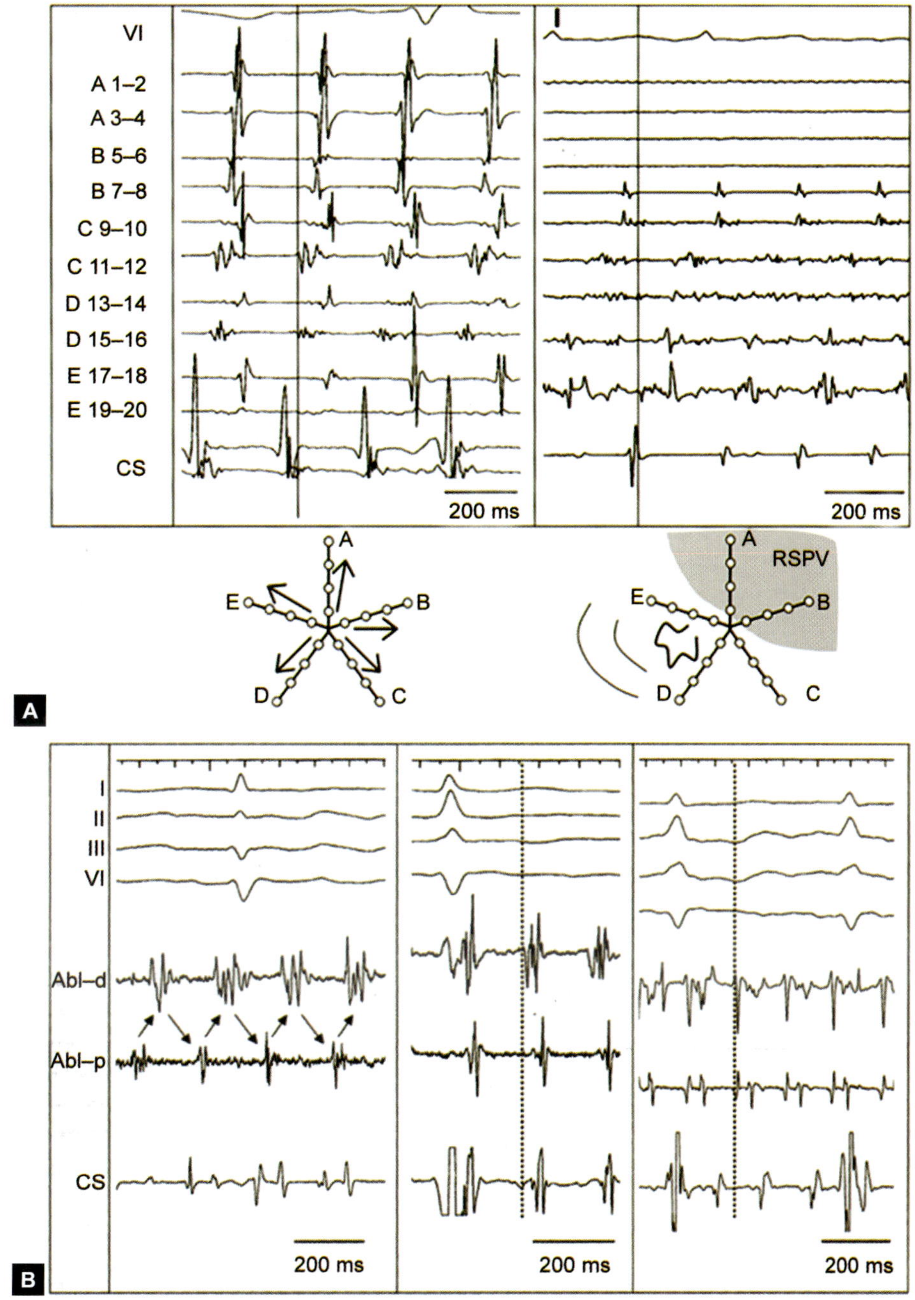

Figures 23.6A and B: (A) Two examples of activation mapping at the source location showing either discrete site of early activation (mean cycle length, 188 ms; bipole D15–16 on the left) or area of prolonged electrograms spanning all the cycle length (mean cycle length, 200 ms; right panel) contiguous to isolated right superior PV (bipoles A and B). The percentage of cycle length covered by local electrograms is 36% and 100%, respectively. Left, the earliest site can be defined within the mapping field with activation spreading from internal (3–4, 7–8, 11–12, 15–16, 19–20) to external bipoles (1–2, 5–6, 9–10, 13–14, 17–18) (before spreading to the surrounding atria). Right, in contrast, the earliest site cannot be defined within the mapping field (however, the remaining atria is activated centrifugally from this area); (B) Electrograms at the ablation site. Left, alternating electrical activity between proximal and distal bipoles of the ablation catheter (arrows), potentially indicating a rotating wave. Middle, distal-to-proximal activation sequence. Right, synchronous activation
Source: Permission to reproduce the figure obtained from Haïssaguerre M, et al. Circulation. 2006;113:616-25.

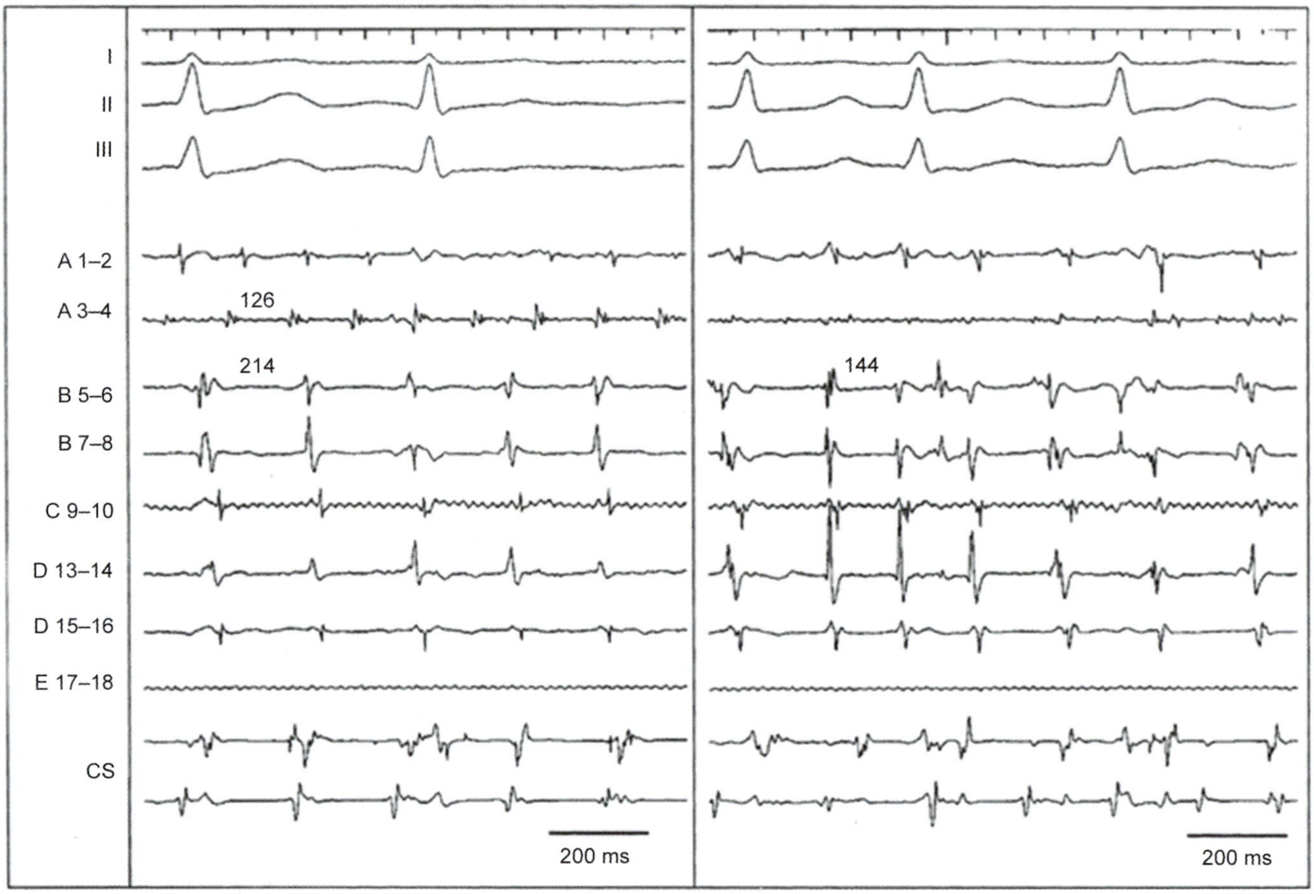

Figure 23.7: Gradient of high-frequency activity recorded in the posterior LA. In both, the bipole A3–4 demonstrates the most rapid activity. Left, activity at bipole A3–4 has a mean cycle length of 126 ms; the immediately surrounding bipoles are much slower, with a mean cycle length of 214 ms. Right, the activity in A3–4 is faster and/or split with the surrounding local activity having a cycle length of 144 ms
Source: Permission to reproduce the figure obtained from Haïssaguerre M, et al. Circulation. 2006;113:616-25.

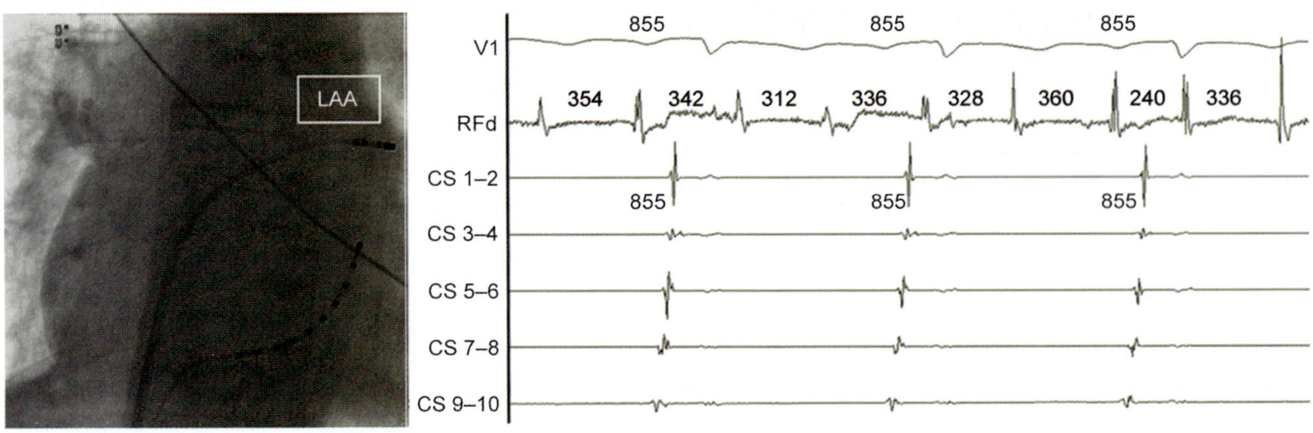

Figure 23.8: Persistence of tachyarrhythmia, albeit slowed down by local ablation, inside the left atrial appendage (LAA) following restoration of sinus rhythm in the atria

activity potentially indicative of focal sources.[31] Sahadevan et al.[31] in an epicardial mapping study of nine patients with chronic AF observed regional short-cycle length activity in seven of these and speculated that this may represent the presence of a focal driver as one mechanism of AF. However, Allessie and coworkers[29,30] consider that the vast majority (90.5%) of focal fibrillatory waves in longstanding persistent AF are due to epicardial breakthrough from waves travelling in deeper layers of atrial tissue and not due to a focal mechanism. They hypothesize that endocardial-epicardial dissociation allowed the breakthrough of these focal waves, which become the equivalent of multiple focal sources. In a goat model of AF, Eckstein et al[32] showed that both the incidence and degree of endocardial-epicardial dissociation increases with increasing AF duration and complexity of AF substrate.

Cuculich et al.[33] imaged AF noninvasively using inverse solution (called ECGI) in 26 patients. There were three main coexisting patterns of activity maintaining AF: wavelets, foci and rotors. The wavelets were the most common (24/26 patients; 92%) and at least 2 simultaneous wavelets (range, 1 to 5) were visible at a time-instant. Single wave macroreentry was rare. The rotor pattern was the least common (4/26 patients; 15%) and was observed in the posterior left atrium and occasionally in the right atrium. The rotors were short lived and seen only in patients with nonparoxysmal AF. Focal discharges frequently occurred near the PVs (18/26 patients; 69%) especially in paroxysmal AF. Non-PV focal sites like posterior left atrium, coronary sinus, lateral right atrium, or vena cavae were also common (16/26 patients; 62%) and were predominantly seen executing role of AF maintenance in nonparoxysmal AF. The number of activities increased with the duration of AF with most complex activities observed in longstanding persistent AF. Relatively fewer activities were seen in paroxysmal AF.

RECENT ADVANCES IN MAPPING AF MECHANISMS

Phase-based computational analysis is the most recently used technique to map clinical AF and decipher its mechanisms. This technique has been applied to electrical signals acquired using high-density contact tools like multielectrode basket catheters, invasively[34] or reconstructed by inversing 252-lead surface ECG on CT-derived biatrial geometry, noninvasively.[35,36] The phase-analysis maps detected localized sources of two types: (1) focal, when a wavefront originated from a point or an area and propagated centrifugally; (2) reentry, either rotor when a wave fully rotated (full phase progression) around a functional center-point, or anatomical when a full rotation occurred around a small anatomical structure (like thoracic vein ostium) **(Figures 23.9A and B)**. The AF-driving characteristic of localized sources was validated by AF termination during ablation of foci and reentries.

Narayan et al.[34] used a 64-electrode basket catheter and a customized software to endocardially map focal sources (rotors and focal impulses) in patients with persistent and paroxysmal AF. Localized rotors (70%) or focal (30%) impulses were detected in the majority (98%) of patients with a mean of 2.1 ± 1.0 sources per patient. AF sources were stable and long lasting and were found in a variety of left and right atrial regions. Targeted ablation at the center of these focal sources resulted in AF termination in 86% of cases.

On the other hand, the noninvasive maps of AF[35,36] showed constantly changing, dynamic beat-to-beat wave fronts and varying spatiotemporal behavior of driver activities (reentries and focal discharges). Reentries were not sustained (median, 2.6 rotations lasting 449 ± 89 ms), meandered substantially but recurred repetitively in the same region.[36] These findings bore resemblance to those obtained in animal experiments.[37] Widely spread 4720 drivers were identified noninvasively in 103 patients with persistent AF: 3802 (80.5%) reentries and 918 (19.5%) focal breakthroughs; most of them co-localized. Of these, 69% reentries and 71% foci were in the left atrium. Rotors and focal drivers were predominantly located in the pulmonary vein antral regions and adjacent inferoposterior left atrial wall in patients without prior LA ablation. However, with longer AF duration, multiple drivers were located at extrapulmonary venous sites. Driver ablation alone terminated 75% and 15% of persistent and long-lasting AF, respectively. The complexity of AF drivers and the number of targeted driver regions increased with the duration of continuous AF: 2 in patients presenting in sinus rhythm, 3 in AF lasting 1 to 3 months, 4 in AF lasting 4 to 6 months, and 6 in AF lasting longer. The termination rate sharply declined after 6 months.[36]

Noninvasive mapping of paroxysmal AF[38] revealed that the antral pulmonary veins and the adjoining posterior LA harbored localized drivers in nearly 90% of patients, which was in concurrence with the team's seminal finding[14] two decades earlier. Among the observed localized drivers, 74% were reentrant and 26% were focal drivers. Additionally nonpulmonary vein foci were also found in 50% patients. Pulmonary vein driver ablation terminated paroxysmal AF in 15/17 (88%) patients. The remaining 2 patients required additional ablation of non-PV drivers to terminate AF.

Of note, there are some intriguing differences in observations made by these two phase-mapping techniques.[39] The nature of AF drivers described by Narayan et al[34] with the endocardial phase-mapping technique appears to be entirely different from the one reported by Haissaguerre et al.[36] using noninvasive epicardial mapping system. Narayan et al. suggested that the rotors were stable and long-lasting, even reproduced after an interval of weeks to months, whereas Haissaguerre et al. describe renascent, 2- to 3-rotation rotors that tend to drift over large distances. As such only few studies[22,34] report stable AF sources in the literature compared with the large amount of them demonstrating the role of wandering wavelets or closed-loop reentry.[36,40-43]

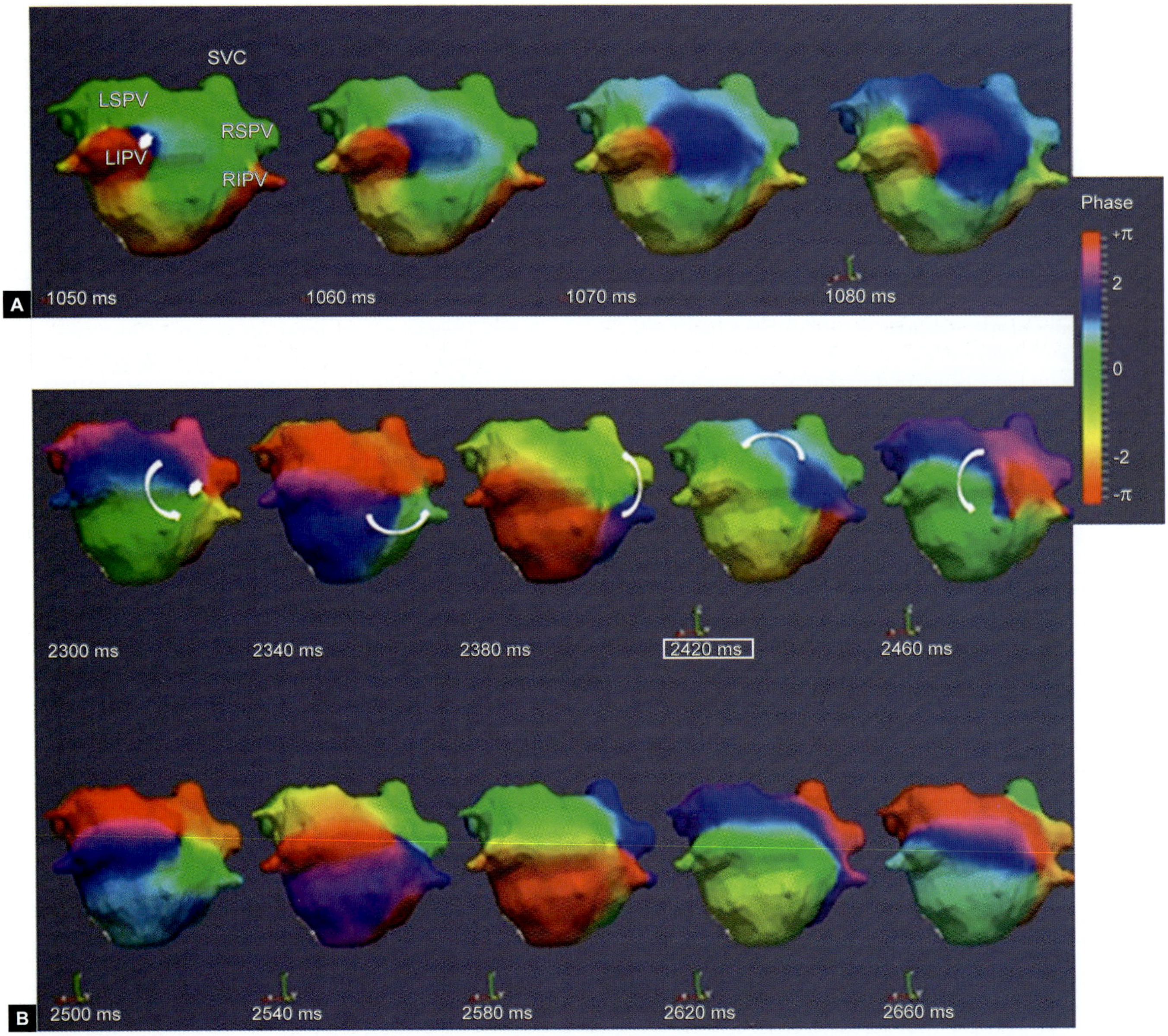

Figures 23.9A and B: Phase mapping showing posterior view of left atrium during paroxysmal AF. (A) Serial snapshots of a single wave emerging out of the left inferior PV (white star) and reaching right veins in 30 ms while it expands radially to the roof and inferior walls; (B) Serial snapshots of two successive rotations (white arrows) of a rotor located near the ostia of right veins. The core of the rotor (white star at the center of rainbow-colored phases of rotor) is seen meandering in a small region in this example. The blue wave indicates the depolarizing front which makes one full rotation in 160 ms. The phases of wave propagation are color-coded using rainbow scale. The blue color represents depolarizing wave and the green represents the end of repolarization. The wavefront can be read by following the blue color. The time (ms) at the bottom of each snapshot represents the moment in the time-window when the snapshot was taken

Abbreviations: LSPV: left superior pulmonary vein; LIPV: left inferior PV; RSPV: right superior PV; RIPV: right inferior PV, SVC: superior vena cava

Source: Permission to reproduce the figure obtained from Haïssaguerre M, et al. J Cardiovasc Electrophysiol. 2013;24:711-7.

On the other hand, in common with the observation made by Narayan et al.[34] using endocardial phase mapping, an endocardial multispline-catheter-based mapping study by Haissaguerre et al.[22] reported stable localized sources (reentries and foci) in the majority of the patients as a mechanism maintaining AF organized by prior linear and pulmonary vein ablations. Could this commonality be because both studies involved *endocardial* mapping remains to be answered in future.

REFERENCES

1. Camm AJ, Kirchhof P, Lip GY, Schotten U, Savelieva I, Ernst S, Van Gelder IC, Al-Attar N, Hindricks G, Prendergast B, Heidbuchel H, Alfieri O, Angelini A, Atar D, Colonna P, De Caterina R, De Sutter J, Goette A, Gorenek B, Heldal M, Hohloser SH, Kolh P, Le Heuzey JY, Ponikowski P, Rutten FH. Guidelines for the management of atrial fibrillation: the Task Force for the Management of Atrial Fibrillation of the European Society of Cardiology (ESC). Europace. 2010;12:1360-420.
2. Calkins H, Kuck KH, Cappato R, Brugada J, Camm AJ, Chen SA, Crijns HJ, Damiano RJ Jr, Davies DW, DiMarco J, Edgerton J, Ellenbogen K, Ezekowitz MD, Haines DE, Haissaguerre M, Hindricks G, Iesaka Y, Jackman W, Jalife J, Jais P, Kalman J, Keane D, Kim YH, Kirchhof P, Klein G, Kottkamp H, Kumagai K, Lindsay BD, Mansour M, Marchlinski FE, McCarthy PM, Mont JL, Morady F, Nademanee K, Nakagawa H, Natale A, Nattel S, Packer DL, Pappone C, Prystowsky E, Raviele A, Reddy V, Ruskin JN, Shemin RJ, Tsao HM, Wilber D; Heart Rhythm Society Task Force on Catheter and Surgical Ablation of Atrial Fibrillation. 2012 HRS/EHRA/ECAS expert consensus statement on catheter and surgical ablation of atrial fibrillation: recommendations for patient selection, procedural techniques, patient management and follow-up, definitions, endpoints, and research trial design: a report of the Heart Rhythm Society (HRS) Task Force on Catheter and Surgical Ablation of Atrial Fibrillation. Developed in partnership with the European Heart Rhythm Association (EHRA), a registered branch of the European Society of Cardiology (ESC) and the European Cardiac Arrhythmia Society (ECAS); and in collaboration with the American College of Cardiology (ACC), American Heart Association (AHA), the Asia Pacific Heart Rhythm Society (APHRS), and the Society of Thoracic Surgeons (STS). Endorsed by the governing bodies of the American College of Cardiology Foundation, the American Heart Association, the European Cardiac Arrhythmia Society, the European Heart Rhythm Association, the Society of Thoracic Surgeons, the Asia Pacific Heart Rhythm Society, and the Heart Rhythm Society. Heart Rhythm. 2012;9:632-696.e21.
3. January CT, Wann LS, Alpert JS, Calkins H, Cigarroa JE, Cleveland JC Jr, Conti JB, Ellinor PT, Ezekowitz MD, Field ME, Murray KT, Sacco RL, Stevenson WG, Tchou PJ, Tracy CM, Yancy CW, Anuary CT, Wann LS, Alpert JS, Calkins H, Cigarroa JE, Cleveland JC Jr, Conti JB, Ellinor PT, Ezekowitz MD, Field ME, Murray KT, Sacco RL, Stevenson WG, Tchou PJ, Tracy CM, Yancy CW. 2014 AHA/ACC/HRS Guideline for the Management of Patients with Atrial Fibrillation: Executive Summary: A Report of the American College of Cardiology/ American Heart Association Task Force on Practice Guidelines and the Heart Rhythm Society. J Am Coll Cardiol. 2014;64: e1-e76.
4. Shah AJ, Liu X, Jadidi AS, Haissaguerre M. Early management of atrial fibrillation: from imaging to drugs to ablation. Nature Reviews Cardiology. 2010;7:345-54.
5. Garrey WE. Auricular fibrillation. Physiol Rev. 1924;4:215-50.
6. Moe GK, Rheinboldt WC, Abildskov JA. A computer model of atrial fibrillation. Am Heart J. 1964;67:200-20.
7. Allessie MA, Bonke FI, Schopman FJ. Circus movement in rabbit atrial muscle as a mechanism of tachycardia. III. The leading circle» concept: a new model of circus movement in cardiac tissue without the involvement of an anatomical obstacle. Circ Res. 1977;41:9-18.
8. Cox JL, Schuessler RB, D'Agostino HJ Jr, Stone CM, Chang BC, Cain ME, Corr PB, Boineau JP. The surgical treatment of atrial fibrillation: development of a definitive surgical procedure. J Thorac Cardiovasc Surg. 1991;101:569-83.
9. Haissaguerre M, Marcus FI, Fischer B, Clementy J. Radiofrequency catheter ablation in unusual mechanisms of atrial fibrillation: report of three cases. J Cardiovasc Electrophysiol. 1994;5:743-51.
10. Haïssaguerre M, Jaïs P, Shah DC, Gencel L, Pradeau V, Garrigues S, Chouairi S, Hocini M, Le Métayer P, Roudaut R, Clémenty J. Right and left atrial radiofrequency catheter therapy of paroxysmal atrial fibrillation. J Cardiovasc Electrophysiol. 1996;7:1132-44.
11. Jais P, Haissaguerre M, Shah DC, Chouairi S, Gencel L, Hocini M, Clementy J. A focal source of atrial fibrillation treated by discrete radiofrequency ablation. Circulation. 1997;95: 572-6.
12. Mandapati R, Skanes A, Chen J, Berenfeld O, Jalife J. Stable microreentrant sources as a mechanism of atrial fibrillation in the isolated sheep heart. Circulation. 2000;101:194-9.
13. Morillo CA, Klein GJ, Jones DL, Guiraudon CM. Chronic rapid atrial pacing. Structural, functional, and electrophysiological characteristics of a new model of sustained atrial fibrillation. Circulation. 1995;91:1588-95.
14. Haissaguerre M, Jais P, Shah DC, Takahashi A, Hocini M, Quiniou G, Garrigue S, Le Mouroux A, Le Metayer P, Clementy J. Spontaneous initiation of atrial fibrillation by ectopic beats originating in the pulmonary veins. N Engl J Med. 1998;339: 659-66.
15. Chen SA, Hsieh MH, Tai CT, Tsai CF, Prakash VS, Yu WC, Hsu TL, Ding YA, Chang MS. Initiation of atrial fibrillation by ectopic beats originating from the pulmonary veins: electrophysiological characteristics, pharmacological responses, and effects of radiofrequency ablation. Circulation 1999;100: 1879-86.
16. Chen SA, Tai CT. Catheter ablation of atrial fibrillation originating from the non-pulmonary vein foci. J Cardiovasc Electrophysiol. 2005;16:229-32.
17. Nattel S. New ideas about atrial fibrillation 50 years on. Nature. 2002;415:219-26.
18. Sanders P, Berenfeld O, Hocini M, Jaïs P, Vaidyanathan R, Hsu LF, Garrigue S, Takahashi Y, Rotter M, Sacher F, Scavée C, Ploutz-Snyder R, Jalife J, Haïssaguerre M. Spectral analysis identifies sites of high-frequency activity maintaining atrial fibrillation in humans. Circulation. 2005;112:789-97.
19. Elvan R, Pride HP, Eble JN, Zipes DP. Radiofrequency catheter ablation of the atria reduces inducibility and duration of atrial fibrillation in dogs. Circulation. 1995;91:2235-44.
20. Schuessler RB, Grayson TM, Bromberg BI, Cox JL, Boineau J. Cholinergically mediated tachyarrhythmias induced by a single extrastimulus in the isolated canine right atrium. Circ Res. 1992;71:1254-67.
21. Scherf D. Studies on auricular tachycardia caused by aconitine administration. Proc Soc Exp Biol Med. 1947;64:233-9.
22. Haissaguerre M, Hocini M, Sanders P, Takahashi Y, Rotter M, Sacher F, Rostock T, Hsu LF, Jonsson A, O'Neill MD, Bordachar P, Reuter S, Roudaut R, Clementy J, Jais P. Localized Sources Maintaining Atrial Fibrillation Organized by Prior Ablation. Circulation. 2006;113:616-25.

23. Allessie M, Ausma J, Schotten U. Electrical, contractile and structural remodeling during atrial fibrillation. Cardiovasc Res. 2002;54:230-46.
24. Burstein B, Nattel S. Atrial fibrosis: mechanisms and clinical relevance in atrial fibrillation. J Am Coll Cardiol. 2008;51:802-9.
25. Jahangir A, Lee V, Friedman PA, Trusty JM, Hodge DO, Kopecky SL, Packer DL, Hammill SC, Shen WK, Gersh BJ. Long-term progression and outcomes with aging in patients with lone atrial fibrillation: a 30-year follow-up study. Circulation. 2007;115:3050-6.
26. Levy S, Maarek M, Coumel P, Guize L, Lekieffre J, Medvedowsky JL, Sebaoun A. Characterization of different subsets of atrial fibrillation in general practice in France: the ALFA study. The College of French Cardiologists. Circulation. 1999;99: 3028-35.
27. Kerr CR, Humphries KH, Talajic M, Klein GJ, Connolly SJ, Green M, Boone J, Sheldon R, Dorian P, Newman D. Progression to chronic atrial fibrillation after the initial diagnosis of paroxysmal atrial fibrillation: results from the Canadian Registry of Atrial Fibrillation. Am Heart J. 2005;149:489-96.
28. de Vos CB, Pisters R, Nieuwlaat R, Prins MH, Tieleman RG, Coelen RJ, van den Heijkant AC, Allessie MA, Crijns HJ. Progression from paroxysmal to persistent atrial fibrillation clinical correlates and prognosis. J Am Coll Cardiol. 2010;55:725-31.
29. de Groot NM, Houben RP, Smeets JL, Boersma E, Schotten U, Schalij MJ, Crijns H, Allessie MA. Electropathological substrate of longstanding persistent atrial fibrillation in patients with structural heart disease: epicardial breakthrough. Circulation. 2010;122:1674-82.
30. Allessie MA, de Groot NM, Houben RP, Schotten U, Boersma E, Smeets JL, Crijns HJ. Electropathological substrate of long-standing persistent atrial fibrillation in patients with structural heart disease: longitudinal dissociation. Circ Arrhythm Electrophysiol. 2010;3:606-15.
31. Sahadevan J, Ryu K, Peltz L, Khrestian CM, Stewart RW, Markowitz AH, Waldo AL. Epicardial mapping of chronic atrial fibrillation in patients: preliminary observations. Circulation. 2004;110:3293-9.
32. Eckstein J, Zeemering D, Linz D, Maesen B, Crijins H, Allessie MA, Schotten U, Verheule S, van Hunnik A. Transmural conduction is the predominant mechanism of breakthrough during atrial fibrillation: evidence from simultaneous endo-epicardial high density activation mapping. Circ Arrhythm Electrophysiol. 2013;6:334-41.
33. Cuculich PS, Wang Y, Lindsay BD, Faddis MN, Schuessler RB, Damiano RJ Jr., Li L, Rudy Y. Noninvasive characterization of epicardial activation in humans with diverse atrial fibrillation patterns. Circulation. 2010;122:1364-72.
34. Narayan SM, Krummen DE, Rappel WJ. Clinical mapping approach to diagnose electrical rotors and focal impulse sources for human atrial fibrillation. J Cardiovasc Electrophysiol. 2012;23:447-54.
35. Haissaguerre M, Hocini M, Shah AJ, Derval N, Sacher F, Jais P, Dubois R. Noninvasive panoramic mapping of human atrial fibrillation mechanisms: a feasibility report. J Cardiovasc Electrophysiol. 2013;24:711-7.
36. Haissaguerre M, Hocini M, Denis A, Shah AJ, Komatsu Y, Yamashita S, Daly M, Amraoui S, Zellerhoff S, Picat MQ, Quotb A, Jesel L, Lim H, Ploux S, Bordachar P, Attuel G, Meillet V, Ritter P, Derval N, Sacher F, Bernus O, Cochet H, Jais P, Dubois R. Driver domains in persistent atrial fibrillation. Circulation. 2014;130:530-8.
37. Skanes AC, Mandapati R, Berenfeld O, Davidenko JM, Jalife J. Spatiotemporal Periodicity During Atrial Fibrillation in the Isolated Sheep Heart. Circulation. 1998;98:1236-48.
38. Lim HS, Zellerhoff S, Hocini M, Derval N, Denis A, Yamashita S, Berte B, Mahida S, Hooks D, Aljefairi N, Shah AJ, Sacher F, Jaïs P, Dubois R, Haïssaguerre M. Noninvasive Mapping to Guide Atrial Fibrillation Ablation. Card Electrophysiol Clin. 2015;7:89-98.
39. Kalifa J, Avula UM. Ablation of driver domains during persistent atrial fibrillation: a call for more understanding. Circulation. 2014;130:525-7.
40. Cox JL, Canavan TE, Schuessler RB, Cain ME, Lindsay BD, Stone C, Smith PK, Corr PB, Boineau JP. The surgical treatment of atrial fibrillation, II: intraoperative electrophysiologic mapping and description of the electrophysiologic basis of atrial flutter and atrial fibrillation. J Thorac Cardiovasc Surg. 1991;101:406–26.
41. Wang Z, Page P, Nattel S. Mechanism of flecainide's antiarrhythmic action in experimental atrial fibrillation. Circ Res. 1992;71:271-87.
42. Konings KT, Kirchhof CJ, Smeets JR, Wellens HJ, Penn OC, Allessie MA. High-density mapping of electrically induced atrial fibrillation in humans. Circulation. 1994;89:1665-80.
43. Kumagai K, Khrestian C, Waldo AL. Simultaneous multisite mapping studies during induced atrial fibrillation in the sterile pericarditis model: insights into the mechanism of its maintenance. Circulation. 1997; 95:511-21.

EDITORS' SUMMARY

Professor Haissaguerre, a pioneer and innovator for contemporary cardiac electrophysiology has traced for us the fundamental principles that underlie atrial fibrillation ablation from his early days through this evolution.

The early studies that led to understanding the role of the thoracic vein triggering atrial fibrillation as well as present ideas on what constitutes the substrate that maintains atrial fibrillation has been carefully outlined. Professor Haissaguerre provides his unique insights into both intracardiac and body surface mapping during atrial fibrillation including potential explanations for the differences in these approaches. When used in conjunction with other chapters in this textbook that look at persistent atrial fibrillation (Chapter 25), atypical atrial flutter (Chapter 22), and cardiac anatomy (Chapter 6), the reader will be well equipped to begin handling the challenges of AF ablation.

CHAPTER 24

Rajiv Mahajan, Darragh Twomey,
Dennis H Lau, Prashanthan Sanders

Atrial Fibrillation Ablation: Pulmonary Vein Isolation Techniques, Strategies and Principles

LIST OF ABBREVIATIONS

AF	Atrial Fibrillation	PVAC	Pulmonary Vein Ablation Catheter
LA	Left Atrium	PVI	Pulmonary Vein Isolation
LMWH	Low Molecular Weight Heparin	RF	Radiofrequency
PV	Pulmonary Vein	WACA	Wide Area Circumferential Ablation

INTRODUCTION

The importance of the spontaneous ectopy in triggering paroxysms of atrial fibrillation (AF) in humans is well recognized. Although a variety of structures (venous or atrial) have been implicated as potential sources of triggers, the pulmonary veins (PVs) are accepted to be the dominant source. Spontaneous activity from these structures can result in a spectrum of atrial arrhythmias ranging from isolated extrasystoles to rapid sustained focal discharges that trigger and participate in maintaining AF in patients with the appropriate substrate. Electrical isolation of the PVs has emerged as cornerstone of the AF ablation procedure, however, some patients may require additional substrate modification and attention to risk factors.[1,2] Emerging data from STAR AF II suggests that PV isolation alone may be as effective without the use of additional substrate modification in persistent AF as well.[3] The technique of PV isolation has evolved from focal 'trigger' ablation to ostial isolation and finally antral/wide circumferential isolation. Current ablation techniques are limited by recovery of PV connections resulting in recurrences after catheter ablation of paroxysmal AF. The introduction of steerable sheaths, contact-force sense technology, improved ablation catheters and possibly higher density mapping have resulted in enhancement of catheter stability, achievement of optimal tissue contact, creation of larger lesions and better identification of residual tissue culminating in improved outcomes of catheter ablation. Alternative energy sources such as cryoablation have also been utilized for AF ablation. This chapter reviews the rationale and various techniques of pulmonary vein isolation in AF ablation.

RATIONALE FOR PULMONARY VEIN ISOLATION

Paroxysms of AF are consistently initiated by spontaneous triggers or extrasystoles arising from several sites including the pulmonary veins (PVs),[4-6] the vein/ligament of Marshall,[7] the coronary sinus,[4] the crista terminalis,[8] the superior vena cava, and the inferior vena cava. However, the vast majority are the result of spontaneous activity originating from the PVs,[9] which may also have a role in the maintenance of AF and in the re-initiation of AF following the cardioversion of persistent AF.[9,10] Spontaneous activity arising from the PVs can manifest in a spectrum of atrial arrhythmias. Single discharges may manifest as isolated extrasystoles, repetitive discharge with a long cycle length may manifest as slow atrial rhythms (even mimicking sinus rhythm), and shorter cycle length discharges may manifest as an atrial tachycardia.[4,11] Rapid sustained focal discharges (sometimes for hours, days or even longer) may drive sustained AF (focal AF- implicating the focus is both the trigger and substrate for AF) or more commonly bursts initiate AF (focally initiated AF) in patients with the appropriate substrate. They may also be responsible for the initiation of isthmus dependent atrial flutter. Elimination of these localized focal triggers provides an attractive target for catheter ablation.

PULMONARY VEIN ABLATION/ ISOLATION TECHNIQUES

Focal Ablation of Pulmonary Vein Triggers

Initially catheter ablation was performed to target the site of earliest endocardial activation during spontaneous ectopy thereby creating focal lesions for the cure of AF. [4,6] The seminal study from Haissaguerre et al.[4] demonstrated that 94% of ectopy originated from the PVs in patients with frequent episodes of drug refractory paroxysmal AF. In this study, the earliest local activity was mapped to a point 2 to 4 cm within the main PV or one of its branches, with depolarization marked by a spike (PV potential) preceding the onset of atrial activation by 35 to 45 ms. Radiofrequency ablation at the site of earliest endocardial activity resulted in acute abolition of atrial ectopy and at 8 ± 6 months 62% remained free of AF without the use of antiarrhythmic agents. This work was confirmed in other studies[6,12] and has become the basis for PV isolation becoming the cornerstone of AF ablation.

Focal ablation was associated with significant incidence of PV stenosis.[4,6] The applicability of PV trigger ablation was also limited by infrequent or even the complete absence of spontaneous ectopy during the procedure in many patients. Provocation maneuvers, both pacing and pharmacological, were unreliable in inducing ectopy. Furthermore, ablation of the induced foci could not exclude other dormant triggers. Several techniques were evolved in an attempt to overcome these limitations including right atrial endocardial activation sequence during ectopy, algorithms to predict the arrhythmogenic PV based on ectopic P-wave morphology with or without QRST subtraction to reveal the morphology of the "P on T" ectopics, utilization of multielectrode mapping catheters to enhance the density of mapping during ectopy, and the mapping of postcardioversion immediate recurrences of AF.[9] Subsequent studies demonstrated that in patients prone to AF, multiple veins and also multiple foci within any given vein may produce spontaneous triggers,[13] necessitating repeat procedures.[12,14] As such this approach evolved to the technique of segmental ostial ablation aimed at electrical isolation of all PVs.

Segmental Pulmonary Vein Isolation

The advent of circumferential mapping catheters made it possible to determine the perimetric distribution and activation sequence of PV activity.[15] PV potentials reflecting local striated muscle have been shown to be present over a variable extent (varying also from one vein to the next) of the perimeter and that PV muscle activation was often sequential from the segment with earliest activation. Therefore, the PVs could be electrically isolated from the left atrium (LA) by ablation of ostial segments. Haissaguerre et al. showed that 73% of patients were free of AF without the use of antiarrhythmic agents at 4 ± 5 months following ablation.[15] Other groups have reported single procedure success rates of approximately 50%.

The earliest left atrial breakthroughs were targeted during segmental ablation. Left atrial to PV breakthroughs (confirmed by ablation) were noted to be most frequent at the bottom of superior PVs (85% prevalence) and the top of inferior PVs (75% prevalence).[16] Electrogram polarity reversal (defined as opposite polarity across adjacent bipoles) has been shown to be a useful additional criterion in combination with earliest activation with 88% sensitivity and 91% specificity to indicate breakthrough sites. Polarity reversal has been found to be restricted to fewer bipoles (2.0 ± 0.4 bipoles) compared with earliest activation (3.4 ± 2.0 bipoles). Shorter radiofrequency application time was required to disconnect PVs displaying wide synchronous activation using polarity reversal compared with using conventional earliest activity (10.3 ± 3.0 min compared to 12.3 ± 3.4 min).[16] The major drawbacks were high PV stenosis rates and transient PV to LA block with segmental ablation which was associated with high recurrence rate as compared to circumferential PV ablation.[17-19]

Wide Antral Isolation

This technique consists of wide circumferential lesions around and outside the pulmonary veins. The initial report described lesions 0.5 cm outside the PV ostia. It has been modified over time with wider circumferential lesions. **Figures 24.1A to C** demonstrates lesion set in ostial, wide antral and single ring ablation for pulmonary vein isolation. Even within the definition of wide antral ablation, there is wide variation in the lesion set ranging from isolation of each vein separately to isolation of ipsilateral PVs. The common features to all current variants are inclusion of the antrum and confirmed electrical isolation. This has been endorsed by the Heart Rhythm Society/European Heart Rhythm Association/European Arrhythmia Society expert consensus statement on catheter and surgical ablation of AF.[20]

Ablation away from the PV ostium in wide antral isolation reduces the risk of PV stenosis.[21] The rationale for wide

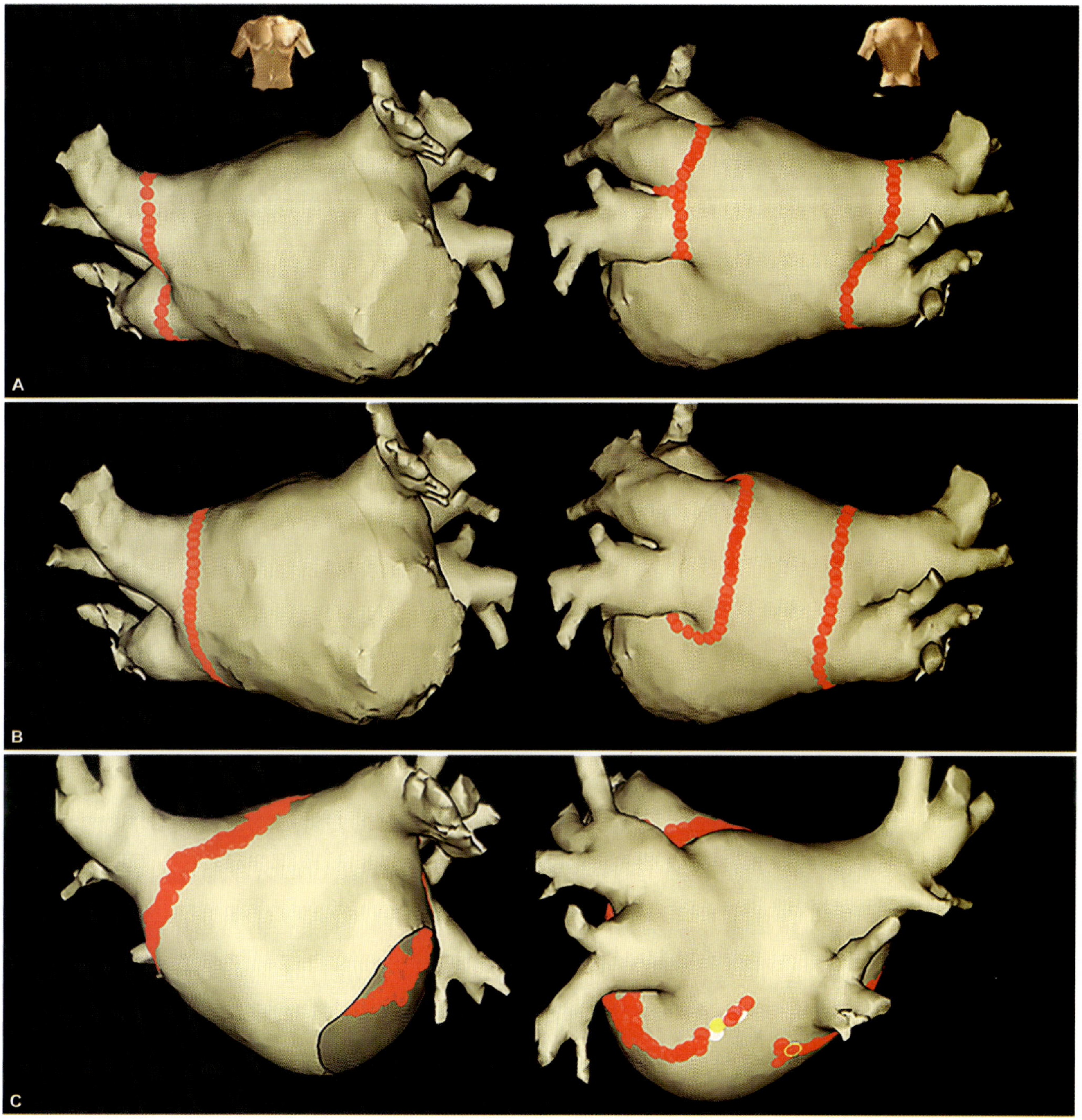

Figures 24.1A to C: Techniques of circumferential AF ablation with (A) Showing ostial ablation; (B) Showing wide antral ablation; and (C) Demonstrating single ring ablation. During single ring isolation in this case, pulmonary vein and posterior wall isolation were achieved before the completion of the inferior segment

antral isolation also stems from experimental studies demonstrating arrhythmogenic potential of PV-LA junctions. Experimental studies have demonstrated that microreentry localized at the PV–LA junction may be critical in maintaining AF.[22-24] Abrupt changes of myocardial fiber orientation at the PV-LA junctions and difference in action potential of PVs and LA are responsible for nonuniform anisotropy and shorter action potential duration, favoring reentry around PV–LA junction and maintaining the AF. Similarly, decremental conduction and conduction blocks with reentry at the PV-LA junction has been demonstrated in human studies.[25,26] Atienza et al. have shown that adenosine accelerates AF drivers, particularly those located at the PV-LA junction.[27,28] Furthermore, wide antral ablation may also lead to concomitant ablation of ganglionic plexuses in the posterior LA.[29]

A recent meta-analysis compared 12 studies with wide antral isolation with segmental ostial ablation.[30] There was greater freedom from overall atrial arrhythmia and AF recurrence with a trend towards increased incidence of left atrial flutter with wide antral isolation. The complication rates were not significantly different between the two groups.

Wide circumferential ablation is facilitated with the use of selective PV angiography, intracardiac echocardiography and 3D electroanatomic mapping systems. Defining the PV ostium has been more of a semantic issue whilst the LA to PV junction is funnel shaped. A double lasso approach was propagated with the rationale that this prevented ostial ablation and facilitated placement of lesions at the antrum.[31] Similarly, intracardiac echocardiogram allow direct visualization of antrum for lesion placement.[32] Registration with CT scans has further improved the understanding of the PV anatomy and facilitated wide circumferential ablation.

Single Ring Isolation (Box Isolation)

This technique incorporates the advantages of wide antral isolation namely, reduced risk of PV stenosis and concomitant isolation of antral tissue. Posterior left atrial wall is considered to play a role in AF genesis.[22,33] Sanders et al. demonstrated the feasibility of posterior wall isolation in patients with chronic AF.[34] Posterior LA isolation resulted in prolongation of the AF cycle length, incremental to the effect of PV isolation, and termination of AF in 20% of patients. At a long-term follow-up, 63% of these patients with chronic AF remained in sinus rhythm at 2 years. More recently, Lim et al. have compared single ring isolation with wide antral isolation and demonstrated reduced recurrence of AF and similar incidence of organized atrial arrhythmias after single ring isolation.[35] They showed that AF-free survival at 2 years was better after single ring isolation (74% [95% CI, 65%–82%]) than wide antral isolation (61% [96% CI, 51%–70%]; p=0.031). Survival free of organized atrial tachyarrhythmia was similar after both single ring and wide antral isolation (67% [57%–75%] versus 64% [54%–72%] respectively at 2 years; p=0.988). Tamborero et al. However, did not find any difference in arrhythmia-free survival after 9.8 ± 4.3 months of follow-up in a randomized comparison involving 120 patients undergoing wide antral isolation with or without additional isolation of the posterior left atrium.[36] However, posterior wall isolation was not achieved in 9% of cases and no distinction was made between AF recurrences and organized atrial arrhythmias.

The approach in our institution has evolved on the same lines and the current approach is to preferentially isolate the pulmonary veins *en bloc* with a single ring lesion set when feasible. This is supplemented (if required) with additional segmental ablation in the posterior wall away from the esophagus. Limiting the ablation on the posterior left atrium may intuitively reduce the risk of left atrial-esophageal fistula.

INTERPRETING ELECTROGRAMS DURING PV ISOLATION

The proximity of the LA to the PVs inevitably results in fusion of their respective potentials as recorded on the circumferential mapping catheter. Failure to recognize persisting far-field atrial potentials on the circumferential mapping catheter is a source of frequent confusion and prolonged and unnecessary ablation. This is particularly evident in the left PVs during sinus rhythm, which produces a synchronous wavefront with the LA or LA appendage. Distal coronary sinus or left atrial appendage pacing to first capture the LA unmasks and separates the left PV potentials, facilitating the recognition of PV potentials during ablation.[37] Changing to differing pacing sites (coronary sinus, left atrial appendage or posterior LA) anticipates far-field components of these potentials allowing their recognition as atrial in origin. In the left superior PV, this is particularly common in the anterior bipoles, which fall in time with the posterior wall of the left atrial appendage.[38] In the left inferior PV, atrial potentials also persist on the superior or anterior poles, in time with the anterior LA. Similar double or triple component electrograms are frequently recorded in the anterior right superior PV. Based on three-dimensional electroanatomic activation maps of the various surrounding structures, the initial component of the electrogram coincided with P-wave onset with identical timing with the adjacent superior vena cava.

STRATEGIES TO ACHIEVE DURABLE PULMONARY VEIN ISOLATION

Electrical isolation of the PVs (elimination or dissociation of PV potentials, entry and exit block) provides a defined procedural endpoint for pulmonary vein isolation. Reports of the immediate procedural success have ranged from 94% to 100%, however half the veins recover within 60 minutes of isolation.[39] The most common etiology for AF recurrence and need for redo ablation procedure is PV reconnection and is postulated to be secondary to transient electrical block due to tissue edema.[39] Cappato et al. reported pulmonary vein reconnection rate as high as 82% after the index ablation.[19] After reablation, a third procedure in symptomatic patients again demonstrated repeat reconnection in two-thirds of reisolated veins. Nanthakumar et al. similarly described reconnection in 42 of 51 previously isolated veins in 15 patients with recurrent symptoms after a first ablation procedure for paroxysmal AF.[40] All patients had 2 or more reconnected veins. An extrapulmonary vein trigger was noted in one patient only. Furthermore, Gerstenfeld demonstrated that triggers induced by isoproterenol were located in the reconnected pulmonary veins.[17] Pulmonary vein reconnection is also responsible for a good proportion of late recurrence along with progression of atrial substrate.[19,41]

Recent studies have provided insights into the role of stability and contact force in creating transmural lesions and hence durable electrical isolation. The multicenter TOCCATA trial demonstrated the feasibility and safety of the tacticath catheter. The study demonstrated that tissue-catheter force-time integral was a predictor for arrhythmia free survival. The authors showed a reduced recurrence rate of 31% with >1000 g-s contact force as compared to a recurrence rate of 75% with <500 g-s contact force.[42] The EFFICAS-1 trial confirmed increased presence of gaps with <20 g-s initial force and <400 g-s contact force-time integral.[43] Similarly, the use of steerable sheaths has been shown to improve the durability of pulmonary vein isolation.

Rigorous assessment of pulmonary vein isolation has been shown to improve the durability of pulmonary vein isolation **(Figures 24.2A to C)**. Most center utilize entry block into the pulmonary vein as assessed with a circular catheter as a criterion for electrical isolation. The exit block is demonstrated by pacing inside the pulmonary veins and assessing for exit into the left atrium.[31,44,45] This test is cumbersome due to difficulty in capturing the tissue inside the pulmonary veins and has not gained wide acceptance. As a result, the utility of exit block has not been evaluated in prospective studies. The acute recovery of the pulmonary veins has been systematically evaluated in studies.[39] Wang et al. undertook an intervention study based on the waiting period after pulmonary vein isolation.[46] They randomized 90 patients to a waiting period of zero (control arm), 30 or 60 minutes with subsequent reablation of recovered pulmonary veins. They reported that 30% of veins recovered acutely, mostly within 30 minutes, and demonstrated improved arrhythmia free outcome in the two groups with a waiting period (61% versus 84% versus 87%, respectively, p = 0.04). Based on this evidence, Heart Rhythm Society guidelines recommend a waiting period of 30 minutes after pulmonary vein isolation.

The role of adenosine in assessing dormant pulmonary veins was initially described in 2004. Two independent groups showed that adenosine could unmask dormant pulmonary vein conduction in 25–35% of isolated pulmonary veins.[47,48] Furthermore, other single center studies have shown that the outcome of ablation was improved by elimination of dormant pulmonary vein conduction.[49-51] Indeed, adenosine-provoked pulmonary vein conduction had a positive predictive value of 90% and a negative predictive value of 15% for recurrent pulmonary vein conduction during a repeat procedure.[52] The number of pulmonary veins reconnection after adenosine administration is similar to the percentage of PVs reconnecting after a 30-minute wait time. Adenosine infusion and 30 minutes wait time are associated with reconduction in 15% and 19% of pulmonary veins, with moderate agreement between the two methods. Yamane et al. evaluated time- and adenosine-provoked pulmonary vein reconduction in 75 patients to guide ablation. They reported a high success rate of 92% (without antiarrhythmic drugs) after a single procedure at 12 months.[53]

STRATEGIES TO REDUCE COMPLICATIONS OF ATRIAL FIBRILLATION ABLATION

The serious complications of AF ablation are cardiac tamponade, pulmonary vein stenosis, perioperative stroke and LA-esophageal fistula.[54] The use of echo-guided transseptal puncture and force-sensing technology improve the safety of the procedure and reduce the risk of cardiac tamponade. The incidence of pulmonary vein stenosis has decreased after transition from segmental approach to wide antral ablation as described above. The risk of periprocedural thromboembolism has diminished by performing catheter ablation for AF under therapeutic warfarin.[55] A multicenter observational study has demonstrated 0.6% rate of periprocedural thromboembolism in patients undergoing ablation with continuation of warfarin as compared to 1% risk of periprocedural thromboembolism in the group that discontinued warfarin (OR 0.54[0.32–0.89], p = 0.017).[56] This was in the absence of significant increase in major bleeding (1.1% versus 0.8%). This has been confirmed in a large pooled analysis of over 27,000 patients demonstrating a marked reduction in peri-procedural thromboembolic risk (OR = 0.10, p<0.001) with catheter ablation undertaken under therapeutic warfarin as compared to warfarin interrupted with low-molecular-weight heparin (LMWH) bridging.[57] Again, there was no significant increase in periprocedural major bleeding with therapeutic warfarin. More recently, a randomized trial has confirmed that performing catheter ablation of AF without warfarin discontinuation reduces the occurrence of periprocedural stroke and minor bleeding complications compared with bridging with LMWH.[58] This study showed a reduced risk of 0.25% of stroke on warfarin compared to 3.7% stroke risk in the group with warfarin discontinuation and bridging LMWH. The experience with the uninterrupted novel anticoagulant agents has been less consistent with regards to safety.

Atrioesophageal fistula remains a rare but often fatal complication of catheter ablation for AF. The incidence of atrioesophageal fistula varies from 0.01 to 0.2% in different series[55,59-62] with an estimated mortality of 40–80%.[60,61,63] Lower body mass index,[64] rise in esophageal temperature beyond 38.5 to 39.5°C,[65,66] sensitherm temperature probe,[66] gastroesophageal reflux,[67] power > 25 Watts[68] on posterior left atrium and general anesthesia[69] have been reported to be associated with esophageal injury after ablation. Reduced power during ablation on the posterior wall,[68,70] use of esophageal contrast or temperature monitoring,

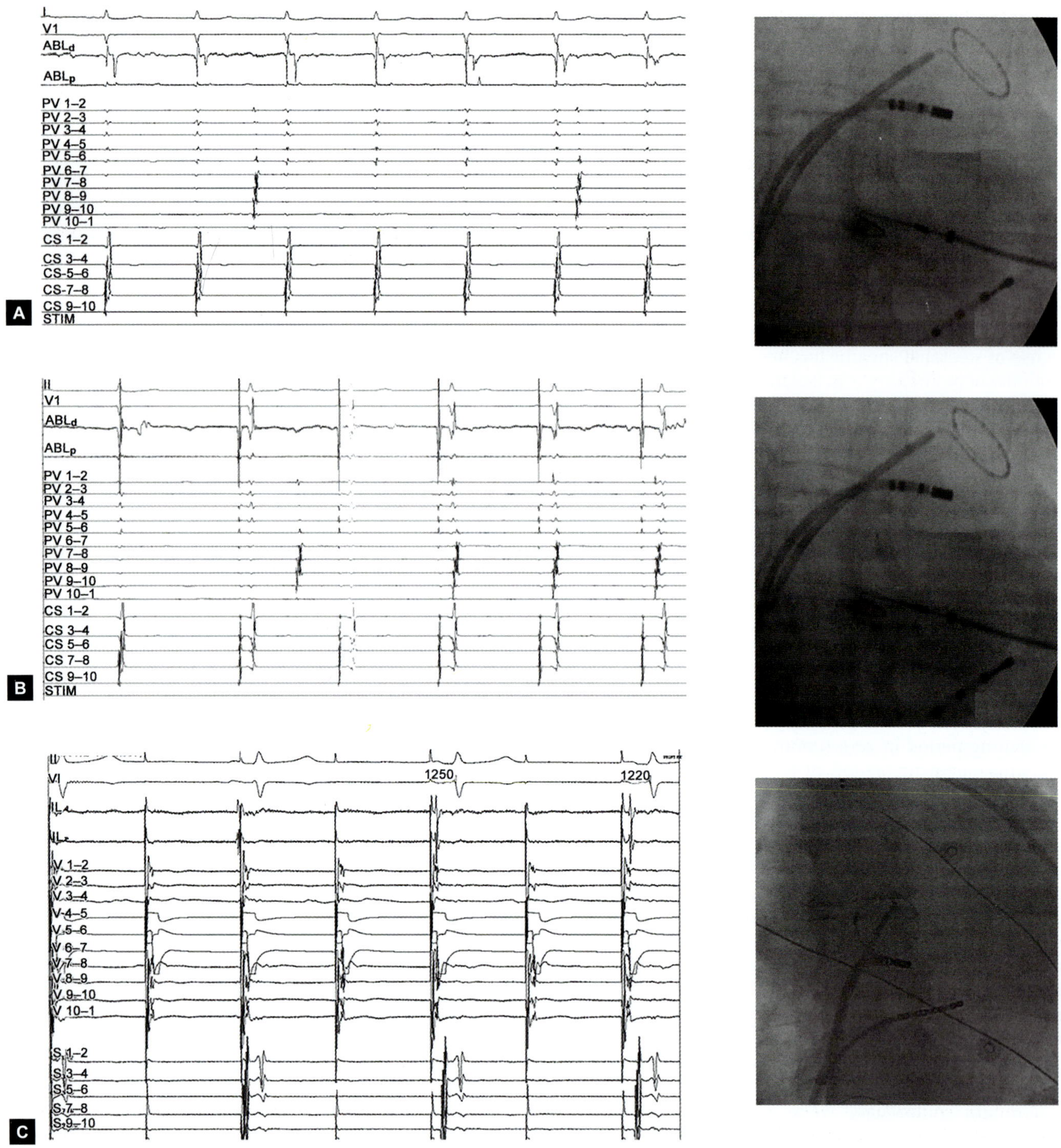

Figures 24.2A to C: (A) Demonstrates both entry and exit block from the pulmonary vein (PV). The circular mapping catheter positioned in the left superior pulmonary vein demonstrates absence of conduction into the pulmonary vein. Dissociated rhythm also confirms exit block; (B) Shows resumption of conduction following adenosine administration requiring further ablation; (C) Demonstrates pacing from the lasso catheter placed on the posterior left atrium. The atrial tissue is captured but there is exit block out of the isolated single ring lesion set. I, V1 representing surface ECG, Abl representing ablation catheter, PV represents circular mapping catheter and CS represents decapolar catheter positioned in the coronary sinus (CS)

postprocedure proton pump inhibitors[67] and mechanical displacement of esophagus[71] have been the strategies that have been advocated to reduce this dreaded complication. Force sensing catheters may help reduce esophageal injury during ablation on the posterior wall. Recently, there has been a concern that the esophageal temperature probe may work as a sink for RF energy causing heating and lesions in the esophagus.

NEW TOOLS FOR AF ABLATION

'One-shot' pulmonary vein ablation systems have been developed in response to the need for quicker AF ablation procedures with potentially shorter learning curves. Two distinct groups of technologies exist, multielectrode radiofrequency (RF) catheters, and balloon-based systems.

Multielectrode Ablation Catheters for Pulmonary Vein Isolation

The first commercially available multielectrode PV isolation (PVI) catheter was the pulmonary vein ablation catheter (PVAC) system (Medtronic Inc., Minneapolis, MN, USA). A steerable, over-the-wire, circular multipolar catheter is delivered to the left atrium through a single transseptal sheath. Pulmonary vein angiography allows visualization of the venous os and negates the need for electroanatomical mapping. Several overlapping duty-cycled RF lesions are then applied to each PV to achieve electrical isolation. The second generation of circular ablation catheter, the nMARQ system (Biosense Webster Inc, Diamond Bar, California) uses the same principle, but incorporates open irrigation and is compatible with the Carto 3 mapping system.

Early retrospective studies of PVAC ablation suggested success rates similar to conventional PVI, with one multicenter study demonstrating 60% freedom from AF after a median follow-up of 20 months, although this protocol did allow one repeat procedure.[72] In another study, a 61% success rate was shown in a mixed paroxysmal and persistent cohort over a mean follow-up period of 12.2 months.[73] Procedure times appeared to be relatively short, with median durations of 135 and 155 minutes. A subsequent randomized study showed a success rate of 72% at a mean of 254 days, in comparison to 68% with standard RF.[74] The only prospective randomized controlled trial of PVAC in patients with paroxysmal AF in comparison with standard RF wide area circumferential ablation (WACA), included 188 patients and demonstrated comparable success rates between the groups at 6 months (78% PVAC vs 77% WACA) and 12 months (60% PVAC, 56% WACA) with 16% shorter procedural duration in the PVAC group.[75] A stroke rate of 2% in the PVAC group (vs 0% WACA) was not statistically significant but was highlighted by the authors.

The second generation of the circular catheters was examined in a feasibility study of 39 patients with paroxysmal AF. Using this catheter system, 98% of PVs could be acutely isolated with a mean procedure duration of 86 ± 29 minutes. Single and multiple procedure success rates over a mean follow-up period of 140 ± 75 days were 66 and 77%, respectively.[76] A recent multicenter study examined 374 patients undergoing nMARQ ablation and demonstrated PVI in 99.6% of targeted PVs with a procedure time for PV isolation only of 1.9 ± 0.7 hours (fluoroscopy 24 ± 14 minutes) and 65% single procedure AF free survival in both paroxysmal and persistent AF groups.[77] A randomized controlled trial of nMARQ, comparing the technology with standard point-to-point RF ablation, began recruitment in 2013.

Postprocedural MRI studies of patients undergoing AF ablation have shown the rate of silent cerebral emboli to be higher in patients undergoing PVAC ablation than with other ablation modalities. Gaita et al. demonstrated a cerebral microemboli rate of 38.9% in those treated with PVAC, in comparison to 8.3% with standard RF ablation and 5.6% with cryoablation.[78] These results were replicated in a multicenter trial, where PVAC ablation caused microemboli in 37.5% of patients, with significantly lower rates with standard irrigated RF ablation (7.4%) and cryoablation (4.3%).[79] Ablation through overlapped proximal and distal electrodes may contribute to embolic risk.[80]

The second generation of circular multielectrode ablation catheters incorporated irrigation, to improve lesion delivery as well as reduce char formation and subsequent cerebrovascular complication, however concerns regarding silent ischemic cerebral events may not be completely alleviated. One study demonstrated MRI lesions in 33% of 43 patients undergoing PVI with nMARQ,[81] another did not find any lesion in 25 patients.[82] Neither study compared these findings with those due to existing technologies. Unsurprisingly, atrioesophageal fistula formation remains a potential complication with this technique.[83]

Balloon-based Technologies for PVI

Balloon-based ablation has been developed to potentially allow delivery of a true 'single shot' ablation lesion to each pulmonary vein. Cryoablation has predominated; laser and ultrasound balloon ablation techniques have also been developed, but less well studied. The Arctic Front system (Medtronic Inc., Minneapolis, MN, USA) consists of an 'over-the-wire' cryoballoon with a 23 or 28 mm diameter with a central lumen permitting distal placement of a circular mapping catheter, allowing real time assessment of PV conduction. In its first iteration, four refrigerant injection jets created a ring of cooling centerd on the balloon's equator. This cooling system was modified in a second-generation balloon, where 8 jets were used in a more distal position, creating a uniform freezing area on the distal half of the balloon.

The first generation system was studied in the STOP-AF trial, which randomized 245 patients with paroxysmal AF to treatment with cryoablation (n = 163) or antiarrhythmic drug therapy (n = 82).[84] All 4 major PVs were isolated in 97.6% of patients, as were 21 of 21 left common PVs and 10 of 13 right middle PVs. However, only 83% of these were using the cryoballoon alone, the remainder required additional focal cryoablation. Median procedure time was 371 minutes (including 30 minutes re-evaluation time), with a mean fluoroscopy time of 63 minutes. Single procedure success rate was 57.7%, including 8% of patients receiving previously ineffective antiarrhythmic drugs. The protocol allowed one further cryoablation procedure within 12 months, after which 69.9% of patients were free from AF, also including 8% requiring medical treatment. Only 7.3% of patients in the antiarrhythmic drug group were free from AF at the end of the study period.

The second-generation system has limited but promising outcome data. A trial of 42 patients with paroxysmal AF recently reported a one-year, single procedure, drug-free success rate of 83%.[85] Additionally, all PVs were isolated using the cryoballoon only. Two other trials of 50 and 55 patients showed similar success rates (84% and 83.6%), and significant improvement when compared with the first generation system (66% and 63.9%).[86,87] The 'fire and ice' trial is currently recruiting and aims to demonstrate non-inferiority of cryoablation when compared with RF ablation.

The most commonly seen complication of cryoablation has been phrenic nerve palsy, particularly with right-sided PV ablation. In the STOP-AF trial, this occurred in 11.2% of cases; half were asymptomatic and 89% showed complete resolution over a mean of 144 days. The procedural stroke rate in this trial was 0.4%. Initial studies of the second-generation balloon found very high rates of phrenic nerve palsy, with a 19% incidence in one trial, albeit with full resolution in all cases.[88] Subsequent studies have shown no significant differences between first and second-generation balloons, with rates as low as 3.5%.[89] Cryoablation was initially thought to be associated with a lower incidence of atrioesophageal fistula formation; the first 5000 cases worldwide were performed without the dreaded complication. However, studies demonstrated significant esophageal ulceration following cryoablation in 17% of patients.[90] Subsequent case reports reported fistula formation following the use of both first and second-generation systems.[91-93] Esophageal temperature monitoring may be useful, lower temperatures have been shown to predict ulceration.[94]

CONCLUSION AND FUTURE DIRECTIONS

The PV isolation remains the cornerstone of AF ablation. The technique has evolved considerably in the last decade improving outcome and reducing serious complications. Current guidelines recommend wide antral pulmonary vein isolation with confirmation of electrical isolation. Contact force technology, steerable sheaths and rigorous assessment of pulmonary vein isolation have improved the durability of pulmonary vein isolation. The novel ablation tools are being developed with the aim to achieve durable and safe pulmonary vein isolation and at the same time reduce procedure time and improve the learning curve for AF ablation.

REFERENCES

1. Pathak RK, Middeldorp ME, Meredith M, Mehta AB, Mahajan R, Wong CX, Twomey D, Elliott AD, Kalman JM, Abhayaratna WP, Lau DH, Sanders P. Long-term effect of goal-directed weight management in an atrial fibrillation cohort: A long-term follow-up study (LEGACY). J Am Coll Cardiol. 2015;65: 2159-69.
2. Pathak RK, Middeldorp M, Lau D, Mehta AB, Mahajan R, Twomey D, Alasady M, Hanley L, Antic NA, McEvoy RD, Kalman JM, Abhayaratna WP, Sanders P. Aggressive risk factor reduction study for atrial fibrillation and implications for the outcome of ablation: The ARREST-AF Cohort Study. J Am Coll Cardiol. 2014;64:2222-31.
3. Verma A, Jiang CY, Betts TR, Chen J, Deisenhofer I, Mantovan R, Macle L, Morillo CA, Haverkamp W, Weerasooriya R, Albenque JP, Nardi S, Menardi E, Novak P, Sanders P, Investigators SAI. Approaches to catheter ablation for persistent atrial fibrillation. N Engl J Med. 2015;372:1812-22.
4. Haissaguerre M, Jais P, Shah DC, Takahashi A, Hocini M, Quiniou G, Garrigue S, Le Mouroux A, Le Metayer P, Clementy J. Spontaneous initiation of atrial fibrillation by ectopic beats originating in the pulmonary veins. N Engl J Med. 1998;339: 659-66.
5. Jais P, Hocini M, Hsu LF, Sanders P, Scavee C, Weerasooriya R, Macle L, Raybaud F, Garrigue S, Shah DC, Le Metayer P, Clementy J, Haissaguerre M. Technique and results of linear ablation at the mitral isthmus. Circulation. 2004;110: 2996-3002.
6. Chen SA, Hsieh MH, Tai CT, Tsai CF, Prakash VS, Yu WC, Hsu TL, Ding YA, Chang MS. Initiation of atrial fibrillation by ectopic beats originating from the pulmonary veins: electrophysiological characteristics, pharmacological responses, and effects of radiofrequency ablation. Circulation. 1999;100:1879-86.
7. Hwang C, Wu TJ, Doshi RN, Peter CT, Chen PS. Vein of marshall cannulation for the analysis of electrical activity in patients with focal atrial fibrillation. Circulation. 2000;101:1503-5.
8. Chen SA, Tai CT, Yu WC, Chen YJ, Tsai CF, Hsieh MH, Chen CC, Prakash VS, Ding YA, Chang MS. Right atrial focal atrial fibrillation: electrophysiologic characteristics and radiofrequency catheter ablation. J Cardiovasc Electrophysiol. 1999;10:328-35.
9. Lau CP, Tse HF, Ayers GM. Defibrillation-guided radiofrequency ablation of atrial fibrillation secondary to an atrial focus. J Am Coll Cardiol. 1999;33:1217-26.
10. Todd DM, Fynn SP, Hobbs WJ, Fitzpatrick AP, Garratt CJ. Prevalence and significance of focal sources of atrial arrhythmia in patients undergoing cardioversion of persistent atrial fibrillation. J Cardiovasc Electrophysiol. 2000;11: 616-22.

11. Mahajan R, Lim HS, Lau DH, Sanders P. Left superior pulmonary vein rhythm masquerading as sinus rhythm. Indian Pacing Electrophysiol J. 2011;11:20-3.
12. Gerstenfeld EP, Guerra P, Sparks PB, Hattori K, Lesh MD. Clinical outcome after radiofrequency catheter ablation of focal atrial fibrillation triggers. J Cardiovasc Electrophysiol. 2001;12:900-8.
13. Hocini M, Haissaguerre M, Shah D, Jais P, Peng JT, Yamane T, Deisenhofer I, Garrigue S, Fuimaono K, Pike R, Clementy J. Multiple sources initiating atrial fibrillation from a single pulmonary vein identified by a circumferential catheter. Pacing Clin Electrophysiol. 2000;23:1828-31.
14. Sanders P, Morton JB, Deen VR, Davidson NC, Sparks PB, Vohra JK, Kalman JM. Immediate and long-term results of radiofrequency ablation of pulmonary vein ectopy for cure of paroxysmal atrial fibrillation using a focal approach. Intern Med J. 2002;32:202-7.
15. Haissaguerre M, Shah DC, Jais P, Hocini M, Yamane T, Deisenhofer I, Chauvin M, Garrigue S, Clementy J. Electrophysiological breakthroughs from the left atrium to the pulmonary veins. Circulation. 2000;102:2463-5.
16. Yamane T, Shah DC, Jais P, Hocini MM, Deisenhofer I, Choi KJ, Macle L, Clementy J, Haissaguerre M. Electrogram polarity reversal as an additional indicator of breakthroughs from the left atrium to the pulmonary veins. J Am Coll Cardiol. 2002;39:1337-44.
17. Gerstenfeld EP, Callans DJ, Dixit S, Zado E, Marchlinski FE. Incidence and location of focal atrial fibrillation triggers in patients undergoing repeat pulmonary vein isolation: implications for ablation strategies. J Cardiovasc Electrophysiol. 2003;14:685-90.
18. Verma A, Kilicaslan F, Pisano E, Marrouche NF, Fanelli R, Brachmann J, Geunther J, Potenza D, Martin DO, Cummings J, Burkhardt JD, Saliba W, Schweikert RA, Natale A. Response of atrial fibrillation to pulmonary vein antrum isolation is directly related to resumption and delay of pulmonary vein conduction. Circulation. 2005;112:627-35.
19. Cappato R, Negroni S, Pecora D, Bentivegna S, Lupo PP, Carolei A, Esposito C, Furlanello F, De Ambroggi L. Prospective assessment of late conduction recurrence across radiofrequency lesions producing electrical disconnection at the pulmonary vein ostium in patients with atrial fibrillation. Circulation. 2003;108:1599-604.
20. Calkins H, Kuck KH, Cappato R, Brugada J, Camm AJ, Chen S-A, Crijns HJG, Damiano RJ, Davies DW, DiMarco J, Edgerton J, Ellenbogen K, Ezekowitz MD, Haines DE, Haissaguerre M, Hindricks G, Iesaka Y, Jackman W, Jalife J, Jais P, Kalman J, Keane D, Kim Y-H, Kirchhof P, Klein G, Kottkamp H, Kumagai K, Lindsay BD, Mansour M, Marchlinski FE, McCarthy PM, Mont JL, Morady F, Nademanee K, Nakagawa H, Natale A, Nattel S, Packer DL, Pappone C, Prystowsky E, Raviele A, Reddy V, Ruskin JN, Shemin RJ, Tsao H-M, Wilber∧ D, Calkins H, Kuck KH, Cappato R, Chen S-A, Prystowsky EN, Kuck KH, Natale A, Haines DE, Marchlinski FE, Calkins H, Davies DW, Lindsay BD, Damiano R, Packer DL, Brugada J, Camm AJ, Crijns HJG, DiMarco J, Edgerton J, Ellenbogen K, Ezekowitz MD, Haissaguerre M, Hindricks G, Iesaka Y, Jackman WM, Jais P, Jalife J, Kalman J, Keane D, Kim Y-H, Kirchhof P, Klein G, Kottkamp H, Kumagai K, Mansour M, Marchlinski F, McCarthy P, Mont JL, Morady F, Nademanee K, Nakagawa H, Nattel S, Pappone C, Raviele A, Reddy V, Ruskin JN, Shemin RJ, Tsao H-M, Wilber D, Ad N, Cummings J, Gillinov AM, Heidbuchel H, January C, Lip G, Markowitz S, Nair M, Ovsyshcher IE, Pak H-N, Tsuchiya T, Shah D, Siong TW, Vardas PE. 2012 HRS/EHRA/ECAS Expert Consensus Statement on Catheter and Surgical Ablation of Atrial Fibrillation: Recommendations for Patient Selection, Procedural Techniques, Patient Management and Follow-up, Definitions, Endpoints, and Research Trial Design: A report of the Heart Rhythm Society (HRS) Task Force on Catheter and Surgical Ablation of Atrial Fibrillation. Developed in partnership with the European Heart Rhythm Association (EHRA), a registered branch of the European Society of Cardiology (ESC) and the European Cardiac Arrhythmia Society (ECAS); and in collaboration with the American College of Cardiology (ACC), American Heart Association (AHA), the Asia Pacific Heart Rhythm Society (APHRS), and the Society of Thoracic Surgeons (STS). Endorsed by the governing bodies of the American College of Cardiology Foundation, the American Heart Association, the European Cardiac Arrhythmia Society, the European Heart Rhythm Association, the Society of Thoracic Surgeons, the Asia Pacific Heart Rhythm Society, and the Heart Rhythm Society. Europace. 2012;14:528-606.
21. Yamane T, Date T, Kanzaki Y, Inada K, Matsuo S, Shibayama K, Miyanaga S, Miyazaki H, Sugimoto K, Mochizuki S. Segmental pulmonary vein antrum isolation using the "large-size" lasso catheter in patients with atrial fibrillation. Circ J. 2007;71:753-60.
22. Skanes AC, Mandapati R, Berenfeld O, Davidenko JM, Jalife J. Spatiotemporal periodicity during atrial fibrillation in the isolated sheep heart. Circulation. 1998;98:1236-48.
23. Arora R, Verheule S, Scott L, Navarrete A, Katari V, Wilson E, Vaz D, Olgin JE. Arrhythmogenic substrate of the pulmonary veins assessed by high-resolution optical mapping. Circulation. 2003;107:1816-21.
24. Hocini M, Ho SY, Kawara T, Linnenbank AC, Potse M, Shah D, Jais P, Janse MJ, Haissaguerre M, De Bakker JM. Electrical conduction in canine pulmonary veins: electrophysiological and anatomic correlation. Circulation. 2002;105:2442-8.
25. Kumagai K, Ogawa M, Noguchi H, Yasuda T, Nakashima H, Saku K. Electrophysiologic properties of pulmonary veins assessed using a multielectrode basket catheter. J Am Coll Cardiol. 2004;43:2281-9.
26. Jais P, Hocini M, Macle L, Choi KJ, Deisenhofer I, Weerasooriya R, Shah DC, Garrigue S, Raybaud F, Scavee C, Le Metayer P, Clementy J, Haissaguerre M. Distinctive electrophysiological properties of pulmonary veins in patients with atrial fibrillation. Circulation. 2002;106:2479-85.
27. Atienza F, Almendral J, Moreno J, Vaidyanathan R, Talkachou A, Kalifa J, Arenal A, Villacastin JP, Torrecilla EG, Sanchez A, Ploutz-Snyder R, Jalife J, Berenfeld O. Activation of inward rectifier potassium channels accelerates atrial fibrillation in humans: evidence for a reentrant mechanism. Circulation. 2006;114:2434-42.
28. Atienza F, Jalife J. Reentry and atrial fibrillation. Heart Rhythm. 2007;4:S13-6.
29. Verma A, Saliba WI, Lakkireddy D, Burkhardt JD, Cummings JE, Wazni OM, Belden WA, Thal S, Schweikert RA, Martin DO, Tchou PJ, Natale A. Vagal responses induced by endocardial left atrial autonomic ganglion stimulation before and after pulmonary vein antrum isolation for atrial fibrillation. Heart Rhythm. 2007;4:1177-82.

30. Proietti R, Santangeli P, Di Biase L, Joza J, Bernier ML, Wang Y, Sagone A, Viecca M, Essebag V, Natale A. Comparative effectiveness of wide antral versus ostial pulmonary vein isolation: a systematic review and meta-analysis. Circ Arrhythm Electrophysiol. 2014;7:39-45.
31. Ouyang F, Bansch D, Ernst S, Schaumann A, Hachiya H, Chen M, Chun J, Falk P, Khanedani A, Antz M, Kuck KH. Complete isolation of left atrium surrounding the pulmonary veins: new insights from the double-Lasso technique in paroxysmal atrial fibrillation. Circulation. 2004;110:2090-6.
32. Verma A, Marrouche NF, Natale A. Pulmonary vein antrum isolation: intracardiac echocardiography-guided technique. J Cardiovasc Electrophysiol. 2004;15:1335-40.
33. Mandapati R, Skanes A, Chen J, Berenfeld O, Jalife J. Stable microreentrant sources as a mechanism of atrial fibrillation in the isolated sheep heart. Circulation. 2000;101:194-9.
34. Sanders P, Hocini M, Jais P, Sacher F, Hsu LF, Takahashi Y, Rotter M, Rostock T, Nalliah CJ, Clementy J, Haissaguerre M. Complete isolation of the pulmonary veins and posterior left atrium in chronic atrial fibrillation. Long-term clinical outcome. Eur Heart J. 2007;28:1862-71.
35. Lim TW, Koay CH, See VA, McCall R, Chik W, Zecchin R, Byth K, Seow SC, Thomas L, Ross DL, Thomas SP. Single-ring posterior left atrial (box) isolation results in a different mode of recurrence compared with wide antral pulmonary vein isolation on long-term follow-up: longer atrial fibrillation-free survival time but similar survival time free of any atrial arrhythmia. Circ Arrhythm Electrophysiol. 2012;5:968-77.
36. Tamborero D, Mont L, Berruezo A, Matiello M, Benito B, Sitges M, Vidal B, de Caralt TM, Perea RJ, Vatasescu R, Brugada J. Left atrial posterior wall isolation does not improve the outcome of circumferential pulmonary vein ablation for atrial fibrillation: a prospective randomized study. Circ Arrhythm Electrophysiol. 2009;2:35-40.
37. Hocini M, Shah DC, Jais P, Haissaguerre M, Peng JT, Yamane T, Deisenhofer I, Garrigue S, Clementy J. Concealed left pulmonary vein potentials unmasked by left atrial stimulation. Pacing Clin Electrophysiol. 2000;23:1832-5.
38. Shah D, Haissaguerre M, Jais P, Hocini M, Yamane T, Macle L, Choi KJ, Clementy J. Left atrial appendage activity masquerading as pulmonary vein potentials. Circulation. 2002;105:2821-5.
39. Cheema A, Dong J, Dalal D, Marine JE, Henrikson CA, Spragg D, Cheng A, Nazarian S, Bilchick K, Sinha S, Scherr D, Almasry I, Halperin H, Berger R, Calkins H. Incidence and time course of early recovery of pulmonary vein conduction after catheter ablation of atrial fibrillation. J Cardiovasc Electrophysiol. 2007;18:387-91.
40. Nanthakumar K, Plumb VJ, Epstein AE, Veenhuyzen GD, Link D, Kay GN. Resumption of electrical conduction in previously isolated pulmonary veins: rationale for a different strategy? Circulation. 2004;109:1226-9.
41. Sotomi Y, Inoue K, Ito N, Kimura R, Toyoshima Y, Masuda M, Doi A, Iwakura K, Okamura A, Koyama Y, Date M, Fujii K. Cause of very late recurrence of atrial fibrillation or flutter after catheter ablation for atrial fibrillation. Am J Cardiol. 2013;111:552-6.
42. Reddy VY, Shah D, Kautzner J, Schmidt B, Saoudi N, Herrera C, Jais P, Hindricks G, Peichl P, Yulzari A, Lambert H, Neuzil P, Natale A, Kuck KH. The relationship between contact force and clinical outcome during radiofrequency catheter ablation of atrial fibrillation in the TOCCATA study. Heart Rhythm. 2012;9:1789-95.
43. Neuzil P, Reddy VY, Kautzner J, Petru J, Wichterle D, Shah D, Lambert H, Yulzari A, Wissner E, Kuck KH. Electrical reconnection after pulmonary vein isolation is contingent on contact force during initial treatment: results from the EFFICAS I study. Circ Arrhythm Electrophysiol. 2013;6:327-33.
44. Gerstenfeld EP, Dixit S, Callans D, Rho R, Rajawat Y, Zado E, Marchlinski FE. Utility of exit block for identifying electrical isolation of the pulmonary veins. J Cardiovasc Electrophysiol. 2002;13:971-9.
45. Essebag V, Baldessin F, Reynolds MR, McClennen S, Shah J, Kwaku KF, Zimetbaum P, Josephson ME. Non-inducibility post-pulmonary vein isolation achieving exit block predicts freedom from atrial fibrillation. Eur Heart J. 2005;26:2550-5.
46. Wang XH, Liu X, Sun YM, Gu JN, Shi HF, Zhou L, Hu W. Early identification and treatment of PV re-connections: role of observation time and impact on clinical results of atrial fibrillation ablation. Europace. 2007;9:481-6.
47. Arentz T, Macle L, Kalusche D, Hocini M, Jais P, Shah D, Haissaguerre M. "Dormant" pulmonary vein conduction revealed by adenosine after ostial radiofrequency catheter ablation. J Cardiovasc Electrophysiol. 2004;15:1041-7.
48. Tritto M, De Ponti R, Salerno-Uriarte JA, Spadacini G, Marazzi R, Moretti P, Lanzotti M. Adenosine restores atrio-venous conduction after apparently successful ostial isolation of the pulmonary veins. Eur Heart J. 2004;25:2155-63.
49. Hachiya H, Hirao K, Takahashi A, Nagata Y, Suzuki K, Maeda S, Sasaki T, Kawabata M, Isobe M, Iesaka Y. Clinical implications of reconnection between the left atrium and isolated pulmonary veins provoked by adenosine triphosphate after extensive encircling pulmonary vein isolation. J Cardiovasc Electrophysiol. 2007;18:392-8.
50. Kumagai K, Naito S, Nakamura K, Hayashi T, Fukazawa R, Sato C, Takemura N, Miki Y, Fuke E, Tanaka Y, Hori Y, Goto K, Iwamoto J, Aonuma K, Oshima S, Taniguchi K. ATP-induced dormant pulmonary veins originating from the carina region after circumferential pulmonary vein isolation of atrial fibrillation. J Cardiovasc Electrophysiol. 2010;21:494-500.
51. Matsuo S, Yamane T, Date T, Inada K, Kanzaki Y, Tokuda M, Shibayama K, Miyanaga S, Miyazaki H, Sugimoto K, Mochizuki S. Reduction of AF recurrence after pulmonary vein isolation by eliminating ATP-induced transient venous re-conduction. J Cardiovasc Electrophysiol. 2007;18:704-8.
52. Gula LJ, Massel D, Leong-Sit P, Gray C, Fox DJ, Segal OR, Krahn AD, Yee R, Klein GJ, Skanes AC. Does adenosine response predict clinical recurrence of atrial fibrillation after pulmonary vein isolation? J Cardiovasc Electrophysiol. 2011;22:982-6.
53. Yamane T, Matsuo S, Date T, Lellouche N, Hioki M, Narui R, Ito K, Tanigawa S, Yamashita S, Tokuda M, Yoshida H, Inada K, Shibayama K, Miyanaga S, Miyazaki H, Abe K, Sugimoto K, Yoshimura M. Repeated provocation of time- and ATP-induced early pulmonary vein reconnections after pulmonary vein isolation: eliminating paroxysmal atrial fibrillation in a single procedure. Circ Arrhythm Electrophysiol. 2011;4:601-8.
54. Gupta A, Perera T, Ganesan A, Sullivan T, Lau DH, Roberts-Thomson KC, Brooks AG, Sanders P. Complications of catheter ablation of atrial fibrillation: a systematic review. Circ Arrhythm Electrophysiol. 2013;6:1082-8.
55. Cappato R, Calkins H, Chen SA, Davies W, Iesaka Y, Kalman J, Kim YH, Klein G, Natale A, Packer D, Skanes A. Prevalence and

causes of fatal outcome in catheter ablation of atrial fibrillation. J Am Coll Cardiol. 2009;53:1798-803.

56. Di Biase L, Burkhardt JD, Mohanty P, Sanchez J, Horton R, Gallinghouse GJ, Lakkireddy D, Verma A, Khaykin Y, Hongo R, Hao S, Beheiry S, Pelargonio G, Dello Russo A, Casella M, Santarelli P, Santangeli P, Wang P, Al-Ahmad A, Patel D, Themistoclakis S, Bonso A, Rossillo A, Corrado A, Raviele A, Cummings JE, Schweikert RA, Lewis WR, Natale A. Periprocedural stroke and management of major bleeding complications in patients undergoing catheter ablation of atrial fibrillation: the impact of periprocedural therapeutic international normalized ratio. Circulation. 2010;121:2550-6.
57. Santangeli P, Di Biase L, Horton R, Burkhardt JD, Sanchez J, Al-Ahmad A, Hongo R, Beheiry S, Bai R, Mohanty P, Lewis WR, Natale A. Ablation of atrial fibrillation under therapeutic warfarin reduces periprocedural complications: evidence from a meta-analysis. Circ Arrhythm Electrophysiol. 2012;5: 302-11.
58. Di Biase L, Burkhardt JD, Santangeli P, Mohanty P, Sanchez JE, Horton R, Gallinghouse GJ, Themistoclakis S, Rossillo A, Lakkireddy D, Reddy M, Hao S, Hongo R, Beheiry S, Zagrodzky J, Rong B, Mohanty S, Elayi CS, Forleo G, Pelargonio G, Narducci ML, Dello Russo A, Casella M, Fassini G, Tondo C, Schweikert RA, Natale A. Periprocedural stroke and bleeding complications in patients undergoing catheter ablation of atrial fibrillation with different anticoagulation management: results from the Role of Coumadin in Preventing Thromboembolism in Atrial Fibrillation (AF) Patients Undergoing Catheter Ablation (COMPARE) randomized trial. Circulation. 2014;129: 2638-44.
59. Dagres N, Kottkamp H, Piorkowski C, Doll N, Mohr F, Horlitz M, Kremastinos DT, Hindricks G. Rapid detection and successful treatment of esophageal perforation after radiofrequency ablation of atrial fibrillation: lessons from five cases. J Cardiovasc Electrophysiol. 2006;17:1213-5.
60. Ghia KK, Chugh A, Good E, Pelosi F, Jongnarangsin K, Bogun F, Morady F, Oral H. A nationwide survey on the prevalence of atriesophageal fistula after left atrial radiofrequency catheter ablation. J Interv Card Electrophysiol. 2009;24:33-6.
61. Dagres N, Hindricks G, Kottkamp H, Sommer P, Gaspar T, Bode K, Arya A, Husser D, Rallidis LS, Kremastinos DT, Piorkowski C. Complications of atrial fibrillation ablation in a high-volume center in 1,000 procedures: still cause for concern? J Cardiovasc Electrophysiol. 2009;20:1014-9.
62. Ren JF, Lin D, Marchlinski FE, Callans DJ, Patel V. Esophageal imaging and strategies for avoiding injury during left atrial ablation for atrial fibrillation. Heart Rhythm. 2006;3:1156-61.
63. Chavez P, Messerli FH, Casso Dominguez A, Aziz EF, Sichrovsky T, Garcia D, Barrett CD, Danik S. Atriesophageal fistula following ablation procedures for atrial fibrillation: systematic review of case reports. Open Heart. 2015;2:e000257.
64. Yamasaki H, Tada H, Sekiguchi Y, Igarashi M, Arimoto T, Machino T, Ozawa M, Naruse Y, Kuroki K, Tsuneoka H, Ito Y, Murakoshi N, Kuga K, Hyodo I, Aonuma K. Prevalence and characteristics of asymptomatic excessive transmural injury after radiofrequency catheter ablation of atrial fibrillation. Heart Rhythm. 2011;8:826-32.
65. Singh SM, d'Avila A, Doshi SK, Brugge WR, Bedford RA, Mela T, Ruskin JN, Reddy VY. Esophageal injury and temperature monitoring during atrial fibrillation ablation. Circ Arrhythm Electrophysiol. 2008;1:162-8.
66. Muller P, Dietrich JW, Halbfass P, Abouarab A, Fochler F, Szollosi A, Nentwich K, Roos M, Krug J, Schade A, Mugge A, Deneke T. Higher incidence of esophageal lesions after ablation of atrial fibrillation related to the use of esophageal temperature probes. Heart Rhythm. 2015;12:1464-9.
67. Zellerhoff S, Lenze F, Eckardt L. Prophylactic proton pump inhibition after atrial fibrillation ablation: is there any evidence? Europace. 2011;13:1219-21.
68. Martinek M, Bencsik G, Aichinger J, Hassanein S, Schoefl R, Kuchinka P, Nesser HJ, Purerfellner H. Esophageal damage during radiofrequency ablation of atrial fibrillation: impact of energy settings, lesion sets, and esophageal visualization. J Cardiovasc Electrophysiol. 2009;20:726-33.
69. Di Biase L, Saenz LC, Burkhardt DJ, Vacca M, Elayi CS, Barrett CD, Horton R, Bai R, Siu A, Fahmy TS, Patel D, Armaganijan L, Wu CT, Kai S, Ching CK, Phillips K, Schweikert RA, Cummings JE, Arruda M, Saliba WI, Dodig M, Natale A. Esophageal capsule endoscopy after radiofrequency catheter ablation for atrial fibrillation: documented higher risk of luminal esophageal damage with general anesthesia as compared with conscious sedation. Circ Arrhythm Electrophysiol. 2009;2:108-12.
70. Tilz RR, Chun KR, Metzner A, Burchard A, Wissner E, Koektuerk B, Konstantinidou M, Nuyens D, De Potter T, Neven K, Furnkranz A, Ouyang F, Schmidt B. Unexpected high incidence of esophageal injury following pulmonary vein isolation using robotic navigation. J Cardiovasc Electrophysiol. 2010;21: 853-8.
71. Chugh A, Rubenstein J, Good E, Ebinger M, Jongnarangsin K, Fortino J, Bogun F, Pelosi F, Jr., Oral H, Nostrant T, Morady F. Mechanical displacement of the esophagus in patients undergoing left atrial ablation of atrial fibrillation. Heart Rhythm. 2009;6:319-22.
72. Scharf C, Boersma L, Davies W, Kanagaratnam P, Peters NS, Paul V, Rowland E, Grace A, Fynn S, Dang L, Oral H, Morady F. Ablation of persistent atrial fibrillation using multielectrode catheters and duty-cycled radiofrequency energy. J Am Coll Cardiol. 2009;54:1450-6.
73. Beukema RP, Beukema WP, Smit JJ, Ramdat Misier AR, Delnoij PP, Wellens H, Elvan A. Efficacy of multi-electrode duty-cycled radiofrequency ablation for pulmonary vein disconnection in patients with paroxysmal and persistent atrial fibrillation. Europace. 2010;12:502-7.
74. Bittner A, Monnig G, Zellerhoff S, Pott C, Kobe J, Dechering D, Milberg P, Wasmer K, Eckardt L. Randomized study comparing duty-cycled bipolar and unipolar radiofrequency with point-by-point ablation in pulmonary vein isolation. Heart Rhythm. 2011;8:1383-90.
75. McCready J, Chow AW, Lowe MD, Segal OR, Ahsan S, de Bono J, Dhaliwal M, Mfuko C, Ng A, Rowland ER, Bradley RJ, Paisey J, Roberts P, Morgan JM, Sandilands A, Yue A, Lambiase PD. Safety and efficacy of multipolar pulmonary vein ablation catheter vs. irrigated radiofrequency ablation for paroxysmal atrial fibrillation: a randomized multicentre trial. Europace. 2014;16:1145-53.
76. Zellerhoff S, Daly M, Lim HS, Denis A, Komatsu Y, Jesel L, Derval N, Sacher F, Cochet H, Knecht S, Yiem S, Hocini M, Haissaguerre M, Jais P. Pulmonary vein isolation using a circular, open irrigated mapping and ablation catheter (nMARQ): a report on feasibility and efficacy. Europace. 2014;16:1296-303.
77. Mahida S, Hooks DA, Nentwich K, Ng GA, Grimaldi M, Shin DI, Derval N, Sacher F, Berte B, Yamashita S, Denis A, Hocini M,

Deneke T, Haissaguerre M, Jais P. nMARQ Ablation for Atrial Fibrillation: Results from a Multicentre Study. J Cardiovasc Electrophysiol. 2015;26:724-9.

78. Gaita F, Leclercq JF, Schumacher B, Scaglione M, Toso E, Halimi F, Schade A, Froehner S, Ziegler V, Sergi D, Cesarani F, Blandino A. Incidence of silent cerebral thromboembolic lesions after atrial fibrillation ablation may change according to technology used: comparison of irrigated radiofrequency, multipolar nonirrigated catheter and cryoballoon. J Cardiovasc Electrophysiol. 2011;22:961-8.
79. Herrera Siklody C, Deneke T, Hocini M, Lehrmann H, Shin DI, Miyazaki S, Henschke S, Fluegel P, Schiebeling-Romer J, Bansmann PM, Bourdias T, Dousset V, Haissaguerre M, Arentz T. Incidence of asymptomatic intracranial embolic events after pulmonary vein isolation: comparison of different atrial fibrillation ablation technologies in a multicenter study. J Am Coll Cardiol. 2011;58:681-8.
80. Wieczorek M, Lukat M, Hoeltgen R, Condie C, Hilje T, Missler U, Hirsch J, Scharf C. Investigation into causes of abnormal cerebral MRI findings following PVAC duty-cycled, phased RF ablation of atrial fibrillation. J Cardiovasc Electrophysiol. 2013;24:121-8.
81. Deneke T, Schade A, Muller P, Schmitt R, Christopoulos G, Krug J, Szollosi G, Mugge A, Kerber S, Nentwich K. Acute safety and efficacy of a novel multipolar irrigated radiofrequency ablation catheter for pulmonary vein isolation. J Cardiovasc Electrophysiol. 2014;25:339-45.
82. Scaglione M, Caponi D, Anselmino M, Di Clemente F, Blandino A, Ferraris F, Di Donna P, Ebrille E, Halimi F, Leclercq JF, Iunco C, Vaudagna C, Cesarani F, Gaita F. Pulmonary vein isolation with a new multipolar irrigated radiofrequency ablation catheter (nMARQ): feasibility, acute and short-term efficacy, safety, and impact on postablation silent cerebral ischemia. J Cardiovasc Electrophysiol. 2014;25:1299-305.
83. Deneke T, Schade A, Diegeler A, Nentwich K. Esophago-pericardial fistula complicating atrial fibrillation ablation using a novel irrigated radiofrequency multipolar ablation catheter. J Cardiovasc Electrophysiol. 2014;25:442-3.
84. Packer DL, Kowal RC, Wheelan KR, Irwin JM, Champagne J, Guerra PG, Dubuc M, Reddy V, Nelson L, Holcomb RG, Lehmann JW, Ruskin JN, Investigators SAC. Cryoballoon ablation of pulmonary veins for paroxysmal atrial fibrillation: first results of the North American Arctic Front (STOP AF) pivotal trial. J Am Coll Cardiol. 2013;61:1713-23.
85. Chierchia GB, Di Giovanni G, Ciconte G, de Asmundis C, Conte G, Sieira-Moret J, Rodriguez-Manero M, Casado R, Baltogiannis G, Namdar M, Saitoh Y, Paparella G, Mugnai G, Brugada P. Second-generation cryoballoon ablation for paroxysmal atrial fibrillation: 1-year follow-up. Europace. 2014;16:639-44.
86. Di Giovanni G, Wauters K, Chierchia GB, Sieira J, Levinstein M, Conte G, de Asmundis C, Baltogiannis G, Saitoh Y, Ciconte G, Julia J, Mugnai G, Irfan G, Brugada P. One-year follow-up after single procedure Cryoballoon ablation: a comparison between the first and second generation balloon. J Cardiovasc Electrophysiol. 2014;25:834-9.
87. Furnkranz A, Bordignon S, Dugo D, Perotta L, Gunawardene M, Schulte-Hahn B, Nowak B, Schmidt B, Chun JK. Improved 1-year clinical success rate of pulmonary vein isoiation with the second-generation cryoballoon in patients with paroxysmal atrial fibrillation. J Cardiovasc Electrophysiol. 2014;25:840-4.
88. Casado-Arroyo R, Chierchia GB, Conte G, Levinstein M, Sieira J, Rodriguez-Manero M, di Giovanni G, Baltogiannis Y, Wauters K, de Asmundis C, Sarkozy A, Brugada P. Phrenic nerve paralysis during cryoballoon ablation for atrial fibrillation: a comparison between the first- and second-generation balloon. Heart Rhythm. 2013;10:1318-24.
89. Metzner A, Rausch P, Lemes C, Reissmann B, Bardyszewski A, Tilz R, Rillig A, Mathew S, Deiss S, Kamioka M, Toennis T, Lin T, Ouyang F, Kuck KH, Wissner E. The incidence of phrenic nerve injury during pulmonary vein isolation using the second-generation 28 mm cryoballoon. J Cardiovasc Electrophysiol. 2014;25:466-70.
90. Ahmed H, Neuzil P, d'Avila A, Cha YM, Laragy M, Mares K, Brugge WR, Forcione DG, Ruskin JN, Packer DL, Reddy VY. The esophageal effects of cryoenergy during cryoablation for atrial fibrillation. Heart Rhythm. 2009;6:962-9.
91. Stockigt F, Schrickel JW, Andrie R, Lickfett L. Atriesophageal fistula after cryoballoon pulmonary vein isolation. J Cardiovasc Electrophysiol. 2012;23:1254-7.
92. Lim HW, Cogert GA, Cameron CS, Cheng VY, Sandler DA. Atriesophageal fistula during cryoballoon ablation for atrial fibrillation. J Cardiovasc Electrophysiol. 2014;25:208-13.
93. Kawasaki R, Gauri A, Elmouchi D, Duggal M, Bhan A. Atriesophageal fistula complicating cryoballoon pulmonary vein isolation for paroxysmal atrial fibrillation. J Cardiovasc Electrophysiol. 2014;25:787-92.
94. Furnkranz A, Bordignon S, Schmidt B, Bohmig M, Bohmer MC, Bode F, Schulte-Hahn B, Nowak B, Dignass AU, Chun JK. Luminal esophageal temperature predicts esophageal lesions after second-generation cryoballoon pulmonary vein isolation. Heart Rhythm. 2013;10:789-93.

EDITORS' SUMMARY

Dr Mahajan, Professor Sanders, and colleagues provide for us a logical and practical historical approach to define where we are in terms of pulmonary vein isolation today. They concisely describe the revolutionary rationale for pulmonary vein isolation and then describe the evolution of this procedure from point/trigger ablation to a single lesion set encircling all four pulmonary veins and the posterior wall (which is also the pulmonary vein embryologically) in one contiguous lesion set.

They describe the difficulty of defining the pulmonary vein ostium exactly, and while largely semantic, the electrophysiologist must accurately estimate this site to avoid ablation within the vein and the risk of pulmonary vein stenosis (Asirvatham SJ. Methods to identify the pulmonary vein ostium. Heart Rhythm. 2005;2:1090-3).

They provide their insights into how best we create lasting pulmonary vein isolation and assess for both entrance and exit block. The unique anatomy of the pulmonary veins can make assessment of when ablation is complete difficult (entrance block vs. appearance of continued conduction from signals arising from nearby sites) (Asirvatham SJ. Pulmonary vein-related maneuvers: Part I. Heart Rhythm, 2007;4:538-44 and Asirvatham SJ. Pacing maneuvers for nonpulmonary vein sources: Part II. Heart Rhythm. 2007;4:681-5).

The early student of electrophysiology would do well to carefully review the figures and the unbiased, meticulous writing explaining what is now the most common procedure in the electrophysiology laboratory before performing the procedure themselves.

CHAPTER 25

Tilman Maurer, Erik Wissner, Karl-Heinz Kuck

Atrial Fibrillation Ablation: Substrate Modification and Other Strategies

LIST OF ABBREVIATIONS

AF	Atrial Fibrillation	LAA	Left Atrial Appendage
AV	Atrioventricular	PVI	Pulmonary Vein Isolation
CFAE	Complex Fractionated Atrial Electrograms	RAA	Right Atrial Appendage
GP	Ganglionated Plexi	RF	Radiofrequency
LA	Left Atrium		

INTRODUCTION

The identification of the pulmonary veins as an important source of initiation and maintenance of atrial fibrillation[1] has made the electrical isolation of the pulmonary veins the cornerstone of the interventional therapy for paroxysmal and persistent atrial fibrillation.[2,3] The pathophysiology of pulmonary vein triggers and the technical approach of pulmonary vein isolation are discussed in other chapters of this book.

In addition to triggers originating from the pulmonary veins, pulmonary vein isolation will also affect less frequent trigger sites at the antral aspect of the pulmonary vein ostia.[4] Deployment of an antral circumferential lesion set around the pulmonary veins will result in substrate modification, thereby reducing the critical mass required for the maintenance of atrial fibrillation. Furthermore, epicardial autonomic plexi located at the pulmonary vein ostia that play an important role in the initiation and perpetuation of atrial fibrillation[5] may be encompassed by wide circumferential pulmonary vein isolation.[6]

The reported success rates for stand-alone pulmonary vein isolation in patients with persistent atrial fibrillation are generally lower than for paroxysmal atrial fibrillation. One-year freedom from recurrent atrial arrhythmia ranges from 37% to 59%.[7,8] To improve the outcome of catheter ablation in patients with non-paroxysmal atrial fibrillation, a variety of additional ablation strategies have been proposed. Deployment of linear lesion sets, ablation of complex fractionated atrial electrograms (CFAE), ablation of ganglionated plexi (GP), and ablation of rotors within the left and right atrium all aim to modify the substrate required to maintain (persistent) atrial fibrillation. The aforementioned techniques will be discussed in detail below.

LINEAR ATRIAL ABLATION

Circumferential pulmonary vein isolation has become the standard interventional treatment for paroxysmal atrial fibrillation.[2] However, in patients presenting with persistent atrial fibrillation, challenges remain due to high recurrence rates after pulmonary vein isolation alone. In addition, the occurrence of left atrial (reentrant) tachycardias has led to the adoption of alternative strategies in order to improve outcomes.

Early on in the history of atrial fibrillation therapy, numerous surgical procedures were developed culminating in an approach that created an electrical maze in the left atrium by performing multiple transmural incisions to prevent atrial reentry and thereby the perpetuation of atrial fibrillation.[9] The success of surgically deployed linear lesion sets (maze procedure) led to the adoption of the same strategy during catheter ablation of atrial fibrillation. To improve clinical efficacy, linear ablation is most commonly performed following circumferential isolation of the pulmonary veins and/or ablation of CFAE.[10-13] Linear ablation may interrupt macro- and micro reentrant circuits, target arrhythmogenic foci other than the pulmonary veins or autonomic GP and debulk the left atrium. Furthermore, rotor anchor points may also be affected.

Deployment of left atrial linear lesion sets may represent an important step towards conversion of atrial fibrillation to sinus rhythm either directly or through an intermediate step converting atrial fibrillation to an atrial tachycardia.[14] Macro-reentry as the underlying mechanism of these emerging atrial tachycardias may require linear ablation itself.[15] However, gap formation along linear lesions can result in regions of slow conduction, which may promote reentry and the development of iatrogenic atrial tachycardias.[11] Hence, bidirectional conduction block confirmed by mapping and pacing maneuvers as discussed below, is a mandatory prerequisite for successful long-term outcome. Left atrial tachycardias may be seen in up to 40% of patients undergoing catheter ablation for persistent atrial fibrillation.[12] It remains an ongoing discussion whether the development of atrial tachycardias during follow-up should be considered a partial procedural success, since the outcome of a repeat procedure for atrial tachycardia offers superior results to re-ablation of persistent atrial fibrillation.[16]

The most common sites for linear atrial ablation are (1) the *mitral isthmus line*, connecting the left inferior pulmonary vein ostium with the mitral annulus, (2) the *left atrial roof line* connecting the superior aspects of wide circumferential lesion sets around the ipsilateral pulmonary veins and (3) the *anterior line* connecting the anterior mitral annulus with the wide circumferential lesion set around the septal pulmonary veins. Ablation of the *right atrial cavotricuspid isthmus* is usually limited to patients with documented episodes of cavotricuspid-dependent atrial flutter or if atrial flutter is induced during the procedure. It is not routinely performed in patients presenting with persistent atrial fibrillation because of limited additional value during long-term follow-up.[17,18]

General Considerations on Left Atrial Linear Ablation

After transseptal puncture, a 3-dimensional mapping system (Carto 3, Biosense Webster or EnSite Velocity, St. Jude Medical) is commonly used to reconstruct the geometry of the left atrium. Particular attention is drawn to anatomical landmarks such as the pulmonary veins, the left atrial appendage (LAA) and the mitral annulus and detailed visualization may be enhanced by selective angiography of the pulmonary veins and/or the LAA. While ablation can be performed under fluoroscopic guidance only, it may be associated with longer procedure and increased fluoroscopy times. Use of a 3-dimensional mapping system will also allow for activation mapping of an atrial tachycardia that can occur during the procedure in order to identify its mechanism. Diagnostic catheters are placed in stable positions at locations according to the targeted ablation area (e.g. coronary sinus and/or the LAA) as anatomic landmarks and the activation registered is closely monitored during ablation since changes in activation may occur due to successful block or change in the tachycardia circuit. Catheter ablation is usually performed using an irrigated-tip catheter.

Mitral Isthmus Line

The mitral isthmus extends from the lateral mitral annulus to the ostium of the left inferior pulmonary vein **(Figure 25.1)**. The distance measures approximately 3.5 cm and myocardial thickness varies considerably along

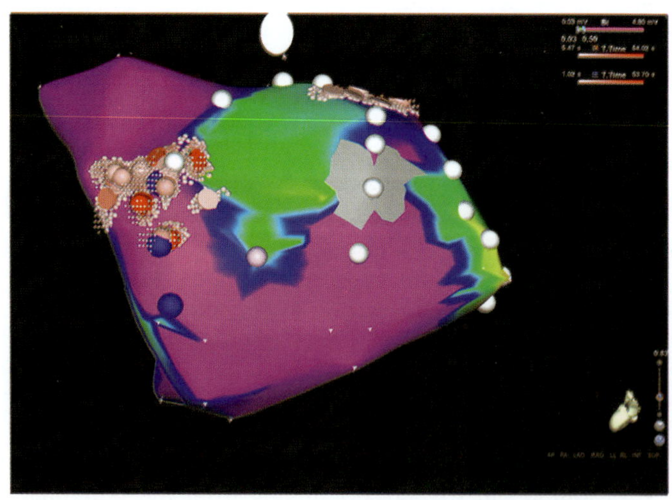

Figure 25.1: Posteroanterior view of an electroanatomical left atrial bipolar voltage map of a patient presenting with a perimitral macroreentry tachycardia (Carto 3, Biosense Webster). Normal voltage amplitude of >0.5 mV is shown in purple. White points mark a line around the ipsilateral pulmonary vein ostia. Pacing sites with perfect entrainment and short postpacing interval are marked in blue, demonstrating perimitral flutter (additional pacing was performed at the anterior mitral annulus). Red points denote sites of radiofrequency ablation. A mitral isthmus line was deployed, connecting the mitral annulus with the ostium of the inferior pulmonary vein. Furthermore, a roof line connects the circumferential lesion sets encircling the ipsilateral septal and lateral pulmonary veins at the superior aspect

its course. At the level of the pulmonary vein ostium myocardial thickness may reach 7.7 mm (average 3 mm) and tapers towards the mitral annulus (average of 1.2 mm).[19]

During ablation, catheter stability is observed examining the local electrograms and the catheter position on the 3-dimensional mapping system and during intermittent fluoroscopy in order to prevent inadvertent catheter displacement into the pulmonary vein or the left atrial appendage. Energy delivery is set to 35–40 Watts with a continuous flow rate of 17–30 mL/min targeting a maximal temperature of 43°C. Radiofrequency energy delivery should result in a wide separation of the local electrogram.

To evaluate conduction block via the mitral isthmus line, a multipolar diagnostic catheter is positioned within the coronary sinus and a spiral mapping catheter placed within the LAA. In case of bidirectional conduction block, pacing distal from the mitral isthmus line from the LAA will result in a proximal to distal propagation sequence within the coronary sinus. Alternatively, pacing proximal from the mitral isthmus line will demonstrate a distal to proximal activation sequence within the coronary sinus before reaching the LAA. Differential pacing helps to discriminate conduction block from slow conduction across the mitral isthmus line: As the site of pacing (e.g. from the coronary sinus catheter) is gradually moved away from the mitral isthmus line, the stimulus-to-electrogram interval on the opposite side of the ablation line will decrease in case of conduction block and increase in the presence of slow conduction.[20,21] Bidirectional conduction block remains crucial, as incomplete block may be associated with recurrent atrial tachycardia.

At times, complete conduction block may be difficult to achieve by endocardial ablation alone. Epicardial ablation within the distal coronary sinus will often result in bidirectional conduction block across the mitral isthmus.[20] Overall, bidirectional block can be achieved in 92% of patients.[20] In order to avoid damage to the left circumflex artery during epicardial ablation within the coronary sinus, power should be limited and the ablation catheter pointed towards the endocardial layer.

It has been proposed that the blood flow within the left circumflex artery and the coronary sinus may act as a heat sink, thereby limiting transmural lesion formation. Temporary occlusion of venous blood at the level of the mitral isthmus using an air-filled coronary sinus balloon may facilitate transmural lesion formation during ablation.[22] Alternatively, a superior mitral isthmus line may overcome the need for epicardial ablation and potential complications. The mitral isthmus tapers in muscle thickness towards the LAA. Hence, following angiographic visualization of the LAA, endocardial ablation at the level of the superior mitral isthmus connecting the lateral pulmonary veins immediately inferior along the base of the LAA with the mitral annulus will often result in bidirectional isthmus block without the need for additional epicardial ablation.

Roof Line

The roof line connects the circumferential lesion sets encircling the ipsilateral septal and lateral pulmonary veins at the superior aspect. Ablation at the roof is performed using power settings limited to 20–30 W using 17–20 mL/min of saline irrigation with a maximum temperature of 43°C.

Conduction block should be assessed during sinus rhythm. During pacing from the LAA, activation across the posterior left atrial wall will spread from an inferior to superior direction. Differential pacing helps to exclude areas of slow conduction. Complete conduction block will result in widely split double potentials along the ablation line.[21]

Anterior Line

The anterior line connects the circumferential lesion set around the septal pulmonary veins with the anterior mitral annulus **(Figure 25.2)**. An alternative approach to the mitral isthmus line, complete conduction block across the anterior line will terminate perimitral flutter due to macro-reentry around the mitral valve annulus. A prerequisite for successful deployment of an anterior line is that the voltage in this area of the left atrium is abnormal, e.g. an atrial voltage <0.5 mV as seen during CARTO (Biosense Webster Inc.) mapping. By contrast, normal voltage amplitude will signify that the septal atrial tissue in this region is too thick to penetrate during irrigated ablation. As an alternative approach, the modified anterior line connects the anterior

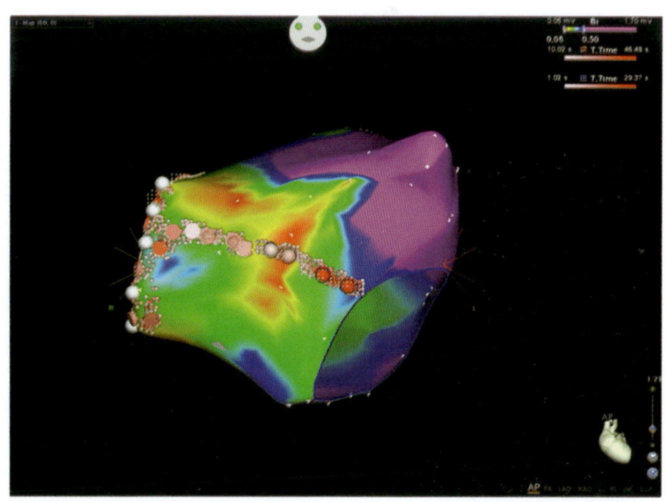

Figure 25.2: Anteroposterior view of an electroanatomical left atrial bipolar voltage map (Carto 3, Biosense Webster). The red points indicate areas of radiofrequency ablation. An anterior line has been deployed, connecting the circumferential lesion set around the septal pulmonary veins with the anterior mitral annulus. Please note the abnormal voltage of the anterior left atrial wall as only areas coded in purple exhibit a normal bipolar voltage of >0.5 mV

mitral annulus with the superior aspect of the circumferential lesion set around the left pulmonary veins.[23] This line resulted in acute success in 88% of 77 patients undergoing ablation for perimitral atrial flutter and persistence of bidirectional block could be demonstrated in 58% of patients during a repeat ablation procedure.[24] Another recent study showed that anterior mitral line and mitral isthmus (posterior) line had a similar success rate in patients with perimitral flutter or persistent atrial fibrillation, though anterior mitral line was associated with significantly shorter procedure time without need for ablation inside the coronary sinus.[25]

Complete conduction block across the anterior line will result in widely split potentials along the entirety of the ablation line and a delay in LAA activation.[24,26] Differential pacing immediately inferoseptal as compared to more cranial from the anterior line will demonstrate greater conduction delay into the LAA.

ABLATION OF COMPLEX FRACTIONATED ATRIAL ELECTROGRAMS

Mapping of complex fractionated atrial electrograms (CFAE) is performed during atrial fibrillation after detailed electroanatomical 3-dimensional reconstruction of the left atrium, the coronary sinus and the right atrium **(Figures 25.3A and B)**. In patients presenting in sinus rhythm, atrial fibrillation is induced by high rate atrial pacing sometimes facilitated by infusion of intravenous isoproterenol.

CFAE are defined as: 1) atrial fractionated electrograms composed of two deflections or more, and/or perturbation of the baseline with continuous deflection of a prolonged activation complex over a 10 second recording period or 2) atrial electrograms with a very short cycle length (≤120 ms) averaged over a 10-second recording period.[27] Furthermore, these electrograms are usually expected to be of low voltage (≤0.15 mV). CFAE are hypothesized to represent areas of fibrillatory wavelet reentry and if targeted and eliminated by catheter ablation should terminate atrial fibrillation.[27] For automatic CFAE mapping, each of the currently available electroanatomical mapping systems provides user-defined mapping algorithms.

CFAE sites appear to be stationary in the individual patient, displaying high temporal and spatial stability.[28,29] Yet, CFAE distribution varies among individuals. CFAE can be found predominantly in the left atrium with a preference for the left atrial roof, the interatrial septum, the mitral annulus and the pulmonary vein ostia. Approximately 15% of CFAE are located in right atrium, involving the septal region, the proximal coronary sinus, the crista terminalis and the cavotricuspid isthmus.[29] Interestingly, patients presenting with paroxysmal atrial fibrillation have a higher prevalence of CFAE in the region of the pulmonary vein antra, whereas patients with persistent atrial fibrillation demonstrate more equal distribution of CFAE sites throughout the left atrium.[30]

Complex Fractionated Atrial Electrograms Ablation Procedure

Complex fractionated atrial electrograms (CFAE) ablation is performed during atrial fibrillation using an irrigated-tip catheter and targets to interrupt the perpetuation of atrial fibrillation by eliminating reentry paths.[27] Primary target areas for ablation may comprise sites displaying a greater percentage of continuous activity or a temporal activation gradient between the distal and proximal pole of the ablation catheter >70 ms, as these sites are more likely to be associated with slowing or termination of atrial

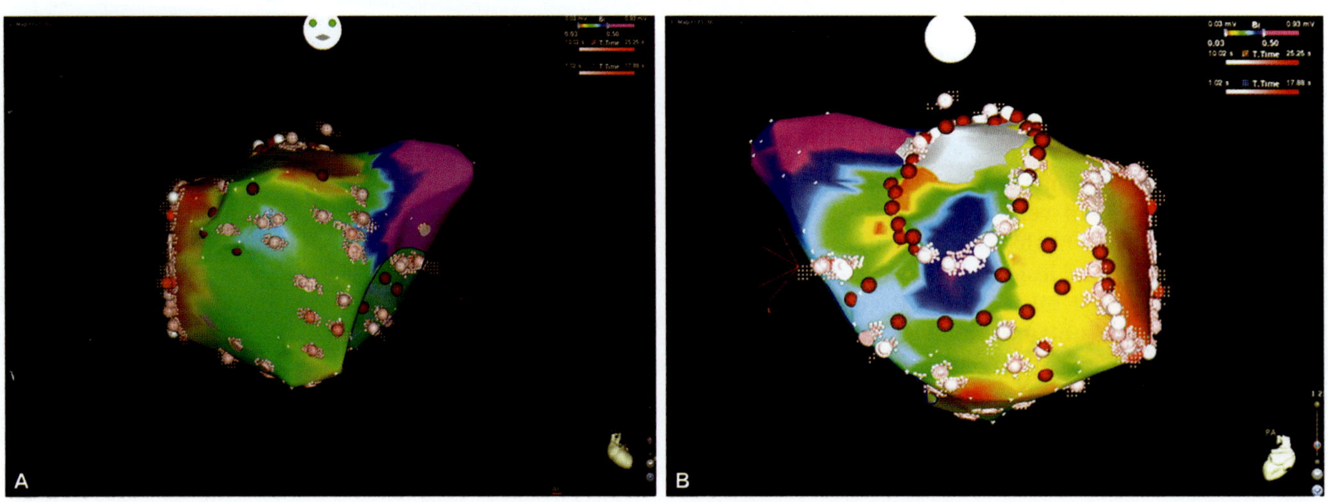

Figures 25.3A and B: Anteroposterior and posteroanterior view of an electroanatomical left atrial bipolar voltage map of a patient presenting with persistent atrial fibrillation (Carto 3, Biosense Webster). Normal voltage amplitude of >0.5 mV is shown in purple. Red points mark sites of radiofrequency ablation. Two wide area circumferential antral lesion sets were deployed around the ipsilateral pulmonary vein ostia. Furthermore, sites displaying complex fractionated atrial electrograms (CFAE) in the anterior and posterior wall were targeted for catheter ablation

fibrillation during focal ablation.[31] Local energy delivery is continued until the fractionated component of the local electrogram is lost or the local electrogram is eliminated. Ablation is started in the left atrium and may be continued within the coronary sinus and the right atrium. Previous studies have reported targeting 64 ± 36 ablation sites per patient,[27] using a mean of 36 ± 13 minutes of energy delivery.[32] Circumferential antral pulmonary vein isolation can decrease the number of areas demonstrating CFAE. Therefore, if a combined approach is pursued, pulmonary vein isolation should be performed first to reduce the total amount of radiofrequency energy delivered.[33]

The procedural endpoint for ablation of persistent atrial fibrillation is either the elimination of all CFAE or conversion of atrial fibrillation to sinus rhythm. If atrial fibrillation converts into an atrial tachycardia, the latter is mapped and ablated.[27,32] Conversion to sinus rhythm may be associated with prolonged procedure times. For paroxysmal atrial fibrillation, the endpoint for CFAE ablation is non-inducibility of atrial fibrillation.

Outcome of CFAE Ablation

The results of CFAE ablation have varied widely between studies. In the original single-center publication, CFAE ablation alone without pulmonary vein isolation in 121 patients with paroxysmal or persistent atrial fibrillation resulted in termination of atrial fibrillation in 95% of the patients demonstrating freedom from atrial fibrillation in 91% of patients after ≤2 procedures at 1-year follow up.[27] Subsequent studies showed only modest short-term outcome following ablation of CFAE alone. Additionally, pulmonary vein tachycardias were more commonly documented in patients presenting for a repeat ablation procedure.[32,34] These findings suggest that CFAE ablation alone is not a feasible approach for the treatment of atrial fibrillation. On the other hand, ablation of CFAE as an adjuvant strategy in combination with antral pulmonary vein isolation or other linear ablation strategies may potentially be of value in treating patients with persistent atrial fibrillation, especially if presenting recurrent atrial fibrillation following catheter ablation.[29] Combining CFAE ablation with antral pulmonary vein isolation in patients with persistent atrial fibrillation demonstrated superior outcome compared to CFAE ablation or pulmonary vein isolation alone.[34,35] This benefit could not be shown for patients with paroxysmal atrial fibrillation.[36]

It is noteworthy that extensive elimination of CFAE, particularly in those with long-standing persistent atrial fibrillation, may encompass large areas of the left atrial endocardium. This, in turn, may increase the risk for periprocedural complications, the development of iatrogenic arrhythmias, prolong procedure as well as fluoroscopy times and may impair the transport function of the left atrium. Since some CFAE sites may result from passive activation, ablation at all identified sites may not be necessary. Yet, whether certain subtypes of CFAE, such as those exhibiting continuous fractionation or particular types of activation gradients, are more important than others, has yet to be proven.[29]

GANGLIONATED PLEXI ABLATION

Autonomic inputs to the atria arise from the extrinsic (central) nervous system and from the intrinsic cardiac autonomic nervous system. Experimental and clinical data suggests, that the autonomic nervous system plays an important role in the initiation and maintenance of atrial fibrillation.[5] Embedded in epicardial fat pads and the ligament of Marshall lay clusters of ganglia and interconnecting neurons, which innervate the heart. The GP contain afferent neurons from the atrial myocardium and the central nervous system as well as efferent cholinergic and adrenergic neurons. Autonomic parasympathetic tone shortens action potential duration and thereby decreases the refractory period of the pulmonary vein myocytes.[37,38] The autonomic nervous system may also be important for the generation of complex fractionated activity observed during atrial fibrillation.[39]

Localization of Atrial Ganglionated Plexi

Typically, the majority of GP within the left and right atrium are located in predefined regions along the pulmonary vein antrum, the crux of the heart and at the junction between right atrium and superior vena cava.[40-42] The superior left GP is located at the roof of the left atrium, medial to the left superior pulmonary vein and often extends towards the medial aspect of the left atrial appendage. The anterior right GP is located anterior to the ostium of the right superior pulmonary vein and extends inferiorly into the region anterior of the right inferior pulmonary vein. Two additional plexi are located at the posteroinferior aspect of the left atrium, each 1 to 3 cm below the right and left inferior pulmonary vein, respectively.

In vivo localization and mapping of GP utilizes high-frequency stimulation delivered from an ablation catheter (20 Hz, 10–150 V, pulse-width 1–10 ms). For better tolerance the patient is deeply sedated. Each plexus contains parasympathetic and sympathetic innervation. Stimulation of up to 5 seconds typically induces an immediate vagal response, which is defined as an 50% increase in the R-R-interval during atrial fibrillation, induction of second or third-degree AV block during sinus rhythm and/or hypotension (>20 mm Hg decrease in systolic blood pressure). Terminating stimulation will result in complete resolution. Furthermore, local stimulation of a GP may produce remote effects such as pulmonary vein depolarization or electrogram fractionation at a distant site, implying active communication among ganglia.[5] High-frequency stimulation during sinus rhythm may induce atrial fibrillation, which commonly is non-sustained. Areas with parasympathetic response are marked on the electroanatomical left atrial map. Stimulation of more than 8 seconds will elicit a delayed sympathetic response, which may conceal the parasympathetic response by facilitating AV conduction or increasing blood pressure. Pacing the inferior ganglia may result in ventricular capture and induction of ventricular fibrillation. A safety margin of 2 cm distant from ventricular myocardium has been proposed.[42]

Ablation of Ganglionated Plexi

Following endocardial ablation of the target GP using an irrigated-tip catheter, high-frequency stimulation is repeated until all vagal response is eliminated. Typically, 3 to 8 applications of 30–60 s in duration are required per site to eliminate any parasympathetic response during repeat stimulation. There is evidence that the AV block witnessed during stimulation maneuvers is driven by the GP located within the fat pad at the crux of the heart between the inferior vena cava and coronary sinus ostium, which, in turn receives innervation from the inferior right GP. Ablating these ganglia first may impair the vagal response evoked by high frequency stimulation to evaluate the endpoint of ablation. Therefore, ablation of GP should follow a predefined order to minimize the loss of any subsequent vagal response. Initially, the Marshall tract GP is targeted followed by the left superior, anterior right, inferior left, and finally, the inferior right GP.[5,43,44]

Alternatively, an anatomical-based approach without use of high-frequency stimulation has shown comparable results in one study,[45] targeting sites for ablation as derived from anatomical studies in human and animal hearts.[46] Since the exact location of GP varies between individuals a more extensive ablation approach is used. The procedural endpoint includes elimination of local electrical activity (peak-to-peak bipolar electrogram <0.1 mV) in target areas and abolition of all vagal response during RF energy delivery.[45,47]

Outcome

Targeting GP during ablation may reduce pulmonary vein firing and subsequent inducibility of atrial fibrillation.[5] A recent clinical study in patients with paroxysmal atrial fibrillation compared pulmonary vein isolation to stand alone GP ablation versus a combined strategy.[48] After two years of follow-up, superior results were documented for the combined approach (74% freedom from atrial fibrillation) without an increase in adverse events versus 56% for pulmonary vein isolation and 48% for GP ablation alone.[48] Similarly, in patients with persistent or long-standing persistent atrial fibrillation comparing a strategy of GP ablation versus linear ablation in addition to pulmonary vein isolation demonstrated better success rates for the former approach during a 3-year follow-up (49% vs. 34%) resulting in a lower rate of subsequent left atrial tachycardias.[49] Since the aforementioned results represent single-center experiences, additional studies are warranted to confirm the benefit of adjuvant GP ablation.

ROTOR ABLATION

The ablation wavelet a hypothesis states that atrial fibrillation results from the presence of multiple, independent and chaotic wavelets propagating through the left and right atrium. The perpetuation of these wavelets requires a minimum of coexisting wavelets, a shortened atrial refractory time, areas of slow conduction and a critical mass of excitable atrial tissue.[50] Mapping of atrial electrograms during atrial fibrillation demonstrates distinct patterns of complexity and frequency: single potentials (indicating rapid uniform conduction), double potentials (representing conduction block) and highly fractionated electrograms or activation with a very short cycle length (complex fractionated atrial electrograms, CFAE). CFAE may represent areas of slowed conduction, wavefront collision or anchor points for reentrant circuits.[51] It has to be noted that fractionated electrical activity may also be recorded at sites of autonomic innervation (see section on GP above),[5] while electrical activity displaying a shortened cycle length may represent drivers or localized sources for atrial fibrillation.[52,53] In contrast to focal sources where activation spreads centrifugally, localized sources sustaining atrial fibrillation have been defined as rotors if their activity is rotational around a core.[54] From the outer perimeter of these rotors, spiraling waves of varying direction and propagation velocity emanate, resulting in electrogram fractionation. Studies in animal models and humans have demonstrated that stable, self-sustained rotors can exist in the atria and that high-frequency activation by such rotors can result in complex patterns of activation seen in atrial fibrillation.[55] To determine the local dominant frequency of activation and thereby identify sites with the highest periodic activity, power spectral analysis is performed using the fast Fourier transform.[56] Initial studies during open-heart surgery utilizing the aforementioned technique could document areas of regular and rapid activation while the rest of the atria was activated in a passive manner.[57] Later, endocardial mapping using multipolar catheters revealed that localized sources activated the remaining atrium centrifugally during persistent atrial fibrillation.[54,58] Importantly, these sites did not correlate with sites exhibiting CFAE.[59,60]

A first study comparing catheter ablation in patients presenting with paroxysmal or persistent atrial fibrillation with or without modulation of focal sources and rotors accompanied by conventional pulmonary vein isolation showed an average of 2.1 rotors in 97% of patients.[61] The majority of rotors were identified in the left atrium (76%) and a higher number of sources per patient were identified in persistent than paroxysmal atrial fibrillation (median 2 vs. 1). Targeting focal sources and rotors for ablation before pulmonary vein isolation resulted in slowing or termination of atrial fibrillation in 44% and 56% of patients, respectively. Patients undergoing a combined approach demonstrated higher freedom from atrial fibrillation after a 3-year follow-up than patients undergoing pulmonary vein isolation alone.[62] These encouraging results await confirmation by other study groups.[63]

Intracardiac recording of rotors and focal sources will require the use of a 64-electrode basket catheter. Individual electrode splines may not equally distribute across the entirety of the endocardial atrial surface or lack contact along certain areas within a dilated atrium. Non-invasive mapping systems have recently been introduced that forgo the need for additional invasive catheter placement.[64,65] As of today, two non-invasive mapping systems are available [Amycard, EP Solutions SA **(Figures 25.4 and 25.5)** and ECVUE, CardioInsight]. Both require unipolar electrodes to be placed on the patient's torso. The electrocardiographic data collected is combined with the anatomical information gathered by a CT- or MRI scan providing information on the anatomy and relative electrode position. These systems provide high-resolution electrocardiographic maps[65] and, in case of the Amycard system, have the capability to discriminate endocardial from epicardial sources.[64] An ongoing multicenter study is currently evaluating non-invasive mapping of drivers for persistent atrial fibrillation. In a preliminary analysis, acute termination of atrial fibrillation during ablation was seen in 64% of patients undergoing rotor ablation alone, in 66% of patients with additional pulmonary vein isolation and in 73% of patients undergoing pulmonary vein isolation and additional ablation of linear lesions. After a follow-up period of 6 ± 3 months, 83% of patients were free from recurrent atrial fibrillation.[66]

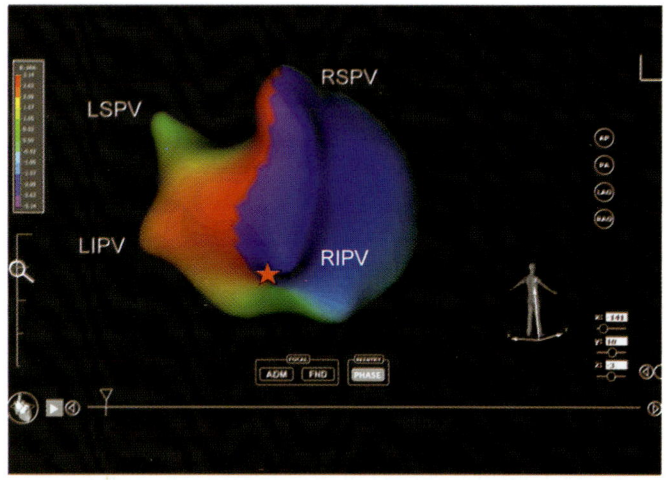

Figure 25.4: Using a non-invasive mapping system (Amycard, EP-Solutions) electrocardiographic data collected by unipolar electrodes placed on the patients torso is combined with anatomical information gathered by a CT- or MRI scan providing information on the anatomy and relative electrode position. Here, a reconstruction of the left atrium is shown. After power spectral analysis was performed using the fast Fourier transform a rotor was visualized. The rotor core (*) is located in the inferior left atrium in proximity to the right pulmonary vein ostium

Abbreviations: LSPV, left superior pulmonary vein; RSPV, right superior pulmonary vein; LIPV, left inferior pulmonary vein; RIPV, right inferior pulmonary vein

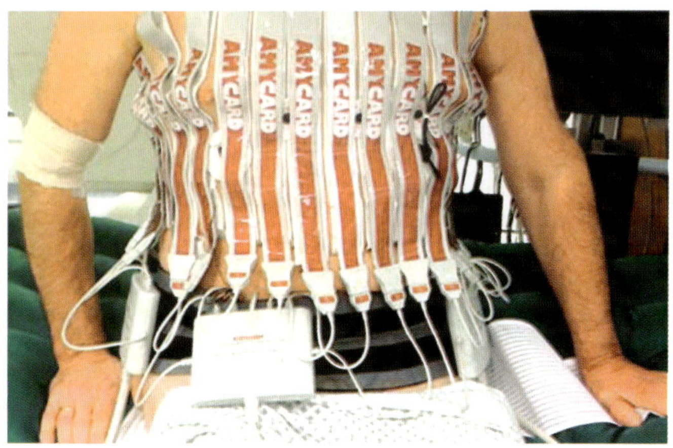

Figure 25.5: A patient has been equipped with 224 unipolar electrodes for non-invasive electroanatomical mapping (Amycard, EP-Solutions)

COMBINED ABLATION APPROACH

For patients presenting with persistent atrial fibrillation, catheter ablation shows superior results regarding freedom from arrhythmia recurrence compared to medical treatment alone.[67] Yet, the optimal ablation strategy remains unclear. Various studies examined a combination of some of the aforementioned ablation techniques with respect to improving the results of the interventional therapy for persistent atrial fibrillation.

The Stepwise Ablation Approach

The stepwise ablation approach targets structures contributing to the initiation and perpetuation of atrial fibrillation in a sequential manner.[12,14,68] The objectives during radiofrequency ablation are isolation of the pulmonary veins, CFAE ablation and linear ablation of the LA roof and mitral isthmus. During each ablative step the average atrial fibrillation cycle-length is monitored at a site remote from the ablation target such as the coronary sinus or the left and/or right atrial appendage. Successful completion of each step will result in an increase in the average cycle-length[69,70] until a critical prolongation is reached and the atria can no longer sustain the fibrillatory process.[14] Finally, conversion to sinus rhythm, or, more often (87% of the patients), to one or multiple atrial tachycardias is seen.[12] These tachycardias are then mapped and ablated according to the methods discussed in the other chapters.

If stepwise ablation within the left atrium fails to terminate AF, the right atrium may be targeted for ablation.[14] The right atrium may serve as a dominant driver if the average cycle-length within the right atrial appendage (RAA) exceeds the cycle-length in the LAA by more than 20 ms or single long beats in the LAA or coronary sinus are not accompanied by the RAA. Possible targets for ablation in the right atrium are the cavotricuspid isthmus and those areas exhibiting CFAE. The superior vena cava is identified as an arrhythmogenic source if high-frequency activity is recorded from within the vessel, making it a target for electrical isolation. Termination of persistent atrial fibrillation is the desired procedural endpoint.[12] After restoration of sinus rhythm, all previously deployed lesions are evaluated for persistent conduction block. This is of particular importance since iatrogenic atrial tachycardias are the main cause for arrhythmia recurrence.[12] Patients who fail termination during the stepwise ablation approach typically present with a shorter baseline average atrial fibrillation cycle-length (130 ± 14 vs. 156 ± 23 ms).[68] Use of the stepwise approach, results in long fluoroscopy times of 84 ± 30 minutes and an average procedure duration of 264 ± 77 minutes.[12] As the average atrial fibrillation cycle-length decreases at time of presentation, fluoroscopy and procedure duration would increase.[14]

After 5 years of follow-up, freedom from recurrent atrial arrhythmias after a single and a mean of 2.1 procedures off antiarrhythmic drugs was 16.8% and 62.9%, respectively.[71] The main predictors for arrhythmia recurrence were failure to terminate atrial fibrillation during the index procedure, a left atrial diameter 6.8% an continuous atrial fibrillation >18 months and structural heart disease.[71]

STAR AF 2

Substrate and Trigger Ablation for Reduction of Atrial Fibrillation Part 2 (STAR AF 2), the largest randomized multicenter trial so far, compared three strategies for ablation of persistent atrial fibrillation. In this study, 589 patients undergoing a first ablation procedure for drug-refractory persistent AF were randomized to pulmonary vein isolation (PVI) alone versus PVI plus CFAE ablation versus PVI plus linear ablation. After 18-month of follow-up, no statistical differences could be shown between the groups. The percentage of patients free from recurrent atrial fibrillation in the PVI only group, PVI plus CFAE group and PVI plus linear ablation group was 59%, 49% and 46% (p-value 0.15) respectively. After a repeat ablation utilizing the same ablation strategy results were similar [(72% for PVI alone, 60% for PVI plus CFAE and 58% for PVI plus lines (p-value 0.18)]. However, the addition of CFAE or linear ablation increased procedure as well as fluoroscopy time.[72]

REFERENCES

1. Haissaguerre M, Jais P, Shah DC, Takahashi A, Hocini M, Quiniou G, Garrigue S, Le Mouroux A, Le Metayer P, Clementy J. Spontaneous initiation of atrial fibrillation by ectopic beats originating in the pulmonary veins. N Engl J Med. 1998;339: 659-66.
2. Calkins H, Kuck KH, Cappato R, Brugada J, Camm AJ, Chen SA, Crijns HJ, Damiano RJ, Jr., Davies DW, DiMarco J, Edgerton J, Ellenbogen K, Ezekowitz MD, Haines DE, Haissaguerre M, Hindricks G, Iesaka Y, Jackman W, Jalife J, Jais P, Kalman J, Keane D, Kim YH, Kirchhof P, Klein G, Kottkamp H, Kumagai K, Lindsay BD, Mansour M, Marchlinski FE, McCarthy PM, Mont JL, Morady F, Nademanee K, Nakagawa H, Natale A, Nattel S, Packer DL, Pappone C, Prystowsky E, Raviele A, Reddy V, Ruskin JN, Shemin RJ, Tsao HM, Wilber D. 2012 HRS/EHRA/ ECAS Expert Consensus Statement on Catheter and Surgical Ablation of Atrial Fibrillation: recommendations for patient selection, procedural techniques, patient management and follow-up, definitions, endpoints, and research trial design. Europace. 2012;14:528-606.
3. Raviele A, Natale A, Calkins H, Camm JA, Cappato R, Ann Chen S, Connolly SJ, Damiano R, Jr R DEP, Edgerton JR, Haissaguerre M, Hindricks G, Ho SY, Jalife J, Kirchhof P, Kottkamp H, Kuck KH, Marchlinski FE, Packer DL, Pappone C, Prystowsky E, Reddy VK, Themistoclakis S, Verma A, Wilber DJ, Willems S. Venice Chart international consensus document on atrial fibrillation ablation: 2011 update. J Cardiovasc Electrophysiol. 2012;23:890-923.
4. Lin WS, Tai CT, Hsieh MH, Tsai CF, Lin YK, Tsao HM, Huang JL, Yu WC, Yang SP, Ding YA, Chang MS, Chen SA. Catheter ablation of paroxysmal atrial fibrillation initiated by non-pulmonary vein ectopy. Circulation. 2003;107:3176-83.
5. Nakagawa H, Scherlag BJ, Patterson E, Ikeda A, Lockwood D, Jackman WM. Pathophysiologic basis of autonomic ganglionated plexus ablation in patients with atrial fibrillation. Heart Rhythm. 2009;6:S26-34.
6. Vaitkevicius R, Saburkina I, Rysevaite K, Vaitkeviciene I, Pauziene N, Zaliunas R, Schauerte P, Jalife J, Pauza DH. Nerve supply of the human pulmonary veins: an anatomical study. Heart Rhythm. 2009;6:221-8.
7. Brooks AG, Stiles MK, Laborderie J, Lau DH, Kuklik P, Shipp NJ, Hsu LF, Sanders P. Outcomes of long-standing persistent atrial fibrillation ablation: a systematic review. Heart Rhythm. 2010;7:835-46.
8. Verma A. Late-Breaking Clinical Trial: Optimal method and outcomes of catheter ablation of persistent AF: The STAR AF 2 trial., in Presented at the ESC on September 1st, 2014.
9. Cox JL, Schuessler RB, D'Agostino HJ, Jr., Stone CM, Chang BC, Cain ME, Corr PB, Boineau JP. The surgical treatment of atrial fibrillation III. Development of a definitive surgical procedure. J Thorac Cardiovasc Surg. 1991;101:569-83.
10. Oral H, Chugh A, Lemola K, Cheung P, Hall B, Good E, Han J, Tamirisa K, Bogun F, Pelosi F, Jr., Morady F. Noninducibility of atrial fibrillation as an end point of left atrial circumferential ablation for paroxysmal atrial fibrillation: a randomized study. Circulation. 2004;110:2797-801.
11. Ernst S, Ouyang F, Lober F, Antz M, Kuck KH. Catheter-induced linear lesions in the left atrium in patients with atrial fibrillation: an electroanatomic study. J Am Coll Cardiol. 2003;42:1271-82.
12. Haissaguerre M, Hocini M, Sanders P, Sacher F, Rotter M, Takahashi Y, Rostock T, Hsu LF, Bordachar P, Reuter S, Roudaut R, Clementy J, Jais P. Catheter ablation of long-lasting persistent atrial fibrillation: clinical outcome and mechanisms of subsequent arrhythmias. J Cardiovasc Electrophysiol. 2005; 16:1138-47.

13. Knecht S, Hocini M, Wright M, Lellouche N, O'Neill MD, Matsuo S, Nault I, Chauhan VS, Makati KJ, Bevilacqua M, Lim KT, Sacher F, Deplagne A, Derval N, Bordachar P, Jais P, Clementy J, Haissaguerre M. Left atrial linear lesions are required for successful treatment of persistent atrial fibrillation. Eur Heart J. 2008;29:2359-66.
14. O'Neill MD, Jais P, Takahashi Y, Jonsson A, Sacher F, Hocini M, Sanders P, Rostock T, Rotter M, Pernat A, Clementy J, Haissaguerre M. The stepwise ablation approach for chronic atrial fibrillation--evidence for a cumulative effect. J Interv Card Electrophysiol. 2006;16:153-67.
15. Chae S, Oral H, Good E, Dey S, Wimmer A, Crawford T, Wells D, Sarrazin JF, Chalfoun N, Kuhne M, Fortino J, Huether E, Lemerand T, Pelosi F, Bogun F, Morady F, Chugh A. Atrial tachycardia after circumferential pulmonary vein ablation of atrial fibrillation: mechanistic insights, results of catheter ablation, and risk factors for recurrence. J Am Coll Cardiol. 2007;50:1781-7.
16. Ammar S, Hessling G, Reents T, Fichtner S, Wu J, Zhu P, Kathan S, Estner HL, Jilek C, Kolb C, Haller B, Deisenhofer I. Arrhythmia type after persistent atrial fibrillation ablation predicts success of the repeat procedure. Circ Arrhythm Electrophysiol. 2011;4:609-14.
17. Scharf C, Veerareddy S, Ozaydin M, Chugh A, Hall B, Cheung P, Good E, Pelosi F, Jr., Morady F, Oral H. Clinical significance of inducible atrial flutter during pulmonary vein isolation in patients with atrial fibrillation. J Am Coll Cardiol. 2004;43: 2057-62.
18. Wazni O, Marrouche NF, Martin DO, Gillinov AM, Saliba W, Saad E, Klein A, Bhargava M, Bash D, Schweikert R, Erciyes D, Abdul-Karim A, Brachman J, Gunther J, Pisano E, Potenza D, Fanelli R, Natale A. Randomized study comparing combined pulmonary vein-left atrial junction disconnection and cavotricuspid isthmus ablation versus pulmonary vein-left atrial junction disconnection alone in patients presenting with typical atrial flutter and atrial fibrillation. Circulation. 2003;108:2479-83.
19. Becker AE. Left atrial isthmus: anatomic aspects relevant for linear catheter ablation procedures in humans. J Cardiovasc Electrophysiol. 2004;15:809-12.
20. Jais P, Hocini M, Hsu LF, Sanders P, Scavee C, Weerasooriya R, Macle L, Raybaud F, Garrigue S, Shah DC, Le Metayer P, Clementy J, Haissaguerre M. Technique and results of linear ablation at the mitral isthmus. Circulation. 2004;110: 2996-3002.
21. Jais P, Hocini M, O'Neill MD, Klein GJ, Knecht S, Sheiiro M, Arentes L, Kodali S, Clementy J, Haissaguerre M. How to perform linear lesions. Heart Rhythm. 2007;4:803-9.
22. D'Avila A, Thiagalingam A, Foley L, Fox M, Ruskin JN, Reddy VY. Temporary occlusion of the great cardiac vein and coronary sinus to facilitate radiofrequency catheter ablation of the mitral isthmus. J Cardiovasc Electrophysiol. 2008;19: 645-50.
23. Tzeis S, Luik A, Jilek C, Schmitt C, Estner HL, Wu J, Reents T, Fichtner S, Kolb C, Karch MR, Hessling G, Deisenhofer I. The modified anterior line: an alternative linear lesion in perimitral flutter. J Cardiovasc Electrophysiol. 2010;21:665-70.
24. Ammar S, Luik A, Hessling G, Bruhm A, Reents T, Semmler V, Buiatti A, Kathan S, Hofmann M, Kolb C, Schmitt C, Deisenhofer I. Ablation of perimitral flutter: acute and long-term success of the modified anterior line. Europace. 2015;17:447-52.
25. Huemer M, Wutzler A, Parwani AS, Attanasio P, Matsuda H, Blaschke F, Boldt LH, Haverkamp W. Comparison of the anterior and posterior mitral isthmus ablation lines in patients with perimitral annulus flutter or persistent atrial fibrillation. J Interv Card Electrophysiol. 2015;44:119-29.
26. Sanders P, Jais P, Hocini M, Hsu LF, Scavee C, Sacher F, Rotter M, Takahashi Y, Pasquie JL, Shah DC, Garrigue S, Clementy J, Haissaguerre M. Electrophysiologic and clinical consequences of linear catheter ablation to transect the anterior left atrium in patients with atrial fibrillation. Heart Rhythm. 2004;1: 176-84.
27. Nademanee K, McKenzie J, Kosar E, Schwab M, Sunsaneewitayakul B, Vasavakul T, Khunnawat C, Ngarmukos T. A new approach for catheter ablation of atrial fibrillation: mapping of the electrophysiologic substrate. J Am Coll Cardiol. 2004;43:2044-53.
28. Scherr D, Dalal D, Cheema A, Nazarian S, Almasry I, Bilchick K, Cheng A, Henrikson CA, Spragg D, Marine JE, Berger RD, Calkins H, Dong J. Long- and short-term temporal stability of complex fractionated atrial electrograms in human left atrium during atrial fibrillation. J Cardiovasc Electrophysiol. 2009;20:13-21.
29. Singh JP, Ptaszek LM, Verma A. Elusive atrial substrate: complex fractionated atrial electrograms and beyond. Heart Rhythm. 2010;7:1886-90.
30. Tada H, Yoshida K, Chugh A, Boonyapisit W, Crawford T, Sarrazin JF, Kuhne M, Chalfoun N, Wells D, Dey S, Veerareddy S, Billakanty S, Wong WS, Kalra D, Kfahagi A, Good E, Jongnarangsin K, Pelosi F, Jr., Bogun F, Morady F, Oral H. Prevalence and characteristics of continuous electrical activity in patients with paroxysmal and persistent atrial fibrillation. J Cardiovasc Electrophysiol. 2008;19:606-12.
31. Takahashi Y, O'Neill MD, Hocini M, Dubois R, Matsuo S, Knecht S, Mahapatra S, Lim KT, Jais P, Jonsson A, Sacher F, Sanders P, Rostock T, Bordachar P, Clementy J, Klein GJ, Haissaguerre M. Characterization of electrograms associated with termination of chronic atrial fibrillation by catheter ablation. J Am Coll Cardiol. 2008;51:1003-10.
32. Oral H, Chugh A, Good E, Wimmer A, Dey S, Gadeela N, Sankaran S, Crawford T, Sarrazin JF, Kuhne M, Chalfoun N, Wells D, Frederick M, Fortino J, Benloucif-Moore S, Jongnarangsin K, Pelosi F, Jr., Bogun F, Morady F. Radiofrequency catheter ablation of chronic atrial fibrillation guided by complex electrograms. Circulation. 2007;115:2606.
33. Roux JF, Gojraty S, Bala R, Liu CF, Dixit S, Hutchinson MD, Garcia F, Lin D, Callans DJ, Riley M, Marchlinski F, Gerstenfeld EP. Effect of pulmonary vein isolation on the distribution of complex fractionated electrograms in humans. Heart Rhythm. 2009;6:156-60.
34. Verma A, Mantovan R, Macle L, De Martino G, Chen J, Morillo CA, Novak P, Calzolari V, Guerra PG, Nair G, Torrecilla EG, Khaykin Y. Substrate and Trigger Ablation for Reduction of Atrial Fibrillation (STAR AF): a randomized, multicentre, international trial. Eur Heart J. 2010;31:1344-56.
35. Li WJ, Bai YY, Zhang HY, Tang RB, Miao CL, Sang CH, Yin XD, Dong JZ, Ma CS. Additional ablation of complex fractionated atrial electrograms after pulmonary vein isolation in patients with atrial fibrillation: a meta-analysis. Circ Arrhythm Electrophysiol. 2011;4:143-8.
36. Di Biase L, Elayi CS, Fahmy TS, Martin DO, Ching CK, Barrett C, Bai R, Patel D, Khaykin Y, Hongo R, Hao S, Beheiry S,

Pelargonio G, Dello Russo A, Casella M, Santarelli P, Potenza D, Fanelli R, Massaro R, Wang P, Al-Ahmad A, Arruda M, Themistoclakis S, Bonso A, Rossillo A, Raviele A, Schweikert RA, Burkhardt DJ, Natale A. Atrial fibrillation ablation strategies for paroxysmal patients: randomized comparison between different techniques. Circ Arrhythm Electrophysiol. 2009;2:113-9.

37. Patterson E, Po SS, Scherlag BJ, Lazzara R. Triggered firing in pulmonary veins initiated by in vitro autonomic nerve stimulation. Heart Rhythm. 2005;2:624-31.
38. Scherlag BJ, Yamanashi W, Patel U, Lazzara R, Jackman WM. Autonomically induced conversion of pulmonary vein focal firing into atrial fibrillation. J Am Coll Cardiol 2005;45:1878-86.
39. Lin J, Scherlag BJ, Zhou J, Lu Z, Patterson E, Jackman WM, Lazzara R, Po SS. Autonomic mechanism to explain complex fractionated atrial electrograms (CFAE). J Cardiovasc Electrophysiol. 2007;18:1197-205.
40. Pauza DH, Skripka V, Pauziene N, Stropus R. Morphology, distribution, and variability of the epicardiac neural ganglionated subplexuses in the human heart. Anat Rec. 2000;259:353-82.
41. Lachman N, Syed FF, Habib A, Kapa S, Bisco SE, Venkatachalam KL, Asirvatham SJ. Correlative anatomy for the electrophysiologist, part II: cardiac ganglia, phrenic nerve, coronary venous system. J Cardiovasc Electrophysiol. 2011;22:104-10.
42. Po SS, Nakagawa H, Jackman WM. Localization of left atrial ganglionated plexi in patients with atrial fibrillation. J Cardiovasc Electrophysiol. 2009;20:1186-9.
43. Malcolme-Lawes LC, Lim PB, Wright I, Kojodjojo P, Koa-Wing M, Jamil-Copley S, Dehbi HM, Francis DP, Davies DW, Peters NS, Kanagaratnam P. Characterization of the left atrial neural network and its impact on autonomic modification procedures. Circ Arrhythm Electrophysiol. 2013;6:632-40.
44. Edgerton JR, Jackman WM, Mack MJ. Minimally invasive pulmonary vein isolation and partial autonomic denervation for surgical treatment of atrial fibrillation. J Interv Card Electrophysiol. 2007;20:89-93.
45. Pokushalov E, Romanov A, Shugayev P, Artyomenko S, Shirokova N, Turov A, Katritsis DG. Selective ganglionated plexi ablation for paroxysmal atrial fibrillation. Heart Rhythm. 2009;6:1257-64.
46. Scherlag BJ, Hou YL, Lin J, Lu Z, Zacharias S, Dasari T, Niu G, Ghias M, Patterson E, Jackman WM, Lazzara R, Po SS. An acute model for atrial fibrillation arising from a peripheral atrial site: evidence for primary and secondary triggers. J Cardiovasc Electrophysiol. 2008;19:519-27.
47. Oral H, Chugh A, Yoshida K, Sarrazin JF, Kuhne M, Crawford T, Chalfoun N, Wells D, Boonyapisit W, Veerareddy S, Billakanty S, Wong WS, Good E, Jongnarangsin K, Pelosi F, Jr., Bogun F, Morady F. A randomized assessment of the incremental role of ablation of complex fractionated atrial electrograms after antral pulmonary vein isolation for long-lasting persistent atrial fibrillation. J Am Coll Cardiol. 2009;53:782-9.
48. Katritsis DG, Pokushalov E, Romanov A, Giazitzoglou E, Siontis GC, Po SS, Camm AJ, Ioannidis JP. Autonomic denervation added to pulmonary vein isolation for paroxysmal atrial fibrillation: a randomized clinical trial. J Am Coll Cardiol. 2013;62:2318-25.
49. Pokushalov E, Romanov A, Katritsis DG, Artyomenko S, Shirokova N, Karaskov A, Mittal S, Steinberg JS. Ganglionated plexus ablation vs linear ablation in patients undergoing pulmonary vein isolation for persistent/long-standing persistent atrial fibrillation: a randomized comparison. Heart Rhythm. 2013;10:1280-6.
50. Moe GK, Abildskov JA. Atrial fibrillation as a self-sustaining arrhythmia independent of focal discharge. Am Heart J. 1959;58:59-70.
51. Konings KT, Smeets JL, Penn OC, Wellens HJ, Allessie MA. Configuration of unipolar atrial electrograms during electrically induced atrial fibrillation in humans. Circulation. 1997;95:1231-41.
52. Mandapati R, Skanes A, Chen J, Berenfeld O, Jalife J. Stable microreentrant sources as a mechanism of atrial fibrillation in the isolated sheep heart. Circulation. 2000;101:194-9.
53. Sanders P, Berenfeld O, Hocini M, Jais P, Vaidyanathan R, Hsu LF, Garrigue S, Takahashi Y, Rotter M, Sacher F, Scavee C, Ploutz-Snyder R, Jalife J, Haissaguerre M. Spectral analysis identifies sites of high-frequency activity maintaining atrial fibrillation in humans. Circulation. 2005;112:789-97.
54. Narayan SM, Krummen DE, Rappel WJ. Clinical mapping approach to diagnose electrical rotors and focal impulse sources for human atrial fibrillation. J Cardiovasc Electrophysiol. 2012;23:447-54.
55. Jalife J, Berenfeld O, Mansour M. Mother rotors and fibrillatory conduction: a mechanism of atrial fibrillation. Cardiovasc Res. 2002;54:204-16.
56. Berenfeld O, Mandapati R, Dixit S, Skanes AC, Chen J, Mansour M, Jalife J. Spatially distributed dominant excitation frequencies reveal hidden organization in atrial fibrillation in the Langendorff-perfused sheep heart. J Cardiovasc Electrophysiol. 2000;11:869-79.
57. Sahadevan J, Ryu K, Peltz L, Khrestian CM, Stewart RW, Markowitz AH, Waldo AL. Epicardial mapping of chronic atrial fibrillation in patients: preliminary observations. Circulation. 2004;110:3293-9.
58. Haissaguerre M, Hocini M, Sanders P, Takahashi Y, Rotter M, Sacher F, Rostock T, Hsu LF, Jonsson A, O'Neill MD, Bordachar P, Reuter S, Roudaut R, Clementy J, Jais P. Localized sources maintaining atrial fibrillation organized by prior ablation. Circulation. 2006;113:616-25.
59. Narayan SM, Shivkumar K, Krummen DE, Miller JM, Rappel WJ. Panoramic electrophysiological mapping but not electrogram morphology identifies stable sources for human atrial fibrillation: stable atrial fibrillation rotors and focal sources relate poorly to fractionated electrograms. Circ Arrhythm Electrophysiol. 2013;6:58-67.
60. Ghoraani B, Dalvi R, Gizurarson S, Das M, Ha A, Suszko A, Krishnan S, Chauhan VS. Localized rotational activation in the left atrium during human atrial fibrillation: relationship to complex fractionated atrial electrograms and low-voltage zones. Heart Rhythm. 2013;10:1830-8.
61. Narayan SM, Krummen DE, Shivkumar K, Clopton P, Rappel WJ, Miller JM. Treatment of atrial fibrillation by the ablation of localized sources: CONFIRM (Conventional Ablation for Atrial Fibrillation with or without Focal Impulse and Rotor Modulation) trial. J Am Coll Cardiol. 2012;60:628-36.
62. Narayan SM, Baykaner T, Clopton P, Schricker A, Lalani GG, Krummen DE, Shivkumar K, Miller JM. Ablation of rotor and

focal sources reduces late recurrence of atrial fibrillation compared with trigger ablation alone: extended follow-up of the CONFIRM trial (Conventional Ablation for Atrial Fibrillation with or without Focal Impulse and Rotor Modulation). J Am Coll Cardiol. 2014;63:1761-8.
63. Kuck KH, Wissner E. A FIRM grip on atrial fibrillation. J Am Coll Cardiol. 2012;60:637-8.
64. Revishvili AS, Wissner E, Lebedev DS, Lemes C, Deiss S, Metzner A, Kalinin VV, Sopov OV, Labartkava EZ, Kalinin AV, Chmelevsky M, Zubarev SV, Chaykovskaya MK, Tsiklauri MG, Kuck KH. Validation of the mapping accuracy of a novel non-invasive epicardial and endocardial electrophysiology system. Europace. 2015;17:1282-8.
65. Haissaguerre M, Hocini M, Shah AJ, Derval N, Sacher F, Jais P, Dubois R. Noninvasive panoramic mapping of human atrial fibrillation mechanisms: a feasibility report. J Cardiovasc Electrophysiol. 2013;24:711-7.
66. Knecht S. Preliminary data from the AFACART (Non-invasive mapping before ablation for atrial fibrillation) study, in 10th International Symposium on Catheter Ablation Techniques. 2014: Paris, France.
67. Wynn GJ, Das M, Bonnett LJ, Panikker S, Wong T, Gupta D. Efficacy of catheter ablation for persistent atrial fibrillation: a systematic review and meta-analysis of evidence from randomized and nonrandomized controlled trials. Circ Arrhythm Electrophysiol. 2014;7:841-52.
68. Haissaguerre M, Sanders P, Hocini M, Takahashi Y, Rotter M, Sacher F, Rostock T, Hsu LF, Bordachar P, Reuter S, Roudaut R, Clementy J, Jais P. Catheter ablation of long-lasting persistent atrial fibrillation: critical structures for termination. J Cardiovasc Electrophysiol. 2005;16:1125-37.
69. Haissaguerre M, Sanders P, Hocini M, Hsu LF, Shah DC, Scavee C, Takahashi Y, Rotter M, Pasquie JL, Garrigue S, Clementy J, Jais P. Changes in atrial fibrillation cycle length and inducibility during catheter ablation and their relation to outcome. Circulation. 2004;109:3007-13.
70. Calo L, Lamberti F, Loricchio ML, De Ruvo E, Colivicchi F, Bianconi L, Pandozi C, Santini M. Left atrial ablation versus biatrial ablation for persistent and permanent atrial fibrillation: a prospective and randomized study. J Am Coll Cardiol. 2006;47:2504-12.
71. Scherr D, Khairy P, Miyazaki S, Aurillac-Lavignolle V, Pascale P, Wilton SB, Ramoul K, Komatsu Y, Roten L, Jadidi A, Linton N, Pedersen M, Daly M, O'Neill M, Knecht S, Weerasooriya R, Rostock T, Manninger M, Cochet H, Shah AJ, Yeim S, Denis A, Derval N, Hocini M, Sacher F, Haissaguerre M, Jais P. Five-year outcome of catheter ablation of persistent atrial fibrillation using termination of atrial fibrillation as a procedural endpoint. Circ Arrhythm Electrophysiol. 2015;8:18-24.
72. Verma A, Jiang CY, Betts TR, Chen J, Deisenhofer I, Mantovan R, Macle L, Morillo CA, Haverkamp W, Weerasooriya R, Albenque JP, Nardi S, Menardi E, Novak P, Sanders P. Approaches to catheter ablation for persistent atrial fibrillation. N Engl J Med. 2015;372:1812-22.

EDITORS' SUMMARY

Drs Maurer and Wißner and Professor Karl-Heinz Kuck provide in this chapter a well-explained, encompassing, and instructive description of the present approaches for complex atrial fibrillation ablation (see also Chapter 23).

The chapter includes a discussion of how to construct a complete ablation line and troubleshooting difficulties when trying to execute a sometimes difficult maneuver. The complex approaches and options for ablating persistent atrial fibrillation are presented in a summary and algorithm advocating a possible step-wise approach for AF ablation. In addition, the authors discuss in a lucid manner mapping approaches to identify arrhythmogenic substrate during atrial fibrillation and provide a balanced consideration of the merit and limitation of each of these approaches.

CHAPTER 26

Amar Upadhyay, Raja J Selvaraj

Atrioventricular Junction Ablation for Rate Control in Atrial Fibrillation

LIST OF ABBREVIATIONS

AF	Atrial Fibrillation	AV	Atrioventricular

INTRODUCTION

Atrial fibrillation (AF) is the most common sustained arrhythmia[1] in the general population and is associated with significant morbidity. The two important causes of AF-related morbidity are the rapid heart rate and increased risk of thromboembolism. Amelioration of symptoms due to the rapid heart rate can be achieved by correcting the rhythm itself (rhythm control) or by lowering the rate while the patient remains in atrial fibrillation (rate control). Although it seems logical that correcting the rhythm should be better, randomized controlled trials[2,3] have failed to prove an advantage for a rhythm control strategy over rate control only. Therefore, rate control remains an important therapeutic option for patients with AF.

In most patients, rate control can be achieved with the use of drugs such as beta blockers, calcium channel blockers or digoxin. However, in a few patients use of drugs may not achieve adequate rate control or the patient may not tolerate drugs in the required doses. In such patients, ablation of the atrioventricular (AV) junction can be a useful nonpharmacological approach to rate control. Ablation can be performed to modify AV conduction with slowing of ventricular rate or to produce complete AV conduction block with subsequent pacemaker implantation.

APPLIED ANATOMY OF THE ATRIOVENTRICULAR NODE

The AV node was discovered after meticulous research by Tawara.[4] Anatomically, it is a subendocardial structure located in the inferoposterior region of the atrial septum at the midpoint of the Koch's triangle and joins the penetrating bundle of His on the membranous portion of the interventricular septum near the apex of the Koch's triangle.

At the apex of the triangle of Koch, whose boundaries are formed by the ostium of the coronary sinus, the tendon of Todaro and the tricuspid annulus, the AV node continues distally as the His bundle which travels through the central fibrous body where it is related to the annuli of mitral, tricuspid and aortic valves. Although three[5] and possibly multiple[6] inputs have been described, in the most widely accepted model, there are two major inputs into the AV node.[7] The posterior input, located between the coronary sinus ostium and tricuspid annulus, corresponds to the slow pathway, while the anterior input corresponds to the fast pathway. While the slow pathway has a slower conduction velocity, it also has a shorter refractory period which means it is capable of allowing conduction of more impulses in a shorter period of time.

ATRIOVENTRICULAR JUNCTION MODIFICATION

Modification of the AV junction was first described by Williamson et al.[8] as an alternative to AV junction ablation causing complete AV block as it does not result in life-long dependence on a pacemaker. Due to its shorter refractory period, the slow pathway plays the dominant role in facilitating rapid conduction of impulses to the ventricle during atrial fibrillation. Thus, ablation of the slow pathway should allow reduction in ventricular rate. In fact, this has also been demonstrated in a mathematical model.[9] On the other hand, ablation of the fast pathway results in previously concealed slow pathway beats to be conducted with no effect on the ventricular rate.[10] Ablation of the slow pathway to modify the AV conduction and slow the ventricular rate has been termed AV junction modification.

This procedure is useful in patients who are refractory or intolerant to drugs for rate control. The major advantage over AV junction ablation is preservation of AV conduction, possibly avoiding the need for pacemaker implantation. Usually the radiofrequency ablation is performed with a 4 mm tip, nonirrigated ablation catheter positioned in the posterior septal region on the tricuspid annulus, similar to slow pathway ablation for atrioventricular nodal reentrant tachycardia. Ablation can be performed in sinus rhythm or during atrial fibrillation and is begun posteriorly, at the level of the coronary sinus ostium with subsequent ablations delivered more anteriorly and superiorly if required. A location with an AV ratio of less than 0.5 is targeted and slowing of ventricular rate during AF is observed for during ablation. When a good response is seen, radiofrequency energy at 20–40 W is delivered for 60 seconds. Endpoint of the procedure is a mean heart rate of 120 bpm during a steady state isoproterenol infusion at 4 µg per minute. When performed in sinus rhythm, presence of slow pathway potential can be used to identify site for ablation and accelerated junctional rhythm can be used as a marker of successful ablation. Acute success is achieved in about 70% of patients.[8,11] Ablation should be avoided at a location with a visible His signal and should be stopped immediately if there is abrupt prolongation of RR intervals. Still, about 10% of patients are likely to develop heart block and require permanent pacing.[12]

Apart from the risk of AV block, the concerns with this procedure have been the variability of response and the partial recovery of conduction during long-term follow-up in some patients. It has been hypothesized that a reason for poor response in some patients may be the absence of a dual AV nodal physiology. The presence of bimodal pattern of RR distribution in a 24-hour ambulatory ECG recording has been considered to indicate dual AV nodal physiology in patients in atrial fibrillation. The patients with this pattern may have a better success rate with AV junction modification compared to those who do not show the pattern.[13] During long-term follow-up, while resting rates continued to be low, the maximal rate during exercise gradually increased reaching almost baseline levels,[8] suggesting recovery of conduction. Late clinical recurrence with rapid ventricular rates during AF were seen in about 10% of patients with an initially successful procedure.[11,14]

ATRIOVENTRICULAR JUNCTION ABLATION

Ablation to interrupt conduction from the atrium to the ventricle is an alternative means of achieving control of the ventricular rate during atrial fibrillation. Since conduction is interrupted, these patients require implantation of a permanent pacemaker for ventricular pacing. This was first described by Scheinman and colleagues in 1982 using direct current.[15] With the use of radiofrequency energy, the success rate and safety of the procedure have improved significantly.

Candidates for AV junction ablation include:[16, 17]

1. Inadequate rate control with drugs and rhythm control not achievable.
2. Drug refractory patients with rate-related cardiomyopathy.
3. Patients with ICD having inappropriate shock due to rapid ventricular rate, not controlled with drugs.
4. Patients with AF having CRT-P or CRT-D device and inadequate biventricular pacing due to rapid intrinsic ventricular rates. The procedure may also be performed at the time of implantation of these devices to ensure adequate biventricular pacing.

The procedure is usually performed with a 4 mm tip catheter inserted through a femoral approach. Attempt is made to target the compact AV node above the level of the His bundle so that a more stable and narrow escape rhythm is achieved **(Figure 26.1)**. If patient does not have a pacemaker already, a temporary pacing lead is preferably positioned in the right ventricle before the procedure.

The ablation catheter is positioned to record a His bundle electrogram at the superomedial tricuspid annulus **(Figure 26.2)**. From here, the catheter is pulled slightly towards the atrium and inferiorly to achieve a larger atrial signal and small or absent His signal **(Figures 26.3 and 26.4)**. An accelerated junctional rhythm is usually seen during energy delivery if the procedure is performed during sinus rhythm. The development of AV block is reflected by appearance of slow regular junctional or ventricular escape rhythm or ventricular pacing **(Figure 26.5)**. If AV block is seen within 10 seconds, ablation may be completed for 60 seconds at a power of 30 to 50 W. Acute success is obtained

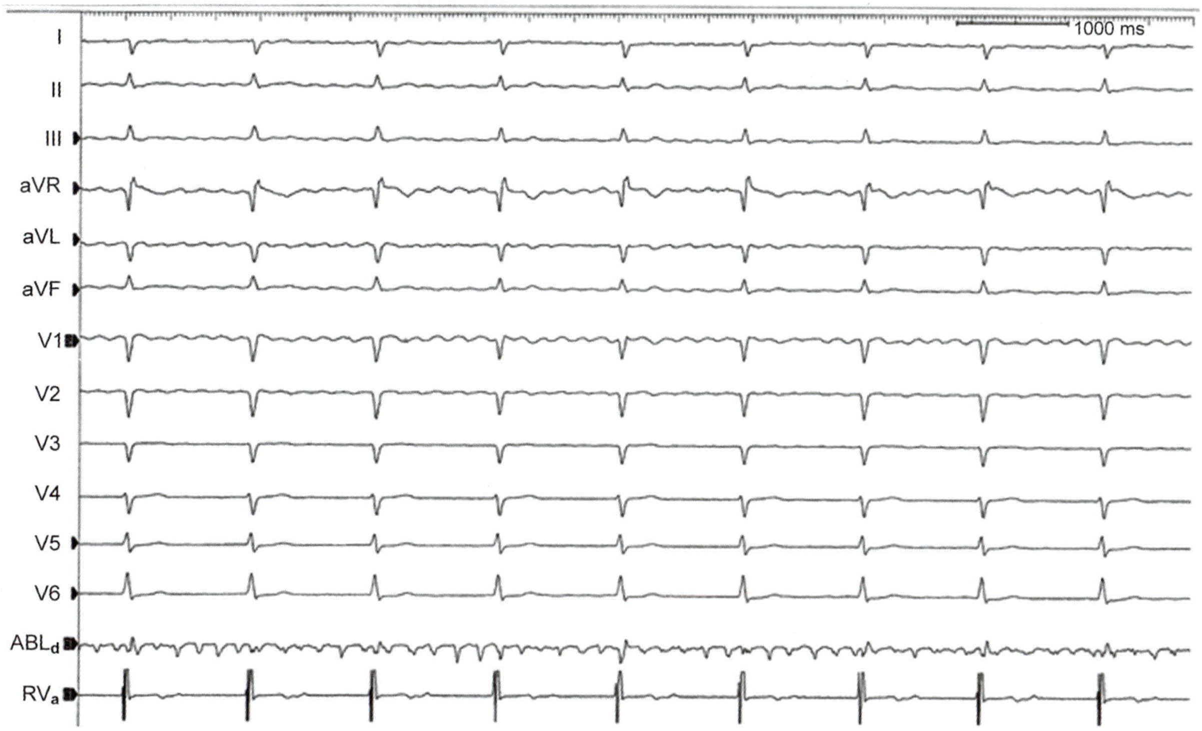

Figure 26.1: Regular narrow QRS junctional escape rhythm after AV nodal ablation in a patient with prosthetic mitral valve and long-standing atrial fibrillation with uncontrolled ventricular rate. The figure shows 12-lead ECG followed by ablation distal (ABL$_d$) and right ventricular (RV$_a$) signals displayed at a speed of 25 mm/s

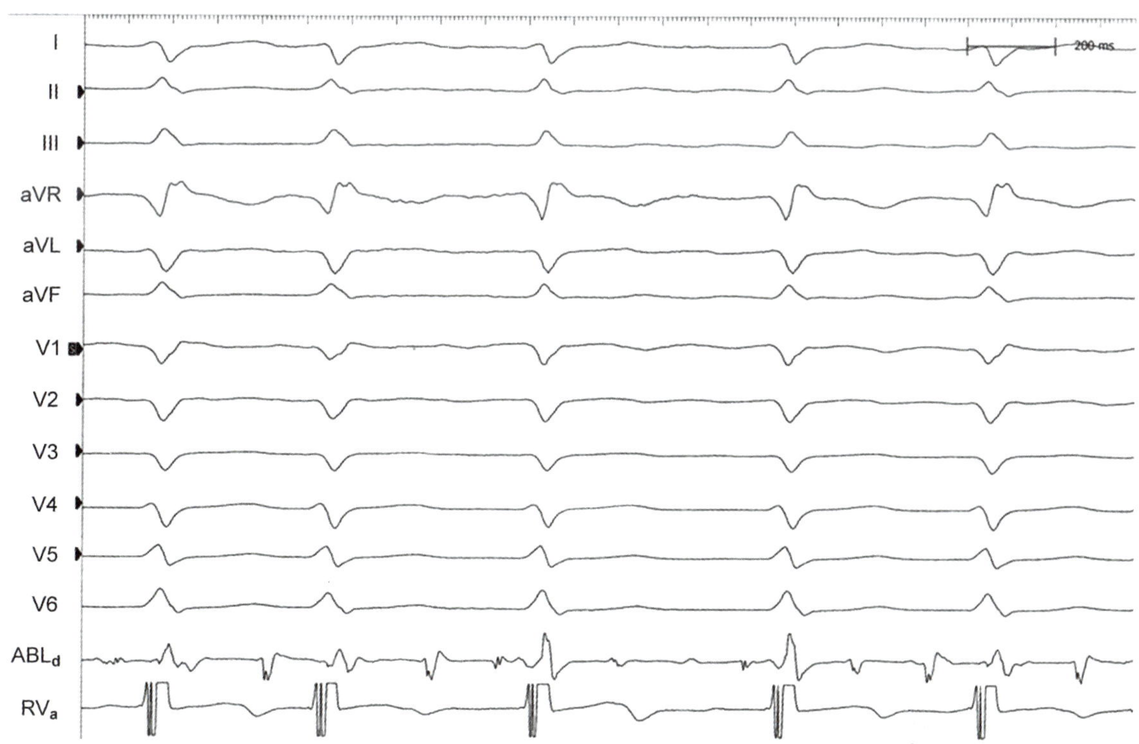

Figure 26.2: His bundle signal seen in the distal ablation recording at a speed of 100 mm/s while attempting AV junctional ablation in the same patient as in Figure 26.1

The abbreviations are same as in Figure 26.1

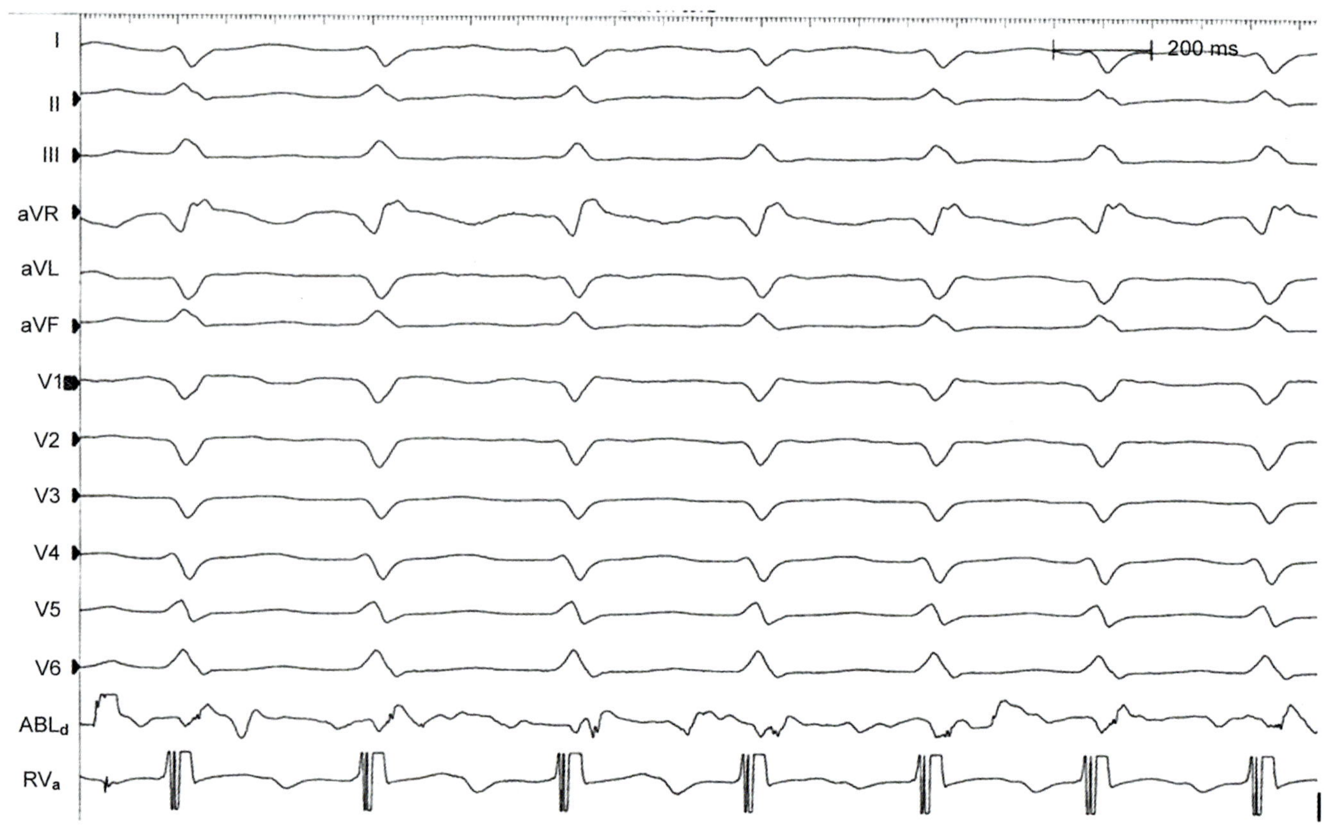

Figure 26.3: The ablation signals at the site of AV junctional ablation of the same patient as in Figure 26.1. Display speed 100 mm/s. Abbreviations as in Figure 26.1

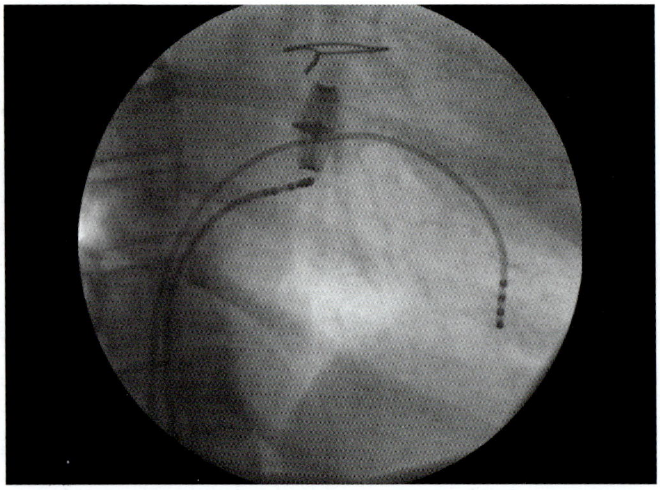

Figure 26.4: Right anterior oblique view showing the position of the ablation catheter for AV junctional ablation of the same patient shown in Figure 26.1. Also visible are the prosthetic mitral valve and a quadripolar catheter at right ventricular apex being used for temporary pacing

in close to 100% of patients. In the small number of patients in whom initial attempts are unsuccessful, switching to a left-sided approach may be better than persisting with attempts from the right side.[18]

Significant improvement in quality of life, exercise duration and symptoms have been documented in patients undergoing AV junction ablation and this procedure is superior to drug therapy alone in patients with refractory symptoms.[19,20] Many patients with atrial fibrillation and persistent high ventricular rates also have left ventricular dysfunction and improvement in ejection fraction is noted after AV junction ablation and pacing.[21]

Sudden death was noted in early reports in 2–5% of patients undergoing AV junction ablation.[22] Among the different possible mechanisms, most accepted now is increased dispersion of refractoriness due to the sudden change in heart rate after ablation. It has become accepted standard practice now to use a higher pacing rate for first few months after the ablation and this has been shown to result in abolition of early sudden deaths related to the ablation.[23] The pacing rate is typically set at 90 beats per

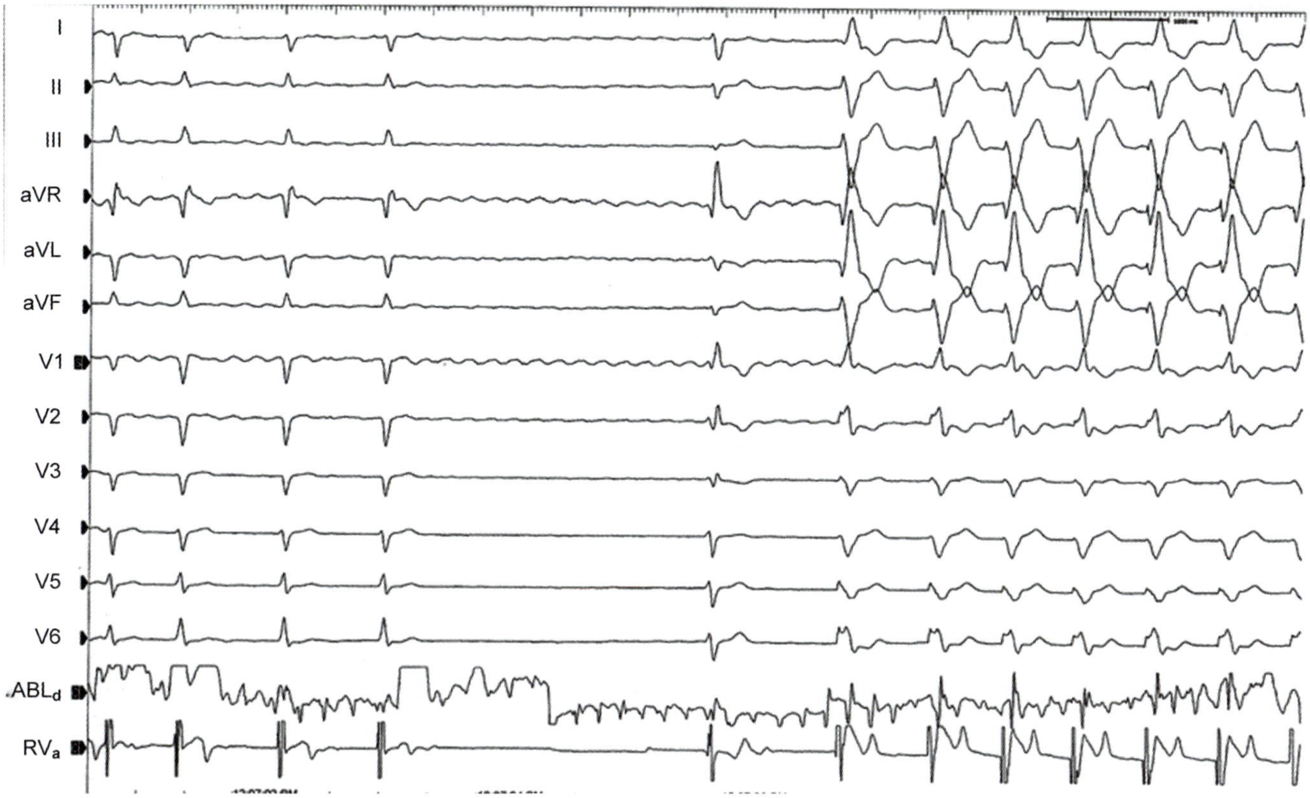

Figure 26.5: Radiofrequency ablation at the site shown in Figure 26.4 results in sudden bradycardia due to development of complete AV block. A single relatively narrow QRS escape beat is seen following which ventricular pacing is started while the radiofrequency energy application is continued. Display speed 25 mm/s
Abbreviations as in Figure 26.1

minute immediately after ablation and reduced by 10 beats per minute monthly until a final lower rate of 60 beats per minute is achieved.

There has been debate about the choice of pacing mode after AV junction ablation. In patients with long-standing persistent or permanent AF, VVIR pacing is sufficient. In paroxysmal atrial fibrillation, dual chamber pacing is shown to be clearly superior to single chamber ventricular pacing in terms of symptomatic benefit.[24] Among dual chamber pacing, there is an option of VDD (no atrial pacing) or DDD pacing modes. It was assumed that dispersion of atrial repolarization, and supraventricular ectopics due to bradycardia serve as electrophysiological substrates for initiation and maintenance of atrial fibrillation and that these could be reduced by atrial-based pacing. However, in a study comparing DDDR and VDD modes, no benefit could be demonstrated for DDDR pacing in preventing recurrence of paroxysmal AF or delaying the development of permanent AF.[25] Moreover, progression to permanent AF is also seen in a large proportion of these patients after one year. Therefore, VDD mode appears sufficient for most patients with paroxysmal AF who undergo AV junction ablation.

CONCLUSION

A strategy of rate control is reasonable in many patients with paroxysmal or persistent atrial fibrillation. For a majority of these patients, adequate rate control can be achieved by drugs alone. However, for patients whose rate is not controlled with drugs, radiofrequency ablation to either modify AV conduction or to completely interrupt AV conduction are possible strategies, especially when they are not candidates for rhythm control. AV junction ablation with permanent pacing, the 'Ablate and Pace' strategy is preferred now because of the more consistent response and high success rate. These patients experience significant symptomatic improvement with increased effort tolerance and often improvement of left ventricular function as well in comparison to patients where drugs therapy alone is continued.

REFERENCES

1. Go AS, Hylek EM, Phillips KA, Chang Y, Henault LE, Selby JV, Singer DE. Prevalence of diagnosed atrial fibrillation in adults: national implications for rhythm management and stroke

prevention: the Anticoagulation and Risk Factors in Atrial Fibrillation (ATRIA) Study. JAMA. 2001;285:2370-5.

2. Wyse DG, Waldo AL, DiMarco JP, Domanski MJ, Rosenberg Y, Schron EB, Kellen JC, Greene HL, Mickel MC, Dalquist JE, Corley SD. A comparison of rate control and rhythm control in patients with atrial fibrillation. N Engl J Med. 2002;347: 1825-33.
3. Van Gelder IC, Hagens VE, Bosker HA, Kingma JH, Kamp O, Kingma T, Said SA, Darmanata JI, Timmermans AJ, Tijssen JG, Crijns HJ. A comparison of rate control and rhythm control in patients with recurrent persistent atrial fibrillation. N Engl J Med. 2002;347:1834-40.
4. Tawara S. Das Reizleitungssystem des Säugetierhezens. Verlag von Gustav Fischer, Jena. 1906.
5. Inoue S, Becker AE. Posterior extensions of the human compact atrioventricular node: a neglected anatomic feature of potential clinical significance. Circulation. 1998;97:188-93.
6. Antz M, Scherlag BJ, Otomo K, Pitha J, Tondo C, Patterson E, et al. Evidence for multiple atrio-AV nodal inputs in the normal dog heart. J Cardiovasc Electrophysiol. 1998;9:395-408.
7. Meijler FL, Janse MJ. Morphology and electrophysiology of the mammalian atrioventricular node. Physiol Rev. 1988;68:608-47.
8. Williamson BD, Man KC, Daoud E, Niebauer M, Strickberger SA, Morady F. Radiofrequency catheter modification of atrioventricular conduction to control the ventricular rate during atrial fibrillation. N Engl J Med. 1994;331:910-7.
9. Climent AM, Guillem MS, Zhang Y, Millet J, Mazgalev TN. Functional mathematical model of dual pathway AV nodal conduction. Am J Physiol Heart Circ Physiol. 2011;300: H1393-401.
10. Zhang Y, Mazgalev TN. Ventricular rate control during atrial fibrillation and AV node modifications: past, present, and future. Pacing Clin Electrophysiol. 2004;27:382-93.
11. Carbucicchio C, Tondo C, Fassini G, Riva S, Agostoni P, Galli C, Della Bella P. Modulation of the atrioventricular node conduction to achieve rate control in patients with atrial fibrillation: long-term results. Pacing Clin Electrophysiol. 1999; 22:442-52.
12. Feld GK. Radiofrequency catheter ablation versus modification of the AV node for control of rapid ventricular response in atrial fibrillation. J Cardiovasc Electrophysiol. 1995;6:217-28.
13. Rokas S, Gaitanidou S, Chatzidou S, Pamboucas C, Achtipis D, Stamatelopoulos S. Atrioventricular node modification in patients with chronic atrial fibrillation: role of morphology of RR interval variation. Circulation. 2001;103:2942-8.
14. Morady F, Hasse C, Strickberger SA, Man KC, Daoud E, Bogun F, Goyal R, Harvey M, Knight BP, Weiss R, Bahu M. Long-term follow-up after radiofrequency modification of the atrioventricular node in patients with atrial fibrillation. J Am Coll Cardiol. 1997;29:113-21.
15. Scheinman MM, Morady F, Hess DS, Gonzalez R. Catheter-induced ablation of the atrioventricular junction to control refractory supraventricular arrhythmias. JAMA. 1982;248:851-5.
16. Betts TR. Atrioventricular junction ablation and pacemaker implant for atrial fibrillation: still valid treatment in appropriately selected patients. Europace. 2008;10:425-32.
17. January CT, Wann LS, Alpert JS, Calkins H, Cigarroa JE, Cleveland JC, Jr., Conti JB, Ellinor PT, Ezekowitz MD, Field ME, Murray KT, Sacco RL, Stevenson WG, Tchou PJ, Tracy CM, Yancy CW. 2014 AHA/ACC/HRS guideline for the management of patients with atrial fibrillation: a report of the American College of Cardiology/American Heart Association Task Force on practice guidelines and the Heart Rhythm Society. Circulation. 2014;130:e199-267.
18. Kalbfleisch SJ, Williamson B, Man KC, Vorperian V, Hummel JD, Calkins H, Strickberger SA, Langberg JJ, Morady F. A randomized comparison of the right- and left-sided approaches to ablation of the atrioventricular junction. Am J Cardiol. 1993;72:1406-10.
19. Brignole M, Gianfranchi L, Menozzi C, Alboni P, Musso G, Bongiorni MG, Gasparini M, Raviele A, Lolli G, Paparella N, Acquarone S. Assessment of atrioventricular junction ablation and DDDR mode-switching pacemaker versus pharmacological treatment in patients with severely symptomatic paroxysmal atrial fibrillation: a randomized controlled study. Circulation. 1997;96:2617-24.
20. Wood MA, Brown-Mahoney C, Kay GN, Ellenbogen KA. Clinical outcomes after ablation and pacing therapy for atrial fibrillation : a meta-analysis. Circulation. 2000;101:1138-44.
21. Twidale N, Sutton K, Bartlett L, Dooley A, Winstanley S, Heddle W, Hassam R, Koutsounis H. Effects on cardiac performance of atrioventricular node catheter ablation using radiofrequency current for drug-refractory atrial arrhythmias. Pacing Clin Electrophysiol. 1993;16:1275-84.
22. Ozcan C, Jahangir A, Friedman PA, Hayes DL, Munger TM, Rea RF, Lloyd MA, Packer DL, Hodge DO, Gersh BJ, Hammill SC, Shen WK. Sudden death after radiofrequency ablation of the atrioventricular node in patients with atrial fibrillation. J Am Coll Cardiol. 2002;40:105-10.
23. Wang RX, Lee HC, Hodge DO, Cha YM, Friedman PA, Rea RF, Munger TM, Jahangir A, Srivathsan K, Shen WK. Effect of pacing method on risk of sudden death after atrioventricular node ablation and pacemaker implantation in patients with atrial fibrillation. Heart Rhythm. 2013;10:696-701.
24. Marshall HJ, Harris ZI, Griffith MJ, Holder RL, Gammage MD. Prospective randomized study of ablation and pacing versus medical therapy for paroxysmal atrial fibrillation: effects of pacing mode and mode-switch algorithm. Circulation. 1999;99:1587-92.
25. Gillis AM, Connolly SJ, Lacombe P, Philippon F, Dubuc M, Kerr CR, Yee R, Rose MS, Newman D, Kavanagh KM, Gardner MJ, Kus T, Wyse DG. Randomized crossover comparison of DDDR versus VDD pacing after atrioventricular junction ablation for prevention of atrial fibrillation. The atrial pacing peri-ablation for paroxysmal atrial fibrillation (PA (3)) study investigators. Circulation. 2000;102:736-41.

EDITORS' SUMMARY

With the advent of targeted trigger and substrate ablation for atrial fibrillation, the frequency with which we do AV node ablation as part of an ablate and pace strategy has significantly declined. We anticipate that with further improvements in the science of energy delivery and our fundamental understanding of atrial fibrillation, AV node ablation may become a rare procedure for a future generation of electrophysiologists.

The details of the anatomic location of the compact AV node and the associated signals recorded at sites where we successfully ablate this structure as detailed by Dr Selvaraj in this chapter remain important in contemporary electrophysiology. This is because while we may not target the structure frequently in the future, we need to be thorough with its location to avoid inadvertent damage of the AV node when performing a variety of other procedures including AV node reentry ablation, atrial flutter ablation, septal atrial tachycardia ablation, and supravalvular ventricular tachycardia ablation.

As explained in the text, despite our advances in the development of recording electrodes and mapping systems, there is no discernible potential that we can record at this time from the AV node itself. Thus, a combination of appreciating the detailed anatomy of the triangle of Koch and recordings from the structures that we can map and represent neighbors of the AV node (septal atrial electrogram and far-field His bundle recording) remain the best estimates of where this structure is located and energy delivery avoided.

CHAPTER 27

Antonio Sorgente, Riccardo Cappato

Atrial Fibrillation Ablation: Clinical Studies, Efficacy and Complications

LIST OF ABBREVIATIONS

AAD	Antiarrhythmic Drugs	PVI	Pulmonary Vein Isolation
AF	Atrial Fibrillation	RCT	Randomized Controlled Trial
CFAE	Complex Fractionated Atrial Electrograms	RF	Radiofrequency
NOAC	Novel Oral Anticoagulant		

INTRODUCTION

Catheter ablation of atrial fibrillation (AF) is a well-known non-pharmacologic treatment option in patients with drug-refractory AF.[1] A huge amount of literature has been produced in the last years to testify the usefulness and the reliability of this technique in the extremely complex scenario of cardiac electrophysiology. A number of reviews on the same topic have demonstrated how catheter ablation of AF is a valid treatment modality although extremely high between-study heterogeneity has to be remarked in this context.

The concept behind this procedure stands on the finding that AF, which remains a very complex arrhythmia whose causes and mechanisms are currently under investigation, can be triggered inside pulmonary veins.[2,3] Pulmonary veins have muscular sleeves which extend into the left atrium and which help to regulate blood flow towards the left cardiac chambers. Interesting histopathological observations have allowed the discovery of P cells, transitional cells and Purkinje cells in these myocardial muscle extensions and these cells combine perfectly with the hypothesis that pulmonary veins are potential sources of rapid electrical activity triggering AF.[4] A large amount of publications have demonstrated that electrical isolation of pulmonary veins achieved with whichever energy source (i.e. radiofrequency vs cryothermal vs laser energy) reduces the burden of AF in patients affected by this arrhythmia more than the antiarrhythmic drugs.[5,6]

CLINICAL STUDIES

Just sticking to the results of randomized controlled trials (RCT), at present if we interrogate the most popular scientific literature databases (i.e. Pubmed, Embase, Web of Science and Cochrane) for "catheter ablation of atrial fibrillation", more than 300 studies can be easily retrieved, not taking into account also the increasing number of meta-analysis already published on the topic. The first RCTs have tried to test the general hypothesis that pulmonary vein isolation is more efficacious than antiarrhythmic drugs (AAD) in preventing recurrences of AF. Piccini et al. have conducted a specific meta-analysis on the topic that was published in Circulation Arrhythmia and Electrophysiology.[7] The primary endpoint tested in this study was freedom from recurrent AF at 12 months follow-up. Using a random-effects modeling according to intention to treat, 6 trials were included with a total of 693 patients with AF treated with pulmonary vein isolation (PVI) or, in turn, with AAD. PVI was associated with significantly increased odds of freedom from AF at 12 months of follow-up (77% versus 29%; odds ratio 9.74; 95% CI, 3.98 to 23.87). Taking apart the studies which also enrolled patients with persistent AF, this benefit in terms of maintenance of sinus rhythm was even greater (odds ratio 15.78; 95% CI, 10.07 to 24.73). Moreover, the authors also found a reduction in hospitalizations for cardiovascular causes (14 versus 93 per 100 person-years; rate ratio 0.15; 95% CI, 0.10 to 0.23). Unsurprisingly, 17% of the patients who underwent a catheter ablation needed a repeat procedure within the 12-month follow-up. Finally, the rate of major complications in the invasive arm of the meta-analysis was of 2.6% (completely in line with the rate of complications of other invasive procedures) against a rate of reported adverse events associated with AAD therapy of 8%. These data find partial confirmation in another meta-analysis by Calkins et al.[8] published in the same journal in the same year that included both RCT and non-RCT. Taking into account an average follow-up of 14 months, the overall success for AAD was 52% (95% CI, 47% to 57%) against a single procedure success rate of catheter ablation of AF off AAD therapy of 57% (50% to 64%). Obviously, the on-AAD success rate of catheter ablation was higher—71% (65% to 77%) after multiple or uncertain number of procedures.

After the spread of this technique in the common clinical practice, more data has been cumulated on the long-term outcome also in terms of recurrence of AF after catheter ablation. Recently, in 2013, a systematic review and meta-analysis by Ganesan et al. has grouped the data from 19 studies with a follow-up ≥3 years.[9] After pooling all the data together, mean follow-up was of ≥24 months after the index procedure. In terms of single procedure efficacy, the results were in line with the ones of the previously cited studies: single procedure freedom from atrial arrhythmia for patients with paroxysmal AF at long-term follow-up was 54.1% (95% CI 44.4% to 63.4%), whereas it was obviously worse for non-paroxysmal AF (41.8%, 95% CI 25.2% to 60.5%). Multiple procedures expectedly were associated with a longer term success rate: the overall freedom from atrial arrhythmias was 79.8% (95% CI 75.0% to 83.8%), without a great difference between paroxysmal AF and non-paroxysmal AF. To testify the great heterogeneity of this study, after performing a meta-regression among the major variables recognized universally as predictive of AF recurrence (such as persistent AF, left ventricular systolic dysfunction or heart failure, structural or valvular heart disease and duration of AF), none of them were statistically significant. The authors of this meta-analysis evidenced also a relationship between the experience of the operator and the success rate of the procedure itself, meaning that usually the most important publications on the topic are provided by the most experienced cardiac electrophysiologists and that there's no real data on the performance of low volume centers.

EFFICACY OF AF ABLATION PROCEDURES

Pulmonary vein isolation is a consolidated technique to address drug refractory paroxysmal AF. It is established that the results of this technique in patients with non-paroxysmal AF are less consistent than the results obtained in patient with paroxysmal AF.[1] Therefore, a number of alternative options in terms of sources or targets of ablation itself have been proposed in the clinical practice in substitution or more often in addition to pulmonary vein isolation, often without a clear pathophysiological prerequisite. One of these targets are the so-called complex fractioned atrial electrograms (CFAE), proposed for the first time by Nademanee and his coworkers[10] as the electrophysiological correlates of drivers or rotors of persistent AF and the anatomical correlates of ganglionated plexi, which seem to have a role in the perpetuation of AF itself. CFAEs are defined as "low-voltage atrial electrograms (ranging from 0.04 to 0.25 mV) that have fractionated electrograms composed of two deflections or more, and/or have a perturbation of the baseline with continuous deflection of a prolonged activation complex". Nademanee et al. demonstrated that ablation of CFAE were efficacious in restoring sinus rhythm in patients with both paroxysmal and non-paroxysmal AF,[11] with 87% of them free of atrial arrhythmias recurrence at an averaged follow-up of 839 ± 493 days. Henceforth, this ablation technique has been applied in a number of clinical studies, generally in addition to pulmonary vein isolation. The results of CFAE ablation have been stressed out in a recent meta-analysis by Wu et al.[12] Unifying the data coming from 11 studies which share additional CFAE ablation as common technique to treat patients with both paroxysmal and non-paroxysmal AF, these authors demonstrated that CFAE ablation, in addition to pulmonary vein isolation, reduces recurrence of atrial tachy-arrhythmias after a single procedure (pooled RR 0.73; 95% CI 0.61, 0.88; p = 0.0007) at ≥3-month follow-up compared to pulmonary vein isolation alone. More in particular, additional CFAE ablation reduced recurrence rate in non-paroxysmal AF (RR 0.68; 95% CI 0.47, 0.99; p = 0.05), without any significant effect on patients with paroxysmal AF (RR 0.79; 95% CI 0.59, 1.06; p = 0.12). This partial benefit in terms of recurrence of non-paroxysmal AF was counterbalanced by a higher incidence of post-procedural atrial tachycardias (RR 1.77; 95% CI 1.02, 3.07; P = 0.04), increased mean procedural times (245.4 + 75.7 vs. 189.5 + 62.3 min, p <0.001), mean fluoroscopy (72.1 + 25.6 vs. 59.5 + 19.3 min, p <0.001), and mean RF energy application times (75.3 + 38.6 vs. 53.2 + 27.5 min, p <0.001). Very recently, Verma et al.[13] have tried to figure out if a more selective approach in CFAE ablation (i.e. CFAE showing a continuous electrical activity and absence of isoelectric segments for more than 75% of their duration) can reduce the length of these procedures and impact the outcome in terms of atrial arrhythmias recurrence. This selective approach reduced fluoroscopy times resulting in a similar incidence of acute AF termination, but unfortunately, at 1 year follow-up freedom from AF/atrial flutter/atrial tachycardia recurrence and need for a repeat procedure were significantly higher than in patients treated with the traditional and generalized CFAE ablation.

An innovative curative approach to non-paroxysmal AF has recently been proposed by Narayan et al.,[14] who hypothesized that ablation of AF substrates (the so-called electrical rotors or focal sources) with the help of a special three-dimensional electro-anatomical mapping system can ensure better and longer arrhythmia-free survival in these patients than ablation of pulmonary and non-pulmonary veins triggers. The CONFIRM (Conventional Ablation for Atrial Fibrillation with or without Focal Impulse and Rotor Modulation)[15] trial enrolled 92 patients with high burden paroxysmal AF or persistent AF and randomized them in a 2-arm 1:2 design, by ablation at sources (FIRM-guided) followed by conventional ablation, mainly pulmonary vein isolation (n = 36), or conventional ablation alone (n = 71; FIRM-blinded). AF termination or slowing of its average cycle length was obtained in about 85% of active arm whereas this objective was reached out only in 20% of FIRM-blinded patients. Interestingly, ablation of sources of AF in addition to pulmonary vein isolation ensured a better outcome at a median follow-up of 273 days (interquartile range: 132 to 681 days) after a single procedure (82.4% vs. 44.9%; p <0.001). No differences in adverse events between groups were reported. Recently, a continuation of the follow-up on the same patients to about 3 years has granted another publication to the same group of authors: superiority of rotor ablation in addition to pulmonary vein isolation was confirmed after a median follow-up of 890 days (interquartile range: 224 to 1,563 days) both in terms of AF and of atrial arrhythmias recurrences. Even if the results of these studies are encouraging, a drawback of this ablation technique is that it needs special electroanatomical mapping system and therefore time and training would be needed before getting more consistent and reliable data.

In the last few years, considering the huge amount of data produced on the superiority of AF ablation over antiarrhythmic drugs, catheter ablation of AF has been proposed also as first-line treatment of patients with paroxysmal AF. Two major randomized clinical trials merited publication in New England Journal of Medicine and Journal of the American Medical Association (JAMA) respectively, targeting this topic. The Medical ANtiarrhythmic Treatment of Radiofrequency Ablation in Atrial Fibrillation (MANTRA-AF) enrolled overall 297 patients with paroxysmal AF and randomized them in a 1:1 fashion to the AAD therapy vs catheter ablation.[16] No difference throughout all the study was found between active or conservative treatment, even if the cumulative burden of AF was reduced in the ablation arm at 24 months follow-up (90th percentile, 9% vs. 18%; p = 0.007). Noteworthy, in the ablation group, there was one death related to a periprocedural stroke and 3 cases of cardiac tamponade. The Radiofrequency Ablation vs Antiarrhythmic Drugs as First-line Treatment of Paroxysmal Atrial Fibrillation (RAAFT-2) trial[17] enrolled 127 drug treatment naive patients with paroxysmal AF and randomized them to AF ablation vs traditional AAD therapy. Patients in the active arm (i.e., AF ablation) had a lower atrial arrhythmia recurrence rate compared to the patients enrolled in the conservative arm (54% vs 72%) at 24 months follow-up. The cost of this reduction in atrial recurrence rate was the occurrence of 4 episodes of cardiac tamponade, fortunately without any death or stroke. The authors concluded that catheter ablation of AF could be proposed as first-line therapy taking into consideration in any case a high rate of atrial arrhythmias recurrence. Take-home message of these 2 trials is that AF catheter ablation can probably reduce the burden of atrial arrhythmias recurrences with a non-negligible rate of major complications.

COMPLICATIONS OF AF ABLATION

Indeed, despite the cited positive results of catheter ablation of AF, complications associated with this procedure cannot and shouldn't be neglected or ignored. The various complications associated with AF ablation as well as their management have been well described.[1] Complications of AF ablation may range from local (mostly related to the percutaneous access that precedes catheter ablation) to life-threatening conditions. According to the most recent international guidelines on AF ablation,[1] "a major complication is defined as a complication that results in permanent injury or death, requires intervention for treatment, or prolongs or requires hospitalization".

A recent worldwide survey focusing on the methods, efficacy and safety of AF catheter ablation[18] revealed that its clinical indications have progressively widened. Nowadays, AF ablation is increasingly offered to larger patient populations presenting with greater degrees of comorbidity. This could explain the lower than expected procedural success rates but similar complication rates despite improvements in techniques and operators' experience. In the above mentioned worldwide survey, major complications were reported to occur in 4.5% of patients: death accounted for 0.15% whereas atrio-esophageal fistula for 0.04%. Among the other major complications, cardiac tamponade accounted for 1.31%, stroke for 0.23%, transient ischemic attack for 0.71% and PV stenosis requiring surgical or percutaneous dilation for another 0.29% of all procedures. Femoral pseudoaneurysms occurred in 0.93% of all interventions whereas arterio-venous fistulae were reported to occur in 0.54% of all procedures.

Shah et al.[19] recently reported on the safety of AF ablation in the real world. Out of about 4,000 patients undergoing a first AF ablation procedure between 2005 and 2008 in the State of California, 5% experienced periprocedural complications, which were mostly vascular, with 9% requiring readmission within 30 days. Elderly, females and patients who had already experienced hospitalization for AF were more prone to develop a complication compared to the remainder of the population. There was also a higher probability of complications in centers with less experience. Overall, there was a high rate of all-cause and arrhythmia-related hospitalizations (38.5% and 21.7%, respectively).

Among all the complications described for catheter ablation of AF, one of the most investigated in the recent years is the occurrence of periprocedural thromboembolic events. Usually, this complication takes place more often in patients with persistent AF and with elevated CHAD2VASc scores.[20] Evidence has been built on this topic over the years and what appears of paramount importance in this context is to ensure an adequate anticoagulation all along the catheter ablation procedure. In a recently published study,[21] Di Biase et al. compared 2 different anticoagulation strategies related to catheter ablation of AF: one arm underwent ablation procedure under full anticoagulation with warfarin (INR was mostly included between 2 and 3) whereas the other group of patients interrupted warfarin treatment 2 to 3 days before the procedure and switched to weight adjusted low molecular weight heparin. Anticoagulation with warfarin was restarted or the night of the procedure in both arms with patients in the interrupted warfarin arm being administered low molecular weight heparins together with oral anticoagulation until the INR was >2. The study enrolled overall 1,584 patients and demonstrated that the incidence of thromboembolic events in the 48 hours after ablation are significantly reduced using the uninterrupted warfarin protocol (0.25% vs 5% total events including transient ischemic attack (TIA) and strokes, $p<0.001$), without any increase in hemorrhagic complications.

The introduction of the novel oral anticoagulants (NOACs) in the treatment of AF have further complicated this scenario, with cardiac electrophysiologists facing another conundrum about the safety of these new drugs in the context of catheter ablation of AF. A recent meta-analysis published by Hohnloser and Camm[22] shed light on the use of at least the first NOAC introduced in the clinical practice, i.e. dabigatran. Summarizing the data of 10 observational studies on the topic with a total of 3,648 included patients, these authors evidenced no significant difference in thromboembolic events, major and minor bleeding between dabigatran and warfarin [odds ratio (OR) 2.38, 95% confidence interval (CI) 0.82–6.85, P = n.s.]. However, considering the significantly high heterogeneity across the studies included in the meta-analysis, the authors advocated the need for a well-designed large-scale clinical trial/s to assess more consistently the reliability of dabigatran and other NOACs in the peri-procedural management of anticoagulation.

CONCLUSION

In conclusion, catheter ablation of AF is an established treatment option for drug-refractory AF. Outcome of this procedure is highly variable, with patient selection playing a major role. Patients with paroxysmal AF respond better to this treatment than patients with non-paroxysmal AF. Given the non-negligible chance of complications and the considerably high incidence of atrial arrhythmia recurrence, at the moment catheter ablation of AF should be discouraged as first-line therapy. Further studies are warranted to deepen our knowledge on the mechanisms which stand behind AF in order to pursue more reliable and safer ablation techniques and treatments for this complex and common arrhythmia.

REFERENCES

1. Calkins H, Kuck KH, Cappato R, Brugada J, Camm AJ, Chen SA, Crijns HJ, Damiano RJ, Jr., Davies DW, DiMarco J, Edgerton J, Ellenbogen K, Ezekowitz MD, Haines DE, Haissaguerre M, Hindricks G, Iesaka Y, Jackman W, Jalife J, Jais P, Kalman J, Keane D, Kim YH, Kirchhof P, Klein G, Kottkamp H, Kumagai K, Lindsay BD, Mansour M, Marchlinski FE, McCarthy PM, Mont JL, Morady F, Nademanee K, Nakagawa H, Natale A, Nattel S, Packer DL, Pappone C, Prystowsky E, Raviele A, Reddy V, Ruskin JN, Shemin RJ, Tsao HM, Wilber D. 2012 HRS/EHRA/ECAS Expert Consensus Statement on Catheter and Surgical Ablation of Atrial Fibrillation: recommendations for patient selection, procedural techniques, patient management and follow-up, definitions, endpoints, and research trial design. Europace. 2012;14:528-606.
2. Haissaguerre M, Jais P, Shah DC, Takahashi A, Hocini M, Quiniou G, Garrigue S, Le Mouroux A, Le Metayer P, Clementy J. Spontaneous initiation of atrial fibrillation by ectopic beats originating in the pulmonary veins. N Engl J Med. 1998;339: 659-66.
3. Jais P, Haissaguerre M, Shah DC, Chouairi S, Gencel L, Hocini M, Clementy J. A focal source of atrial fibrillation treated by discrete radiofrequency ablation. Circulation. 1997;95:572-6.
4. Perez-Lugones A, McMahon JT, Ratliff NB, Saliba WI, Schweikert RA, Marrouche NF, Saad EB, Navia JL, McCarthy PM, Tchou P, Gillinov AM, Natale A. Evidence of specialized conduction cells in human pulmonary veins of patients with atrial fibrillation. J Cardiovasc Electrophysiol. 2003;14: 803-9.
5. Sorgente A, Chierchia GB, Capulzini L, Yazaki Y, Muller-Burri A, Bayrak F, Sarkozy A, de Asmundis C, Paparella G, Brugada B. Atrial fibrillation ablation: a single center comparison between remote magnetic navigation, cryoballoon and conventional manual pulmonary vein isolation. Indian Pacing Electrophysiol J. 2010;10:486-95.
6. Xu J, Huang Y, Cai H, Qi Y, Jia N, Shen W, Lin J, Peng F, Niu W. Is cryoballoon ablation preferable to radiofrequency ablation for treatment of atrial fibrillation by pulmonary vein isolation? A meta-analysis. PLoS One. 2014;9:e90323.
7. Piccini JP, Lopes RD, Kong MH, Hasselblad V, Jackson K, Al-Khatib SM. Pulmonary vein isolation for the maintenance of sinus rhythm in patients with atrial fibrillation: a meta-analysis

of randomized, controlled trials. Circ Arrhythm Electrophysiol. 2009;2:626-33.

8. Calkins H, Reynolds MR, Spector P, Sondhi M, Xu Y, Martin A, Williams CJ, Sledge I. Treatment of atrial fibrillation with antiarrhythmic drugs or radiofrequency ablation: two systematic literature reviews and meta-analyses. Circ Arrhythm Electrophysiol. 2009;2:349-61.
9. Ganesan AN, Shipp NJ, Brooks AG, Kuklik P, Lau DH, Lim HS, Sullivan T, Roberts-Thomson KC, Sanders P. Long-term outcomes of catheter ablation of atrial fibrillation: a systematic review and meta-analysis. J Am Heart Assoc. 2013;2: e004549.
10. Nademanee K, Lockwood E, Oketani N, Gidney B. Catheter ablation of atrial fibrillation guided by complex fractionated atrial electrogram mapping of atrial fibrillation substrate. J Cardiol. 2010;55:1-12.
11. Nademanee K, Schwab MC, Kosar EM, Karwecki M, Moran MD, Visessook N, Michael AD, Ngarmukos T. Clinical outcomes of catheter substrate ablation for high-risk patients with atrial fibrillation. J Am Coll Cardiol. 2008;51:843-9.
12. Wu SH, Jiang WF, Gu J, Zhao L, Wang YL, Liu YG, Zhou L, Gu JN, Xu K, Liu X. Benefits and risks of additional ablation of complex fractionated atrial electrograms for patients with atrial fibrillation: a systematic review and meta-analysis. Int J Cardiol. 2013;169:35-43.
13. Verma A, Sanders P, Champagne J, Macle L, Nair GM, Calkins H, Wilber DJ. Selective complex fractionated atrial electrograms targeting for atrial fibrillation study (SELECT AF): a multicenter, randomized trial. Circ Arrhythm Electrophysiol. 2014;7:55-62.
14. Narayan SM, Baykaner T, Clopton P, Schricker A, Lalani GG, Krummen DE, Shivkumar K, Miller JM. Ablation of rotor and focal sources reduces late recurrence of atrial fibrillation compared with trigger ablation alone: extended follow-up of the CONFIRM trial (Conventional Ablation for Atrial Fibrillation With or Without Focal Impulse and Rotor Modulation). J Am Coll Cardiol. 2014;63:1761-8.
15. Narayan SM, Krummen DE, Shivkumar K, Clopton P, Rappel WJ, Miller JM. Treatment of atrial fibrillation by the ablation of localized sources: CONFIRM (Conventional Ablation for Atrial Fibrillation With or Without Focal Impulse and Rotor Modulation) trial. J Am Coll Cardiol. 2012;60:628-36.
16. Cosedis Nielsen J, Johannessen A, Raatikainen P, Hindricks G, Walfridsson H, Kongstad O, Pehrson S, Englund A, Hartikainen J, Mortensen LS, Hansen PS. Radiofrequency ablation as initial therapy in paroxysmal atrial fibrillation. N Engl J Med. 2012;367:1587-95.
17. Morillo CA, Verma A, Connolly SJ, Kuck KH, Nair GM, Champagne J, Sterns LD, Beresh H, Healey JS, Natale A. Radiofrequency ablation vs antiarrhythmic drugs as first-line treatment of paroxysmal atrial fibrillation (RAAFT-2): a randomized trial. JAMA. 2014;311:692-700.
18. Cappato R, Calkins H, Chen SA, Davies W, Iesaka Y, Kalman J, Kim YH, Klein G, Natale A, Packer D, Skanes A, Ambrogi F, Biganzoli E. Updated worldwide survey on the methods, efficacy, and safety of catheter ablation for human atrial fibrillation. Circ Arrhythm Electrophysiol. 2010;3:32-8.
19. Shah RU, Freeman JV, Shilane D, Wang PJ, Go AS, Hlatky MA. Procedural complications, rehospitalizations, and repeat procedures after catheter ablation for atrial fibrillation. J Am Coll Cardiol. 2012;59:143-9.
20. Spragg DD, Dalal D, Cheema A, Scherr D, Chilukuri K, Cheng A, Henrikson CA, Marine JE, Berger RD, Dong J, Calkins H. Complications of catheter ablation for atrial fibrillation: incidence and predictors. J Cardiovasc Electrophysiol. 2008;19:627-31.
21. Di Biase L, Burkhardt JD, Santangeli P, Mohanty P, Sanchez JE, Horton R, Gallinghouse GJ, Themistoclakis S, Rossillo A, Lakkireddy D, Reddy M, Hao S, Hongo R, Beheiry S, Zagrodzky J, Rong B, Mohanty S, Elayi CS, Forleo G, Pelargonio G, Narducci ML, Dello Russo A, Casella M, Fassini G, Tondo C, Schweikert RA, Natale A. Periprocedural stroke and bleeding complications in patients undergoing catheter ablation of atrial fibrillation with different anticoagulation management: results from the Role of Coumadin in Preventing Thromboembolism in Atrial Fibrillation (AF) Patients Undergoing Catheter Ablation (COMPARE) randomized trial. Circulation. 2014;129:2638-44.
22. Hohnloser SH, Camm AJ. Safety and efficacy of dabigatran etexilate during catheter ablation of atrial fibrillation: a meta-analysis of the literature. Europace. 2013;15:1407-11.

EDITORS' SUMMARY

While the technical fundamentals of AF ablation including the biophysics, image integration, and mapping have been discussed elsewhere, in this chapter, Drs Sorgente and Cappato succinctly describe our present state of knowledge from the few but important clinical studies we have available to base our recommendations on. In addition, the authors, who are pioneers in compiling outcomes and complications from AF ablation, summarize their work in the available literature on adverse outcomes during and following an ablation procedure. This summary will be useful for clinicians as well as electrophysiologists when recommending procedures and alternatives to patients and assessing them after an AF ablation procedure is done.

CHAPTER 28

Matthew C Henn, Matthew R Schill,
Chawannuch Ruaengsri, Richard B Schuessler,
Ralph J Damiano Jr

Surgical Ablation for Atrial Fibrillation

LIST OF ABBREVIATIONS

AF	Atrial Fibrillation	PV	Pulmonary Vein
AV	Atrioventricular	PVI	Pulmonary Vein Isolation
CMIV	Cox-Maze IV Procedure	RF	Radiofrequency
CMP	Cox-Maze Procedure	SA	Sinoatrial
GP	Ganglionated Plexus		

INTRODUCTION

Over the past several decades, surgical ablation has become an important treatment option for refractory and debilitating cardiac arrhythmias. Surgical ablation technology has rapidly evolved and has revolutionized therapies for the most common cardiac arrhythmia, atrial fibrillation (AF). Though indications for surgical ablation have narrowed, surgery remains an important and effective treatment option. This chapter will focus on the historical aspects, technique, and results of surgical ablation for atrial fibrillation.

Medical treatment of AF has had many shortcomings including both the inefficacy and unwanted side effects of many antiarrhythmic drugs.[1] Furthermore, initial attempts aimed at providing rate control failed to prevent the hemodynamic and thromboembolic sequelae of AF. These shortcomings led to the development of catheter and surgical ablation in the 1980s. The early attempts to develop a surgical procedure were abandoned because of their inability to eliminate the three-detrimental sequelae of AF: (a) debilitating symptoms, (b) loss of synchronous atrioventricular (AV) contraction resulting in ventricular dysfunction, and (c) stasis of blood flow in the left atrium, resulting in thromboembolism.[2,3] After almost a decade of experimental studies, the Maze procedure was introduced in 1987.[4] It has gone through several modifications and has become the gold standard for the treatment of AF.

EARLY SURGICAL ABLATION

The Left Atrial Isolation Procedure

In 1980, Dr James Cox at Duke University developed the *left atrial isolation,* the first surgical procedure designed specifically to eliminate AF. This procedure confined AF to the left atrium, allowing the remainder of the heart to be in sinus rhythm.[5] This reestablished a regular ventricular rate and normal hemodynamics, but failed to address the thromboembolic risk of left atrial stasis. Furthermore, it did not address patients in whom the AF originated in the right atrium. This procedure was only performed in a single patient but represented a step towards an effective technique.

Catheter Ablation of the Atrioventricular Node—His Bundle Complex

In 1982, Scheinman and colleagues first described *catheter fulguration of the His bundle,* a procedure that electrically isolated the atria from the ventricles, controlling the irregular ventricular rhythm associated with AF and other refractory supraventricular arrhythmias.[6] While effective, a side effect of this procedure was that it resulted in heart block and bradycardia, requiring all patients to receive a permanent ventricular pacemaker to achieve a normal ventricular rate. Furthermore, this procedure did not alleviate the hemodynamic compromise due to AV dyssynchrony and the risk of thromboembolism associated with AF. Despite these limitations, AV node ablation continues to be commonly used for patients with medically refractory AF.

The Corridor Procedure

In 1985, Guiraudon and associates developed the *corridor procedure,* which sought to isolate a strip of atrial septum including both the sinoatrial (SA) and atrioventricular (AV) nodes to allow the SA node to pace both ventricles.[7, 8] The corridor procedure had many of the same shortcomings as AV node ablation; it neither prevented thromboembolism nor prevented AV dyssynchrony. It did have the advantage of preserving physiologic AV conduction. Each atrium, however remained in fibrillation or developed its own asynchronous intrinsic rhythm due to electrical isolation. The corridor procedure was abandoned because of these shortcomings.

The Atrial Transection Procedure

While the initial interventional procedures were aimed at confining AF to the atria, the *atrial transection procedure* devised by Dr James Cox and associates in 1985 was the first procedure that attempted to terminate AF.[9,10] Using a canine model, they found that a single long incision around both atria and down into the septum would terminate AF. This atrial transection procedure effectively prevented AF or atrial flutter in animals. Unfortunately, this procedure was ineffective in humans and was quickly abandoned, but it represented a transitional step toward the Cox-Maze procedure.

THE COX-MAZE PROCEDURE

The first successful curative intervention for AF was the Cox-Maze procedure (CMP). After extensive animal studies, the CMP was introduced clinically in 1987 by Dr James Cox.[9,11] The CMP was designed based on the theory that macro-reentrant circuits cause and propagate AF. The CMP was conceived to interrupt such macro-reentrant circuits, eliminating the ability of the atrium to sustain flutter or fibrillate (**Figure 28.1**).[11] The CMP restored sinus rhythm as well as AV synchrony, reducing the risk of stroke and thromboembolism.[12] The original CMP consisted of multiple surgical incisions across both atria that allowed for a pathway for the sinus impulse to reach the AV node. It permitted depolarization of most of the atrial myocardium resulting in preservation of atrial contractile function in animals and in most patients.[13] Moreover, the left atrial appendage was removed to further reduce the risk of thromboembolism.

The Maze II was developed because the initial Maze procedure had problems with late chronotropic incompetence and a high incidence of pacemaker implantation. This was quickly abandoned because of its technical difficulty and was replaced by the Maze III procedure (**Figure 28.2**).[14,15]

The Cox-Maze III procedure soon became the gold standard for the surgical treatment of AF. The procedure is often called the cut-and-sew Maze, and the surgical results of the Cox-Maze III were excellent, with over 90% of patients free from symptomatic AF at late follow up.[16-19] However, it also was technically difficult and required a lengthy period of aortic cross-clamping, which limited its widespread adoption.

Over the last two decades, the introduction of ablation devices to replace many of the atrial incisions has dramatically changed the surgical treatment of AF. These devices

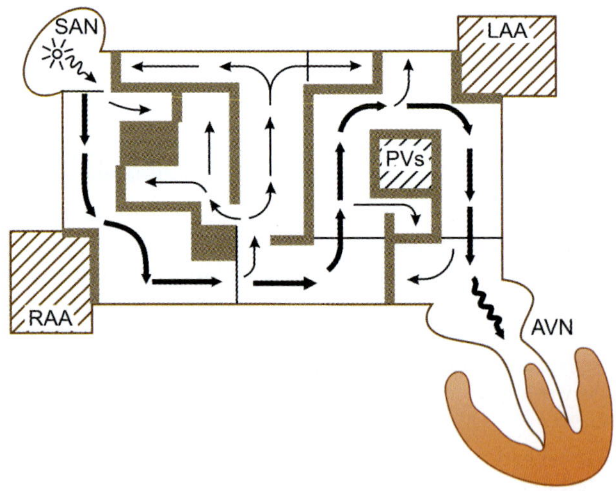

Figure 28.1: Original conceptual design of the Cox-Maze procedure for atrial fibrillation. Both atrial appendages were excised, and the pulmonary veins were isolated. (Reproduced with permission from Cox JL, Canavan TE, Schuessler RB, et al. The surgical treatment of atrial fibrillation II. Intraoperative electrophysiologic mapping and description of the electrophysiologic basis of atrial flutter and atrial fibrillation. J Thorac Cardiovasc Surg. 1991;101:406-26)
Abbreviations: AVN, atrioventricular node; LAA, left atrial appendage; PVs, pulmonary veins; RAA, right atrial appendage; SAN, sinoatrial node

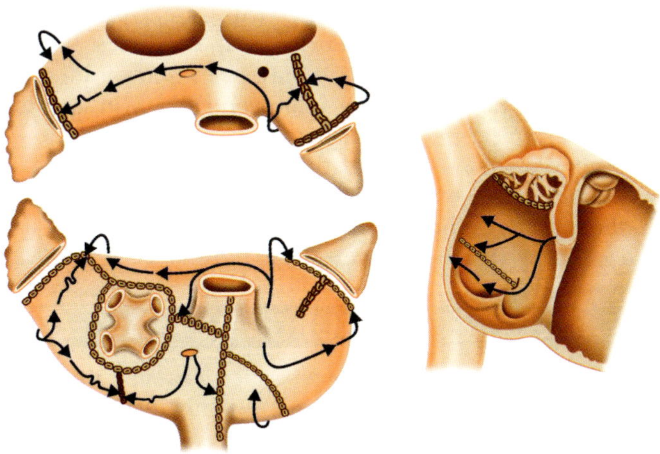

Figure 28.2: Two-dimensional drawing depicting the atrial incisions of the Cox-Maze III procedure

From: Cox JL, Boineau JP, Schuessler RB, et al. Modification of the Maze procedure for atrial flutter and atrial fibrillation I. Rationale and surgical results. J Thorac Cardiovasc Surg. 1995;110:473-84

have simplified the Cox-Maze procedure and have allowed for more widespread adoption.[20] Modern ablation technology has allowed surgeons to treat AF with reduced morbidity and mortality and has allowed the development of less invasive approaches.

SURGICAL ABLATION TECHNOLOGY

The development and evolution of surgical ablation technology has allowed for the transformation of the cut-and-sew Cox-Maze III into the technically easier, shorter, and less invasive Cox-Maze IV. When ablation technology was introduced, the goal was to replace as many of the original incision lines of the Cox-Maze III as possible. An ablation technology had to have three key characteristics in order to replicate a surgical incision. First, a device had to create a line of reliable bidirectional conduction block. A pattern of lesions with these properties can prevent AF, either through blocking macro- or micro-reentrant circuits or by isolating focal triggers. Only transmural ablation lesions produce reliable conduction block, as even small gaps in ablation lines retain the ability to conduct both sinus and fibrillatory impulses. Our laboratory and others have demonstrated this in animal models.[21-23] Second, the ablation device had to be safe. Safety requires that the device delivers a precise dose of energy in order to minimize both inadequate ablation and potential injury to nearby vital structures such as the coronary arteries, veins, and valves caused by excessive ablation. Finally, the ablation device had to make AF surgery simpler and require less time to perform than the cut-and-sew technique. This requires the device to create lesions rapidly and have adequate length and flexibility to facilitate minimally invasive approaches.

Several ablation technologies have been developed, and each has its relative advantages and disadvantages. Two ablation technologies are currently in widespread clinical use: cryoablation and radiofrequency ablation.

Cryoablation

Cryoablation technology creates ablation lines by freezing myocardial tissue. Cryoablation preserves the myocardial fibrous skeleton and collagen structure, making it one of the safest energy sources available. These devices work by pumping a liquid refrigerant to the tip of a device where it undergoes evaporation, and in the process absorbing heat from the tissue in contact with the tip. This causes intracellular and extracellular water to freeze. The resulting ice crystals disrupt the plasma membrane and cause early cell death via lysis. Lesions also expand due to induced apoptosis. The size of the lesion produced depends on the thermal conductivity and temperature of both the probe and the tissue.[24]

Two commercially available sources of cryothermal energy are in clinical use in cardiac surgery. Nitrous oxide-based devices are manufactured by AtriCure (Cincinnati, OH). Devices using argon have been developed and are currently distributed by Medtronic (Minneapolis, MN). The minimum temperature that can be produced by an ablation device is limited by the thermodynamic properties of the refrigerant used. At 1 atmosphere of pressure, nitrous oxide is capable of cooling tissue to –89.5°C, whereas argon can cool tissue to –185.7°C. Nitrous oxide-based cryoablation has a long history of clinical use with a well-defined efficacy and is generally safe except around the coronary arteries.[25,26] Experimental and clinical studies have shown intimal hyperplasia and coronary artery stenosis after cryoablation.[26-28] One disadvantage of cryoablation is the relatively long time required to create transmural lesions (2 to 3 minutes). There is also difficulty in creating lesions on the beating heart from an epicardial approach because the circulating blood acts as a heat sink, limiting the minimum temperature that can be reached.[29] Furthermore, freezing of intra-atrial blood poses a potential risk of thromboembolism.

The nitrous oxide technology can be used with both the rigid, reusable and the flexible, disposable probes. In our institution, we favor the rigid probes because of their ease of use and cost-effectiveness. The argon technology is available only as a flexible, disposable ablation device.

Radiofrequency Energy

Radiofrequency (RF) energy has been used for many years by cardiac electrophysiologists and surgeons to ablate cardiac tissue.[30] Resistive RF energy can be delivered using unipolar or bipolar electrodes. These electrodes may be dry or irrigated. With unipolar RF technology, energy is dispersed between the electrode tip and an indifferent electrode, usually a grounding pad applied to the patient. In bipolar RF technology, alternating current is passed between two closely approximated electrodes, usually embedded in the jaws of a clamp. Lesion size depends on the electrode-tissue contact area, the interface temperature, the amount of power applied, and the duration of energy delivery. Several factors can limit the depth of the lesion, potentially preventing successful creation of a transmural lesion with conduction block. These include char formation, epicardial fat, myocardial and endocavitary blood flow, and tissue thickness.

Several unipolar RF ablation devices have been developed. These include dry devices, irrigated devices and suction-assisted devices. These devices have had limited applicability in cardiac surgery. Dry unipolar RF can create transmural lesions on the arrested heart in animals with sufficiently long ablation times, but this has not been reproducible in humans. In one study, after 2-minute endocardial ablations during mitral valve surgery, only 20% of the lesions were transmural.[31] Epicardial ablation on the beating heart with unipolar RF has been even less successful. Animal studies have shown that epicardial unipolar RF is incapable of creating transmural lesions on the beating heart.[32,33] Epicardial RF ablation in humans resulted in only a 10% rate of transmural lesion creation.[34] Convection caused by circulating blood has been felt to explain the failure of epicardial unipolar RF ablation on the beating heart.[35,36] This has led industry to add both irrigation and suction. Although these additions have improved depth of penetration, no unipolar RF device has been shown by independent laboratories to be capable of reliably creating transmural lesions on the beating heart.[37]

To overcome the deficiencies of unipolar RF ablation, bipolar RF clamps were developed. The electrodes are embedded in the jaws of a clamp to focus the delivery of energy. Shielding the electrodes from the circulating blood pool improves lesion quality, shortens the time required for lesion formation and limits collateral injury. Multiple studies have shown bipolar RF ablation to be capable of creating transmural lesions on the beating heart in both animals and humans with short ablation times.[38-40] Bipolar RF devices are currently sold by two companies in the United States (AtriCure, West Chester, OH and Medtronic, Minneapolis, MN). The Medtronic device is irrigated. Both devices have shown similar experimental and clinical efficacy.

Bipolar RF energy also has a more favorable safety profile when compared with unipolar RF. Numerous clinical complications of unipolar RF devices have been reported, including coronary artery injuries, stroke and esophageal perforation leading to atrioesophageal fistula.[41-44] There have been no collateral injuries reported after bipolar RF technology despite its widespread clinical use.

Innovation continues within the field of RF ablation technology, including the development of unipolar-bipolar hybrid devices. The Cobra Fusion™ (AtriCure, West Chester, OH) is a suction-assisted device that combines bipolar and unipolar RF. This device has been shown in early experimental reports to have improved efficacy in creating transmural epicardial lesions on the beating heart.[45]

Other modalities of energy delivery including microwave, laser, and ultrasound technology have been used clinically, but limitations of these technologies have led to limited use and withdrawal of these devices from the market.[36,46-50]

INDICATIONS FOR SURGICAL ABLATION

A recent consensus statement described current indications for surgical ablation of AF.[1] These presently include: (a) All symptomatic patients with documented AF undergoing other cardiac surgical procedures; (b) selected asymptomatic patients with AF undergoing cardiac surgery in which the ablation can be performed with minimal risk in experienced centers; and (c) stand-alone AF ablation should be considered for symptomatic patients with atrial fibrillation who either prefer a surgical approach, have failed one or more attempts at catheter ablation, or are not candidates for catheter ablation.

There is still controversy regarding the referral of patients for surgery with medically refractory, symptomatic AF in lieu of catheter ablation. Programs involved in the surgical and interventional treatment of AF should develop a team approach to these patients, including both electrophysiologists and surgeons, to ensure appropriate patient selection. Treatment should also be tailored to individual patients, and clinical decisions should take into account institutional experience and outcomes with surgical and catheter ablation.

Some relative indications for surgery were not included in the consensus statement. The first is a contraindication to long-term anticoagulation in patients with persistent AF and a high risk for stroke ($CHADS_2$ score ≥2). Up to one-third of patients with AF screened for participation in clinical trials of warfarin are deemed ineligible for chronic anticoagulation, mainly because of a high perceived risk for bleeding complications. In one study, the annual rate of intracranial hemorrhage in anticoagulated patients with AF was 0.9% per year, and the overall major bleeding complication rate was 2.3% per year. The stroke rate without anticoagulation following the Cox-Maze procedure has been remarkably low, even in high-risk patients. At our institution, only 6 of 433 patients had a stroke after a mean follow-up of 6.9 ± 5.1 years. There was no difference in stroke rate in those patients with CHADS scores above or below 2.[51] This low risk of stroke after the Cox-Maze procedure has also been noted in other series.[12, 52, 53] The low stroke risk is likely due both to the high rate of restoration of sinus rhythm as well as the removal of the left atrial appendage. Surgical ablation of AF with amputation of the left atrial appendage also should be considered in patients with chronic AF who have suffered a cerebrovascular accident despite adequate anticoagulation, as these patients are at high risk for future neurologic events.

SURGICAL TECHNIQUES

There are several procedures that are currently performed to surgically treat AF: the Cox-Maze IV procedure (CMIV), left atrial lesion sets, pulmonary vein isolation (PVI), and hybrid ablations.

The Cox-Maze IV Procedure

At our institution, bipolar RF energy and cryoablation have been used to replace most of the surgical incisions of the Cox-Maze III procedure. Our current RF ablation-assisted procedure, termed the Cox-Maze IV, was introduced in 2002 and recapitulates the lesion set of the Cox-Maze III **(Figures 28.3A and B)**.[54] Our clinical results have shown that this modified procedure replicates the high success rate of the Cox-Maze III procedure while significantly reducing operative time and lowering complication rates.[55,56]

The Cox-Maze IV procedure requires cardiopulmonary bypass which is achieved via central or femoral cannulation. The operation can be done either through a traditional median sternotomy or a less invasive (5 cm) right mini-thoracotomy. In a sternotomy approach, the right and left pulmonary veins (PVs) are bluntly dissected. If the patient is in AF, amiodarone is administered and the patient is electrically cardioverted. Pacing thresholds are obtained from each pulmonary vein. Using a bipolar RF ablation device, the PVs are isolated by ablating a cuff of atrial tissue surrounding the right and left PVs. Proof of electrical isolation is confirmed after ablation by demonstrating exit block from each PV.

The right atrial lesion set is performed on the beating heart. A bipolar RF clamp is used to create most of the lesions. A unipolar device (cryoablation has been our favored technology) is used to make the ablation lines endocardially down to the tricuspid annulus because of the difficulty of clamping in this area **(Figures 28.3A and B)**. Cryoablation is also safer than RF in the vicinity of valve tissue.

The remaining left-sided lesions **(Figures 28.3A and B)** are performed on the arrested heart. First, the left atrial appendage is amputated and an ablation is performed through the amputated left atrial appendage into one of the left PVs. A standard left atriotomy is performed and extended inferiorly around the right inferior PV and superiorly onto the dome of the left atrium. Connecting lesions are made with the bipolar RF device into the left superior and inferior pulmonary veins and a final ablation is performed down toward the mitral annulus. Our group has shown that a "box lesion" isolating the entire posterior left atrium with ablation lines into both left pulmonary veins resulted in a better drug-free freedom from AF at 12 months and 5 years than a single connecting lesion.[57,58] Cryoablation is used to connect the lesion to the mitral annulus and to complete the left atrial isthmus line.

The procedure has been altered to allow performance via a right mini-thoracotomy incision. This approach has been described in previous publication[59] from our group.

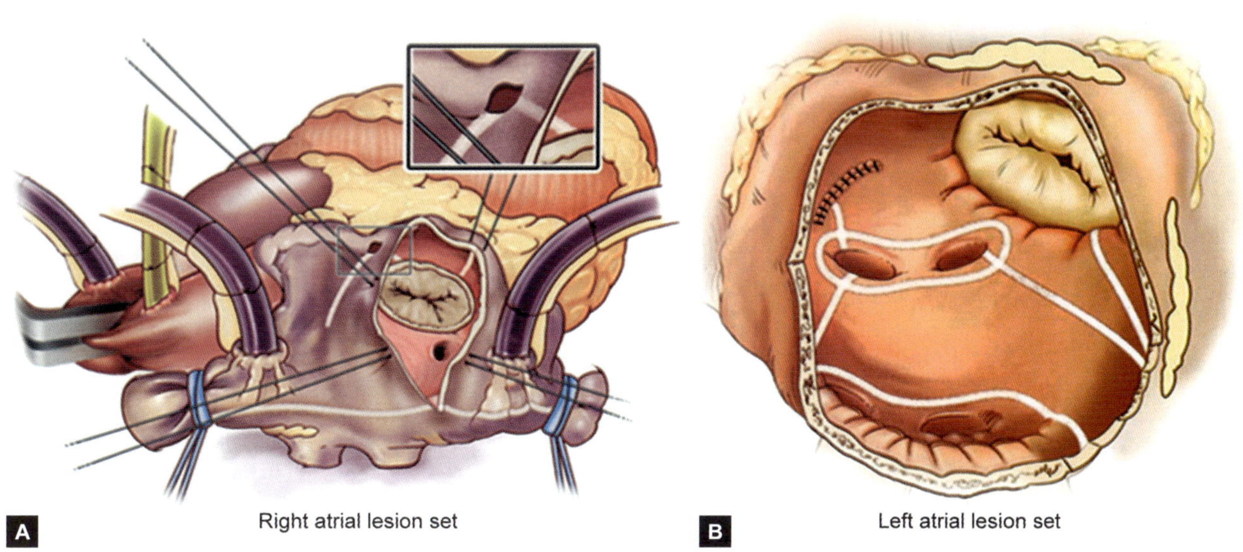

Figures 28.3A and B: Standard right and left atrial lesions sets utilized for the Cox-Maze IV procedure. In the right atrium (RA) (A) radiofrequency (RF) ablation lines (white lines) extend from superior vena cava (SVC) to inferior vena cava (IVC) and along the RA free wall down to tricuspid valve annulus. In the left atrium (B), all ablation lines are performed with a bipolar radiofrequency clamp except for an endocardial cryoablation at the mitral annulus and an epicardial cryoablation over the coronary sinus

From: Weimar T, Bailey MS, Watanabe Y, et al. The Cox-Maze IV procedure for lone atrial fibrillation: a single center experience in 100 consecutive patients. J Interv Card Electrophysiol. 2011;31:47-54

Femoral cannulation is used and a high definition 5 mm 30-degree endoscope is employed to aid in visualization. Only the right PVs are isolated since there is no epicardial access to the left PVs. The right atrial lesion set is performed through three purse-string sutures with no atriotomy. **(Figure 28.4)**. The left atrial lesions set requires the use of cryoablation to complete the isolation of the left PVs and posterior left atrium **(Figure 28.5)**. Finally, the left atrial appendage is oversewn from the endocardial side instead of being excised.

The Cox-Maze IV Procedure Surgical Results

The Cox-Maze III procedure has had excellent long-term results. In our series at Washington University, 97% of 198 consecutive patients who underwent the procedure with a mean follow-up of 5.4 years were free from symptomatic AF. Eighty percent of stand-alone patients and 75% of concomitant ablation patients were also free of antiarrhythmic drugs at late follow-up. There was no difference in the cure rates between patients undergoing a stand-alone Cox-Maze procedure and those undergoing concomitant procedures.[16] Similar results have been obtained from other institutions around the world with the traditional "cut-and-sew" method.[17,19,60] However, most patients did not have electrocardiographic follow-up or prolonged monitoring to assess their rhythm.

Our results from patients who underwent the Cox-Maze IV procedure have been encouraging as well. In a prospective, single-center trial from our institution, 91% of patients at the 6-month follow-up were free from AF.[38] The Cox-Maze IV procedure had significantly shortened the mean cross-clamp times for a lone Cox-Maze from 93 ± 34 minutes for the Cox-Maze III to 47 ± 26 minutes for the Cox-Maze IV ($p < 0.001$).[38] A propensity analysis performed by our group has shown that there was no significant difference in the freedom from AF at 3, 6, or 12 months between the appropriately matched Cox-Maze III and IV groups.[56] A more recent prospective cohort study from our institution in 100 consecutive patients who underwent a stand-alone Cox-Maze IV procedure demonstrated postoperative freedom from AF at 93%, 90%, and 90% at 6, 12, and 24 months, respectively.[54] A report of over two decades of experience at our institution with both the Cox-Maze III and Cox-Maze IV procedures showed no difference in freedom from AF and a significantly decreased major complication rate.[61]

The Cox-Maze IV procedure worked as well in patients with paroxysmal as for longstanding persistent AF. Our most recent report of Cox-Maze IV data reviewed 576 consecutive patients who underwent this procedure between

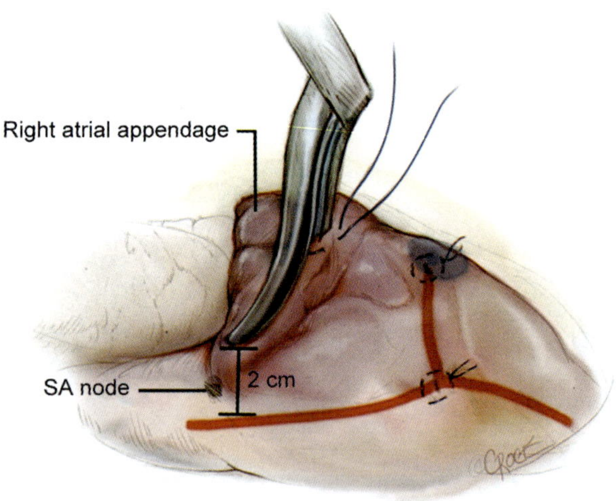

Figure 28.4: Completion of the right atrial lesion set using a bipolar RF clamp. The clamp has been previously placed through a purse-string suture to create lesions toward the SVC, IVC and tricuspid valve. The tricuspid valve annulus is cryoablated via a second purse-string suture. The clamp is then placed through a third purse-string suture at the base of the right atrial appendage. A gap of at least two centimeters must be left between the SVC and right atrial appendage ablation lines to prevent injury to the sinoatrial node

From: Robertson JO, Saint LL, Leidenfrost JE, Damiano RJ Jr. Illustrated techniques for performing the Cox-Maze IV procedure through a right mini-thoracotomy. Ann Cardiothoracic Surg. 2014;3:105-16

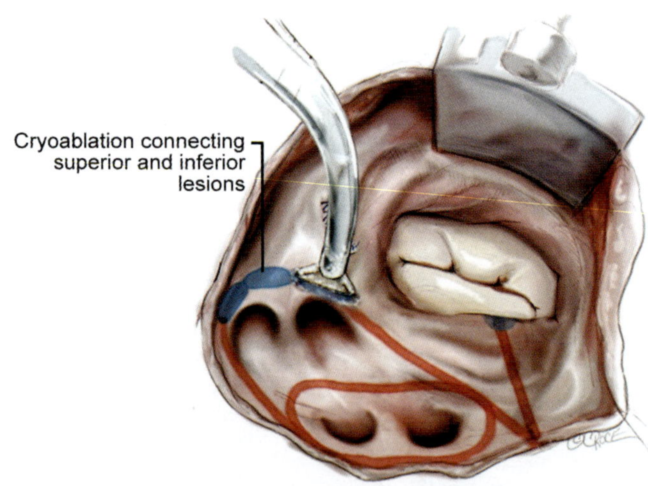

Figure 28.5: Completion of the left atrial lesion set using a cryosurgical probe. A right-sided pulmonary vein isolation, a lesion to the mitral valve annulus, and a "box lesion" connecting the two sets of pulmonary veins and isolating the posterior left atrial wall have been performed with a bipolar RF clamp. Due to the difficulty of epicardial access to the left pulmonary veins via a right thoracotomy, the left-sided pulmonary vein isolation is performed via endocardial cryoablation

From: Robertson JO, Saint LL, Leidenfrost JE, Damiano RJ Jr. Illustrated techniques for performing the Cox-Maze IV procedure through a right mini-thoracotomy. Ann Cardiothoracic Surg. 2014;3:105-16

January 2002 and September 2014. All patients were followed with ECGs or prolonged monitoring. Our 12-month freedom from AF was 93%, with 85% of patients were also off all antiarrhythmic drugs, while our 5-year freedom from AF was 78%, with 66% of patients also off all antiarrhythmic drugs. When comparing those with paroxysmal AF to those with persistent AF, freedom from AF on and off AADs was not significantly different at any time point.[58] Our five-year results were similar to those of other groups as well.[62]

However, our results and others' were significantly better than two recent prospective multicenter trials that both showed only a 66% freedom from AF at 9 or 12 months follow-up.[63,64] However, these studies did not require standardized ablation techniques and included institutions with variable experience with surgical ablation. Many of the patients did not undergo a complete Maze lesion set in these trials.

The Cox-Maze procedure has also been successful in reducing the incidence of stroke. In patients undergoing the Cox-Maze procedure, the preoperative incidence of neurological events has been high due to inherent risk in patients with AF. In a report from our institution, 57 out of 433 patients (13%) had experienced a neurological event before surgery. Despite this, there were only six neurological events during long-term follow-up (mean, 6.6 ± 5.0 years) in this cohort. The long-term stroke rate after the Cox-Maze procedure has been 0.2% per year despite the fact that the great majority of patients had discontinued their anti-coagulation.[51]

The Cox-Maze procedure has been increasingly used as a concomitant procedure.[20] Previous studies from our institution and others have documented high rates of restoration of sinus rhythm without increasing morbidity following concomitant procedures including coronary artery bypass, mitral valve surgery, tricuspid valve surgery, and aortic valve surgery.[64-73] Current clinical practice guidelines recommend considering surgical ablation in all patients with AF undergoing concomitant cardiac procedures,[1] and a biatrial Cox-Maze IV lesion set is recommended in most cases.

In an effort to decrease operative morbidity, a minimally invasive Cox-Maze IV lesion set has been introduced through a right mini-thoracotomy.[74,75] This has become our preferred approach in selected patients. In both the stand-alone Cox-Maze IV and concomitant population, this approach has been shown to be equally effective at restoring sinus rhythm while significantly decreasing major complication rates, operative mortality, ICU length of stay, and hospital length of stay when compared to a traditional sternotomy approach.[76]

Left Atrial Procedures

A number of centers around the world have advocated performing ablation confined to the left atrium only to cure AF. This concept is supported by the fact that the majority of paroxysmal AF appears to originate from the PVs and the posterior left atrium. A left atrial lesion set typically involves pulmonary vein isolation, often with a lesion to the mitral annulus as well as removal of the left atrial appendage. One advantage of avoiding right atrial lesions is a potentially lower rate of postoperative pacemaker implantation.[77] Many ablation technologies have been used to create these lesion sets with varied degrees of success.[43,78-85] However, Gillinov and colleagues published a large series demonstrating that the omission of the left atrial isthmus lesion resulted in a significantly higher incidence of recurrent AF in patients with persistent AF.[86] To complete this lesion, it is critical to also ablate the coronary sinus in line with the endocardial lesion. In addition, our clinical results have shown that isolation of the entire posterior left atrium is associated with improved outcomes compared with isolation of the pulmonary veins alone. Isolating the entire posterior left atrium significantly improved our drug-free freedom from AF at 6 months (54% versus 79%, p = 0.011) and 5 years (66% versus 33%, p = 0.017) in retrospective analyses.[57,58]

There have been no randomized trials of surgical left atrial ablation compared with biatrial ablation (i.e. Cox-Maze procedure). Because of this, the importance of the right atrial lesions of the traditional Cox-Maze procedure are difficult to precisely determine. A meta-analysis of the literature by Barnett and Ad revealed that a biatrial lesion set resulted in a significantly higher late freedom from AF when compared with a left atrial lesion set alone (87% versus 73%, $p = 0.05$).[87] This is not surprising considering the results of intraoperative mapping of patients with atrial fibrillation. Both our group and others have shown that AF can originate from the right atrium in 10 to 30% of cases.[88-90]

Of the specific left atrial lesions of the Cox-Maze procedure, it is difficult to determine the importance of each ablation line. All surgeons agree on the importance of isolating the pulmonary veins. Moreover, omitting the lesion to the mitral annulus leaves the patient at risk for the development of late left atrial flutter. In a randomized trial, Gaita and coauthors examined pulmonary vein isolation alone versus two alternate lesion sets that both included ablation of the left atrial isthmus. In this study, normal sinus rhythm off antiarrhythmic drugs at 2-year follow-up was only seen in 25% in the PVI group versus 59% and 65% in the left atrial lesion groups (p <0.006).[79]

It is our opinion that a complete left atrial Cox-Maze lesion set is needed to ensure a high success rate.

Pulmonary Vein Isolation

Pulmonary vein isolation (PVI) is an attractive therapeutic strategy due to its simplicity. PVI can be performed without the need for cardiopulmonary bypass and utilizing minimally invasive techniques via either thoracoscopy or minithoracotomy. PVI can also be easily and quickly added to other cardiac surgical procedures (e.g. coronary bypass graft or a valve procedure). Based on the original report of Haissaguerre, it has been well documented that the triggers for paroxysmal AF originate from the pulmonary veins in the majority of cases.[91] However, it is important to remember that up to 30% of triggers may originate outside the pulmonary veins.[92] In an attempt to increase efficacy, some investigators have added ablation of the ganglionic plexus (GP).[93-95] However, our group has shown experimentally that animals rapidly reinnervate their atria following GP ablation, and there has been no clear clinical documentation of efficacy of GP ablation.[96]

The pulmonary veins can be isolated separately or as a box. The most common approach for treatment of lone AF uses an endoscopic, port-based approach to minimize incision size and pain for the patient. At our center, bipolar RF clamps are favored to isolate the pulmonary veins, but unipolar radiofrequency, cryoablation, and high-intensity focused ultrasound devices have also been used.[48,97,98] Accumulating data suggest that a box isolation of the entire posterior left atrium is the more effective strategy.[57,58,99]

Patient preparation begins with double-lumen endotracheal intubation. A transesophageal echocardiogram is performed to confirm the absence of thrombus in the left atrial appendage. If a thrombus is found, the procedure is either aborted or converted to an open procedure, in which the risk of systemic thromboembolism from left atrial clot can be minimized. External defibrillator pads are placed on the patient and the patient is positioned with the right side turned upward 45 to 60 degrees and the right arm positioned above the head to expose the right axilla.

An initial port for the thoracoscopic camera is placed at the sixth intercostal space. Under thoracoscopic vision, a small working port can then be placed in either the third or fourth intercostal space at the midaxillary line depending on surgeon preference and patient anatomy. The right phrenic nerve is identified to avoid injury to this structure. An incision is made in the pericardium, anterior and parallel to the phrenic nerve, to expose the heart from the superior vena cava to the diaphragm. Through this pericardiotomy, the space above and below the right pulmonary veins is dissected to allow enough room for insertion of a specialized thoracoscopic dissector. This includes opening into the oblique sinus and dissecting the space between the right superior PV and the right pulmonary artery. The dissector and a guiding sheath is introduced through a second port, either lateral or medial to the scope port, and guided into the space between the right superior pulmonary vein and right pulmonary artery. After the dissector is carefully removed from the chest, the sheath remains in place as a guide for the insertion of the bipolar RF clamp. At this point, the patient is cardioverted into sinus rhythm so that pacing thresholds can be obtained. As with a Cox-Maze IV procedure, it is critical to document pacing thresholds from the pulmonary veins before isolation. Some surgeons also use the opportunity provided by surgical exposure to test and ablate ganglionated plexus but there are no data to support this practice and it is not performed at our institution.

The sheath is attached to the lower jaw of a bipolar RF clamp. The clamp is introduced into the chest, and the left atrium surrounding the pulmonary veins is clamped and ablated. After confirmation of exit block by pacing, the instruments are removed from the right chest and the right chest ports are closed.

The approach to the left chest is similar to the right. The patient is repositioned such that the left chest is elevated 45 to 60 degrees and the left arm is held up to expose the left axilla. A port for the thoracoscopic camera is placed in the sixth intercostal space, slightly more posterior than on the right side. With thoracoscopic visualization, a left-sided working port is created in the third or fourth intercostal space. The left phrenic nerve is identified, and the pericardium is opened posterior to the course of the nerve. The ligament of Marshall is identified and divided. The dissector is then introduced through a second port, also in the sixth intercostal space. This port site is placed to allow for a straight-line introduction of the dissector around the pulmonary veins. The guiding sheath is used to position the RF clamp around the left pulmonary veins, and they are isolated. Again, exit block is confirmed with pacing.

The procedure is not complete until the left atrial appendage has been addressed. Historically, this has been done by stapling across the base of the left atrial appendage with an endoscopic stapler. This requires careful surgical technique and attention because it can result in tears and bleeding.[100] Clip devices have been designed to address this difficulty, and they are used exclusively at our center because of their improved efficacy and safety when compared to staplers.[101,102] A multicenter trial of a clip device (AtriClip, Atricure, West Chester, Ohio) in 2011 enrolled 71 patients.[103] Imaging follow-up showed a 98.4% rate of successful occlusion. After ablation of the left pulmonary veins and exclusion of the left atrial appendage, the left side of the pericardium is closed. The ports are then removed, and the left chest is closed.

Pulmonary Vein Isolation: Surgical Results

The results of PVI alone have been variable and have been dependent on patient selection and the energy source utilized. In the first report of surgical PVI, Wolf and colleagues reported that 91% of patients undergoing a video-assisted bilateral PVI and left atrial appendage exclusion were free from AF at three months follow-up.[104] However, this was a small study with very limited follow-up. Edgerton et al. reported on 57 patients undergoing PVI with GP ablation with more thorough follow-up and found 82% of their patients with paroxysmal AF to be free from AF at 6 months, with 74% off antiarrhythmic drugs.[105] However, no results were presented at one year, which is the minimal acceptable follow-up period.

Subsequent studies have shown encouraging results in patients with paroxysmal AF. In a study involving 21 patients with paroxysmal AF undergoing PVI with GP ablation, McClelland et al. reported 88% freedom from AF at 1 year without antiarrhythmic drugs.[94] A larger, single-center trial recently reported a 65% single procedure success at 1 year in a series of 45 patients undergoing PVI with GP ablation, including patients with persistent and paroxysmal AF.[106] A multicenter trial reported 87% sinus rhythm rate in a more diverse patient population, including some patients with longstanding persistent AF; however, those patients with longstanding persistent AF had a 71% incidence of sinus rhythm.[107] The FAST trial, a more recent multicenter randomized trial, compared 63 patients who received linear antral pulmonary vein isolation by way of catheter ablation and 61 patients who received bipolar RF PVI and GP ablation. Most patients had paroxysmal AF. At 1 year, freedom from left atrial arrhythmias >30 seconds evaluated by a 7 day Holter without antiarrhythmic drugs was 66% for surgical ablation vs 36% for catheter ablation ($p = 0.002$).[108]

In patients with persistent or longstanding persistent AF, the results of PVI have been poor. In a study from Edgerton and his group, only 35% of 28 patients were free from AF and antiarrhythmic drugs at 6 months follow-up.[109] Long-term data for PVI with GP ablation are equally disappointing. One group reported 139 patients with up to five years of follow-up: freedom from AF and antiarrhythmic drugs was 52, 28, and 29% for paroxysmal, persistent, and long-standing persistent AF.[110] With concomitant procedures, the success rate of PVI also has been low. Of 23 patients undergoing mitral valve surgery or coronary revascularization with concomitant PVI, only half of patients were free from AF at a follow-up of 57 ± 37 months.[111] Another recent series compared patients undergoing cardiac surgery with concomitant PVI and showed only a modest improvement in freedom from AF at 1 year (78% PVI, 73% untreated PAF, with fewer patients in the PVI group (77% vs. 82% control) off antiarrhythmic drugs.[112] In the setting of mitral valve disease, Tada and colleagues report only 17% freedom from AF and antiarrhythmic drugs in their series of 66 patients undergoing PVI.[113] In patients undergoing aortic valve replacement and PVI, freedoms from AF and antiarrhythmic drugs was only 50% at two years at our institution.[72]

Hybrid Ablations

Although the Cox-Maze procedure has achieved high rates of success and recent technological advances have made it easier to perform through less invasive incisions, it still requires cardiopulmonary bypass. In order to lessen the invasiveness of surgical ablation, a number of groups around the world have begun performing extended epicardial ablation with the aid of unipolar and/or bipolar RF and cryoablation probes, which can be placed through thoracoscopic ports. However, these probes have not been able to achieve the same degree of transmurality achieved with bipolar clamps.[37] This led to the idea of combining both endocardial ablation via transcatheter techniques and epicardial ablation via surgical techniques in a "hybrid" approach. This has the advantage of being able to perform a more complete lesion set with better and more transmural lesion formation with minimal morbidity, while using a thoracoscopic approach.

Though specific lesion sets and approaches have varied greatly from institution to institution, initial results have been promising.[114,115] In one study, 78 consecutive patients underwent thoracoscopic hybrid ablation and 74% were free of AF off antiarrhythmic drugs without further ablations at 24 months follow up.[116] These are excellent results and comparable to a full Cox-Maze procedure. Another group utilized a similar lesion set via a pericardioscopic hybrid approach in 101 consecutive patients, and demonstrated freedom from AF in 66% at one year.[117] Lastly, a recent meta-analysis including nine studies demonstrated a freedom from AF between 63 and 93% at 6 months.[118] However, with increasing experience with these newer procedures, important safety concerns including high rates of conversion to sternotomy and re-operation for bleeding have been reported, particularly at less experienced centers.[119]

Though new minimally invasive and hybrid techniques have yet to be standardized, they hold promise and require continued clinical investigation to determine their precise role. Careful patient selection is advised.

CONCLUSION

The ideal surgical procedure for AF would be a minimally invasive operation that does not require cardiopulmonary bypass. Such a procedure should preserve normal atrial physiology, have minimal morbidity, and a have a high success rate. Achieving this goal will require a better understanding of the mechanism of AF in individual patients, and tailoring of treatment approaches. This more patient-specific surgical approach would have significant advantages and prevent both over-ablation and under-ablation in certain patient subgroups. This will require better preoperative diagnostics to identify mechanisms of AF. Non-invasive ECG imaging has a great potential in this arena.[120]

In conclusion, the development of ablation technologies over the past two decades has dramatically changed the field of AF surgery. The replacement of surgical incisions with ablation lines has transformed a complex, technically demanding procedure into one accessible to the majority of surgeons. More importantly, these new ablation technologies have facilitated minimally invasive approaches, prompting efforts to develop simpler procedures that can be performed epicardially on the beating heart. However, surgeons must remember that the Cox-Maze IV procedure has excellent efficacy in these patients and can be performed using a small thoracotomy with low morbidity.[76] It is imperative for surgeons trying new procedures to carefully follow their results and to publish them in peer-reviewed journals.[121] For surgeons performing AF ablation, it is mandatory to adhere to the recently published guidelines for follow-up of patients and for determining success or failure.[1] As we learn more about the mechanisms of AF and develop improved preoperative diagnostic technologies capable of precisely identifying mechanisms, it may become possible to tailor specific lesion sets and ablation modalities to individual patients, making the surgical treatment of AF more effective and available to an even larger population of the patients.

REFERENCES

1. Calkins H, Kuck KH, Cappato R, Brugada J, Camm AJ, Chen SA, Crijns HJ, Damiano RJ, Jr., Davies DW, DiMarco J, Edgerton J, Ellenbogen K, Ezekowitz MD, Haines DE, Haissaguerre M, Hindricks G, Iesaka Y, Jackman W, Jalife J, Jais P, Kalman J, Keane D, Kim YH, Kirchhof P, Klein G, Kottkamp H, Kumagai K, Lindsay BD, Mansour M, Marchlinski FE, McCarthy PM, Mont JL, Morady F, Nademanee K, Nakagawa H, Natale A, Nattel S, Packer DL, Pappone C, Prystowsky E, Raviele A, Reddy V, Ruskin JN, Shemin RJ, Tsao HM, Wilber D. 2012 HRS/EHRA/ECAS expert consensus statement on catheter and surgical ablation of atrial fibrillation: recommendations for patient selection, procedural techniques, patient management and follow-up, definitions, endpoints, and research trial design: a report of the Heart Rhythm Society (HRS) Task Force on Catheter and Surgical Ablation of Atrial Fibrillation. Developed in partnership with the European Heart Rhythm Association (EHRA), a registered branch of the European Society of Cardiology (ESC) and the European Cardiac Arrhythmia Society (ECAS); and in collaboration with the American College of Cardiology (ACC), American Heart Association (AHA), the Asia Pacific Heart Rhythm Society (APHRS), and the Society of Thoracic Surgeons (STS). Endorsed by the governing bodies of the American College of Cardiology Foundation, the American Heart Association, the European Cardiac Arrhythmia Society, the European Heart Rhythm Association, the Society of Thoracic Surgeons, the Asia Pacific Heart Rhythm Society, and the Heart Rhythm Society. Heart Rhythm. 2012;9:632-96 e21.
2. Sherman DG, Kim SG, Boop BS, Corley SD, Dimarco JP, Hart RG, Haywood LJ, Hoyte K, Kaufman ES, Kim MH, Nasco E, Waldo AL. Occurrence and characteristics of stroke events in the Atrial Fibrillation Follow-up Investigation of Sinus Rhythm Management (AFFIRM) study. Arch Intern Med. 2005;165:1185-91.
3. Wolf PA, Abbott RD, Kannel WB. Atrial fibrillation as an independent risk factor for stroke: the Framingham Study. Stroke. 1991;22:983-8.
4. Cox JL, Schuessler RB, D'Agostino HJ, Jr., Stone CM, Chang BC, Cain ME, Corr PB, Boineau JP. The surgical treatment of atrial fibrillation III. Development of a definitive surgical procedure. J Thorac Cardiovasc Surg. 1991;101:569-83.
5. Williams JM, Ungerleider RM, Lofland GK, Cox JL. Left atrial isolation: new technique for the treatment of supraventricular arrhythmias. J Thorac Cardiovasc Surg. 1980;80:373-80.
6. Scheinman MM, Morady F, Hess DS, Gonzalez R. Catheter-induced ablation of the atrioventricular junction to control refractory supraventricular arrhythmias. JAMA. 1982;248:851-5.
7. Guiraudon GN, Campbell CS, Jones DL, McLellan DG, MacDonald JL. Combined Sino-atrial Node Ventricular Node Isolation: A Surgical Alternative to AV Node Ablation in Patients with Atrial Fibrillation. Circulation. 1985;72:111-220.
8. Defauw JJ, Guiraudon GM, van Hemel NM, Vermeulen FE, Kingma JH, de Bakker JM. Surgical therapy of paroxysmal atrial fibrillation with the "corridor" operation. Ann Thorac Surg. 1992;53:564-70; discussion 71.
9. Cox JL. The surgical treatment of atrial fibrillation. IV. Surgical technique. J Thorac Cardiovasc Surg. 1991;101:584-92.
10. Smith PK, Holman WL, Cox JL. Surgical treatment of supraventricular tachyarrhythmias. Surg Clin North Am. 1985; 65:553-70.
11. Cox JL, Canavan TE, Schuessler RB, Cain ME, Lindsay BD, Stone C, Smith PK, Corr PB, Boineau JP. The surgical treatment of atrial fibrillation. II. Intraoperative electrophysiologic mapping and description of the electrophysiologic basis of atrial flutter and atrial fibrillation. J Thorac Cardiovasc Surg. 1991;101:406-26.
12. Cox JL, Ad N, Palazzo T. Impact of the maze procedure on the stroke rate in patients with atrial fibrillation. J Thorac Cardiovasc Surg. 1999;118:833-40.
13. Feinberg MS, Waggoner AD, Kater KM, Cox JL, Lindsay BD, Perez JE. Restoration of atrial function after the maze procedure for patients with atrial fibrillation. Assessment by Doppler echocardiography. Circulation. 1994;90:II285-92.
14. Cox JL, Boineau JP, Schuessler RB, Jaquiss RD, Lappas DG. Modification of the maze procedure for atrial flutter and atrial fibrillation I. Rationale and surgical results. J Thorac Cardiovasc Surg. 1995;110:473-84.
15. Cox JL, Jaquiss RD, Schuessler RB, Boineau JP. Modification of the maze procedure for atrial flutter and atrial fibrillation II. Surgical technique of the maze III procedure. J Thorac Cardiovasc Surg. 1995;110:485-95.
16. Prasad SM, Maniar HS, Camillo CJ, Schuessler RB, Boineau JP, Sundt TM, 3rd, Cox JL, Damiano RJ, Jr. The Cox Maze III procedure for atrial fibrillation: long-term efficacy in patients undergoing lone versus concomitant procedures. J Thorac Cardiovasc Surg. 2003;126:1822-8.
17. McCarthy PM, Gillinov AM, Castle L, Chung M, Cosgrove D, 3rd. The Cox-Maze procedure: the Cleveland Clinic experience. Semin Thorac Cardiovasc Surg. 2000;12:25-9.
18. Raanani E, Albage A, David TE, Yau TM, Armstrong S. The efficacy of the Cox-Maze procedure combined with mitral valve surgery: a matched control study. Eur J Cardiothorac Surg. 2001;19:438-42.
19. Schaff HV, Dearani JA, Daly RC, Orszulak TA, Danielson GK. Cox-Maze procedure for atrial fibrillation: Mayo Clinic experience. Semin Thorac Cardiovasc Surg. 2000;12:30-7.
20. Gammie JS, Haddad M, Milford-Beland S, Welke KF, Ferguson TB, Jr., O'Brien SM, Griffith BP, Peterson ED. Atrial fibrillation correction surgery: lessons from the Society of Thoracic Surgeons National Cardiac Database. Ann Thorac Surg. 2008;85:909-14.
21. Inoue H, Zipes DP. Conduction over an isthmus of atrial myocardium in vivo: a possible model of Wolff-Parkinson-White syndrome. Circulation. 1987;76:637-47.
22. Ishii Y, Nitta T, Sakamoto S, Tanaka S, Asano G. Incisional atrial reentrant tachycardia: experimental study on the conduction

property through the isthmus. J Thorac Cardiovasc Surg. 2003;126:254-62
23. Melby SJ, Lee AM, Zierer A, Kaiser SP, Livhits MJ, Boineau JP, Schuessler RB, Damiano RJ, Jr. Atrial fibrillation propagates through gaps in ablation lines: implications for ablative treatment of atrial fibrillation. Heart Rhythm. 2008;5:1296-301.
24. Melby SJ, Lee AM, Damiano RJ. Advances in surgical ablation devices for atrial fibrillation. In: Wang PJ, editor. New Arrhythmia Technologies. Blackwell Futura; 2005. pp. 233-41.
25. Gage AM, Montes M, Gage AA. Freezing the canine thoracic aorta in situ. J Surg Res. 1979;27:331-40.
26. Holman WL, Ikeshita M, Ungerleider RM, Smith PK, Ideker RE, Cox JL. Cryosurgery for cardiac arrhythmias: acute and chronic effects on coronary arteries. Am J Cardiol. 1983;51: 149-55.
27. Watanabe H, Hayashi J, Aizawa Y. Myocardial infarction after cryoablation surgery for Wolff-Parkinson-White syndrome. Jpn J Thorac Cardiovasc Surg. 2002;50:210-2.
28. Manasse E, Colombo P, Roncalli M, Gallotti R. Myocardial acute and chronic histological modifications induced by cryoablation. Eur J Cardiothorac Surg. 2000;17:339-40.
29. Aupperle H, Doll N, Walther T, Kornherr P, Ullmann C, Schoon HA, Mohr FW. Ablation of atrial fibrillation and esophageal injury: effects of energy source and ablation technique. J Thorac Cardiovasc Surg. 2005;130:1549-54.
30. Viola N, Williams MR, Oz MC, Ad N. The technology in use for the surgical ablation of atrial fibrillation. Semin Thorac Cardiovasc Surg. 2002;14:198-205.
31. Santiago T, Melo JQ, Gouveia RH, Martins AP. Intra-atrial temperatures in radiofrequency endocardial ablation: histologic evaluation of lesions. Ann Thorac Surg. 2003;75: 1495-501.
32. Thomas SP, Guy DJ, Boyd AC, Eipper VE, Ross DL, Chard RB. Comparison of epicardial and endocardial linear ablation using handheld probes. Ann Thorac Surg. 2003;75:543-8.
33. Hoenicke EM, Strange RG, Patel H, Prophet GA, Damiano RJ. Initial experience with epicardial radiofrequency ablation catheter in an ovine model: moving towards an endoscopic maze procedure. J Am Coll Surg. 2000;191:S9-10.
34. Santiago T, Melo J, Gouveia RH, Neves J, Abecasis M, Adragao P, Martins AP. Epicardial radiofrequency applications: in vitro and in vivo studies on human atrial myocardium. Eur J Cardiothorac Surg. 2003;24:481-6; discussion 6.
35. Gaynor SL, Byrd GD, Diodato MD, Ishii Y, Lee AM, Prasad SM, Gopal J, Schuessler RB, Damiano RJ, Jr. Microwave ablation for atrial fibrillation: dose-response curves in the cardioplegia-arrested and beating heart. Ann Thorac Surg. 2006;81:72-6.
36. Melby SJ, Zierer A, Kaiser SP, Schuessler RB, Damiano RJ, Jr. Epicardial microwave ablation on the beating heart for atrial fibrillation: the dependency of lesion depth on cardiac output. J Thorac Cardiovasc Surg. 2006;132:355-60.
37. Schuessler RB, Lee AM, Melby SJ, Voeller RK, Gaynor SL, Sakamoto S, Damiano RJ, Jr. Animal studies of epicardial atrial ablation. Heart Rhythm. 2009;6:S41-5.
38. Gaynor SL, Diodato MD, Prasad SM, Ishii Y, Schuessler RB, Bailey MS, Damiano NR, Bloch JB, Moon MR, Damiano RJ, Jr. A prospective, single-center clinical trial of a modified Cox-Maze procedure with bipolar radiofrequency ablation. J Thorac Cardiovasc Surg. 2004;128:535-42.
39. Prasad SM, Maniar HS, Diodato MD, Schuessler RB, Damiano RJ, Jr. Physiological consequences of bipolar radiofrequency energy on the atria and pulmonary veins: a chronic animal study. Ann Thorac Surg. 2003;76:836-41; discussion 41-2.
40. Prasad SM, Maniar HS, Schuessler RB, Damiano RJ, Jr. Chronic transmural atrial ablation by using bipolar radiofrequency energy on the beating heart. J Thorac Cardiovasc Surg. 2002;124:708-13.
41. Demaria RG, Page P, Leung TK, Dubuc M, Malo O, Carrier M, Perrault LP. Surgical radiofrequency ablation induces coronary endothelial dysfunction in porcine coronary arteries. Eur J Cardiothorac Surg. 2003;23:277-82.
42. Gillinov AM, Pettersson G, Rice TW. Esophageal injury during radiofrequency ablation for atrial fibrillation. J Thorac Cardiovasc Surg. 2001;122:1239-40.
43. Kottkamp H, Hindricks G, Autschbach R, Krauss B, Strasser B, Schirdewahn P, Fabricius A, Schuler G, Mohr FW. Specific linear left atrial lesions in atrial fibrillation: intraoperative radiofrequency ablation using minimally invasive surgical techniques. J Am Coll Cardiol. 2002;40:475-80.
44. Doll N, Borger MA, Fabricius A, Stephan S, Gummert J, Mohr FW, Hauss J, Kottkamp H, Hindricks G. Esophageal perforation during left atrial radiofrequency ablation: Is the risk too high? J Thorac Cardiovasc Surg. 2003;125:836-42.
45. Saint LL, Lawrance CP, Okada S, Kazui T, Robertson JO, Schuessler RB, Damiano RJ, Jr. Performance of a novel bipolar/monopolar radiofrequency ablation device on the beating heart in an acute porcine model. Innovations (Phila) 2013;8:276-83.
46. Groh MA, Binns OA, Burton HG, 3rd, Champsaur GL, Ely SW, Johnson AM. Epicardial ultrasonic ablation of atrial fibrillation during concomitant cardiac surgery is a valid option in patients with ischemic heart disease. Circulation. 2008;118:S78-82.
47. Klinkenberg TJ, Ahmed S, Ten Hagen A, Wiesfeld AC, Tan ES, Zijlstra F, Van Gelder IC. Feasibility and outcome of epicardial pulmonary vein isolation for lone atrial fibrillation using minimal invasive surgery and high intensity focused ultrasound. Europace. 2009;11:1624-31.
48. Mitnovetski S, Almeida AA, Goldstein J, Pick AW, Smith JA. Epicardial high-intensity focused ultrasound cardiac ablation for surgical treatment of atrial fibrillation. Heart Lung Circ. 2009;18:28-31.
49. Nakagawa H, Antz M, Wong T, Schmidt B, Ernst S, Ouyang F, Vogtmann T, Wu R, Yokoyama K, Lockwood D, Po SS, Beckman KJ, Davies DW, Kuck KH, Jackman WM. Initial experience using a forward directed, high-intensity focused ultrasound balloon catheter for pulmonary vein antrum isolation in patients with atrial fibrillation. J Cardiovasc Electrophysiol. 2007;18:136-44.
50. Ninet J, Roques X, Seitelberger R, Deville C, Pomar JL, Robin J, Jegaden O, Wellens F, Wolner E, Vedrinne C, Gottardi R, Orrit J, Billes MA, Hoffmann DA, Cox JL, Champsaur GL. Surgical ablation of atrial fibrillation with off-pump, epicardial, high-intensity focused ultrasound: results of a multicenter trial. J Thorac Cardiovasc Surg. 2005;130:803-9.
51. Pet M, Robertson JO, Bailey M, Guthrie TJ, Moon MR, Lawton JS, Rinne A, Damiano RJ, Jr., Maniar HS. The impact of CHADS2 score on late stroke after the Cox-Maze procedure. J Thorac Cardiovasc Surg. 2013;146:85-9.
52. Gillinov AM, Sirak J, Blackstone EH, McCarthy PM, Rajeswaran J, Pettersson G, Sabik FJ, 3rd, Svensson LG, Navia JL, Cosgrove DM, Marrouche N, Natale A. The Cox-Maze procedure in mitral valve disease: predictors of recurrent atrial fibrillation. J Thorac Cardiovasc Surg. 2005;130:1653-60.

53. Ad N, Cox JL. The Maze procedure for the treatment of atrial fibrillation: a minimally invasive approach. J Card Surg. 2004;19:196-200.
54. Weimar T, Bailey MS, Watanabe Y, Marin D, Maniar HS, Schuessler RB, Damiano RJ, Jr. The Cox-Maze IV procedure for lone atrial fibrillation: a single center experience in 100 consecutive patients. J Interv Card Electrophysiol. 2011;31: 47-54.
55. Mokadam NA, McCarthy PM, Gillinov AM, Ryan WH, Moon MR, Mack MJ, Gaynor SL, Prasad SM, Wickline SA, Bailey MS, Damiano NR, Ishii Y, Schuessler RB, Damiano RJ, Jr. A prospective multicenter trial of bipolar radiofrequency ablation for atrial fibrillation: early results. Ann Thorac Surg. 2004;78:1665-70.
56. Lall SC, Melby SJ, Voeller RK, Zierer A, Bailey MS, Guthrie TJ, Moon MR, Moazami N, Lawton JS, Damiano RJ, Jr. The effect of ablation technology on surgical outcomes after the Cox-Maze procedure: a propensity analysis. J Thorac Cardiovasc Surg. 2007;133:389-96.
57. Voeller RK, Bailey MS, Zierer A, Lall SC, Sakamoto S, Aubuchon K, Lawton JS, Moazami N, Huddleston CB, Munfakh NA, Moon MR, Schuessler RB, Damiano RJ, Jr. Isolating the entire posterior left atrium improves surgical outcomes after the Cox-Maze procedure. J Thorac Cardiovasc Surg. 2008;135:870-7.
58. Henn MC, Lancaster TS, Miller JR, Sinn LA, Schuessler RB, Moon MR, Melby SJ, Maniar HS, Damiano RJ, Jr. Late outcomes after the Cox-Maze IV procedure for atrial fibrillation. J Thorac Cardiovasc Surg. 2015;150:1168-76, 78 e1-2.
59. Robertson JO, Saint LL, Leidenfrost JE, Damiano RJ, Jr. Illustrated techniques for performing the Cox-Maze IV procedure through a right mini-thoracotomy. Ann Cardiothorac Surg. 2014;3: 105-16.
60. Arcidi JM, Jr., Doty DB, Millar RC. The Maze procedure: the LDS Hospital experience. Semin Thorac Cardiovasc Surg. 2000;12:38-43.
61. Weimar T, Schena S, Bailey MS, Maniar HS, Schuessler RB, Cox JL, Damiano RJ, Jr. The Cox-Maze procedure for lone atrial fibrillation: a single-center experience over 2 decades. Circ Arrhythm Electrophysiol, 2012;5:8-14.
62. Ad N, Holmes SD, Stone LE, Pritchard G, Henry L. Rhythm course over 5 years following surgical ablation for atrial fibrillation. Eur J Cardiothorac Surg. 2015;47:52-8; discussion 8.
63. Damiano RJ, Jr. Badhwar V, Acker MA, Veeragandham RS, Kress DC, Robertson JO, Sundt TM. The CURE-AF trial: a prospective, multicenter trial of irrigated radiofrequency ablation for the treatment of persistent atrial fibrillation during concomitant cardiac surgery. Heart Rhythm. 2014;11:39-45.
64. Gillinov AM, Gelijns AC, Parides MK, DeRose JJ, Jr., Moskowitz AJ, Voisine P, Ailawadi G, Bouchard D, Smith PK, Mack MJ, Acker MA, Mullen JC, Rose EA, Chang HL, Puskas JD, Couderc JP, Gardner TJ, Varghese R, Horvath KA, Bolling SF, Michler RE, Geller NL, Ascheim DD, Miller MA, Bagiella E, Moquete EG, Williams P, Taddei-Peters WC, O'Gara PT, Blackstone EH, Argenziano M. Surgical ablation of atrial fibrillation during mitral-valve surgery. N Engl J Med. 2015;372:1399-409.
65. Stulak JM, Sundt TM, 3rd, Dearani JA, Daly RC, Orsulak TA, Schaff HV. Ten-year experience with the Cox-maze procedure for atrial fibrillation: how do we define success? Ann Thorac Surg. 2007;83:1319-24.
66. Saint LL, Damiano RJ, Jr. Cuculich PS, Guthrie TJ, Moon MR, Munfakh NA, Maniar HS. Incremental risk of the Cox-Maze IV procedure for patients with atrial fibrillation undergoing mitral valve surgery. J Thorac Cardiovasc Surg. 2013;146: 1072-7.
67. Saint LL, Bailey MS, Prasad S, Guthrie TJ, Bell J, Moon MR, Lawton JS, Munfakh NA, Schuessler RB, Damiano RJ, Jr. Maniar HS. Cox-Maze IV results for patients with lone atrial fibrillation versus concomitant mitral disease. Ann Thorac Surg. 2012;93:789-94; discussion 94-5.
68. Lawrance CP, Henn MC, Miller JR, Sinn LA, Schuessler RB, Damiano RJ, Jr. Comparison of the stand-alone Cox-Maze IV procedure to the concomitant Cox-Maze IV and mitral valve procedure for atrial fibrillation. Ann Cardiothorac Surg. 2014;3:55-61.
69. Damiano RJ, Jr. Gaynor SL, Bailey M, Prasad S, Cox JL, Boineau JP, Schuessler RP. The long-term outcome of patients with coronary disease and atrial fibrillation undergoing the Cox maze procedure. J Thorac Cardiovasc Surg. 2003;126:2016-21.
70. Ad N, Holmes SD, Massimiano PS, Pritchard G, Stone LE, Henry L. The effect of the Cox-Maze procedure for atrial fibrillation concomitant to mitral and tricuspid valve surgery. J Thorac Cardiovasc Surg. 2013;146:1426-34; discussion 34-5.
71. Abreu Filho CA, Lisboa LA, Dallan LA, Spina GS, Grinberg M, Scanavacca M, Sosa EA, Ramires JA, Oliveira SA. Effectiveness of the maze procedure using cooled-tip radiofrequency ablation in patients with permanent atrial fibrillation and rheumatic mitral valve disease. Circulation. 2005;112:I20-5.
72. Henn MC, Lawrance CP, Sinn LA, Miller JR, Schuessler RB, Moon MR, Melby SJ, Maniar HS, Damiano RJ, Jr. Effectiveness of Surgical Ablation in Patients with Atrial Fibrillation and Aortic Valve Disease. Ann Thorac Surg. 2015;100:1253-9; discussion 9-60.
73. Ad N, Henry L, Hunt S, Holmes SD. Do we increase the operative risk by adding the Cox-Maze III procedure to aortic valve replacement and coronary artery bypass surgery? J Thorac Cardiovasc Surg. 2012;143:936-44.
74. Saint LL, Lawrance CP, Leidenfrost JE, Robertson JO, Damiano RJ, Jr. How I do it: minimally invasive Cox-Maze IV procedure. Ann Cardiothorac Surg. 2014;3:117-9.
75. Lee AM, Clark K, Bailey MS, Aziz A, Schuessler RB, Damiano RJ, Jr. A minimally invasive Cox-Maze procedure: operative technique and results. Innovations (Phila) 2010;5:281-6.
76. Lawrance CP, Henn MC, Miller JR, Sinn LA, Schuessler RB, Maniar HS, Damiano RJ, Jr. A minimally invasive Cox-Maze IV procedure is as effective as sternotomy while decreasing major morbidity and hospital stay. J Thorac Cardiovasc Surg. 2014;148:955-61; discussion 62-2.
77. Phan K, Xie A, Tsai YC, Kumar N, La Meir M, Yan TD. Biatrial ablation vs. left atrial concomitant surgical ablation for treatment of atrial fibrillation: a meta-analysis. Europace, 2015;17:38-47.
78. Fasol R, Meinhart J, Binder T. A modified and simplified radiofrequency ablation in patients with mitral valve disease. J Thorac Cardiovasc Surg. 2005;129:215-7.
79. Gaita F, Riccardi R, Caponi D, Shah D, Garberoglio L, Vivalda L, Dulio A, Chiecchio A, Manasse E, Gallotti R. Linear cryoablation of the left atrium versus pulmonary vein cryoisolation in patients with permanent atrial fibrillation and valvular heart disease: correlation of electroanatomic mapping and long-term clinical results. Circulation. 2005;111:136-42.
80. Imai K, Sueda T, Orihashi K, Watari M, Matsuura Y. Clinical analysis of results of a simple left atrial procedure

for chronic atrial fibrillation. Ann Thorac Surg. 2001;71: 577-81.
81. Knaut M, Spitzer SG, Karolyi L, Ebert HH, Richter P, Tugtekin SM, Schuler S. Intraoperative microwave ablation for curative treatment of atrial fibrillation in open heart surgery—the MICRO-STAF and MICRO-PASS pilot trial. MICROwave Application in Surgical treatment of Atrial Fibrillation. MICROwave Application for the Treatment of Atrial Fibrillation in Bypass-Surgery. Thorac Cardiovasc Surg. 1999;47(Suppl 3): 379-84.
82. Kondo N, Takahashi K, Minakawa M, Daitoku K. Left atrial maze procedure: a useful addition to other corrective operations. Ann Thorac Surg. 2003;75:1490-4.
83. Schuetz A, Schulze CJ, Sarvanakis KK, Mair H, Plazer H, Kilger E, Reichart B, Wildhirt SM. Surgical treatment of permanent atrial fibrillation using microwave energy ablation: a prospective randomized clinical trial. Eur J Cardiothorac Surg. 2003;24:475-80; discussion 80.
84. Sie HT, Beukema WP, Misier AR, Elvan A, Ennema JJ, Haalebos MM, Wellens HJ. Radiofrequency modified maze in patients with atrial fibrillation undergoing concomitant cardiac surgery. J Thorac Cardiovasc Surg. 2001;122:249-56.
85. Benussi S, Nascimbene S, Agricola E, Calori G, Calvi S, Caldarola A, Oppizzi M, Casati V, Pappone C, Alfieri O. Surgical ablation of atrial fibrillation using the epicardial radiofrequency approach: mid-term results and risk analysis. Ann Thorac Surg. 2002;74:1050-6; discussion 7.
86. Illinov AM, McCarthy PM, Blackstone EH, Rajeswaran J, Pettersson G, Sabik JF, Svensson LG, Cosgrove DM, Hill KM, Gonzalez-Stawinski GV, Marrouche N, Natale A. Surgical ablation of atrial fibrillation with bipolar radiofrequency as the primary modality. J Thorac Cardiovasc Surg. 2005;129:1322-9.
87. Barnett SD, Ad N. Surgical ablation as treatment for the elimination of atrial fibrillation: a meta-analysis. J Thorac Cardiovasc Surg. 2006;131:1029-35.
88. Nitta T, Ishii Y, Miyagi Y, Ohmori H, Sakamoto S, Tanaka S. Concurrent multiple left atrial focal activations with fibrillatory conduction and right atrial focal or reentrant activation as the mechanism in atrial fibrillation. J Thorac Cardiovasc Surg. 2004;127:770-8.
89. Sahadevan J, Ryu K, Peltz L, Khrestian CM, Stewart RW, Markowitz AH, Waldo AL. Epicardial mapping of chronic atrial fibrillation in patients: preliminary observations. Circulation. 2004;110:3293-9.
90. Schuessler RB, Kay MW, Melby SJ, Branham BH, Boineau JP, Damiano RJ, Jr. Spatial and temporal stability of the dominant frequency of activation in human atrial fibrillation. J Electrocardiol. 2006;39:S7-12.
91. Haissaguerre M, Jais P, Shah DC, Takahashi A, Hocini M, Quiniou G, Garrigue S, Le Mouroux A, Le Metayer P, Clementy J. Spontaneous initiation of atrial fibrillation by ectopic beats originating in the pulmonary veins. N Engl J Med. 1998;339: 659-66.
92. Lee SH, Tai CT, Hsieh MH, Tsao HM, Lin YJ, Chang SL, Huang JL, Lee KT, Chen YJ, Cheng JJ, Chen SA. Predictors of non-pulmonary vein ectopic beats initiating paroxysmal atrial fibrillation: implication for catheter ablation. J Am Coll Cardiol. 2005;46:1054-9.
93. Doll N, Pritzwald-Stegmann P, Czesla M, Kempfert J, Stenzel MA, Borger MA, Mohr FW. Ablation of ganglionic plexi during combined surgery for atrial fibrillation. Ann Thorac Surg. 2008;86:1659-63.
94. McClelland JH, Duke D, Reddy R. Preliminary results of a limited thoracotomy: new approach to treat atrial fibrillation. J Cardiovasc Electrophysiol. 2007;18:1289-95.
95. Mehall JR, Kohut RM, Jr. Schneeberger EW, Taketani T, Merrill WH, Wolf RK. Intraoperative epicardial electrophysiologic mapping and isolation of autonomic ganglionic plexi. Ann Thorac Surg. 2007;83:538-41.
96. Sakamoto S, Schuessler RB, Lee AM, Aziz A, Lall SC, Damiano RJ, Jr. Vagal denervation and reinnervation after ablation of ganglionated plexi. J Thorac Cardiovasc Surg. 2010;139: 444-52.
97. Geuzebroek GS, Ballaux PK, van Hemel NM, Kelder JC, Defauw JJ. Medium-term outcome of different surgical methods to cure atrial fibrillation: is less worse? Interact Cardiovasc Thorac Surg. 2008;7:201-6.
98. Reyes G, Benedicto A, Bustamante J, Sarraj A, Nuche JM, Alvarez P, Duarte J. Restoration of atrial contractility after surgical cryoablation: clinical, electrical and mechanical results. Interact Cardiovasc Thorac Surg. 2009;9:609-12.
99. Bisleri G, Rosati F, Bontempi L, Curnis A, Muneretto C. Hybrid approach for the treatment of long-standing persistent atrial fibrillation: electrophysiological findings and clinical results. Eur J Cardiothorac Surg. 2013;44:919-23.
100. Healey JS, Crystal E, Lamy A, Teoh K, Semelhago L, Hohnloser SH, Cybulsky I, Abouzahr L, Sawchuck C, Carroll S, Morillo C, Kleine P, Chu V, Lonn E, Connolly SJ. Left Atrial Appendage Occlusion Study (LAAOS): results of a randomized controlled pilot study of left atrial appendage occlusion during coronary bypass surgery in patients at risk for stroke. Am Heart J. 2005;150:288-93.
101. Salzberg SP, Gillinov AM, Anyanwu A, Castillo J, Filsoufi F, Adams DH. Surgical left atrial appendage occlusion: evaluation of a novel device with magnetic resonance imaging. Eur J Cardiothorac Surg. 2008;34:766-70.
102. Salzberg SP, Plass A, Emmert MY, Desbiolles L, Alkadhi H, Grunenfelder J, Genoni M. Left atrial appendage clip occlusion: early clinical results. J Thorac Cardiovasc Surg. 2010;139: 1269-74.
103. Ailawadi G, Gerdisch MW, Harvey RL, Hooker RL, Damiano RJ, Jr., Salamon T, Mack MJ. Exclusion of the left atrial appendage with a novel device: early results of a multicenter trial. J Thorac Cardiovasc Surg. 2011;142:1002-9, 9 e1.
104. Wolf RK, Schneeberger EW, Osterday R, Miller D, Merrill W, Flege JB, Jr., Gillinov AM. Video-assisted bilateral pulmonary vein isolation and left atrial appendage exclusion for atrial fibrillation. J Thorac Cardiovasc Surg. 2005;130:797-802.
105. Edgerton JR, Jackman WM, Mack MJ. Minimally invasive pulmonary vein isolation and partial autonomic denervation for surgical treatment of atrial fibrillation. J Interv Card Electrophysiol. 2007;20:89-93.
106. Han FT, Kasirajan V, Kowalski M, Kiser R, Wolfe L, Kalahasty G, Shepard RK, Wood MA, Ellenbogen KA. Results of a minimally invasive surgical pulmonary vein isolation and ganglionic plexi ablation for atrial fibrillation: single-center experience with 12-month follow-up. Circ Arrhythm Electrophysiol. 2009;2:370-7.
107. Beyer E, Lee R, Lam BK. Point: Minimally invasive bipolar radiofrequency ablation of lone atrial fibrillation: early multicenter results. J Thorac Cardiovasc Surg. 2009;137:521-6.
108. Boersma LV, Castella M, van Boven W, Berruezo A, Yilmaz A, Nadal M, Sandoval E, Calvo N, Brugada J, Kelder J, Wijffels M, Mont L. Atrial fibrillation catheter ablation versus surgical

ablation treatment (FAST): a 2-center randomized clinical trial. Circulation, 2012;125:23-30.

109. Edgerton JR, Edgerton ZJ, Weaver T, Reed K, Prince S, Herbert MA, Mack MJ. Minimally invasive pulmonary vein isolation and partial autonomic denervation for surgical treatment of atrial fibrillation. Ann Thorac Surg. 2008;86:35-8; discussion 9.
110. Zheng S, Li Y, Han J, Zhang H, Zeng W, Xu C, Jia Y, Wang J, Guo K, Jiao Y, Meng X. Long-term results of a minimally invasive surgical pulmonary vein isolation and ganglionic plexi ablation for atrial fibrillation. PLoS One 2013;8:e79755.
111. Melby SJ, Zierer A, Bailey MS, Cox JL, Lawton JS, Munfakh N, Crabtree TD, Moazami N, Huddleston CB, Moon MR, Damiano RJ, Jr. A new era in the surgical treatment of atrial fibrillation: the impact of ablation technology and lesion set on procedural efficacy. Ann Surg. 2006;244:583-92.
112. McCarthy PM, Manjunath A, Kruse J, Andrei AC, Li Z, McGee EC, Jr., Malaisrie SC, Lee R. Should paroxysmal atrial fibrillation be treated during cardiac surgery? J Thorac Cardiovasc Surg. 2013;146:810-23.
113. Tada H, Ito S, Naito S, Hasegawa Y, Kurosaki K, Ezure M, Kaneko T, Oshima S, Taniguchi K, Nogami A. Long-term results of cryoablation with a new cryoprobe to eliminate chronic atrial fibrillation associated with mitral valve disease. Pacing Clin Electrophysiol. 2005;28(Suppl 1):S73-7.
114. Mahapatra S, LaPar DJ, Kamath S, Payne J, Bilchick KC, Mangrum JM, Ailawadi G. Initial experience of sequential surgical epicardial-catheter endocardial ablation for persistent and long-standing persistent atrial fibrillation with long-term follow-up. Ann Thorac Surg. 2011;91:1890-8.
115. Krul SP, Pison L, La Meir M, Driessen AH, Wilde AA, Maessen JG, De Mol BA, Crijns HJ, de Groot JR. Epicardial and endocardial electrophysiological guided thoracoscopic surgery for atrial fibrillation: a multidisciplinary approach of atrial fibrillation ablation in challenging patients. Int J Cardiol. 2014;173:229-35.
116. Pison L, Gelsomino S, Luca F, Parise O, Maessen JG, Crijns HJ, La Meir M. Effectiveness and safety of simultaneous hybrid thoracoscopic and endocardial catheter ablation of lone atrial fibrillation. Ann Cardiothorac Surg. 2014;3:38-44.
117. Gehi AK, Mounsey JP, Pursell I, Landers M, Boyce K, Chung EH, Schwartz J, Walker TJ, Guise K, Kiser AC. Hybrid epicardial-endocardial ablation using a pericardioscopic technique for the treatment of atrial fibrillation. Heart Rhythm, 2013;10: 22-8.
118. Gelsomino S, Van Breugel HN, Pison L, Parise O, Crijns HJ, Wellens F, Maessen JG, La Meir M. Hybrid thoracoscopic and transvenous catheter ablation of atrial fibrillation. Eur J Cardiothorac Surg. 2014;45:401-7.
119. Je HG, Shuman DJ, Ad N. A systematic review of minimally invasive surgical treatment for atrial fibrillation: a comparison of the Cox-Maze procedure, beating-heart epicardial ablation, and the hybrid procedure on safety and efficacy. Eur J Cardiothorac Surg. 2015;48:531-40; discussion 40-1.
120. Cuculich PS, Wang Y, Lindsay BD, Faddis MN, Schuessler RB, Damiano RJ, Jr. Li L, Rudy Y. Noninvasive characterization of epicardial activation in humans with diverse atrial fibrillation patterns. Circulation. 2010;122:1364-72.
121. McCulloch P, Altman DG, Campbell WB, Flum DR, Glasziou P, Marshall JC, Nicholl J, Aronson JK, Barkun JS, Blazeby JM, Boutron IC, Clavien PA, Cook JA, Ergina PL, Feldman LS, Maddern GJ, Reeves BC, Seiler CM, Strasberg SM, Meakins JL, Ashby D, Black N, Bunker J, Burton M, Campbell M, Chalkidou K, Chalmers I, de Leval M, Deeks J, Grant A, Gray M, Greenhalgh R, Jenicek M, Kehoe S, Lilford R, Littlejohns P, Loke Y, Madhock R, McPherson K, Meakins J, Rothwell P, Summerskill B, Taggart D, Tekkis P, Thompson M, Treasure T, Trohler U, Vandenbroucke J. No surgical innovation without evaluation: the IDEAL recommendations. Lancet, 2009;374:1105-12.

EDITORS' SUMMARY

No conversation with a patient that we counsel on best treatment approaches for symptomatic atrial fibrillation can be complete without discussing the option of surgical ablation. Electrophysiologists are often poorly equipped to carry out this conversation with lack of familiarity of the various approaches available and the paucity of data in the published literature on more recent minimally invasive surgical and hybrid approaches.

One of the leading groups in the field of surgical ablation led by Professor Damiano has provided for this textbook an outstanding historical and clinically practical summary of the rationale and existing approaches for surgical ablation.

As the authors state, the poor and, sometimes abysmal results, for eliminating persistent atrial fibrillation with catheter-based procedures, needs to be acknowledged. At the same time, the limitations for surgical approaches, particularly, newer techniques in trying to obtain the excellent results of the Cox-Maze III procedure remains an unknown in terms of large, randomized trials.

The specific sections on hybrid procedures and the technical details and operative differences among the commonly employed procedures will be of great value when thoroughly studied by practitioners of invasive electrophysiology.

CHAPTER 29

Edward P Walsh

Atrial Arrhythmias in Congenital Heart Disease and Postcardiac Surgery

LIST OF ABBREVIATIONS

AF	Atrial Fibrillation	ICD	Implantable Cardioverter-Defibrillator
CHD	Congenital Heart Disease	LA	Left Atrium
IART	Intra-atrial Reentrant Tachycardia	RA	Right Atrium

INTRODUCTION

Atrial pathology comes in many forms, but a universal consequence is disruption of normal conduction patterns giving rise to various atrial tachyarrhythmias, including macroreentrant circuits, focal tachycardias, and fibrillation. Often the situation becomes further complicated by concomitant sinus node dysfunction resulting in the tachy-brady syndrome. Although these arrhythmias are usually not immediately life-threatening, the negative impact on hemodynamic status and the potential for thromboembolic complications can have a profound effect on long-term patient outcomes.

This chapter will review atrial arrhythmias that develop following cardiac surgery for congenital heart disease (CHD) and several other anatomic cardiac conditions (**Table 29.1**). Most emphasis will be placed on CHD since the classic operations employed for these defects can result in discrete conduction corridors that serve as a natural laboratory for the study of atrial muscle reentry. The CHD population is

Table 29.1: Common postoperative atrial tachyarrhythmia mechanisms according to type of surgery, age at surgery, and follow-up timing

Types of operation (age at surgery)	*Acute Postoperative*	*Intermediate follow-up*	*Long-term follow-up*
CHD (infant)	EAT (+)	—	IART (+)
CHD (child)	—	IART (+)	IART (+)
CHD (Adolescent and young adult)	IART (+), AF (+)	IART (++), Focal (+), AF (+)	IART (++), Focal (+), AF (++)
Other cardiac surgery (Adult)	AF (+++)	IART (+), AF (++)	AF (++)

(+) occasional; (++) moderately frequent; (+++) very frequent
Abbreviations: AF, atrial fibrillation, CHD, surgery for congenital heart disease; EAT, automatic ectopic atrial tachycardia; Focal, focal atrial tachycardia (triggered or microreentry); IART, intra-atrial macroreentrant tachycardia (including atrial flutter)

also unique in the sense that most surgical interventions are performed at young ages before decades of degenerative remodeling have rendered the atria vulnerable to fibrillation, resulting in a much different profile for postoperative rhythm disturbances compared to elderly patients in whom atrial fibrillation (AF) predominates.

ATRIAL ARRHYTHMIAS IN PATIENTS WITH CONGENITAL HEART DISEASE

Beginning with the first successful closure of a patent ductus arteriosus by Dr Robert Gross in 1938,[1] the fields of pediatric cardiology and cardiac surgery became sharply focused on devising hemodynamic interventions that might allow CHD patients to survive beyond infancy and early childhood. A remarkable series of advances in surgical and catheterization techniques progressively satisfied this goal, to the point that it is rare nowadays to encounter a CHD lesion that cannot be managed in a fashion that permits survival into adulthood. However, this improved longevity has exposed a host of late complications, central among which are cardiac arrhythmias.

Atrial tachycardias are the most common arrhythmias observed in the CHD population.[2] They are a major source of morbidity, and may occasionally contribute to sudden cardiac death. Bouchardy et al.[3] found in a large cohort of adults with CHD that the prevalence of some type of atrial tachycardia was 15%, with a lifetime risk of 50% regardless of severity of the CHD lesion. Atrial arrhythmias were associated with a 50% increase in mortality, a two-fold increased risk of heart failure or stroke, and a three-fold higher risk of requiring some major cardiac intervention. They also complicate implantable cardioverter defibrillator (ICD) use in this population by triggering inappropriate shocks for rapidly-conducted supraventricular rhythms.[4] Patients with transposition of the great arteries following Mustard or Senning operations, and single ventricle patients with a Fontan circulation, have the highest atrial tachycardia burden, but even simple atrial septal defect closure can be linked to tachyarrhythmias during extended follow-up. Fortunately, multiple refinements in the surgical approach to CHD over the last few decades have markedly improved rhythm prognosis. Transposition is now managed with direct arterial switch rather than large atrial baffles, and the Fontan operation is now being performed with modifications that redirect caval blood directly to the pulmonary arteries, thereby bypassing the right atrium (RA) and avoiding the massive atrial distension characteristic of the older style atriopulmonary Fontan connection. Most importantly, CHD surgery is now being performed at much younger ages with definitive repairs rather than palliative procedures, which may spare atrial myocardium years of exposure to cyanosis and the hemodynamic stress that predisposes to later arrhythmia development. Still, there is a large and growing population of adult survivors repaired in the old manner who are actively struggling with the arrhythmogenic consequences of the earlier forms of surgery.[5]

Intra-atrial Reentrant Tachycardia

Most atrial tachycardias in CHD patients involve macro-reentrant circuits located in RA tissue anterior to the crista terminalis. These can include typical atrial flutter with a peritricuspid circuit through the cavotricuspid isthmus, as well as novel circuits related to atriotomy incisions, caval cannulation sites, surgical patches, and other scarred regions. Multiple circuits will often be present in the same patient. The label "intra-atrial reentrant tachycardia" (IART) has been widely adopted as a collective term to encompass all possible locations for the macroreentrant circuits found in CHD patients.

It is unusual to encounter IART in the immediate post-operative period in young patients. It does not typically surface until a decade or more after repair, suggesting that a period of atrial remodeling may be needed until conduction velocity slows sufficiently for reentry to sustain. Cycle lengths for IART circuits tend to be longer than conventional atrial flutter (on the order of 250–350 ms), which permits a rapid ventricular response that can easily approach 1:1 when catecholamines become elevated.[6]

Similar to the management of AF, precautions against thromboembolic complications are necessary whenever IART duration is protracted or uncertain. Anticoagulation according to standard guidelines and/or screening for intracardiac thrombi with transesophageal echocardiography are recommended if IART duration exceeds 48 hours.[7] Acute termination can be achieved reliably with electrical cardioversion, overdrive atrial pacing from the esophagus,[8] or overdrive pacing from an implanted pacemaker or ICD. Pharmacologic conversion can also be successful in select cases, but the limited data on acute drug therapy have not been sufficiently compelling in terms of success and risk[9] to recommend this as a standard approach.

Prevention of IART recurrence is a major challenge, and unfortunately, IART does not respond well to chronic antiarrhythmic drugs. More than 60% of patients will experience one or more sustained recurrences within 2 years even when using Class I and Class III agents.[10] Catheter ablation has thus emerged as a first-line therapy for IART at many centers caring for CHD patients.

Catheter ablation has been applied to IART since the early 1990s.[11] Among the most helpful lessons from the initial experience was that predictable patterns existed for circuit location according to the underlying CHD lesion and method used for surgical repair.[12] In patients with simple 4-chamber CHD whose repair involved a lateral atriotomy incision (e.g. isolated atrial or ventricular septal defect closure, tetralogy of Fallot repair), the most common circuit will to be found around the tricuspid annulus through the cavotricuspid isthmus similar to conventional atrial flutter

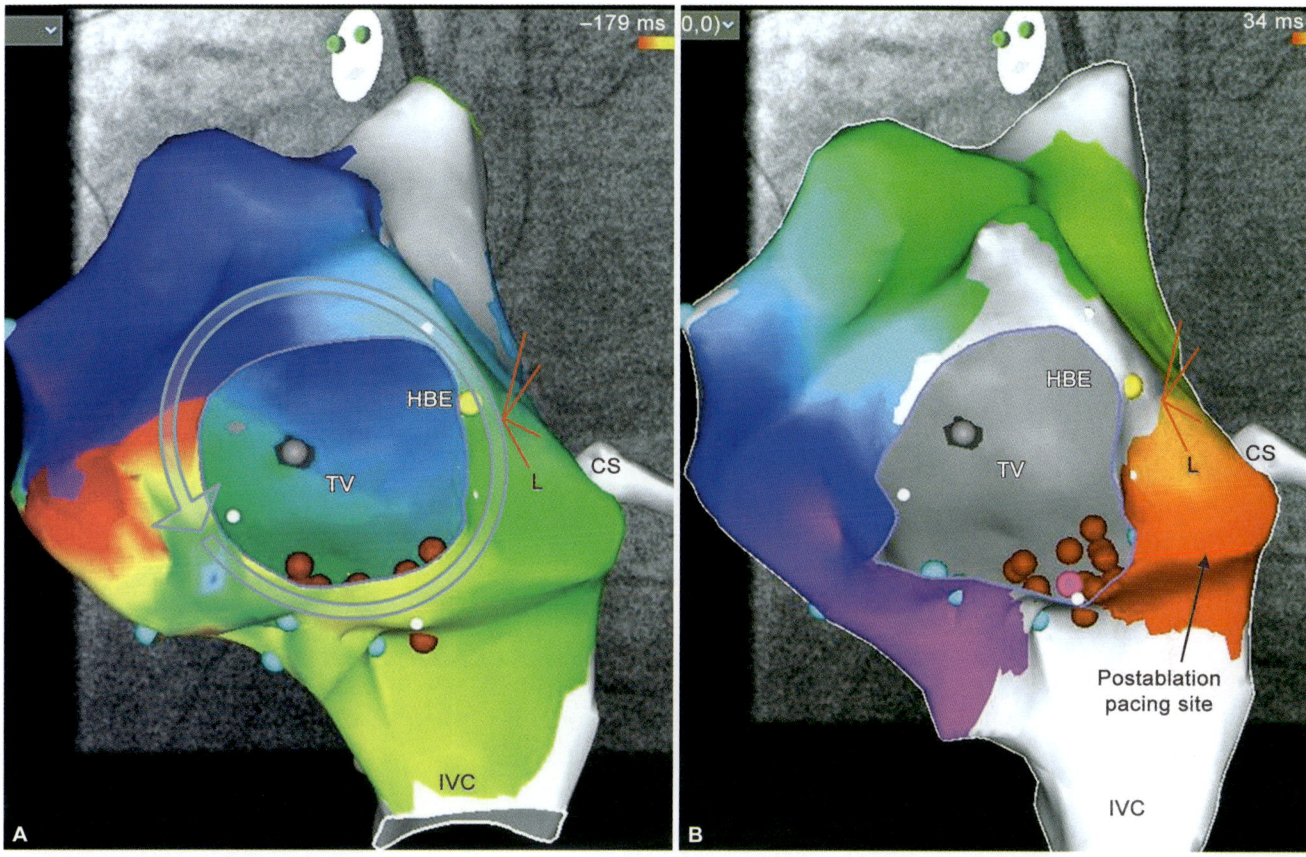

Figures 29.1A and B: Intra-atrial reentrant tachycardia in a 43-year-old who underwent repair of tetralogy of Fallot as a child. (A) Activation map showing counterclockwise macroreentry around the tricuspid valve (TV) through the cavo-tricuspid isthmus. Positions of the coronary sinus (CS), the inferior vena cava (IVC) and the His bundle recording site (HBE) are marked; (B) Following ablation (red dots) at the cavo-tricuspid isthmus, pacing from the medial aspect of the isthmus confirms medial-lateral conduction block

(Figures 29.1A and B), but this is further complicated by a figure-of-eight or dual loop configuration with an outer loop circuit around the atriotomy scar on the lateral RA wall.[13] Effective ablation usually requires interruption of both loops by creating a line of conduction block through the isthmus, as well as through the narrow corridor between the lower edge of the atriotomy scar and the inferior vena cava. The atriotomy can be localized by high-density substrate mapping along the lateral RA wall, looking for a vertical line of split potentials positioned between the crista terminalis and the lateral edge of the tricuspid ring (**Figure 29.2**).

For patients who have undergone the Mustard or Senning operations for transposition, the typical IART circuit likewise involves the cavotricuspid isthmus, but in these cases the true isthmus is located on the pulmonary venous side of the atrial baffle.[12,14] Entry into the pulmonary venous atrium is almost always required for successful ablation of IART in this form of CHD. This can be accomplished using a retrograde aortic approach back through the tricuspid valve, or by transbaffle puncture.[15] Tip control with conventional catheters is somewhat awkward when attempting the retrograde approach, but centers equipped with magnetic navigation systems have used this technology to good advantage in such cases.[16] Most other centers have developed a strong preference for the transbaffle technique **(Figures 29.3A and B)**. Both methods are associated with a high success rate in the Mustard and Senning populations.

The least predictable IART circuits involve patients with a single ventricle who have undergone some variations of the Fontan operation. The surgical design for this operation has evolved over the years, and the different designs vary in terms of their arrhythmogenic potential and circuit location(s). The traditional Fontan operation utilized a RA-pulmonary artery anastomosis that resulted in dramatic RA dilation with an IART incidence as high as 40%, usually involving multiple circuits in atypical locations.[12,17,18] Acute ablation success and freedom from recurrence tends to be lower in this group than in any other CHD category, prompting some centers to advocate a surgical approach for conversion to the one of the newer Fontan designs, along with excision of redundant

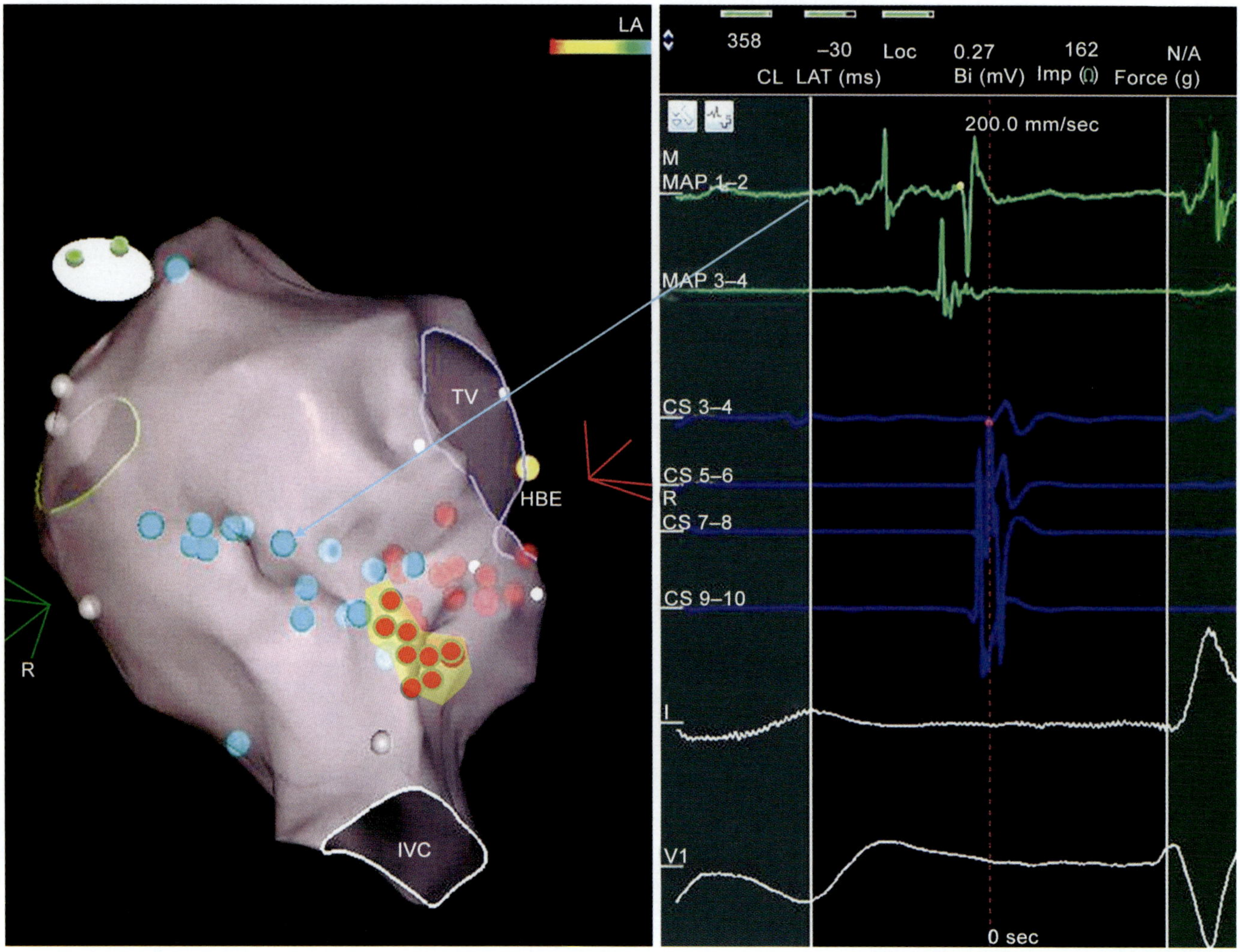

Figure 29.2: Substrate map to identify the lateral atriotomy scar in the same tetralogy patient shown in Figure 29.1. A line of split potentials (electrogram example shown) was identified on the lateral right atrial wall (blue dots). The lower edge of this line was connected to the inferior vena cava (IVC) with an empiric set of radiofrequency applications (red dots highlighted in yellow) to prevent macroreentry on the lateral wall Abbreviations as Figure 29.1

RA tissue and a cryosurgical maze.[19] Newer Fontan designs bypass the RA using either a lateral tunnel or an extracardiac conduit for a direct caval connection to the pulmonary arteries, thereby avoiding RA dilation and resulting in a reduction of the IART incidence to <10%.[20] However, for the occasional patient who does develop IART in a more modern Fontan design, circuits are likely to be located on the pulmonary venous side of the tunnel or conduit (**Figures 29.4A and B**), requiring complex techniques for transseptal access.[21,22]

Clear registration of anatomic details is essential for successful IART mapping in all forms of CHD. Procedures are best performed using 3D electroanatomic mapping systems,[23] augmenting the spatial shell geometry by merging one or more additional imaging modalities (MRI, CT, intracardiac echo, angiography). Creation of a substrate maps in baseline rhythm is a helpful starting exercise to locate low-voltage areas and split potentials corresponding to scars and patches that may participate in IART circuits.[24] Efforts must also be made to locate position of the His bundle electrogram as precisely as possible since the atrioventricular conduction tissues can be anatomically displaced in certain forms of CHD.[25,26] Activation mapping and entrainment maneuvers can then be performed during induced IART to characterize the circuit according to standard methodology for macroreentry (**Figure 29.5**), which in turn guides selection of the most likely critical corridors for ablation lesions (**Figure 29.6**). Achieving effective lines of conduction block in atrial tissue of some CHD patients can be difficult owing to increased wall thickness,[27] but irrigated-tip ablation catheters, long deflectable vascular sheaths, contact-force sensing, and intracardiac echocardiography

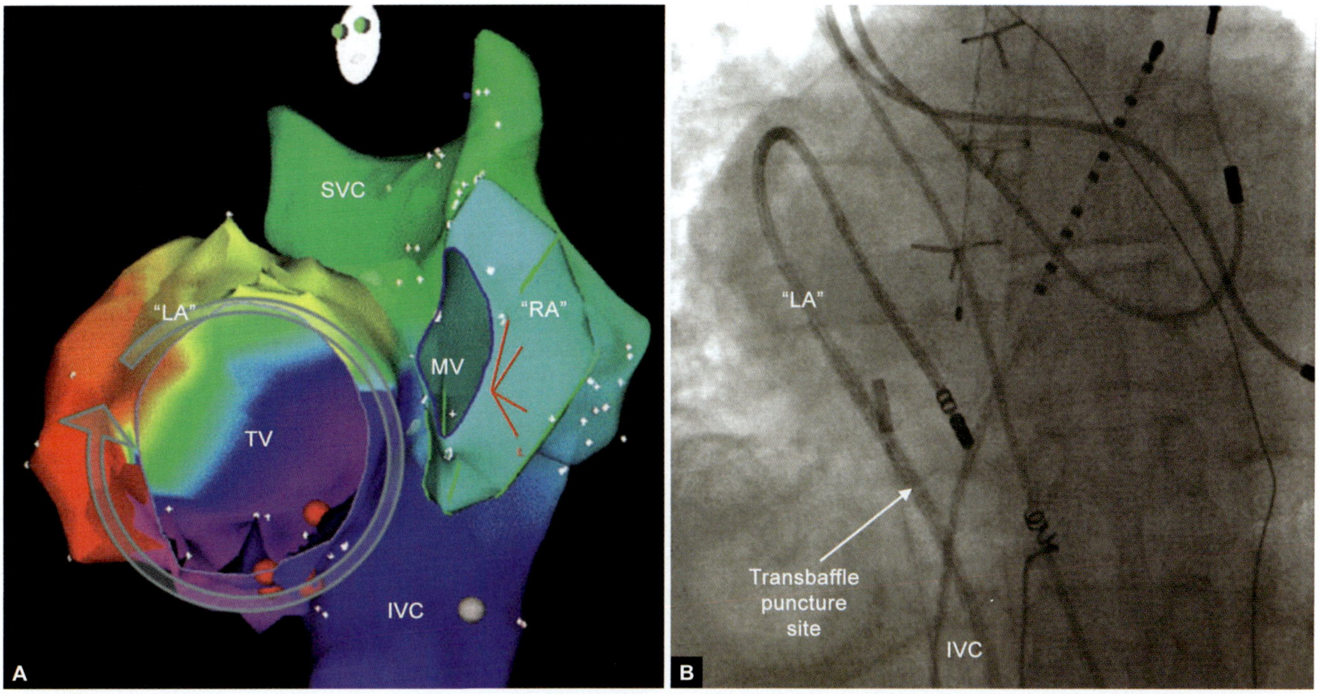

Figures 29.3A and B: Intra-atrial reentrant tachycardia in a 31-year-old who underwent a Mustard operation for transposition of the great arteries. (A) Electroanatomic map showing the systemic venous return from the superior and inferior vena cava (SVC & IVC) which is redirected into the neo-right atrium ("RA") towards the mitral valve (MV). The pulmonary veins return to the neo-left atrium ("LA"). The tachycardia circuit involves clockwise macroreentry around the tricuspid valve (TV). The cavo-tricuspid isthmus was the effective ablation target, but in order to reach this area, the catheter tip had to be positioned in the "LA"; (B) Transbaffle puncture was performed from the IVC into the "LA", allowing successful ablation of the cavo-tricuspid isthmus

are among the many improvements in recent years that have helped address this challenge.[23]

Success rates for IART ablation continue to improve with advances in mapping technology, more effective lesion creation, and expanded procedural experience.[11,22,28-33] Acute success can now be achieved in roughly 85% of cases, though the recurrence rate still remains relatively high (10–30%), especially for the Fontan subgroup. Still, these outcomes are far superior to the degree of control possible with drug therapy, and will hopefully improve further with additional refinements in technology.

Many CHD patients who develop IART also suffer from sinus node dysfunction that is likely a consequence of direct trauma to the node or its arterial supply during surgery.[34] This is especially true for patients who have undergone Mustard, Senning, Glenn, and Fontan operations.[35] Chronotropic incompetence not only interferes with the ability to safely prescribe AV nodal blocking agents and other antiarrhythmic drugs, but may actually increase the frequency of IART episodes. Several studies have demonstrated that restoration of physiologic atrial rates with permanent pacemaker implant can reduce (and sometimes eliminate) future IART episodes.[36,37] Pacemakers can also be used to manually overdrive IART episodes, or if the device is equipped with antitachycardia features, can be programmed in select patients to automatically attempt overdrive pacing to terminate atrial reentry.[36,38] Sinus node dysfunction in CHD patients with IART is ranked as a Class IIa indication for permanent pacemaker implant according to the ACC/AHA/HRS guidelines for device-based therapy of cardiac rhythm abnormalities.[39] However, decisions regarding permanent pacemaker implant in CHD patients can never be made casually. Unusual venous connections and small patient size may make lead insertion difficult,[40] and in cases where residual intracardiac shunting is present, transvenous leads may be contraindicated because of the thromboembolic risk.[41] Open-chest procedures for epicardial implant are thus required in many of these patients.

Focal Atrial Tachycardia in CHD

Intermittent bursts of atrial tachycardias with nonsinus P-wave morphology and variable rates characterized by "warm-up & cool-down" can be observed in the *early* postoperative period in some infants following surgery for cyanotic CHD lesions, especially those who have undergone

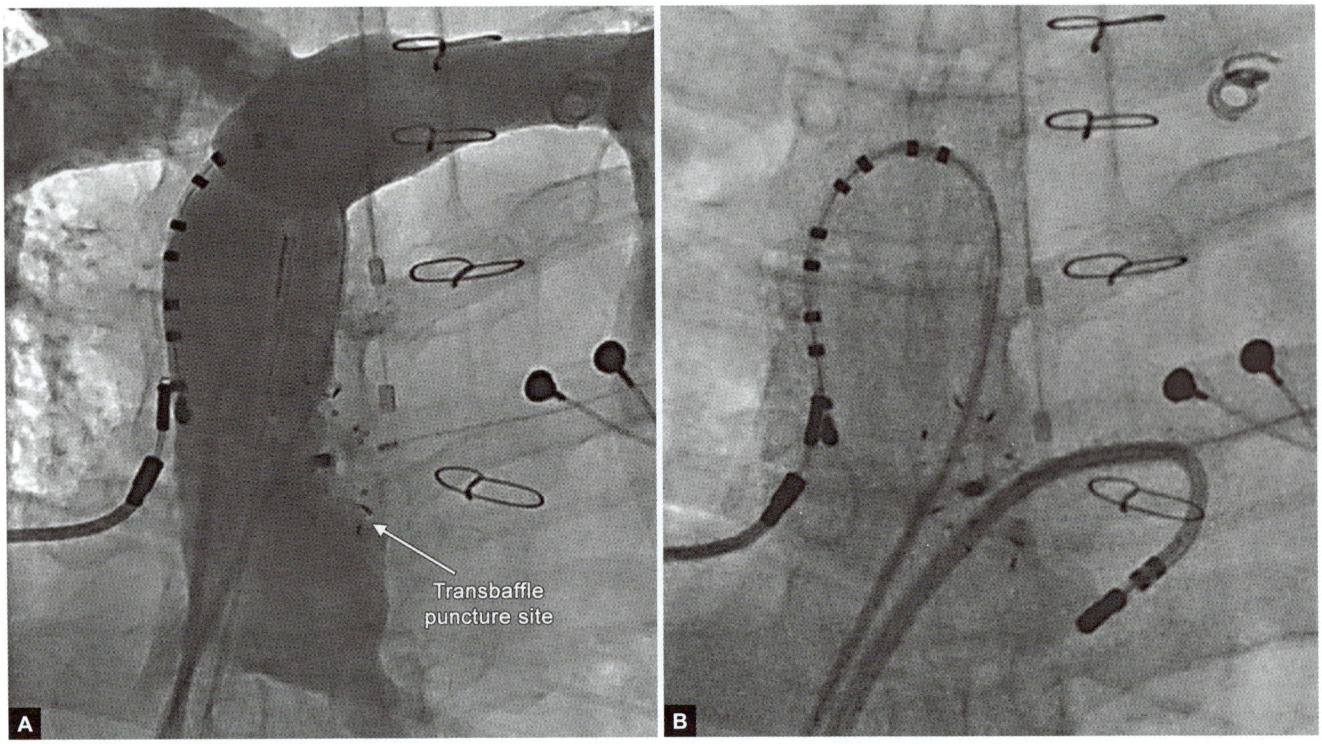

Figures 29.4A and B: Ablation for intra-atrial reentrant tachycardia in a patient with single ventricle who has undergone a lateral tunnel Fontan operation. (A) Angiogram showing how the lateral tunnel drains to the pulmonary arteries, with no evidence of baffle leak into the left atrium. Note there is septal occlusion device which was placed many years prior to close a surgical fenestration. The tachycardia circuit was in the left atrium; (B) Transbaffle puncture was performed at the lower edge of the occlusion device, and the ablation catheter tip is positioned at the site of successful ablation for this circuit

preoperative balloon atrial septostomy.[42] Associated postoperative factors include hypokalemia and high-dose catecholamine infusions. The clinical behavior of this tachycardia suggests a focus of abnormal automaticity, and a mechanistic label of automatic ectopic atrial tachycardia appears to be appropriate. This arrhythmia can usually be controlled with potassium repletion or simple beta-blocker therapy, and typically resolves completely within a matter of days.

A different type of focal atrial tachycardia can be seen as a *late* arrhythmia many years after surgical repairs of CHD. It has clinical features and an electrocardiographic pattern that are indistinguishable from IART, though the tachycardia appears to emanate from a point-source when intracardiac mapping is performed. It can usually be initiated and terminated with programmed stimulation or bursts of rapid atrial pacing, operates at fairly fixed cycle lengths, and responds promptly to direct current cardioversion. Characteristics such as these would tend to implicate either localized triggered activity or a small area of microreentry as the underlying mechanism.[43] Precision mapping reveals radial propagation away from a discrete epicenter that is usually located near the edge of a scar zone or surgical suture line (**Figure 29.7**). The local electrogram can appear fractionated with long-duration electrical activity preceding the onset of the electrocardiographic P-wave.[44] Ablation efforts can either be focused on the point of earliest activation, or on the creation of a peripheral boundary line to isolate the abnormal site. Tachycardia will sometimes terminate promptly with a single well positioned radiofrequency application, confirming the focal nature of this disorder. Ablation success rates for late-onset focal tachycardia in CHD are on the order of 90%, and recurrences are uncommon. Focal atrial tachycardias account for roughly 5-10% of all atrial tachycardias targeted for catheter ablation in CHD patients, and are encountered most frequently in those with single ventricle who have undergone the Fontan operation, usually as a secondary tachycardia along with circuits of more conventional macroreentrant IART.

Atrial Fibrillation in CHD

Late-onset AF is being encountered with increasing frequency in the CHD population as a growing number of these patients advance into adulthood. The most common underlying lesions include congenital aortic valve disease,

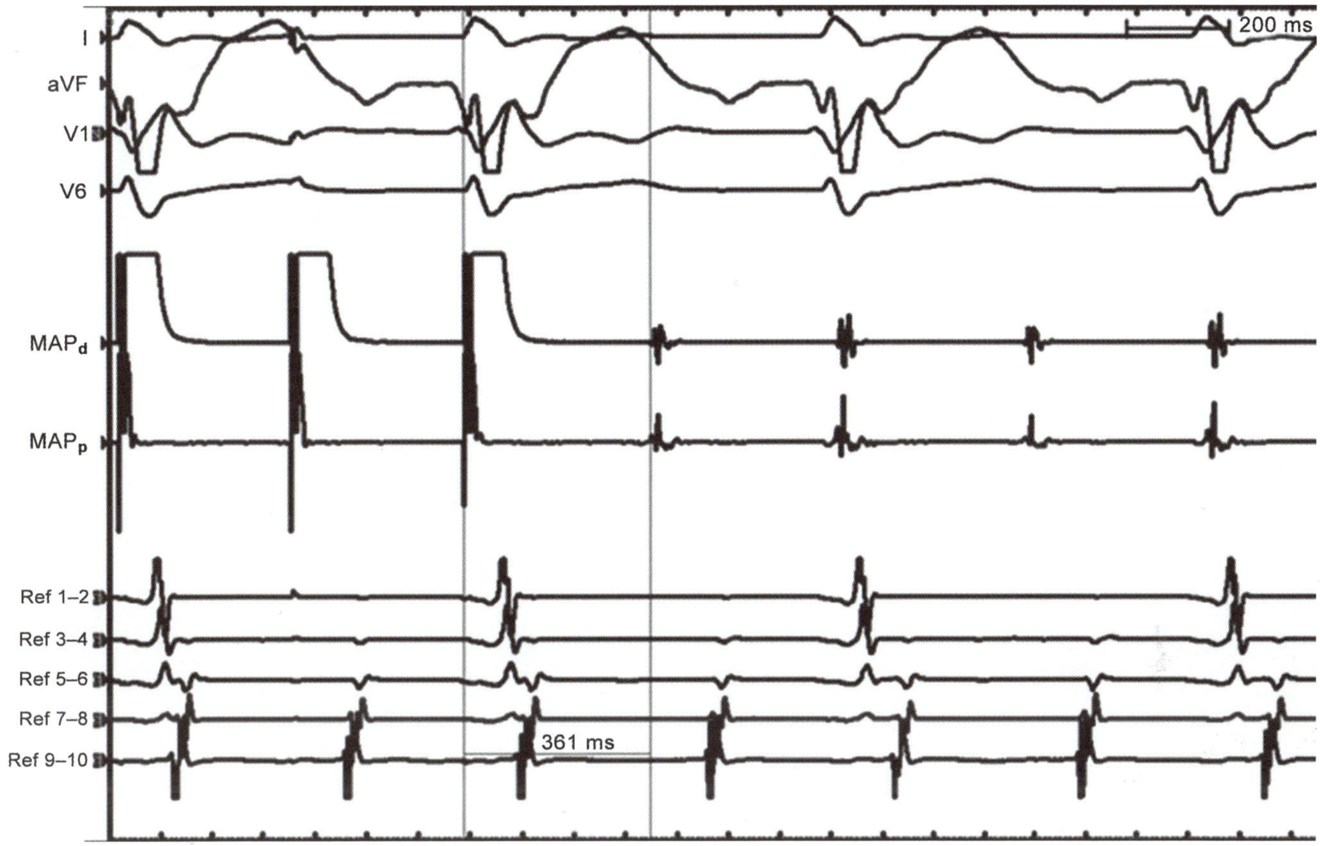

Figure 29.5: Standard entrainment maneuvers used to confirm location of intra-atrial reentrant tachycardia. The catheter tip in this case was positioned in circuit near the entrance to the zone of slow conduction. Note perfect concealed entrainment with considerable delay between the stimulus and surface P-wave. The postpacing interval was identical to the tachycardia cycle length. In addition, the stimulus to P-wave delay was identical to the electrogram to P-wave timing on the mapping catheter

mitral valve disease, palliated single ventricle, and large defects of the atrial septum.[45] These congenital lesions are logical triggers for AF since they all contribute to left atrial (LA) dilation, but the list is gradually expanding to include varieties of CHD that were previously regarded as exclusively affecting the right heart. For example, it was recently reported that up to 23% of patients will develop AF many years after straightforward atrial septal defect closure,[46] and as many as 30% of CHD patients who have undergone prior successful IART ablation may present at some later time with AF.[47] Clearly, AF is emerging as a growing concern as more CHD patients survive to middle age. The average age of onset was reported as 49 years in a recent multicenter study,[48] well below the typical age of AF onset seen in the general population. Simply put, the atrial septum cannot be viewed as an impervious barrier to histopathologic changes. It appears that any atrial insult, in combination with advancing age, can ultimately lead down a path towards AF.

Mapping in CHD patients reveals an AF pattern similar to other forms of heart disease. The most rapid and irregular fibrillatory activity is usually found within the LA in the vicinity of the pulmonary veins, with passive propagation to the RA through Bachmann's bundle and the lower atrial septum. Occasionally, atrial activity recorded from the surface electrocardiogram and the RA endocardium can look deceptively regular and organized if left-to-right conduction is limited by surgical barriers (e.g. scarring from a large atrial septal patch), causing diagnostic confusion with IART on occasion. However, direct recordings from the coronary sinus and LA endocardium will clarify the true nature of the more rapid left-sided generator.

General management of AF in CHD should adhere to standard ACC/AHA/HRS guidelines[7] in terms of anticoagulation, electrical cardioversion, and antiarrhythmic drugs. It is quite rare that CHD patients will be able to tolerate permanent AF with rate-control alone for long periods. Many have borderline hemodynamic status to begin with, and the loss of AV synchrony tends to produce intolerable symptoms. The published experience with catheter therapy for AF in the CHD population remains limited, but because the efficacy of pharmacologic therapy in maintaining sinus rhythm is so imperfect, efforts are now underway at several

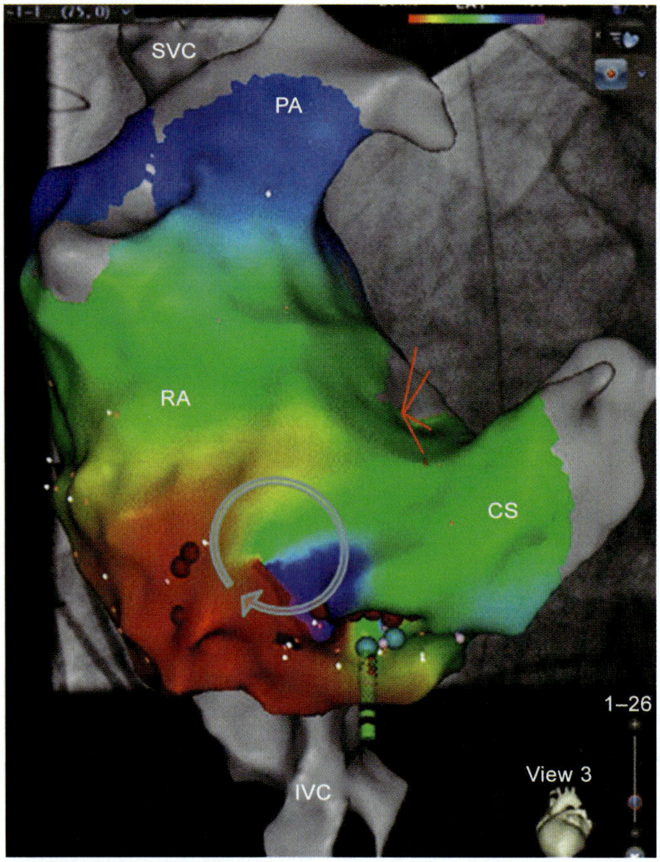

Figure 29.6: Intra-atrial reentrant tachycardia in a 28-year-old who underwent an old-style atriopulmonary Fontan operation for tricuspid atresia. A dilated right-atrium (RA) is connected to the pulmonary arteries (PA). Positions of the superior and inferior vena cava (SVC & IVC), as well as a very dilated coronary sinus (CS) are shown. The electroanatomic map indicates an unusual circuit location in the low RA near the mouth of CS

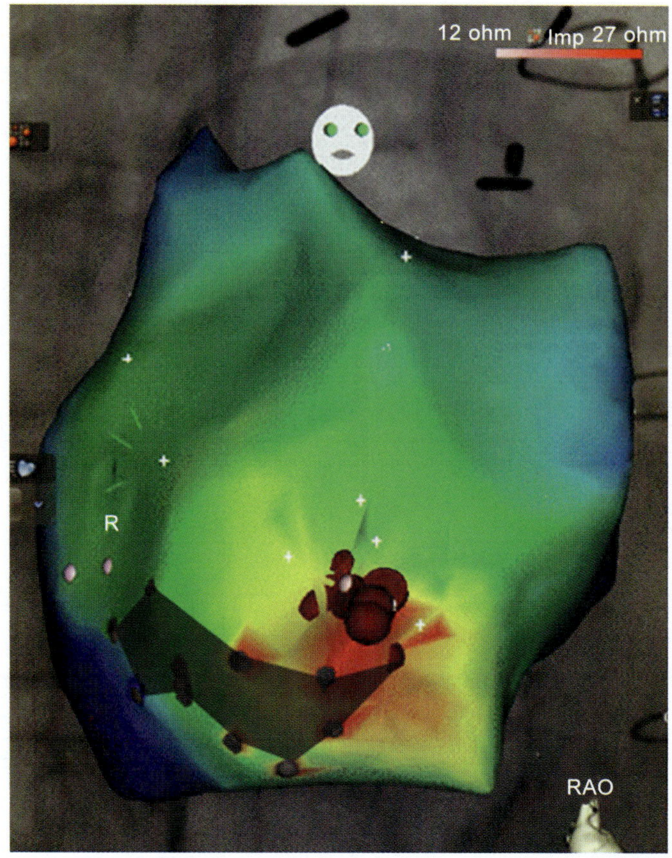

Figure 29.7: Electroanatomic map of focal atrial tachycardia in a 33-year-old who has undergone an atriopulmonary Fontan operation for single ventricle. Earliest activation (red zone) was located on the anterior wall of a very dilated right atrium, near a region of scar (gray dots and gray shaded region). Ablation in the region of earliest atrial activation successfully eliminated this tachycardia

centers to explore transcatheter pulmonary vein isolation in carefully selected patients.[49-52] Most published experience to date has involved relatively simple lesions such as atrial septal defects, though the technique is being gradually expanded to more complex anatomy (**Figure 29.8**). Trans-septal access to the LA can be more challenging than usual due to the presence of patches and septal occlusion devices,[50] but these can be crossed successfully in nearly all instances using the assistance of radiofrequency energy delivered through the needle tip.[21] Case volume is still limited and selection criteria are still being developed, but long-term success has been reported in up to 76% of CHD patients with simple 4-chamber CHD.[49] The experience remains too anecdotal for meaningful outcome analysis in more complicated lesions.

Surgical therapy also plays a role in AF management for CHD patients. If the patient is returning to the operating room for hemodynamic reasons, it may be possible to address AF with an intraoperative maze procedure.[53] Most CHD patients in whom this has been attempted fall into the categories of either Ebstein's anomaly (undergoing a Cone procedure) or single ventricle (undergoing revision of a Fontan procedure). Cryoablation encircling the pulmonary veins is the most commonly used technique, and a RA lesion set is typically added as well to address IART. Transient recurrences are seen occasionally in the early postoperative period, but the long-term freedom from AF recurrence appears to be excellent at intermediate follow-up after a surgical maze.[54,55]

ATRIAL ARRHYTHMIAS FOLLOWING OTHER CARDIAC SURGERY

Apart from the CHD population, most other cardiac surgical procedures are performed in adults who are middle-aged or older, and for whom AF is by far the most common

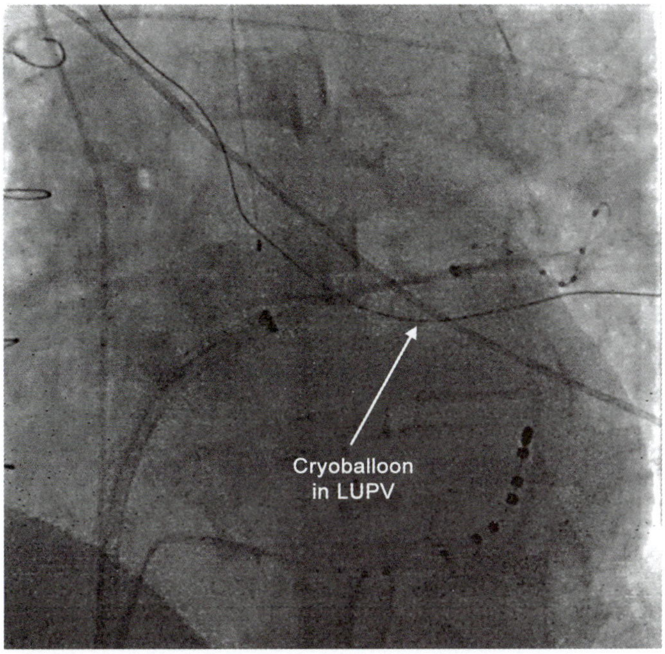

Figure 29.8: Catheter positions during successful pulmonary vein isolation procedure in a 28-year-old with aortic valve and sub-valve stenosis, who developed recurrent atrial fibrillation that could not be controlled with medical therapy. The inflated cryoballoon is located in the left upper pulmonary vein (LUPV) region

postoperative atrial arrhythmia. Occasional patients undergoing valve replacement surgery may present with macroreentrant atrial tachycardias, but even when the presenting tachycardia appears to be organized IART, some risk of AF usually coexists. This was demonstrated clearly in a 2013 report describing catheter ablation for right-sided IART in 21 subjects who had undergone prior mitral valve replacement through a right atrial incision for rheumatic disease.[56] Although ablation successfully eliminated IART, 75% of these patients still had recurrent tachycardias in the form of AF or some other a left-sided substrate soon thereafter. This experience is not surprising in light of the well-known occurrence of AF in nonpostoperative adults undergoing ablation for atrial flutter; even when flutter ablation is acutely successful, AF will emerge as a new clinical issue in more than 50% of cases over 5 years of follow-up.[57]

Early postoperative AF is an extremely common occurrence in adult patients undergoing cardiac surgery as well as some noncardiac thoracic procedures.[58,59] The reported incidence is 15–40% after coronary artery bypass, 35–50% after valve replacement, and up to 60% after combined coronary bypass and valve replacement. The peak time of onset is on the second postoperative day. It is usually a self-limited condition with a mean duration of 12 hours, but a subset of patients will have recurrent and/or sustained episodes. The window of atrial instability stretches out to about the sixth postoperative week, after which more than 90% of patients are in stable sinus rhythm. It is difficult to measure how much direct impact early postoperative AF has on longer-term rhythm status since all of these patients have pre-existent cardiac pathology that could predispose them to future AF events even if they had not undergone surgery.

Despite its transient nature, postoperative AF is associated with increased length of hospital stay, thromboembolic complications, and increased overall operative mortality.[60] Its cause appears to be multifactorial, with potential triggers involving a combination of direct surgical trauma, inflammatory and oxidative stress, ischemia, disruption of autonomic innervation, and elevated catecholamines.[61] There is a long list of associated risk factors which includes advanced age, left ventricular dysfunction, obesity, chronic obstructive pulmonary disease, metabolic syndrome, atrial enlargement on electrocardiogram, and others.[62] Of interest, postoperative AF may involve a somewhat different electrophysiologic mechanism than conventional AFl; some studies suggest it is not prevented or eliminated by traditional pulmonary vein isolation,[63] possibly indicating a more diffuse atrial process.

Extensive efforts have been made to develop strategies for prevention of postoperative AF. Clinical trials involving thousands of subjects have investigated a wide variety of approaches, such as: (1) Prophylactic administration of beta-blockers and other antiarrhythmic drugs,[64] (2) Atrial pacing to prevent sinus pauses and other atrial irregularities,[65] (3) Creation of a posterior pericardiotomy incision to prevent pericardial fluid accumulation,[66] (4) Anterior fat pad preservation to minimize disruption of autonomic ganglia,[67] (5) Tight perioperative glucose control,[68] and (6) A wide assortment of agents to combat inflammation and oxidative stress including steroids, statins, fish oil, colchicine, and vitamins.[69-71] All these options have shown benefits in selected studies, but because postoperative AF is such a multifactorial problem, none has proven universally effective.

CONCLUSION

Maintenance of sinus atrial rhythm optimizes hemodynamics, reduces thromboembolic events, decreases overall mortality, improves a patient's quality of life, and reduces medical costs. Whenever cardiac surgical procedures become necessary to address a grave anatomic concern like CHD or serious acquired heart disease, the electrical equilibrium of atrial tissue is put to the test, and atrial rhythm disorders can develop as a result. A large arsenal of treatment options has evolved to address postoperative atrial tachycardias, but all are palliative, and none actually restores intra-atrial conduction back to its normal state. There is some hope that the current generation of CHD patients may escape degenerative atrial changes thanks to modern surgical approaches that emphasize earlier repair with less direct mechanical insult to atrial myocardium.

REFERENCES

1. Gross RE. Surgical management of the patent ductus arteriosus, with summary of four surgically treated cases. Ann Surg. 1939;110:321-56.
2. Walsh EP. Interventional electrophysiology in patients with congenital heart disease. Circulation. 2007;115:3224-34.
3. Bouchardy J, Therrien J, Pilote L, Ionescu-Ittu R, Martucci G, Bottega N, Marelli AJ. Atrial arrhythmias in adults with congenital heart disease. Circulation. 2009;120:1679-86.
4. Love BA, Barrett KS, Alexander ME, Bevilacqua LM, Epstein MR, Triedman JK, Walsh EP, Berul CI. Supraventricular arrhythmias in children and young adults with implantable cardioverter defibrillators. J Cardiovasc Electrophysiol. 2001;12:1097-101.
5. Kumar S, Tedrow UB, Triedman JK. Arrhythmias in adult congenital heart disease: diagnosis and management. Cardiol Clin. 2015;33:571-88.
6. Walsh EP. Arrhythmias in patients with congenital heart disease. Card Electrophysiol Rev. 2002;6:422-30.
7. January CT, Wann LS, Alpert JS, Calkins H, Cigarroa JE, Cleveland JC, Jr., Conti JB, Ellinor PT, Ezekowitz MD, Field ME, Murray KT, Sacco RL, Stevenson WG, Tchou PJ, Tracy CM, Yancy CW. 2014 AHA/ACC/HRS guideline for the management of patients with atrial fibrillation: executive summary: a report of the American College of Cardiology/American Heart Association Task Force on practice guidelines and the Heart Rhythm Society. Circulation. 2014;130:2071-104.
8. Rhodes LA, Walsh EP, Saul JP. Conversion of atrial flutter in pediatric patients by transesophageal atrial pacing: a safe, effective, minimally invasive procedure. Am Heart J. 1995;130:323-7.
9. Hoyer AW, Balaji S. The safety and efficacy of ibutilide in children and in patients with congenital heart disease. Pacing Clin Electrophysiol. 2007;30:1003-8.
10. Triedman JK. Atrial reentrant tachycardias. In: Walsh EP, Saul JP, Triedman JK (Eds). Cardiac arrhythmias in children and young adults with congenital heart disease. Philadelphia, Lippincott Williams and Wilkins; 2001. pp. 137-60.
11. Triedman JK, Bergau DM, Saul JP, Epstein MR, Walsh EP. Efficacy of radiofrequency ablation for control of intraatrial reentrant tachycardia in patients with congenital heart disease. J Am Coll Cardiol. 1997;30:1032-8.
12. Collins KK, Love BA, Walsh EP, Saul JP, Epstein MR, Triedman JK. Location of acutely successful radiofrequency catheter ablation of intraatrial reentrant tachycardia in patients with congenital heart disease. Am J Cardiol. 2000;86:969-74.
13. Mah DY, Alexander ME, Cecchin F, Walsh EP, Triedman JK. The electroanatomic mechanisms of atrial tachycardia in patients with tetralogy of Fallot and double outlet right ventricle. J Cardiovasc Electrophysiol. 2011;22:1013-7.
14. Kanter RJ, Papagiannis J, Carboni MP, Ungerleider RM, Sanders WE, Wharton JM. Radiofrequency catheter ablation of supraventricular tachycardia substrates after Mustard and Senning operations for d-transposition of the great arteries. J Am Coll Cardiol. 2000;35:428-41.
15. Perry JC1, Boramanand NK, Ing FF. "Transseptal" technique through atrial baffles for 3-dimensional mapping and ablation of atrial tachycardia in patients with d-transposition of the great arteries. J Interv Card Electrophysiol. 2003;9:365-9.
16. Ernst S, Babu-Narayan SV, Keegan J, Horduna I, Lyne J, Till J, Kilner PJ, Pennell D, Rigby ML, Gatzoulis MA. Remote-controlled magnetic navigation and ablation with 3D image integration as an alternative approach in patients with intra-atrial baffle anatomy. Circ Arrhythm Electrophysiol. 2012;5:131-9.
17. Fishberger SB, Wernovsky G, Gentles TL, Horduna I, Lyne J, Till J, Kilner PJ, Pennell D, Rigby ML, Gatzoulis MA. Factors that influence the development of atrial flutter after the Fontan operation. J Thorac Cardiovasc Surg. 1997;113:80-6.
18. Cecchin F, Johnsrude CL, Perry JC, Friedman RA. Effect of age and surgical technique on symptomatic arrhythmias after the Fontan procedure. Am J Cardiol. 1995;76:386-91.
19. Mavroudis C, Backer CL, Deal BJ, Johnsrude C, Strasburger J. Total cavopulmonary conversion and maze procedure for patients with failure of the Fontan operation. J Thorac Cardiovasc Surg. 2001;122:863-71.
20. Stamm C, Friehs I, Mayer JE Jr, Zurakowski D, Triedman JK, Moran AM, Walsh EP, Lock JE, Jonas RA, Del Nido PJ. Long-term results of the lateral tunnel Fontan operation. J Thorac Cardiovasc Surg. 2001;121:28-41.
21. Esch JJ, Triedman JK, Cecchin F, Alexander ME, Walsh EP. Radiofrequency-assisted transseptal perforation for electrophysiology procedures in children and adults with repaired congenital heart disease. Pacing Clin Electrophysiol. 2013;36:607-11.
22. Correa R, Sherwin ED, Kovach J, Mah DY, Alexander ME, Cecchin F, Walsh EP, Triedman JK, Abrams DJ. Mechanism and ablation of arrhythmia following total cavopulmonary connection. Circ Arrhythm Electrophysiol. 2015;8:318-25.
23. Triedman JK, Alexander MA, Love BA, Collins KK, Berul CI, Bevilacqua LM, Walsh EP. Influence of patient factors and ablative technologies on outcomes of radiofrequency ablation of intra-atrial tachycardia in patients with congenital heart disease. J Am Coll Cardiol. 2002;39:1827-35.
24. Love BA, Collins KK, Walsh EP, Triedman JK. Electroanatomic characterization of conduction barriers in sinus/atrially paced rhythm and association with intra-atrial reentrant tachycardia circuits following congenital heart disease surgery. J Cardiovasc Electrophysiol. 2001;12:17-25.
25. Anderson RH, Ho SY. The disposition of the conduction tissues in congenitally malformed hearts with reference to their embryological development. J Perinat Med. 1991;19(Suppl 1):201-6.
26. Anderson RH, Brown NA, Moorman AF. The sinus node, isomerism, and heterotaxy. Cardiovasc Pathol. 2013;22:243-4.
27. Wolf CM, Seslar SP, den Boer K, Juraszek AL, McGowan FX, Cowan DB, Del Nido P, Triedman JK, Berul CI, Walsh EP. Atrial remodeling after the Fontan operation. Am J Cardiol. 2009;104:1737-42.
28. Blaufox AD, Numan MT, Laohakunakorn P, Knick B, Paul T, Saul JP. Catheter tip cooling during radiofrequency ablation of intra-atrial reentry: effects on power, temperature, and impedance. J Cardiovasc Electrophysiol. 2002;13:783-7.
29. de Groot NM, Schalij MJ, Zeppenfeld K, Blom NA, Van der Velde ET, Van der Wall EE. Voltage and activation mapping: how the recording technique affects the outcome of catheter ablation procedures in patients with congenital heart disease. Circulation. 2003;108:2099-106.
30. Tanner H, Lukac P, Schwick N, Fuhrer J, Pedersen AK, Hansen PS, Delacretaz E. Irrigated-tip catheter ablation of intraatrial reentrant tachycardia in patients late after surgery of congenital heart disease. Heart Rhythm. 2004;1:268-75.

31. Lukac P, Pedersen AK, Mortensen PT, Jensen HK, Hjortdal V, Hansen PS. Ablation of atrial tachycardia after surgery for congenital and acquired heart disease using an electroanatomic mapping system: Which circuits to expect in which substrate? Heart Rhythm. 2005;2:64-72.
32. Ueda A, Suman-Horduna I, Mantziari L, Gujic M, Marchese P, Ho SY, Babu-Narayan SV, Ernst S. Contemporary outcomes of supraventricular tachycardia ablation in congenital heart disease: a single-center experience in 116 patients. Circ Arrhythm Electrophysiol. 2013;6:606-13.
33. Anguera I, Dallaglio P, Macías R, Jimenez-Candil J, Peinado R, Garcia-Seara J, Arcocha MF, Herreros B, Quesada A, Hernandez-Madrid A, Alvarez M, Filgueiras D, Matia R, Cequier A, Sabate X. Long-term outcome after ablation of right atrial tachyarrhythmias after the surgical repair of congenital and acquired heart disease. Am J Cardiol. 2015;115:1705-13.
34. Flinn CJ, Wolff GS, Dick M, 2nd, Campbell RM, Borkat G, Casta A, Hordof A, Hougen TJ, Kavey RE, Kugler J, et al. Cardiac rhythm after the Mustard operation for complete transposition of the great arteries. N Engl J Med. 1984;310:1635-8.
35. Manning PB, Mayer JE Jr, Wernovsky G, Fishberger SB, Walsh EP. Staged operation to Fontan increases the incidence of sinoatrial node dysfunction. J Thorac Cardiovasc Surg. 1996;111:833-9.
36. Rhodes LA, Walsh EP, Gamble WJ, Triedman JK, Saul JP. Benefits and potential risks of atrial antitachycardia pacing after repair of congenital heart disease. Pacing Clin Electrophysiol. 1995;18:1005-16.
37. Drago F, Silvetti MS, Grutter G, De Santis A. Long term management of atrial arrhythmias in young patients with sick sinus syndrome undergoing early operation to correct congenital heart disease. Europace. 2006;8:488-94.
38. Stephenson EA, Casavant D, Tuzi J, Alexander ME, Law I, Serwer G, Strieper M, Walsh EP, Berul CI. Efficacy of atrial antitachycardia pacing using the Medtronic AT500 pacemaker in patients with congenital heart disease. Am J Cardiol. 2003;92:871-6.
39. Epstein AE, DiMarco JP, Ellenbogen KA, Estes NA, 3rd, Freedman RA, Gettes LS, Gillinov AM, Gregoratos G, Hammill SC, Hayes DL, Hlatky MA, Newby LK, Page RL, Schoenfeld MH, Silka MJ, Stevenson LW, Sweeney MO, Smith SC, Jr., Jacobs AK, Adams CD, Anderson JL, Buller CE, Creager MA, Ettinger SM, Faxon DP, Halperin JL, Hiratzka LF, Hunt SA, Krumholz HM, Kushner FG, Lytle BW, Nishimura RA, Ornato JP, Riegel B, Tarkington LG, Yancy CW. ACC/AHA/HRS 2008 Guidelines for Device-Based Therapy of Cardiac Rhythm Abnormalities: a report of the American College of Cardiology/American Heart Association Task Force on Practice Guidelines (Writing Committee to Revise the ACC/AHA/NASPE 2002 Guideline Update for Implantation of Cardiac Pacemakers and Antiarrhythmia Devices) developed in collaboration with the American Association for Thoracic Surgery and Society of Thoracic Surgeons. J Am Coll Cardiol. 2008;51:e1-62.
40. Walsh EP, Cecchin F. Recent advances in pacemaker and implantable defibrillator therapy for young patients. Curr Opin Cardiol. 2004;19:91-6.
41. Khairy P, Landzberg MJ, Gatzoulis MA, Mercier LA, Fernandes SM, Cote JM, Lavoie JP, Fournier A, Guerra PG, Frogoudaki A, Walsh EP, Dore A. Transvenous pacing leads and systemic thromboemboli in patients with intracardiac shunts: a multicenter study. Circulation. 2006;113:2391-7.
42. Rosales AM1, Walsh EP, Wessel DL, Triedman JK. Postoperative ectopic atrial tachycardia in children with congenital heart disease. Am J Cardiol. 2001;88:1169-72.
43. Seslar SP, Alexander ME, Berul CI, Cecchin F, Walsh EP, Triedman JK. Ablation of non-automatic focal atrial tachycardia in children and adults with congenital heart disease. J Cardiovasc Electrophysiol. 2006;17:359-65.
44. de Groot NM, Zeppenfeld K, Wijffels MC, Chan WK, Blom NA, Van der Wall EE, Schalij MJ. Ablation of focal atrial arrhythmia in patients with congenital heart defects after surgery: role of circumscribed areas with heterogeneous conduction. Heart Rhythm. 2006;3:526-35.
45. Kirsh JA, Walsh EP, Triedman JK. Prevalence of and risk factors for atrial fibrillation and intraatrial reentrant tachycardia among patients with congenital heart disease. Am J Cardiol. 2002;90:338-40.
46. Katritsis DG. Transseptal puncture through atrial septal closure devices. Heart Rhythm. 2011;8:1676-7.
47. Teh AW, Medi C, Lee G, Rosso R, Sparks PB, Morton JB, Kistler PM, Halloran K, Vohra JK, Kalman JM. Long-term outcome following ablation of atrial flutter occurring late after atrial septal defect repair. Pacing Clin Electrophysiol. 2011;34:431-5.
48. Teuwen CP, Ramdjan TT, Götte M, Brundel BJ, Evertz R, Vriend JW, Molhoek SG, Dorman HG, van Opstal JM, Konings TC, van der Voort P, Delacretaz E, Houck C, Yaksh A, Jansz LJ, Witsenburg M, Roos-Hesselink JW, Triedman JK, Bogers AJ, de Groot NM. Time course of atrial fibrillation in patients with congenital heart defects. Circ Arrhythm Electrophysiol. 2015;8:1065-72.
49. Lakkireddy D, Rangisetty U, Prasad S, Verma A, Biria M, Berenbom L, Pimentel R, Emert M, Rosamond T, Fahmy T, Patel D, Di Biase L, Schweikert R, Burkhardt D, Natale A. Intracardiac echo-guided radiofrequency catheter ablation of atrial fibrillation in patients with atrial septal defect or patent foramen ovale repair: A feasibility, safety, and efficacy study. J Cardiovasc Electrophysiol. 2008;19:1137-42.
50. McCready JW, Moon JC, Chow AW. Right to left shunt following radiofrequency catheter ablation of atrial fibrillation in a patient with complex congenital heart disease. Europace. 2010;12:289-90.
51. Philip F, Muhammad KI, Agarwal S, Natale A, Krasuski RA. Pulmonary vein isolation for the treatment of drug-refractory atrial fibrillation in adults with congenital heart disease. Congenit Heart Dis. 2012;7:392-9.
52. Sherwin ED, Triedman JK, Walsh EP. Update on interventional electrophysiology in congenital heart disease: evolving solutions for complex hearts. Circ Arrhythm Electrophysiol. 2013;6:1032-40.
53. Jang WS, Kim WH, Choi K, Nam J, Choi ES, Lee JR, Kim YJ, Kwon BS, Kim GB, Bae EJ. The mid-term surgical results of Fontan conversion with antiarrhythmia surgery. Eur J Cardiothorac Surg. 2014;45:922-7.
54. Backer CL, Tsao S, Deal BJ, Mavroudis C. Maze procedure in single ventricle patients. Semin Thorac Cardiovasc Surg Pediatr Card Surg Annu. 2008;1:44-8.
55. Mavroudis C, Deal BJ, Backer CL, Tsao S. Arrhythmia surgery in patients with and without congenital heart disease. Ann Thorac Surg. 2008;86:857-68.

56. Chen H, Yang B, Ju W, Zhang F, Gu K, Li M, Wang J, Cao K, Chen M. Long-term outcome following ablation of atrial tachycardias occurring after mitral valve replacement in patients with rheumatic heart disease. Pacing Clin Electrophysiol. 2013;36:795-802.
57. Gilligan DM, Zakaib JS, Fuller I, Shepard RK, Dan D, Wood MA, Clemo HF, Stambler BS, Ellenbogen KA. Long-term outcome of patients after successful radiofrequency ablation for typical atrial flutter. Pacing Clin Electrophysiol. 2003;26:53-8.
58. Yadava M, Hughey AB, Crawford TC. Postoperative atrial fibrillation: incidence, mechanisms, and clinical correlates. Cardiol Clin. 2014;32:627-36.
59. Joshi KK, Tiru M, Chin T, Fox MT, Stefan MS. Postoperative atrial fibrillation in patients undergoing non-cardiac non-thoracic surgery: A practical approach for the hospitalist. Hosp Pract. 2015;43:235-44.
60. Lahtinen J, Biancari F, Salmela E, Mosorin M, Satta J, Rainio P, Rimpilainen J, Lepojarvi M, Juvonen T. Postoperative atrial fibrillation is a major cause of stroke after on-pump coronary artery bypass surgery. Ann Thorac Surg. 2004;77:1241-4.
61. Zakkar M, Ascione R, James AF, Angelini GD, Suleiman MS. Inflammation, oxidative stress and postoperative atrial fibrillation in cardiac surgery. Pharmacol Ther. 2015;154:13-20.
62. Raiten JM, Ghadimi K, Augoustides JG, Ramakrishna H, Patel PA, Weiss SJ, Gutsche JT. Atrial fibrillation after cardiac surgery: clinical update on mechanisms and prophylactic strategies. J Cardiothorac Vasc Anesth. 2015;29:806-16.
63. Kiaii B, Fox S, Chase L, Fernandes M, Stitt LW, Guo R, Quantz M, Chu MW, Koka P, McClure RS, McKenzie FN, Klein GJ, Novick RJ, Skanes AC. Postoperative atrial fibrillation is not pulmonary vein dependent: results from a randomized trial. Heart Rhythm. 2015;12:699-705.
64. Turagam MK, Downey FX, Kress DC, Sra J, Tajik AJ, Jahangir A. Pharmacological strategies for prevention of postoperative atrial fibrillation. Expert Rev Clin Pharmacol. 2015;8:233-50.
65. Shea J, Sodhi G, Najam F, Solomon AJ. Does the addition of atrial pacing to amiodarone reduce the incidence of post-operative atrial fibrillation: a pilot study. J Thorac Cardiovasc Surg. 2014;148:1752-3.
66. Kuralay E, Ozal E, Demirkili U, Tatar H. Effect of posterior pericardiotomy on postoperative supraventricular arrhythmias and late pericardial effusion. J Thorac Cardiovasc Surg. 1999; 118:492-5.
67. Cummings JE, Gill I, Akhrass R, Dery M, Biblo LA, Quan KJ. Preservation of the anterior fat pad paradoxically decreases the incidence of postoperative atrial fibrillation in humans. J Am Coll Cardiol. 2004;43:994-1000.
68. Chishaki A, Chishaki H. Postoperative high blood glucose—a potentially treatable marker related to atrial fibrillation after coronary artery bypass grafting. Circ J. 2015;79:45-6.
69. Viviano A, Kanagasabay R, Zakkar M. Is perioperative corticosteroid administration associated with a reduced incidence of postoperative atrial fibrillation in adult cardiac surgery? Interact Cardiovasc Thorac Surg. 2014;18:225-9.
70. Yoo D, Vinten-Johansen J, Schmarkey LS. Adhesive epicardial corticosteroids prevent postoperative atrial fibrillation. Circ Arrhythm Electrophysiol. 2010;3:505-10.
71. Worden JC, Asare K. Postoperative atrial fibrillation: role of inflammatory biomarkers and use of colchicine for its prevention. Pharmacotherapy. 2014;34:1167-73.

SECTION E

Ventricular Tachyarrhythmias

CHAPTER 30

George Shaw, David Callans

Introduction to Ventricular Arrhythmias

LIST OF ABBREVIATIONS

ARVC	Arrhythmogenic Right Ventricular Cardiomyopathy	LV	Left Ventricle
AV	Atrioventricular	PVC	Premature Ventricular Contraction
CCB	Calcium Channel Blocker	SAECG	Signal Averaged Electrocardiogram
EP	Electrophysiology	VA	Ventriculoatrial
ICD	Implantable Cardioverter-Defibrillator	VT	Ventricular Tachycardia

INTRODUCTION

Sudden cardiac death is a leading cause of mortality, with an incidence of 300,000 to 450,000 deaths per year in the United States alone.[1] And while most people who suffer sudden cardiac death have coronary disease, only a small fraction suffers myocardial infarction precipitating their demise. Ventricular ectopy can also contribute to heart failure. Recognizing, understanding the pathophysiology, and knowing the treatment options for these arrhythmias is paramount to making a dent in this sobering statistic. But this is also a fascinating field, rich in complexity and nuance of forms and mechanisms and treatments. First one must recognize ventricular arrhythmias, and though they are usually wide complex rhythms on 12 lead ECG, this task is sometimes more challenging than expected. The urgency of evaluation and intervention is then dependent on the patient's symptom severity and risk of deterioration. This chapter will review the broad range of disease processes that originate distal to the atrioventricular (AV) node, ranging from rare premature ventricular contractions (PVCs) to ventricular tachycardia (VT) and fibrillation. The goal here is not to overwhelm but to help the reader approach a complex but rewarding field.

ETIOLOGY AND PATHOPHYSIOLOGY

Ventricular ectopy can occur by many mechanisms. The presence of prior ischemia and scar affects the likelihood by which a wide complex rhythm is in fact VT, and the likely mechanism. VT can be broadly classified in disorders of impulse conduction and disorders of impulse formation. Reentrant mechanisms are perhaps the best known of these and are disorders of impulse conduction. Reentrant arrhythmias rely on electrical wavefronts traveling around a functional or anatomic block. These are rather common in patients with old infarcts who now have areas of infarcted tissues or regions of diseased tissue with slow conduction. They can also been seen in patients with previous surgery, infiltrative diseases (including some infectious processes), and connective tissue disorders, such as arrhythmogenic right ventricular cardiomyopathy (ARVC).

Structurally normal hearts can also sustain ventricular tachycardia via a reentrant mechanism, usually utilizing the native conduction system. Examples include bundle branch reentrant VT and fascicular VT.

Abnormalities of impulse formation describes the mechanism by which premature ventricular depolarizations frequently occur, which may serve as triggers for ventricular fibrillation and many sustained VT episodes. Impulse formation includes the concepts of both automaticity and triggered activity. Normal automaticity is seen in the conduction system of healthy individuals. Abnormal automaticity can be seen in both healthy and diseased myocardium. Unlike normal automaticity, abnormal automaticity is usually calcium dependent, not sodium dependent (and therefore poorly responsive to sodium channel blockade), and it cannot be suppressed by overdrive pacing. Worse, abnormal automaticity is often exacerbated by pacing and by adrenergic stimulation, so overdrive pacing can exacerbate arrhythmias leading to requirement of cardioversion or defibrillation, resulting in rapid and dramatic decompensation. This highlights the importance of considering underlying ventricular pathophysiology—abnormal impulse formation versus conduction—when formulating a treatment plan.

Triggered activity also falls under the rubric of abnormal impulse formation. Triggered activity commonly manifests as benign premature contractions, classically caffeine-induced, but it can be critically important in certain forms of PVC-triggered ventricular tachycardia (particularly outflow tract VT) or fibrillation episodes.

ECG EVALUATION AND DIFFERENTIAL DIAGNOSIS

Wide complex tachycardia on 12-lead ECG can be ventricular or supraventricular in origin. Similarly, though rare, narrow complex tachycardias can be VT originating from the His-Purkinje system. It is important to make as accurate a diagnosis as possible with the information available. Though it is true that a wide complex rhythm is most likely ventricular tachycardia in the setting of known coronary disease and structural heart disease, any such rhythm must be distinguished from other wide complex rhythms including baseline or rate-dependent aberrant conduction and ventricular preexcitation via an accessory pathway. In the urgent setting, such a rhythm should be treated as ventricular tachycardia by default.

Ventricular tachycardia is definitively diagnosed on 12-lead ECG only by evidence of atrioventricular dissociation (possibly manifested by capture beats). Such ECG features are more often found in textbooks than in clinical encounters. If one does not have direct evidence of AV dissociation, then diagnosing ventricular tachycardia requires accumulating evidence from the patient's history and ECG to support the diagnosis of either supraventricular versus ventricular tachycardia. Fortunately there exist additional morphologic criteria to support the diagnosis of VT. The Brugada criteria are the most well-known of such schema, though others exist.[2] Instead of following such schema, however, it would be wise to consider the physiology of normal ventricular depolarization and how changes in the surface ECG may or may not be consistent with normal depolarization.

A northwest or extreme axis of the QRS in the frontal plane (negative in I and II) is most likely VT. When evaluating wide complex rhythms with a right bundle branch block morphology, the following features are highly suggestive of ventricular tachycardia: monophasic R, Rsr', or qR in V1; QRS wider than 140 ms; S wave greater than the R in V6. Consider that these features suggest ventricular depolarization predominantly toward the right shoulder, away from the apex. When evaluating a left bundle branch block morphology rhythm, the following criteria suggest VT: overall QRS wider than 160 ms; an initial r wave in V1 longer than 40 ms; notched S downstroke in V1; time from the beginning of the QRS complex to the maximum S wave deflection longer than 80 ms (the intrinsicoid deflection).[3] The findings suggest myocardial depolarization through diseased tissue far away from the His-Purkinje system. Much like an extreme axis, concordance (either positive or negative) in the precordial leads also suggests VT, because these activation patterns suggest initial ventricular activation far away from the native conduction system. It can't be overemphasized that morphologic criteria are imperfect and exceptions can be found to every rule.

If the diagnosis remains elusive, clinical observations and maneuvers during stable tachycardia may be helpful. Physical examination (cannon A waves in the jugular pulse or marked variation in the intensity of the first heart sound) can sometimes allow diagnosis of AV dissociation that is not apparent in the ECG. Carotid massage or Valsalva maneuvers may terminate the tachycardia, suggesting an AV node dependent mechanism, or increase the degree the AV block revealing AV or VA dissociation. AHA/ACC/HRS Advanced Cardiac Life Support guidelines instruct adenosine administration as a next step. However, adenosine can precipitate hypotension and compensatory adrenergic surge, as well as coronary steal and hemodynamic compromise in an already tenuous patient. Adenosine should be avoided if at all possible for the purpose of diagnosis of a wide QRS tachycardia.

TYPES OF VENTRICULAR ARRHYTHMIAS

Ventricular arrhythmia can manifest in many different ways, ranging from rare premature ventricular depolarizations to triggered ventricular fibrillation. The specific arrhythmias and underlying pathophysiology guide medical and interventional treatments, including evaluation for an implantable pacemaker or defibrillator. More information about each of the following arrhythmias will be discussed in subsequent chapters.

Premature Ventricular Contractions

Infrequent, isolated premature ventricular depolarizations are rarely themselves a problem, though they may be a marker of more significant disease. Premature ventricular contractions (PVCs), even just 5% of total beats, can cause significant symptoms or contribute to cardiomyopathy and heart failure. Ablation of PVCs can alleviate symptoms and reverse cardiomyopathy. It is also important to note that PVCs can also be a reproducible trigger for ventricular tachycardia or fibrillation. Such cases are not common, and they usually occur in the setting of a structurally abnormal heart, but it is important to recognize that in these patients the PVC may be the primary target to eliminate.

Nonsustained Ventricular Tachycardia

Nonsustained ventricular tachycardia, being longer than three beats and self-terminating within 30 seconds, is evaluated somewhat differently than sustained VT. Patients with nonsustained VT require evaluation for structural heart disease. Many patients with nonsustained VT are asymptomatic. Those patients, if they have an otherwise normal heart, are at no increased risk of sudden death and may require no further evaluation. If they have documented structural heart disease, however, they require an evaluation for myocardial ischemia with consideration for revascularization. Similarly, medications and electrolytes must be reviewed to correct any proarrhythmic effects. An electrophysiology (EP) study may help guide subsequent management in some cases. Two landmark trials, MUSTT[4] and MADIT I[5], demonstrated mortality benefit in patients given implantable cardioverter-defibrillators (ICDs) if they had structural heart disease, nonsustained VT, and inducible VT during an EP study. These criteria are rarely considered now because they have been superseded by later studies that demonstrated mortality benefit in patients with left ventricular systolic dysfunction regardless of known clinical or inducible ventricular arrhythmias.

Sustained Monomorphic Ventricular Tachycardia

Sustained monomorphic VT can be seen in many settings most common of which is coronary artery disease and healed infarct. This is also the scenario where we have the most data for medical treatment and primary and secondary prevention with ICDs. An interventional approach is sometimes needed, however, due to recurrent or medication-refractory VT. New presentations of VT should prompt a complete evaluation, even if the patient has known coronary disease, to evaluate for active ischemia, proarrhythmic medications, electrolyte abnormalities or new nonischemic cardiomyopathy.

Dilated cardiomyopathy is notable due to the challenge of finding an underlying etiology. Underlying causes include common problems such as ischemic heart disease or viral myocarditis and more unusual genetic or infectious causes such as lamin A/C deficiency or Chagas disease. The differential is very broad and must be guided by a patient's presentation and history.[6] Frequently, no underlying etiology for dilated cardiomyopathy can be found and therapy is empirical. EP studies are not adequate to risk stratify patients, and medication therapy does not adequately mitigate the risk of sudden cardiac death, hence, an ICD is often indicated.

Infiltrative diseases, such as sarcoidosis and amyloidosis, can create focal or diffuse infiltrates almost anywhere. In the conduction system, these processes may lead to sinus node dysfunction or heart block.[7] In the ventricular myocardium, these processes may lead to irritable foci or an anatomic region of block, creating functional scenarios for both automatic and reentrant VT. Interestingly, these processes are oftentimes treatable with a reasonable expectation for improvement in myocardial and conduction system function. There is much yet to be learned about the pathology and optimal management of these processes.

Arrhythmogenic right ventricular cardiomyopathy (ARVC) is a genetic, autosomal dominant, desmosomal disorder resulting in gradual fibro-fatty tissue replacement in the heart. It is usually identified first in the right ventricle primarily because the right ventricle is relatively thin walled, however the process affects both the right and the left ventricles.[8] Ablation in these patients can often relieve incessant VT and patients can do quite well.[9]

Outflow tract ventricular tachycardias are an interesting form of idiopathic VT. They are a form of triggered or automatic VT related to delayed afterdepolarizations.[10] Though outflow tract VT is rarely sustained or life-threatening, it can be highly symptomatic and contribute to cardiomyopathy. These rhythms are frequently provoked by exercise, stress or anxiety, or by stimulants like caffeine. As the mechanism is dependent on intracellular calcium release, outflow tract VT is typically terminated by intravenous adenosine, and it may be treated successfully with beta blockers or calcium channel antagonists. Radiofrequency ablation is often curative as well, and should be considered in patients with symptoms despite medical therapy.

Fascicular ventricular tachycardia—also known as idiopathic left VT and Bellhasen VT—is similarly due to a triggered mechanism[11] related to calcium loading and can be acutely responsive to calcium channel blockers (CCB).[12] This VT is classically associated with the left ventricular (LV) Purkinje fibers, and as such typically has a right bundle branch block pattern in VT. If one is unsure of the diagnosis, however, CCBs should be avoided due to mortality associated with these agents in VT.

Polymorphic Ventricular Tachycardia

Polymorphic VT is a form of VT with multiple circuits or foci, resulting in multiple wide complex morphologies during a single event. Torsade de pointes is a classic example: pause-dependent polymorphic VT associated with prolonged QT interval. Another example is a bidirectional VT, classically associated with digoxin toxicity or catecholaminergic polymorphic VT.[13] Fortunately, digoxin toxicity is seen rarely in the current practice. Besides these specific examples, it is important to remember that polymorphic VT is most commonly associated with acute myocardial ischemia, and therefore patients with polymorphic VT must be evaluated promptly for active ischemia and revascularized if indicated.[14] After this, consideration should be given to medication overdoses or interactions, electrolyte abnormalities, and genetic abnormalities such as long QT syndrome. Carefully review of available telemetry and intracardiac electrocardiograms for the possibility of PVC-triggered polymorphic VT is essential. ICD implantation is usually indicated in cases of polymorphic VT[15] if no treatable and reversible cause is responsible; antiarrhythmic medications sometimes play an adjunctive role.

NONINVASIVE EVALUATION OF VENTRICULAR ARRHYTHMIAS

When a patient presents acutely with wide complex tachyarrhythmia, they should be evaluated for hemodynamic stability and managed as per the familiar advanced cardiac life support guidelines. If a patient is hemodynamically unstable, cardioversion or defibrillation should be performed immediately. If the patient is stable, one may have the luxury of considering a differential diagnosis, including supraventricular tachycardia with aberrancy or preexcitation versus ventricular tachycardia. Obtaining a 12-lead ECG of the arrhythmia can be very valuable later for diagnostic evaluation and procedural planning. Having diagnosed ventricular tachycardia, it is important to consider active myocardial ischemia and refer the patient for emergent cardiac catheterization if coronary ischemia is likely. Ultimately a patient with newly diagnosed ventricular tachycardia will need some form of evaluation for coronary disease—usually coronary angiography but it could also include coronary CT or stress testing—in addition to substrate evaluation and arrhythmia burden. Transthoracic echocardiography and cardiac MRI effectively evaluate overall cardiac function, relative wall motion abnormalities, valvular dysfunction, and possible infiltrative processes, all of which are important when evaluating a patient and considering therapeutic interventions. Arrhythmia burden can also be helpful, for example when deciding between medical and ablative interventions.

Holter test, external loop and implantable loop monitors can all provide information pertinent to ventricular arrhythmias, such as PVC and VT frequency, VT initiation characteristics, and heart rate variability. Ambulatory monitors are often superior to hospital-based evaluations when diagnosing arrhythmias.[16] Holter monitors are usually worn for 24 to 48 hours and are appropriate for patients with frequent ectopy. Externally-worn loop monitors are usually worn for 7 to 30 days, and implantable loop monitors can maintain battery power for as long as three years. Loop monitors are superior to event monitors because they are always recording data and activating the device prompts the monitor to save data for several seconds before, during and after activation. Event monitors start saving data only after device activation and therefore usually miss arrhythmia activation. On the other hand, loop monitors must be worn at all times to record information. Event recorders are comparatively very small and convenient—some connect to regular mobile telephones—making event recorders preferable to many patients. Companies are constantly bringing new ever-more-convenient devices to market.

Signal-averaged ECG (SAECG) is useful in identifying subtle surface ECG signals that result from delayed conduction through diseased myocardium affected by inflammation, scar and fibrosis.[17] A signal-averaged ECG analyzes the QRS complex over many beats, enhancing the signal-to-noise ratio and revealing characteristics indicative of arrhythmogenic substrate.[18] These data can be used for risk stratification, diagnosis (e.g. suspected ARVC, for example), and for treatment decisions (e.g. monitoring for chemotherapy toxicity). Regarding risk stratification, international guidelines concur that SAECG is primarily useful in identifying patient at low risk for sudden cardiac death.[19]

CONCLUSION

Ventricular arrhythmias encompass a wide range of presentations from benign PVCs to life-threatening ventricular tachycardia and ventricular fibrillation. The underlying etiologies and mechanisms that lead to such an array of clinical presentations are even more diverse and fascinating. This chapter has touched on mechanisms of these arrhythmias, the associated clinical pathology and the range of ventricular tachyarrhythmias. Subsequent chapters will delve into more detail about each of these topics.

REFERENCES

1. Zheng ZJ, Croft JB, Giles WH, Mensah GA. Sudden cardiac death in the United States, 1989 to 1998. Circulation. 2001;104: 2158-63.
2. Brugada P, Brugada J, Mont L, Smeets J, Andries EW. A new approach to the differential diagnosis of a regular tachycardia with a wide QRS complex. Circulation. 1991;83:1649-59.
3. Lau EW, Pathamanathan RK, Ng GA, Cooper J, Skehan JD, Griffith MJ. The Bayesian approach improves the electrocardiographic diagnosis of broad complex tachycardia. Pacing Clin Electrophysiol. 2000;23:1519-26.
4. Buxton AE, Fisher JD, Josephson ME, Lee KL, Pryor DB, Prystowsky EN, Simson MB, DiCarlo L, Echt DS, Packer D, et al. Prevention of sudden death in patients with coronary artery disease: the Multicenter Unsustained Tachycardia Trial (MUSTT). Prog Cardiovasc Dis. 1993;36:215-26.

5. Moss AJ, Hall WJ, Cannom DS, Daubert JP, Higgins SL, Klein H, Levine JH, Saksena S, Waldo AL, Wilber D, Brown MW, Heo M. Improved survival with an implanted defibrillator in patients with coronary disease at high risk for ventricular arrhythmia. Multicenter Automatic Defibrillator Implantation Trial Investigators. N Engl J Med. 1996;335:1933-40.
6. Felker GM, Thompson RE, Hare JM, Hruban RH, Clemetson DE, Howard DL, Baughman KL, Kasper EK. Underlying causes and long-term survival in patients with initially unexplained cardiomyopathy. N Engl J Med. 2000;342:1077-84.
7. Reisinger J, Dubrey SW, Lavalley M, Skinner M, Falk RH. Electrophysiologic abnormalities in AL (primary) amyloidosis with cardiac involvement. J Am Coll Cardiol. 1997;30:1046-51.
8. Sen-Chowdhry S, Lowe MD, Sporton SC, McKenna WJ. Arrhythmogenic right ventricular cardiomyopathy: clinical presentation, diagnosis, and management. Am J Med. 2004; 117:685-95.
9. Marchlinski FE, Zado E, Dixit S, Gerstenfeld E, Callans DJ, Hsia H, Lin D, Nayak H, Russo A, Pulliam W. Electroanatomic substrate and outcome of catheter ablative therapy for ventricular tachycardia in setting of right ventricular cardiomyopathy. Circulation. 2004; 110:2293-8.
10. Lerman BB, Belardinelli L, West GA, Berne RM, DiMarco JP. Adenosine-sensitive ventricular tachycardia: evidence suggesting cyclic AMP-mediated triggered activity. Circulation. 1986;74:270-80.
11. Zipes DP, Foster PR, Troup PJ, Pedersen DH. Atrial induction of ventricular tachycardia: reentry versus triggered automaticity. Am J Cardiol. 1979;44:1-8.
12. Belhassen B, Rotmensch HH, Laniado S. Response of recurrent sustained ventricular tachycardia to verapamil. Br Heart J. 1981;46:679-82.
13. Priori SG, Napolitano C, Memmi M, Colombi B, Drago F, Gasparini M, DeSimone L, Coltorti F, Bloise R, Keegan R, Cruz Filho FE, Vignati G, Benatar A, DeLogu A. Clinical and molecular characterization of patients with catecholaminergic polymorphic ventricular tachycardia. Circulation. 2002;106: 69-74.
14. Kelly P, Ruskin JN, Vlahakes GJ, Buckley MJ, Jr., Freeman CS, Garan H. Surgical coronary revascularization in survivors of prehospital cardiac arrest: its effect on inducible ventricular arrhythmias and long-term survival. J Am Coll Cardiol. 1990;15:267-73.
15. Epstein AE, DiMarco JP, Ellenbogen KA, Estes NA, 3rd, Freedman RA, Gettes LS, Gillinov AM, Gregoratos G, Hammill SC, Hayes DL, Hlatky MA, Newby LK, Page RL, Schoenfeld MH, Silka MJ, Stevenson LW, Sweeney MO, Smith SC, Jr., Jacobs AK, Adams CD, Anderson JL, Buller CE, Creager MA, Ettinger SM, Faxon DP, Halperin JL, Hiratzka LF, Hunt SA, Krumholz HM, Kushner FG, Lytle BW, Nishimura RA, Ornato JP, Riegel B, Tarkington LG, Yancy CW. ACC/AHA/HRS 2008 Guidelines for Device-Based Therapy of Cardiac Rhythm Abnormalities: a report of the American College of Cardiology/American Heart Association Task Force on Practice Guidelines (Writing Committee to Revise the ACC/AHA/NASPE 2002 Guideline Update for Implantation of Cardiac Pacemakers and Antiarrhythmia Devices): developed in collaboration with the American Association for Thoracic Surgery and Society of Thoracic Surgeons. Circulation, 2008;117:e350-408.
16. Giada F, Gulizia M, Francese M, Croci F, Santangelo L, Santomauro M, Occhetta E, Menozzi C, Raviele A. Recurrent unexplained palpitations (RUP) study comparison of implantable loop recorder versus conventional diagnostic strategy. J Am Coll Cardiol. 2007;49:1951-6.
17. Farrell TG, Bashir Y, Cripps T, Malik M, Poloniecki J, Bennett ED, Ward DE, Camm AJ. Risk stratification for arrhythmic events in postinfarction patients based on heart rate variability, ambulatory electrocardiographic variables and the signal-averaged electrocardiogram. J Am Coll Cardiol. 1991;18: 687-97.
18. Kulakowski P, Malik M, Poloniecki J, Bashir Y, Odemuyiwa O, Farrell T, Staunton A, Camm J. Frequency versus time domain analysis of signal-averaged electrocardiograms. II. Identification of patients with ventricular tachycardia after myocardial infarction. J Am Coll Cardiol. 1992;20:135-43.
19. Zipes DP, Camm AJ, Borggrefe M, Buxton AE, Chaitman B, Fromer M, Gregoratos G, Klein G, Moss AJ, Myerburg RJ, Priori SG, Quinones MA, Roden DM, Silka MJ, Tracy C, Smith SC, Jr., Jacobs AK, Adams CD, Antman EM, Anderson JL, Hunt SA, Halperin JL, Nishimura R, Ornato JP, Page RL, Riegel B, Blanc JJ, Budaj A, Dean V, Deckers JW, Despres C, Dickstein K, Lekakis J, McGregor K, Metra M, Morais J, Osterspey A, Tamargo JL, Zamorano JL. ACC/AHA/ESC 2006 guidelines for management of patients with ventricular arrhythmias and the prevention of sudden cardiac death: a report of the American College of Cardiology/American Heart Association Task Force and the European Society of Cardiology Committee for Practice Guidelines (Writing Committee to Develop Guidelines for Management of Patients With Ventricular Arrhythmias and the Prevention of Sudden Cardiac Death). J Am Coll Cardiol. 2006;48:e247-346.

EDITORS' SUMMARY

Success with managing ventricular tachycardia involves a comprehensive and organized approach that includes clinical investigation, management of the underlying structural heart disease, detailed knowledge of the pros and cons of various mapping approaches (entrainment, substrate, activation), and expert knowledge of the biophysics of energy delivery to minimize thromboembolic complications and enhance success. Drs Shaw and Callans in this chapter provide an overview of ventricular tachycardia that will be an excellent start guiding the EP and ablation student towards obtaining the necessary knowledge and tools to manage ventricular tachycardia patients.

CHAPTER 31

Jianqing Li, Mark E Josephson

Monomorphic Ventricular Tachycardia: Mechanisms and Etiology

LIST OF ABBREVIATIONS

AV	Atrioventricular	PCL	Paced Cycle Length
BBR	Bundle Branch Reentry	PES	Programmed Electrical Stimulation
CAD	Coronary Artery Disease	RBBB	Right Bundle Branch Block
cAMP	Cyclic Adenosine Monophosphate	RB	Right Bundle
CICR	Calcium-induced Calcium Release	RVOT	Right Ventricular Outflow Tract
DAD	Delayed Afterdepolarization	SA	Sinoatrial
EAD	Early Afterdepolarization	SERCA	Sarcoplasmic Reticulum Calcium Adenosine Triphosphatase
HPS	His-Purkinje System	SF	Safety Factor
IVC	Inferior Vena Cava	SR	Sarcoplasmic Reticulum
LAFB	Left Anterior Fascicular Block	TCL	Tachycardia Cycle Length
LBBB	Left Bundle Branch Block	VES	Ventricular Extrastimulus
LB	Left Bundle	VF	Ventricular Fibrillation
LPFB	Left Posterior Fascicular Block	VT	Ventricular Tachycardia
NCX	Sodium-calcium Exchanger		

INTRODUCTION

The mechanisms of cardiac arrhythmias can be categorized into disorders of impulse formation (automaticity and triggered activity), impulse conduction (reentry), or a combination of both. Similarly, the different forms of monomorphic ventricular tachycardia (VT) can be grouped by their underlying mechanisms.

Having a clear understanding of the underlying mechanism is extremely important and helpful in the diagnosis and treatment of the different ventricular arrhythmias. Medical and surgical therapy of the ventricular tachycardias can be precisely targeted if we can correctly identify their underlying etiology.

AUTOMATICITY

Automaticity refers to the ability of a cardiac cell to spontaneously depolarize, reach threshold potential, and initiate an impulse in the absence of external stimulation.

This is a normal property of pacemaker cells such as sinus node, atrioventricular (AV) node, and the His-Purkinje system (HPS).

The mechanism for spontaneous depolarization in phase 4 of the action potential for the sinoatrial (SA) node is still controversial. However, most evidence suggests that a combination of I_f and Ca^{+2} current is responsible for the rise in the membrane potential to threshold at -40 mV and onset of action potential.[1,2] I_f current is an inward current carried largely by Na^+ and to a lesser extent K^+ ions. The Na^+/Ca^{+2} exchanger (NCX) has also been found to provide a substantial contribution during the late diastolic phase by allowing more Na^+ entry into the cell.[3-5] NCX is activated by submembrane spontaneous rhythmic local Ca^{+2} release from the sarcoplasmic reticulum (SR) via ryanodine receptors; such rhythmic release of calcium by the SR is referred to an "intracellular calcium" clock and it helps to form the overall pacemaker clock.[6]

The likelihood of reaching threshold potential by pacemaker cells is affected by (1) maximal diastolic membrane potential (2) rate of spontaneous depolarization (slope of phase 4 of the action potential) and (3) the threshold potential for initiation of action potential.

Normal pacemaker cells reach -40 mV of threshold potential by slow depolarization of these cells in phase 4. Once threshold potential is reached, Ca^{+2} influx initiates phase 0 of the action potential. Normal atrial and ventricular tissues do not have spontaneous diastolic depolarization and do not initiate spontaneous impulses.

ABNORMAL AUTOMATICITY

Abnormal automaticity refers to impulse formation in cells that do not normally exhibit automaticity.

Even though the I_f current exists in normal ventricular myocytes, range of activation of the I_f current is much more negative at -120 to -170 mV and it is inactive at normal resting ventricular myocyte membrane potentials of -85 to -95 mV. As a result, ventricular myocytes normally are not capable of spontaneous depolarization and do not have normal automaticity. However, when ventricular myocytes reach membrane potential of -70 to -30 mV, spontaneous depolarization can occur and this is known as depolarization-induced-automaticity or abnormal automaticity. A similar phenomenon occurs in Purkinje fibers and spontaneous depolarization occurs at -60 mV or less.[7]

The upstroke of the action potential (Phase 0) of an abnormal automatic focus can be initiated by Na^+ or Ca^{+2} inwards currents. At membrane potentials between -70 and -50 mV, Na channels are functional and allow Na^+ entry into the cell to initiate the action potential. Na channels are inactive between membrane potentials of -50 to -30 mV, and action potential initiation is driven by Ca^{+2}.

The sinus node is the dominant pacemaker in the heart and maintains its dominance over subsidiary pacemakers by overdrive suppression. During sinus rhythm, subsidiary pacemakers are activated faster than their intrinsic spontaneous depolarization frequency. Na^+ entry into the cell occurs with each depolarization and the Na^+/K^+ exchange pump is activated by an increase in intracellular Na concentration. Na^+/K^+ exchange pump is an electrogenic pump that extrudes Na^+ ion out of the cell and moves K^+ into the cell and generates a net outward current. With this hyperpolarization current, the cell membrane becomes more negative and keeps the I_f current in the subsidiary pacemakers inactive. An accelerated stimulation of pacemaker cells can be simulated by overdrive pacing. With overdrive pacing, there is transient suppression due to hyperpolarization of cell membrane followed by resumption of the automatic focus post pacing **(Figure 31.1A)**.[8]

In abnormal automaticity, depolarization of the cell is driven mostly by Ca^{+2}, not Na^+ at depolarized resting cell membrane potential. The hyperpolarized current does not exist since depolarization is not Na^+ mediated; as a result, overdrive suppression does not take place and the abnormal automatic rhythm is not affected by overdrive pacing **(Figure 31.1B)**.

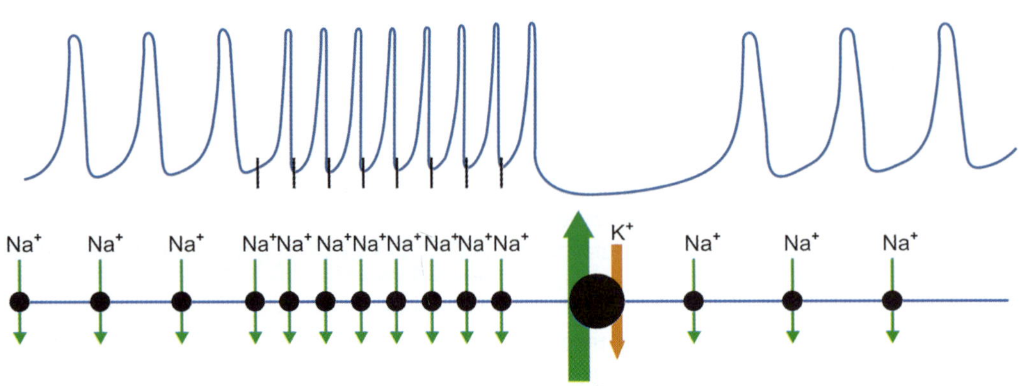

Figure 31.1A: Overdrive suppression of normal automaticity

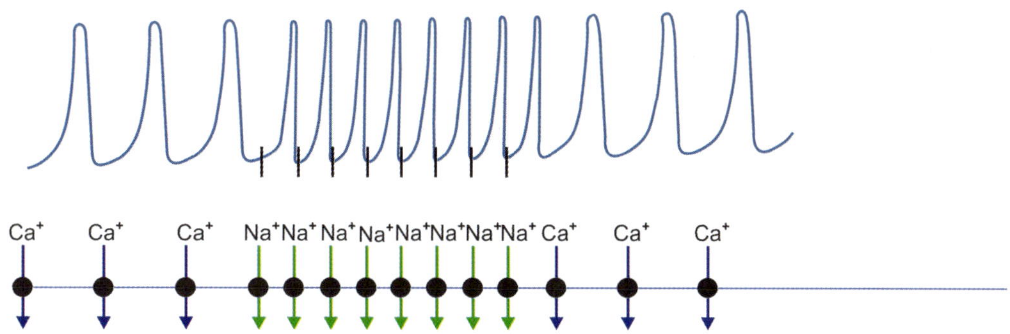

Figure 31.1B: No overdrive suppression in abnormal automaticity

Ventricular Tachycardias due to Abnormal Automaticity

With ischemia and infarction, there is a loss of cell membrane integrity and the resting membrane potentials in the ischemic tissues are partially depolarized. At elevated resting membrane potentials, either Ca^{+2} or Na^{+} entry into the cell will initiate action potentials and lead to spontaneous depolarization. Accelerated idioventricular rhythms that occur post reperfusion are due to abnormal automaticity in the damaged myocytes. A similar phenomenon can occur in other damaged myocytes.

Uncoupling of cells by fibrosis or infarction around pacemaker sites can lead to loss of the inhibitory electrotonic influences between nonpacemaker cells and pacemaker cells. With the loss of adjacent inhibitory influence, latent pacemakers can initiate spontaneous depolarization and impulse formation.

TRIGGERED ACTIVITY

Triggered activities are caused by afterdepolarizations that are able to reach threshold to generate another action potential and further impulse formation. There are two types of afterdepolarizations, *early* and *delayed* afterdepolarizations that occur during different phases of the action potential.

Early afterdepolarizations (EADs) occur during phase 2 and phase 3 of the action potential and are results of prolonged action potential duration and late inward calcium currents. EADs often lead to polymorphic VT and ventricular fibrillation (VF), not sustained monomorphic VTs.

Delayed afterdepolarizations (DAD) occur after repolarization of the action potential is completed and are results of intracellular calcium overload.

Under normal conditions, excitation contraction coupling occurs with each action potential generation. During the plateau phase of the action potential (phase 2), voltage dependent L-type calcium channels open and allow calcium to enter the cell to counteract the exit of potassium outside the cell. The influx of calcium (I_{CaL}) triggers the release of calcium from the sarcoplasmic reticulum (SR) in a process known as Ca^{2+}-induced Ca^{2+} release (CICR). Calcium then binds to the actin-myosin complex and initiates myocyte contraction. The increased cytosolic calcium concentration at the same time activates the NCX on the cell membrane and extrudes 2 Ca^{2+} to the extracellular space for 3 Na^{+} ions into the cell. This results in a net positive current into the cell. During repolarization, calcium is then sequestered back into the SR by the SR Ca^{2+} adenosine triphosphatase (SERCA). This recurrent process of calcium entry and exit from the cytosol occurs with each action potential **(Figure 31.2)**.

Catecholamines initiate DADs by binding to the β-adrenergic receptor and activating adenyl cyclase which then leads to an increase in intracellular cyclic adenosine monophosphate (cAMP) and increase in I_{CaL}.[9] As mentioned earlier, an increase in I_{CaL} leads to the release of Ca^{2+} from the SR and activation of the NCX. The net positive inward current then generates the DAD. If the resultant DAD reaches threshold potential, an action potential is triggered. The triggered activity can further initiate DADs leading to repetitive action potentials and tachycardia.[10]

The higher the amplitude of the DAD generated, the more likely it will reach threshold potential and lead to impulse formation. The cycle length of the preceding action potentials, the membrane potential at the time of DAD initiation, and the action potential duration directly affect the amplitude the DAD.

Rapid pacing is the most successful method of initiating sustained triggered activity due to DADs. At shorter pacing cycle lengths, there is less time allowed for calcium sequestration back into the SR by SERCA and the cytosolic calcium concentration is higher. This leads to a higher concentration

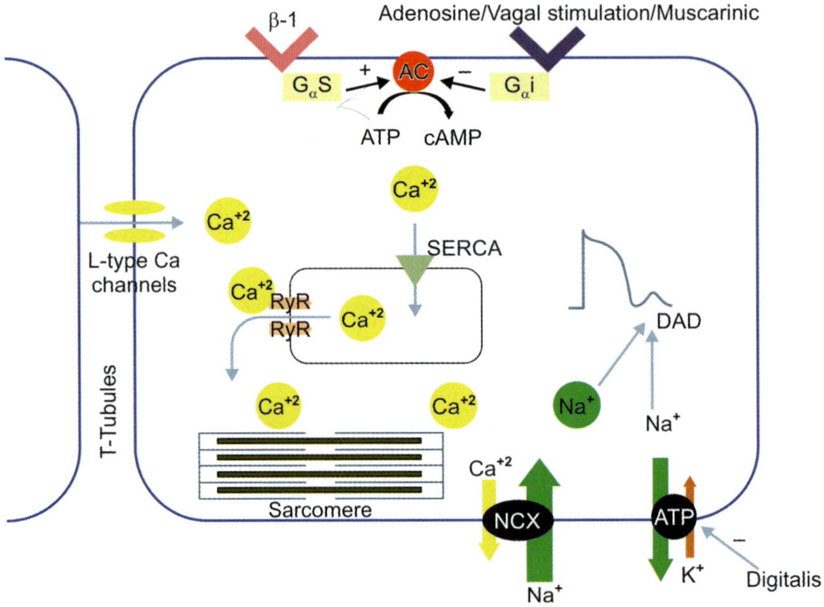

Figure 31.2: Calcium fluxes into and out of a cell

Abbreviations: Na^+, sodium ion; Ca^{+2}, calcium ion; K^+, potassium ion; AC, adenylate cyclase; ATP, adenosine triphosphate; cAMP, cyclic adenosine monophosphate; DAD, delayed afterdepolarization; SERCA, sarcoplasmic reticulum calcium adenosine triphosphatase; NCX, sodium calcium exchanger

gradient driving the NCX with a higher influx of Na^+ into the cell and causing a steeper upstroke and higher amplitude of the DAD. As a result, the DAD is more likely to reach threshold potential **(Figures 31.3A to C)**. In addition, the coupling interval between the last stimulated beat and the DAD is directly proportional to the pacing cycle length preceding the DAD. The coupling interval between the last stimulated beat and the first DAD initiated decreases as the preceding pacing cycle length decreases.[11] There is a critical point in which DADs are no longer able to reach threshold with faster pacing or shorter pacing cycle length. This is a result of activation of the Na^+/K^+ ATPase by the inward Na current initiating the DAD, leading to hyperpolarization of the cell membrane and inability of the DAD to reach threshold potential **(Figure 31.3D)**.[12]

Once a triggered rhythm is initiated, a period of quiescence is necessary to reinitiate the triggered rhythm. Thus, the ability to initiate, terminate and reinitiate in sequence is uncommon. In addition, sustained triggered activity accelerates following initiation before reaching a stable cycle length.

Catecholamine or drugs that increase cAMP are frequently required to initiate sustained rhythmic activity. Triggered activity is often seen during reperfusion after myocardial ischemia due to intracellular calcium overload. Disorders of calcium trafficking into and out of the SR can also lead to cytosolic calcium overload and DADs. Vagal maneuvers, beta blockers, calcium channel blockers, and adenosine can terminate triggered activity by decreasing sympathetic tone, activation of cAMP, calcium channel blockade, and ultimately intracellular calcium concentration.[13,14]

Outflow Tract Triggered Monomorphic Ventricular Tachycardia

Outflow tract VTs are the most commonly encountered ventricular arrhythmias due to triggered activity mediated by catecholamine-induced DADs and they are cAMP-dependent. There is evidence that cellular mutations in areas of the right ventricular outflow tract (RVOT) may be responsible for the mechanism of arrhythmia origin in the RVOT. Samples of myocytes from the arrhythmic focus in the RVOT obtained from a patient with RVOT VT showed a somatic mutation in the G binding protein (Gαi2) that leads to an excessive increase in cAMP level by beta-adrenergic stimulation which was not present in other areas of the myocardium.[15] These findings suggest that alterations in the cAMP dependent transduction pathway may be the cause of arrhythmia genesis in the outflow tracts.

Because activation of adenylyl cyclase and I_{CaL} is critical for the development of cAMP-mediated triggered activity, the triggered arrhythmia is sensitive to a constellation of electropharmacologic perturbations: beta-blockade, calcium channel blockade (verapamil), vagal maneuvers, and adenosine **(Figure 31.2)**.[14]

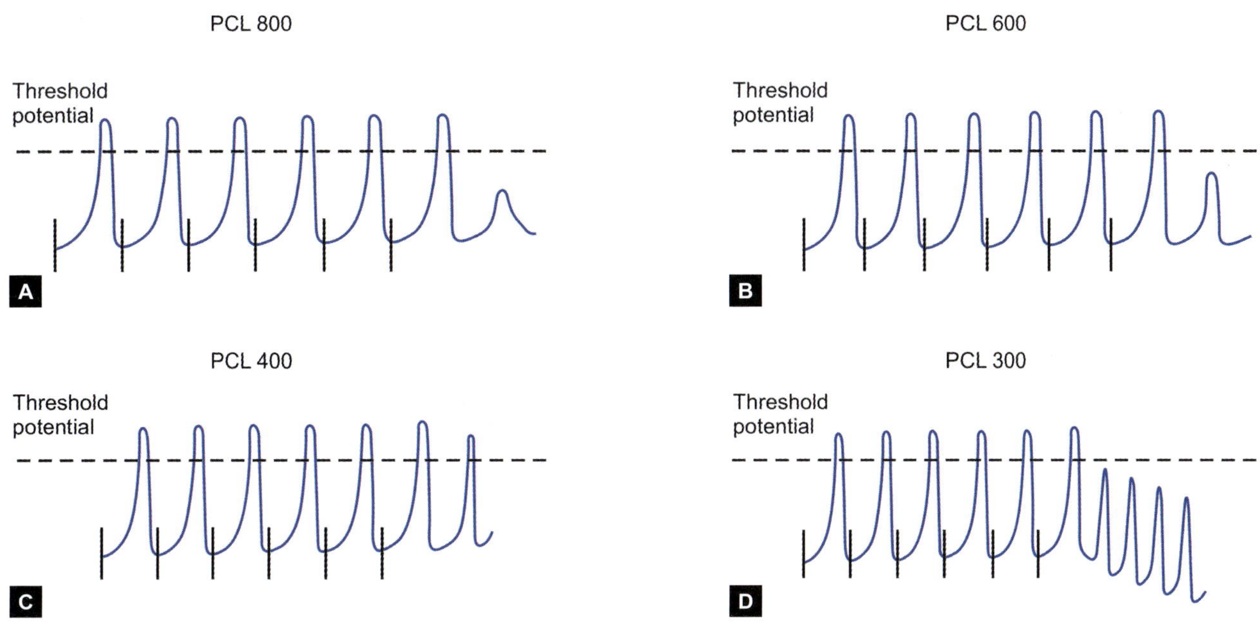

Figures 31.3A to D: Triggered activity. See text for details

Triggered Activity due to Digitalis Toxicity

Digitalis binds to the Na^+/K^+ ATPase and prevents active Na removal from the cytosol. As a result, intracellular Na concentration increases and activates the Na^+/Ca^{+2} exchanger leading an influx of Ca^{+2} into the cytoplasm. The rise of Ca^{+2} leads to DAD and triggered activity and initiation of monomorphic VT. Since the etiology of DADs and triggered activity are independent of adenyl cyclase and cAMP, adenosine has no effect on digitalis induced triggered arrhythmias **(Figure 31.2)**.

Interestingly, there is also a bigeminal pattern of the triggered ventricular tachycardia due to digitalis toxicity. In a model of ouabain toxic canine Purkinje fibers, a bigeminy pattern due to alternans in the afterdepolarization was observed. The action potentials during the bigeminal rhythm had alternating maximal diastolic potential, *dV/dt* of the DAD upstroke, action potential duration, and cycle length. This may be due to the fact that DADs are voltage-dependent, with individual afterdepolarizations varying in amplitude depending on the membrane potential at which they are initiated. The alternans pattern in maximal diastolic potential can be considered a likely modulator of the amplitude and the slope of the ascending limbs of the afterdepolarizations, thereby contributing to the bigeminal pattern.[16]

Based on a rabbit model, this bigeminal pattern occurs first in one of the fascicles of the HPS. When the heart rate exceeded the threshold for bigeminy at the first site in the HPS, ventricular bigeminy developed, causing the heart rate to accelerate and exceed the threshold for bigeminy at the second site. Thus, the triggered beat from the first site induced a triggered beat from the second site. The triggered beat from the second site next reciprocated by inducing a triggered beat from the first site, and so forth. Bigeminy from two sites produced bidirectional VT and polymorphic VT occurs if triggered activity occurs in 3 or more sites.[17]

REENTRY

The most common mechanism for monomorphic VT in patients with structural heart disease is reentry.

Reentry refers to the concept of circular propagation of an electrical wavefront such that the head of the impulse continuously revolves around an area of either *anatomic or functional block* (or *obstacle*) and meets that tail of the wavefront forming the circuit.

In order to reentry to occur, there must be a *trigger* and substrate for initiation. The trigger may be a premature impulse or impulse generated by dispersion of refractoriness in the tissue. Such trigger will then need to cause *unidirectional block* and *slow conduction* to allow recovery of conduction in the previously blocked tissue for reentry to occur.

In order to sustain reentry, the wavelength of the circuit must be less than the path length of the circuit such that there is an area excitable by the head of the wavefront to allow continuation of the circuit without reaching fully unexcitable tissue and abolishing the wavefront. The area of excitable tissue between the head and the tail of the circuit allowing the continuation of the circuit is known as the *excitable gap.*

Substrate

In the case of monomorphic ventricular tachycardia, the substrate is most often the scars located in areas with wall motion abnormalities due to myocardial infarction, infiltrative diseases, or viral infections. In contrast to scars formed in ischemic heart disease, pathophysiologic substrate of nonischemic cardiomyopathies are less well defined.

In the case of myocardial infarction, the electrophysiological consequences include abnormalities in conduction and refractoriness, heterogeneity of conduction and refractoriness, enhanced automaticity, and areas of inexcitability. These cellular changes lead to reentry and arrhythmia formation.

The myocardial remodeling process provides the anatomic and functional barriers required for reentry. Myocardial infarction leads to separation of the myocytes by collagen formation in the extracellular matrix and scar formation.[18] Anatomic evaluation of tissues removed from sites of VT origin and sites remote from VT demonstrated viable myocardium embedded within the scar. [19-21] In addition, the uncoupling of the myocytes as a result of extracellular collagen deposition and fibrosis leads to slow conduction and anisotropic conduction of the wavefronts due to loss of gap junction communications.[18]

In normal myocardium, electrical impulses propagate from one myocyte to the next via the gap junctions located on the cell membrane. The gap junctions are composed of a channel from one cell in communication with another channel from the adjacent cell, these channels are known as connexons.[22] The predominant connexon in ventricular myocardium is composed of individual units of connexin43.[23,24] The alignment of these gap junction on the cell membrane leads to differential resistivity of the cellular current conduction.

The resistivity of gap functional cell membrane is several orders higher in magnitude than the cytoplasmic intracellular resistivity. The conduction velocity in the direction *parallel* to the myocardial fiber axis is three times more rapid than in the *transverse* direction and it is attributed to the lower resistivity of the myocardium in the longitudinal than the transverse direction. This preferential conduction of wavefront is known as *uniform anisotropy*.

In infarcted tissue, there is lateralization of gap junctions (Connexon 43) and destruction by apoptosis.[25] With the lost and lateralization of connexons, there is decreased gap junction conductance and increased intercellular resistance leading to nonuniform anisotropy, slow conduction, conduction block, and facilitation of reentry.[26] The lines of block created by the gap junction disruption of the myocytes in the border zones and the myocardial bridges formed by viable myocardium within the scar forms the channels of the reentrant circuit.[27]

The fiber disarray resulting from fibrosis and tissue remodeling can also lead to activation delay due to source-sink mismatch in electrical current conduction. The activation wavefront generated by a small strand of myocardium within the infarct will encounter higher resistance in the larger muscle bundle downstream leading to activation delay, providing slow conduction, conduction block, and facilitation of reentry.

In a canine model, decreased side to side cell connections by fibrosis leads to an increase of path length and the number of intercellular junctions traversed by the wavefront moving in the transverse direction in a zig-zag manner.[28] This has been shown in ex-vivo human hearts as well.

The clinical and electrophysiological manifestations of these cellular abnormalities are represented by abnormal endocardial electrograms identified during endocardial mapping. These abnormal electrograms are low in amplitude, fractionated, prolonged in duration, and often occur at the end of the QRS. In contrast to patients with nonsustained VT, patients with sustained monomorphic VT have the higher numbers of abnormal electrograms involving more areas of the myocardium. These abnormal electrograms most often are located in the area of the endocardium where bipolar voltages are between 0.1–0.5 mV.[29-34]

Mechanism of Slow Conduction

Action potential propagation and conduction velocity in cardiac tissues are determined by source–sink relationships. An excited cardiac cell acts as the source of electric charge for depolarization of neighboring unexcited cells towards their excitation threshold. The unexcited cell serves as the sink of the electrical charge. In order for action potential to propagate, there must be sufficient electrical charge provided by the source cell to the sink cell to reach membrane threshold potential. The *Safety Factor* (SF) of conduction refers to the relationship between the source and the sink and defines the likelihood of action potential propagation. The safety factor can be considered as the ratio of charge generated by the source cell to the charge consumed by the sink cell. Conduction block occurs if $SF<1$. Factors such as cell membrane excitability, gap junction conductance, and tissue structure can affect the safety factor and conduction success.[35]

Reduced Membrane Excitability

During acute ischemia, acidosis and increased intracellular calcium can lead to decreased gap junction conductance without a change in number and location of connexins.[36] With decreased ion channel conductance, there is slow propagation of the electric signal and slow conduction.

In addition, the cell membrane is partially depolarized in ischemic and infarcted tissues. Sodium channels responsible for phase 0 of the action potential are partially deactivated in depolarized cellular membranes at –40 mV leading to a reduced inward I_{Na} current.[37,38] As a result, dV/dt of the action potential upstroke, conduction velocity, and SF are reduced.[35] This phenomenon is more prominent during the acute ischemic phase and has been shown in experimental models of cellular conduction.

Besides a decrease in function of partially activated Na channels, there is a 30% reduction of Na current density in dog myocytes originating from infarcted tissue.[39] Similar observations were found in explanted human hearts from patients with end stage heart failure.[40] In addition to a reduced dV/dt of phase 0 of the action potential, decreased Na channels expression leads to a 17% increase in effective refractory period of the action potential duration and slow conduction.[41]

Slow Conduction due to Decreased Cell-cell Coupling

Electrical remodeling secondary to uncoupling of myocytes due to lateralization and loss of connexon 43 leads to nonuniform anisotropy and slow conduction.[27,42,43]

The safety factor for conduction is higher for transverse propagation than longitudinal propagation in nonuniform anisotropic tissue. In nonuniform anisotropic atrial muscles, there is a decrease in conduction in both the longitudinal and transverse direction with premature stimulation. With more premature stimulation, longitudinal propagation either terminates or proceeds in a slow discontinuous manner relative to transverse propagation. With the delay in longitudinal conduction, tissue recovery from refractoriness occurs and allows reentry to takes place.[44-47]

Slow Conduction due to Tissue Structure

Based on studies on spiral wave reentry in cardiac muscle, the concept of convex wavefront curvature was shown to be one of the causes of slow conduction. The greater the curvature, the slower the conduction. In a figure of 8 reentrant circuit, the greatest curvature occurs around the pivot points at the end of the lines of block as the reentrant wavefront emerges from the relatively narrow central common pathway into a larger mass of myocardium.[48-50] Source-sink mismatch between small and larger area of myocardium leads to conduction delay.

Fiber disarray within scar tissue produces a high degree of tissue discontinuity and branch points between small and big fibers. Slow conduction takes place at branch points with source-sink mismatch between small and large fiber bundles. As the propagating source of electrical charge from the small fiber encounters the downstream large fiber, the local current is dispersed laterally (transversely) in a slow circuitous manner to activate side branching cells leading to slow conduction.[51,52]

Mechanism of Unidirectional Block

As mentioned earlier, cellular uncoupling due to electrical remodeling after myocardial infarction, impedance mismatch due to structural remodeling and fibrosis, and inhomogeneity of membrane excitation and refractoriness can lead to unidirectional block during wavefront propagation.

There is a critical window in which cellular membrane excitation by a premature stimulus can lead to unidirectional block.[53-55] For example, an earlier premature stimulus may cause block in both orthodromic and antidromic direction of the reentry circuit due to encroachment of the refractory period. Similarly, a later premature stimulus may lead to recovery of tissue excitability and conduction in both limbs of the reentry circuit and no reentry can occur. In this critical window of prematurity, the premature stimulus will encroach on the absolute refractory period and cause unidirectional block in one direction of the circuit and simultaneous conduction down the opposite direction to allow reentry to occur.

Myocardial infarction can lead to abnormalities in refractoriness and unidirectional block; however, abnormalities of conduction are likely more important in the genesis of sustained uniform VT. Comparing to a patient with structurally normal heart and a patient with long QT syndrome, a patient with coronary artery disease and sustained ventricular arrhythmias has normal dispersion of refractoriness but marked abnormal ventricular activation which produces the consequent dispersion of total recovery in the left ventricle. The greater these abnormalities, the more likely uniform tachycardia are initiated spontaneously or induced.[56]

Central Area of Block or Obstacle

The central area of block for maintaining reentry can be anatomic or functional.

Anatomical block is the result of barriers caused by scar formation or anatomic barriers such as the mitral annulus, tricuspid valve, or inferior vena cava (IVC).

In the case of functional block, enhanced nonuniformity of conduction and conduction block were most evident in the transverse direction, particularly at sites of inhomogeneous gap junction distribution, intercellular clefts, and non-myocytes in the border between fully unexcitable infarcted tissues and viable myocardium. The alteration in the spatial organization of gap junctions impedes the conduction of wavefront in the transverse direction and forms lines of block in anisotropic reentrant circuits.[27]

Excitable Gap

The excitable gap refers to the excitable area between the head of the propagating impulse and tail of the preceding wavefront around the reentry circuit. In order for the circulating impulse to continue propagation within the circuit, there must an area of excitable tissue in front of the propagating wavefront, otherwise the propagating wavefront will encounter totally refractory tissue, thereby abolishing the wavefront. The tissue within the excitable gap can be fully excitable or partially excitable to sustain reentry.

The excitable gap of a reentry circuit has both *temporal* (time during the cycle length that the circuit is excitable) and *spatial* (length of the circuit that is excitable at a given time) properties.

The *spatial excitable gap* is determined by the wavelength of the tachycardia. The wavelength of the tachycardia refers to the distance travelled by the impulse and it is a product of conduction velocity and refractoriness of the tissue. In order to sustain reentry, the wavelength of the tachycardia must be less than the path length of the circuit. The difference between the wavelength and path length of the tachycardia is known as the spatial excitable gap. Slowing of conduction and shortening of the refractoriness of the tissue can decrease the wavelength and increase the spatial excitable gap for continuous reentry. Based on the previously published evaluation of the excitable gaps in a canine model, the spatial extent of the excitable gap changes markedly in different locations of the circuit and ranges from 5 to 55% of the circuit length.

The *temporal excitable gap* refers to the time during the tachycardia cycle length that the circuit is excitable by a premature stimulus. It is best illustrated by plotting the coupling interval of the premature stimulus against the return cycle length **(Figure 31.4)**.

The dashed line **(Figure 31.4)** is the line of unity representing the absence of reset with the premature stimulus; in other words, the premature stimulus fails to reset and advance the circuit. There is a critical window of prematurity in which the circuit is reset and the return cycle after the premature stimulus is advanced known as the *zone of reset* and it is represented as the points below the line of unity. The timing of the return cycle is determined by the prematurity of the stimulus, refractoriness of the tissue, and conduction velocity of the tissue.

It is important to note that the temporal excitable gap of the circuit varies in different parts of the circuit. For example, part of circuit may be excited by the premature stimulus delivered up to 79 ms earlier whereas other part of the circuit may be blocked by a premature stimulus delivered only 7 ms earlier. Some of the factors causing the difference of the temporal excitable gap duration are anisotropic conduction due to different fiber orientation and subsequent conduction velocity and site of stimulation. In the canine infarct model, conduction velocity is slowest at the turning point of the circuit such as the exit and entrance sites. This occurs due to the change of direction of conduction from parallel to the line of block to the transverse direction relative to the myocardial fiber orientation at these sites. As a result,

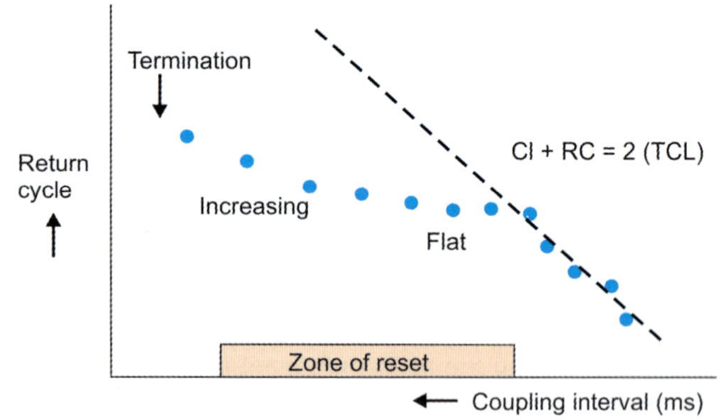

Figure 31.4: Temporal excitable gap. See text for details.
Abbreviations: CI, coupling interval; RC, return cycle length; TCL, tachycardia cycle length

the temporal excitable gap will be shorter at sites of conduction delay.[57]

CHARACTERISTICS OF REENTRY

Initiation

The ability to *reproducibly* initiate the tachycardia by programmed electrical stimulation (PES) is the characteristic of both reentry and triggered activity; however, the responses to PES are different between the two mechanisms. The relationship of the coupling interval between the premature stimulation and the first beat of the tachycardia is helpful in distinguishing the two mechanisms. In reentry arrhythmias, the coupling interval between the premature stimulation and the first beat of the tachycardia are inversely related. In contrast, the coupling interval between the premature stimulation and the first beat of the tachycardia in a triggered rhythm have a direct relationship. As the pacing cycle length decreases, coupling interval between the last stimulated beat and the first beat of the triggered tachycardia decreases.

On the other hand, as the coupling interval between S1-S2 decreases with programmed extrastimuli, the interval between S2-S3 increases as S2 encroaches on refractory tissue in a reentrant rhythm. In other words, there is an inverse relationship between the premature stimulus and the first return beat of the reentrant tachycardia.[58]

The response of triggered activity due to DADs to programmed extrastimuli is more variable and can demonstrate a flat resetting response, a shortening of the return cycle, or termination of the tachycardia.

In addition, site specificity of PES for initiation of the ventricular tachycardia is observed in reentrant VT. Approximately 20% of the reentrant VTs are initiated by PES at the RVOT and 2–5% are initiated by PES from the left ventricle only. This was not observed in triggered rhythms in the the studies that looked into it.[59,60]

Resetting

Resetting a tachycardia refers to the advancement of the subsequent beat and continuation of the original rhythm by a premature stimulus.[61]

In the case of an automatic focus, a premature stimulus enters the origin of the automatic focus, prematurely depolarizes the focus, and resets the clock of the automatic focus such that the subsequent beat occurs at the same prematurity equivalent to the prematurity of the premature stimulus (under the condition of fully excitable tissue surrounding the exit of the automatic focus such that there is no delay in the exit of the focus). Fusion between the premature stimulus and the wavefront of the tachycardia is not possible in resetting of an automatic focus because in order for resetting to occur, the premature beat has to activate the automatic site before it exits the automatic focus and activate the surrounding myocardium. The same concept applies to triggered rhythms. In contrast, *resetting with fusion* is diagnostic of reentry.

In a reentrant circuit with a separate entrance and exit **(Figure 31.5A)**, the premature stimulus collides with the wavefront exiting the circuit antidromically and results in fusion of the wavefronts. At the same time, the premature stimulus is able to enter the circuit and advance or delay the subsequent beat, i.e., reset the circuit in the orthodromic direction. Since resetting involves delivery of a single premature stimulus (N^{th} stimulus), the subsequent beat (N+1) following the fusion of the premature stimulus with native wavefront (N-1) will have the same QRS morphology as that of the tachycardia.

In order for fusion to occur, there must be a separate entrance and exit of the reentrant circuit. The coupling interval between the return cycle (N+1) beat and the fused beat depends on the distance between the entrance and exit. If the entrance and exit are farther apart, the return cycle (N+1) beat will occur earlier than if the entrance and exit are closer together **(Figures 31.5B and C)**.

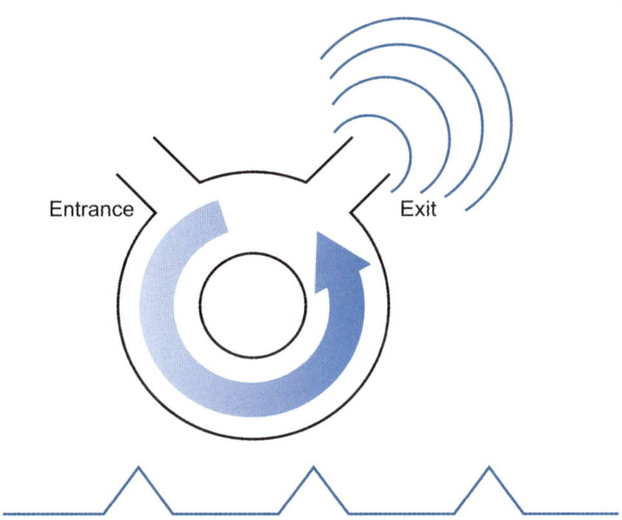

Figure 31.5A: Reentrant circuit of a ventricular tachycardia with separate entrance and exit sites

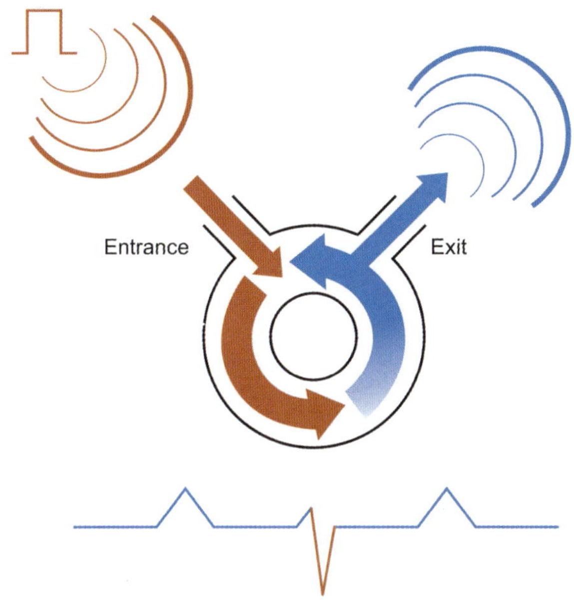

Figure 31.5B: Resetting of a ventricular tachycardia by a premature stimulus with fusion in the surface ECG

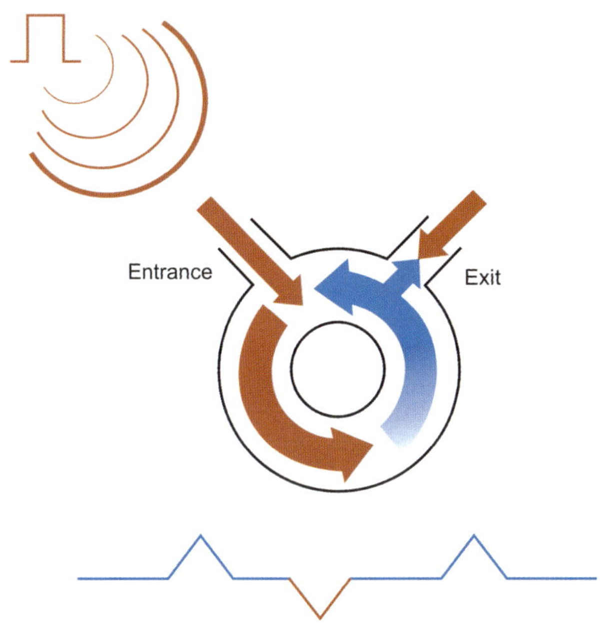

Figure 31.5C: Resetting of a ventricular tachycardia with a premature stimulus without fusion in the surface ECG

Fusion can be observed on the ECG as well as in the intracardiac recordings. For fusion to occur on the surface ECG, enough myocardium must be activated by the native wavefront exiting the circuit before collision with the wavefront generated by the premature stimulus. In addition, the entrance and exit of the circuit must be wide apart in order for surface ECG fusion to occur **(Figure 31.5B)**. If the entrance and exit are close together, the wavefront generated by the premature stimulus would enter both the entrance and exit at approximately the same time and no fusion on the surface ECG is seen.

Local fusion refers to fusion of local presystolic activity in the VT reentrant circuit before it is able to reach the exit such that intracardiac fusion is present without surface ECG fusion **(Figure 31.5C)**.

Resetting Response Curves

Response patterns during resetting are helpful in distinguishing the different sustained ventricular arrhythmia mechanisms. The response patterns are characterized by plotting the return cycle versus the coupling interval of the extrastimulus producing resetting at the site of stimulation.

There are 4 types of responses to resetting: *flat, increasing, decreasing*, or *mixed*.

A *flat* response is defined by the presence of a return cycle that is constant (less than 10 ms difference) over a ≥ 30 ms range of coupling intervals. An *increasing* response pattern is defined as an increase in return cycle as the coupling interval of the extrastimuli is decreased. A *decreasing* response pattern shows the opposite: a decrease in return cycle with decreasing coupling interval of the extrastimuli. A *mixed* response refers to a flat response at long coupling intervals and an increasing response at shorter coupling intervals. A flat or decreasing curve is expected for triggered rhythms due to DAD **(Figure 31.6)**.

Although a flat response pattern can theoretically be seen in automatic, triggered, and reentrant arrhythmias, a flat response pattern with return cycles *shorter* than the tachycardia cycle length (TCL) is only possible in reentry.

A flat response curve in human VT is most compatible with reentry and suggests the presence of (1) a fully excitable gap (2) fixed entrance and exit of the circuit (3) fixed conduction time to and from the entrance and exit of the circuit to the site of stimulation.

Reentrant arrhythmias can have increasing response to extrastimulation. This response pattern is observed in 1/3 of the VTs studied[62,63] and it is likely due to encroachment of refractory tissue and slowed conduction within the circuit by the extrastimulus (encroaching on phase 3 of the action potential). This gradual increase in return cycle over a long range of decreasing coupling intervals has not been observed in triggered rhythms.

Another feature that distinguishes a reentrant arrhythmia and triggered rhythm is the site specificity of PES for resetting of the tachycardia.[64,65] Triggered activity may be reset to produce flat response curves at 100% to 110% of the TCL or a decreasing return cycle with a direct relationship to the coupling interval. These responses have no stimulation site specificity whereas, the resetting curve may change

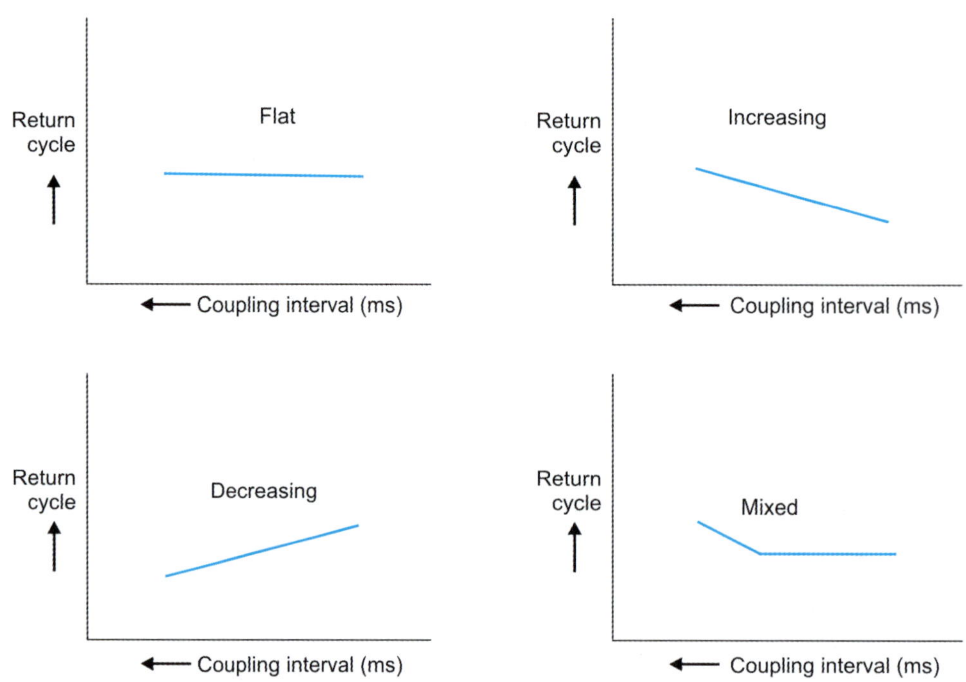

Figure 31.6: Resetting response patterns to the extrastimuli in ventricular tachycardia

depending on the site of stimulation in a reentrant arrhythmias due to anisotropic conduction of the stimulation wavefront.

Entrainment

Entrainment is the continuous resetting of the reentrant circuit by ≥ 2 consecutive premature stimulus. We refer to the first stimulus in a train that resets the circuit as the Nth stimulus. Resetting refers to advancement of the subsequent beat and continuation of the original rhythm by the Nth premature stimulus. Entrainment occurs when N+1 premature stimulus collides with the Nth wavefront in the antidromic direction and conducts in the orthodromic direction without termination of the tachycardia. Since the Nth beat is already reset by the Nth premature stimulus, entrainment by the N+1 stimulus refers to resetting of the already reset circuit by the Nth stimulus.

This has important implications. Only the first stimulus that resets the tachycardia (N^{th} stimulus) interacts with the tachycardia and all subsequent stimuli in the pacing train interact with the reset circuit. Resetting defines characteristics of the original circuit whereas entrainment shows characteristics of the reset circuit. The duration of the excitable gap, conduction velocity within the circuit and refractoriness of the tissue within the circuit are different with entrainment and resetting. Resetting is the only method of defining the original circuit.

The following criteria are used to recognize the presence of entrainment: (1) fixed fusion of the paced complexes at any cycle length (2) fixed progressive fusion at decreasing paced cycle length (PCL) (i.e. the QRS morphology progressively looks more similar to the purely paced QRS complex as the PCL is decreased) (3) resumption of the tachycardia with return cycle equal to TCL at cessation of pacing.

Termination

Reentrant arrhythmias can be terminated by both PES and overdrive pacing.

With earlier delivery of an extrastimulus in a reentrant tachycardia, the extrastimulus encroaches on the refractory tissue and *abruptly* terminates the tachycardia. This abrupt termination of tachycardia by PES distinguishes reentry from triggered activity. Termination by either extrastimuli or overdrive pacing can be abrupt in a triggered rhythm but is often preceded by several afterdepolarizations of increased cycle lengths, i.e. gradual slowing of the triggered rhythm before termination.[11,66-68]

Analyzing the resetting response curve of a reentrant tachycardia would show a flat component followed by an increasing component before termination of the tachycardia. In other words, resetting should be observed before termination of a reentrant tachycardia.

The tachycardia cycle length seems to be the main determinant of whether the tachycardia can be terminated by some form of programmed stimulation, pacing, or cardioversion. Slower tachycardias with TCL >300 ms are more likely to be terminated by single ventricular extrastimulus (VES). If a reentrant tachycardia can be terminated by single or double VES, it can also be terminated by overdrive pacing.

Again, the site of stimulation influences the likelihood of terminating reentrant arrhythmias. Changing the site of stimulation may modify the ability of the stimulated impulse to reach the tachycardia site in time to terminate it. This site specific response to termination may be demonstrated in 15–20% of the cases of reentry. Approximately 40% of the VTs demonstrate different resetting curve with RV apical and RVOT stimulation. This change in response depending on the site of stimulation in a reentrant arrhythmia is likely due to anisotropic conduction of the stimulation wavefront.

TYPES OF REENTRANT VENTRICULAR ARRHYTHMIAS

Infarct-related Scar

In our experience, patients with sustained monomorphic VT have the lowest ejection fraction. The extent of the infarction and perhaps a location involving the septum may be the two important prognostic factors associated with these malignant ventricular arrhythmias.[69,70]

About 30% of patients present with their first episode of sustained uniform VT within the first year following myocardial infarction.[58] Previous data suggest a consistent 3–5% per year incidence of VT occurring over the following 15 years. Since the widespread usage of thrombolysis and primary angioplasties, the incidence has decreased to less than 1% per year.[71]

As mentioned above, the cellular remodeling, changes in electrical coupling, and abnormalities of tissue conduction and refractoriness as a result of the infarct provide the substrate for reentry. In addition, gap junction remodeling and cellular apoptosis leads to nonuniform anisotropy, slow conduction, and areas of block for initiation and continuation of reentry.

Reentrant circuits typically arise from areas of fibrosis containing bundles of surviving myocardium. Areas of fibrosis provide the anatomical and functional barriers to form the channels with entrance, common central pathway, and exit of the reentrant circuit.

A reentrant circuit in patients with myocardial infarction has several components: entrance, central common pathway/isthmus, exit, outer loop, and inner loop. This is best depicted in **Figure 31.7**. The wavefront of the ventricular tachycardia encounters lines of block (fixed or functional) usually in parallel orientation to the long axis of the ventricle and enters the entrance of the circuit where the greatest curvature and slowest conduction take place. The wavefront then conducts down the central isthmus. By the time the wavefront reaches the exit of the circuit, it will depolarize

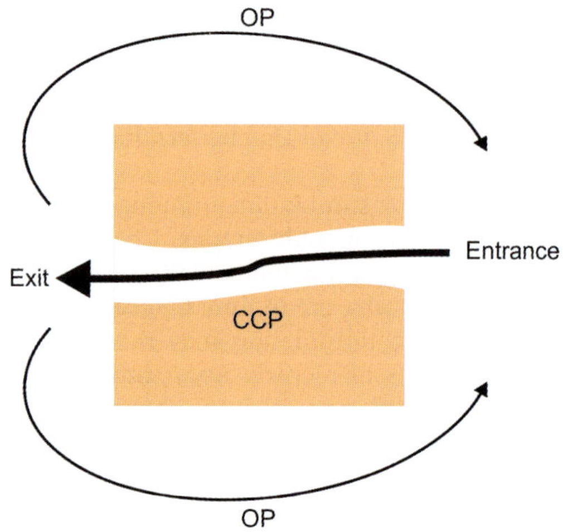

Figure 31.7: Hypothetical figure of eight reentrant circuit of ventricular tachycardia in a patient with prior infarction. The barriers represent areas of anatomical or functional block

Abbreviations: CCP, common central pathway/isthmus; OP, outer pathway/loop

the recovered myocardium and continue conduction along the outer loop to complete the reentrant circuit.

Historically, conduction velocity in the isthmus was considered the slowest such that the wavefront which is confined by the anatomic and functional barriers on each side conducts down the protected central isthmus slowly to allow recovery of tissue distal and outside the central protected zone. This slow conduction provides the delay required for recovery of refractory tissue and reentry.[72,73] Recent data based on both animal and human studies using catheters with small electrodes and closer interelectrode distance showed a very different picture. High-resolution mapping using catheters with small electrodes and closer interelectrode distance allowed more accurate activation mapping and demonstrated that the conduction velocity in the central isthmus is nearly normal whereas the area of slowest conduction actually occurs at the entrance followed by the exit of the reentrant circuit where the greatest curvature takes place. In addition, the high-resolution mapping allowed better definition of the true substrate and circuit of infarct-related VT. In contrast to the common belief that the barriers of the circuit are anatomic areas of fixed block, the borders of the central isthmus is functional due to pseudoblock. Such pseudoblock is a result of anisotropic conduction from a combination of fibrosis, impedance mismatch, gap junction remodeling, and ion channel dysfunction.[74,75]

Bundle Branch Reentry and Interfascicular Reentry

Reentry within the His-Purkinje system can lead to sustained macroreentrant monomorphic VT. Sustained bundle branch reentry (BBR) VT is uncommon and it is rarely the sole inducible monomorphic VT. The patients with BBR VT often have multiple intramyocardial VTs as well.

In most patients with BBR VT, incomplete or complete left bundle branch block (LBBB) pattern with HV ≥65 ms during sinus rhythm is usually present and typically the BBR VT has LBBB morphology. With a premature ventricular stimulus, there is a *unidirectional retrograde block* of the right bundle (RB), followed by slow conduction of the premature stimulus across the septum, conduction up the left bundle (LB), and antegrade conduction down the RB to complete the reentrant circuit. The prolonged VH interval provides the slow conduction criteria for reentry to occur. It is noteworthy that the underlying substrate for BBR VT lies in *conduction delay*, not block, in the bundle branches. If true block is present in either bundle branches, BBR would not be possible.

The HV interval during BBR VT may be longer or shorter than the HV interval during sinus rhythm depending on the site of His recording. If the His electrogram is recorded distally, the HV interval is equal to or longer than the HV interval during sinus rhythm. On the other hand, if the His electrogram is recorded more proximally, the HV interval should be shorter than the HV interval recorded during sinus rhythm; however, a HV interval more than 15 ms shorter than the HV interval during sinus rhythm is never observed in BBR, but rather the rule in *interfascicular* reentry.

The excitable gap in BBR exists within the HPS and is determined by HPS refractoriness.

VT due to *interfascicular reentry* is most commonly seen in patients with coronary artery disease (CAD), specifically those with anterior infarct, RB branch block (RBBB), and either left anterior fascicular block (LAFB) or left posterior fascicular block (LPFB). In these patients, RBBB is complete and bidirectional; hence, BBR VT does not occur. In the case of interfascicular VT, the slow conduction takes place in the presumed "blocked" fascicle which is actually slowly conducting in sinus rhythm relative to the "healthy" fascicle. A premature stimulus (atrial or ventricular) leads to block in the slowly conducting fascicle and conduction down the other hemifascicle giving rise to the same QRS morphology as sinus rhythm, and then reenters the blocked hemifascicle to induce reentrant VT. In this case, the HV interval is at least 40 ms shorter than the HV interval during sinus rhythm.[58]

Verapamil Sensitive Ventricular Tachycardia

One type of idiopathic VT that occurs in patients with structurally normal hearts is Verapamil Sensitive or Fascicular VT. There are three subtypes of verapamil sensitive VT: (1) "left posterior fascicular" VT with RBBB and LAFB morphology (2) "left anterior fascicular" VT with RBBB and LPFB morphology (3) upper fascicular VT with narrow QRS and normal or right axis.

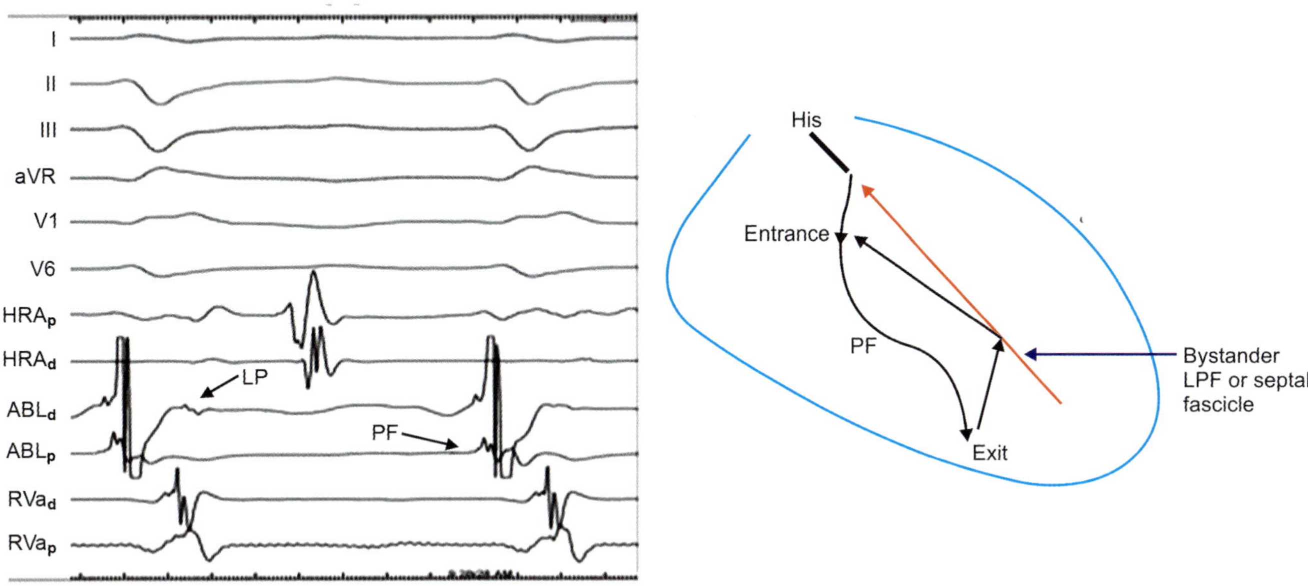

Figure 31.8: Verapamil sensitive ventricular tachycardia
From top to bottom in the left panel are—surface ECG leads, I, II, III, aVR, V1 and V6; high right atrium proximal (HRA_p) and distal (HRA_d); ablation distal (ABL_d) and proximal (ABL_p); right ventricular apex distal (RVa_d) and proximal (RVa_p)
Abbreviations: LP, late potential; LPF, left posterior fascicle; PF, abnormal verapamil sensitive Purkinje fiber

The so called "left posterior fascicular" VT accounts for 90% of the verapamil sensitive VTs. The tachycardia is characterized by RBBB and superior axis suggesting an exit near the left posterior fascicle. Endocardial mapping during ventricular tachycardia showed earliest site of activation in the region of the inferoposterior or inferoapical LV septum and was associated with early Purkinje activation. Some investigators suggest this activation is over the posterior fascicle despite the fact that early activity is on the septum.[76] So far, evidences point to a reentrant mechanism using the abnormal verapamil-sensitive fibers as the antegrade limb of the reentrant circuit.[77] The retrograde limb is uncertain, although it appears to connect to the HPS. It is unlikely that the HPS is critical since the VT can be entrained from the atrium with complete normalization of the QRS and HV with resumption of the tachycardia on cessation of pacing.[78]

False tendons or fibromuscular bands that extend from the posterior inferior LV to the basal septum have been reported to be part of the reentrant circuit. Histological analysis of the false tendons in one of the patients showed Purkinje fibers oriented parallel to the long axis of the tendon and inserting into the endocardium.[79] However, false tendons are present in a high percentage of patients without verapamil sensitive fascicular VT and the direct cause-effect relation between the two remains unclear.[80,81]

The mechanism of the verapamil sensitive fascicular VT is most consistent with reentry based on the ability to initiate and terminate by atrial and ventricular premature stimulus, reset and entrainment with fusion, and presence of an inverse relationship between the coupling interval of the initiating VES or PCL and the first beat of the tachycardia.[82]

In sinus rhythm, the impulse conducts down both the retrograde limb of the reentrant circuit and the abnormal fiber; however, the abnormal fiber is activated retrogradely by the retrograde limb of the circuit due to slow antegrade conduction. With premature stimulation, unidirectional block occurs in the retrograde limb of the reentrant circuit and the abnormal fiber is activated antegradely. Due to the slow conduction of the abnormal fiber, the retrograde limb of the reentrant circuit recovers and is engaged at the distal end by the abnormal fiber and conduct retrogradely to complete the circuit. The left posterior fascicle or other more distal Purkinje fibers are passively engaged and conducts to generate the QRS with RBBB and LAFB morphology as well as responsible for retrograde His bundle activation that is usually seen **(Figure 31.8)**.

The tissue exhibits slow, decremented conduction, that is verapamil sensitive, along the midseptum.[83] Hence, the tachycardia slows and terminates in response to verapamil. Even though both outflow tract VTs and fascicular VTs are based on a calcium dependent mechanism, adenyl cyclase induced increase in cAMP and subsequent Ca^{+2} overload is responsible for triggered outflow tract VTs whereas fascicular VTs are due to a slow inward Ca^{+2} current for arrhythmia initiation. The ability to terminate the outflow tract triggered tachycardia but not fascicular VT with adenosine theoretically is a helpful way to distinguish the two arrhythmias; however, no systemic evaluation of the effects of adenosine on the "fascicular VTs" have been done.

REFERENCES

1. Mangoni ME, Nargeot J. Genesis and regulation of the heart automaticity. Physiol Rev. 2008;88:919-82.
2. Barbuti A, Baruscotti M, DiFrancesco D. The pacemaker current: from basics to the clinics. J Cardiovasc Electrophysiol. 2007;18:342-7.
3. Lakatta EG. A paradigm shift for the heart's pacemaker. Heart Rhythm. 2010;7:559-64.
4. Venetucci LA, Trafford AW, O'Neill SC, Eisner DA. The sarcoplasmic reticulum and arrhythmogenic calcium release. Cardiovasc Res. 2008;77:285-92.
5. DiFrancesco D. The role of the funny current in pacemaker activity. Circ Res. 2010;106:434-46.
6. Maltsev VA, Lakatta EG. Dynamic interactions of an intracellular Ca^{2+} clock and membrane ion channel clock underlie robust initiation and regulation of cardiac pacemaker function. Cardiovasc Res. 2008;77:274-84.
7. NS Peters CC, AL Wit. Arrythmogenic mechanisms: automaticity, triggered activity, and reentry. In: DP Zipes JJ (Ed). Cardiac Electrophysiology: from cell to bedside, 3rd edn. 2000: Saunders; 2000.
8. Dangman KH, Hoffman BF. Studies on overdrive stimulation of canine cardiac Purkinje fibers: maximal diastolic potential as a determinant of the response. J Am Coll Cardiol. 1983;2: 1183-90.
9. Han X, Ferrier GR. Contribution of Na(+)-Ca^{2+} exchange to stimulation of transient inward current by isoproterenol in rabbit cardiac Purkinje fibers. Circ Res. 1995;76:664-74.
10. Wit AL, Cranefield PF. Triggered activity in cardiac muscle fibers of the simian mitral valve. Circ Res. 1976;38:85-98.
11. Johnson N, Danilo P, Jr., Wit AL, Rosen MR. Characteristics of initiation and termination of catecholamine-induced triggered activity in atrial fibers of the coronary sinus. Circulation. 1986;74:1168-79.
12. Wit AL, Cranefield PF, Gadsby DC. Electrogenic sodium extrusion can stop triggered activity in the canine coronary sinus. Circ Res. 1981;49:1029-42.
13. Lerman BB, Wesley RC, Jr., DiMarco JP, Haines DE, Belardinelli L. Antiadrenergic effects of adenosine on His-Purkinje automaticity. Evidence for accentuated antagonism. J Clin Invest. 1988;82:2127-35.
14. Lerman BB. Mechanism of outflow tract tachycardia. Heart Rhythm. 2007;4:973-6.
15. Lerman BB, Dong B, Stein KM, Markowitz SM, Linden J, Catanzaro DF. Right ventricular outflow tract tachycardia due to a somatic cell mutation in G protein subunitalphai2. J Clin Invest. 1998;101:2862-8.
16. Kieval RS, Johnson NJ, Rosen MR. Triggered activity as a cause of bigeminy. J Am Coll Cardiol. 1986;8:644-7.
17. Baher AA, Uy M, Xie F, Garfinkel A, Qu Z, Weiss JN. Bidirectional ventricular tachycardia: ping pong in the His-Purkinje system. Heart Rhythm. 2011;8:599-605.
18. Icardo JM, Colvee E. Collagenous skeleton of the human mitral papillary muscle. Anat Rec. 1998;252:509-18.
19. Josephson ME, Wit AL. Fractionated electrical activity and continuous electrical activity: fact or artifact? Circulation. 1984;70:529-32.
20. Gardner PI, Ursell PC, Fenoglio JJ, Jr., Wit AL. Electrophysiologic and anatomic basis for fractionated electrograms recorded from healed myocardial infarcts. Circulation. 1985;72:596-611.
21. de Bakker J, Janse M. Pathophysiologic correlates of ventricular tachycardia in hearts with a healed infarct. In: Zipes DP, Jalife J., ed. Cardiac electrophysiology: from cell to bedside. Philadelphia: WB Saunders; 2000.
22. Beyer EC, Paul DL, Goodenough DA. Connexin family of gap junction proteins. J Membr Biol. 1990;116:187-94.
23. Beyer EC, Paul DL, Goodenough DA. Connexin43: a protein from rat heart homologous to a gap junction protein from liver. J Cell Biol. 1987;105:2621-9.
24. Davis LM, Rodefeld ME, Green K, Beyer EC, Saffitz JE. Gap junction protein phenotypes of the human heart and conduction system. J Cardiovasc Electrophysiol. 1995;6: 813-22.
25. Smith JH, Green CR, Peters NS, Rothery S, Severs NJ. Altered patterns of gap junction distribution in ischemic heart disease. An immunohistochemical study of human myocardium using laser scanning confocal microscopy. Am J Pathol. 1991;139: 801-21.
26. Peters NS, Coromilas J, Severs NJ, Wit AL. Disturbed connexin43 gap junction distribution correlates with the location of reentrant circuits in the epicardial border zone of healing canine infarcts that cause ventricular tachycardia. Circulation. 1997;95:988-96.
27. Peters NS, Wit AL. Myocardial architecture and ventricular arrhythmogenesis. Circulation. 1998;97:1746-54.
28. de Bakker JM, Wittkampf FH. The pathophysiologic basis of fractionated and complex electrograms and the impact of recording techniques on their detection and interpretation. Circ Arrhythm Electrophysiol. 2010;3:204-13.
29. Cassidy DM, Vassallo JA, Miller JM, Poll DS, Buxton AE, Marchlinski FE, Josephson ME. Endocardial catheter mapping in patients in sinus rhythm: relationship to underlying heart disease and ventricular arrhythmias. Circulation. 1986;73: 645-52.
30. Vassallo JA, Cassidy DM, Marchlinski FE, Miller JM, Buxton AE, Josephson ME. Abnormalities of endocardial activation pattern in patients with previous healed myocardial infarction and ventricular tachycardia. Am J Cardiol. 1986;58:479-84.
31. Cassidy DM, Vassallo JA, Marchlinski FE, Buxton AE, Untereker WJ, Josephson ME. Endocardial mapping in humans in sinus rhythm with normal left ventricles: activation patterns and characteristics of electrograms. Circulation. 1984;70:37-42.
32. Cassidy DM, Vassallo JA, Buxton AE, Doherty JU, Marchlinski FE, Josephson ME. Catheter mapping during sinus rhythm: relation of local electrogram duration to ventricular tachycardia cycle length. Am J Cardiol. 1985;55:713-6.
33. Untereker WJ, Spielman SR, Waxman HL, Horowitz LN, Josephson ME. Ventricular activation in normal sinus rhythm: abnormalities with recurrent sustained tachycardia and a history of myocardial infarction. Am J Cardiol. 1985;55:974-9.
34. Kienzle MG, Miller J, Falcone RA, Harken A, Josephson ME. Intraoperative endocardial mapping during sinus rhythm: relationship to site of origin of ventricular tachycardia. Circulation. 1984;70:957-65.
35. Shaw RM, Rudy Y. Ionic mechanisms of propagation in cardiac tissue. Roles of the sodium and L-type calcium currents during reduced excitability and decreased gap junction coupling. Circ Res. 1997;81:727-41.
36. Ek-Vitorin JF, Calero G, Morley GE, Coombs W, Taffet SM, Delmar M. PH regulation of connexin43: molecular analysis of the gating particle. Biophys J. 1996;71:1273-84.

37. Downar E, Janse MJ, Durrer D. The effect of acute coronary artery occlusion on subepicardial transmembrane potentials in the intact porcine heart. Circulation. 1977;56:217-24.
38. Kleber AG, Janse MJ, Wilms-Schopmann FJ, Wilde AA, Coronel R. Changes in conduction velocity during acute ischemia in ventricular myocardium of the isolated porcine heart. Circulation. 1986;73:189-98.
39. Maltsev VA, Sabbab HN, Undrovinas AI. Down-regulation of sodium current in chronic heart failure: effect of long-term therapy with carvedilol. Cell Mol Life Sci. 2002;59:1561-8.
40. Borlak J, Thum T. Hallmarks of ion channel gene expression in end-stage heart failure. FASEB J. 2003;17:1592-608.
41. Baba S, Dun W, Cabo C, Boyden PA. Remodeling in cells from different regions of the reentrant circuit during ventricular tachycardia. Circulation. 2005;112:2386-96.
42. Kieken F, Mutsaers N, Dolmatova E, Virgil K, Wit AL, Kellezi A, Hirst-Jensen BJ, Duffy HS, Sorgen PL. Structural and molecular mechanisms of gap junction remodeling in epicardial border zone myocytes following myocardial infarction. Circ Res. 2009;104:1103-12.
43. Macia E, Dolmatova E, Cabo C, Sosinsky AZ, Dun W, Coromilas J, Ciaccio EJ, Boyden PA, Wit AL, Duffy HS. Characterization of gap junction remodeling in epicardial border zone of healing canine infarcts and electrophysiological effects of partial reversal by rotigaptide. Circ Arrhythm Electrophysiol. 2011;4:344-51.
44. Luke RA, Saffitz JE. Remodeling of ventricular conduction pathways in healed canine infarct border zones. J Clin Invest. 1991;87:1594-602.
45. Spach MS, Miller WT, 3rd, Geselowitz DB, Barr RC, Kootsey JM, Johnson EA. The discontinuous nature of propagation in normal canine cardiac muscle. Evidence for recurrent discontinuities of intracellular resistance that affect the membrane currents. Circ Res. 1981;48:39-54.
46. Spach MS, Dolber PC, Heidlage JF. Influence of the passive anisotropic properties on directional differences in propagation following modification of the sodium conductance in human atrial muscle. A model of reentry based on anisotropic discontinuous propagation. Circ Res. 1988;62:811-32.
47. Spach MS, Josephson ME. Initiating reentry: the role of nonuniform anisotropy in small circuits. J Cardiovasc Electrophysiol. 1994;5:182-209.
48. Fast VG, Kleber AG. Role of wavefront curvature in propagation of cardiac impulse. Cardiovasc Res. 1997;33:258-71.
49. Fast VG, Kleber AG. Block of impulse propagation at an abrupt tissue expansion: evaluation of the critical strand diameter in 2- and 3-dimensional computer models. Cardiovasc Res. 1995;30:449-59.
50. Cabo C, Pertsov AM, Baxter WT, Davidenko JM, Gray RA, Jalife J. Wave-front curvature as a cause of slow conduction and block in isolated cardiac muscle. Circ Res. 1994;75:1014-28.
51. Kucera JP, Rudy Y. Mechanistic insights into very slow conduction in branching cardiac tissue: a model study. Circ Res. 2001;89:799-806.
52. Kucera JP, Kleber AG, Rohr S. Slow conduction in cardiac tissue, II: effects of branching tissue geometry. Circ Res. 1998;83:795-805.
53. Quan W, Rudy Y. Unidirectional block and reentry of cardiac excitation: a model study. Circ Res. 1990;66:367-82.
54. Shaw RM, Rudy Y. The vulnerable window for unidirectional block in cardiac tissue: characterization and dependence on membrane excitability and intercellular coupling. J Cardiovasc Electrophysiol. 1995;6:115-31.
55. Starmer CF, Biktashev VN, Romashko DN, Stepanov MR, Makarova ON, Krinsky VI. Vulnerability in an excitable medium: analytical and numerical studies of initiating unidirectional propagation. Biophys J. 1993;65:1775-87.
56. Vassallo JA, Cassidy DM, Kindwall KE, Marchlinski FE, Josephson ME. Nonuniform recovery of excitability in the left ventricle. Circulation. 1988;78:1365-72.
57. Peters NS, Coromilas J, Hanna MS, Josephson ME, Costeas C, Wit AL. Characteristics of the temporal and spatial excitable gap in anisotropic reentrant circuits causing sustained ventricular tachycardia. Circ Res. 1998;82:279-93.
58. Josephson ME. Clinical Cardiac Electrophysiology: Techniques and Interpretations. 4th edn. Philadelphia: Lippincott Williams and Wilkins; 2008.
59. Doherty JU, Kienzle MG, Waxman HL, Buxton AE, Marchlinski FE, Josephson ME. Programmed ventricular stimulation at a second right ventricular site: an analysis of 100 patients, with special reference to sensitivity, specificity and characteristics of patients with induced ventricular tachycardia. Am J Cardiol. 1983;52:1184-9.
60. Robertson JF, Cain ME, Horowitz LN, Spielman SR, Greenspan AM, Waxman HL, Josephson ME. Anatomic and electrophysiologic correlates of ventricular tachycardia requiring left ventricular stimulation. Am J Cardiol. 1981;48:263-8.
61. Josephson ME, Almendral J, Callans DJ. Resetting and entrainment of reentrant ventricular tachycardia associated with myocardial infarction. Heart Rhythm. 2014;11:1239-49.
62. Josephson ME, Almendral JM, Buxton AE, Marchlinski FE. Mechanisms of ventricular tachycardia. Circulation. 1987;75:III41-7.
63. Almendral JM, Stamato NJ, Rosenthal ME, Marchlinski FE, Miller JM, Josephson ME. Resetting response patterns during sustained ventricular tachycardia: relationship to the excitable gap. Circulation. 1986;74:722-30.
64. Rosenthal ME, Stamato NJ, Almendral JM, Marchlinski FE, Buxton AE, Miller JM, Josephson ME. Influence of the site of stimulation on the resetting phenomenon in ventricular tachycardia. Am J Cardiol. 1986;58:970-6.
65. Callans DJ, Zardini M, Gottlieb CD, Josephson ME. The variable contribution of functional and anatomic barriers in human ventricular tachycardia: an analysis with resetting from two sites. J Am Coll Cardiol. 1996;27:1106-11.
66. Peters N, Cabo C, Wit AL. Arrythmogenic mechanisms: Automaticity, triggered activity, and reentry. Cardiac Electrophysiology: from cell to bedside. Chapter 40. Philadelphia: WB Saunders; 2000.
67. Brugada P, Wellens HJJ. Cardiac arrhythmias : where to go from here? Mount Kisco, N.Y.: Futura Pub. Co.; 1987.
68. Cranefield PF, Aronson RS. Cardiac arrhythmias: the role of triggered activity and other mechanisms. Mount Kisco, N.Y.: Futura Pub. Co.; 1988.
69. Bolick DR, Hackel DB, Reimer KA, Ideker RE. Quantitative analysis of myocardial infarct structure in patients with ventricular tachycardia. Circulation. 1986;74:1266-79.
70. Adhar GC, Larson LW, Bardy GH, Greene HL. Sustained ventricular arrhythmias: differences between survivors of cardiac arrest and patients with recurrent sustained ventricular tachycardia. J Am Coll Cardiol. 1988;12:159-65.

71. Wyse DG, Friedman PL, Brodsky MA, Beckman KJ, Carlson MD, Curtis AB, Hallstrom AP, Raitt MH, Wilkoff BL, Greene HL Life-threatening ventricular arrhythmias due to transient or correctable causes: high risk for death in follow-up. J Am Coll Cardiol. 2001;38:1718-24.
72. Cabo C, Yao J, Boyden PA, Chen S, Hussain W, Duffy HS, Ciaccio EJ, Peters NS, Wit AL. Heterogeneous gap junction remodeling in reentrant circuits in the epicardial border zone of the healing canine infarct. Cardiovasc Res. 2006;72:241-9.
73. Ciaccio EJ. Localization of the slow conduction zone during reentrant ventricular tachycardia. Circulation. 2000;102: 464-9.
74. Josephson ME, Anter E. Substrate mapping for ventricular tachycardia: assumptions and misconceptions. JACC: Clin Electrophysiol. 2015;1:341-52.
75. Anter E, Tschabrunn CM, Buxton AE, Josephson ME. High-resolution mapping of post-infarction reentrant ventricular tachycardia: electrophysiological characterization of the circuit. Circulation. (accepted for publication).
76. Nakagawa H, Beckman KJ, McClelland JH, Wang X, Arruda M, Santoro I, Hazlitt HA, Abdalla I, Singh A, Gossinger H, Sweidan R, Hirao K, Widman L, Pitha JV, Lazzara R, Jackman WM. Radiofrequency catheter ablation of idiopathic left ventricular tachycardia guided by a Purkinje potential. Circulation. 1993; 88:2607-17.
77. Nogami A, Naito S, Tada H, Taniguchi K, Okamoto Y, Nishimura S, Yamauchi Y, Aonuma K, Goya M, Iesaka Y, Hiroe M. Demonstration of diastolic and presystolic Purkinje potentials as critical potentials in a macroreentry circuit of verapamil-sensitive idiopathic left ventricular tachycardia. J Am Coll Cardiol. 2000;36:811-23.
78. Morishima I, Nogami A, Tsuboi H, Sone T. Negative participation of the left posterior fascicle in the reentry circuit of verapamil-sensitive idiopathic left ventricular tachycardia. J Cardiovasc Electrophysiol. 2012;23:556-9.
79. Suwa M, Yoneda Y, Nagao H, Sakai Y, Nakayama Y, Hirota Y, Kawamura K, Iwa T. Surgical correction of idiopathic paroxysmal ventricular tachycardia possibly related to left ventricular false tendon. Am J Cardiol. 1989;64:1217-20.
80. Thakur RK, Klein GJ, Sivaram CA, Zardini M, Schleinkofer DE, Nakagawa H, Yee R, Jackman WM. Anatomic substrate for idiopathic left ventricular tachycardia. Circulation. 1996;93: 497-501.
81. Lin FC, Wen MS, Wang CC, Yeh SJ, Wu D. Left ventricular fibromuscular band is not a specific substrate for idiopathic left ventricular tachycardia. Circulation. 1996;93:525-8.
82. Okumura K, Yamabe H, Tsuchiya T, Tabuchi T, Iwasa A, Yasue H. Characteristics of slow conduction zone demonstrated during entrainment of idiopathic ventricular tachycardia of left ventricular origin. Am J Cardiol. 1996;77:379-83.
83. Tsuchiya T, Okumura K, Honda T, Iwasa A, Ashikaga K. Effects of verapamil and lidocaine on two components of the re-entry circuit of verapamil-senstitive idiopathic left ventricular tachycardia. J Am Coll Cardiol. 2001;37:1415-21.

EDITORS' SUMMARY

Drs Josephson and Li have provided what will be an enduring reference for students of electrophysiology looking for a concise yet comprehensive introduction to ventricular tachycardia. The sections on mechanisms of ventricular arrhythmia are applicable for a variety of areas in cardiac electrophysiology and contain simple, easy to understand explanations along with appropriate references for complex phenomena difficult for the student to learn themselves.

The section in this chapter that explains what "substrate" for arrhythmia means is insightful and will make the chapters on cardiac mapping (See Chapters 8 and 9) more relevant.

The introductory explanation to the fundamentals of resetting and entrainment will make a perfect preface to the detailed entrainment chapter in this textbook (See Chapter 43). Uniquely high in teaching value is Dr Josephson's explanation of verapamil sensitive ventricular tachycardia as well as the mechanism of triggered activity. This chapter along with the sections on entrainment, diagnostic maneuvers for supraventricular tachycardia, and the principles of cardiac mapping constitute a series within this textbook that will be the cornerstone for any specialized instruction in invasive electrophysiology.

CHAPTER 32

Adam Lee, Haris M Haqqani

Ventricular Tachycardia in Ischemic and Nonischemic Cardiomyopathy: Reentrant Circuits, Mapping Techniques and Ablation Strategies

LIST OF ABBREVIATIONS

3D	Three-dimensional	LAVA	Local Abnormal Ventricular Activity
BBRVT	Bundle Branch Reentrant Ventricular Tachycardia	LBBB	Left Bundle Branch Block
CAD	Coronary Artery Disease	LV	Left Ventricle
CMR	Cardiac Magnetic Resonance	MI	Myocardial Infarction
CT	Computed Tomography	NOAC	Novel Oral Anticoagulant
CTCA	Computed Tomography Coronary Angiogram	PPI	Postpacing Interval
DCM	Dilated Cardiomyopathy	PTSD	Post-traumatic Stress Disorder
E-IDC	Electrograms with Isolated Delayed Components	PVC	Premature Ventricular Complex
ECG	Electrocardiogram	RBBB	Right Bundle Branch Block
ECMO	Extracorporeal Membrane Oxygenation	RCA	Right Coronary Artery
EGM	Electrogram	RF	Radiofrequency
EUS	Electrically Unexcitable Scar	RV	Right Ventricle
GA	General Anesthesia	SCD	Sudden Cardiac Death
IABP	Intra-aortic Balloon Pump	TCL	Tachycardia Cycle Length
ICD	Implantable Cardioverter-Defibrillator	TEE	Transesophageal Echocardiography
ICE	Intracardiac Echocardiography	TTE	Transthoracic Echocardiogram
IP	Isolated Potential	VT	Ventricular Tachycardia
LAD	Left Anterior Descending		

INTRODUCTION

Ventricular tachycardia (VT) in the setting of structural heart is a prognostically significant arrhythmia that can lead to sudden cardiac death (SCD). This can occur in two broad settings: VT that arises in the post-myocardial infarction (MI) context, i.e. ischemic cardiomyopathy and VT that arises in patients with nonischemic dilated cardiomyopathy (DCM).

Despite advances in the secondary prevention of coronary artery disease (CAD) and improved focus on risk factor modification in recent decades, CAD remains the leading cause of death in middle and high income countries.[1] Myocardial infarction (MI) that arises in the setting of CAD leads to the formation of scar that acts as the substrate for reentrant VT whilst causing left ventricular (LV) systolic dysfunction. Sudden cardiac death or presumed arrhythmic death is the leading cause of mortality in patients with CAD.[2] Additionally, CAD is the underlying etiology in the majority of the patients who present with SCD.[3]

In contrast, nonischemic DCM refers to myocardial disease and dysfunction that are not due to MI. This umbrella term comprises multiple different underlying etiologies including sarcoidosis, viral myocarditis, Chagas disease, laminopathy and ectopy-mediated cardiomyopathy. Some of these specific entities are addressed in other chapters and the discussion here will focus predominantly on idiopathic DCM. It is important to recognize that some patients with DCM have coexisting CAD that has not caused MI scar formation, the so-called mixed myopathy group.[4]

In patients with CAD and DCM, the role of the implantable cardioverter defibrillator (ICD) in addressing the risk of SCD is now well established both for patients that have suffered VT or cardiac arrest (secondary prevention) as well as those who are at significant risk of but have not yet had VT (primary prevention).[5] Although ICDs can terminate acute VT, they are unable to prevent the occurrence of arrhythmias and thus, serve to reduce the risk of SCD rather than modify the VT substrate. High-voltage shocks from ICDs are painful and known to be associated with significant morbidity, particularly psychological, with up to 20% of patients who have experienced shocks developing post-traumatic stress disorder (PTSD).[6,7] Recent studies have also associated ICD shocks, both appropriate and inappropriate, with increased mortality.[8,9]

The role of medical therapy in the prevention of VT is limited. Beta-blockers and angiotensin converting enzyme inhibitors are the cornerstone of therapy in patients with LV systolic dysfunction. Though these agents reduce the risk of SCD,[2,10-14] the residual arrhythmic risk in some patients, particularly in those with more advanced LV dysfunction, remains high. With the exception of amiodarone, a drug with significant extracardiac toxicity, most other membrane active antiarrhythmic agents have a limited role in these patients due to their negative inotropic and proarrhythmic effects.

Catheter ablation has an important adjunctive role in the management of VT in patients with ischemic or non-ischemic cardiomyopathy. At present, catheter ablation is usually considered a 'last resort' therapy often in the setting of electrical storm following maximal antiarrhythmic therapy (including long-term amiodarone use).[15] In addition to improving quality of life through reduced shock burden, recent data suggests a prognostic benefit from prophylactic ablation prior to the onset of clinical VT.[16]

PATHOPHYSIOLOGY

Broadly speaking, both reentrant and focal mechanisms may be responsible for sustained monomorphic VT in patients with structural heart disease but the former is operative in the vast majority of cases.[17,18] The substrate for reentry in these patients is usually myocardial scar but other structures such as valve annuli and the His-Purkinje system may also serve as components of the reentry circuitry.[19]

Coronary Artery Disease

In the setting of an acute coronary syndrome, ischemia can result in abnormal automaticity or triggered activity from injured Purkinje cells which may degenerate into polymorphic VT or VF.[20] Focal VT can also occur in the post-infarct setting. These arrhythmias were thought to arise from structures such as diseased Purkinje fibers[21,22] or infarcted papillary muscles.[23] Recent data, however, suggests that focal VT may arise from any region of the infarcted heart and may account for up to 9% of VTs in the postinfarct setting.[24] Nonetheless, the majority of VTs arising in the postinfarct setting are due to macroreentrant circuits.[18,25,26] Early electrophysiological and surgical studies established the close relationship between VT circuits and the infarct scar.[27] Subendocardial resection of this substrate eliminated VT in patients who survived the perioperative period.[28]

An acute coronary occlusion leads to MI in a specific territory corresponding to the distribution of the affected major epicardial vessel. The process of myocardial necrosis is predominantly subendocardial as the epicardial location of the major coronary arteries results in a gradient of injury from the endocardium to the epicardium during an acute coronary occlusion.[29] Extended periods of coronary occlusions (as occurs in ST-elevation MI) do, however, result in larger, transmural infarcts. As such, patients with post-MI scar VT have predominantly endocardial-based scars in predictable locations.

Infarction results in loss of myocytes with replacement by noncontractile fibrous collagen. This process, however, is patchy and heterogeneous and results in surviving bundles of myocytes within the regions of dense fibrous tissue. Such myofibril bundles may organize into conducting channels that can form protected diastolic isthmuses during VT. The surviving myocytes within these bundles are poorly coupled electrically due to the presence of interstitial fibrosis and gap junction dysfunction. This results in slow circuitous wavefront propagation through scar and also leads to the potential for unidirectional conduction block due to impedance mismatch.[30] Whilst dense scar may form anatomic barriers that constrain the VT circuit's diastolic isthmus, functional barriers due to heterogeneous refractoriness and wavefront curvature are also important in scar-related reentrant VT.[31]

Clearly the presence of myocardial scar, in itself, is insufficient to cause VT. Many patients with severe left ventricular dysfunction due to widespread scar never develop VT. Compared to post-MI patients without spontaneous clinical VT, patients with equally severe ischemic cardiomyopathy and LV systolic dysfunction show quantitatively and qualitatively different electrophysiologic substrate with smaller areas of electrogram attenuation and a reduced density of abnormal electrograms within the scarred regions.[32]

Dilated Cardiomyopathy

Although the majority of monomorphic VT in DCM is also due to myocardial reentry,[17] the precise mechanisms underlying VT in this context are less well understood compared to the post-MI setting. One of the reasons for this is the lack of an extensive history of surgical investigations that defined the electrophysiology of VT and its precise substrate as occurred with post-MI VT. Also, the process of myocyte loss (by necrosis, apoptosis or both) and fibrosis is more complex in DCM with an unpredictable time course of injury and healing. Fibrosis is seldom seen in confluent surface sheets in this condition as it is after infarct healing and instead occurs predominantly as interstitial and replacement fibrosis in a more patchy and diffuse manner. Nevertheless, DCM patients with VT do show regions of more dense fibrosis but unlike postinfarct patients, in whom the scar is subendocardially based, the substrate in DCM is more variable with a much higher prevalence of biventricular epicardial and intramural scarring.[17,33,34] However, the characteristic feature of the VT substrate in nonischemic cardiomyopathies, regardless of its transmural distribution in any given patient, is its predilection to involve the basal periannular regions.[17,35]

Given that intramural and epicardial substrate are much more common in DCM patients compared to postinfarct settings,[36] an endocardial ablation strategy alone may be insufficient to successfully eliminate all VT circuits.[17] In DCM patients with failed endocardial ablation and suspected epicardial VT exits, the extent of substrate abnormality on the epicardium exceeds that found on the endocardium and endocardial voltage mapping may be largely normal.[33]

In DCM, as discussed later in this chapter, it is particularly important to exclude His-Purkinje system reentry as the cause of any induced VTs.[21] This is due to a predilection to involve this tissue early in the process of diffuse fibrosis, often manifest as left bundle branch block (LBBB). Bundle-branch reentry VT is the most common variant of His-Purkinje reentry seen and its recognition is vital in view of its usually rapid rate and relative ease of elimination with catheter ablation.

PROCEDURAL PLANNING

Ablation of scar-related VT in the context of advanced structural heart disease is a complex procedure performed in an often sick cohort of patients who frequently have poor hemodynamic reserve. There is thus, the consequent potential for significant complications, both cardiac and noncardiac.[37] As such, meticulous attention to detail must be maintained throughout to optimize patient outcomes.

Assessment of Clinical VTs

Prior to the procedure, all efforts should be made to obtain tracings of the patient's clinical arrhythmias. The ideal record of a clinical VT is the 12-lead electrocardiogram (ECG) as these allow for prediction of the location of the scar substrate from which the VT wavefront exits and also allow for easy identification of the clinical arrhythmia if multiple VTs are induced during the EP study. However, many patients will have rapid arrhythmia termination by their ICD and hence 12 lead ECGs of clinical VTs may be difficult to obtain. In these cases, stored ICD electrograms or multilead telemetry tracings may be helpful; valuable information such as electrogram (EGM) morphology and VT cycle length can be obtained from these strips. Additionally, features of the resting 12 lead ECG, particularly regional Q-waves in patients with CAD, can point towards the underlying substrate.

In the setting of focal VT, the surface QRS morphology localizes the point source of origin of the arrhythmia from which centripetal wavefront propagation activates the ventricles. Most focal VT occurs in structurally normal hearts and the ECG is a particularly accurate mapping tool in this context in the absence of scar and distortion of cardiac chamber geometry.[38] In reentrant scar-related VT, however, the surface QRS morphology represents the exit site of the VT circuit as the activation emerges from the constrained diastolic isthmus and depolarizes the remainder of the myocardium, thus generating the QRS. Other components of reentrant VT circuits which may be better targets for ablation (such as the central isthmus) may be located in areas remote from the exit site. Multiple algorithms exist for predicting scar-related VT exit sites, all generated from series of patients with post-infarct VT,[39-41] though their use has been extrapolated in the setting of DCM. Briefly, a right bundle branch block (RBBB)-like morphology (dominant R wave in V1) suggests a left ventricle free wall exit site, whilst a left bundle branch block (LBBB)-like morphology (dominant Q or S wave in V1) usually suggests an exit from the interventricular septum or the right ventricle. If the VT originates from the LV, three additional dimensional axes can be determined. Firstly, leads V4 and aVR differentiate basal from apical exits; negative complexes in V4/aVR suggest an apical exit, whilst positive complexes suggest a basal one. Secondly, as the anterior LV wall is located superiorly, an inferior axis (positive complexes in II, III, aVF) suggests an anterior exit, whilst a superior axis (negative complexes in II, aVF) localizes to the inferior wall. Finally, leads I and aVL can distinguish septal (positive complexes) from lateral wall (negative complexes) **(Figure 32.1)**. As a general rule, most patients with scar VT in the setting of CAD have VT arising

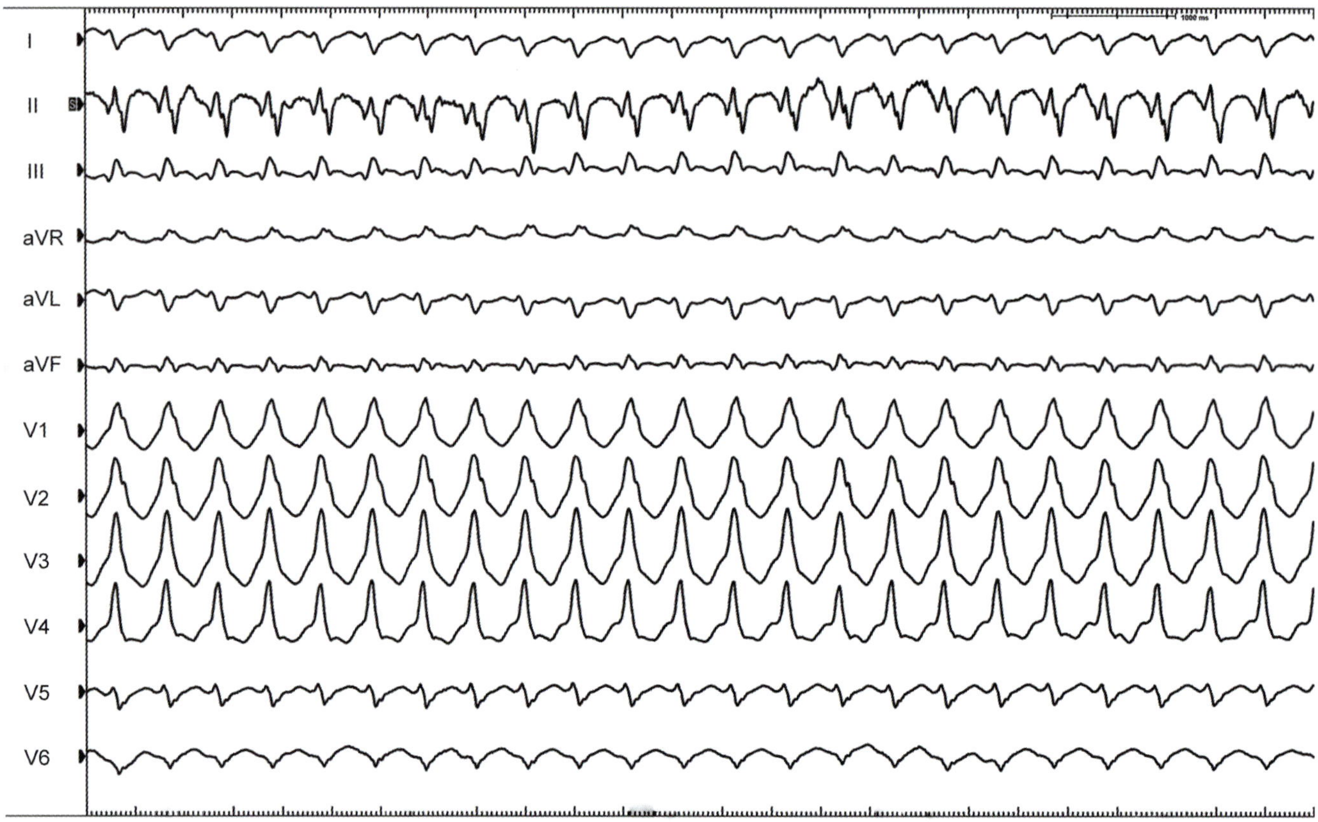

Figure 32.1: VT from basolateral scar. A clinical VT occurring in a patient with an ischemic cardiomyopathy referred for ablation due to recurrent ICD shocks. The VT morphology implies a basal (positive QRS in V4, aVR) and lateral (negative I, aVL) exit site. There is discordance in the inferior leads (negative II, positive III, aVF). The VT was successfully ablated in the region of the basal inferolateral scar

from the left ventricle. The right ventricle can be involved following inferior infarction involving the right coronary artery (RCA) prior to the acute marginal branch,[42] but VT arising from the RV in the setting of CAD is rare.

In patients with DCM, preprocedural identification of epicardial exit sites of clinical VTs is important in predicting epicardial substrate but also the need for pericardial access to facilitate ablation on the epicardium.[17,33] This has implications for procedural planning; a decision may be made to access the pericardial space up front prior to initiation of systemic anticoagulation.[43] Although, the substrate in post-infarct VT is mostly subendocardial, transmural infarction (often involving the posterior LV wall) can result in epicardial substrate, though the area of epicardial scarring tends to be much less than the corresponding endocardial segments.[44] Thus, though less commonly required than in patients with DCM, epicardial ablation may be required in a subset of postinfarct patients.[45,46]

Criteria have been developed that aid in predicting epicardial exit sites based on the surface QRS morphology of VTs.[47-50] Though, these are derived from series of patients without CAD; their use has been extrapolated for use in patients with postinfarction VT. Interval criteria that relate to the onset of the surface QRS rely on the later engagement of the His-Purkinje system with epicardial exits as compared to endocardial ones, resulting in a more 'slurred' QRS. These include a pseudo-delta wave of ≥34 ms, an intrinsicoid deflection of ≥ 85 ms, an RS complex duration of ≥ 121 ms or a maximal deflection index of ≥ 0.59 **(Figure 32.2)**. Morphology criteria rely on the presence or absence of Q-waves in specific leads reflecting the local underlying transmural myocardial depolarization. A Q-wave in lead I suggests an epicardial exit at the basal or apical superior LV, whilst Q-waves in the inferior leads (II, III, aVF) suggest an epicardial exit from the basal or apical inferior LV. Despite the suggestion of an epicardial exit site, it should be remembered that other critical components of the VT circuit may be located elsewhere, including the midmyocardium or endocardium, where they may be better targets for ablation.

Imaging

Preoperative imaging studies are important for procedural planning. Echocardiography is a readily available modality

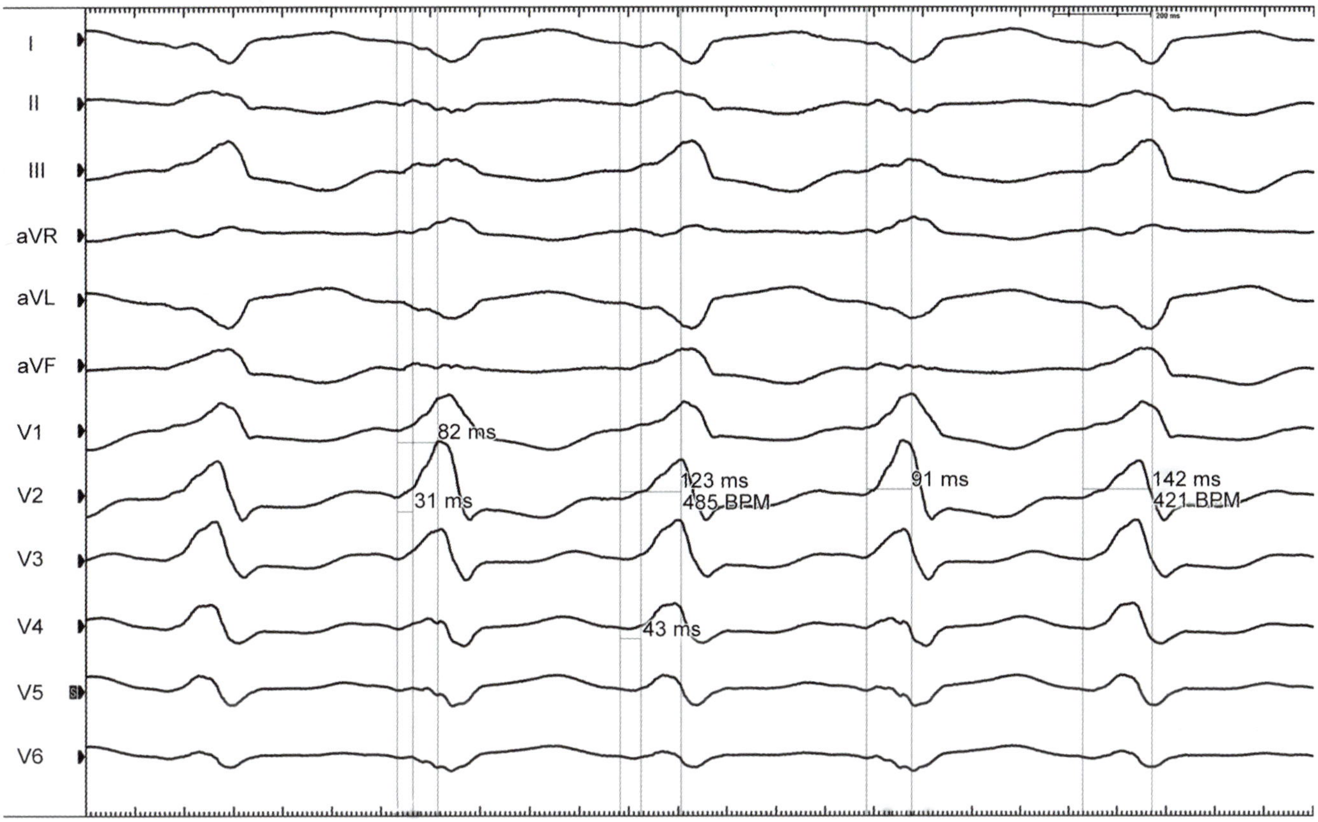

Figure 32.2: **VT with epicardial and endocardial exit sites.** VT occurring in a 73-year-old male with dilated cardiomyopathy (LVEF 33%) with 'alternans' phenomena. The VT circuits utilize a shared isthmus with alternative exit sites on a beat by beat basis. The two QRS morphologies have similar vectorial axes; this represented alternating endocardial and epicardial exits from a presumptive intramural substrate. The 1st, 3rd and 5th beats demonstrate a pseudo-delta wave of 43 ms, an intrinsicoid deflection of 123 ms and an RS complex interval of 142 ms; all features suggestive of an epicardial exit

and gives immediate information with regards to systolic and diastolic function, valvular function and regional wall motion abnormalities. In patients with significant LV dysfunction, a transthoracic echocardiogram (TTE) with contrast is useful to exclude an LV thrombus, particularly if a cardiac magnetic resonance (CMR) imaging study is contraindicated.[51,52] An LV thrombus is traditionally considered a contraindication to instrumentation of the LV endocavity, however, the procedure may still be feasible if the thrombus has organized.[53] Transesophageal echocardiography (TEE) is useful in patients with atrial fibrillation or flutter to exclude a left atrial appendage thrombus as the likelihood of performing cardioversion or defibrillation during a VT study is high. Additionally, presence of severe aortic atheroma diagnosed on TEE may guide towards a transseptal rather than retrograde aortic approach to access the LV endocardium.

CMR is now available in most tertiary centers; such imaging allows direct visualization of myocardial scar whilst also offering an assessment of valvular and overall LV function.[54] The tissue resolution of CMR allows for the precise delineation of the target substrate as late gadolinium enhancement can localize scar as subendocardial, epicardial or transmural.[55,56] This is of particular utility in patients with DCM, in whom the planned ablation approach may be adjusted according to the location of scar. The ability to perform or interpret CMR may, however, be limited by severe renal impairment with the consequential risk of nephrogenic systemic sclerosis,[57] and the presence of implantable cardiac devices. Most patients with structural heart disease presenting for a scar-VT ablation procedure usually already have an ICD in situ. Although, current guidelines suggest that an MRI can often be performed even in the presence of non-MRI conditional devices under strict safety conditions,[58] such scans may currently result in suboptimal imaging due to magnetic susceptibility artifacts.[59]

Intracardiac echocardiography (ICE) is of potentially great utility as a real-time imaging modality during scar-VT ablation procedures. It allows direct visualization of catheter contact, valvular location, endocavitary structures (such as papillary muscles) and lesion formation during ablation.[60] **(Figure 32.3)**. Additionally, ICE allows direct visualization of the interatrial septum during transseptal access. Immediate

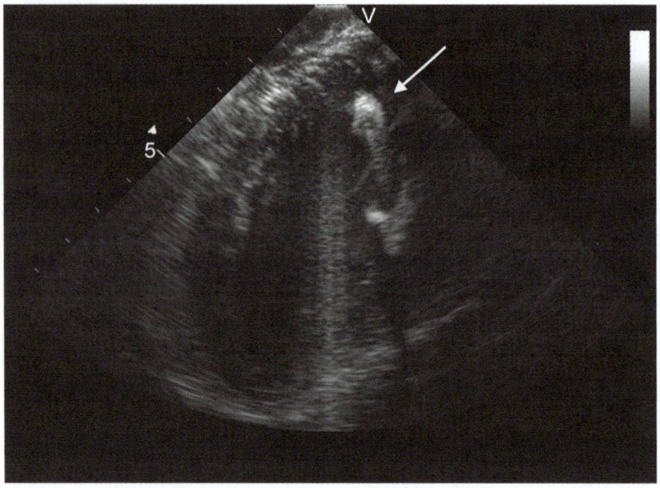

Figure 32.3: Intracardiac echocardiography demonstrating radiofrequency lesion. The left ventricle visualized on intracardiac echocardiography (ICE). The arrow points to a lesion easily visualized following ablation resulting in a 'steam pop'

recognition of complications such as steam pop and cardiac perforation is one of the particular advantages of ICE.[61]

In patients with postinfarct VT, the most recent assessment of coronary arterial status should be sought. In the absence of symptoms of ischemia, a functional study or a computed tomography coronary angiogram (CTCA) may suffice, however, if in doubt, an invasive diagnostic coronary angiogram should be performed. Although coronary revascularization does not alter the arrhythmic substrate,[62,63] any nonrevascularized ischemic territories should be addressed to minimize procedural risk.

Three-dimensional (3D) electroanatomical mapping systems provide immense benefits including reduced radiation exposure, integration with preacquired cardiac chamber imaging (with CT or MRI) and real time integration with ICE or fluoroscopy. They allow for the ability to project electrogram information acquired from roving mapping catheters into 3D color-coded maps. This enables easy visualization of the chamber geometry, the VT circuit, the underlying substrate and lesion delivery during the procedure. The use of such mapping systems is now routine during these procedures.

Anesthesia

Scar-related VT ablation procedures are complex, usually prolonged and involve repeated induction of often poorly tolerated VTs in patients with marginal hemodynamic reserve. The anesthetic agents required for patient tolerance are themselves cardiodepressors.[64] Additionally, the use of open-irrigation catheters in these patients with poor LV systolic function may result in pulmonary edema.[65] As such, preprocedural optimization of their clinical volume status is critical to procedural safety.

The choice of anesthetic strategy lies between general anesthesia (GA) and conscious sedation and both have their own particular limitations. GA may impose a greater hemodynamic stress, may limit the inducibility of VT and may render those that are inducible nonmappable due to poor hemodynamic tolerance. However, if epicardial access or a predominantly substrate-based ablation is planned, GA offers significant benefits in regards to patient tolerance for what is often a long procedure.[66] GA potentially improves catheter stability by removing unwanted patient movement and allows controlled apnea if required.[67] Conscious sedation maximizes the chance of inducing VTs with the least possible hemodynamic compromise to allow for entrainment mapping. However, significant doses of sedative are still generally required for patient tolerance. Both strategies have demonstrated comparable safety.[68]

In patients at particular high risk of hemodynamic decompensation, particularly those with severely dilated left ventricles, consideration for mechanical circulatory support should be entertained. This most often involves an intra-aortic balloon pump (IABP), but percutaneous LV support devices (such as the Impella) or even extracorporeal membrane oxygenation (ECMO) are sometimes considered.[69,70]

Vascular Access and Periprocedural Medications

Vascular access should be planned prior to the procedure according to the context and patient-specific factors. In both postinfarct VT and VT in the setting of DCM, LV endocardial mapping is generally performed requiring femoral arterial access if a retrograde approach is undertaken. In DCM, access to the right ventricle (RV) endocardium is often also required, necessitating additional femoral venous access above that required for the usual diagnostic catheter set. If IABP use is planned, contralateral femoral arterial access is required. Similarly, if the use of ICE is planned, additional femoral venous access should be attained. Short sheaths can be initially introduced; these can be switched to longer preformed sheaths depending on clinical requirement.

Access to the LV endocardium can be obtained either via a transseptal or retrograde aortic route depending on patient factors and operator preference. The retrograde aortic route provides better catheter contact in the basal anterior and inferoseptal, basal inferior and basolateral segments, whilst the transseptal route provides better contact on the mid-anteroseptum, the midlateral and apical segments.[71] For the retrograde aortic route, a long braided sheath can be used to overcome femoral tortuosity and to provide better catheter support. The presence of mechanical mitral valve prosthesis precludes transseptal access to the LV endocardium and the presence of a mechanical aortic valve prosthesis or severe peripheral arterial disease precludes retrograde aortic access. In the rare occurrence of both mitral and aortic mechanical prostheses ("no entry ventricle") a primary epicardial procedure can be attempted though adhesions will need to be negotiated.[72] If endocardial access is absolutely required, access has rarely been reported by transapical punctures[73] or transseptal punctures of the interventricular septum.[74]

Periprocedural management of antiarrhythmic and anticoagulant medications must be decided on well prior to the day of the procedure. For elective patients, it is best that antiarrhythmic agents be withheld for 3–5 half lives, though this is clearly not practical for amiodarone. Cessation 1–2 weeks prior to the day of procedure is generally acceptable for most drugs. As arterial access is required in most cases, patients on anticoagulation with warfarin or a novel oral anticoagulant (NOAC) should have their agents withheld. Even if a transseptal procedure is planned, cessation of anticoagulation allows for arterial access in case backup retrograde access or mechanical hemodynamic support is required. Warfarin should be withheld 5 days prior and the INR should be < 1.3 on the day of the procedure. NOACs should be withheld for at least 24 hours; patients with renal impairment may require cessation up to 5 days prior.[75] Bridging anticoagulation may be required in high-risk patients such as those with mechanical mitral valves.

MAPPING AND ABLATION

The gold standard approach to mapping the circuit of any reentrant arrhythmia is with the use of entrainment. In scar-VT ablation, however, the majority of VTs induced are not mappable by entrainment for various reasons, chiefly hemodynamic nontolerability. For this reason, the alternative approach of substrate mapping is frequently utilized. This involves identifying the scar regions in the ventricle and localizing the 'footprints' of the VT circuits during baseline rhythm.

Induction of VT is usually attempted with programmed stimulation from the right ventricle. Multiple induction protocols exist;[76-78] up to four extrastimuli are placed at progressively shortening coupling intervals with at least 2 drive train rates (600 ms and 400 ms). The protocol may need to be repeated at a second pacing site (RV apex or RV outflow tract) if no VT was induced at the initial site. VT may also occur spontaneously or with ectopy-induced during catheter manipulation.

Prior to mapping of myocardial scar VTs, bundle branch reentrant VT (BBRVT) should be excluded as a mechanism of a clinical or induced VT. Although, traditionally associated with DCM where it occurs in up to 11% of patients, BBRVT can occasionally occur in the setting of postinfarct VT, especially if there is evidence of His-Purkinje disease.[21] The typical and most common form of BBRVT involves reentry utilizing the left bundle as the retrograde limb and the right bundle as the anterograde limb; it presents with a rapid wide complex tachycardia (> 200 bpm) with a typical LBBB morphology. It is important to have a catheter recording the His potential as this signal is critical for the diagnosis of BBRVT. Characteristic features include a long HV during tachycardia (exceeding that of the HV during sinus rhythm), H-H intervals predicting V-V intervals during tachycardia wobble, and entrainment from RV apex indicating proximity to the circuit (postpacing interval minus tachycardia cycle length <30 ms). The importance of diagnosing this rhythm early during the study lies in the ease of cure; ablation of the right bundle is generally curative.[79] A reverse form of BBRVT utilizing the same circuit in the opposite direction and interfascicular reentrant VT (due to reentry between the left posterior and left anterior hemifascicles) are less common.[21]

Entrainment Mapping

When a particular reentrant VT circuit can be defined by entrainment, that particular VT is considered mappable. For this to be possible; the VT must be inducible, it must be sustained and monomorphic and have a stable cycle length. It must tolerate perturbation by overdrive pacing without changing morphology or cycle length. Most importantly, the VT must be hemodynamically tolerated. For these reasons, only the minority of VTs are mappable. Nonetheless, a strategy of targeting mappable VTs first is often adopted, particularly if any of these VTs are clinical arrhythmias.

Entrainment mapping enables the precise delineation of components of a VT circuit including critical regions such as the diastolic isthmus.[80-83] As the circuit is mapped during VT, functional as well as anatomical barriers and preferential conduction are accounted for. A reentrant circuit can be disrupted by transecting any component of the circuit. Nonetheless, it is the diastolic corridor or isthmus which is usually the narrowest component and hence the most likely to be blocked by the minimum amount of ablation. Indeed some VTs may terminate with one radiofrequency (RF) lesion applied to these critical regions.[80] Additionally, this isthmus may be shared between multiple circuits; thus allowing the disruption of multiple circuits with the fewest lesions.[84]

The 12 lead morphology of the mappable VT should be analyzed for localization of the VT exit site to focus mapping efforts to this region. An electroanatomic voltage map of the involved ventricle is useful to aid in visualizing the dense region of scar and its border zones. Once the ablation is placed in a candidate region of VT circuitry (ascertained based on the 12 lead morphology of the VT), overdrive pacing should be performed at a rate 10–30 ms faster than the tachycardia cycle length and with an output that is twice the diastolic threshold at a pulse width of 1–2 ms; high outputs are often required in areas of scar. The pacing cycle length should not be excessively short as this risks introducing decrement into a part of the circuit; this is more likely to change functional barriers and render postpacing measurements less valid. Using excessive output risks capturing surrounding areas of myocardium unrelated to the tachycardia circuit. Although the vast majority of VTs in patients with structural heart disease are reentrant in nature, this should be confirmed by demonstrating fixed fusion at a constant pacing cycle length, with progressive fusion at faster pacing rates.[85,86] The last beat of the pacing train is entrained but not fused.

For ventricular overdrive pacing of VT to offer useful information about the current location of the pacing (mapping) catheter relative to the circuit, the tachycardia must continue following pacing cessation without any disturbance to the VT cycle length or morphology. Successful entrainment should be confirmed by ensuring the tachycardia accelerated to the paced cycle length during pacing; the response to and following pacing can then be analyzed.

The first metric to be measured is the difference between postpacing interval (PPI) and tachycardia cycle length (TCL). The PPI is the time measured from the last pacing stimulus to the first return electrogram on the mapping catheter channel. This difference reflects the proximity of the catheter to the VT circuit. Pacing within the circuit will result in the orthodromic wavefront traversing the circuit once and, following pacing cessation, return to the pacing site with a PPI exactly matching the TCL (assuming no decrement due to relative refractoriness within the circuit at the faster pacing rate relative to the TCL). Pacing outside the circuit requires the stimulus to reach the circuit's excitable gap, traverse the circuit, then exit the gap before returning to the pacing site. The excess time, or difference between PPI and TCL, therefore represents the transit time between the circuit and the pacing site. Whilst, in theory, the PPI should equal the TCL if the catheter is within the circuit, a difference of up to 30 ms is accepted as 'in the circuit' to allow for potential decrement due to pacing at a shorter cycle length and the large size of the recording bipole relative to components of the VT circuit.

The second factor to be considered is the QRS morphology during entrainment. During entrainment, there is constant fusion between the myocardium depolarized by the orthodromic wavefront and that depolarized in the antidromic direction by the pacing stimulus prior to its collision with the head of the orthodromic wavefront of the previous cycle. The important distinction to note here is the presence of concealed versus manifest fusion. In the case of pacing within a constrained diastolic isthmus (or a protected adjacent bystander), the antidromic wavefront propagated by the stimulus does not contribute to the QRS morphology if the orthodromic wavefront of the previous cycle has reached the entrance to the isthmus prior to the antidromic wavefront exiting this site. In this case, the two wavefronts will collide within the isthmus and the QRS morphology will look identical to that of the tachycardia. This is termed 'concealed fusion' and its presence places the catheter within a protected component of the VT circuit, either the common isthmus or an adjacent bystander.

The final metric of consideration is the comparison between the time between the stimulus to QRS onset (stim-QRS) during overdrive pacing and the time from the pacing site electrogram to QRS onset (EGM-QRS) during tachycardia. This measure is of use once it is confirmed that the catheter is within the circuit (PPI–TCL <30 ms) and that it is potentially within the protected diastolic isthmus (concealed fusion). In this situation the stim-QRS and EGM-QRS should be equivalent. This time therefore, reflects the distance from the catheter to the orthodromic exit out of the protected isthmus. Stim-QRS/EGM-QRS times should be compared to the TCL. Short times, which indicate catheter proximity to the isthmus exit, are traditionally defined as a stim-QRS/EGM-QRS time of < 30% of the TCL and are termed 'exit sites'. Long stim-QRS/EGM-QRS times indicate a proximal position within the protected isthmus, are defined as 50–70% of the TCL and are termed 'entrance sites'. Central locations within the isthmus are defined as stim-QRS/EGM-QRS times of 30–50% of the TCL. If the stim-QRS/EGM-QRS is particularly long (> 70% of the TCL), then the catheter tip is probably within an 'inner loop' which is a protected pathway connected and in parallel to the diastolic isthmus; ablation here would be unlikely to terminate the tachycardia.

Site of VT termination by a pacing stimulus that does not result in global ventricular capture represents a critical component of the circuit. Such a site indicates the pacing catheter to be within the protected diastolic isthmus as the VT is disrupted without the orthodromic wavefront exiting. These sites are excellent targets for ablation.[87]

A summary of potential catheter locations relative to a VT circuit and the expected parameter values are outlined in **Table 32.1**. Examples of this are demonstrated in **Figures 32.4 to 32.6**.

The central portion of the protected diastolic isthmus is the primary target of entrainment mapping; this is often the narrowest critical segment of the tachycardia circuit and ablation at a site meeting the above criteria, particularly if an isolated potential is seen at this site, will often result in VT termination with minimal ablation.[88] Failure of termination despite ideal entrainment parameters may occur in the setting of inadequate lesion formation, the presence of a wide isthmus requiring multiple lesions to transect the circuit or the presence of deep intramural or epicardial isthmus components which arise beyond the depth of the endocardial ablation lesion.

Substrate Mapping

Since most VTs are unmappable, alternative ablation strategies are often required to find areas in sinus rhythm that have the potential to form VT circuits. Such a strategy, whilst requiring more extensive lesion formation, has the additional benefit of targeting not only inducible clinical tachycardias, but also the substrate underlying non-inducible tachycardias and potential future tachycardias. These strategies, collectively, come under the umbrella term 'substrate mapping'[89] and have been shown to result in

Table 32.1: Responses to entrainment mapping and the corresponding sites in relation to the entrained VT

Site	*Description*	*PPI–TCL (ms)*	*Concealed Fusion*	*Stim-QRS/TCL (or EGM-QRS/TCL)*
Exit site	Near the exit of the critical protected isthmus	< 30	Yes	< 30%
Central isthmus	Within the central zone of the critical protected isthmus	< 30	Yes	30–50%
Entrance site	Near the entrance to the critical protected isthmus	< 30	Yes	51–70%
Inner loop	Within a protected limb parallel to and adjoining the critical isthmus at the entrance and exit sites	< 30	Yes	> 70%
Adjacent bystander	Within a blind cul-de-sac connected to the critical isthmus	> 30	Yes	Variable
Outer loop	Within a part of the VT circuit but outside of the protected isthmus	< 30	No	Variable
Remote bystander ("out of the circuit")	Site unrelated to VT	> 30	No	Variable

Abbreviations: EGM, electrogram; PPI, postpacing interval; TCL, tachycardia cycle length; VT, ventricular tachycardia

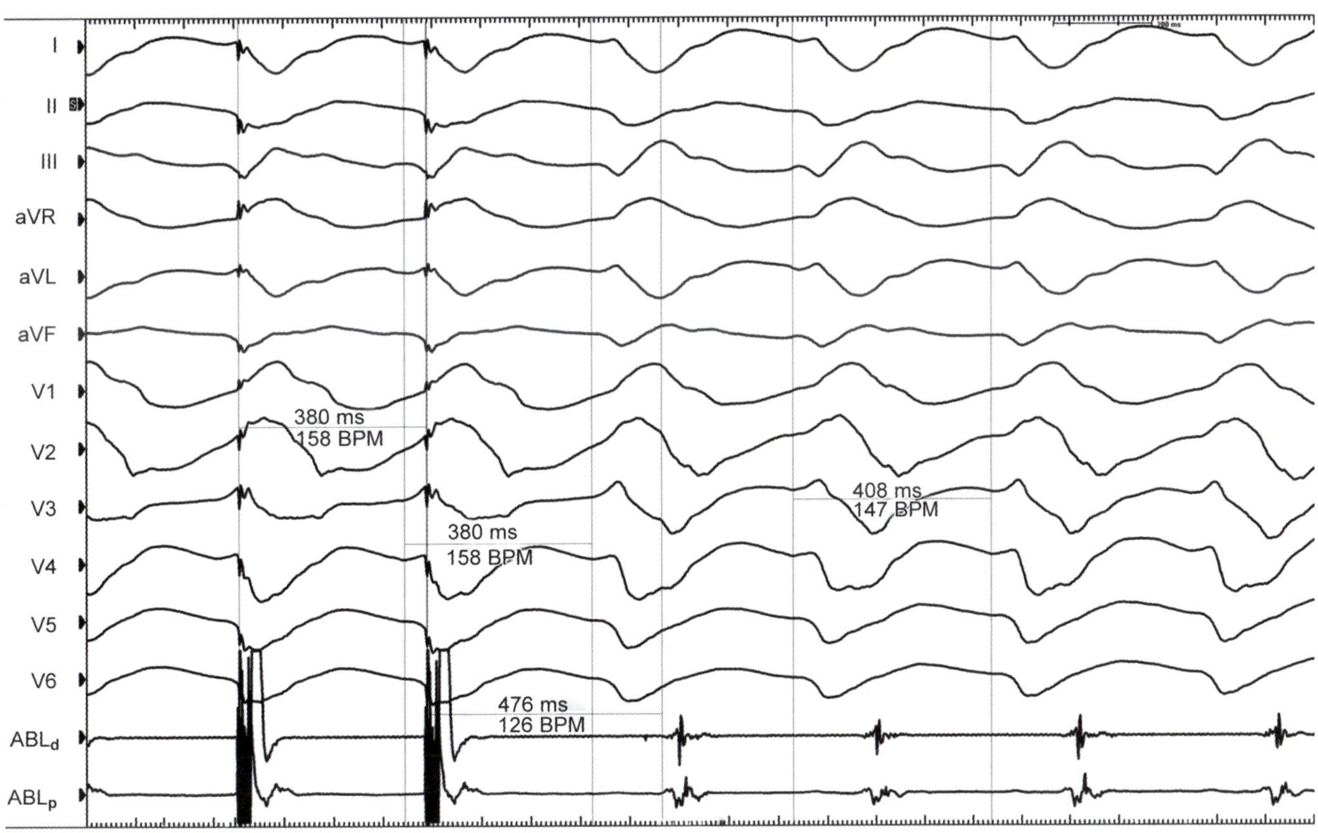

Figure 32.4: Entrainment with manifest fusion from a site not in the reentrant circuit. Entrainment of a mappable VT in a 71-year-old male with an ischemic cardiomyopathy (LVEF 31%). There is acceleration of the tachycardia to the pacing drive train (380 ms). The paced QRS morphology differs from that of VT indicating manifest fusion. The fusion can be specifically appreciated in this case with the stimulus artifacts occurring after the onset of the QRS. The last accelerated QRS is entrained but not fused as there is no further antidromic wavefront for it to extinguish with. This manifest fusion in the presence of continuous tachycardia reset (to the paced cycle length) is diagnostic of reentry as the VT mechanism. The postpacing interval minus tachycardia cycle length (PPI–TCL) is 476–408 = 68 ms. The catheter is thus, neither in the protected isthmus nor in the VT circuit ("out of the circuit")

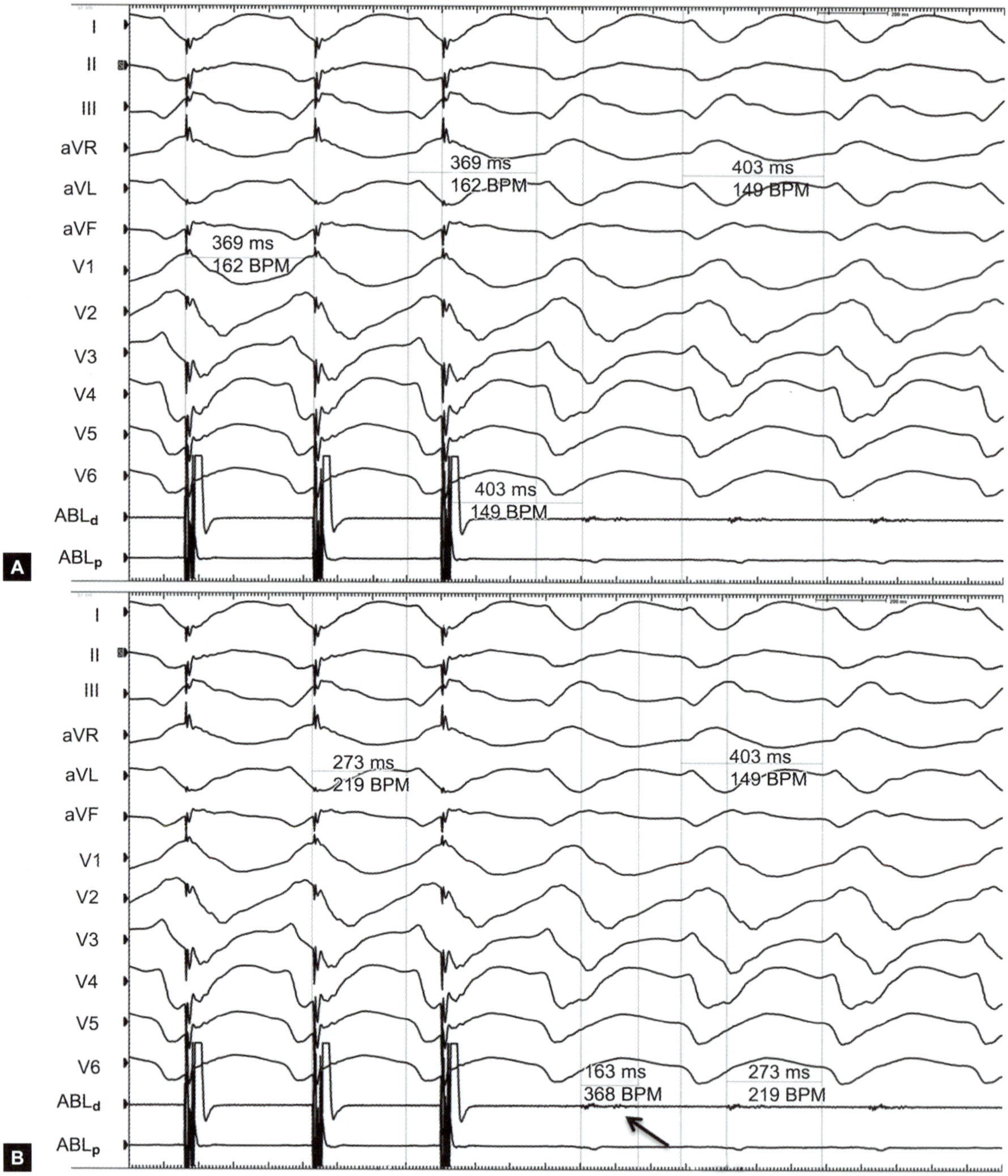

Figures 32.5A and B: Entrainment with concealed fusion. (A) Entrainment of the same VT as Figure 32.4 from a different site. The tachycardia is accelerated to the pacing drive train (370 ms). The paced QRS morphology is identical to that of VT indicating concealed fusion. The PPI–TCL is 403–403 = 0 ms. Thus, the catheter is within the constrained isthmus of the VT circuit; (B) The stim-QRS/EGM-QRS value is 273 ms which is (273/403) = 68% of the TCL suggesting an entrance site location within the isthmus. Also note the low voltage, highly fractionated and prolonged (163 ms) electrogram on the mapping catheter at the site of entrainment (arrow)

superior outcomes when compared to a strategy of entrainment mapping of clinical VTs alone.[90]

In scar-related VT, the cornerstone of substrate mapping involves creation of a voltage map of the involved ventricle. In patients with postinfarct VT, this is most often the LV endocardium. Patients with DCM often require RV endocardial and epicardial mapping in addition. Voltage mapping involves using a mapping catheter to systematically ascertain peak to peak bipolar voltages over the ventricular endocardial surface. On the basis of considerable animal

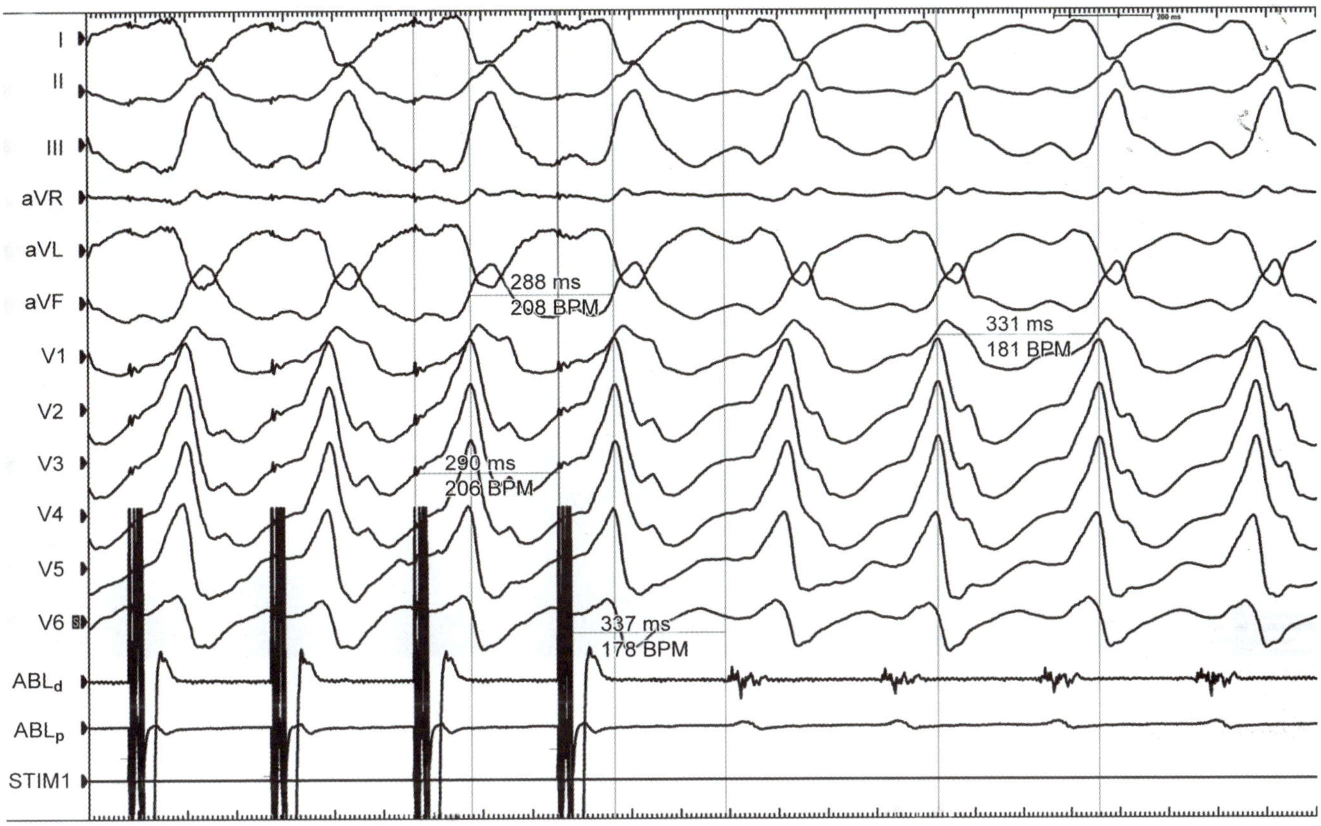

Figure 32.6: Entrainment with manifest fusion in an outer loop site. VT in a 59-year-old male with an ischemic cardiomyopathy (LVEF 42%) and a basolateral aneurysm. Pacing has accelerated the tachycardia to the paced cycle length (290 ms). There are subtle differences between the paced QRS and the VT QRS (most evident in lead III and aVR) indicating manifest fusion. The PPI–TCL is 337–331 = 6 ms. This indicates that the catheter is in the circuit, but not within the constrained isthmus ("outer loop"). The fact that the QRS morphology is only subtly different from that of VT suggests close proximity to the isthmus exit site

and human data, areas with voltage > 1.5 mV are defined as normal, whilst those with voltages < 0.5 mV are defined as dense scar.[91-93] Areas with intermediate voltages 0.5–1.5 mV are considered the 'border zone' and are characteristically found at the edge of infarct zones **(Figures 32.7A and B)**. Failure to capture despite high output pacing (up to an output of 20 mA at 10 ms) define areas of electrically unexcitable scar (EUS).[94,95]

Of particular relevance in patients with DCM, is the utility of endocardial unipolar voltage mapping in identifying substrate beyond the endocardium. The larger field of view afforded by the unipolar window allows for delineation of intramural and epicardial substrate.[96] Normal unipolar electrograms values have been defined as > 8.27 mV in the left ventricle[96] and > 5.5 mV in the right ventricular free wall.[97] This is particularly useful in determining the potential need for epicardial access or for employment of techniques to address intramural scar.

Pace-mapping plays a different role in scar VT as compared to focal VT cases where a perfect pace-map approximates the point source of origin of the arrhythmia. Rather, the purpose of pace-mapping during sinus rhythm in patients with scar VT is to search for areas of slow conduction, some of which may form conduction channels that can become constrained isthmuses during VT. High output pacing may be required to achieve capture in these extensive scarred regions. The aim is to capture the surviving myocytes within the scar allowing orthodromic propagation to form a QRS that is similar to any VT utilizing the same isthmus. Progressively lengthening stim-QRS times with identical QRS morphologies indicates closer proximity to the central portions of the isthmus; a stim-QRS of > 40 ms with a perfect pace map is an excellent target for ablation[62] **(Figure 32.8** and **Table 32.2)**. It should be noted that functional barriers and inner loop sites may change between sinus rhythm and VT. Thus, a perfect pace map may not necessarily reflect a critical isthmus site; conversely pacing within a critical isthmus in sinus rhythm may not reproduce the QRS of the clinical VT.

The presence of multiple pacemap morphologies at a single drive train cycle length at a stable pacing site implies that the catheter is at a location that may be a common

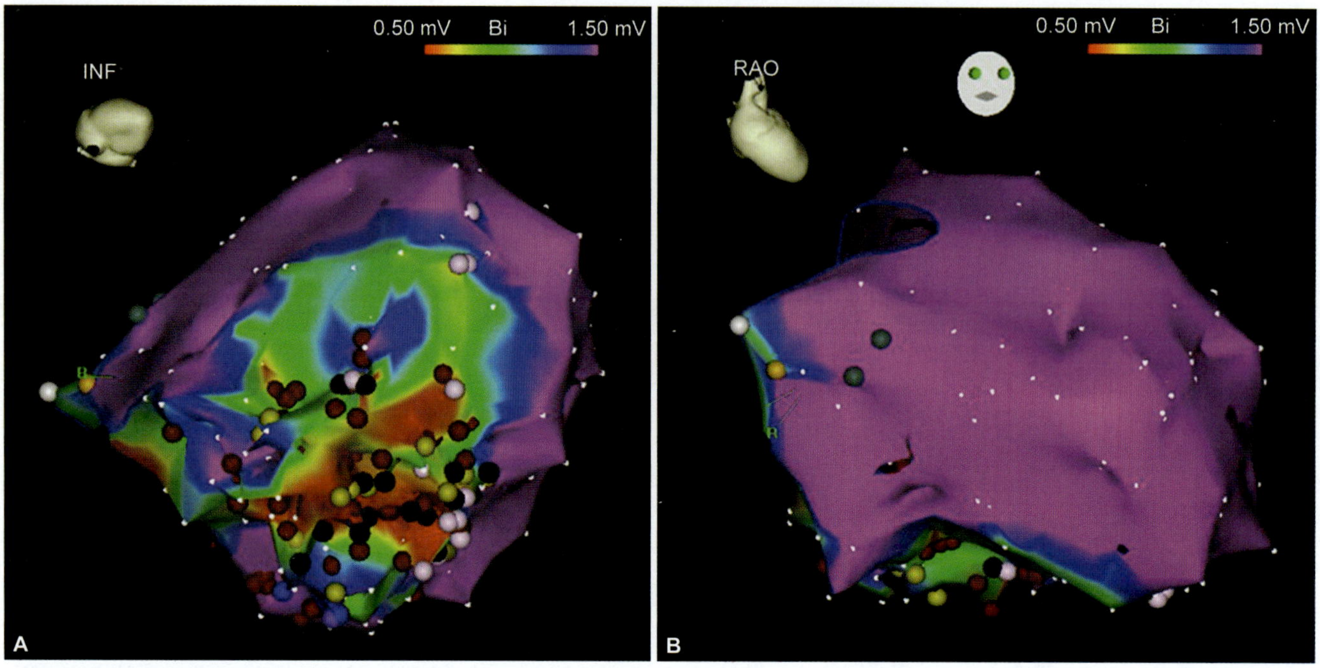

Figures 32.7A and B: Endocardial bipolar voltage map of the left ventricle. An endocardial voltage map of the left ventricle in a patient with an inferior infarct. (A) An inferior (INF) view illustrates the area of dense scar (red) surrounded by scar border zone (non-purple intermediate colors) that encompass the inferior surface of the LV. Isolated potentials are marked with black dots. Ablation lesions are marked with red dots; (B) The right anterior oblique (RAO) view demonstrates preserved voltages of the unaffected anteroapical walls

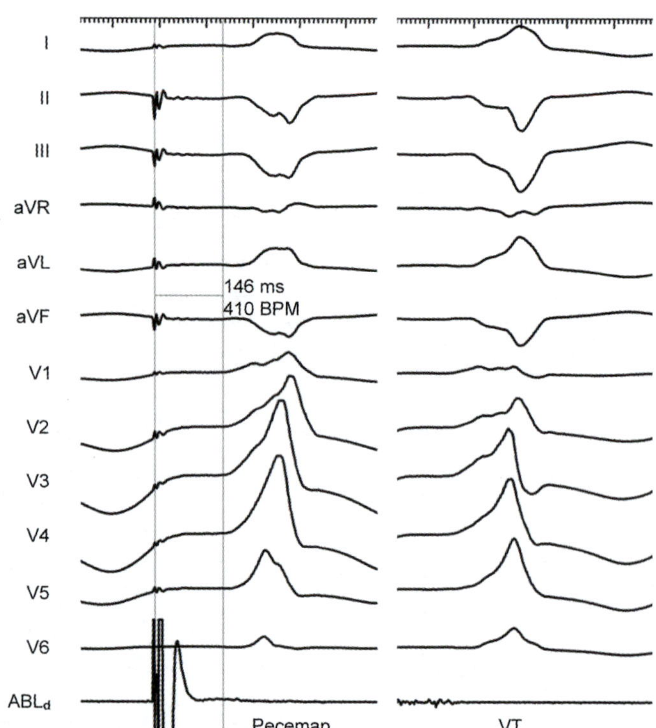

Figure 32.8: Pace-mapping during sinus rhythm. Pace-mapping in a 77-year-old male with an ischemic cardiomyopathy (LVEF 27%). The long stim-QRS of 146 ms suggests that the catheter is within an area of slow conduction; the paced morphology is similar but not identical to the clinical VT. This may represent the constrained isthmus of the VT, though differences in functional barriers during VT and sinus rhythm alter the QRS exit morphology. This is a good site for ablation

isthmus to multiple VT circuits with multiple different exit sites. Pace-mapping that initiates VT, especially with a functional delay as manifest by a long Stim-QRS interval, also suggests that the catheter is positioned within a critical isthmus. Both multiple exit sites during pacing and pace-mapping induction may be specific sites for critical isthmuses and thus, represent good targets for ablation[98] (**Figure 32.9** and *see* **Table 32.2**).

Conducting channels can also be defined during substrate mapping by adjusting the voltage thresholds defining 'scar' on the bipolar electrograms. Most conduction channels are identified when the lower threshold is reduced to ≤ 0.2 mV[99,100] where they can be seen as a zone of relatively higher voltage within the dense background scar. The specificity of this relatively low-resolution technique is limited with no more than around 30% of such conduction channels being related to critical VT isthmuses, with the rest forming bystander sites.[101] The presence of isolated potentials within a channel, however, makes it more likely to be a clinically relevant channel.

Table 32.2: Ablation targets during substrate mapping

Sites with isolated potentials
Sites of good pacemap match with long stim-QRS (> 40 ms)
Sites of pacemap with initiation of VT
Multiple exit sites at a single pacemap site
Conducting channels

Cell to cell conduction through healthy myocardium is rapid enough that only one electrogram per beat is seen by a mapping bipole, comprised of a summation of the myocyte depolarizations detected by the bipolar 'antenna'. However, in the presence of dense scar with surviving bundles of myocytes, the electrogram is often fractionated and prolonged in duration.[102,103] In areas of profoundly compromised electrical coupling, there is a separate near field component distinct from the main electrogram that is often but not always separated by an isoelectric period. These near field electrograms represent very slowly conducting surviving myocytes within potential critical isthmuses and are referred to as isolated potentials (IPs)[103-105] (**Figure 32.10**). They are often also termed late potentials[106] since they usually occur late after completion of the QRS,

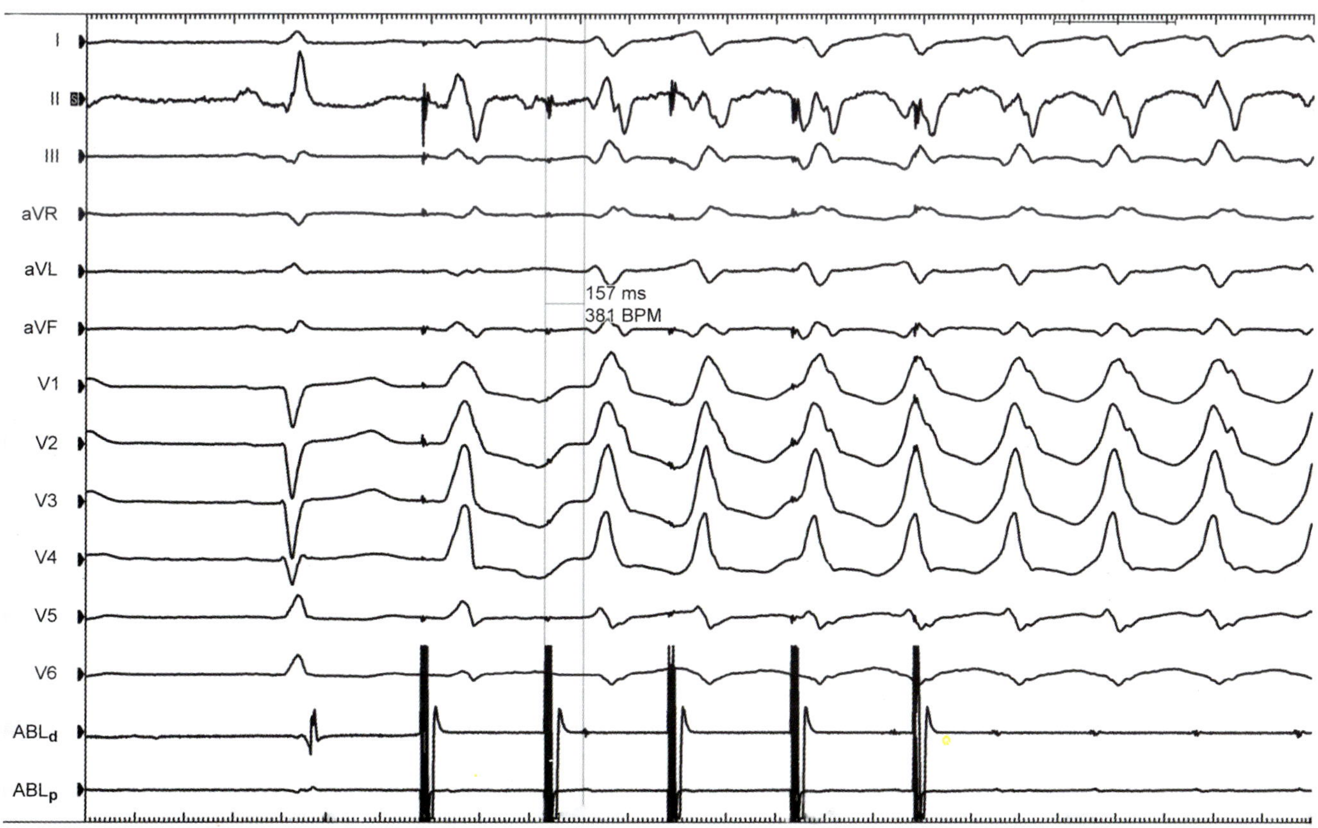

Figure 32.9: Initiation of VT during pace-mapping. Pace-mapping via the ablation catheter initiates VT on the 2nd beat with an identical paced QRS morphology to the induced VT. The stim-QRS delay (157 ms) on the 2nd beat suggestive of conduction delay and presumptive unidirectional block that initiates tachycardia. This is suggestive of a critical isthmus location and is a good site for ablation

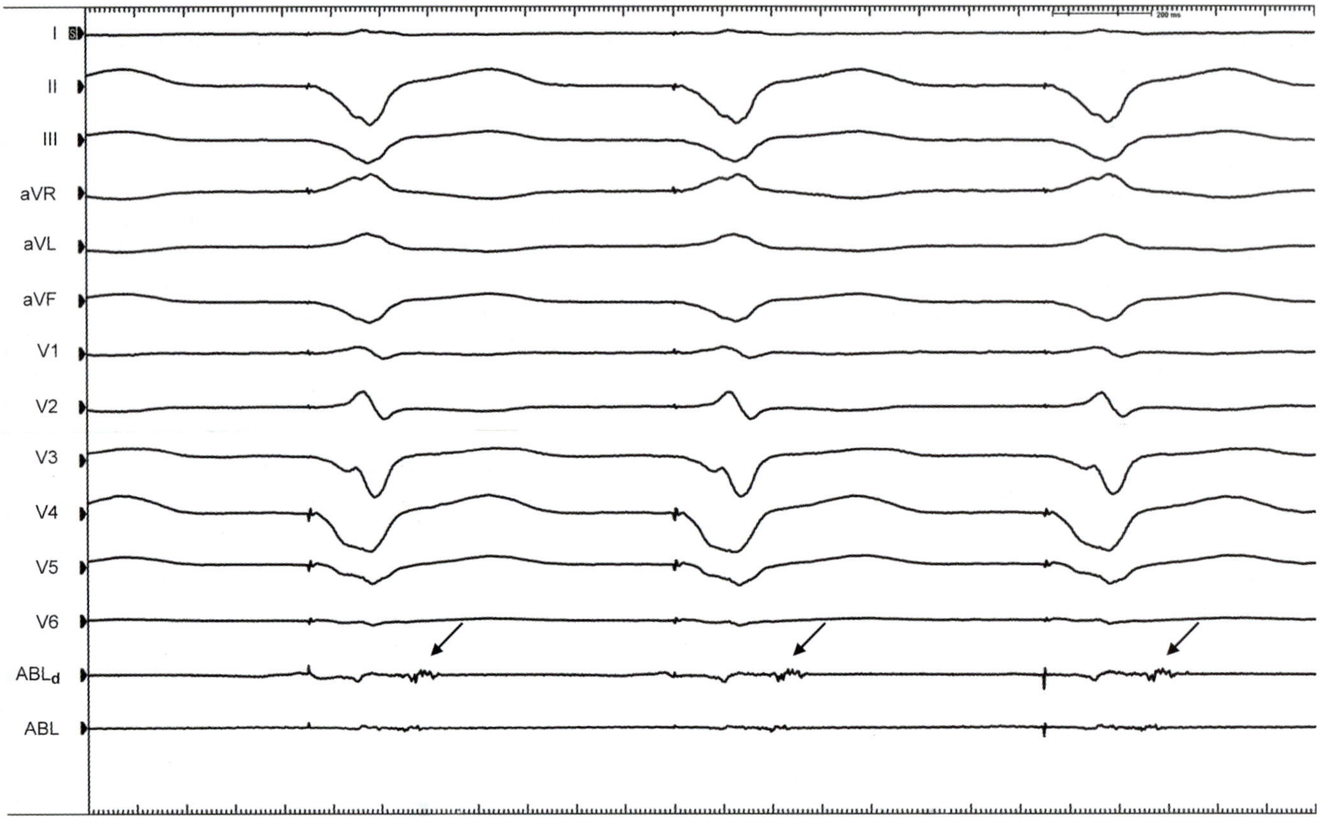

Figure 32.10: Substrate mapping showing isolated potentials. Mapping during right ventricular apical pacing (in a pacing-dependent patient). The arrow points to an isolated potential—a sharp, high frequency component that is clearly distinct from the remainder of the far field electrogram. These should be targeted for ablation

but they may actually occur at time after the far field signal, and sometimes during the QRS. Visualizing them during substrate mapping is often dependent on the wavefront vector activating scar, and mapping during right ventricular pacing may disclose more IPs than during sinus rhythm.[107] Other terms used to describe this concept include 'local abnormal ventricular activity' (LAVA)[108] or 'electrograms with isolated delayed components' (E-IDC).[107] Isolated potentials may represent potential isthmus sites of both current and future VTs and thus, are appropriate ablation targets (*see* **Table 32.2**). Again, entrainment and pace-mapping can be performed in these regions to clarify their relation to clinical VTs. However, not all isolated potentials represent isthmus sites and many may be related to adjacent bystander regions and thus, not participate in tachycardia.

Epicardial Mapping

Although, mapping and ablation of scar VT in the post-infarct setting is usually successfully accomplished via an endocardial only approach, there is a need for early epicardial mapping in certain patients. This is particularly true in the DCM population, where involvement of the midmyocardial and epicardial layers by the diffuse and heterogeneous scar is common. In patients who have failed a prior endocardial ablation, the majority have significant epicardial substrate that requires ablation for arrhythmic control.[33,109,110] Epicardial substrate can rarely be successfully modified from the endocardium.[111] Suspicion for epicardial substrate based on the underlying disease process, epicardial scar seen on CMR and epicardial VT morphology clues may be influential in adopting an early epicardial approach.[43] In patients with VT in the setting of postinfarct scar, an epicardial substrate may be present in up to 10% of cases;[112] there is increasing evidence that epicardial mapping and ablation may be beneficial in some of these patients despite the predominantly subendocardially-based substrate.[45,113]

In cases of idiopathic VT, particularly in cases of premature ventricular complexes (PVCs) arising from the LV summit, the epicardium can be mapped via the coronary venous system.[114] However, this route has limited utility in scar-related VT cases due to geographical restriction and inability to deliver adequate power due to high impedances via this approach. As such, access to the epicardium occurs via the pericardial space. Traditionally this was achieved using the 'Sosa technique',[115] though more recently a 'needle in needle' technique has been described which reduces the risk of inadvertent RV puncture and hemopericardium.[116,117] These techniques are described in the detail in another chapter **(Chapter 47)** of this book. A history of open heart surgery is important in patients being considered for epicardial mapping. Pericardial adhesions make access and navigation within this space difficult though not impossible.[118,119]

Mapping the epicardium poses several unique challenges. The presence of epicardial fat, which is particularly thick overlying grooves containing the major coronary arteries, attenuates the underlying electrogram signal. However, unlike true scar, the morphology of such signals is normal and they do not demonstrate the splitting, fractionation or isolated components characteristic of scar electrograms.[33,120] This fat-related voltage attenuation reduces the accepted reference range for the normal peak-to-peak bipolar electrogram. The definition of dense scar remains <0.5 mV, but normal myocardium is defined at a lower value of >1.0 mV[33] **(Figures 32.11A to C)**. It is important not to define epicardial substrate solely on the basis of low voltage, however, but to look instead for the zones of confluent abnormal electrograms within low voltage areas. Ablation in the pericardial space has the potential to injure the epicardial coronary arteries or the phrenic nerve. Coronary angiography is needed to confirm an arterial distance of at least 5 mm (ideally 10 mm) from potential ablation sites[121] prior to energy delivery. Proximity to the phrenic nerve can be confirmed with high output pacing at potential ablation sites. If ablation is required at these sites, techniques to raise the phrenic nerve off the epicardium including the instillation of air and saline or the placement of a balloon may be employed.[122,123]

Ablation

Having created an electroanatomical substrate map, defined potential isthmuses through pace-mapping, identified potential conducting channels and mapped isolated potentials, an ablation strategy is then planned. Such strategies include linear ablations connecting potential isthmuses within scar border zones to areas of scar (either EUS or valvular apparatus), linear ablations within scar border zones or linear ablation across conduction channels.[16,91,124] Entrances to conducting channels can be targeted in a strategy termed '*scar dechanneling*'.[125] This may result in modification of adjacent interconnected areas with improved VT control.[126] A more extensive (and time consuming) strategy involves abolition of all or as many IPs as possible.[108,127-129] The ultimate form of this strategy is termed '*scar homogenization*' and involves abolition of all abnormal electrograms within areas of scar.[45] This theoretically targets as many VT circuits as possible (both current and those with the future potential to facilitate arrhythmias). Recently, a strategy of core isolation of critical VT circuitry components has been described.[130] In a manner, analogous to pulmonary vein isolation, the concept involves applying circumferential lesions to disconnect an area harboring critical VT components from the remainder of the myocardium.

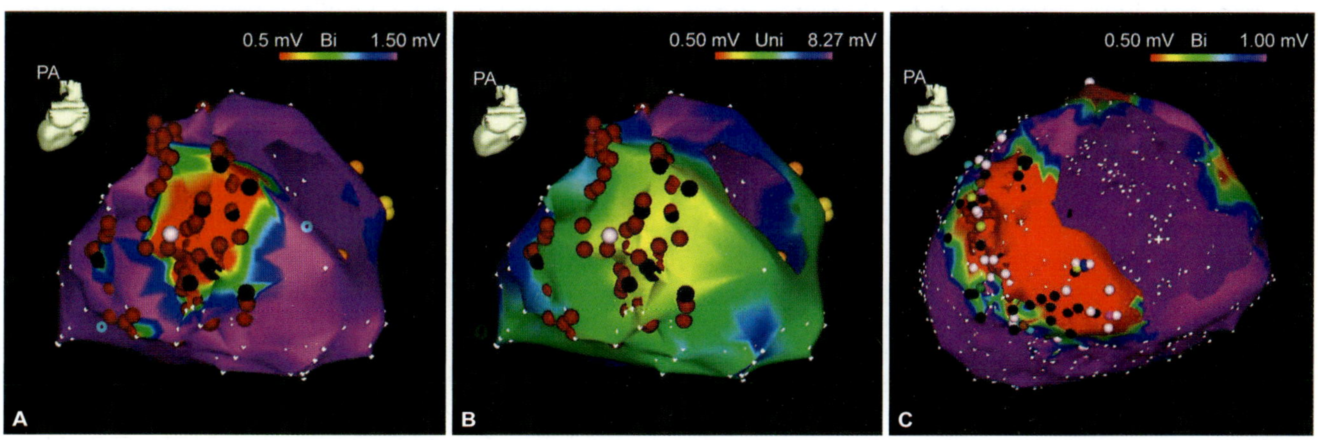

Figures 32.11A to C: Endocardial (bipolar and unipolar) and epicardial voltage maps. (A) An endocardial bipolar voltage map of a patient with dilated cardiomyopathy as seen from the posterior-anterior (PA) view. The substrate abnormality is confined to the typical pattern of the basal paravalvular regions; (B) The same endocardial map with unipolar settings demonstrates a much larger involved area. This suggests mid-myocardial or epicardial involvement that extends far beyond the affected endocardial territory; (C) The corresponding epicardial bipolar voltage map in the same patient confirms involvement of the basal paravalvular region beyond the area suggested by the endocardial bipolar map. Note the area of epicardial involvement is less than that portrayed by the unipolar endocardial map suggesting extensive intramural substrate not detected by either the endocardial or epicardial bipolar maps. Extensive ablation was performed in this epicardial region targeting isolated potentials and areas of fractionation

Ablation should be performed with an open irrigated RF ablation catheter which results in the production of larger, deeper lesions.[131] Large series have demonstrated good efficacy with such catheters.[132,133] Such catheters also reduce the incidence of thrombus formation, when compared to solid tip catheters.[134,135] The initial power should be set at 30 W, though this can be up titrated to 50 W if adequate impendence drops are not achieved at lower powers. Temperature limitation with irrigated catheters is typically set to around 43°C although tip electrode cooling is highly efficient with current generation irrigation platforms incorporating multiple internal and external irrigation ports. An impedance drop of approximately 10 Ω targeted to suggest adequate catheter contact and current delivery. Contact-force catheters provide immediate feedback of not only catheter contact but also the vector of contact. In the absence of adequate contact force, a significant proportion of applications does not result in any lesion formation.[136] This is particularly important during epicardial ablation where an inward vector is required to prevent wasted energy delivery to the pericardium.[137] Predictors of lesion formation include clean termination of VT (without ectopy), loss of isolated potentials, significant change in the local electrogram and/or noncapture at high output when capture was possible preablation.

The presence of intramural septal substrate poses a unique problem in the DCM population. Endocardial ablation from either the RV or LV may be ineffective due to the substrate being beyond the depth of the lesions created by current RF ablation technology. If sequential septal ablation from both ventricles is inadequate in controlling VT, a number of novel strategies can be considered. Bipolar ablation between two ablation catheter that 'sandwich' the septum between the RV and LV has been found to result in more transmural lesions than sequential ablations.[138,139] Use of an RF catheter with an extendable needle to allow deeper myocardial penetration has been shown to result in larger and deeper lesions.[140] This has shown promise in addressing intramural substrate in early human trials.[141] Transcoronary ethanol ablation involving the injection of ethanol into a subselected septal branch of the left anterior descending (LAD) artery in order to induce a localized infarct can be used to target deep septal substrate. This has been shown to be feasible and effective, particularly in patients who have failed an initial RF ablation.[142-144] A similar technique utilizing coil embolization has been recently reported.[145]

As isolated potentials and isthmuses are found in areas of dense noncontractile scar, myocardial damage and worsening systolic function are rarely seen despite extensive ablation. Given the extensive endocardial denudation, a period of anticoagulation initially with intravenous heparin (after confirmation of adequate access site hemostasis) followed by warfarin or a NOAC is administered for 4–6 weeks postprocedure in patients who have had extensive LV endocardial ablation to prevent thromboembolic events.

Procedural Endpoints

The optimal procedural endpoint in scar VT ablation is not clearly defined. Traditionally, noninducibility of clinical VTs has been used as an endpoint in this setting. Patients with no inducible VT at the end of the case have better VT free survival than those with inducible nonclinical VTs who in turn do better than those in whom the clinical VT remains inducible.[146] Recent studies have suggested that the best long-term outcomes may be achieved with targeted abolition of isolated potentials or a complete scar homogenization strategy[90,108] **(Table 32.3)**. Scar-related VT ablation is usually not a curative procedure, notwithstanding the tremendously positive impact it may have on patients with frequent ICD shocks or VT episodes. Incomplete ablation or substrate progression means repeat procedures are not uncommonly required, especially in patients with a larger scar burden.[147]

Table 32.3: Outcome Data in contemporary substrate ablation studies

Study	*Year*	*No. of patients*	*Epicardial access (%)*	*Ablation targets (% achieved)*	*VT non-inducibility (%)*	*VT recurrence (%)*	*Median follow-up (months)*
Jais P et al.[108]	2012	56 ICM, 14 NICM	30%	LAVA (70%)	NA	46%	22
Di Biase L et al.[45]	2012	43 ICM	100%	Abnormal electrograms	100%	19%	21
Vergara P et al.[128]	2012	41 ICM, 23 NICM	42%	Isolated potentials (84%)	25/35 (71%)	20%	13
Arenal A et al.[127]	2013	59 ICM	NA	Isolated potentials (97%) and conduction channels (83%)	20/32 (62%)	42%	39
Berruezo A et al.[125]	2015	75 ICM, 26 NICM	27%	Conducting channels (84%) + residual inducible VT (73%)	78%	27%	21
Di Biase L et al.[90]	2015	58 ICM	10%	Abnormal electrograms (84%)	100%	16%	12

Abbreviations: ICM, ischemic cardiomyopathy; NICM, nonischemic cardiomyopathy; LAVA, local abnormal ventricular activities; VT, ventricular tachycardia

REFERENCES

1. Lopez AD, Mathers CD, Ezzati M, Jamison DT, Murray CJ. Global and regional burden of disease and risk factors, 2001: systematic analysis of population health data. Lancet. 2006;367:1747-57.
2. Effect of metoprolol CR/XL in chronic heart failure: Metoprolol CR/XL Randomised Intervention Trial in Congestive Heart Failure (MERIT-HF). Lancet. 1999;353:2001-7.
3. Zheng ZJ, Croft JB, Giles WH, Mensah GA. Sudden cardiac death in the United States, 1989 to 1998. Circulation. 2001;104: 2158-63.
4. Aldhoon B, Tzou WS, Riley MP, Lin D, Callans DJ, Hutchinson MD, Dixit S, Garcia FC, Zado ES, Marchlinski FE. Nonischemic cardiomyopathy substrate and ventricular tachycardia in the setting of coronary artery disease. Heart Rhythm. 2013;10: 1622-7.
5. Russo AM, Stainback RF, Bailey SR, Epstein AE, Heidenreich PA, Jessup M, Kapa S, Kremers MS, Lindsay BD, Stevenson LW. ACCF/HRS/AHA/ASE/HFSA/SCAI/SCCT/SCMR 2013 appropriate use criteria for implantable cardioverter-defibrillators and cardiac resynchronization therapy: a report of the American College of Cardiology Foundation appropriate use criteria task force, Heart Rhythm Society, American Heart Association, American Society of Echocardiography, Heart Failure Society of America, Society for Cardiovascular Angiography and Interventions, Society of Cardiovascular Computed Tomography, and Society for Cardiovascular Magnetic Resonance. J Am Coll Cardiol. 2013;61:1318-68.
6. Ladwig KH, Baumert J, Marten-Mittag B, Kolb C, Zrenner B, Schmitt C. Post-traumatic stress symptoms and predicted mortality in patients with implantable cardioverter-defibrillators: results from the prospective living with an implanted cardioverter-defibrillator study. Arch Gen Psychiatry. 2008;65:1324-30.
7. Passman R, Subacius H, Ruo B, Schaechter A, Howard A, Sears SF, Kadish A. Implantable cardioverter defibrillators and quality of life: results from the defibrillators in nonischemic cardiomyopathy treatment evaluation study. Arch Intern Med. 2007;167:2226-32.
8. Gasparini M, Proclemer A, Klersy C, et al. Effect of long-detection interval vs standard-detection interval for implantable cardioverter-defibrillators on antitachycardia pacing and shock delivery: The advance iii randomized clinical trial. JAMA. 2013;309:1903-11.
9. Moss AJ, Schuger C, Beck CA, Brown MW, Cannom DS, Daubert JP, Estes NA, 3rd, Greenberg H, Hall WJ, Huang DT, Kautzner J, Klein H, McNitt S, Olshansky B, Shoda M, Wilber D, Zareba W. Reduction in inappropriate therapy and mortality through ICD programming. N Engl J Med. 2012;367: 2275-83.
10. The Cardiac Insufficiency Bisoprolol Study II (CIBIS-II): a randomised trial. Lancet. 1999;353:9-13.
11. Flather MD, Shibata MC, Coats AJ, Van Veldhuisen DJ, Parkhomenko A, Borbola J, Cohen-Solal A, Dumitrascu D, Ferrari R, Lechat P, Soler-Soler J, Tavazzi L, Spinarova L, Toman J, Bohm M, Anker SD, Thompson SG, Poole-Wilson PA, Investigators S. Randomized trial to determine the effect of nebivolol on mortality and cardiovascular hospital admission in elderly patients with heart failure (SENIORS). Eur Heart J. 2005;26:215-25.
12. Packer M, Coats AJ, Fowler MB, Katus HA, Krum H, Mohacsi P, Rouleau JL, Tendera M, Castaigne A, Roecker EB, Schultz MK, DeMets DL. Carvedilol Prospective Randomized Cumulative Survival Study G. Effect of carvedilol on survival in severe chronic heart failure. N Engl J Med. 2001;344:1651-8.
13. Flather MD, Yusuf S, Kober L, Pfeffer M, Hall A, Murray G, Torp-Pedersen C, Ball S, Pogue J, Moye L, Braunwald E. Long-term ACE-inhibitor therapy in patients with heart failure or left-ventricular dysfunction: a systematic overview of data from individual patients. ACE-Inhibitor Myocardial Infarction Collaborative Group. Lancet. 2000;355:1575-81.
14. Sogaard P, Gotzsche CO, Ravkilde J, Norgaard A, Thygesen K. Ventricular arrhythmias in the acute and chronic phases after acute myocardial infarction. Effect of intervention with captopril. Circulation. 1994;90:101-7.
15. Frankel DS, Mountantonakis SE, Robinson MR, Zado ES, Callans DJ, Marchlinski FE. Ventricular tachycardia ablation remains treatment of last resort in structural heart disease: argument for earlier intervention. J Cardiovasc Electrophysiol. 2011;22:1123-8.
16. Reddy VY, Reynolds MR, Neuzil P, Richardson AW, Taborsky M, Jongnarangsin K, Kralovec S, Sediva L, Ruskin JN, Josephson ME. Prophylactic catheter ablation for the prevention of defibrillator therapy. N Engl J Med. 2007;357:2657-65.
17. Soejima K, Stevenson WG, Sapp JL, Selwyn AP, Couper G, Epstein LM. Endocardial and epicardial radiofrequency ablation of ventricular tachycardia associated with dilated cardiomyopathy: the importance of low-voltage scars. J Am Coll Cardiol. 2004;43:1834-42.
18. de Bakker JM, van Capelle FJ, Janse MJ, Wilde AA, Coronel R, Becker AE, Dingemans KP, van Hemel NM, Hauer RN. Reentry as a cause of ventricular tachycardia in patients with chronic ischemic heart disease: electrophysiologic and anatomic correlation. Circulation. 1988;77:589-606.
19. Caceres J, Jazayeri M, McKinnie J, Avitall B, Denker ST, Tchou P, Akhtar M. Sustained bundle branch reentry as a mechanism of clinical tachycardia. Circulation. 1989;79:256-70.
20. Arnar DO, Bullinga JR, Martins JB. Role of the Purkinje system in spontaneous ventricular tachycardia during acute ischemia in a canine model. Circulation. 1997;96:2421-9.
21. Lopera G, Stevenson WG, Soejima K, Maisel WH, Koplan B, Sapp JL, Satti SD, Epstein LM. Identification and ablation of three types of ventricular tachycardia involving the His-purkinje system in patients with heart disease. J Cardiovasc Electrophysiol. 2004;15:52-8.
22. Szumowski L, Sanders P, Walczak F, Hocini M, Jais P, Kepski R, Szufladowicz E, Urbanek P, Derejko P, Bodalski R, Haissaguerre M. Mapping and ablation of polymorphic ventricular tachycardia after myocardial infarction. J Am Coll Cardiol. 2004;44:1700-6.
23. Bogun F, Desjardins B, Crawford T, Good E, Jongnarangsin K, Oral H, Chugh A, Pelosi F, Morady F. Post-infarction ventricular arrhythmias originating in papillary muscles. J Am Coll Cardiol. 2008;51:1794-802.
24. Das MK, Scott LR, Miller JM. Focal mechanism of ventricular tachycardia in coronary artery disease. Heart Rhythm. 2010;7: 305-11.
25. Wellens HJ, Duren DR, Lie KI. Observations on mechanisms of ventricular tachycardia in man. Circulation. 1976;54:237-44.
26. Downar E, Harris L, Mickleborough LL, Shaikh N, Parson ID. Endocardial mapping of ventricular tachycardia in the intact

human ventricle: evidence for reentrant mechanisms. J Am Coll Cardiol. 1988;11:783-91.
27. de Bakker JM, Janse MJ, Van Capelle FJ, Durrer D. Endocardial mapping by simultaneous recording of endocardial electrograms during cardiac surgery for ventricular aneurysm. J Am Coll Cardiol. 1983;2:947-53.
28. Miller JM, Kienzle MG, Harken AH, Josephson ME. Subendocardial resection for ventricular tachycardia: predictors of surgical success. Circulation. 1984;70:624-31.
29. Engblom H, Carlsson MB, Hedstrom E, Heiberg E, Ugander M, Wagner GS, Arheden H. The endocardial extent of reperfused first-time myocardial infarction is more predictive of pathologic Q waves than is infarct transmurality: a magnetic resonance imaging study. Clin Physiol Funct Imaging. 2007;27:101-8.
30. de Bakker JM, van Capelle FJ, Janse MJ, Tasseron S, Vermeulen JT, de Jonge N, Lahpor JR. Slow conduction in the infarcted human heart. 'Zigzag' course of activation. Circulation. 1993;88:915-26.
31. Callans DJ, Zardini M, Gottlieb CD, Josephson ME. The variable contribution of functional and anatomic barriers in human ventricular tachycardia: an analysis with resetting from two sites. J Am Coll Cardiol. 1996;27:1106-11.
32. Haqqani HM, Kalman JM, Roberts-Thomson KC, Balasubramaniam RN, Rosso R, Snowdon RL, Sparks PB, Vohra JK, Morton JB. Fundamental differences in electrophysiologic and electroanatomic substrate between ischemic cardiomyopathy patients with and without clinical ventricular tachycardia. J Am Coll Cardiol. 2009;54:166-73.
33. Cano O, Hutchinson M, Lin D, Garcia F, Zado E, Bala R, Riley M, Cooper J, Dixit S, Gerstenfeld E, Callans D, Marchlinski FE. Electroanatomic substrate and ablation outcome for suspected epicardial ventricular tachycardia in left ventricular nonischemic cardiomyopathy. J Am Coll Cardiol. 2009;54: 799-808.
34. Haqqani HM, Tschabrunn CM, Tzou WS, Dixit S, Cooper JM, Riley MP, Lin D, Hutchinson MD, Garcia FC, Bala R, Verdino RJ, Callans DJ, Gerstenfeld EP, Zado ES, Marchlinski FE. Isolated septal substrate for ventricular tachycardia in nonischemic dilated cardiomyopathy: incidence, characterization, and implications. Heart Rhythm. 2011;8:1169-76.
35. Hsia HH, Callans DJ, Marchlinski FE. Characterization of endocardial electrophysiological substrate in patients with nonischemic cardiomyopathy and monomorphic ventricular tachycardia. Circulation. 2003;108:704-10.
36. Behairy NH, Mansour SM. Pattern of delayed myocardial enhancement: A key to differentiate ischemic and non-ischemic cardiomyopathies. Egyptian J Radiol Nucl Med. 2014;45:53-60.
37. Bohnen M, Stevenson WG, Tedrow UB, Michaud GF, John RM, Epstein LM, Albert CM, Koplan BA. Incidence and predictors of major complications from contemporary catheter ablation to treat cardiac arrhythmias. Heart Rhythm. 2011;8:1661-6.
38. Josephson ME, Callans DJ. Using the twelve-lead electrocardiogram to localize the site of origin of ventricular tachycardia. Heart Rhythm. 2005;2:443-6.
39. Miller JM, Marchlinski FE, Buxton AE, Josephson ME. Relationship between the 12-lead electrocardiogram during ventricular tachycardia and endocardial site of origin in patients with coronary artery disease. Circulation. 1988;77: 759-66.
40. Segal OR, Chow AW, Wong T, Trevisi N, Lowe MD, Davies DW, Della Bella P, Packer DL, Peters NS. A novel algorithm for determining endocardial VT exit site from 12-lead surface ECG characteristics in human, infarct-related ventricular tachycardia. J Cardiovasc Electrophysiol. 2007;18:161-8.
41. Kuchar DL, Ruskin JN, Garan H. Electrocardiographic localization of the site of origin of ventricular tachycardia in patients with prior myocardial infarction. J Am Coll Cardiol. 1989;13:893-903.
42. Bowers TR, O'Neill WW, Pica M, Goldstein JA. Patterns of coronary compromise resulting in acute right ventricular ischemic dysfunction. Circulation. 2002;106:1104-9.
43. Della Bella P, Brugada J, Zeppenfeld K, Merino J, Neuzil P, Maury P, Maccabelli G, Vergara P, Baratto F, Berruezo A, Wijnmaalen AP. Epicardial ablation for ventricular tachycardia: a European multicenter study. Circ Arrhythm Electrophysiol. 2011;4:653-9.
44. Cesario DA, Vaseghi M, Boyle NG, Fishbein MC, Valderrabano M, Narasimhan C, Wiener I, Shivkumar K. Value of high-density endocardial and epicardial mapping for catheter ablation of hemodynamically unstable ventricular tachycardia. Heart Rhythm. 2006;3:1-10.
45. Di Biase L, Santangeli P, Burkhardt DJ, Bai R, Mohanty P, Carbucicchio C, Dello Russo A, Casella M, Mohanty S, Pump A, Hongo R, Beheiry S, Pelargonio G, Santarelli P, Zucchetti M, Horton R, Sanchez JE, Elayi CS, Lakkireddy D, Tondo C, Natale A. Endo-epicardial homogenization of the scar versus limited substrate ablation for the treatment of electrical storms in patients with ischemic cardiomyopathy. J Am Coll Cardiol. 2012;60:132-41.
46. Sarkozy A, Tokuda M, Tedrow UB, Sieria J, Michaud GF, Couper GS, John R, Stevenson WG. Epicardial ablation of ventricular tachycardia in ischemic heart disease. Circ Arrhythm Electrophysiol. 2013;6:1115-22.
47. Berruezo A, Mont L, Nava S, Chueca E, Bartholomay E, Brugada J. Electrocardiographic recognition of the epicardial origin of ventricular tachycardias. Circulation. 2004;109:1842-7.
48. Bazan V, Gerstenfeld EP, Garcia FC, Bala R, Rivas N, Dixit S, Zado E, Callans DJ, Marchlinski FE. Site-specific twelve-lead ECG features to identify an epicardial origin for left ventricular tachycardia in the absence of myocardial infarction. Heart Rhythm. 2007;4:1403-10.
49. Valles E, Bazan V, Marchlinski FE. ECG criteria to identify epicardial ventricular tachycardia in nonischemic cardiomyopathy. Circ Arrhythm Electrophysiol. 2010;3:63-71.
50. Daniels DV, Lu YY, Morton JB, Santucci PA, Akar JG, Green A, Wilber DJ. Idiopathic epicardial left ventricular tachycardia originating remote from the sinus of Valsalva: electrophysiological characteristics, catheter ablation, and identification from the 12-lead electrocardiogram. Circulation. 2006;113:1659-66.
51. Mansencal N, Nasr IA, Pilliere R, Farcot JC, Joseph T, Lacombe P, Dubourg O. Usefulness of contrast echocardiography for assessment of left ventricular thrombus after acute myocardial infarction. Am J Cardiol. 2007;99:1667-70.
52. Weinsaft JW, Kim RJ, Ross M, Krauser D, Manoushagian S, LaBounty TM, Cham MD, Min JK, Healy K, Wang Y, Parker M, Roman MJ, Devereux RB. Contrast-enhanced anatomic imaging as compared to contrast-enhanced tissue characterization for detection of left ventricular thrombus. JACC Cardiovasc Imaging. 2009;2:969-79.
53. Rao HB, Yu R, Chitnis N, Do D, Boyle NG, Shivkumar K, Bradfield JS. Ventricular Tachycardia Ablation in the Presence of Left Ventricular Thrombus: Safety and Efficacy. J Cardiovasc Electrophysiol; 2015.

54. Perez-David E, Arenal A, Rubio-Guivernau JL, del Castillo R, Atea L, Arbelo E, Caballero E, Celorrio V, Datino T, Gonzalez-Torrecilla E, Atienza F, Ledesma-Carbayo MJ, Bermejo J, Medina A, Fernandez-Aviles F. Noninvasive identification of ventricular tachycardia-related conducting channels using contrast-enhanced magnetic resonance imaging in patients with chronic myocardial infarction: comparison of signal intensity scar mapping and endocardial voltage mapping. J Am Coll Cardiol. 2011;57:184-94.
55. Andreu D, Ortiz-Perez JT, Boussy T, Fernandez-Armenta J, de Caralt TM, Perea RJ, Prat-Gonzalez S, Mont L, Brugada J, Berruezo A. Usefulness of contrast-enhanced cardiac magnetic resonance in identifying the ventricular arrhythmia substrate and the approach needed for ablation. Eur Heart J. 2014;35:1316-26.
56. Bogun FM, Desjardins B, Good E, Gupta S, Crawford T, Oral H, Ebinger M, Pelosi F, Chugh A, Jongnarangsin K, Morady F. Delayed-enhanced magnetic resonance imaging in nonischemic cardiomyopathy: utility for identifying the ventricular arrhythmia substrate. J Am Coll Cardiol. 2009;53:1138-45.
57. Marckmann P, Skov L, Rossen K, Dupont A, Damholt MB, Heaf JG, Thomsen HS. Nephrogenic systemic fibrosis: suspected causative role of gadodiamide used for contrast-enhanced magnetic resonance imaging. J Am Soc Nephrol. 2006;17: 2359-62.
58. Brignole M, Auricchio A, Baron-Esquivias G, Bordachar P, Boriani G, Breithardt OA, Cleland J, Deharo JC, Delgado V, Elliott PM, Gorenek B, Israel CW, Leclercq C, Linde C, Mont L, Padeletti L, Sutton R, Vardas PE. 2013 ESC guidelines on cardiac pacing and cardiac resynchronization therapy: the task force on cardiac pacing and resynchronization therapy of the European Society of Cardiology (ESC). Developed in collaboration with the European Heart Rhythm Association (EHRA). Europace. 2013;15:1070-118.
59. Gotte MJ, Russel IK, de Roest GJ, Germans T, Veldkamp RF, Knaapen P, Allaart CP, van Rossum AC. Magnetic resonance imaging, pacemakers and implantable cardioverter-defibrillators: current situation and clinical perspective. Neth Heart J. 2010;18:31-7.
60. Hussein A, Jimenez A, Ahmad G, Mesubi O, Klein T, Gurm G, Beck H, Shams O, See V, Saliaris A, Shorofsky S, Dickfeld T. Assessment of ventricular tachycardia scar substrate by intracardiac echocardiography. Pacing Clin Electrophysiol. 2014;37:412-21.
61. Jongbloed MR, Bax JJ, van der Burg AE, Van der Wall EE, Schalij MJ. Radiofrequency catheter ablation of ventricular tachycardia guided by intracardiac echocardiography. Eur J Echocardiogr. 2004;5:34-40.
62. Brunckhorst CB, Stevenson WG, Soejima K, Maisel WH, Delacretaz E, Friedman PL, Ben-Haim SA. Relationship of slow conduction detected by pace-mapping to ventricular tachycardia re-entry circuit sites after infarction. J Am Coll Cardiol. 2003;41:802-9.
63. Mondesert B, Khairy P, Schram G, Shohoudi A, Talajic M, Andrade JG, Dubuc M, Guerra PG, Macle L, Roy D, Dyrda K, Thibault B, Barrero M, Diaz A, Kouz S, McNicoll S, Nowakowska D, Rivard L. Impact of revascularization in patients with sustained ventricular arrhythmias, prior myocardial infarction and preserved left ventricular ejection fraction. Heart Rhythm, 2016.
64. Vatner SF. Effects of anesthesia on cardiovascular control mechanisms. Environ Health Perspect. 1978;26:193-206.
65. Hwang ES, Pak HN, Park SW, Park JS, Joung B, Choi D, Lee MH, Kim YH. Risks and benefits of an open irrigation tip catheter in intensive radiofrequency catheter ablation in patients with non-paroxysmal atrial fibrillation. Circ J. 2010;74: 644-9.
66. Ashley ME. Anaesthesia for electrophysiology procedures in the cardiac catheter laboratory. Contin Educ Anaesth Crit Care Pain. 2012;12:230-6.
67. Di Biase L, Conti S, Mohanty P, Bai R, Sanchez J, Walton D, John A, Santangeli P, Elayi CS, Beheiry S, Gallinghouse GJ, Mohanty S, Horton R, Bailey S, Burkhardt JD, Natale A. General anesthesia reduces the prevalence of pulmonary vein reconnection during repeat ablation when compared with conscious sedation: results from a randomized study. Heart Rhythm. 2011;8:368-72.
68. Wutzler A, Mueller A, Loehr L, Huemer M, Parwani AS, Attanasio P, Blaschke F, Storm C, Boldt LH, Haverkamp W. Minimal and deep sedation during ablation of ventricular tachycardia. Int J Cardiol. 2014;172:161-4.
69. Bunch TJ, Darby A, May HT, Ragosta M, Lim DS, Taylor AM, DiMarco JP, Ailawadi G, Revenaugh JR, Weiss JP, Mahapatra S. Efficacy and safety of ventricular tachycardia ablation with mechanical circulatory support compared with substrate-based ablation techniques. Europace. 2012;14:709-14.
70. Reddy YM, Chinitz L, Mansour M, Bunch TJ, Mahapatra S, Swarup V, Di Biase L, Bommana S, Atkins D, Tung R, Shivkumar K, Burkhardt JD, Ruskin J, Natale A, Lakkireddy D. Percutaneous left ventricular assist devices in ventricular tachycardia ablation: multicenter experience. Circ Arrhythm Electrophysiol. 2014;7:244-50.
71. Tilz RR, Makimoto H, Lin T, Rillig A, Metzner A, Mathew S, Deiss S, Wissner E, Rausch P, Kamioka M, Heeger C, Kuck KH, Ouyang F. In vivo left-ventricular contact force analysis: comparison of antegrade transseptal with retrograde trans-aortic mapping strategies and correlation of impedance and electrical amplitude with contact force. Europace. 2014;16: 1387-95.
72. Soejima K, Nogami A, Sekiguchi Y, Harada T, Satomi K, Hirose T, Ueda A, Miwa Y, Sato T, Nishio S, Shirai Y, Kowase S, Murakoshi N, Kunugi S, Murata H, Nitta T, Aonuma K, Yoshino H. Epicardial catheter ablation of ventricular tachycardia in no entry left ventricle: mechanical aortic and mitral valves. Circ Arrhythm Electrophysiol. 2015;8:381-9.
73. Hsieh CH, Thomas SP, Ross DL. Direct transthoracic access to the left ventricle for catheter ablation of ventricular tachycardia. Circ Arrhythm Electrophysiol. 2010;3:178-85.
74. Vaseghi M, Macias C, Tung R, Shivkumar K. Percutaneous interventricular septal access in a patient with aortic and mitral mechanical valves: a novel technique for catheter ablation of ventricular tachycardia. Heart Rhythm. 2013;10:1069-73.
75. Heidbuchel H, Verhamme P, Alings M, Antz M, Diener HC, Hacke W, Oldgren J, Sinnaeve P, Camm AJ, Kirchhof P. Updated European Heart Rhythm Association Practical Guide on the use of non-vitamin K antagonist anticoagulants in patients with non-valvular atrial fibrillation. Europace. 2015;17: 1467-507.
76. Hummel JD, Strickberger SA, Daoud E, Niebauer M, Bakr O, Man KC, Williamson BD, Morady F. Results and efficiency of programmed ventricular stimulation with four extrastimuli

compared with one, two, and three extrastimuli. Circulation. 1994;90:2827-32.
77. Morady F, Kadish A, de Buitleir M, Kou WH, Calkins H, Schmaltz S, Rosenheck S, Sousa J. Prospective comparison of a conventional and an accelerated protocol for programmed ventricular stimulation in patients with coronary artery disease. Circulation. 1991;83:764-73.
78. Zaman S, Kumar S, Narayan A, Sivagangabalan G, Thiagalingam A, Ross DL, Thomas SP, Kovoor P. Induction of ventricular tachycardia with the fourth extrastimulus and its relationship to risk of arrhythmic events in patients with post-myocardial infarct left ventricular dysfunction. Europace. 2012;14:1771-7.
79. Balasundaram R, Rao HB, Kalavakolanu S, Narasimhan C. Catheter ablation of bundle branch reentrant ventricular tachycardia. Heart Rhythm. 2008;5:S68-72.
80. El-Shalakany A, Hadjis T, Papageorgiou P, Monahan K, Epstein L, Josephson ME. Entrainment/mapping criteria for the prediction of termination of ventricular tachycardia by single radiofrequency lesion in patients with coronary artery disease. Circulation. 1999;99:2283-9.
81. Morady F, Kadish A, Rosenheck S, Calkins H, Kou WH, De Buitleir M, Sousa J. Concealed entrainment as a guide for catheter ablation of ventricular tachycardia in patients with prior myocardial infarction. J Am Coll Cardiol. 1991;17:678-89.
82. Stevenson WG, Friedman PL, Sager PT, Saxon LA, Kocovic D, Harada T, Wiener I, Khan H. Exploring postinfarction reentrant ventricular tachycardia with entrainment mapping. J Am Coll Cardiol. 1997;29:1180-9.
83. Stevenson WG, Khan H, Sager P, Saxon LA, Middlekauff HR, Natterson PD, Wiener I. Identification of reentry circuit sites during catheter mapping and radiofrequency ablation of ventricular tachycardia late after myocardial infarction. Circulation. 1993;88:1647-70.
84. Bogun F, Li YG, Groenefeld G, Hohnloser SH, Schuger C, Oral H, Pelosi F, Knight B, Strickberger SA, Morady F. Prevalence of a shared isthmus in postinfarction patients with pleiomorphic, hemodynamically tolerated ventricular tachycardias. J Cardiovasc Electrophysiol. 2002;13:237-41.
85. Almendral J. Resetting and entrainment of reentrant arrhythmias: part II: informative content and practical use of these responses. Pacing Clin Electrophysiol. 2013;36:641-61.
86. Almendral J, Caulier-Cisterna R, Rojo-Alvarez JL. Resetting and entrainment of reentrant arrhythmias: part I: concepts, recognition, and protocol for evaluation: surface ECG versus intracardiac recordings. Pacing Clin Electrophysiol. 2013;36:508-32.
87. Bogun F, Hohnloser SH, Bender B, Li YG, Groenefeld G, Pelosi F, Oral H, Knight B, Strickberger SA, Morady F. Mechanism of ventricular tachycardia termination by pacing at left ventricular sites in patients with coronary artery disease. J Interv Card Electrophysiol. 2002;6:35-41.
88. Bogun F, Bahu M, Knight BP, Weiss R, Paladino W, Harvey M, Goyal R, Daoud E, Man KC, Strickberger SA, Morady F. Comparison of effective and ineffective target sites that demonstrate concealed entrainment in patients with coronary artery disease undergoing radiofrequency ablation of ventricular tachycardia. Circulation. 1997;95:183-90.
89. Santangeli P, Marchlinski FE. Substrate mapping for unstable ventricular tachycardia. Heart Rhythm. 2016;13:569-83.
90. Di Biase L, Burkhardt JD, Lakkireddy D, Carbucicchio C, Mohanty S, Mohanty P, Trivedi C, Santangeli P, Bai R, Forleo G, Horton R, Bailey S, Sanchez J, Al-Ahmad A, Hranitzky P, Gallinghouse GJ, Pelargonio G, Hongo RH, Beheiry S, Hao SC, Reddy M, Rossillo A, Themistoclakis S, Dello Russo A, Casella M, Tondo C, Natale A. Ablation of Stable VTs Versus Substrate Ablation in Ischemic Cardiomyopathy: The VISTA Randomized Multicenter Trial. J Am Coll Cardiol. 2015;66:2872-82.
91. Marchlinski FE, Callans DJ, Gottlieb CD, Zado E. Linear ablation lesions for control of unmappable ventricular tachycardia in patients with ischemic and nonischemic cardiomyopathy. Circulation. 2000;101:1288-96.
92. Codreanu A, Odille F, Aliot E, Marie PY, Magnin-Poull I, Andronache M, Mandry D, Djaballah W, Regent D, Felblinger J, de Chillou C. Electroanatomic characterization of post-infarct scars comparison with 3-dimensional myocardial scar reconstruction based on magnetic resonance imaging. J Am Coll Cardiol. 2008;52:839-42.
93. Deneke T, Muller KM, Lemke B, Lawo T, Calcum B, Helwing M, Mugge A, Grewe PH. Human histopathology of electroanatomic mapping after cooled-tip radiofrequency ablation to treat ventricular tachycardia in remote myocardial infarction. J Cardiovasc Electrophysiol. 2005;16:1246-51.
94. Sarrazin JF, Kuehne M, Wells D, Chalfoun N, Crawford T, Boonyapisit W, Good E, Chugh A, Oral H, Jongnarangsin K, Pelosi F, Morady F, Bogun F. High-output pacing in mapping of postinfarction ventricular tachycardia. Heart Rhythm. 2008;5:1709-14.
95. Soejima K, Stevenson WG, Maisel WH, Sapp JL, Epstein LM. Electrically unexcitable scar mapping based on pacing threshold for identification of the reentry circuit isthmus: feasibility for guiding ventricular tachycardia ablation. Circulation. 2002;106:1678-83.
96. Hutchinson MD, Gerstenfeld EP, Desjardins B, Bala R, Riley MP, Garcia FC, Dixit S, Lin D, Tzou WS, Cooper JM, Verdino RJ, Callans DJ, Marchlinski FE. Endocardial unipolar voltage mapping to detect epicardial ventricular tachycardia substrate in patients with nonischemic left ventricular cardiomyopathy. Circ Arrhythm Electrophysiol. 2011;4:49-55.
97. Polin GM, Haqqani H, Tzou W, Hutchinson MD, Garcia FC, Callans DJ, Zado ES, Marchlinski FE. Endocardial unipolar voltage mapping to identify epicardial substrate in arrhythmogenic right ventricular cardiomyopathy/dysplasia. Heart Rhythm. 2011;8:76-83.
98. Tung R, Mathuria N, Michowitz Y, Yu R, Buch E, Bradfield J, Mandapati R, Wiener I, Boyle N, Shivkumar K. Functional pace-mapping responses for identification of targets for catheter ablation of scar-mediated ventricular tachycardia. Circ Arrhythm Electrophysiol. 2012;5:264-72.
99. Arenal A, del Castillo S, Gonzalez-Torrecilla E, Atienza F, Ortiz M, Jimenez J, Puchol A, Garcia J, Almendral J. Tachycardia-related channel in the scar tissue in patients with sustained monomorphic ventricular tachycardias: influence of the voltage scar definition. Circulation. 2004;110:2568-74.
100. Hsia HH, Lin D, Sauer WH, Callans DJ, Marchlinski FE. Anatomic characterization of endocardial substrate for hemodynamically stable reentrant ventricular tachycardia: identification of endocardial conducting channels. Heart Rhythm. 2006;3:503-12.
101. Mountantonakis SE, Park RE, Frankel DS, Hutchinson MD, Dixit S, Cooper J, Callans D, Marchlinski FE, Gerstenfeld EP. Relationship between voltage map "channels" and the location of critical isthmus sites in patients with post-infarction

cardiomyopathy and ventricular tachycardia. J Am Coll Cardiol. 2013;61:2088-95.
102. Cassidy DM, Vassallo JA, Buxton AE, Doherty JU, Marchlinski FE, Josephson ME. The value of catheter mapping during sinus rhythm to localize site of origin of ventricular tachycardia. Circulation. 1984;69:1103-10.
103. Miller JM, Tyson GS, Hargrove WC, 3rd, Vassallo JA, Rosenthal ME, Josephson ME. Effect of subendocardial resection on sinus rhythm endocardial electrogram abnormalities. Circulation. 1995;91:2385-91.
104. Hsia HH, Lin D, Sauer WH, Callans DJ, Marchlinski FE. Relationship of late potentials to the ventricular tachycardia circuit defined by entrainment. J Interv Card Electrophysiol. 2009;26:21-9.
105. Kocovic DZ, Harada T, Friedman PL, Stevenson WG. Characteristics of electrograms recorded at reentry circuit sites and bystanders during ventricular tachycardia after myocardial infarction. J Am Coll Cardiol. 1999;34:381-8.
106. Bogun F, Bahu M, Knight BP, Weiss R, Goyal R, Daoud E, Man KC, Strickberger SA, Morady F. Response to pacing at sites of isolated diastolic potentials during ventricular tachycardia in patients with previous myocardial infarction. J Am Coll Cardiol. 1997;30:505-13.
107. Arenal A, Glez-Torrecilla E, Ortiz M, Villacastin J, Fdez-Portales J, Sousa E, del Castillo S, Perez de Isla L, Jimenez J, Almendral J. Ablation of electrograms with an isolated, delayed component as treatment of unmappable monomorphic ventricular tachycardias in patients with structural heart disease. J Am Coll Cardiol. 2003;41:81-92.
108. Jais P, Maury P, Khairy P, Sacher F, Nault I, Komatsu Y, Hocini M, Forclaz A, Jadidi AS, Weerasooryia R, Shah A, Derval N, Cochet H, Knecht S, Miyazaki S, Linton N, Rivard L, Wright M, Wilton SB, Scherr D, Pascale P, Roten L, Pederson M, Bordachar P, Laurent F, Kim SJ, Ritter P, Clementy J, Haissaguerre M. Elimination of local abnormal ventricular activities: a new end point for substrate modification in patients with scar-related ventricular tachycardia. Circulation. 2012;125:2184-96.
109. Schmidt B, Chun KR, Baensch D, Antz M, Koektuerk B, Tilz RR, Metzner A, Ouyang F, Kuck KH. Catheter ablation for ventricular tachycardia after failed endocardial ablation: epicardial substrate or inappropriate endocardial ablation? Heart Rhythm. 2010;7:1746-52.
110. Schweikert RA, Saliba WI, Tomassoni G, Marrouche NF, Cole CR, Dresing TJ, Tchou PJ, Bash D, Beheiry S, Lam C, Kanagaratnam L, Natale A. Percutaneous pericardial instrumentation for endo-epicardial mapping of previously failed ablations. Circulation. 2003;108:1329-35.
111. Komatsu Y, Daly M, Sacher F, Cochet H, Denis A, Derval N, Jesel L, Zellerhoff S, Lim HS, Jadidi A, Nault I, Shah A, Roten L, Pascale P, Scherr D, Aurillac-Lavignolle V, Hocini M, Haissaguerre M, Jais P. Endocardial ablation to eliminate epicardial arrhythmia substrate in scar-related ventricular tachycardia. J Am Coll Cardiol. 2014;63:1416-26.
112. Verma A, Marrouche NF, Schweikert RA, Saliba W, Wazni O, Cummings J, Abdul-Karim A, Bhargava M, Burkhardt JD, Kilicaslan F, Martin DO, Natale A. Relationship between successful ablation sites and the scar border zone defined by substrate mapping for ventricular tachycardia post-myocardial infarction. J Cardiovasc Electrophysiol. 2005;16:465-71.
113. Izquierdo M, Sanchez-Gomez JM, Ferrero de Loma-Osorio A, Martinez A, Bellver A, Pelaez A, Nunez J, Nunez C, Chorro J, Ruiz-Granell R. Endo-epicardial versus only-endocardial ablation as a first line strategy for the treatment of ventricular tachycardia in patients with ischemic heart disease. Circ Arrhythm Electrophysiol. 2015;8:882-9.
114. Yamada T, McElderry HT, Doppalapudi H, Okada T, Murakami Y, Yoshida Y, Yoshida N, Inden Y, Murohara T, Plumb VJ, Kay GN. Idiopathic ventricular arrhythmias originating from the left ventricular summit: anatomic concepts relevant to ablation. Circ Arrhythm Electrophysiol. 2010;3:616-23.
115. Sosa E, Scanavacca M, d'Avila A, Pilleggi F. A new technique to perform epicardial mapping in the electrophysiology laboratory. J Cardiovasc Electrophysiol. 1996;7:531-6.
116. Kumar S, Bazaz R, Barbhaiya CR, Enriquez AD, Helmbold AF, Chinitz JS, Baldinger SH, Mahida S, McConville JW, Tedrow UB, John RM, Michaud GF, Stevenson WG. "Needle-in-needle" epicardial access: Preliminary observations with a modified technique for facilitating epicardial interventional procedures. Heart Rhythm. 2015;12:1691-7.
117. Gunda S, Reddy M, Pillarisetti J, Atoui M, Badhwar N, Swarup V, DiBiase L, Mohanty S, Mohanty P, Nagaraj H, Ellis C, Rasekh A, Cheng J, Bartus K, Lee R, Natale A, Lakkireddy D. Differences in complication rates between large bore needle and a long micropuncture needle during epicardial access: time to change clinical practice? Circ Arrhythm Electrophysiol. 2015;8:890-5.
118. Killu AM, Ebrille E, Asirvatham SJ, Munger TM, McLeod CJ, Packer DL, Friedman PA, Mulpuru SK. Percutaneous epicardial access for mapping and ablation is feasible in patients with prior cardiac surgery, including coronary bypass surgery. Circ Arrhythm Electrophysiol. 2015;8:94-101.
119. Tschabrunn CM, Haqqani HM, Cooper JM, Dixit S, Garcia FC, Gerstenfeld EP, Callans DJ, Zado ES, Marchlinski FE. Percutaneous epicardial ventricular tachycardia ablation after noncoronary cardiac surgery or pericarditis. Heart Rhythm. 2013;10:165-9.
120. Tung R, Nakahara S, Ramirez R, Lai C, Fishbein MC, Shivkumar K. Distinguishing epicardial fat from scar: analysis of electrograms using high-density electroanatomic mapping in a novel porcine infarct model. Heart Rhythm. 2010;7:389-95.
121. Roberts-Thomson KC, Steven D, Seiler J, Inada K, Koplan BA, Tedrow UB, Epstein LM, Stevenson WG. Coronary artery injury due to catheter ablation in adults: presentations and outcomes. Circulation. 2009;120:1465-73.
122. Di Biase L, Burkhardt JD, Pelargonio G, Dello Russo A, Casella M, Santarelli P, Horton R, Sanchez J, Gallinghouse JG, Al-Ahmad A, Wang P, Cummings JE, Schweikert RA, Natale A. Prevention of phrenic nerve injury during epicardial ablation: comparison of methods for separating the phrenic nerve from the epicardial surface. Heart Rhythm. 2009;6:957-61.
123. Matsuo S, Jais P, Knecht S, Lim KT, Hocini M, Derval N, Wright M, Sacher F, Haissaguerre M. Images in cardiovascular medicine. Novel technique to prevent left phrenic nerve injury during epicardial catheter ablation. Circulation. 2008;117:e471.
124. Soejima K, Suzuki M, Maisel WH, Brunckhorst CB, Delacretaz E, Blier L, Tung S, Khan H, Stevenson WG. Catheter ablation in patients with multiple and unstable ventricular tachycardias after myocardial infarction: short ablation lines guided by reentry circuit isthmuses and sinus rhythm mapping. Circulation. 2001;104:664-9.
125. Berruezo A, Fernandez-Armenta J, Andreu D, Penela D, Herczku C, Evertz R, Cipolletta L, Acosta J, Borras R, Arbelo E,

Tolosana JM, Brugada J, Mont L. Scar dechanneling: new method for scar-related left ventricular tachycardia substrate ablation. Circ Arrhythm Electrophysiol. 2015;8:326-36.

126. Tung R, Mathuria NS, Nagel R, Mandapati R, Buch EF, Bradfield JS, Vaseghi M, Boyle NG, Shivkumar K. Impact of local ablation on interconnected channels within ventricular scar: mechanistic implications for substrate modification. Circ Arrhythm Electrophysiol. 2013;6:1131-8.

127. Arenal A, Hernandez J, Calvo D, Ceballos C, Atea L, Datino T, Atienza F, Gonzalez-Torrecilla E, Eidelman G, Miracle A, Avila P, Bermejo J, Fernandez-Aviles F. Safety, long-term results, and predictors of recurrence after complete endocardial ventricular tachycardia substrate ablation in patients with previous myocardial infarction. Am J Cardiol. 2013;111: 499-505.

128. Vergara P, Trevisi N, Ricco A, Petracca F, Baratto F, Cireddu M, Bisceglia C, Maccabelli G, Della Bella P. Late potentials abolition as an additional technique for reduction of arrhythmia recurrence in scar related ventricular tachycardia ablation. J Cardiovasc Electrophysiol. 2012;23:621-7.

129. Volkmer M, Ouyang F, Deger F, Ernst S, Goya M, Bansch D, Berodt K, Kuck KH, Antz M. Substrate mapping vs. tachycardia mapping using CARTO in patients with coronary artery disease and ventricular tachycardia: impact on outcome of catheter ablation. Europace. 2006;8:968-76.

130. Tzou WS, Frankel DS, Hegeman T, Supple GE, Garcia FC, Santangeli P, Katz DF, Sauer WH, Marchlinski FE. Core isolation of critical arrhythmia elements for treatment of multiple scar-based ventricular tachycardias. Circ Arrhythm Electrophysiol. 2015;8:353-61.

131. Soejima K, Delacretaz E, Suzuki M, Brunckhorst CB, Maisel WH, Friedman PL, Stevenson WG. Saline-cooled versus standard radiofrequency catheter ablation for infarct-related ventricular tachycardias. Circulation. 2001;103:1858-62.

132. Stevenson WG, Wilber DJ, Natale A, Jackman WM, Marchlinski FE, Talbert T, Gonzalez MD, Worley SJ, Daoud EG, Hwang C, Schuger C, Bump TE, Jazayeri M, Tomassoni GF, Kopelman HA, Soejima K, Nakagawa H. Irrigated radiofrequency catheter ablation guided by electroanatomic mapping for recurrent ventricular tachycardia after myocardial infarction: the multicenter thermocool ventricular tachycardia ablation trial. Circulation. 2008;118:2773-82.

133. Tanner H, Hindricks G, Volkmer M, Furniss S, Kuhlkamp V, Lacroix D, C DEC, Almendral J, Caponi D, Kuck KH, Kottkamp H. Catheter ablation of recurrent scar-related ventricular tachycardia using electroanatomical mapping and irrigated ablation technology: results of the prospective multicenter Euro-VT-study. J Cardiovasc Electrophysiol. 2010;21:47-53.

134. Houmsse M, Daoud EG. Biophysics and clinical utility of irrigated-tip radiofrequency catheter ablation. Expert Rev Med Devices. 2012;9:59-70.

135. Waldo AL, Wilber DJ, Marchlinski FE, Stevenson WG, Aker B, Boo LM, Jackman WM. Safety of the open-irrigated ablation catheter for radiofrequency ablation: safety analysis from six clinical studies. Pacing Clin Electrophysiol. 2012;35: 1081-9.

136. Sacher F, Wright M, Derval N, Denis A, Ramoul K, Roten L, Pascale P, Bordachar P, Ritter P, Hocini M, Dos Santos P, Haissaguerre M, Jais P. Endocardial versus epicardial ventricular radiofrequency ablation: utility of in vivo contact force assessment. Circ Arrhythm Electrophysiol. 2013;6: 144-50.

137. Jesel L, Sacher F, Komatsu Y, Daly M, Zellerhoff S, Lim HS, Derval N, Denis A, Ambri W, Ramoul K, Aurillac V, Hocini M, Haissaguerre M, Jais P. Characterization of contact force during endocardial and epicardial ventricular mapping. Circ Arrhythm Electrophysiol. 2014;7:1168-73.

138. Koruth JS, Dukkipati S, Miller MA, Neuzil P, d'Avila A, Reddy VY. Bipolar irrigated radiofrequency ablation: a therapeutic option for refractory intramural atrial and ventricular tachycardia circuits. Heart Rhythm. 2012;9:1932-41.

139. Sivagangabalan G, Barry MA, Huang K, Lu J, Pouliopoulos J, Thomas SP, Ross DL, Thiagalingam A, Kovoor P. Bipolar ablation of the interventricular septum is more efficient at creating a transmural line than sequential unipolar ablation. Pacing Clin Electrophysiol. 2010;33:16-26.

140. Berte B, Cochet H, Magat J, Naulin J, Ghidoli D, Pillois X, Casassus F, Yamashita S, Mahida S, Derval N, Hocini M, Quesson B, Bernus O, Weerasooriya R, Haissaguerre M, Sacher F, Jais P. Irrigated Needle Ablation Creates Larger and More Transmural Ventricular Lesions Compared With Standard Unipolar Ablation in an Ovine Model. Circ Arrhythm Electrophysiol. 2015;8:1498-506.

141. Sapp JL, Beeckler C, Pike R, Parkash R, Gray CJ, Zeppenfeld K, Kuriachan V, Stevenson WG. Initial human feasibility of infusion needle catheter ablation for refractory ventricular tachycardia. Circulation. 2013;128:2289-95.

142. Tokuda M, Sobieszczyk P, Eisenhauer AC, Kojodjojo P, Inada K, Koplan BA, Michaud GF, John RM, Epstein LM, Sacher F, Stevenson WG, Tedrow UB. Transcoronary ethanol ablation for recurrent ventricular tachycardia after failed catheter ablation: an update. Circ Arrhythm Electrophysiol. 2011;4:889-96.

143. Kay GN, Epstein AE, Bubien RS, Anderson PG, Dailey SM, Plumb VJ. Intracoronary ethanol ablation for the treatment of recurrent sustained ventricular tachycardia. J Am Coll Cardiol. 1992;19:159-68.

144. Sacher F, Sobieszczyk P, Tedrow U, Eisenhauer AC, Field ME, Selwyn A, Raymond JM, Koplan B, Epstein LM, Stevenson WG. Transcoronary ethanol ventricular tachycardia ablation in the modern electrophysiology era. Heart Rhythm. 2008;5:62-8.

145. Tholakanahalli VN, Bertog S, Roukoz H, Shivkumar K. Catheter ablation of ventricular tachycardia using intracoronary wire mapping and coil embolization: description of a new technique. Heart Rhythm. 2013;10:292-6.

146. Frankel DS, Mountantonakis SE, Zado ES, Anter E, Bala R, Cooper JM, Deo R, Dixit S, Epstein AE, Garcia FC, Gerstenfeld EP, Hutchinson MD, Lin D, Patel VV, Riley MP, Robinson MR, Tzou WS, Verdino RJ, Callans DJ, Marchlinski FE. Noninvasive programmed ventricular stimulation early after ventricular tachycardia ablation to predict risk of late recurrence. J Am Coll Cardiol. 2012;59:1529-35.

147. Yokokawa M, Desjardins B, Crawford T, Good E, Morady F, Bogun F. Reasons for recurrent ventricular tachycardia after catheter ablation of post-infarction ventricular tachycardia. J Am Coll Cardiol. 2013;61:66-73.

EDITORS' SUMMARY

Among the most challenging mapping and ablation procedures in contemporary electrophysiology is for ablation of ventricular tachycardia in the structurally *abnormal* heart. Patients with sometimes abysmal quality of life because of frequent ICD shocks and failure of antiarrhythmic therapy require our best efforts to control or eliminate this arrhythmia. In the present chapter, Drs Lee and Haqqani have provided a concise and extremely well referenced review of the primary challenges and keys to success with this ablation.

They outline the mapping approach during tachycardia, and their statements used along with the chapter on entrainment mapping will allow for a reasoned approach to mapping VT. Also discussed are methods to manage the hemodynamic consequences of prolonged ventricular tachycardia and the value (including a figure) of intracardiac echocardiography for understanding the substrate and monitoring the patient during these complex procedures.

The authors provide outstanding parallels with regard to substrate mapping both when discrete scar is present and in the setting of an idiopathic dilated cardiomyopathy. The relative value of the voltage map and specific findings of fragmented electrograms and late potentials are discussed in a practical and useable manner.

CHAPTER 33

Hugh Calkins

Ventricular Tachycardia in Arrhythmogenic Right Ventricular Dysplasia/Cardiomyopathy

LIST OF ABBREVIATIONS

AAV	Adeno-associated Virus
ACE	Angiotensin Converting Enzyme
AHA	American Heart Association
ARVD/C	Arrhythmogenic Right Ventricular Dysplasia/Cardiomyopathy
DSC	Desmocollin
DSG	Desmoglein
DSP	Desmoplakin
EPS	Electrophysiology Study
ICD	Implantable Cardioverter-Defibrillator
JUP	Plakoglobin
LBBB	Left Bundle Branch Block
LV	Left Ventricle
MET	Metabolic Equivalent
NSVT	Non-sustained Ventricular Tachycardia
PKP	Plakophilin
PLN	Phospholamban
PVC	Premature Ventricular Contraction
RVOT	Right Ventricular Outflow Tract
RV	Right Ventricle
RYR	Ryanodine Receptor
SAECG	Signal Averaged Electrocardiogram
SCD	Sudden Cardiac Death
TFC	Task Force Criteria
TGFβ	Transforming Growth Factor Beta
TMEM43	Transmembrane Protein 43
TTN	Titin
TWI	T-wave inversion
VArr	Ventricular Arrhythmias
VF	Ventricular Fibrillation
VT	Ventricular Tachycardia

INTRODUCTION

Arrhythmogenic right ventricular dysplasia/cardiomyopathy (ARVD/C) is an inherited cardiomyopathy that is characterized by ventricular arrhythmias, an increased risk of sudden death, and abnormalities of right (and less commonly left) ventricular structure and function. Although structural involvement of the right ventricle predominates (globally as well as in the United States), a left dominant form is also seen. The pathologic hallmark of ARVD/C is myocyte loss with fibrofatty replacement. Since the first detailed clinical description of the disorder in 1982,[1] significant advances have been made in our understanding of all aspects of this disease. Mutations predominantly in desmosomal proteins have been determined to be the genetic basis of ARVD/C in up to two-thirds of affected individuals.[2,3] There is increasing evidence supporting the relationship between exercise and ARVD/C. It has been observed that exercise causes an earlier onset and more severe arrhythmic and structural disease, suggesting that this is a very important environmental factor for the development and progression of ARVD/C. It has been proposed that exercise and genetic predisposition have an additive effect towards a threshold for ARVD/C pathogenesis. However, there are very few recommendations as to what is the appropriate level of exercise that will not cause triggering of the onset of the disease.

The purpose of this chapter is to provide an overview of ARVD/C and the ventricular arrhythmias that occur in patients with this condition.

CLINICAL PRESENTATION AND NATURAL HISTORY

ARVD/C is an inherited condition with an estimated prevalence of 1 per 5000. Patients usually present during the second to fifth decade of life with palpitations, lightheadedness, syncope, or sudden death.[3,4] Symptoms correlate with the presence of ventricular arrhythmias. Heart failure is an uncommon and late manifestation of the disease. **Flow chart 33.1** summarizes the major presenting clinical features, clinical course, and arrhythmia and survival

Flow chart 33.1: Schematic representation of the presentation, clinical course and outcome in Arrhythmogenic Right ventricular Dysplasia/Cardiomyopathy (ARVD/C) index-patients. The majority presented with sustained ventricular arrhythmias (VArr) and received an implantable cardioverter-defibrillator (ICD) during follow-up

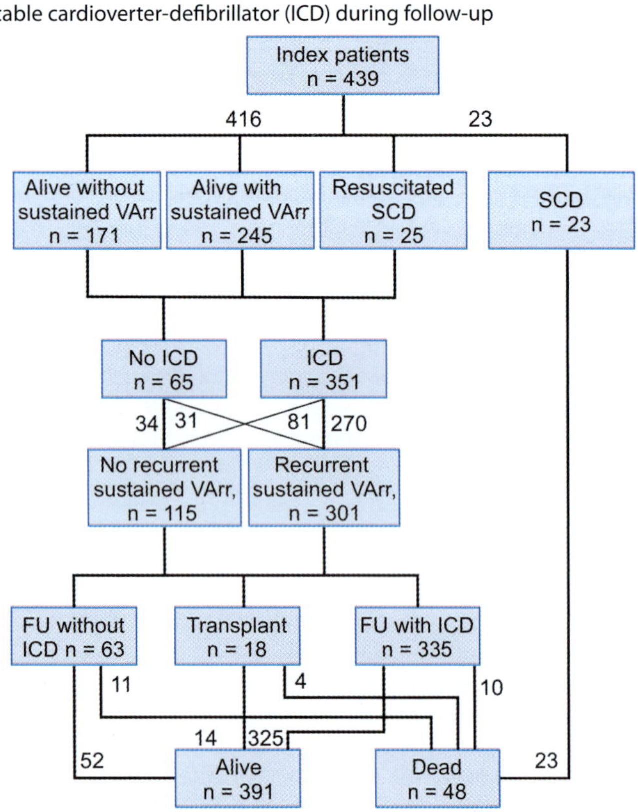

Abbreviations: SCD, sudden cardiac death; FU, follow-up
Reproduced with the permission from Groeneweg J, et al.[3]

outcomes of 439 index-patients drawn from a combined US/Dutch ARVD/C registry.[4] The mean age at presentation was 36±14 years. Most patients (419, 95%) presented with symptoms, and the remaining 20 (5%) were asymptomatic but came to medical attention because of abnormal tests in diverse settings. Forty-eight index-patients (11%) presented with a cardiac arrest among whom 25 were resuscitated and 23 died with the diagnosis established at autopsy (median age at cardiac arrest 25 years, IQR 21, range 13–70). An additional 220 index-patients (50%) presented with a sustained ventricular arrhythmias (VArr). During the clinical disease course, an implantable cardioverter-defibrillator (ICD) was implanted in 212 (87%) of the 245 index-patients with a sustained VArr or resuscitated sudden cardiac death (SCD) and in 139 (81%) of the 171 index-patients presenting without sustained VArr. Sixty-five index-patients did not have an ICD implanted during follow-up (33 with and 32 without sustained VArr at presentation). Sustained VArr during follow-up was seen in more than two-thirds of index-patients (301, 72%). Of the 65 index-patients without an ICD, 31 (48%) experienced a sustained VArr during follow-up.

Among index-patients with an ICD, 10 (3%) died (median follow-up 7 years): 2 of SCD, 3 of heart failure, 2 of a combination of heart failure and arrhythmias, and 3 of non-cardiac causes. Among index-patients without an ICD, 11 (17%) died (median follow- up 5 years): 10 of these 11 patients died of SCD and 1 of heart failure. The SCD incidence was higher in index-patients without an ICD compared to those with an ICD (16% vs. 0.6%, $p < 0.001$). During long-term follow-up, 54 index-patients (13%) developed symptomatic heart failure and 18 (4%) had a cardiac transplantation. Four patients that underwent transplantation died during follow-up. Overall, 391 of the 416 index-patients (94%) who presented alive were alive at last follow-up.

Figures 33.1A and B show the results of Kaplan-Meier survival analysis by age for these 416 index-patients who presented alive for the following outcomes: 1) any ARVD/C related symptoms, 2) sustained VArr, 3) cardiac mortality, and 4) cardiac transplantation. Of particular note is that all patients presented in their teenage years or later (range 10–78 years). The development of symptoms correlated closely with the development of a sustained VArr, with cardiac mortality and the need for cardiac transplantation being low.

Although ARVD/C is predominantly a disease of the right ventricle (RV),[5-8] it is now well established that involvement of the left ventricle may occur, particularly when MR imaging is used to detect subtle abnormalities in left ventricular function and also in patients with advanced disease. Left-dominant arrhythmogenic cardiomyopathy also is defined by early disease of the left ventricle (LV), often affecting the posterolateral LV wall, in the absence of significant right ventricular systolic dysfunction. Left-dominant disease is more commonly seen in patients with desmoplakin (DSP) or phospholamban (*PLN*) mutations.[8]

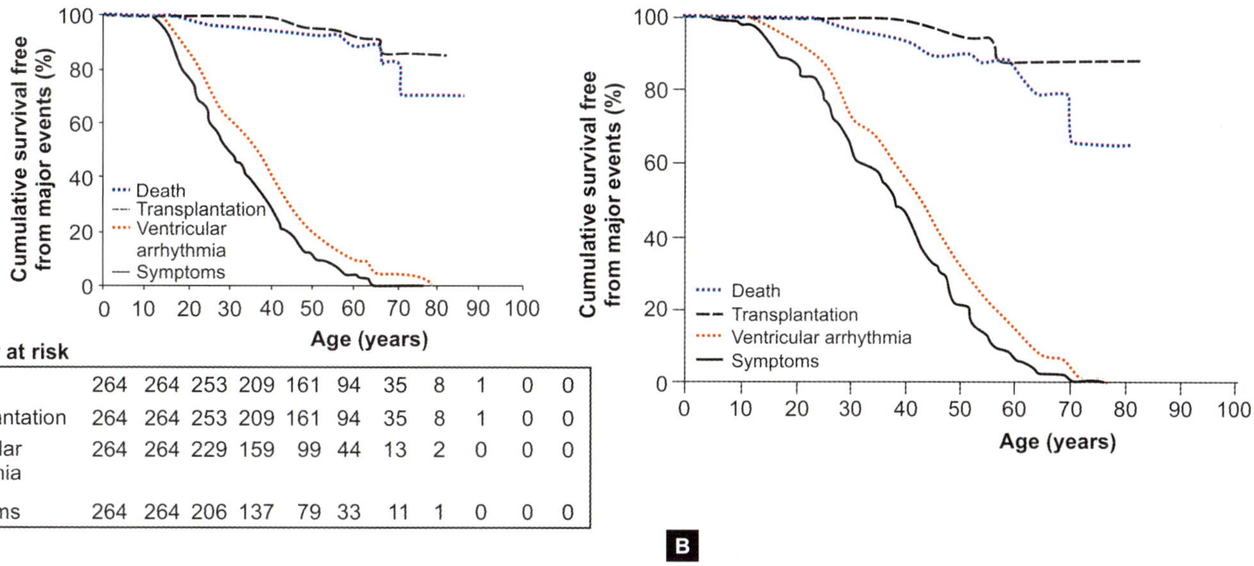

Number at risk

Death	264	264	253	209	161	94	35	8	1	0	0
Transplantation	264	264	253	209	161	94	35	8	1	0	0
Ventricular arrhythmia	264	264	229	159	99	44	13	2	0	0	0
Symptoms	264	264	206	137	79	33	11	1	0	0	0

Figures 33.1A and B: Survival free from any arrhythmogenic right ventricular dysplasia/cardiomyopathy (ARVD/C) related symptoms, sustained ventricular arrhythmias (VArr), cardiac death and cardiac transplantation in ARVD/C index-patients with (A) pathogenic mutations and (B) without identified mutations. Symptoms ($p = 0.005$) and sustained VArr ($p = 0.020$) occurred more often at younger age in index-patients with mutations. Survival free from cardiac death ($p = 0.644$) and transplantation ($p = 0.704$) was similar in both groups. Reproduced with permission from Groeneweg J, et al.[3]

GENETIC BASIS OF ARVD/C

In most cases, ARVD/C is inherited in an autosomal dominant pattern with incomplete age-related penetrance and significant variable expressivity. Among probands diagnosed with this disease, screening of first degree relatives identifies other affected individuals in approximately 50% of cases. In a minority of cases, ARVD/C is inherited in an autosomal recessive pattern as part of a cardiocutaneous syndrome such as Naxos disease or Carvajal syndrome which is also characterized by woolly hair and palmoplantar keratoderma.

Linkage mapping and candidate gene evaluation studies performed in patients with the autosomal dominant form of ARVD/C initially was not productive due to significant variability in the penetrance and expressivity of the disease. It was the investigation of patients with Naxos syndrome, a disease with 100% penetrance by adolescence, that first identified a disease causing mutation: a homozygous deletion of two base pairs found in the plakoglobin (*JUP*) gene located at the 17q21 locus.[9] The gene encodes a key component of desmosomes, which are complex intercellular adhesion structures found in stratified epithelial cells of the skin as well as in myocytes. Desmosomes are composed of three major groups of proteins: Cadherins are transmembrane proteins which provide the actual mechanical coupling between individual cells and include desmoglein and desmocollin. Desmoplakin is a plakin-family protein which serves to anchor the desmosomal structure to the intermediate filaments of the cell. Lastly, Armadillo proteins including plakoglobin and plakophilin link desmoplakin and the cadherin tails.

The identification of defective desmosomal proteins in Naxos syndrome led to studies investigating their role in other arrhythmogenic cardiomyopathies. The Carvajal syndrome, another cardiocutaneous syndrome that has left-dominant arrhythmogenic cardiomyopathy, was shown to be associated with a recessive mutation in desmoplakin (*DSP*).[10] Mutations in desmosomal genes including *DSP*, *DSG2* encoding desmoglein-2, *DSC2* encoding desmocollin-2 and *PKP2* encoding plakophilin-2[2,8] were subsequently identified in families with autosomal-dominant ARVD/C. Mutations in several extra-desmosomal genes such as those encoding transforming growth factor β_3 (*TGF*-β_3), cardiac ryanodine receptor (*RYR2*), Titin (*TTN*), and transmembrane protein 43 (*TMEM43*) have also been implicated in specific types of atypical forms of ARVD/C. In the United States, a desmosomal mutation can be identified in approximately 60% of ARVD/C patients.[3,8]

Bhonsale et al. recently reported the genetic findings of a large trans-atlantic cohort of patients with ARVD/C, selected based on the presence of an ARVD/C related mutation.[8] The study population was derived from the Johns Hopkins ARVD/C registry (259 patients: 102 probands, 157 family members) and the Dutch ARVD/C cohort (318 patients: 128 probands, 190 family members). The registries were statistically similar in terms of sex, race and proband/family member ratios. Men constituted 55% of the overall population with the average age at presentation of 35±17 years.

The majority of participants (463, 80%) carried a single copy of a *PKP2* mutation (164 probands, 299 family members) with significantly fewer heterozygous carriers of mutations in other ARVD/C-associated genes (31 *DSG2*, 31 *PLN*, 19 *DSP*, 8 *DSC2*, 2 *JUP*, and 1 *TMEM43*). Twenty-two individuals (4%) carried two or more pathogenic mutations (compound heterozygote, homozygote, or digenic mutation carriers). Among carriers of single mutations, premature truncating, splice site, and missense mutations were identified in 342 (60%), 130 (23%), and 83 (14%) patients respectively. Patients with sudden cardiac death (SCD)/ventricular fibrillation (VF) at presentation (n = 36) were younger (median 23 vs. 36 years; p <0.001) than those presenting with sustained monomorphic ventricular tachycardia (VT). Amongst 541 subjects presenting alive, over a mean follow-up of 6±7 years, 12 (2%) patients died, 162 (30%) had sustained VT/VF, 78 (14%) manifested left ventricular dysfunction (EF <55%), 28 (5%) experienced heart failure and 10 (2%) required cardiac transplantation. Patients (n = 22; 4%) with >1 mutation had significantly earlier occurrence of sustained VT/VF (mean age 28±12 years), lower VT/VF free survival (p = 0.037), more frequent left ventricular dysfunction (29%), HF (19%) and cardiac transplantation (9%) as compared to those with only one mutation. *DSP* mutation carriers experienced >4 fold occurrence of left ventricular dysfunction (40%) and heart failure (13%) than *PKP2* carriers. Missense mutation carriers had similar death/transplant free survival and VT/VF penetrance (p = 0.137) as compared to those with truncating or splice site mutations.

PATHOPHYSIOLOGIC BASIS OF ARVD/C

The genetics of ARVD/C has provided support for the hypothesis that ARVD/C is a disease of desmosomal dysfunction. The pathogenic mechanisms are not fully clear, but several theories have been advanced. Defective desmosomal proteins may lead to impaired mechanical coupling between individual cells, leading to myocyte uncoupling especially under conditions that increase myocardial strain. The resulting inflammation, fibrosis and adipocytosis may be a non-specific response to injury similar to that seen in other forms of myocardial damage. This pathogenic model can explain the observation that prolonged strenuous exertion, which increases myocardial strain, significantly increases the risk of an earlier clinical onset of the disease and augments the risk of sudden death. It also explains why the RV, which is more distensible than the LV due to its thinner wall and asymmetric shape, is more often involved in ARVD/C especially in its early stages. Furthermore, defects in mechanical coupling of myocytes may also lead to impairment in electrical coupling. Other hypotheses concerning the mechanisms of ARVD/C involve complex intracellular signaling pathways. This remains an active area of investigation.

DIAGNOSTIC CRITERIA FOR ARVD/C AND DIAGNOSTIC APPROACH

Diagnosis of ARVD/C relies upon a scoring system with major and minor criteria based on the demonstration of a combination of defects in RV morphology and function, characteristic depolarization/repolarization ECG abnormalities, characteristic tissue pathology, ventricular arrhythmias, family history, and the results of genetic testing. The original 1994 Task Force Criteria were recently revised to improve upon the subjectivity of some of the original criteria and to increase sensitivity by integrating new knowledge and technology **(Table 33.1)**.[11] These criteria should now be relied on to make a diagnosis of ARVD/C. Patients are diagnosed as having definite ARVD/C if they have "4 points" (a major criteria is equal to two points and a minor criteria is equal to one point); and probable ARVD/C if their score totals to "3 points". The patients with "1 or 2 points are classified as not meeting criteria for ARVD/C.

When considering these guideline recommendations it is important to note that there is no single gold-standard diagnostic test. The initial evaluation of all patients should include a physical exam and clinical history including family history of arrhythmias or sudden death, ECG, signal averaged-ECG (SAECG), 24-hour Holter monitoring, and comprehensive noninvasive imaging of both ventricles. MRI can be of great value but is also a common cause for misdiagnosis.[12] If this noninvasive workup is suggestive but not diagnostic of ARVD/C, further testing should be considered to establish the diagnosis including electrophysiological testing. Although endomyocardial biopsy was used for diagnosis in the past, it is rarely used nowadays. Similarly, right ventriculography is rarely needed due to the availability of high quality echocardiography and MR imaging.

The diagnosis of ARVD/C should be considered in any patient who does not have known heart disease and who presents with frequent premature ventricular contractions (PVCs) or symptomatic ventricular tachycardia, especially if there is left bundle-branch block (LBBB) morphology with superior axis, the LBBB VT ECG pattern is not typical of idiopathic right ventricular outflow tract (RVOT) VT, or if the VT occurs in a patient with T-wave inversion (TWI) in the right precordial leads. The most common conditions that must be considered in the differential diagnosis include idiopathic RVOT VT, VT arising from the aortic root, and cardiac sarcoidosis. Several studies have recently compared the morphology of VT or PVCs with LBBB-inferior axis morphology in patients with idiopathic RVOT VT with patients with ARVD/C. One of these studies confirmed that a QRSd > 120 ms in lead V1 during VT or with PVCs favors the diagnosis of ARVD/C as compared with idiopathic RVOT VT.[13]

Cardiac sarcoidosis should be suspected in patients who have evidence of conduction system abnormalities,

Table 33.1: 2010 Task Force Criteria for the diagnosis of ARVD/C. A major criteria is equal to two points and a minor criteria is equal to one point. Patients are diagnosed as having definite ARVD/C if they have "4 points"; and probable ARVD/C if their score totals to "3 points". The patients with "1 or 2 points" are classified as not meeting criteria for ARVD/C

	Major	*Minor*
I. Global or regional dysfunction and structural alterations		
By 2D Echo	Regional RV akinesia, dyskinesia, or aneurysm • *and* 1 of the following (end-diastole): – PLAX RVOT ≥ 32 mm (corrected for body size [PLAX/BSA] ≥ 19 mm/m²) – PSAX RVOT≥ 36 mm (corrected for body size [PSAX/BSA] ≥ 21 mm/m²) – *or* fractional area change ≤ 33%	Regional RV akinesia or dyskinesia • *and* 1 of the following (end diastole): – PLAX RVOT≥ 29 to ≤ 32 mm (corrected for body size [PLAX/BSA] ≥ 16 to ≤ 19 mm/m²) – PSAX RVOT ≥ 32 to ≤ 36 mm (corrected for body size [PSAX/BSA] ≥ 18 to ≤ 21 mm/m²) – *or* fractional area change > 33% to ≤ 40%
By MRI	Regional RV akinesia or dyskinesia or dyssynchronous RV contraction • *and* 1 of the following: – Ratio of RV end-diastolic volume to BSA ≥ 110 mL/m² (male) or ≥ 100 mL/m² (female) – *or* RV ejection fraction ≤ 40%	Regional RV akinesia or dyskinesia or dyssynchronous RV contraction • *and* 1 of the following: – Ratio of RV end-diastolic volume to BSA ≥ 100 to < 110 mL/m² (male) or ≥90 to <100 mL/m² (female) – *or* RV ejection fraction >40% to ≤ 45%
By RV Angiography	Regional RV akinesia, dyskinesia, or aneurysm	
II. Tissue Characterization of wall	Residual myocytes < 60% by morphometric analysis (or <50% if estimated), with fibrous replacement of the RV free wall myocardium in ≥ 1 sample, with or without fatty replacement of tissue on endomyocardial biopsy	Residual myocytes 60% to 75% by morphometric analysis (or 50% to 65% if estimated), with fibrous replacement of the RV free wall myocardium in ≥1 sample, with or without fatty replacement of tissue on endomyocardial biopsy
III. Repolarization abnormalities	Inverted T waves in right precordial leads (V1, V2, and V3) or beyond in individuals > 14 years of age (in the absence of complete RBBB QRS ≥120 ms)	• Inverted T waves in leads V1 and V2 in individuals > 14 years of age (in the absence of complete RBBB) or in V4, V5, or V6 • Inverted T waves in leads V1, V2, V3, and V4 in individuals >14 years of age in the presence of complete RBBB
IV. Depolarization/ conduction abnormalities	Epsilon wave (reproducible low-amplitude signals between end of QRS complex to onset of the T wave) in the right precordial leads (V1 to V3)	• Late potentials by SAECG in ≥ 1 of 3 parameters in the absence of a QRS duration of ≥ 110 ms on the standard ECG • Filtered QRS duration (fQRS) ≥ 114 ms • Duration of terminal QRS < 40 microV (low-amplitude signal duration) ≥ 38 ms • Root-mean-square voltage of terminal 40 ms ≤ 20 microV • Terminal activation duration of QRS ≥55 ms measured from the nadir of the S wave to the end of the QRS, including R′ in V1, V2, or V3, in the absence of complete RBBB
V. Arrhythmias	Nonsustained or sustained VT of LBBB morphology with superior axis (negative or indeterminate QRS in leads II, III, and aVF and positive in lead aVL)	• Nonsustained or sustained VT of RV outflow configuration, LBBB morphology with inferior axis (positive QRS in leads II, III, and aVF and negative in lead aVL) or of unknown axis • > 500 ventricular extrasystoles per 24 hours (Holter)
VI. Family history	• ARVD/C confirmed in a first-degree relative who meets current Task Force criteria • ARVD/C confirmed pathologically at autopsy or surgery in a first-degree relative • Identification of a pathogenic mutation categorized as associated or probably associated with ARVD/C in the patient under evaluation	• History of ARVD/C in a first-degree relative in whom it is not possible or practical to determine whether the family member meets current Task Force criteria • Premature sudden death (<35 years of age) due to suspected ARVD/C in a first-degree relative • ARVD/C confirmed pathologically or by current Task Force Criteria in second-degree relative

Abbreviations: ARVD/C, Arrhythmogenic right ventricular dysplasia/cardiomyopathy; BSA, body surface area; LBBB, left bundle branch block; PLAX, Parasternal long axis; PSAX, parasternal short axis; RV, right ventricle; PVC, premature ventricular contraction; RBBB, right bundle branch block; RVOT, right ventricular outflow tract; SAECG, signal-averaged ECG; VT, ventricular tachycardia

Adapted from Marcus FI et al.[11]

especially in the presence of other extracardiac symptoms. In rare situations, an endomyocardial biopsy may become necessary to differentiate between the two disorders. The infrequency with which endomyocardial biopsy is required reflects the fact that cardiac sarcoidosis can usually be suspected based on the presence of conduction system abnormalities, mediastinal lymphadenopathy, tissue diagnosis of extracardiac sarcoidosis, or the presence of septal scar.[14]

A minority of ARVD/C patients first present with symptoms of RV systolic heart failure. The differential diagnosis in such patients includes RV infarction or pulmonary hypertension. Dilated cardiomyopathy must be considered if there is evidence of biventricular failure. Patients with dilated cardiomyopathy who have early significant ventricular ectopy should be evaluated for possible biventricular arrhythmogenic cardiomyopathy.

ROLE OF EXERCISE

The observation that there are a disproportionate number of athletes among patients with ARVD/C led to the hypothesis that exercise is an environmental factor in the pathogenesis of this disease. It is believed that the increased cardiac output caused by exercise produces stretching of the RV wall which results in myocyte uncoupling. The resulting myocardial inflammation and cell death leads to fibrosis and adipose tissue deposition that in turn predisposes these patients to cardiac arrhythmias and increases the risk of sudden cardiac death.

One of the first studies to highlight the relationship between exercise and ARVD/C was done by Corrado et al.[15] in the region of Veneto, Italy. They found that young athletes had a five-fold risk of dying of ARVD/C compared to non-athletes. A subsequent study confirmed this finding when they found that implementing a preparticipation screening declined the incidence of sudden cardiovascular death in competitive athletes.[16]

Since then, many studies followed, and their aim has been to determine the role of exercise as a disease modifier in ARVD/C. La Gerche and colleagues[17] were one of the pioneer groups to observe that ARVD/C phenotype can be acquired through intense exercise. They studied 47 athletes with definite or probable ARVD/C. The majority (n = 41) practiced endurance sports (cyclists 72%, distance runners 6%, thriathletes 6%, and kayakers 2%). They identified desmosomal mutations in only 6 athletes and only 2 patients in the group had family history of ARVD/C. They found that the group that performed the most exercise had lower rates of desmosomal mutations, yet many of them met diagnostic criteria for definite or probable ARVD/C. Based on this results they concluded that high intensity endurance exercise may be sufficient to evoke an ARVD/C phenotype, even in mutation negative individuals.

Saverniak and colleagues[18] investigated the impact of exercise on myocardial function. The study included 110 patients, 65 of them with ARVD/C and 45 mutation positive family members. Exercise participation was measured by metabolic equivalent (MET)-minutes per week. Athletes were classified as those participating in vigorous (> = 6 METs) for > = 4 hours/week. The authors found that athletes were more likely to meet diagnostic criteria, they had a lower biventricular function and earlier onset of life threatening ventricular arrhythmias when compared with non-athletes.

Ruwald et al.[19] studied 108 probands that met Task force criteria for ARVD/C diagnosis, and assessed the effects of competitive and recreational sports on age at onset and risk of ventricular arrhythmias or death. Patients self-reported the age at which they initiated the sport and the commonly practiced sport via a questionnaire. They found that the patients engaged in competitive exercise had an earlier presentation of the disease. Moreover, they also had a two-fold increase in the risk of life-threatening arrhythmias and death when compared with inactive patients and those practicing recreational sports.

The Johns Hopkins ARVD/C Program has contributed three important manuscripts that have helped define the link between exercise in ARVD/C patients with and without mutations, as well as examining the important question of a safe exercise threshold.

James et al.[20] were the first to study the role of exercise in ARVD/C patients inheriting a pathogenic desmosomal mutation **(Figure 33.2)**. They evaluated 87 probands and family members from the Johns Hopkins ARVD/C Registry. All patients participated in an exercise interview detailing their exercise history for leisure/recreation, work, and transportation. Participants were classified as an endurance athlete if they performed 50 hours/year or more of vigorous intensity sports with a high dynamic demand as defined by the 36th Bethesda Conference Classification of Sports (Task Force 8).[21] The study had several key findings. First, ARVD/C patients who were endurance athletes became symptomatic at an earlier age. Furthermore, endurance exercise and higher duration of exercise participation were both associated with increasing likelihood of developing manifest ARVD/C. Endurance exercise was also associated with worse survival from a ventricular arrhythmia and heart failure. Lastly, those individuals who continued to participate in the top quartile for hours of annual exercise after presentation had worse survival from first ventricular arrhythmia compared to individuals who reduced their exercise after presentation.

The role of exercise in ARVD/C patients without mutations was subsequently studied by Sawant et al.[22] They assessed the role of duration and intensity of exercise participation among 43 probands without a desmosomal mutation and compared it to 39 probands with desmosomal mutations all of whom met the 2010 task force criteria (TFC). It was

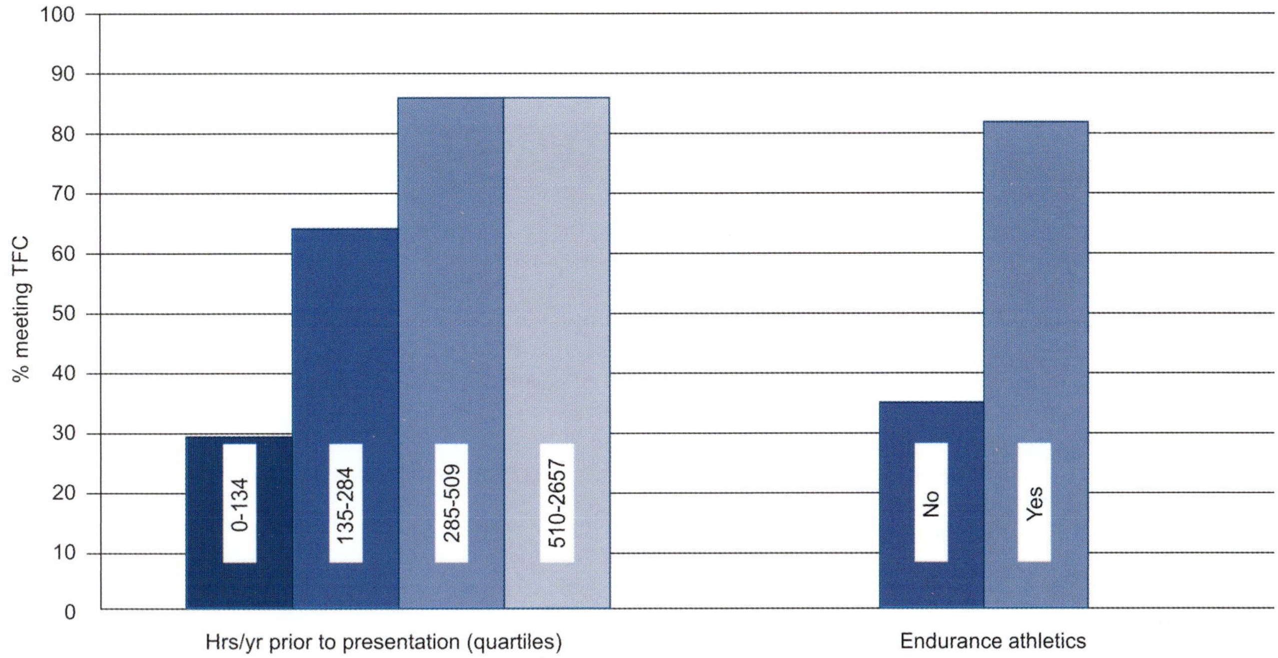

Figure 33.2: Association of exercise history with the likelihood of a diagnosis of arrhythmogenic right ventricular dysplasia/cardiomyopathy (ARVD/C). The likelihood of meeting the ARVD/C diagnostic criteria at last follow-up is associated with increasing hours per year of exercise ($P<0.001$) and participation in endurance athletics ($P<0.001$). Hrs/yr, hours per year; TFC, 2010 Task Force Diagnostic Criteria. Reproduced with Permission of James CA et al.[20]

found that among non-desmosomal mutation patients, those participating in the highest quartile of MET-Hrs/year exercise presented at a significantly earlier age, had worse structural abnormalities on cardiac MRI and significantly poorer survival from ventricular arrhythmia during follow up. Next, exercise participation stratified by mutation status and family history was compared and it was found that although, non-desmosomal ARVD/C patients had done a similar duration of annual exercise as desmosomal carriers; their exercise was significantly more intense, with significantly higher participation in endurance sports and expending greater MET-Hrs/year of exercise as compared to desmosomal patients. Lastly, ARVD/C non-desmosomal patients with no family history performed the highest MET-Hrs/year exercise compared to non-desmosomal patients with family history and desmosomal mutation carriers**.** Since the non-desmosomal patients without family history did the highest intensity exercise, they concluded that exercise may be the key environmental factor driving disease pathogenesis in that sub-group. Interestingly, when they compared annual pre-presentation MET-Hrs and endurance exercise participation during youth (age ≤ 25 years), it was found that higher intensity exercise during youth was associated with earlier age of presentation in both desmosomal and non-desmosomal ARVD/C patients.

Lastly, the Johns Hopkins group assessed the safety of the American Heart Association (AHA) minimum exercise recommendations for overall health (390 to 690 Met/Hr year), for healthy desmosomal mutation carriers.[23] To accomplish this they interviewed 28 family members of 10 probands with a *PKP2* mutation. They reported that probands had done more exercise than family members, and the family members that were athletic had worse outcomes. However, there were no life-threatening ventricular arrhythmias in the healthy carriers that restricted exercise at or below the upper level of the AHA minimum exercise recommendation. Furthermore, at the time of ARVD/C diagnosis and their first ventricular arrhythmia, patients had accumulated 2.8- fold and a 3.5-fold greater Met/Hr exercise than the AHA recommendations respectively. Their conclusion was that, while it is clear that unaffected *PKP2* mutation carriers should refrain from endurance and high intensity exercise, it might be potentially safe for them to practice the minimum exercise for healthy adults recommended by the AHA.

The link between exercise and ARVD has also been advanced through important research in animal models. The production of transgenic animals is a very important tool that has been used to understand ARVD/C. They have helped us not only to understand how desmosomal mutations produce the ARVD/C phenotype but to provide more evidence of the relationship between exercise and the disease.

In 2006, Kirchhof et al.[24] used heterozygous plakoglobin-deficient mice and their wild-type siblings to study whether plakoglobin and training have a functional role in the development of ARVD/C. Endurance training with 8 weeks of daily swimming was used to test the hypothesis. Using murine echocardiography, electrocardiogram, MRI and positron-emission tomography they measured cardiac dimensions and function as well as myocardial glucose uptake. They found that plakoglobin deletion is sufficient to produce an ARVD/C like phenotype. Furthermore, endurance training produced altered RV contractile and electrophysiological function in plakoglobin-deficient mice manifested by increased RV volume, reduced RV function, spontaneous ventricular arrhythmias and prolonged conduction times when compared to their wild-type counterparts.

Another group evaluated the impact of exercise on ARVD/C cardiac manifestations.[25] To accomplish this, they used an adeno-associated virus (AAV)-mediated *PKP2* mutant gene to produce an ARVD/C causing mutation in the cardiac tissue of wild-type mice. Subsequently the mice were divided in two groups, trained and sedentary, and they were euthanized to obtain heart sampling. Via cardiac MR, left and right end-diastolic volume, end-systolic volume, ejection fraction and wall motion abnormalities were assessed. They found that sedentary mice did not have any sign of RV dysfunction. On the contrary, endurance exercise training resulted in RV dysfunction that was similar to the ARVD/C phenotype.

Recently Chelko S et al.[26] looked at disease progression in a mouse model with ARVD/C. They compared desmoglein-2 homozygous, heterozygous and wild type mice by examining the effects that exercise had in the disease. This was done by making mice swim 90 minutes per day, 5 days per week. This resulted in 6/12 homozygous mutant mice surviving to 16 weeks of age, with 6 dying during exercise. With the help of echocardiography and electrocardiography they observed that, the homozygous mice had reduced ejection fraction, longer QRS duration and isovolumetric relaxation and an increased risk of dying from a cardiac arrhythmia when compared to the heterozygous and wild type mice.

In the most recent study using animal models, the investigators generated transgenic mice with overexpression of desmoplakin, wild type and mutant, and compared it to a non-transgenic model.[27] The mice were divided in two groups, sedentary or exposed to a 12 week running regimen. Their results showed that exercise accelerated the development of the disease, manifested by RV dilation and focal fat infiltration in the mutant mice when compared to the wild type and non-transgenic mice. The left ventricular function was not affected in either of the models.

The data raises a critical question of how much exercise can be considered safe in these patients. The answer is that more research is needed to evaluate what is the threshold needed to trigger the onset of ARVD/C. We also need to understand the interaction of genotype and exercise as well as other environmental factors with the potential of triggering the disease. Furthermore, the improved understanding of the molecular mechanisms through which exercise causes the pathological features of ARVD/C is key to improve patient care.

MANAGEMENT

Management of patients with ARVD/C has 4 components. The first is getting the diagnosis correct. The second component involves accurate risk stratification for sudden cardiac death and deciding whether to implant an ICD. The third component of management is minimizing ICD therapies. And the final component of management is preventing progression of the disease. Each of these will be examined in detail.

Establishing an Accurate Diagnosis

As noted above, the first step in management is making the diagnosis. Misdiagnosis of ARVD/C is common due to lack of awareness of the 2010 Task Force Criteria and misinterpretation of MR imaging.

Risk Stratification and Deciding When to Implant an Implantable Cardioverter Defibrillator

Prevention of sudden cardiac death is the primary goal of management. Several studies of ARVD/C patients who received an ICD have reported appropriate interventions during follow-up in more than 50% of patients.[28,29] Predictors of appropriate therapy included a prior sustained ventricular arrhythmia, syncope, and the extent of structural heart disease.

The incidence of appropriate ICD therapy among 84 patients who had an ICD implanted for primary prevention was recently reported.[28] Over a mean follow up of 4.7 ± 3.4 years, appropriate ICD therapy was experienced by 40 (48%) patients of which 16 (19%) received interventions for rapid VT/VF. Proband status, inducibility at electrophysiological study (EPS), presence of non-sustained VT (NSVT), and PVC count >1000/24hrs were identified as significant predictors of appropriate ICD therapy. The 5-year survival free from appropriate ICD therapy for patients with one, two, three and four risk factors was 100%, 83%, 21% and 15%, respectively. Inducibility at EPS and NSVT remained as significant predictors on multivariate analysis. These findings are important as they demonstrate that nearly half of the ARVD/C patients treated with an ICD for primary prevention experienced appropriate ICD interventions. Inducibility at EPS and NSVT are independent strong predictors of appropriate ICD therapy. More frequent ventricular ectopy is associated with progressively more common ICD therapy. Incremental risk of ventricular arrhythmias and ICD therapy was observed in the presence of multiple risk factors.

At present ICD implantation is recommended in all probands who meet Task Force criteria, especially if they have a history of sudden death, sustained VT, arrhythmogenic syncope, or have a high degree of ventricular ectopy and/or NSVT. Clinicians should be more circumspect about recommending implantation of an ICD in a family member who has been diagnosed with ARVD/C as a result of cascade screening. These individuals are being identified at a much earlier stage in their disease than was possible previously. With exercise restriction and the use of a beta blocker, their risk of sudden death appears to be reduced to a level below which placement of an ICD should be routinely advised. If a decision is made not to implant an ICD close monitoring and follow-up are emphasized.

Minimizing Symptoms and Prevent ICD Therapies

Pharmacologic Therapy

Pharmacologic therapy plays an important role in the management of patients with ARVD/C despite the fact that few studies have been done to define the safety and efficacy of pharmacologic therapy in this condition. Beta-blockers are recommended for almost all patients with ARVD/C, which reflects several lines of evidence. First, beta-blockers are the only pharmacologic therapy that has shown to reduce risk of SCD in populations of patients without ARVD/C. Second, the great majority of ventricular arrhythmias and sudden death episodes are triggered by exercise. And third, high dose isoproterenol results in the triggering of VT in patients with ARVD/C.[30,31] ACE inhibitors are also used in most patients with ARVD/C and especially those with evidence of significant disease. Though, there are no published trials in patients with ARVD/C, there is a wealth of data supporting the role of ACE inhibitors in a broader population of patients with cardiomyopathy. When it comes to membrane active antiarrhythmic agents, sotalol and amiodarone are commonly used. In rare cases, flecainide, propafenone, or dofetilide can also be used. For most patients with ARVD/C and symptomatic ventricular arrhythmias and/or ICD therapies we will attempt therapy with at least one antiarrhythmic medication before considering VT ablation.

Catheter Ablation

Catheter ablation is another important option for treatment of patients with ARVD/C who have recurrent VT. It is important to recognize that unlike idiopathic VT where catheter ablation is curative, the role of catheter ablation in patients with ARVD/C is to improve quality of life by decreasing the frequency of episodes of VT.

Three studies have evaluated the outcomes of catheter ablation of VT in patients with ARVD/C.[32-34] In the first study, 24 patients with ARVD/C underwent 48 VT ablation procedures at 29 different electrophysiology centers.[32] The cumulative VT free survival was 75% at 1.5 months, 50% at 5 months, and 25% at 14 months. The immediate success of the procedure had no bearing on recurrence; nor did the use of assisted mapping techniques, or repetition of the procedure.[32] The second study reported on an expanded series of 87 patients who underwent a total of 175 VT ablation procedures.[33] Over a follow-up of 88 + 66 months, the freedom of VT was 47%, 21%, and 15% at 1, 5, and 10 years respectively. The cumulative freedom from VT following epicardial VT ablation was 64% and 45% at 1 and 5 years. Importantly, the burden of VT decreased following ablation from a median of 0.16 VT episodes per month pre-ablation to 0.08 episodes per month post-ablation. Most recently a single center experience with epicardial VT ablation in patients with ARVD/C has been published.[34] It included 30 ARVD/C patients who underwent endo-/epicardial mapping and epicardial catheter ablation of VT. ICD interrogation data were evaluated for VT recurrence. Eight (27%) patients experienced VT recurrence after epicardial RFA and the VT free survival was 83%, 76%, and 70% at 6, 12 and 24 months respectively. A significant reduction of the VT burden was observed and no complications occurred during the procedure. The majority of VT recurrences occurred during the first year after RFA, during exercise, had fast cycle lengths, and required ICD shock for termination.

Exercise Restriction

An important recommendation for patients with ARVD/C is exercise restriction. The association of exercise stems from the observation that SCD in ARVD/C patients often occurred during exertion and that there are a large number of athletes among patients with ARVD/C. There is enough evidence that supports the hypothesis that repeated strenuous exercise, is an important factor that could increase the chance of development of ARVD/C, especially in patients with a mutation.

Recently, an update to the 36th Bethesda Conference Eligibility Recommendations for Competitive Athletes with Cardiovascular Abnormalities' has been published by the AHA and the American College of Cardiology.[35] The current recommendation is to avoid all competitive activities for patients with probable, borderline or definite diagnosis of ARVD/C except for class I-A sports with a low cardiovascular demand (Class III, Level of Evidence C).

A recently ARVD consensus, published by Corrado et al.,[36] concluded that healthy gene carriers should be restricted only from competitive sports (Class IIa).

Multiple studies show that patients with overt disease or at risk for development of ARVD/C, who participate in high intensity exercise can develop the disease earlier and have a more severe clinical course manifested by earlier onset arrhythmias, structural dysfunction, heart failure and need for transplant. Therefore, patients should refrain from practicing high intensity endurance exercise. More research is needed to establish recommendations for at-risk family members.

Prevent Progression

The final consideration in patients with ARVD/C is preventing disease progression.

It is important to note that no studies have examined the extent and rate of progression of ARVD/C. Exercise restriction is a very important tool in preventing disease progression. Evidence supporting this statement was provided in the "Exercise and ARVD/C" section of this chapter.

Cardiac Transplantation

It is rare for patients with ARVD to require cardiac transplantation. The details of 18 ARVD/C patients who underwent cardiac transplantation for ARVD/C has been recently reported.[37] The average age of first ARVD symptoms was 24 ± 13 years and the average age at cardiac transplant was 40 ± 14 years. These patients often had clinical onsets of the disease at a relatively young age. One year after transplantation, survival was 94% and 88% were alive at an average post-transplant follow-up of 6.2 ± 4.8 years.

CONCLUSION

Arrhythmogenic Right Ventricular Dysplasia/Cardiomyopathy (ARVD/C) is an inherited cardiomyopathy characterized clinically by ventricular arrhythmias, sudden death, and structural abnormalities of the right ventricle. Due to significantly variable penetrance and expressivity, the diagnosis of ARVD/C is challenging and requires a multifaceted approach to patient evaluation. Exercise has been widely described as an important environmental factor that contributes to the development of the disease. The observation that there is a disproportionate number of athletes with ARVD/C has led to extensive research in this area in animal models and humans. Multiple studies have shown that among patients with overt disease or at risk for development of ARVD/C, those that participate in high intensity exercise can develop the disease earlier and have a more severe clinical course manifested by earlier onset arrhythmias, structural dysfunction, heart failure and need for transplant.

The management of patients with ARVD/C is primarily aimed at reducing the burden of symptomatic arrhythmias and decreasing the incidence of sudden cardiac death. An important consideration in patients with ARVD/C is preventing disease progression, and this can be accomplished by exercise restriction. In conclusion, there is enough evidence to say that regardless of their genotype, patients with ARVD/C should be restricted from competitive, frequent, high-intensity exercise.

REFERENCES

1. Marcus FI, Fontaine GH, Guiraudon G, Frank R, Laurenceau JL, Malergue C, Grosgogeat Y. Right ventricular dysplasia: a report of 24 adult cases. Circulation. 1982;65:384-98.
2. den Haan AD, Tan BY, Zikusoka MN, Llado LI, Jain R, Daly A, Tichnell C, James C, Amat-Alarcon N, Abraham T, Russell SD, Bluemke DA, Calkins H, Dalal D, Judge DP. Comprehensive desmosome mutation analysis in north americans with arrhythmogenic right ventricular dysplasia/cardiomyopathy. Circ Cardiovasc Genet. 2009;2:428-35.
3. Groeneweg JA, Bhonsale A, James CA, te Riele AS, Dooijes D, Tichnell C, Murray B, Wiesfeld AC, Sawant AC, Kassamali B, Atsma DE, Volders PG, de Groot NM, de Boer K, Zimmerman SL, Kamel IR, van der Heijden JF, Russell SD, Jan Cramer M, Tedford RJ, Doevendans PA, van Veen TA, Tandri H, Wilde AA, Judge DP, van Tintelen JP, Hauer RN, Calkins H. Clinical Presentation, Long-Term Follow-Up, and Outcomes of 1001 Arrhythmogenic Right Ventricular Dysplasia/Cardiomyopathy Patients and Family Members. Circ Cardiovasc Genet. 2015;8:437-46.
4. Dalal D, Nasir K, Bomma C, Prakasa K, Tandri H, Piccini J, Roguin A, Tichnell C, James C, Russell SD, Judge DP, Abraham T, Spevak PJ, Bluemke DA, Calkins H. Arrhythmogenic right ventricular dysplasia: a United States experience. Circulation. 2005;112:3823-32.
5. Jain A, Tandri H, Calkins H, Bluemke DA. Role of cardiovascular magnetic resonance imaging in arrhythmogenic right ventricular dysplasia. J Cardiovasc Magn Reson. 2008;10:32.
6. Rastegar N, Burt JR, Corona-Villalobos CP, Te Riele AS, James CA, Murray B, Calkins H, Tandri H, Bluemke DA, Zimmerman SL, Kamel IR. Cardiac MR findings and potential diagnostic pitfalls in patients evaluated for arrhythmogenic right ventricular cardiomyopathy. Radiographics. 2014;34:1553-70.
7. Rastegar N, Zimmerman SL, Te Riele AS, James C, Burt JR, Bhonsale A, Murray B, Tichnell C, Judge D, Calkins H, Tandri H, Bluemke DA, Kamel IR. Spectrum of Biventricular Involvement on CMR Among Carriers of ARVD/C-Associated Mutations. JACC Cardiovasc Imaging. 2015;8:863-4.
8. Bhonsale A, Groeneweg JA, James CA, Dooijes D, Tichnell C, Jongbloed JD, Murray B, te Riele AS, van den Berg MP, Bikker H, Atsma DE, de Groot NM, Houweling AC, van der Heijden JF, Russell SD, Doevendans PA, van Veen TA, Tandri H, Wilde AA, Judge DP, van Tintelen JP, Calkins H, Hauer RN. Impact of genotype on clinical course in arrhythmogenic right ventricular dysplasia/cardiomyopathy-associated mutation carriers. Eur Heart J. 2015;36:847-55.
9. McKoy G, Protonotarios N, Crosby A, Tsatsopoulou A, Anastasakis A, Coonar A, Norman M, Baboonian C, Jeffery S, McKenna WJ. Identification of a deletion in plakoglobin in arrhythmogenic right ventricular cardiomyopathy with palmoplantar keratoderma and woolly hair (Naxos disease). Lancet. 2000;355:2119-24.
10. Norgett EE, Hatsell SJ, Carvajal-Huerta L, Cabezas JC, Common J, Purkis PE, Whittock N, Leigh IM, Stevens HP, Kelsell DP. Recessive mutation in desmoplakin disrupts desmoplakin-intermediate filament interactions and causes dilated cardiomyopathy, woolly hair and keratoderma. Hum Mol Genet. 2000;9:2761-6.
11. Marcus FI, McKenna WJ, Sherrill D, Basso C, Bauce B, Bluemke DA, Calkins H, Corrado D, Cox MG, Daubert JP, Fontaine G,

Gear K, Hauer R, Nava A, Picard MH, Protonotarios N, Saffitz JE, Sanborn DM, Steinberg JS, Tandri H, Thiene G, Towbin JA, Tsatsopoulou A, Wichter T, Zareba W. Diagnosis of arrhythmogenic right ventricular cardiomyopathy/dysplasia: proposed modification of the task force criteria. Circulation. 2010;121:1533-41.
12. Bomma C, Rutberg J, Tandri H, Nasir K, Roguin A, Tichnell C, Rodriguez R, James C, Kasper E, Spevak P, Bluemke DA, Calkins H. Misdiagnosis of arrhythmogenic right ventricular dysplasia/cardiomyopathy. J Cardiovasc Electrophysiol. 2004;15:300-6.
13. Hoffmayer KS, Bhave PD, Marcus GM, James CA, Tichnell C, Chopra N, Moxey L, Krahn AD, Dixit S, Stevenson W, Calkins H, Badhwar N, Gerstenfeld EP, Scheinman MM. An electrocardiographic scoring system for distinguishing right ventricular outflow tract arrhythmias in patients with arrhythmogenic right ventricular cardiomyopathy from idiopathic ventricular tachycardia. Heart Rhythm. 2013;10:477-82.
14. Philips B, Madhavan S, James CA, te Riele AS, Murray B, Tichnell C, Bhonsale A, Nazarian S, Judge DP, Calkins H, Tandri H, Cheng A. Arrhythmogenic right ventricular dysplasia/cardiomyopathy and cardiac sarcoidosis: distinguishing features when the diagnosis is unclear. Circ Arrhythm Electrophysiol. 2014;7:230-6.
15. Corrado D, Basso C, Rizzoli G, Schiavon M, Thiene G. Does sports activity enhance the risk of sudden death in adolescents and young adults? J Am Coll Cardiol. 2003;42:1959-63.
16. Corrado D, Basso C, Pavei A, Michieli P, Schiavon M, Thiene G. Trends in sudden cardiovascular death in young competitive athletes after implementation of a preparticipation screening program. JAMA. 2006;296:1593-601.
17. La Gerche A, Burns AT, Mooney DJ, Inder WJ, Taylor AJ, Bogaert J, Macisaac AI, Heidbuchel H, Prior DL. Exercise-induced right ventricular dysfunction and structural remodelling in endurance athletes. Eur Heart J. 2012;33:998-1006.
18. Saberniak J, Hasselberg NE, Borgquist R, Platonov PG, Sarvari SI, Smith HJ, Ribe M, Holst AG, Edvardsen T, Haugaa KH. Vigorous physical activity impairs myocardial function in patients with arrhythmogenic right ventricular cardiomyopathy and in mutation positive family members. Eur J Heart Fail. 2014;16:1337-44.
19. Ruwald AC, Marcus F, Estes NA, 3rd, Link M, McNitt S, Polonsky B, Calkins H, Towbin JA, Moss AJ, Zareba W. Association of competitive and recreational sport participation with cardiac events in patients with arrhythmogenic right ventricular cardiomyopathy: results from the North American multidisciplinary study of arrhythmogenic right ventricular cardiomyopathy. Eur Heart J. 2015;36:1735-43.
20. James CA, Bhonsale A, Tichnell C, Murray B, Russell SD, Tandri H, Tedford RJ, Judge DP, Calkins H. Exercise increases age-related penetrance and arrhythmic risk in arrhythmogenic right ventricular dysplasia/cardiomyopathy-associated desmosomal mutation carriers. J Am Coll Cardiol. 2013;62:1290-7.
21. Maron BJ, Zipes DP. Introduction: eligibility recommendations for competitive athletes with cardiovascular abnormalities-general considerations. J Am Coll Cardiol. 2005;45:1318-21.
22. Sawant AC, Bhonsale A, te Riele AS, Tichnell C, Murray B, Russell SD, Tandri H, Tedford RJ, Judge DP, Calkins H, James CA. Exercise has a disproportionate role in the pathogenesis of arrhythmogenic right ventricular dysplasia/cardiomyopathy in patients without desmosomal mutations. J Am Heart Assoc. 2014;3:e001471.
23. Sawant AC, Te Riele AS, Tichnell C, Murray B, Bhonsale A, Tandri H, Judge DP, Calkins H, James CA. Safety of American Heart Association-recommended minimum exercise for desmosomal mutation carriers. Heart Rhythm. 2016;13:199-207.
24. Kirchhof P, Fabritz L, Zwiener M, Witt H, Schafers M, Zellerhoff S, Paul M, Athai T, Hiller KH, Baba HA, Breithardt G, Ruiz P, Wichter T, Levkau B. Age- and training-dependent development of arrhythmogenic right ventricular cardiomyopathy in heterozygous plakoglobin-deficient mice. Circulation. 2006;114:1799-806.
25. Cruz FM, Sanz-Rosa D, Roche-Molina M, Garcia-Prieto J, Garcia-Ruiz JM, Pizarro G, Jimenez-Borreguero LJ, Torres M, Bernad A, Ruiz-Cabello J, Fuster V, Ibanez B, Bernal JA. Exercise triggers ARVC phenotype in mice expressing a disease-causing mutated version of human plakophilin-2. J Am Coll Cardiol. 2015;65:1438-50.
26. Chelko S, Asimaki A, Wei A, DeMazumde D, Bedj D, Wagle R, Amat N, O'Rourke B, Saffitz J, Judje DP. Exercise and mitochondrial respiration in mice with arrhythmogenic cardiomyopathy (abstract). Circulation. 2014;130:A20589.
27. Martherus R, Jain R, Takagi K, Mendsaikhan U, Turdi S, Osinska H, James JF, Kramer K, Purevjav E, Towbin JA. Accelerated cardiac remodeling in desmoplakin transgenic mice in response to endurance exercise is associated with perturbed Wnt/beta-catenin signaling. Am J Physiol Heart Circ Physiol. 2016;310:H174-87.
28. Bhonsale A, James CA, Tichnell C, Murray B, Gagarin D, Philips B, Dalal D, Tedford R, Russell SD, Abraham T, Tandri H, Judge DP, Calkins H. Incidence and predictors of implantable cardioverter-defibrillator therapy in patients with arrhythmogenic right ventricular dysplasia/cardiomyopathy undergoing implantable cardioverter-defibrillator implantation for primary prevention. J Am Coll Cardiol. 2011;58:1485-96.
29. Piccini JP, Dalal D, Roguin A, Bomma C, Cheng A, Prakasa K, Dong J, Tichnell C, James C, Russell S, Crosson J, Berger RD, Marine JE, Tomaselli G, Calkins H. Predictors of appropriate implantable defibrillator therapies in patients with arrhythmogenic right ventricular dysplasia. Heart Rhythm. 2005;2:1188-94.
30. Philips B, Madhavan S, James C, Tichnell C, Murray B, Needleman M, Bhonsale A, Nazarian S, Laurita KR, Calkins H, Tandri H. High prevalence of catecholamine-facilitated focal ventricular tachycardia in patients with arrhythmogenic right ventricular dysplasia/cardiomyopathy. Circ Arrhythm Electrophysiol. 2013;6:160-6.
31. Denis A, Sacher F, Derval N, Lim HS, Cochet H, Shah AJ, Daly M, Pillois X, Ramoul K, Komatsu Y, Zemmoura A, Amraoui S, Ritter P, Ploux S, Bordachar P, Hocini M, Jais P, Haissaguerre M. Diagnostic value of isoproterenol testing in arrhythmogenic right ventricular cardiomyopathy. Circ Arrhythm Electrophysiol. 2014;7:590-7.
32. Dalal D, Jain R, Tandri H, Dong J, Eid SM, Prakasa K, Tichnell C, James C, Abraham T, Russell SD, Sinha S, Judge DP, Bluemke DA, Marine JE, Calkins H. Long-term efficacy of catheter ablation of ventricular tachycardia in patients with arrhythmogenic right ventricular dysplasia/cardiomyopathy. J Am Coll Cardiol. 2007;50:432-40.

33. Philips B, Madhavan S, James C, Tichnell C, Murray B, Dalal D, Bhonsale A, Nazarian S, Judge DP, Russell SD, Abraham T, Calkins H, Tandri H. Outcomes of catheter ablation of ventricular tachycardia in arrhythmogenic right ventricular dysplasia/cardiomyopathy. Circ Arrhythm Electrophysiol. 2012;5:499-505.
34. Philips B, te Riele AS, Sawant A, Kareddy V, James CA, Murray B, Tichnell C, Kassamali B, Nazarian S, Judge DP, Calkins H, Tandri H. Outcomes and ventricular tachycardia recurrence characteristics after epicardial ablation of ventricular tachycardia in arrhythmogenic right ventricular dysplasia/cardiomyopathy. Heart Rhythm. 2015;12:716-25.
35. Maron BJ, Udelson JE, Bonow RO, Nishimura RA, Ackerman MJ, Estes NA, 3rd, Cooper LT, Jr., Link MS, Maron MS. Eligibility and Disqualification Recommendations for Competitive Athletes With Cardiovascular Abnormalities: Task Force 3: Hypertrophic Cardiomyopathy, Arrhythmogenic Right Ventricular Cardiomyopathy and Other Cardiomyopathies, and Myocarditis: A Scientific Statement From the American Heart Association and American College of Cardiology. Circulation. 2015;132:e273-80.
36. Corrado D, Wichter T, Link MS, Hauer RN, Marchlinski FE, Anastasakis A, Bauce B, Basso C, Brunckhorst C, Tsatsopoulou A, Tandri H, Paul M, Schmied C, Pelliccia A, Duru F, Protonotarios N, Estes NM, 3rd, McKenna WJ, Thiene G, Marcus FI, Calkins H. Treatment of Arrhythmogenic Right Ventricular Cardiomyopathy/Dysplasia: An International Task Force Consensus Statement. Circulation. 2015;132: 441-53.
37. Tedford RJ, James C, Judge DP, Tichnell C, Murray B, Bhonsale A, Philips B, Abraham T, Dalal D, Halushka MK, Tandri H, Calkins H, Russell SD. Cardiac transplantation in arrhythmogenic right ventricular dysplasia/cardiomyopathy. J Am Coll Cardiol. 2012;59:289-90.

EDITORS' SUMMARY

One of the world's leading experts in the investigation and treatment of patients with right ventricular cardiomyopathy, Professor Hugh Calkins, has written a marvelously succinct yet detailed approach to the patient being suspected of having ARVC. The clinical presentation and the genetic basis are first described and referenced for those who wish for a more detailed study. Then, the difficult area of diagnosis and applying the published diagnostic criteria is simplified with insights that can only come from the type of vast experience such as the author has. More recent advances including ablation approaches, the role for biopsy, and a look to the future is also described. The section and paragraphs on the interaction of exercise and the course of ARVC by itself would be highly valuable reading to provide a meaningful basis for when we have to counsel patients in this vexing issue.

CHAPTER 34

Daljeet Kaur Saggu, Calambur Narasimhan

Ventricular Tachycardia in Specific Cardiomyopathies: Sarcoidosis and Tuberculosis

LIST OF ABBREVIATIONS

AAD	Antiarrhythmic Drug	LN	Lymph Node
ARVC	Arrhythmogenic Right Ventricular Cardiomyopathy	*MTb*	*Mycobacterium tuberculosis*
ATT	Antitubercular Treatment	NSVT	Nonsustained Ventricular Tachycardia
CHF	Congestive Heart Failure	PCR	Polymerase Chain Reaction
CMP	Cardiomyopathy	PET-CT	Positron Emission Tomography-Computed Tomography
CMR	Cardiac Magnetic Resonance Imaging	PLVT	Pleomorphic Ventricular Tachycardia
CTB	Cardiac Tuberculosis	PMVT	Polymorphic Ventricular Tachycardia
EAM	Electroanatomical Map	PVC	Premature Ventricular Contraction
EMB	Endomyocardial Biopsy	SMVT	Sustained Monomorphic Ventricular Tachycardia
FDG	Fluorodeoxyglucose	TB	Tuberculosis
fQRS	Fragmented QRS	VF	Ventricular Fibrillation
GM	Granulomatous Myocarditis	VT	Ventricular Tachycardia
HPE	Histopathological Examination		
ICD	Implantable Cardioverter-defibrillator		

INTRODUCTION

Cardiomyopathy due to granulomatous myocarditis (GM) as a result of sarcoidosis or tuberculosis is an under-recognized entity. Ventricular tachycardia (VT) with or without ventricular systolic dysfunction may be the presenting feature of GM. These patients generally present without any constitutional symptoms like fever, weight loss and without involvement of other organs, contributing to the delay in diagnosis. Managing VT is challenging in both of these types of GM. Early accurate diagnosis and treatment with disease-specific drugs along with antiarrhythmic drugs is necessary to reduce the morbidity and mortality of this disease. Since the VTs in this entity are treatable, if the diagnosis is made early, GM should be an important diagnostic consideration in patients with VT of unknown origin.

CARDIAC SARCOIDOSIS

Sarcoidosis is a multisystem disease of unknown etiology characterized by histopathological finding of noncaseating granulomas and subsequent scarring.[1,2] In patients with cardiac involvement, the diagnosis of sarcoidosis prior to death is low (26.7%) compared with sarcoid patients with neurological (50%) and pulmonary involvement (59.4%).[3] Cardiac manifestations such as conduction abnormalities, congestive heart failure (CHF), and ventricular arrhythmias are rare, but potentially fatal. Cardiac sarcoidosis is associated with a mortality rate exceeding 40% at 5 years.[4-6] Important causes of death include ventricular arrhythmias and CHF caused by infiltration of the myocardium by granulomas and fibrosis of the heart.[6-10]

CARDIAC TUBERCULOSIS

Cardiac tuberculosis (CTB) is another important cause of GM and is considered to be rare.[11] We believe that CTB is highly under-recognized, especially in countries where tuberculosis (TB) is highly prevalent. There are isolated case reports[12-23] and few case series of cardiac TB.[24-26] Clinical presentation of CTB mimics that of cardiac sarcoidosis and has a poor prognosis if not diagnosed and treated promptly.[14-16,27] Another condition referred to as tuberculous-sarcoidosis[28] has a similar clinical presentation. In this entity, there is evidence of TB like positive tuberculin skin test and positive tubercular polymerase chain reaction (PCR) from the lymph node (LN). However, it is probably a paucibacillary condition and the immunological manifestations overshadow the clinical picture. Clinical response is seen only when steroids are added to the antitubercular treatment (ATT).

The granulomas in these diseases result in myocardial scarring that not only causes abnormalities in the systolic and diastolic function, but also leads to formation of an anatomical substrate for reentrant VT by creating a slow conduction zone in the scarred areas.[6,10,29] Early initiation of disease-specific agents limits the granulomatous inflammation and scarring. This helps to preserve cardiac function and improves clinical outcome.[13,24,30-33]

This chapter discusses the clinical manifestations, management and outcome of patients with cardiac sarcoidosis and CTB presenting with ventricular arrhythmias.

CLINICAL PRESENTATION

Patients present with varying symptoms that may include palpitations, presyncope, syncope, breathlessness, and symptoms of heart failure. Cardiac arrest due to ventricular arrhythmias may be the presenting feature in a few patients. The tachyarrhythmias may vary from frequent premature ventricular contractions (PVCs), nonsustained VT (NSVT), sustained monomorphic VT (SMVT) and incessant VT to polymorphic VT (PMVT) and ventricular fibrillation (VF).[4,6,9,10,34-38] Mohan et al.[24] reported a series of 13 patients with isolated CTB; of which, 11(84%) presented with sustained VT. None of these patients had clinical features or constitutional symptoms suggestive of TB. Thachil et al.[7] reported a series of 14 patients with GM. These patients were relatively young (mean age: 44 ± 11 years) and were referred for evaluation with a diagnosis of VT of unknown origin.

While most patients present with SMVT, Panda et al.[39] reported pleomorphic VT (PLVT) in patients with cardiac sarcoidosis. They observed that pleomorphism in VT can be used as a distinguishing feature between cardiac sarcoidosis and VTs of idiopathic origin. PLVT is defined as VT with more than one morphologically distinct QRS complex occurring during the same episode of VT, but the QRS configuration not changing continuously **(Figures 34.1A to C)**. This is different from PMVT wherein the QRS configuration changes continuously from beat to beat. A patient can have recurrent VT episodes with QRS morphologies that differ from that in the index VT indicating ongoing inflammation in the myocardium at different sites. Shenthar[40] reported bidirectional VT in a patient with cardiac sarcoidosis who presented as incessant VT.

Fragmented QRS (fQRS) **(Figure 34.2)** during sinus rhythm has been shown to be associated with myocardial scar in coronary artery disease, nonischemic cardiomyopathy (CMP), arrhythmogenic right ventricular cardiomyopathy (ARVC) and cardiac sarcoidosis.[41-44] Roukoz et al.[45] reported that in patients with VT and structurally normal heart, the presence of fQRS on baseline ECG is strongly associated with GM and warrants further evaluation. Hence, the presence of pleomorphism or cycle length variability during VT and/or fQRS during sinus rhythm in patients with unexplained VT should raise the suspicion of underlying GM. However, there is currently no data on the sensitivity and specificity of these ECG features in patients with GM.

DIAGNOSIS

The diagnosis of GM can be challenging and may involve various investigations involving imaging, histopathology, microbiology and immunology. The **Flow chart 34.1** outlines our management protocol in patients suspected with GM.

Tuberculin Skin Test

Tuberculin skin test for *Mycobacterium tuberculosis* (MTB) is performed with 5 tuberculin-units of purified protein derivative. A horizontal induration of ≥10 mm at 48 hours at the site of injection is considered a positive result.

Cardiac Imaging

Echocardiography for evaluation of cardiac function should be performed in all cases. A peculiar feature of GM is involvement of basal septum with or without cardiac dysfunction **(Figure 34.3)**. Positron emission tomography-computed tomography with 18-fluorodeoxyglucose (^{18}FDG-PET-CT) and cardiac MRI (CMR) complement each other in the diagnostic work-up of cardiac sarcoidosis and TB. An high uptake of FDG is interpreted as inflammation; whereas matched perfusion and metabolism defect is interpreted

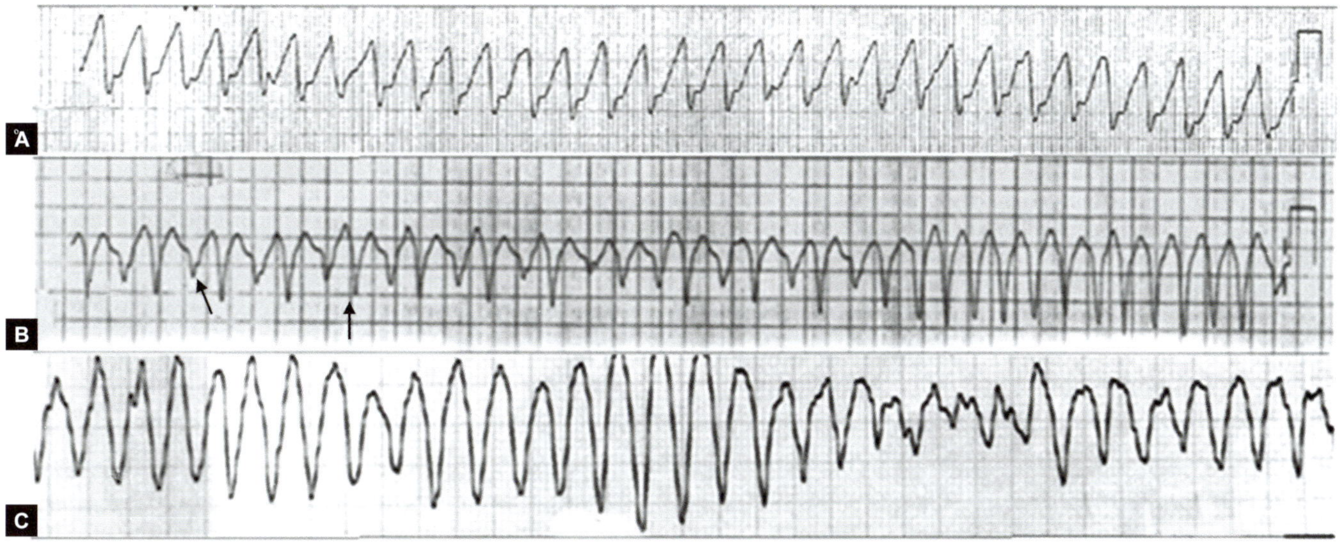

Figures 34.1A to C: (A) Monomorphic tachycardia; (B) Pleomorphic tachycardia (note QRS complexes of different morphologies indicated by the arrow); (C) Polymorphic ventricular tachycardia. See text for details

Adapted from: Daljeet K, Narasimhan C. Cardiac Sarcoidosis/Tuberculosis: Not so uncommon cause of VT/Cardiomyopathy in our country. Medicine Update 2016-1 (Progress in Medicine): Publisher: Jaypee Brothers; Volume 262016: Chapter-283. With permission

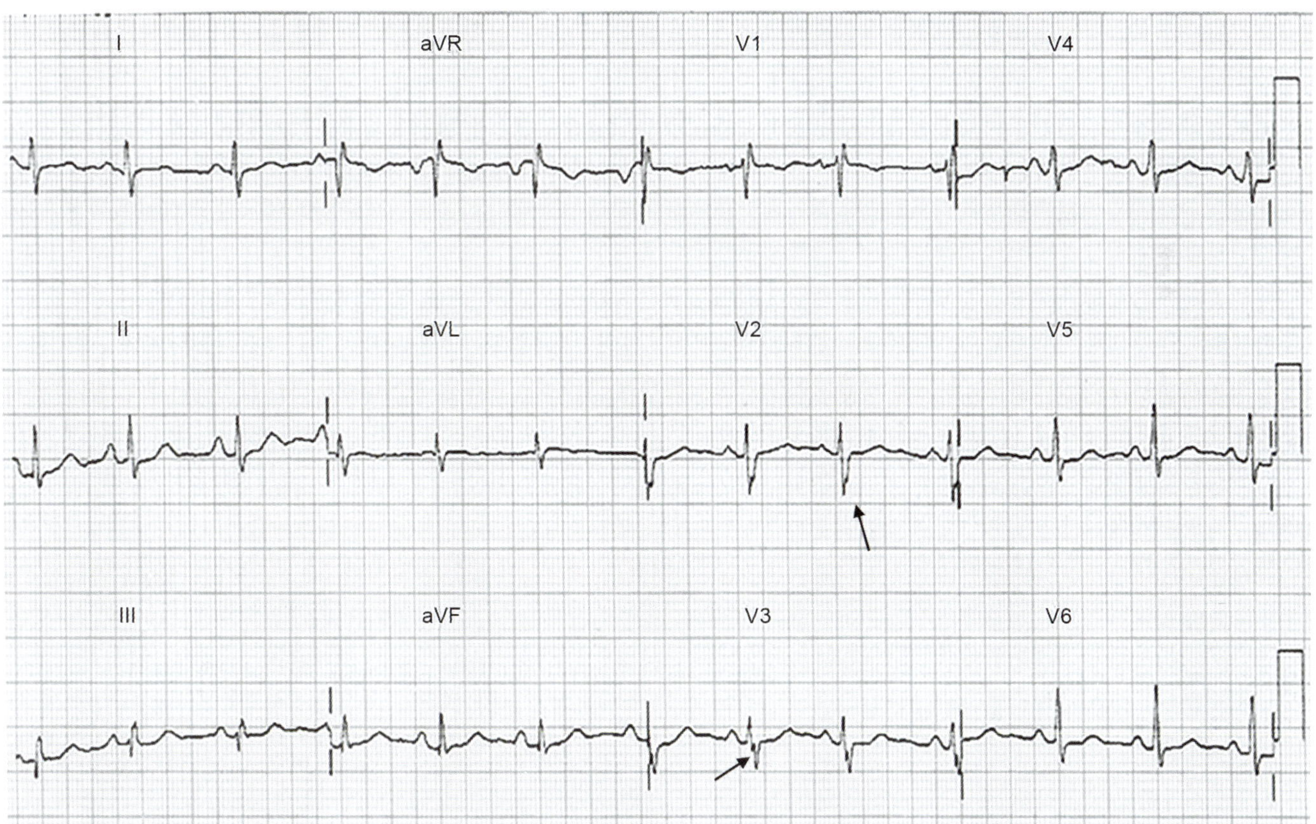

Figure 34.2: Fragmented QRS during sinus rhythm in a patient with cardiac sarcoidosis. The arrows indicate fractionation of QRS complexes

Adapted from: Daljeet K, Narasimhan C. Cardiac Sarcoidosis/Tuberculosis: Not so uncommon cause of VT/Cardiomyopathy in our country. Medicine Update 2016-1 (Progress in Medicine): Publisher: Jaypee Brothers; Volume 262016: Chapter-283. With permission

Flow chart 34.1: Diagnostic and treatment protocol in patients suspected of granulomatous myocarditis

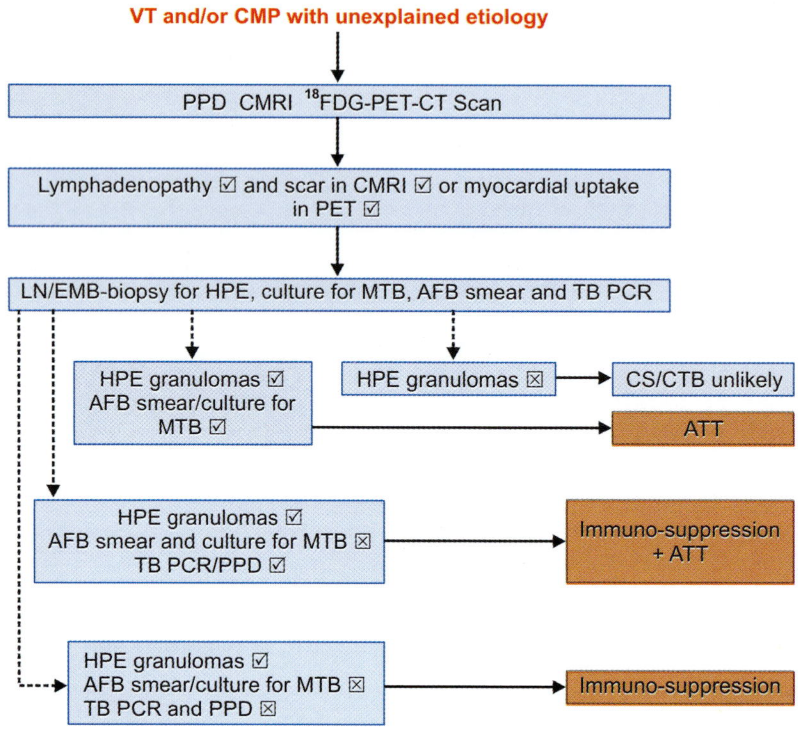

Abbreviations: 18-FDG PET CT scan, 18 fluorodeoxyglucose positron emission tomography in conjunction with computed tomography scan; AFB, acid fast bacilli; ATT, antitubercular therapy; CMP, cardiomyopathy; CMRI, cardiac magnetic resonance imaging; CS, cardiac sarcoidosis; CTB, cardiac tuberculosis; EMB, endomyocardial biopsy; HPE, histopathological examination; LN, lymph node; MTB, *Mycobacterium tuberculosis*; PPD, purified protein derivative; TB PCR, tuberculous polymerase chain reaction; VT, ventricular tachycardia; ☑, denotes present or positive; ☒, denotes absent or negative

Adapted from: Daljeet K, Narasimhan C. Cardiac Sarcoidosis/Tuberculosis: Not so uncommon cause of VT/ Cardiomyopathy in our country. Medicine Update 2016-1 (Progress in Medicine): Publisher: Jaypee Brothers; Volume 262016: Chapter-283. With permission

as scar. ^{18}FDG-PET-CT also helps to identify mediastinal/peripheral LNs if they are affected **(Figure 34.4)** by the disease process. The most involved and amenable LN is chosen for biopsy sampling. Apart from aiding in the diagnosis of the inflammatory phase of cardiac sarcoidosis/TB, ^{18}FDG-PET-CT also helps in the follow-up and surveillance. CMR can demonstrate both scar and myocardial edema; myocardial inflammation presents as increased signal intensity on the T2-weighted images. Patchy mid-myocardial scar not corresponding to a vascular distribution is a hallmark pattern of infiltration of cardiac sarcoidosis and tuberculosis. Myocardial inflammation and scar, both may be present in the same patient; the presence or absence of which guides the treatment regimen **(Flow chart 34.1)**. Therefore, both CMR and PET-CT should be done whenever possible.

Tissue Biopsy

The biopsy of the FDG-avid LNs is more contributory compared to endomyocardial biopsy (EMB). The yield of biopsy using conventional EMB is low in cardiac sarcoidosis/CTB[46] as the involvement in these disease states is patchy and often midmyocardial or/and epicardial preventing sampling of involved sites. Enlarged lymph nodes with FDG uptake documented on ^{18}FDG-PET scan offer an easier site for biopsy enabling histopathological examination (HPE) and further analysis.

Histopathological Diagnosis

All tissue samples should be subjected to HPE, Gram's and acid fast bacilli staining and culture for MTB and fungi. A definitive diagnosis of GM is made by the presence of granuloma in the HPE section of the sampled tissue. A deoxyribonucleic acid PCR detecting the IS6110 sequence of MTB should be performed on all samples. A patient is diagnosed as cardiac sarcoidosis if PCR and culture for MTB are negative and there is no other known cause for a granuloma.

TREATMENT MODALITIES

The optimal management of cardiac sarcoidosis and CTB presenting with ventricular arrhythmias and/or heart failure

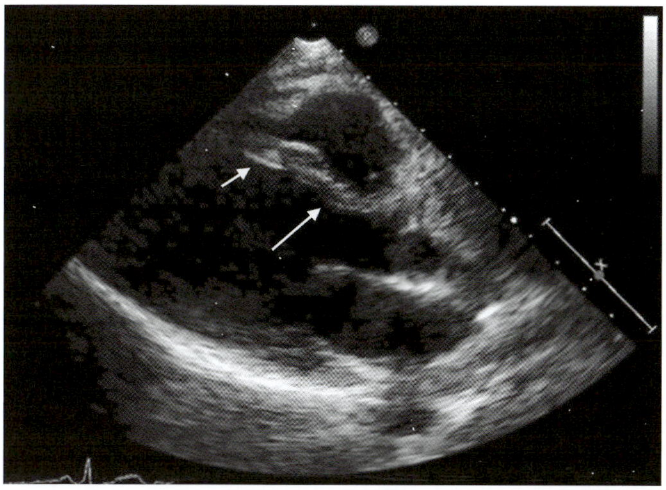

Figure 34.3: Two dimensional echocardiographic parasternal long axis (PLAX) view showing basal septal thinning in a patient with cardiac sarcoidosis; Large arrow showing the basal thin interventricular septum (IVS); small arrow is the normal septum
Adapted from: Daljeet K, Narasimhan C. Cardiac Sarcoidosis/ Tuberculosis: Not so uncommon cause of VT/Cardiomyopathy in our country. Medicine Update 2016-1 (Progress in Medicine): Publisher: Jaypee Brothers; Volume 262016: Chapter-283. With permission

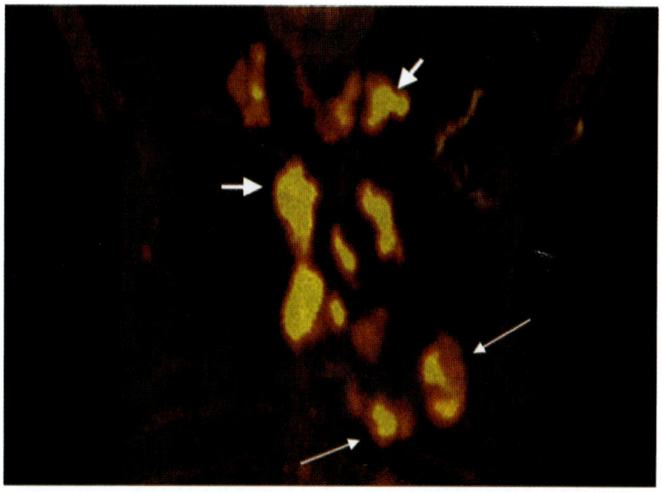

Figure 34.4: Cardiac ^{18}FDG-PET-CT scan showing inflammatory foci in the left ventricular myocardium in the apex, inferior, and anterolateral segments (thin white arrows) and in the mediastinal and cervical lymph nodes (thick white arrows). ^{18}FDG-PET-CT—^{18}fluorodeoxyglucose positron emission tomography and computed tomography
Adapted from: Daljeet K, Narasimhan C. Cardiac Sarcoidosis/ Tuberculosis: Not so uncommon cause of VT/ Cardiomyopathy in our country. Medicine Update 2016-1 (Progress in Medicine): Publisher: Jaypee Brothers; Volume 262016: Chapter-283. With permission

is not well defined. Treatment must be focused both on arrhythmias/heart failure and the underlying disease.

Disease-Specific and Antiarrhythmic Drug Therapy

Corticosteroids are the mainstay of therapy in sarcoidosis and antitubercular agents plus corticosteroids in TB. The therapy with disease-specific agents reduces the disease burden and along with antiarrhythmic drugs (AADs), prevents recurrence of ventricular arrhythmias in more than 50% of patients,[4,30,33,38,47] in the active phase of the disease.

A combined approach to arrhythmia management using disease-specific agents, AADs and catheter ablation may be necessary. All patients presenting with VT should receive implantable cardioverter defibrillator (ICD) device as prophylaxis against sudden death.[38]

Catheter Ablation in Cardiac Sarcoidosis and Tuberculosis

There are few case series describing the electrophysiological characteristics of ventricular arrhythmias associated with cardiac sarcoidosis and isolated case reports describing the same in CTB.[35] Active inflammation and fibrosis both participate in arrhythmogenesis hence, ventricular arrhythmias may be seen in both early inflammatory phase and late scar phase of the disease in GM.[6,7,33] Triggered activity and abnormal automaticity, observed in both cardiac sarcoidosis and CTB is attributed to inflammation. As granulomas might serve as a foci for abnormal automaticity, decrease in arrhythmia burden has been demonstrated after initiating disease specific agents.[13,30,33,34,38,48,49] Induction of reentrant VTs has also been shown during the active phase of disease,[10] which may be due to dispersion of both ventricular activation and recovery processes.

It has been suggested that the mechanism of VT in patients with cardiac sarcoidosis is reentry occurring through surviving myocyte bundles in and around the scar.[10,29] Both these diseases are characterized by myocardial inflammation and interstitial fibrosis which can lead to conduction slowing and macro-reentrant arrhythmias.[29,36,37,50-54] Inducibility of VT with programmed extrastimulation also supports reentrant nature of these ventricular arrhythmias.[37,55] Thus, reentrant substrate is present in both the active and inactive phase. In fact, in contrast to occurrence of atrioventricular block, inducibility of VT may not be associated with disease activity in cardiac sarcoidosis.[33,55-57] Patchy scarring demonstrated by CMR and three-dimensional electroanatomic mapping (EAM) systems is capable of sustaining a large number of reentrant VT circuits. Multiple low voltage areas are identified by EAM that may represent fibrosis or granulomatous inflammation, and VTs have been demonstrated to originate from these abnormal areas.[29,33]

The inducible VT in both cardiac sarcoidosis and tuberculosis can be monomorphic with right or left bundle branch block pattern or may be PLVT **(Figure 34.5)**;

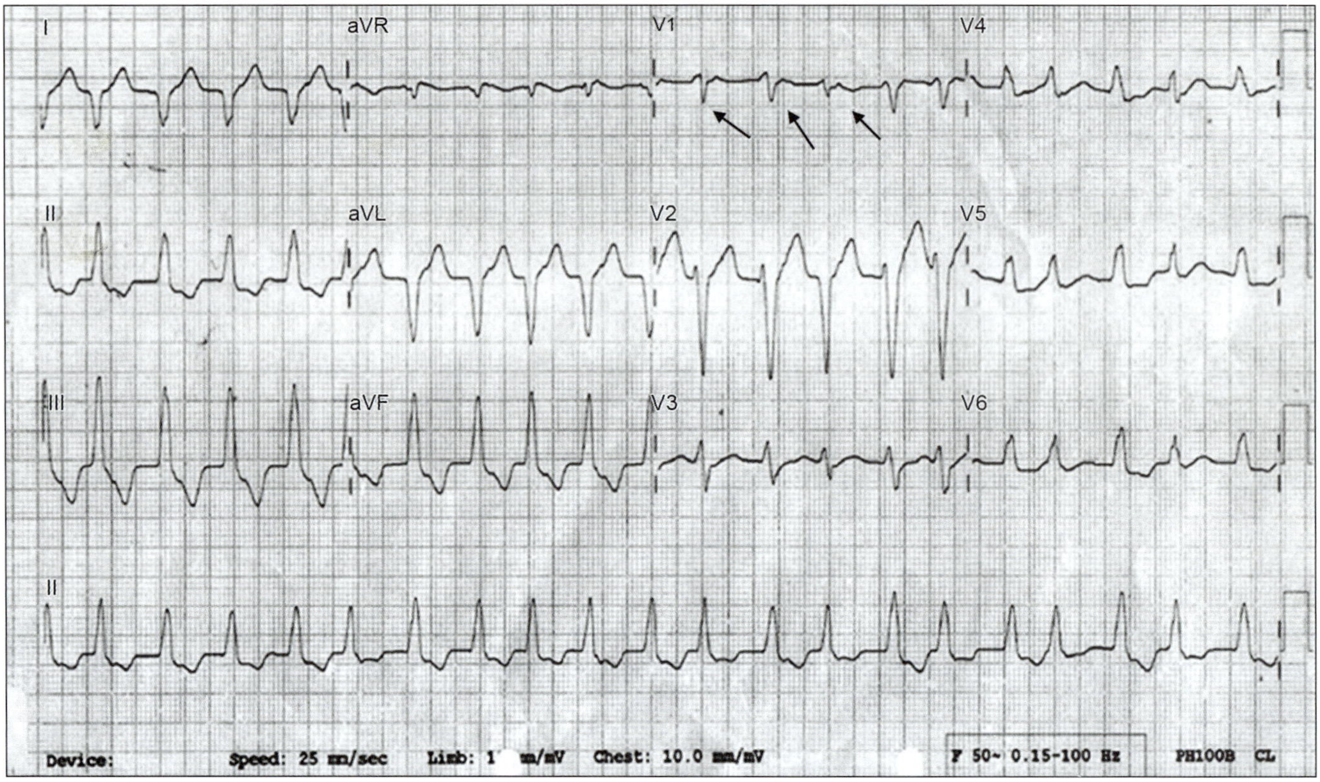

Figure 34.5: Surface ECG of a patient with cardiac sarcoidosis showing pleomorphic ventricular tachycardia. Note the variability in cycle length and changing morphology of QRS complex (black arrows)

even PMVT and VF may also occur.[6,7,10,29,33-39] Naruse et al. demonstrated induction of Purkinje related VTs along with scar related reentry VT in their cohort of patients with sarcoidosis.[38] All patients with Purkinje related VT had some or other form of conduction disease also. Relatively narrow QRS with duration of <170 ms can be used as a marker of Purkinje related VT. Noda et al. demonstrated a critical isthmus between two scar-like areas with a figure of eight pattern macroreentrant VT in a patient with cardiac sarcoidosis.[53] Induction of non-clinical VTs in the electrophysiology laboratory is not uncommon. Multiple morphologies of SMVTs are commonly induced in each patient[6,7,29,34,37,55] that is attributable to diffuse and heterogeneous involvement of the myocardium. More the number of VTs induced, more are the chances of future recurrence.[38]

EAM has demonstrated extensive scarring in both the ventricles and epicardial regions in these disease states.[29,34,37] Abnormal signals in the form of late potentials and fragmented signals in the low voltage areas (< 1.5V) are seen during EAM at sites of both inflammation and fibrosis.[29,33] Epicardial scars overlay and exceed the region of corresponding endocardial scar. Sometimes, epicardial scar may not correspond to the region of endocardial scar **(Figures 34.6A and B)**.[37]

Different authors have reported predominance of different areas of VT origin in cardiac sarcoidosis.[37,51,58] Intramural substrates for VT in the septum or free wall are not uncommon in these patients.[35,37,38] These can be sought by assessing unipolar voltage maps with electrogram amplitude <5.5 mV for the RV free wall[59] and <8.3 mV in the left ventricle or the interventricular septum identifying potential intramural scar.[29] The ablation of these intramural sites is difficult and newer techniques like chemical ablation, needle ablation or bipolar ablation may be needed to eliminate all VT circuits.

It is not uncommon for patients with cardiac sarcoidosis to undergo more than one ablation procedure because of recurrences and induction of multiple morphology VTs. Saurabh et al.[37] performed ablation in 21 patients with cardiac sarcoidosis presenting with VT, and demonstrated that catheter ablation abolished at least one inducible VT in 90% and eliminated VT storm in 78% of patients. Although multiple procedure VT free survival at one year was only 37%, VT control was achievable in majority of patients with fewer AADs compared with preablation. Peri- and postprocedural circulatory support should be strongly considered in these patients because of tendency for advanced heart failure, induction of multiple hemodynamically unstable VTs during the study and need for extensive mapping during the procedure.

Outcome of catheter ablation is also dependent upon stage of disease. Outcome may be better with more localized

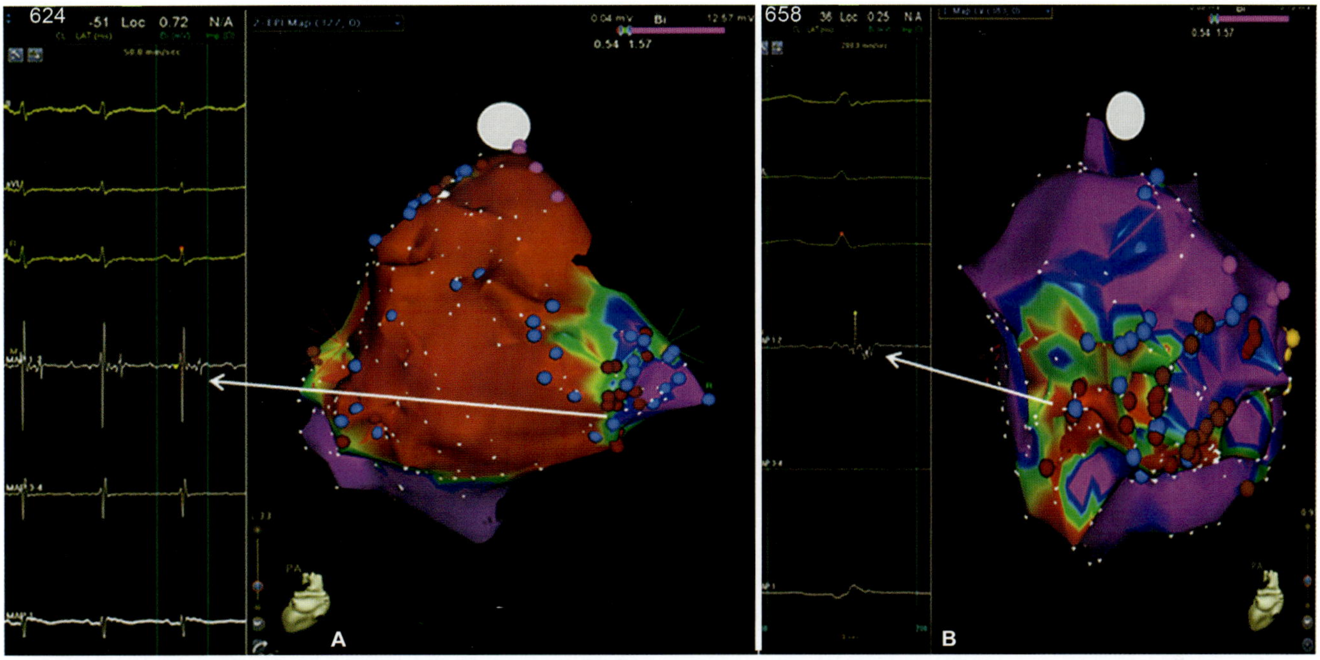

Figures 34.6A and B: PA view of (A) Epicardial and (B) Endocardial bipolar voltage map of LV of a patient with cardiac tuberculosis. Note the extensive low voltage area (red) in the epicardium (A). The corresponding endocardial region shows mostly normal voltage (B). Blue tags represent isolated late potentials (white arrows), red tags represent sites of ablation, brown tags represent fractionated low voltage signals and yellow tag represents His bundle

Abbreviations: PA, posteroanterior view; LV, left ventricle

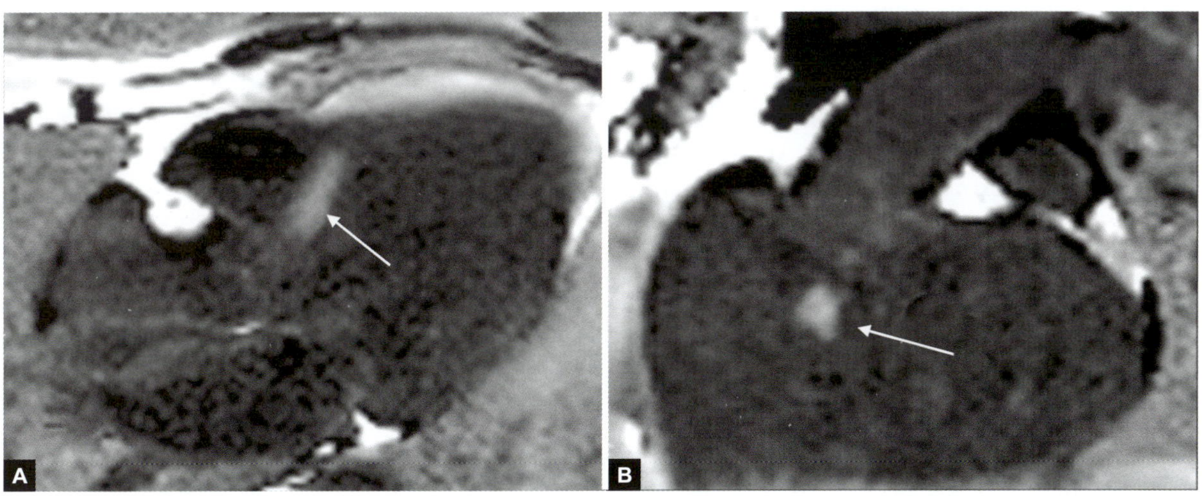

Figures 34.7A and B: Delayed gadolinium enhancement cardiac MRI with arrows showing midmyocardial septal scar (A) in the four chamber view and extending to the RVOT region in the outflow view (B) which are responsible for intramural VT circuits, making catheter ablation difficult

Abbreviations: RVOT, right ventricular outflow tract; VT, ventricular tachycardia

Adapted from: Daljeet K, Narasimhan C. Cardiac Sarcoidosis/Tuberculosis: Not so uncommon cause of VT/Cardiomyopathy in our country. Medicine Update 2016-1 (Progress in Medicine): Publisher: Jaypee Brothers; Volume 262016: Chapter-283. With permission

involvement[58] as compared to extensive myocardial involvement.[37] Catheter ablation is effective in controlling VT storm and eliminating ≥ 1 morphology of VTs, but recurrences are common. The reasons for failure to abolish VTs ventricular arrhythmias—septal intramural circuits **(Figures 34.7A and B)**, extensive scarring with multiple reentry circuits, and/or epicardial site of origin near a major coronary artery or parahisian region prohibiting safe ablation.[37] Thus, catheter ablation should be attempted in patients presenting with recurrent uncontrollable VT or VT storm not responding to immunosuppressive therapy, ATT (for CTB) and AADs.

ICD Implantation

Since many patients may develop life-threatening VT years after initial stabilization[34,38] and VF has been reported in several cases of cardiac sarcoidosis during inactive phase of disease,[29,59,60] it is prudent to implant ICD in all these patients, regardless of the initial response. Thus, disease specific therapy along with AADs and ICD are initially recommended and catheter ablation should be attempted only if patient does not respond to above line of management. Although sarcoidosis has been reported to recur in the transplanted donor heart, transplantation remains the only option in the patient with advanced heart failure.[61-63]

RESPONSE TO THERAPY

Response to therapy is monitored by clinical response as measured by reduction in the number of VT episodes, and improvement in heart failure symptoms. Serial measurement of high-sensitivity C-reactive protein while on disease-specific therapy is helpful and may also guide the duration of steroid or other active drugs in these inflammatory conditions. The resolution of myocardial inflammation on the follow-up PET CT scan and improvement in the left ventricular ejection fraction are good objective indicators of treatment response.

CONCLUSION

VT can be the first or the sole manifestation of GM (cardiac sarcoidosis/TB). The index of suspicion of GM should be high in patients presenting with unexplained VT, especially if there are conduction abnormalities or fQRS during sinus rhythm. Recurrent VTs of different morphologies or multiform premature ventricular contractions, on Holter should arouse suspicion of an underlying GM among such patients. Medical therapy is ineffective in approximately 50% of these patients and catheter ablation is a viable therapeutic option in selected patients with recurrent VT episodes. Despite a combination of medical therapy, ICD and catheter ablation, a significant proportion of patients may not survive or need cardiac transplant, underscoring the need for early diagnosis and intensive treatment in this group of patients.

REFERENCES

1. Baughman RP, Lower EE, du Bois RM. Sarcoidosis. Lancet. 2003;361:1111-8.
2. Thomas KW, Hunninghake GW. Sarcoidosis. JAMA. 2003; 289:3300-3.
3. Sugie T, Hashimoto N, Iwai K. Clinical and autopsy studies on prognosis of sarcoidosis. Nihon Rinsho. 1994;52:1567-70.
4. Bargout R, Kelly RF. Sarcoid heart disease: clinical course and treatment. Int J Cardiol. 2004;97:173-82.
5. Doughan AR, Williams BR. Cardiac sarcoidosis. Heart. 2006;92:282-8.
6. Duke C, Rosenthal E. Sudden death caused by cardiac sarcoidosis in childhood. J Cardiovasc Electrophysiol. 2002;13: 939-42.
7. Thachil A, Christopher J, Sastry BK, Reddy KN, Tourani VK, Hassan A, Raju BS, Narasimhan C. Monomorphic ventricular tachycardia and mediastinal adenopathy due to granulomatous infiltration in patients with preserved ventricular function. J Am Coll Cardiol. 2011;58:48-55.
8. Matsui Y, Iwai K, Tachibana T, Fruie T, Shigematsu N, Izumi T, Homma AH, Mikami R, Hongo O, Hiraga Y, Yamamoto M. Clinicopathological study of fatal myocardial sarcoidosis. Ann N Y Acad Sci. 1976;278:455-69.
9. Winters SL, Cohen M, Greenberg S, Stein B, Curwin J, Pe E, Gomes JA. Sustained ventricular tachycardia associated with sarcoidosis: assessment of the underlying cardiac anatomy and the prospective utility of programmed ventricular stimulation, drug therapy and an implantable antitachycardia device. J Am Coll Cardiol. 1991;18:937-43.
10. Furushima H, Chinushi M, Sugiura H, Kasai H, Washizuka T, Aizawa Y. Ventricular tachyarrhythmia associated with cardiac sarcoidosis: its mechanisms and outcome. Clin Cardiol. 2004; 27:217-22.
11. Sharma SK, Mohan A. Tuberculosis: From an incurable scourge to a curable disease—journey over a millennium. Indian J Med Res. 2013;137:455-93.
12. Kanchan T, Nagesh KR, Lobo FD, Menezes RG. Tubercular granuloma in the myocardium: an autopsy report. Singapore Med J. 2010;51:e15-7.
13. Khurana R, Shalhoub J, Verma A, Assomull R, Prasad SK, Kooner JS, Sethi A. Tubercular myocarditis presenting with ventricular tachycardia. Nat Clin Pract Cardiovasc Med. 2008;5:169-74.
14. Schnitzer R. Myocardial tuberculosis with paroxysmal ventricular tachycardia. Br Heart J. 1947;9:213-9.
15. Agarwal R, Malhotra P, Awasthi A, Kakkar N, Gupta D. Tuberculous dilated cardiomyopathy: an under-recognized entity? BMC Infect Dis. 2005;5:29.
16. Wallis PJ, Branfoot AC, Emerson PA. Sudden death due to myocardial tuberculosis. Thorax. 1984;39:155-6.
17. Bali HK, Wahi S, Sharma BK, Anand IS, Datta BN, Wahi PL. Myocardial tuberculosis presenting as restrictive cardiomyopathy. Am Heart J. 1990;120:703-6.
18. Horn H, Saphir O. The involvement of the myocardium in tuberculosis: A review of the literature and report of three cases. Am Rev Tuberc. 1935;32:492-506.
19. Maeder M, Ammann P, Rickli H, Schoch OD. Fever and night sweats in a 22-year-old man with a mediastinal mass involving the heart. Chest. 2003;124:2006-9.
20. Behr G, Palin HC, Temperly JM. Myocardial tuberculosis. Br Med J. 1977;1:951.
21. Kinare SG. Interesting facets of cardiovascular tuberculosis. Indian J Surg. 1975;37:144-51.
22. Kinare SG, Deshmukh MM. Complete atrioventricular block due to myocardial tuberculosis. Report of a case. Arch Pathol. 1969;88:684-7.

23. Diaz-Peromingo JA, Marino-Callejo AI, Gonzalez-Gonzalez C, Garcia-Rodriguez JF, Ameneiros-Lago ME, Sesma-Sanchez P. Tuberculous myocarditis presenting as long QT syndrome. Eur J Intern Med. 2000;11:340-2.
24. Mohan A, Thachil A, Sundar G, Sastry BK, Hasan A, Sridevi C, Narasimhan C. Ventricular tachycardia and tuberculous lymphadenopathy: sign of myocardial tuberculosis? J Am Coll Cardiol. 2015;65:218-20.
25. Kapoor OP, Mascarenhas E, Rananaware MM, Gadgil RK. Tuberculoma of the heart. Report of 9 cases. Am Heart J. 1973;86:334-40.
26. Rose AG. Cardiac tuberculosis. A study of 19 patients. Arch Pathol Lab Med. 1987;111:422-6.
27. Gulati GS, Kothari SS. Diffuse infiltrative cardiac tuberculosis. Ann Pediatr Cardiol. 2011;4:87-9.
28. Shah JR. Tuberculous Sarcoidosis. Lung India. 2007;24:83-6.
29. Koplan BA, Soejima K, Baughman K, Epstein LM, Stevenson WG. Refractory ventricular tachycardia secondary to cardiac sarcoid: electrophysiologic characteristics, mapping, and ablation. Heart Rhythm. 2006;3:924-9.
30. Yodogawa K, Seino Y, Ohara T, Takayama H, Katoh T, Mizuno K. Effect of corticosteroid therapy on ventricular arrhythmias in patients with cardiac sarcoidosis. Ann Noninvasive Electrocardiol. 2011;16:140-7.
31. Gopi A, Jesuraj ML, Sridevi C, Kalavakolanu S, Christopher J, Lalukota K, Narsimhan C. Reversible ventricular dysfunction due to granulomatous myocarditis. Eur Heart J. 2013; 34(Suppl 1):688-9.
32. Chiu CZ, Nakatani S, Zhang G, Tachibana T, Ohmori F, Yamagishi M, Kitakaze M, Tomoike H, Miyatake K. Prevention of left ventricular remodeling by long-term corticosteroid therapy in patients with cardiac sarcoidosis. Am J Cardiol. 2005;95:143-6.
33. Tung R, Bauer B, Schelbert H, Lynch JP, 3rd, Auerbach M, Gupta P, Schiepers C, Chan S, Ferris J, Barrio M, Ajijola O, Bradfield J, Shivkumar K. Incidence of abnormal positron emission tomography in patients with unexplained cardiomyopathy and ventricular arrhythmias: the potential role of occult inflammation in arrhythmogenesis. Heart Rhythm. 2015;12:2488-98.
34. Uusimaa P, Ylitalo K, Anttonen O, Kerola T, Virtanen V, Paakko E, Raatikainen P. Ventricular tachyarrhythmia as a primary presentation of sarcoidosis. Europace. 2008;10:760-6.
35. Kirchhof P, Eckardt L, Haverkamp W, Baba HA, Seidl KH, Borggrefe TM, Breithardt G. Intracardiac tuberculoma causing "idiopathic" ventricular tachycardia in a patient without detectable heart disease. J Cardiovasc Electrophysiol. 2001;12:118.
36. Latcu DG, Duparc A, Chabbert V, Labarre D, Mondoly P, Maury P, Delay M. Systemic sarcoidosis revealed by ventricular tachycardia: electrocardiography and MRI correspondence. Pacing Clin Electrophysiol. 2007;30:1566-70.
37. Kumar S, Barbhaiya C, Nagashima K, Choi EK, Epstein LM, John RM, Maytin M, Albert CM, Miller AL, Koplan BA, Michaud GF, Tedrow UB, Stevenson WG. Ventricular tachycardia in cardiac sarcoidosis: characterization of ventricular substrate and outcomes of catheter ablation. Circ Arrhythm Electrophysiol. 2015;8:87-93.
38. Naruse Y, Sekiguchi Y, Nogami A, Okada H, Yamauchi Y, Machino T, Kuroki K, Ito Y, Yamasaki H, Igarashi M, Tada H, Nitta J, Xu D, Sato A, Aonuma K. Systematic treatment approach to ventricular tachycardia in cardiac sarcoidosis. Circ Arrhythm Electrophysiol. 2014;7:407-13.
39. Panda S, Kaur D, Lalukota K, Sundar G, Pavri BB, Narasimhan C. Pleomorphism during Ventricular tachycardia: a distinguishing feature between cardiac sarcoidosis and idiopathic VT. Pacing Clin Electrophysiol. 2015;38:694-9.
40. Shenthar J. Unusual incessant ventricular tachycardia: what is the underlying cause and the possible mechanism? Circ Arrhythm Electrophysiol. 2015;8:1507-11.
41. Das MK, Zipes DP. Fragmented QRS: a predictor of mortality and sudden cardiac death. Heart Rhythm. 2009;6:S8-14.
42. Sha J, Zhang S, Tang M, Chen K, Zhao X, Wang F. Fragmented QRS is associated with all-cause mortality and ventricular arrhythmias in patient with idiopathic dilated cardiomyopathy. Ann Noninvasive Electrocardiol. 2011;16:270-5.
43. Peters S, Trummel M, Koehler B. QRS fragmentation in standard ECG as a diagnostic marker of arrhythmogenic right ventricular dysplasia-cardiomyopathy. Heart Rhythm. 2008;5:1417-21.
44. Homsi M, Alsayed L, Safadi B, Mahenthiran J, Das MK. Fragmented QRS complexes on 12-lead ECG: a marker of cardiac sarcoidosis as detected by gadolinium cardiac magnetic resonance imaging. Ann Noninvasive Electrocardiol. 2009;14:319-26.
45. Roukoz H, Shah M, Masilamani LJ, Thachil A, Jayakumar PK, Benditt DG, Narasimhan C. fQRS as a marker of granulomatous disease in patients presenting with ventricular tachycardia and normal left ventricular ejection fraction. Indian Heart J. 2015;67:222-6.
46. Ardehali H, Howard DL, Hariri A, Qasim A, Hare JM, Baughman KL, Kasper EK. A positive endomyocardial biopsy result for sarcoid is associated with poor prognosis in patients with initially unexplained cardiomyopathy. Am Heart J. 2005;150:459-63.
47. Walsh MJ. Systemic sarcoidosis with refractory ventricular tachycardia and heart failure. Br Heart J. 1978;40:931-3.
48. Stees CS, Khoo MS, Lowery CM, Sauer WH. Ventricular tachycardia storm successfully treated with immunosuppression and catheter ablation in a patient with cardiac sarcoidosis. J Cardiovasc Electrophysiol. 2011;22:210-3.
49. Vanga SR, Vacek J, Berenbom L, Lakkireddy DR. Ventricular tachycardia storm—an atypical presentation of sarcoidosis exacerbation. Indian Pacing Electrophysiol J. 2009;9:351-4.
50. Soejima K, Yada H. The work-up and management of patients with apparent or subclinical cardiac sarcoidosis: with emphasis on the associated heart rhythm abnormalities. J Cardiovasc Electrophysiol. 2009;20:578-83.
51. Dechering DG, Kochhauser S, Wasmer K, Zellerhoff S, Pott C, Kobe J, Spieker T, Piers SR, Bittner A, Monnig G, Breithardt G, Wichter T, Zeppenfeld K, Eckardt L. Electrophysiological characteristics of ventricular tachyarrhythmias in cardiac sarcoidosis versus arrhythmogenic right ventricular cardiomyopathy. Heart Rhythm. 2013;10:158-64.
52. Sekiguchi M, Hiroe M, Take M, Hirosawa K. Clinical and histopathological profile of sarcoidosis of the heart and acute idiopathic myocarditis. Concepts through a study employing endomyocardial biopsy. II. Myocarditis. Jpn Circ J. 1980;44: 264-73.
53. Noda T, Suyama K, Shimizu W, Satomi K, Otomo K, Okamura H, Kurita T, Aihara N, Kamakura S. Ventricular tachycardia with figure eight pattern originating from the right ventricle in

a patient with cardiac sarcoidosis. Pacing Clin Electrophysiol. 2004;27:561-2.

54. Santucci PA, Morton JB, Picken MM, Wilber DJ. Electroanatomic mapping of the right ventricle in a patient with a giant epsilon wave, ventricular tachycardia, and cardiac sarcoidosis. J Cardiovasc Electrophysiol. 2004;15:1091-4.
55. Banba K, Kusano KF, Nakamura K, Morita H, Ogawa A, Ohtsuka F, Ogo KO, Nishii N, Watanabe A, Nagase S, Sakuragi S, Ohe T. Relationship between arrhythmogenesis and disease activity in cardiac sarcoidosis. Heart Rhythm. 2007;4:1292-9.
56. Chinushi M, Mezaki T, Aoki Y, Nakagawa I, Washizuka T, Aizawa Y. Demonstration of transient entrainment in monomorphic sustained ventricular tachycardia associated with cardiac sarcoidosis. Jpn Circ J. 2000;64:635-7.
57. Mezaki T, Chinushi M, Washizuka T, Furushima H, Chinushi Y, Ebe K, Okumura H, Aizawa Y. Discrepancy between inducibility of ventricular tachycardia and activity of cardiac sarcoidosis. Requirement of defibrillator implantation for the inactive stage of cardiac sarcoidosis. Intern Med. 2001;40:73
58. Jefic D, Joel B, Good E, Morady F, Rosman H, Knight B, Bogun F. Role of radiofrequency catheter ablation of ventricular tachycardia in cardiac sarcoidosis: report from a multicenter registry. Heart Rhythm. 2009;6:189-95.
59. Stein E, Stimmel B, Siltzbach LE. Clinical course of cardiac sarcoidosis. Ann N Y Acad Sci. 1976;278:470-4.
60. Tornling G, Olsson G, von Unge H. Ventricular fibrillation in myocardial sarcoidosis. Eur J Respir Dis. 1985;66:347-9.
61. Luk A, Lee A, Ahn E, Soor GS, Ross HJ, Butany J. Cardiac sarcoidosis: recurrent disease in a heart transplant patient following pulmonary tuberculosis infection. Can J Cardiol. 2010;26:e273-5.
62. Oni AA, Hershberger RE, Norman DJ, Ray J, Hovaguimian H, Cobanoglu AM, Hosenpud JD. Recurrence of sarcoidosis in a cardiac allograft: control with augmented corticosteroids. J Heart Lung Transplant. 1992;11:367-9.
63. Yager JE, Hernandez AF, Steenbergen C, Persing B, Russell SD, Milano C, Felker GM. Recurrence of cardiac sarcoidosis in a heart transplant recipient. J Heart Lung Transplant. 2005;24:1988-90.

EDITORS' SUMMARY

Although sarcoidosis affecting the heart and producing its protean manifestations has been well described for several decades, it is only recently that far less obvious manifestations, particularly arrhythmias hitherto thought to occur in the structurally normal heart have come to light. A large part of the credit for this increased awareness and the new description of nonsarcoid infectious granulomatous myocarditis is due to the pioneering work from the senior author of this chapter, Dr Calambur Narasimhan. A comprehensive description of the clinical features, intracardiac distribution, and arrhythmic manifestations is provided, and the reader would undoubtedly have enhanced awareness as well as an enthusiasm to strive and find an exact diagnosis in patients with an apparently structurally normal heart and ventricular tachycardia.

CHAPTER 35

Akihiko Nogami

Idiopathic Left Ventricular Tachycardia

LIST OF ABBREVIATIONS

LBBB	Left Bundle Branch Block	RF	Radiofrequency
LF	Left Fascicle	VT	Ventricular Tachycardia
RBBB	Right Bundle Branch Block		

INTRODUCTION

Sustained monomorphic ventricular tachycardia (VT) is most often related to myocardial structural heart disease, including healed myocardial infarction and cardiomyopathies. However, no apparent structural abnormality is identified in about 10% of all sustained monomorphic VTs in the United States[1] and 20% of those in Japan.[2] These VTs are referred to as "idiopathic". Idiopathic VTs usually occur in specific locations and have specific QRS morphologies,[3-8] whereas VTs associated with structural heart disease have a QRS morphology that tends to indicate the location of the scar. Idiopathic VT comprises multiple discrete subtypes that are best differentiated by their mechanism, QRS morphology, and site of origin. The most common idiopathic VT originates from a focus in the outflow tract of the right ventricle, and its mechanism is most likely triggered activity. In idiopathic left VT, four types of VT exist: verapamil-sensitive left fascicular VT (reentry), VT with a focal origin in the distal Purkinje system (abnormal automaticity), left ventricular outflow tract VT, and VT from the mitral annulus (triggered activity, reentry, or automaticity). This chapter focuses on the assessment and nonpharmacologic treatment of verapamil-sensitive left fascicular VT.

CLASSIFICATION AND PATHOPHYSIOLOGY

History and Classification

Verapamil-sensitive fascicular VT is the most common form of idiopathic left VT. It was first recognized as an electrocardiographic entity in 1979 by Zipes and colleagues,[9] who identified the characteristic diagnostic triad: (1) induction with atrial pacing, (2) right bundle branch block (RBBB) and left-axis configuration, and (3) manifestation in patients without structural heart disease. In 1981, Belhassen and associates[10] were the first to demonstrate the verapamil sensitivity of the tachycardia, a fourth identifying feature. Ohe and coworkers[11] reported another type of this tachycardia with RBBB and a right-axis deviation in 1988 and we described the upper septal form of this tachycardia.[12] According to the QRS morphology, verapamil-sensitive left fascicular VT can be classified into three subgroups: (1) left posterior fascicular VT, whose QRS morphology exhibits an RBBB configuration and a superior axis **(Figure 35.1)**; (2) left anterior fascicular VT, whose QRS morphology exhibits an RBBB configuration and right-axis deviation **(Figure 35.2)**; and (3) upper septal fascicular VT, whose QRS morphology

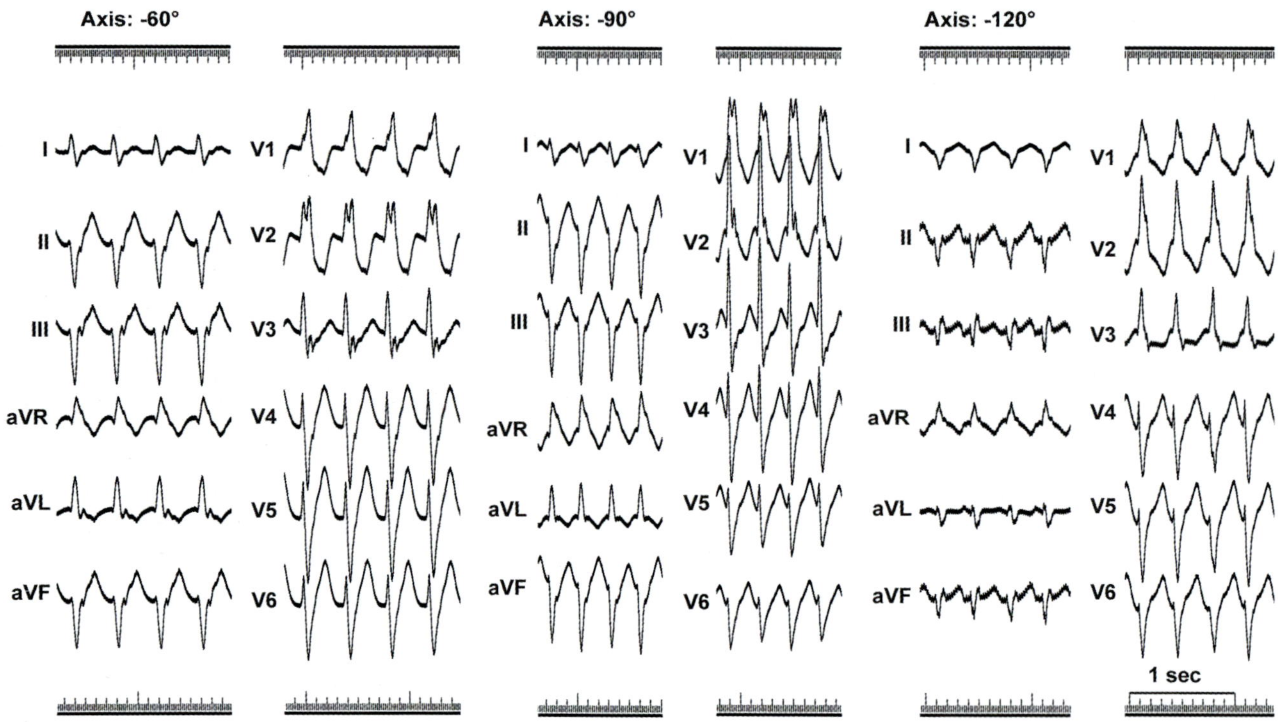

Figure 35.1: Twelve-lead electrocardiograms of verapamil-sensitive left posterior fascicular ventricular tachycardias (VTs). Three different VTs are shown

From: Nogami A. Idiopathic left ventricular tachycardia: assessment and treatment. Card Electrophysiol Rev. 2002;6:448-57

exhibits a narrow QRS configuration and normal or right-axis deviation **(Figures 35.3A and B)**. Left posterior fascicular VT is common, left anterior fascicular VT is uncommon, and left upper septal fascicular VT is very rare.

Substrate and Mechanism

The anatomic basis of this tachycardia has provoked considerable interest. Some data suggest that the tachycardia may originate from a false tendon or fibromuscular band in the left ventricle.[13-15] Suwa and coworkers[14] described a false tendon in the left ventricle of a patient with idiopathic VT in whom the VT was eliminated by surgical resection of the tendon. Using transthoracic and transesophageal echocardiography, Thakur and colleagues[15] found false tendons extending from the posteroinferior left ventricle to the basal septum in 15 of 15 patients with idiopathic left VT but in only 5% of control patients. Maruyama and associates[16] reported a case with the recording of sequential diastolic potentials bridging the entire diastolic period and a false tendon extending from the midseptum to the inferoapical septum. Lin and colleagues[17] found that 17 of 18 patients with idiopathic VT had this fibromuscular band but also found it in 35 of 40 control patients. They concluded that the band was a common echocardiographic finding and was not a specific arrhythmogenic substrate for this tachycardia, although they could not exclude the possibility that the band was a potential substrate of the VT. Small fibromuscular bands, trabeculae carneae, and small papillary muscles cannot be detected by echocardiography. The Purkinje networks in these small anatomic structures are important when considering the mechanism of left fascicular VT. This circuit is not completely defined but may comprise fascicular tissue and ventricular myocardium.

The mechanism of verapamil-sensitive left VT is reentry because it can be induced, entrained, and terminated by programmed ventricle or atrial stimulation. To confirm its reentry circuit and the mechanism, my colleagues and I performed left ventricular septal mapping using an octapolar electrode catheter in 20 patients with left posterior fascicular VT[18] **(Figures 35.4A and B)**. In 15 of 20 patients, two distinct potentials, P1 and P2, were recorded during the VT at the midseptum **(Figures 35.5A and B)**. Although the mid-diastolic potential (P1) was recorded earlier from the proximal rather than the distal electrodes, the fused presystolic Purkinje potential (P2) was recorded earlier from the distal electrodes. During sinus rhythm, recording at the same site demonstrated P2, which was recorded after the His bundle

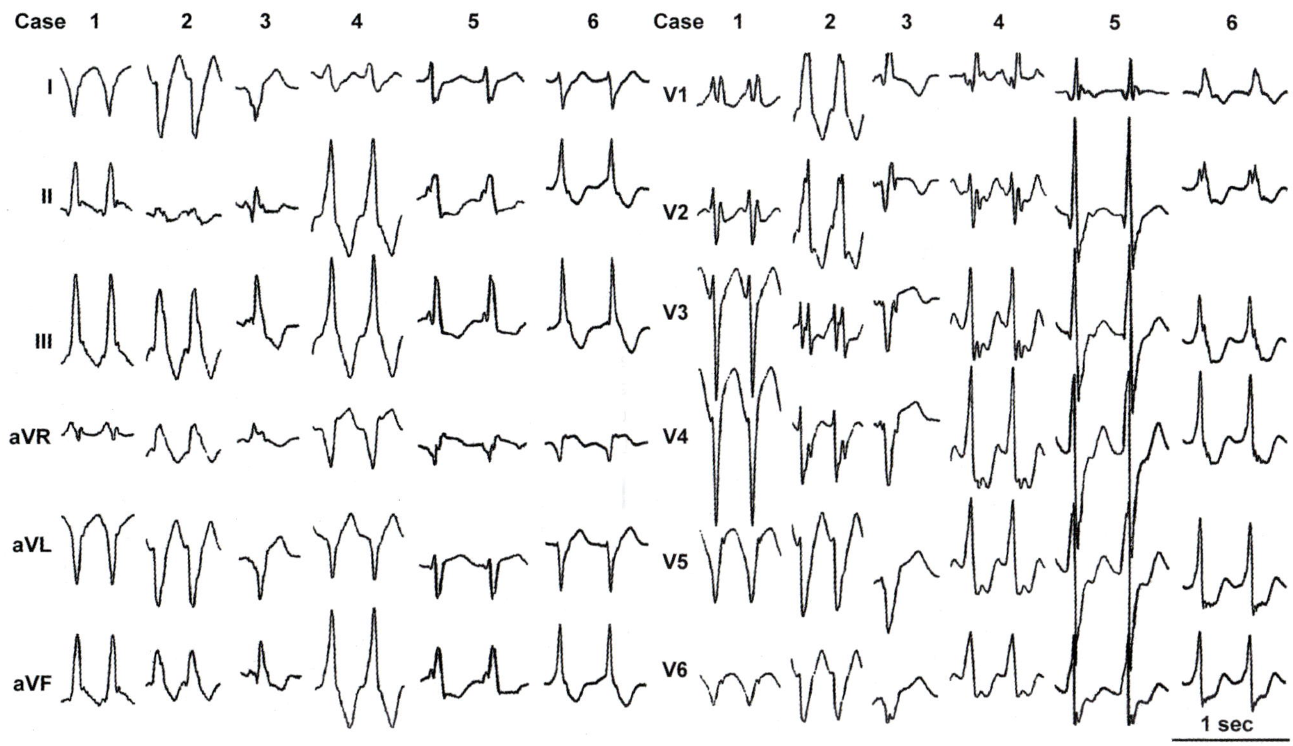

Figure 35.2: Twelve-lead electrocardiograms of verapamil-sensitive left anterior fascicular ventricular tachycardias in six patients
From: Nogami A, Naito S, Tada H, et al. Verapamil-sensitive left anterior fascicular ventricular tachycardia: results of radiofrequency ablation in six patients. J Cardiovasc Electrophysiol. 1998;9:1269-78

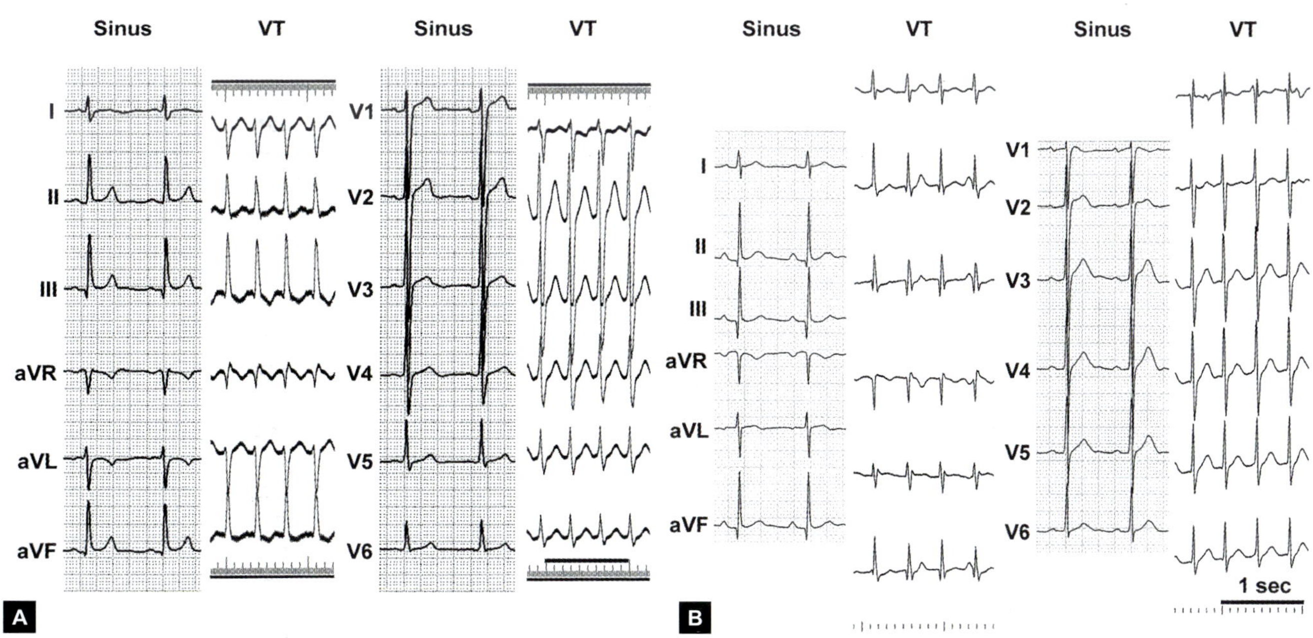

Figures 35.3A and B: Twelve-lead electrocardiograms of verapamil-sensitive left upper septal ventricular tachycardia (VT). (A) The QRS morphology during the VT is narrow (100 ms) and similar to those during sinus rhythm except S-wave in leads I, V5, and V6; (B) VT that appeared 2 years after the initial session for left posterior fascicular ventricular tachycardia demonstrates a narrow QRS complex (90 ms) and normal axis. The QRS morphology during the VT is similar to those during sinus rhythm except rSr′ pattern in lead V1
[(A) From Nogami A. Idiopathic left ventricular tachycardia: assessment and treatment. Card Electrophysiol. Rev. 2002;6:448-57; (B) From Nishiuchi S, Nogami A, Naito S. A case with occurrence of antidromic tachycardia after ablation of idiopathic left fascicular tachycardia: Mechanism of left upper septal ventricular tachycardia. J Cardiovasc Electrophysiol. 2013;24:825-7]

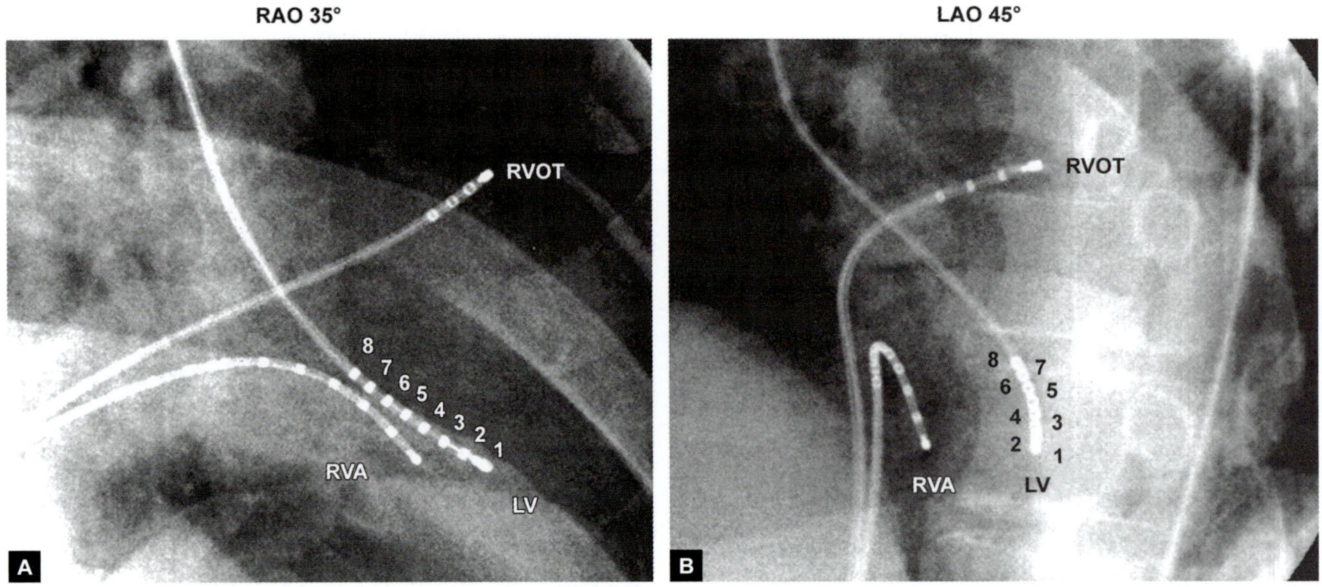

Figures 35.4A and B: Representation of an octapolar electrode catheter positioned at the left ventricular septum as viewed fluoroscopically in the right anterior oblique (RAO) and left anterior oblique (LAO) projections. The distance between electrodes 1 and 8 of the octapolar electrode catheter was approximately 25 mm

Abbreviations: LV, left ventricle; RVA, right ventricular apex; RVOT, right ventricular outflow tract

From: Nogami A, Naito S, Tada H, et al. Demonstration of diastolic and presystolic Purkinje potential as critical potentials on a macroreentry circuit of verapamil-sensitive idiopathic left ventricular tachycardia. J Am Coll Cardiol. 2000;36:811-23

potential and before the onset of the QRS complex; however, the sequence of the P2 was the reverse of that seen during the VT. VT could be entrained from the atrium and from the ventricle. Entrainment pacing from the atrium or ventricle captured P1 orthodromically and reset the VT **(Figures 35.6A to C)**. The interval from the stimulus to P1 was prolonged as the pacing rate increased. These findings demonstrated that P1 is a critical potential in the circuit of the verapamil-sensitive left posterior fascicular VT and suggested the presence of a macroreentry circuit involving the normal Purkinje system and abnormal Purkinje tissue with decremental properties and verapamil sensitivity. Although P1 has proved to be a critical potential in the VT circuit, whether the left posterior fascicle or Purkinje fiber (P2) is involved in the retrograde limb of the reentrant circuit is unclear.[16,19,20] Morishima and associates[20] reported a case with negative participation of the proximal left posterior fascicle to the VT circuit. Although selective capture of left posterior fascicle by sinus beat did not affect the cycle length of VT, the postpacing interval after the entrainment from left ventricular septal myocardium was equal to the cycle length of VT **(Figures 35.7A and B)**. Ouyang and coworkers[21] suggested that idiopathic left VT reentry might be a small macroreentry circuit consisting of one anterograde Purkinje fiber with a Purkinje potential, one retrograde Purkinje fiber with retrograde Purkinje potential, and the ventricular myocardium as the bridge.

Tachycardia Circuit

The hypothesized circuit of left posterior fascicular VT is depicted in **Figures 35.8A** and **35.9**. In this circuit, P1 represents the activation potential in the distal portion of the specialized Purkinje tissue; it has decremental properties and verapamil sensitivity. P2 represents the activation of the left posterior fascicle or Purkinje fiber near the left posterior fascicle and it is a bystander during VT. P1 represents the antegrade limb of the circuit in VT and left ventricular septal muscle is the retrograde limb.

During sinus rhythm, the activation goes from P2 to P1 at the point of the fusion; therefore, P1 is buried in the local ventricular activation **(Figure 35.9A)**. During VT, P1 and P2 activate in the reverse direction **(Figure 35.9B)**. This explains why the activation sequences of P2 are reversed during sinus rhythm and VT. During concealed entrainment from the VT exit (e.g. at a cycle length of 400 ms as in **Figure 35.6A**), P1 is activated orthodromically and the antidromic wavefront blocks, presumably in the connection between P1 and left ventricular septal muscle **(Figure 35.9C)**. The orthodromic wavefront of the preceding (n-1)th beat also blocks in the connection between P1 and left ventricular septal muscle because it encounters the refractoriness created by the antidromic wavefront from the (n)th pacing impulse. The orthodromic wavefront from the last pacing impulse continues the tachycardia with resetting.

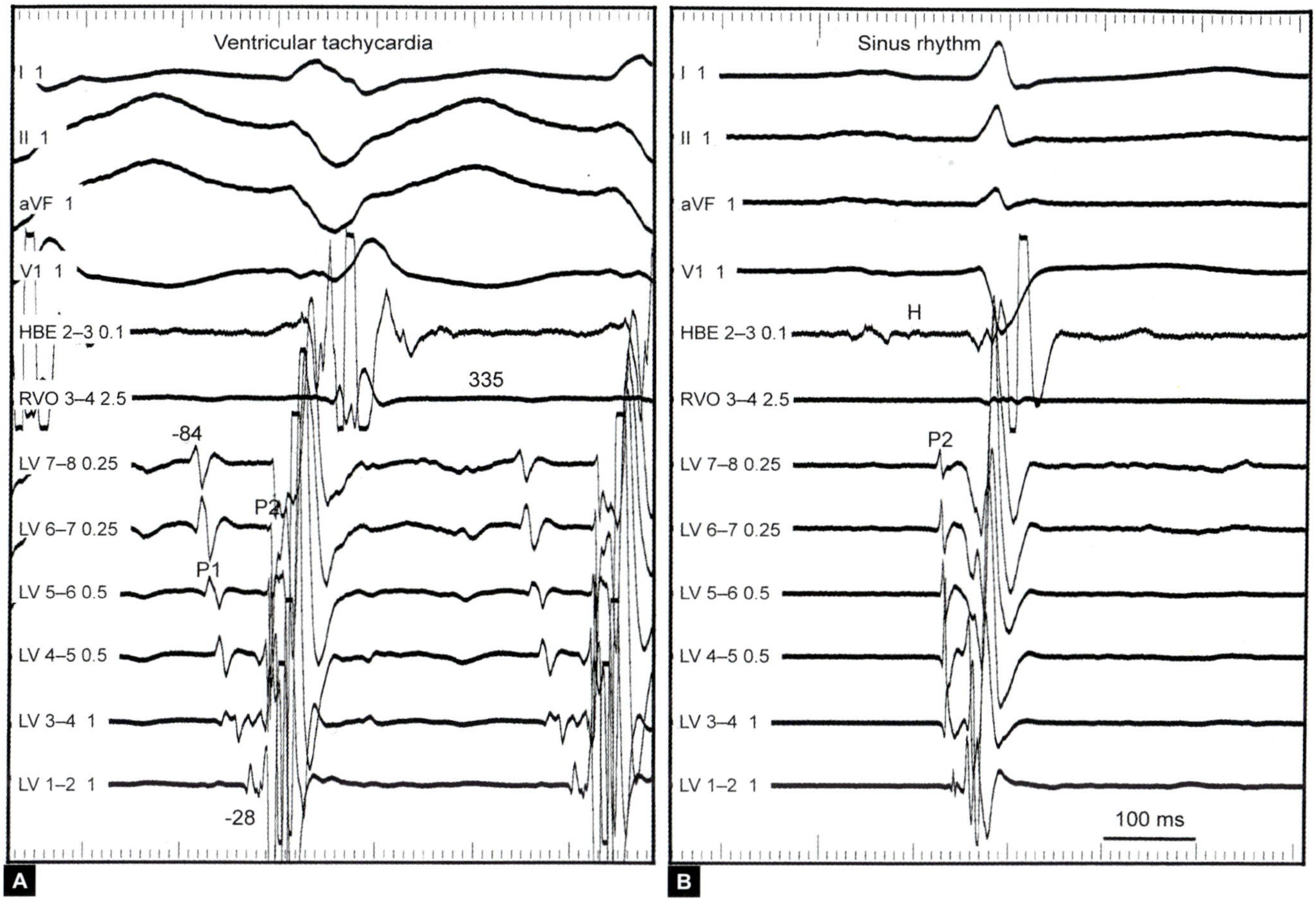

Figures 35.5A and B: Intracardiac recordings from an octapolar electrode catheter. (A) During left posterior fascicular ventricular tachycardia, a diastolic potential (P1) and a presystolic Purkinje potential (P2) were recorded. While P1 was recorded earlier from the proximal rather than the distal electrodes, P2 was recorded earlier from the distal rather than the proximal electrodes; (B) During sinus rhythm, recording at the same site demonstrated that P2 is now recorded before the onset of the QRS complex and is earliest on the proximal electrodes
Abbreviations: HBE, His bundle electrogram; RVO, right ventricular outflow; LV, left ventricle; 7–8, proximal bipole; 1–2, distal bipole; H, His
From: Nogami A, Naito S, Tada H, et al. Demonstration of diastolic and presystolic Purkinje potential as critical potentials on a macroreentry circuit of verapamil-sensitive idiopathic left ventricular tachycardia. J Am Coll Cardiol. 2000;36:811-23

During entrainment pacing with a shorter cycle length (e.g. at 380 ms as in **Figure 35.6B**), the distal portion of P1 activates antidromically, and the antidromic wavefront blocks at the middle portion of P1 in the area of slow conduction **(Figure 35.9D)**. The orthodromic wavefront from the last pacing impulse continues and resets the tachycardia. However, the interval from the last pacing stimulus to the orthodromically activated P1 is prolonged because of rate-dependent conduction delay in the area of slow conduction. During entrainment pacing with an even shorter cycle length or a shorter starting coupling interval (e.g. at a starting coupling interval of 300 ms as in **Figure 35.6C**), P1 activates antidromically, and the antidromic wavefront blocks at the proximal portion of P1 in the area of slow conduction **(Figure 35.9E)**. However, the orthodromic wavefront from the previous paced beat also blocks. It blocks independent of either the collision with, or refractoriness secondary to, the previous antidromic wavefront. Because both the antidromic and the orthodromic wavefronts of the same beat are blocked, the VT is interrupted. Radiofrequency (RF) catheter ablation results in elimination of the conduction between P1 and left ventricular septal muscle. This type of VT can be named as left posterior slow-fast type fascicular VT.

DIAGNOSTIC CRITERIA

Surface Electrocardiogram

Based on the QRS morphology, verapamil-sensitive fascicular VT can be classified into three subgroups. The 12-lead electrocardiogram (ECG) of the left posterior fascicular VT exhibits an RBBB and a superior axis (left-axis deviation or northwest axis) **(Figure 35.1)**. This is the common type

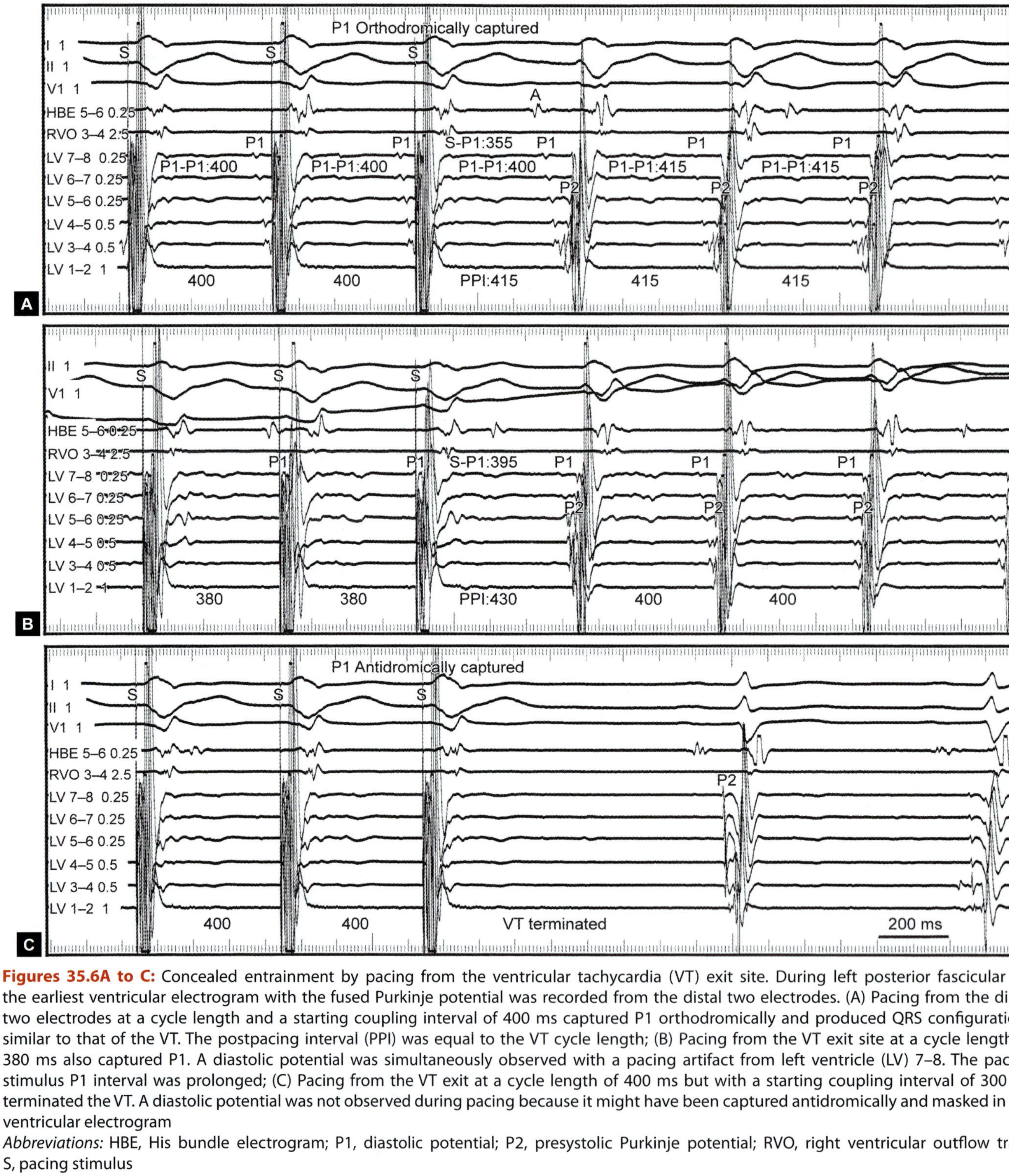

Figures 35.6A to C: Concealed entrainment by pacing from the ventricular tachycardia (VT) exit site. During left posterior fascicular VT, the earliest ventricular electrogram with the fused Purkinje potential was recorded from the distal two electrodes. (A) Pacing from the distal two electrodes at a cycle length and a starting coupling interval of 400 ms captured P1 orthodromically and produced QRS configurations similar to that of the VT. The postpacing interval (PPI) was equal to the VT cycle length; (B) Pacing from the VT exit site at a cycle length of 380 ms also captured P1. A diastolic potential was simultaneously observed with a pacing artifact from left ventricle (LV) 7–8. The pacing stimulus P1 interval was prolonged; (C) Pacing from the VT exit at a cycle length of 400 ms but with a starting coupling interval of 300 ms terminated the VT. A diastolic potential was not observed during pacing because it might have been captured antidromically and masked in the ventricular electrogram

Abbreviations: HBE, His bundle electrogram; P1, diastolic potential; P2, presystolic Purkinje potential; RVO, right ventricular outflow tract; S, pacing stimulus

From: Nogami A, Naito S, Tada H, et al. Demonstration of diastolic and presystolic Purkinje potential as critical potentials on a macroreentry circuit of verapamil-sensitive idiopathic left ventricular tachycardia. J Am Coll Cardiol. 2000; 36:811-23

of verapamil-sensitive fascicular VT and may account for up to 90% of cases. The uncommon type of this VT is a left anterior fascicular VT whose QRS morphology exhibits an RBBB configuration and right-axis deviation **(Figure 35.2)**.[11,22] The last type of VT is an upper septal fascicular VT, whose QRS morphology exhibits a relatively narrow QRS configuration and normal or right-axis deviation **(Figure 35.3)**.[12,23] This type of VT is very rare.

Intracardiac Electrograms

With left posterior fascicular VT, the earliest ventricular activation is recorded from the apical septum, and diastolic potentials are recorded from the midseptum **(Figure 35.5)**. His activation follows QRS onset by 5–30 ms.[24] During sinus rhythm, recording from the same site demonstrates the Purkinje potentials after the His bundle potential and before the onset of the QRS complex.

With left anterior fascicular VT, the earliest ventricular activation is recorded from the anterolateral left ventricle **(Figures 35.10A to C)**, and diastolic potentials are recorded from the midseptum **(Figures 35.11A to C)**. There have been several reports that describe a left VT with an RBBB configuration, right-axis deviation, and a different mechanism. Yeh and colleagues[25] reported four cases with an RBBB configuration and right-axis deviation. This VT was adenosine sensitive and was successfully ablated from the anterobasal left ventricle. The chest leads exhibited an atypical RBBB configuration with wide "R" morphology. Crijns and colleagues[26] reported a case of interfascicular reentrant VT with an RBBB configuration and right-axis deviation (bundle branch reentry tachycardia type B). In their patient, the VT circuit used the anterior fascicle as the anterograde limb and the posterior fascicle as the retrograde limb. Interfascicular VT usually has a His bundle potential recorded in the diastolic phase during the VT as well as posterior fascicular potentials. However, it may be difficult to distinguish between interfascicular VT and intrafascicular VT (verapamil-sensitive left anterior fascicular VT).[22] The diagnostic criteria for reentrant idiopathic left fascicular VT are given in **Table 35.1**.

The differential diagnosis includes supraventricular tachycardias with bifascicular block aberrancy. With left upper septal fascicular VT, the retrograde activation of the His bundle is recorded before the onset of the QRS complex **(Figures 35.12A and B)**. If there is retrograde ventriculoatrial conduction during the tachycardia, it mimics atrioventricular nodal reentry tachycardia or atrioventricular reciprocating tachycardia. The response of these tachycardias to verapamil and the ability to initiate and entrain them by atrial pacing may

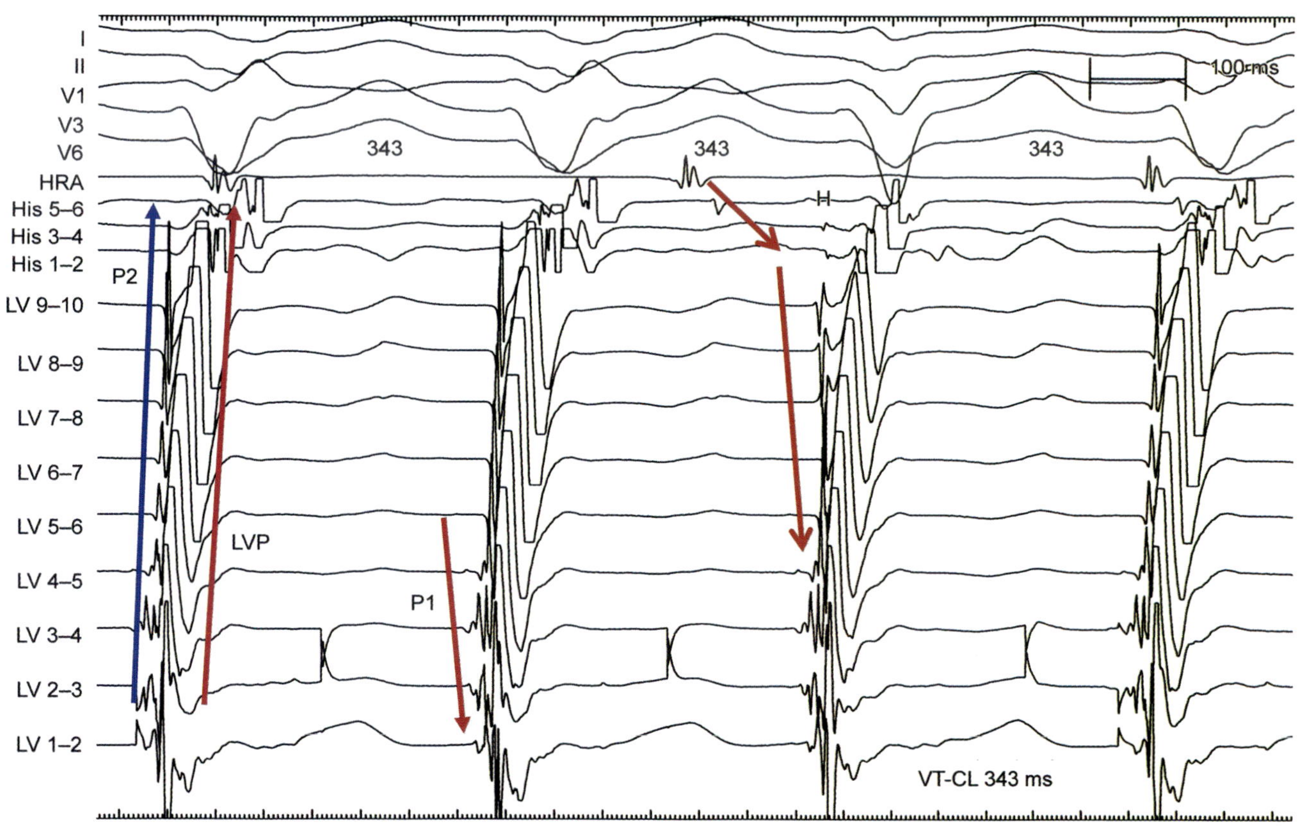

Figure 35.7A

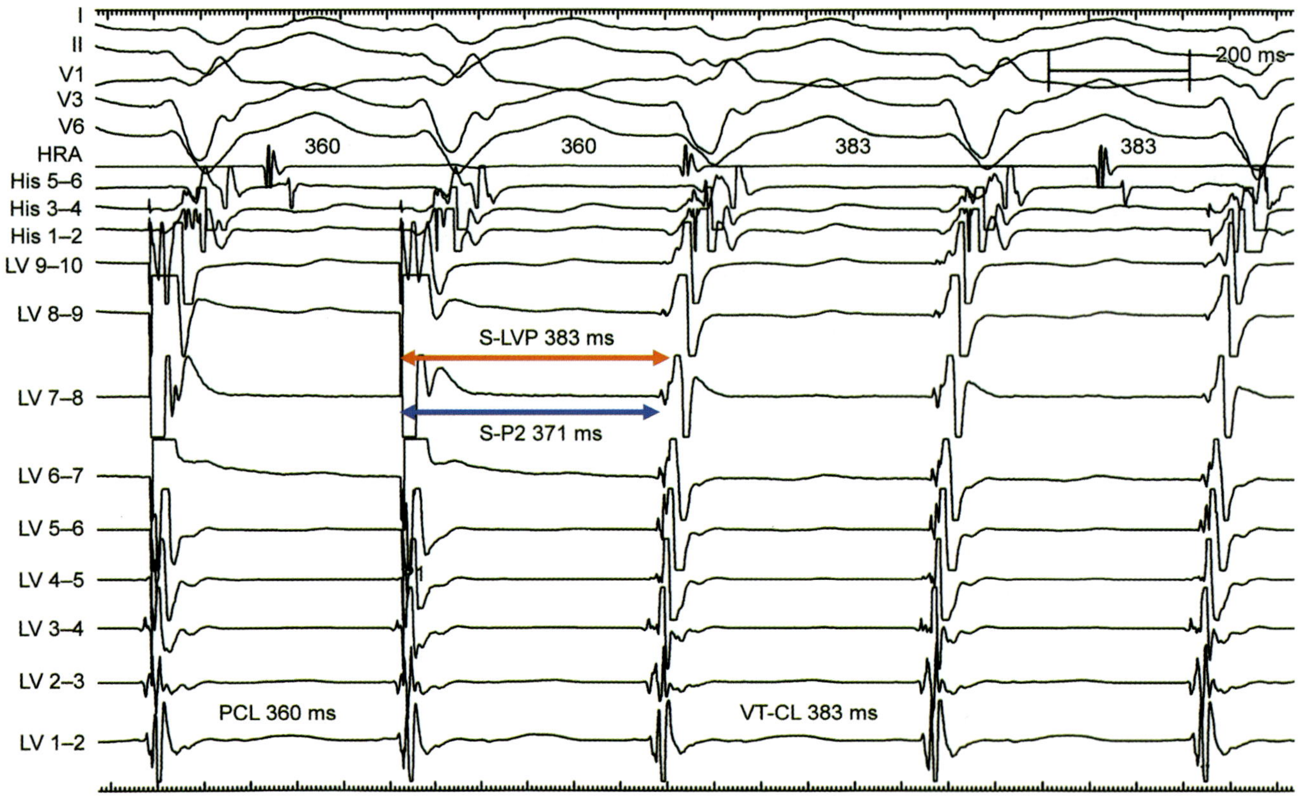

Figure 35.7B

Figures 35.7A and B: Negative participation of the proximal left posterior fascicle to the ventricular tachycardia (VT) circuit. (A) Three sequences of potentials were recorded at the left posterior septum during verapamil-sensitive idiopathic left ventricular tachycardia: diastolic Purkinje potentials (P1) propagating from base to apex and presystolic left posterior fascicular potentials (P2) and systolic left ventricular myocardial potentials (LVP) propagating in the reverse direction. Note that selective capture of the left posterior fascicle by a sinus beat (3rd QRS from left) did not affect the cycle length of VT; (B) During entrainment pacing from LV 7–8, both P2 and LVP were simultaneously captured. Although the postpacing interval of LVP was equal to VTCL, the postpacing interval of P2 was shorter than VTCL

Abbreviations: CL, cycle length; LPF, left posterior fascicle; LVP, left ventricular myocardium potential; PCL, pacing cycle length; S, pacing stimulus

From: Morishima I, Nogami A, Tsuboi H, Sone T. Negative participation of the left posterior fascicle in the reentry circuit of verapamil-sensitive idiopathic left ventricular tachycardia. J Cardiovascular Electrophysiol. 2012;23:556-9

Table 35.1: Diagnostic criteria for idiopathic left fascicular ventricular tachycardia

- Characteristic surface ECG appearance
  - RBBB and superior axis configuration (common type)
  - RBBB and inferior axis configuration (uncommon type)
  - Narrow QRS and inferior axis configuration (rare type)
- Electrophysiological findings
  - Tachycardia dependence on left ventricular fascicular reentry
  - Purkinje potentials and diastolic potentials preceding ventricular activation
  - Changes in tachycardia rate preceded by similar changes in Purkinje and diastolic potentials
  - His activation follows QRS onset (short positive HV in rare type)
  - Induction and entrainment with ventricular and/or atrial pacing
- Drug response
  - Verapamil-sensitive termination or slowing of tachycardia due to conduction slowing or block in fascicular system

Abbreviations: ECG, electrocardiogram; HV, His-to-ventricular; RBBB, right bundle branch block; VT, ventricular tachycardia also lead to diagnostic confusion. To avoid a misdiagnosis, recognition of the retrograde sequence of the His bundle activation and measurement of a shorter His-to-ventricular (HV) interval during the tachycardia than in sinus rhythm is important. An earlier potential than the His bundle potential is recorded from the left ventricular upper septum, where the left bundle potential is recorded during sinus rhythm. VT can be slowed or terminated by the intravenous administration of verapamil; however, it is unresponsive to β-blockers or Valsalva maneuvers. Class Ia and class Ic drugs are also effective. Rare cases of adenosine responsiveness occur, but only if the tachycardia shows catecholamine dependency.

In bundle branch reentry, the His activation precedes activation of the left bundle to produce a RBBB QRS morphology. In idiopathic left VT, the HV interval is shorter (negative) and follows left fascicular activation.

MAPPING AND ABLATION

RF catheter ablation may be considered a potential first-line therapy for patients with idiopathic VT because these VTs can be eliminated by ablation in a high percentage of patients.

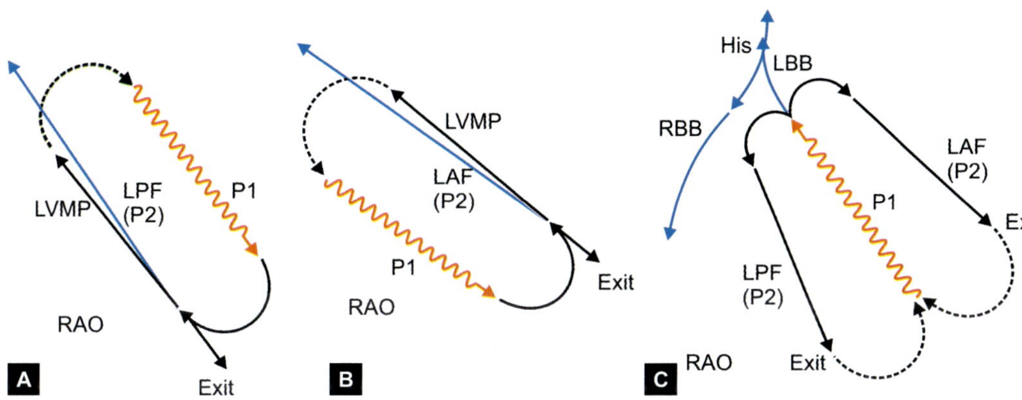

Figures 35.8A to C: Schematic representation of the reentrant circuits in verapamil-sensitive left fascicular ventricular tachycardias (VTs). (A) Left posterior fascicular VT. During the VT, P1 propagates from base to apex, P2 and left ventricular myocardial potentials (LVMP) activate in the reverse direction. The proposed upper turn-around area is shown by the dotted line. The undulating line represents a zone of slow conduction. Although the antegrade limb of the VT circuit consists of P1, the retrograde limb consists of LVMP, but not of P2; (B) Left anterior fascicular VT. During VT, the antegrade limb is the P1, the retrograde limb is the LVMP, and the exit to the ventricular muscle is near the distal portion of left anterior fascicle; (C) Left upper septal VT. P1 represents the activation potential of the specialized Purkinje tissue at left ventricular upper septum. P2 represents the activation of the left anterior and posterior fascicles. Both left anterior and posterior fascicles are the antegrade limbs of the reentrant circuit in VT. This explains why this VT exhibits a narrow QRS configuration and inferior axis

Abbreviations: LAF, left anterior fascicle; LPF, left posterior fascicle; LBB, left bundle branch; LVMP, left ventricular myocardial potential; P1, diastolic potential; P2, presystolic Purkinje potential; RAO, right anterior oblique view; RBB, right bundle branch

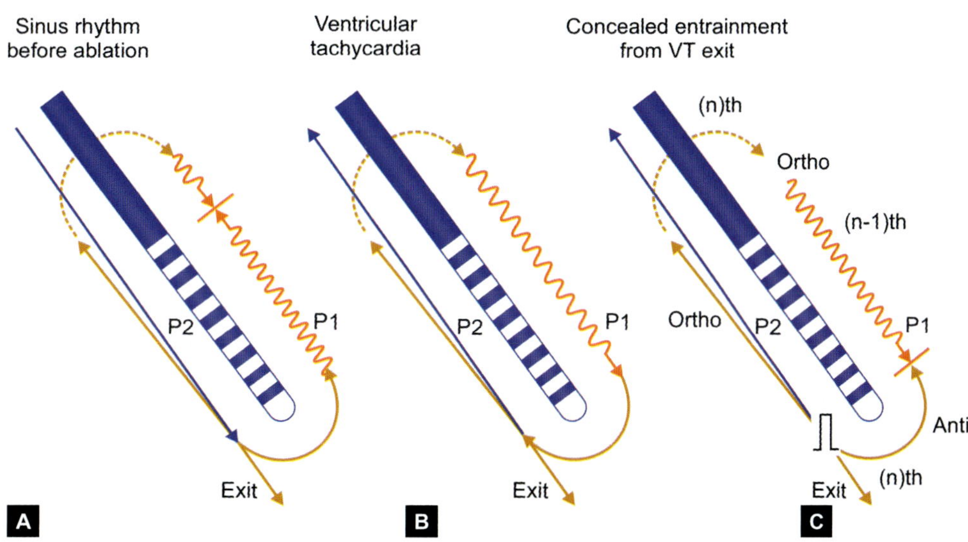

Figures 35.9A to C

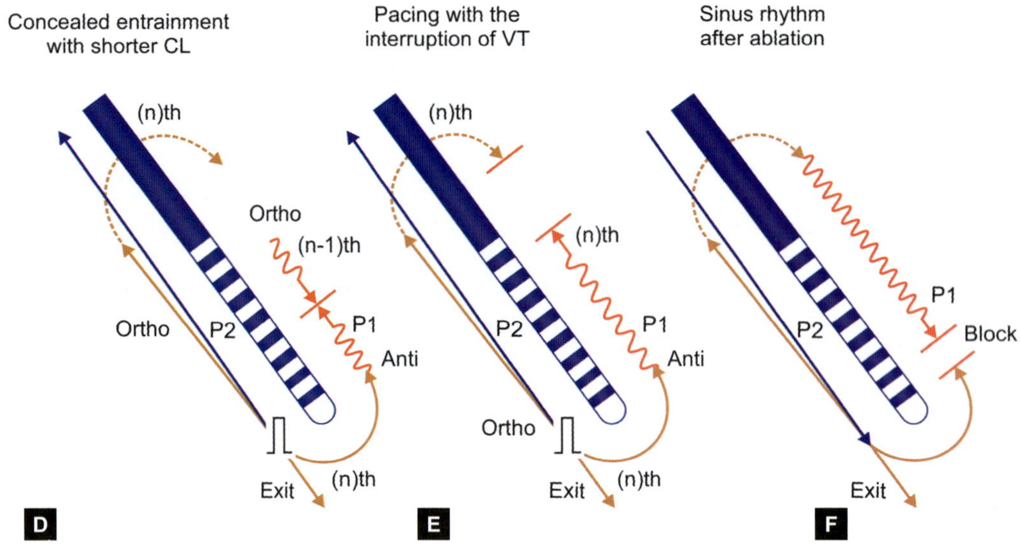

Figures 35.9D to F

Figures 35.9A to F: Schematic representation of the mechanism of left posterior fascicular ventricular tachycardia (VT). See the text for details

Abbreviations: Anti, antidromic wavefront; CL, cycle length; ortho, orthodromic wavefront; P1, diastolic potential; P2, presystolic Purkinje potential; VT, ventricular tachycardia. The dotted lines indicate the ventricular myocardium as the bridge between P1 and left septal myocardium. The undulating line represents a zone of slow conduction

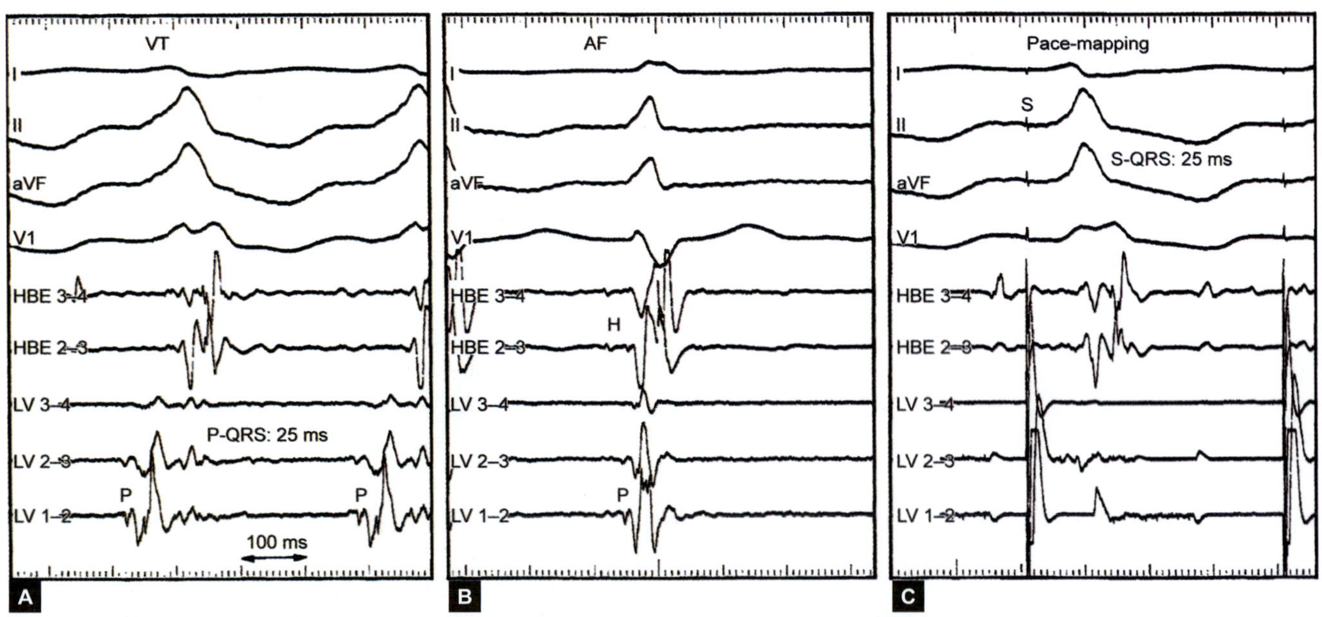

Figures 35.10A to C: Intracardiac electrograms at the ventricular tachycardia (VT) exit site during left anterior fascicular VT. (A) During the VT, the Purkinje potential preceded the QRS (P-QRS) by 25 ms; (B) During the basal rhythm (atrial fibrillation [AF]), a Purkinje potential was recorded after the His bundle potential (H) and before the QRS complex; (C) Pace-mapping at that site produced a similar QRS complex with an interval between the pacing stimulus and QRS (S-QRS) of 25 ms, equal to the P-QRS interval during the VT. The radiofrequency current delivered at that site terminated the VT; however, the VT was still inducible

Abbreviations: HBE, His bundle electrogram; LV, left ventricle

From: Nogami A, Naito S, Tada H, et al. Verapamil-sensitive left anterior fascicular ventricular tachycardia: results of radiofrequency ablation in six patients. J Cardiovasc Electrophysiol. 1998;9:1269-78

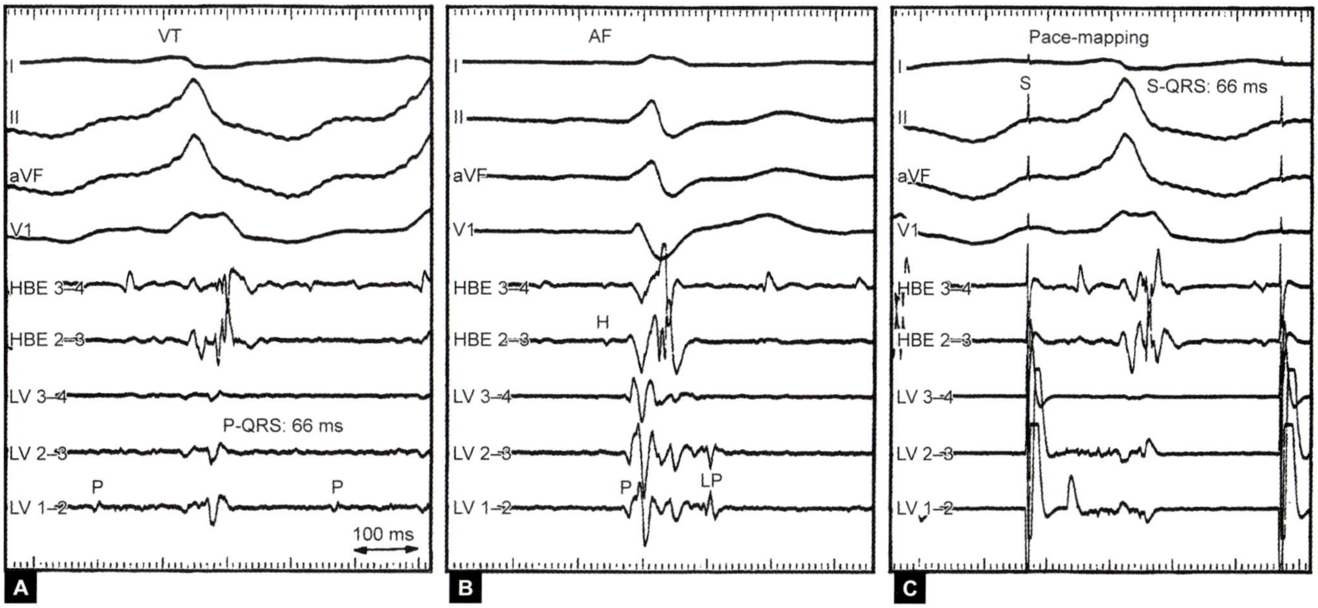

Figures 35.11A to C: (A) Intracardiac electrograms at the zone of slow conduction during left anterior fascicular ventricular tachycardia (VT). (A) During the VT, the Purkinje potential (P) preceded the QRS (P-QRS) by 66 ms; (B) During atrial fibrillation (AF), a Purkinje potential was recorded after the His bundle potential (H) and before the QRS complex, and a late potential (LP) was also recorded after the QRS complex; (C) Pace-mapping at that site produced a similar QRS complex with an interval between the pacing stimulus and QRS (S-QRS) of 66 ms, equal to the P-QRS interval during the VT. The radiofrequency current delivered at that site terminated the VT and suppressed the reinduction of the VT
From: Nogami A, Naito S, Tada H, et al. Verapamil-sensitive left anterior fascicular ventricular tachycardia: results of radiofrequency ablation in six patients. J Cardiovasc Electrophysiol. 1998;9:1269-78

Left Posterior Fascicular Ventricular Tachycardia

Conventional left ventricular septal mapping using a multipolar electrode catheter is useful in patients with left posterior fascicular VT.[18] Electroanatomic activation mapping is not typically required, but the ability to tag catheter positions of interest is often helpful. Two distinct potentials, P1 and P2, can be recorded during the VT from the midseptum **(Figures 35.5A and B)**. Because the diastolic potential (P1) has been proved a critical potential in the VT circuit, this potential can be targeted to cure the tachycardia. Nakagawa and coworkers[24] first reported the importance of Purkinje potentials in the ablation of this VT, and Tsuchiya and associates[27] reported the significance of a late diastolic potential and emphasized the role of late diastolic and presystolic potentials in the VT circuit. However, the successful ablation sites identified by these two research groups were different. Whereas Nakagawa's ablation sites were at the apical-inferior septum of the left ventricle, Tsuchiya's ablation sites were at the basal septal regions close to the main trunk of the left bundle branch. These findings suggest that any P1 during VT can be targeted for catheter ablation. We usually target the apical third of the septum, to avoid the creation of left bundle branch block (LBBB) or atrioventricular block **(Figure 35.13)**.

Using the retrograde aortic approach, the ablation catheter crosses the aortic valve with a tight curve oriented to the right side of the fluoroscopic view in right anterior oblique projection. Once in the left ventricular chamber, the catheter is rotated toward the septum, then the curvature is opened, allowing the tip of the catheter to fall toward the inferior septum toward the apex. In our study, P1 was recorded during the VT in 15 of 20 patients. RF ablation was successfully performed at this site in all 15 patients. During energy application, the P1-QRS interval was gradually prolonged, and the VT was terminated by block between P1 and QRS **(Figure 35.14)**. After termination of the tachycardia, the P1 was noted to occur after the QRS complex during sinus rhythm, whereas the P2 was still observed before the QRS complex. **Figures 35.15A and B** show the potentials during sinus rhythm before and after the successful ablation. After successful ablation, the P1 occurred after the QRS complex, with an identical activation sequence to that observed during the VT. **Figure 35.9F** explains why P1 appears after ablation in the middiastolic period and with the same activation sequence as during the VT. When the distal segment of P1 is ablated, the P1 activation proceeds orthodromically around the circuit and subsequently blocks from a proximal to distal direction during sinus rhythm. The P1 that appears after ablation exhibits decremental properties during atrial pacing or ventricular pacing, or both,

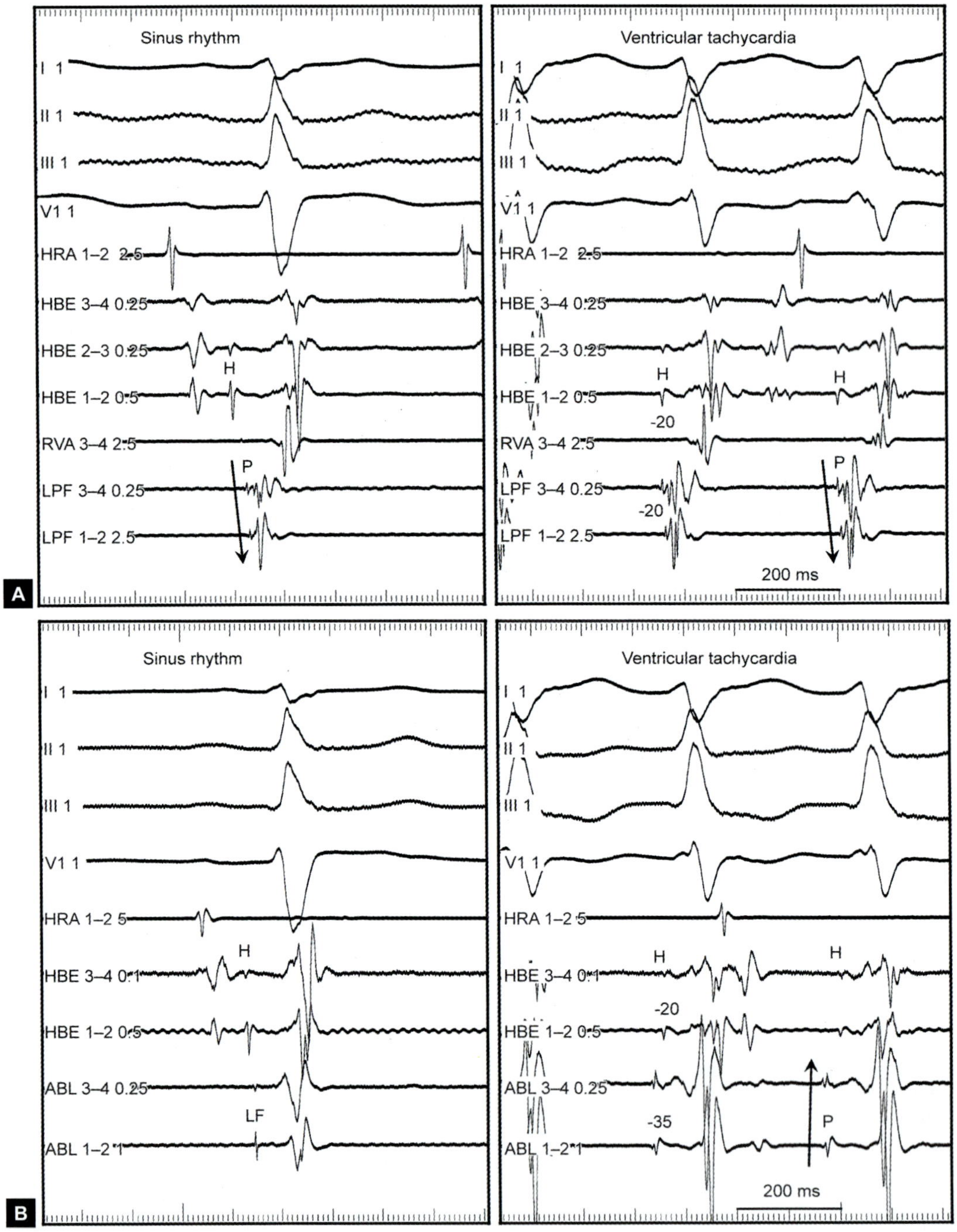

Figures 35.12A and B: Intracardiac electrograms of a left upper septal fascicular ventricular tachycardia (VT). During the VT, there was a retrograde activation of the His bundle (H). The activation sequence of the His bundle potentials was reverse to that during sinus rhythm. The His-ventricular interval is short during the VT. (A) During sinus rhythm, a fused Purkinje potential was recorded at left posterior fascicular (LPF) area. During the VT, recording at the same site also demonstrated a fused Purkinje potential, which preceded the onset of QRS by 20 ms. The activation sequences of Purkinje potentials are similar during sinus rhythm and VT. This site at the left posterior fascicular area is one of exit during VT because a fused presystolic ventricular potential was recorded. And the other exit during VT might be the left anterior fascicular area because the QRS morphology during VT is narrow and exhibited inferior axis; (B) The VT was successfully ablated at the left ventricular upper septum. At that site, a left bundle branch (LF) potential was recorded during sinus rhythm, and the potential preceded the QRS by 35 ms during the VT. The radiofrequency application eliminated the VT without making left bundle branch block or atrioventricular block

Abbreviations: ABL, ablation catheter; HBE, His bundle electrogram; HRA, high right atrium; RVA, right ventricular apex

From: Nogami A. Idiopathic left ventricular tachycardia: assessment and treatment. Card Electrophysiol Rev. 2002;6:448-57

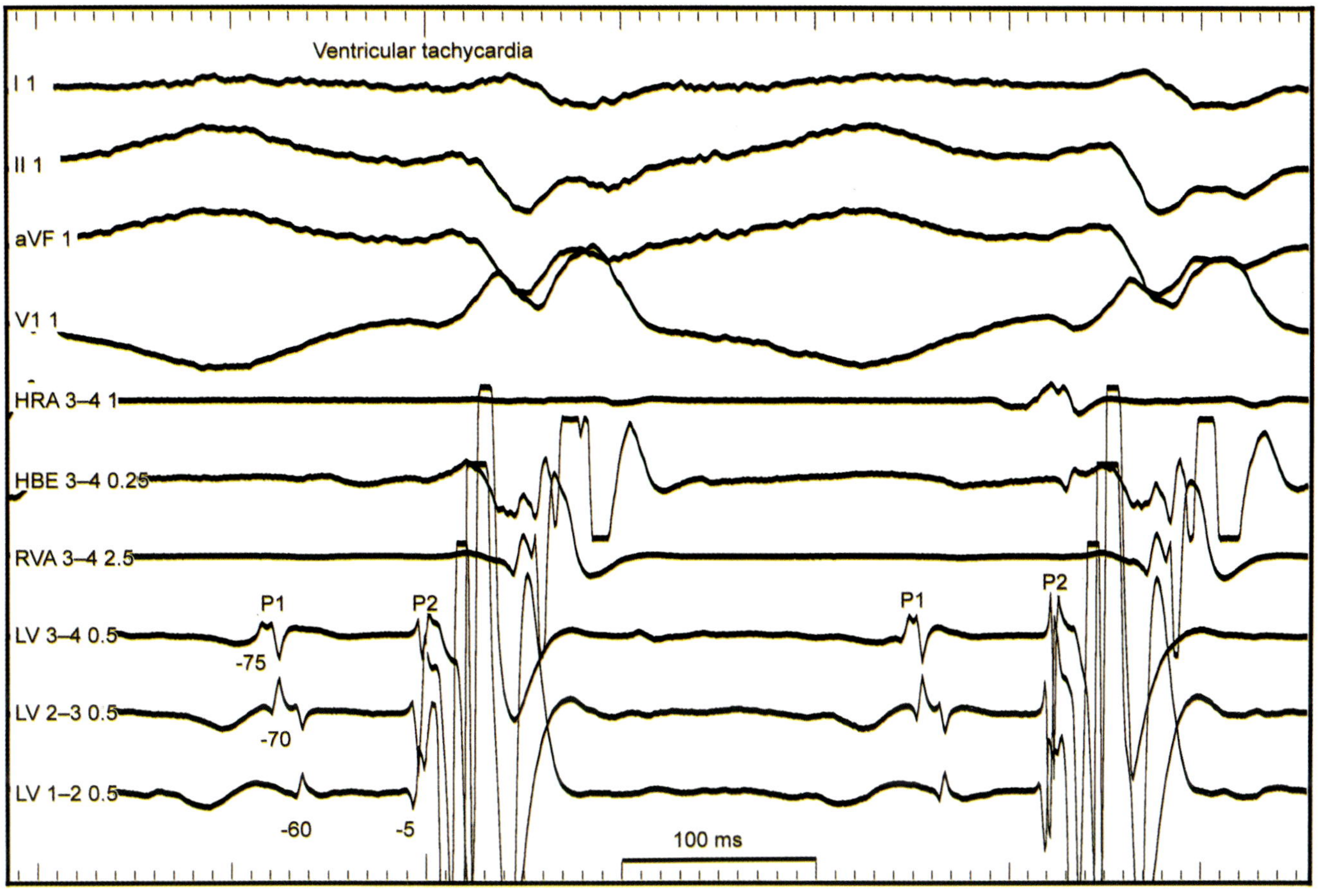

Figure 35.13: Recordings from the site of successful ablation during left posterior fascicular ventricular tachycardia (VT). A diastolic potential (P1) and presystolic Purkinje potential (P2) were recorded in the midseptal area. The proximal two electrodes of the ablation catheter (LV) recorded the diastolic potential (P1) 15 ms earlier than the distal pair of electrodes

Abbreviations: HBE, His bundle electrogram; HRA, high right atrium; RVA, right ventricular apex

From: Nogami A, Naito S, Tada H, et al. Demonstration of diastolic and presystolic Purkinje potential as critical potentials on a macroreentry circuit of verapamil-sensitive idiopathic left ventricular tachycardia. J Am Coll Cardiol. 2000;36:811-23

and the intravenous administration of verapamil significantly prolongs the His-to-P1 interval during sinus rhythm. Pace-mapping at the successful ablation site is usually not good because the selective pacing of P1 is difficult and there is an antidromic activation of the proximal P1 potential. Pace-mapping after successful ablation is sometimes better than before ablation because the antidromic activation of P1 is blocked.[28]

In the remaining 5 of our 20 patients, the diastolic potential (P1) could not be detected, and a single fused P2 was recorded only at the VT exit site. Successful ablation was performed at this site in all 5 patients. We can speculate that the circuit in these patients may have involved less of the Purkinje system or that the area of slow conduction may not have been close to the endocardial surface.

Left Anterior Fascicular Ventricular Tachycardia

Figure 35.2 shows the 12-lead ECGs of verapamil-sensitive left anterior fascicular VTs that we experienced.[22] The mean cycle length of the VT was 390 ± 62 ms, and the mean electrical axis during the VT was 120 ± 16°. Patient 3 also had a typical left posterior fascicular VT. Left ventricular endocardial mapping during left anterior fascicular VT identified the earliest ventricular activation in the anterolateral wall of the left ventricle. RF current delivered to this site suppressed the VT in three patients (patients 1, 2, and 3). The fused Purkinje potential was recorded at that site and preceded the QRS complex by 20 to 35 ms, with pace-mapping exhibiting an optimal match between the paced rhythm and clinical VT.

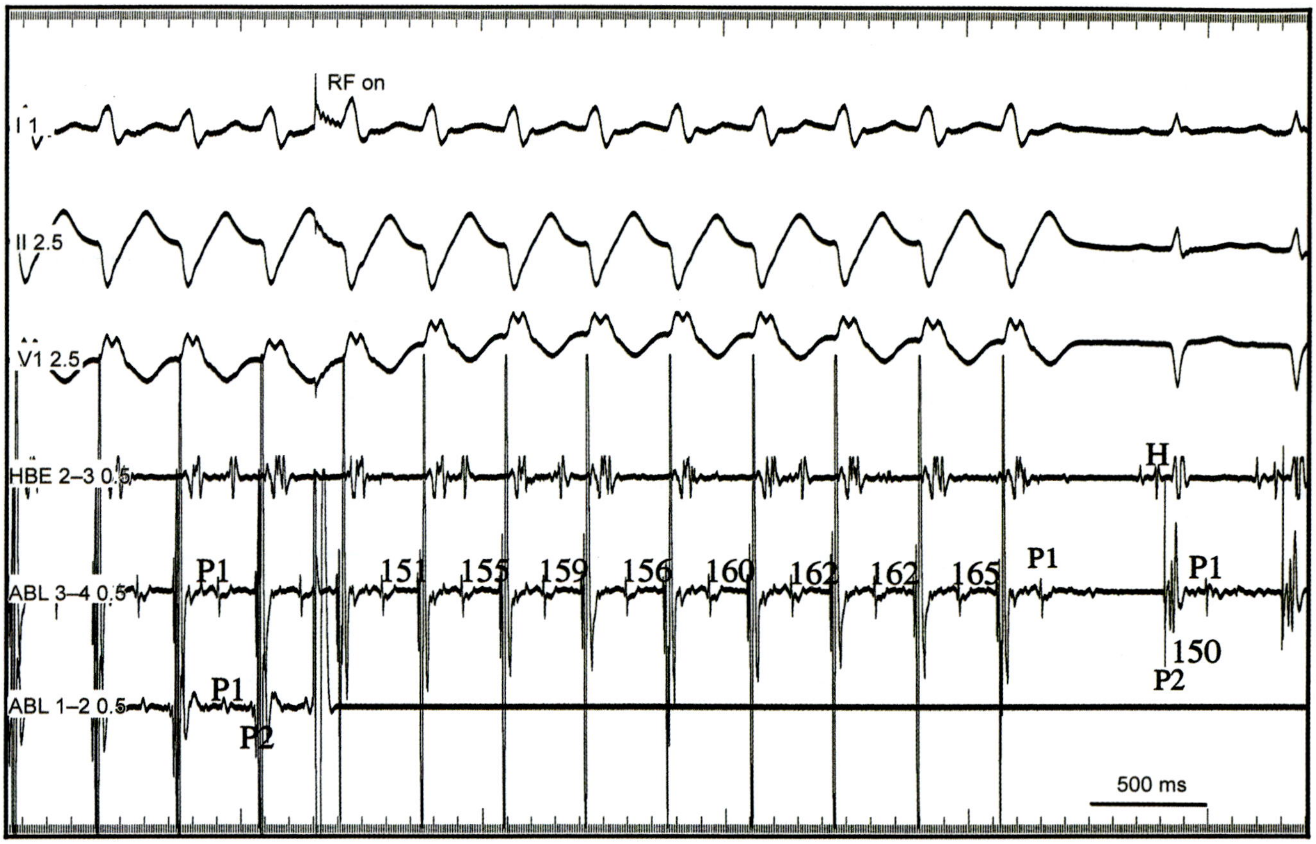

Figure 35.14: An application of radiofrequency (RF) current delivered during left posterior fascicular ventricular tachycardia (VT). During the energy application, the P1-QRS interval gradually prolonged, and the VT was terminated by block between P1 and QRS. After the ablation, the P1 occurred after the QRS complex during sinus rhythm

Abbreviations: ABL, ablation catheter; H, His recording; HBE, His bundle electrogram

From: Nogami A, Naito S, Tada H, et al. Demonstration of diastolic and presystolic Purkinje potential as critical potentials on a macroreentry circuit of verapamil-sensitive idiopathic left ventricular tachycardia. J Am Coll Cardiol. 2000;36:811-23

In the remaining three patients, RF catheter ablation at the site of the earliest ventricular activation was unsuccessful. In these patients, a Purkinje potential was recorded in the diastolic phase during the VT at the midanterior left ventricular septum. The Purkinje potential preceded the QRS during VT by 56 to 66 ms, and catheter ablation at these sites was successful (patients 4, 5, and 6).

Figures 35.10A to C show the intracardiac recording from the VT exit (anterolateral wall) in patient 4. The Purkinje potential preceded the QRS (P-QRS interval) by 25 ms during the VT, and pace-mapping at that site produced a similar QRS complex with an interval between the pacing stimulus and QRS (S-QRS) of 25 ms, equal to the P-QRS interval during VT. RF current delivered at this site terminated the VT; however, the VT was still induced. **Figures 35.11A to C** show the intracardiac recordings from patient 4 at the zone of slow conduction during the VT. The ablation catheter was positioned in the midseptal area, where the diastolic Purkinje potential was recorded. The Purkinje potential was recorded during the VT. Pace-mapping at that site produced a similar QRS complex, with an S-QRS interval of 66 ms, equal to the P-QRS interval during the VT. RF current delivered at this site terminated the VT and suppressed the reinduction of the VT.

One of our patients with the left anterior fascicular VT also had a typical left posterior fascicular VT. Kottkamp and colleagues[29] also reported one patient who had two left VT configurations with right- and left-axis deviation. In this patient, RF catheter ablation delivered to the single site between the left anterior and posterior fascicles successfully eliminated both VTs. This suggests that the antegrade limb is the common pathway.

The circuit of the left anterior fascicular VT was shown in **Figure 35.8B**. In this circuit, P1 represents the activation potential in the proximal portion of the specialized Purkinje tissue with a decremental property. During VT,

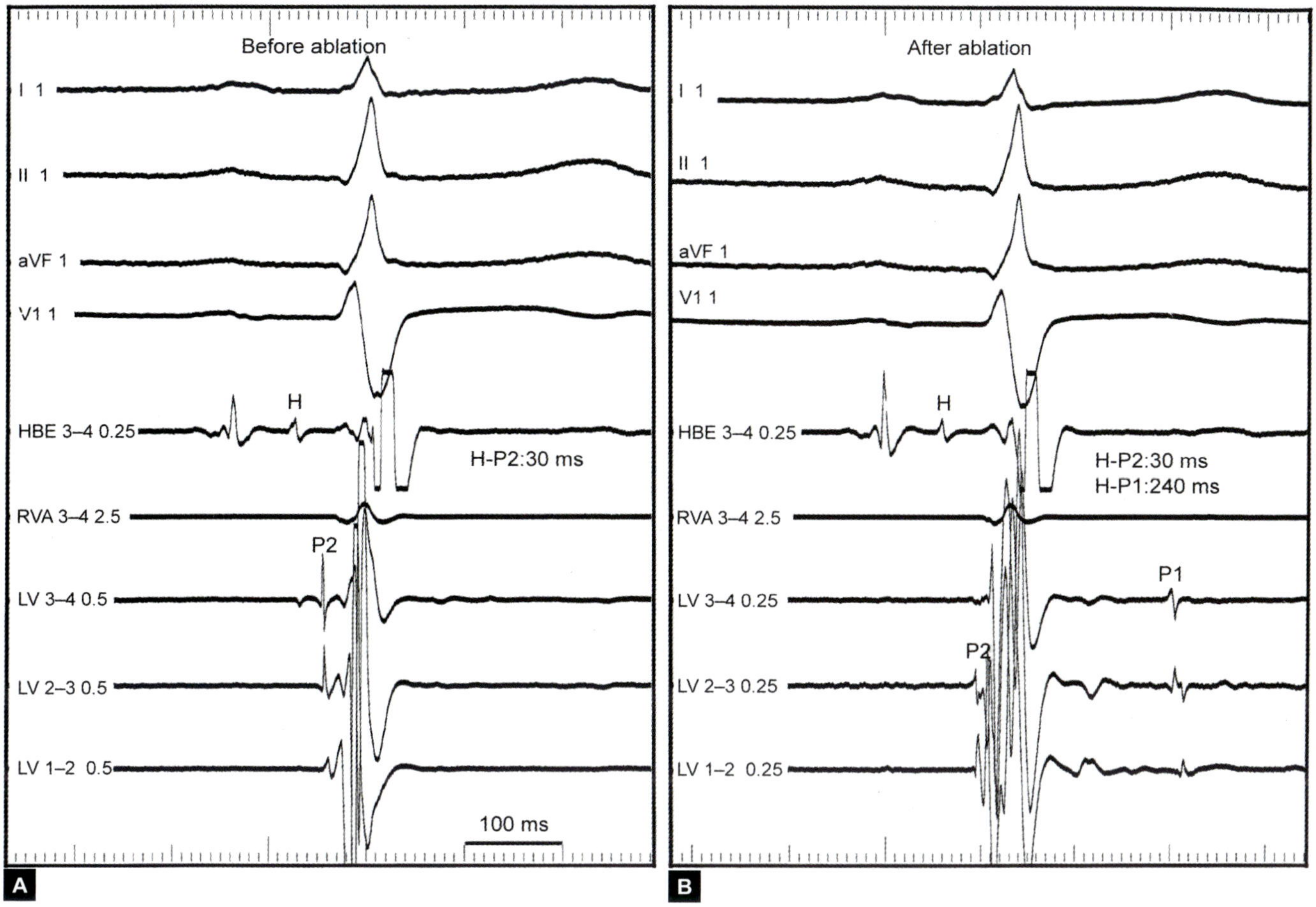

Figures 35.15A and B: Intracardiac recordings during sinus rhythm before and after the successful ablation of left posterior fascicular ventricular tachycardia (VT). (A) Before the ablation, no diastolic potential was observed during sinus rhythm; (B) After the ablation, the P1 occurred after the QRS complex. The activation sequence of P1 was identical to that observed during the VT shown in Figure 35.13

Abbreviations: HBE, His bundle electrogram; LV, left ventricle; RVA, right ventricular apex

From: Nogami A, Naito S, Tada H, et al. Demonstration of diastolic and presystolic Purkinje potential as critical potentials on a macroreentry circuit of verapamil-sensitive idiopathic left ventricular tachycardia. J Am Coll Cardiol. 2000;36:811-23

the antegrade limb is the P1, and the retrograde limb is the left ventricular muscle. This type of VT can be named as left anterior slow-fast type fascicular VT. The circuits of the left anterior and posterior fascicular VTs are mirror images.

Left Upper Septal Fascicular Ventricular Tachycardia

Figures 35.12A and B show the intracardiac electrograms of the upper septal fascicular VT.[12] A fused Purkinje potential was recorded at left posterior fascicular area during sinus rhythm **(Figure 35.12A)**. And during VT, recording at the same site also demonstrated a fused presystolic Purkinje potential, which preceded the onset of QRS by 20 ms. The activation sequences of Purkinje potentials at left posterior fascicular area are similar during sinus rhythm and VT. This site is one of exit during VT because a fused presystolic ventricular potential was recorded. And the other exit site during VT might be left anterior fascicular area because the QRS morphology during VT is quite narrow and exhibited an inferior axis. This VT was successfully ablated at the left ventricular upper septum **(Figure 35.12B)**. At this site, a left bundle branch (left fascicle; LF) potential was recorded during sinus rhythm and the Purkinje potential preceded the QRS by 35 ms during the VT. The RF application eliminated the VT without creating an LBBB or atrioventricular block.

When the P1 is selectively captured during tachycardia, concealed entrainment can be obtained **(Figures 35.16A and B)**.[23] Multipolar electrode catheter on the LV middle septum demonstrates articulate diastolic potential (P1) and presystolic potential (P2) during VT. Activation sequence of

P1 is from distal to proximal, while the activation sequence of P2 is from proximal to distal. These activation sequences of P1 and P2 are reverse pattern of those in left posterior or anterior fascicular VT. Entrainment pacing from the middle septal area with P1 potential selectively captures P1 potential and produces an identical QRS complex to that of the VT with an S-QRS latency of 53 ms, equal to the P1-QRS interval during VT. The difference between the postpacing interval (S-P1) and the VTCL is 10 ms.

The hypothesized VT circuit is depicted in **Figure 35.8C**. In this circuit, P1 represents the activation potential of the specialized Purkinje tissue at left ventricular upper septum. P2 represents the activation of the left anterior and posterior fascicles. Both left anterior and posterior fascicles are the antegrade limbs of the reentrant circuit in VT. This explains why this VT exhibits a narrow QRS configuration and inferior axis. DP represents the common retrograde limb of the circuit in VT and can be ablation target. This type of VT can be named as fast-slow type fascicular VT. The circuit of the left upper septal fascicular VT is the antidromic form of the left anterior and posterior fascicular VTs **(Figures 35.8A to C)**.

End Point of Radiofrequency Ablation

With catheter ablation of verapamil-sensitive idiopathic left VT, no special mapping or ablation system is typically needed. We usually use a quadripolar steerable electrode catheter with or without irrigation. RF energy is delivered using maximum power of 50 W. We deliver RF energy during the tachycardia of left posterior and anterior fascicular VTs. If the VT is terminated or slowed within 15 seconds, additional current is applied for another 60 to 90 seconds. If the initial RF current is ineffective, ablation is directed to a more proximal site with the earlier diastolic potential. If the middiastolic potential cannot be detected, RF current is applied at the VT exit site showing a single fused presystolic Purkinje potential. With upper septal fascicular VT, we deliver RF energy for 30 to 60 seconds during sinus rhythm to avoid atrioventricular block. We perform catheter ablation in this region using a low power output (i.e. 10 W), which can gradually be increased while carefully monitoring for development of a junctional rhythm or atrioventricular block.

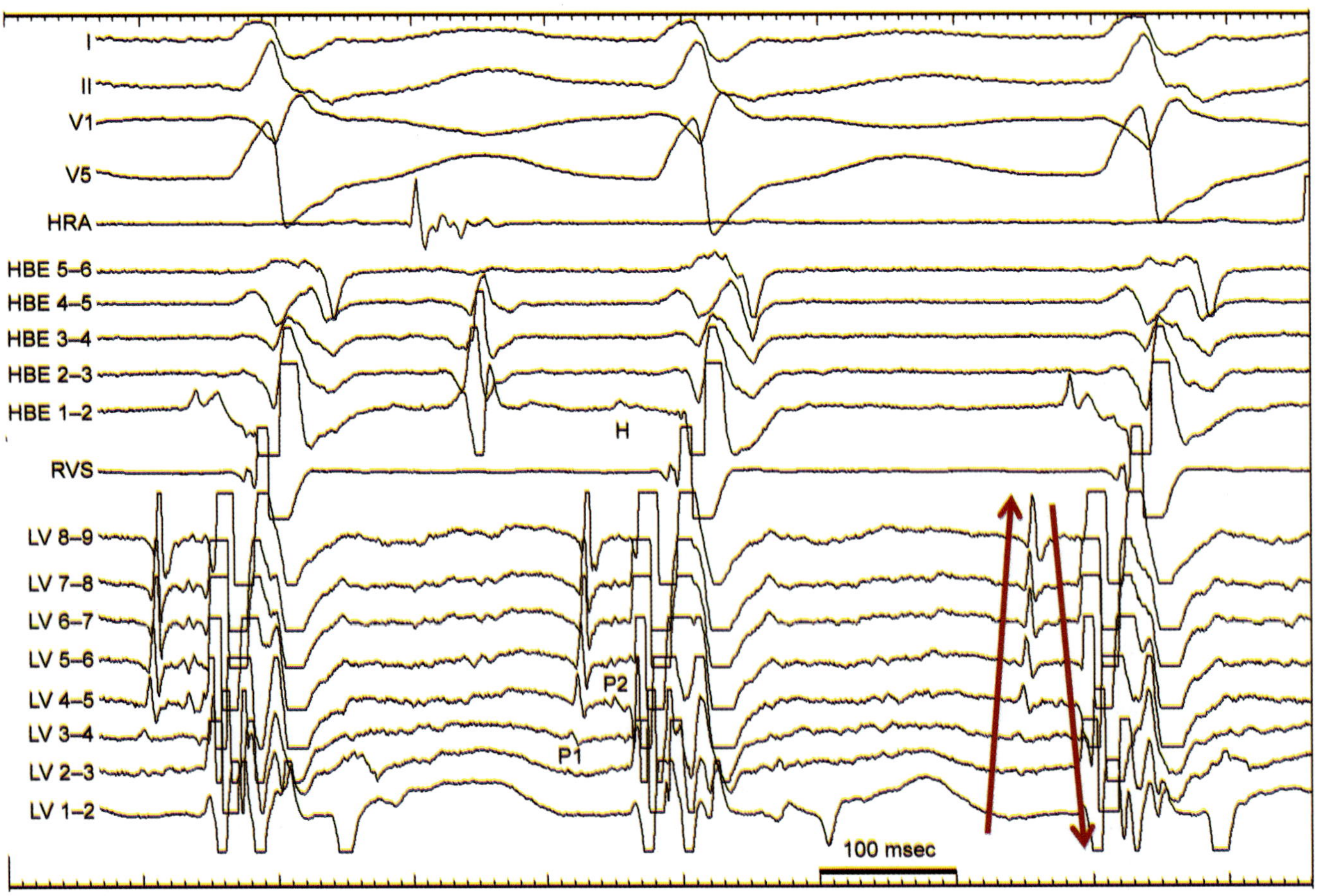

 Figure 35.16A

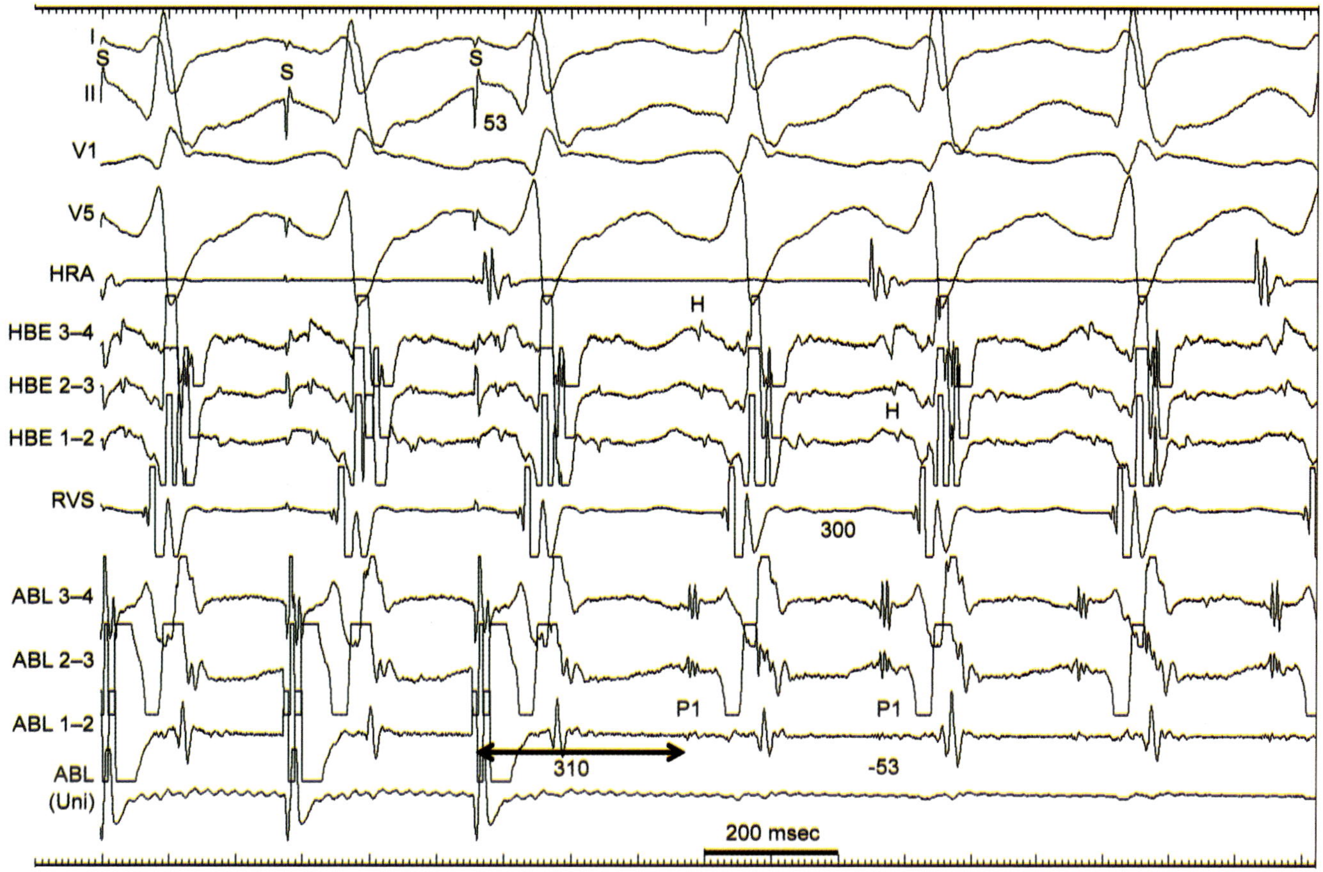

Figure 35.16B

Figures 35.16A and B: Intracardiac recording and entrainment during left upper septal fascicular ventricular tachycardia (VT). (A) Multipolar electrode catheter on the LV midseptum demonstrates articulate diastolic potential (P1) and presystolic potential (P2) during VT. Activation sequence of P1 is from distal to proximal, while the activation sequence of P2 is from proximal to distal; (B) Entrainment pacing from the midseptal area with P1 potential selectively captures P1 potential and produces an identical QRS complex to that of the VT with an S-QRS latency of 53 ms, equal to the P1-QRS interval during VT. The difference between the postpacing interval (S-P1) and the VTCL is 10 ms. RF energy application to the left upper septum slowed and terminated the VT within a few seconds

Abbreviations: ABL, ablation catheter; H, His bundle potential; HRA, high right atrium; LV, left ventricle; P1, diastolic potential; P2, presystolic Purkinje potential; RVS, right ventricular septum; S, stimulation artifact; VTCL, VT cycle length

From: Nishiuchi S, Nogami A, Naito S. A case with occurrence of antidromic tachycardia after ablation of idiopathic left fascicular tachycardia: Mechanism of left upper septal ventricular tachycardia. J Cardiovasc Electrophysiol. 2013;24:825-7

After the ablation, programmed stimulation should be repeated. Other than the noninducibility of VT, there are several electrophysiologic findings that can serve as end points of RF applications for left posterior fascicular VT. After ablation of the distal attachment between P1 and ventricular muscle, P1 appears after the QRS complex **(Figures 35.9F and 35.15)**. However, this phenomenon is not sufficient for an end point because this only indicates conduction block in the direction from the left septal ventricular muscle to P1 only. This unidirectional block can be seen during the baseline state[21] or after an insufficient RF application.[28] To confirm the creation of bidirectional block between P1 and the ventricular muscle, we do atrial pacing with various cycle lengths after the ablation. If there is residual conduction from P1 to the ventricular muscle, a premature ventricular complex (i.e. ventricular echo beat) with a similar QRS morphology as that observed during the VT can be observed repeatedly.

SUCCESS AND RECURRENCE RATES

Our experience at the time of this writing includes 160 patients with left posterior fascicular VT, 30 patients with left anterior fascicular VT, and 8 patients with left upper septal fascicular VT. The success and recurrence rates are 97% and 4%, respectively, for left posterior fascicular VT; 90%

and 11% for left anterior fascicular VT; and 100% and 2.5% for left upper septal fascicular VT.

Aside from the complications that may result from any left ventricular electrophysiologic procedure (e.g. thrombophlebitis, damage to the femoral artery, ventricular perforation), the only complication that has been associated with catheter ablation of idiopathic left VT has been LBBB and atrioventricular block. Tsuchiya and associates[27] reported that 2 patients (12.5%) had transient LBBB after ablation in their series of 16 patients. They targeted the left basal septum, and the LBBB disappeared within 10 minutes without VT recurrence. In our experience, 1 (0.5%) of 198 patients had a transient atrioventricular block. This patient had a left posterior fascicular VT, and the diastolic potential (P1) at the midseptum was targeted for the ablation. Before the ablation, the patient had catheter-induced RBBB. About 15 seconds into the RF delivery, the VT terminated, and second-degree atrioventricular block was observed. The atrioventricular block disappeared immediately after discontinuation of the RF energy delivery.

TROUBLESHOOTING THE DIFFICULT CASE

Inability to reliably induce VT is a formidable obstacle to successful ablation. Isoproterenol facilitates induction of sustained VT in 60% to 70% of those patients without inducible sustained VT at baseline. In some patients, the administration of small doses of class Ia drugs enhances the slow conduction at the specialized Purkinje tissue and facilitates induction of stable sustained VT. Catheter mapping sometimes mechanically suppresses the conduction in the VT circuit ("bump" phenomenon). In such cases, a ventricular echo beat during sinus rhythm or atrial pacing is useful. If premature ventricular complexes with a similar QRS morphology to that observed during the VT are repeatedly seen, activation mapping can be performed. If no ventricular echo beats are inducible, the empirical anatomic approach can be an effective strategy for ablation of left posterior fascicular VT.[30] First, the VT exit site is sought by pace-mapping during sinus rhythm, and RF energy is delivered to that site. Second, a linear lesion is placed at the midseptum, perpendicular to the long-axis of the left ventricle, about 10 to 15 mm proximal to the VT exit. During anatomic linear ablation, P1 suddenly appears after the QRS complex if the ablation site is on the descending limb of the VT circuit. This anatomic approach is also useful in patients in whom diastolic Purkinje potential cannot be recorded during VT. **Figure 35.17** shows activation mapping during VT. Although the earliest myocardial activation site was observed at the inferoapical septum, diastolic potential could not be recorded. RF energy application to this exit site was ineffective. A linear RF lesion about 10 mm proximal to the VT exit was also ineffective. And finally, more proximal linear lesion successfully suppressed the VT.

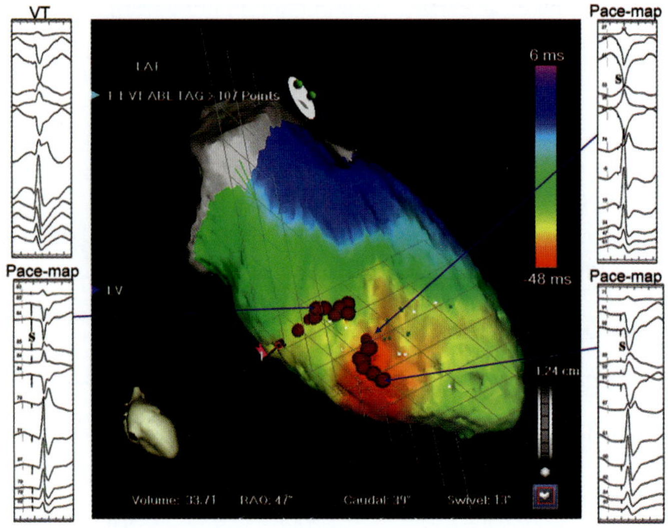

Figure 35.17: Anatomic approach when diastolic Purkinje potential cannot be recorded during ventricular tachycardia (VT). While the earliest myocardial activation site was observed at the inferoapical septum, diastolic potential could not be recorded. First, radiofrequency (RF) energy was delivered to the exit site, but that was ineffective. Second, a linear RF lesion about 10 mm proximal to the VT exit was created, but that was also ineffective. Finally, more proximal linear lesion successfully suppressed VT induction

Abbreviations: LAT, lateral projection; LV, left ventricle; RAO, right anterior oblique projection

If a good electrogram is not found at the septum, one possible reason is poor catheter contact with the septum. The left anterior oblique fluoroscopic view is used to guide the catheter toward the septum, and the right anterior oblique view to guide the catheter posteriorly and toward the apical third of the septum.

If ablation catheter stability is poor during the VT because of excessive heart motion, RF energy can be delivered during sinus rhythm. However, even during sinus rhythm, frequent ventricular premature beats (with a similar QRS morphology to that observed during the VT) and VT are sometimes induced during the RF energy application. In such cases, overdrive pacing or intravenous administration of verapamil is effective for suppressing the ventricular premature beats and VT during the RF energy application. However, after such an infusion, the noninducibility of the VT becomes invalid as an end point for the ablation. Cryoablation of left fascicular VT has been reported in a selected population.[31] Cryoablation is effective given the superficial nature of the reentrant circuit and may offer the advantages of no induction of premature ventricular complexes and extreme catheter stability during ablation.

REFERENCES

1. Lerman BB, Stein KM, Markowitz SM. Mechanism of idiopathic ventricular tachycardia. J Cardiovasc Electrophysiol. 1997;8: 571-83.
2. Okumura K, Tsuchiya T. Idiopathic left ventricular tachycardia: clinical features, mechanism and management. Card Electrophysiol Rev. 2002;6:61-7.
3. Coggins DL, Lee RJ, Sweeney J, Chein WW, Van Hare G, Epstein L, Gonzalez R, Griffin JC, Lesh MD, Scheinman MM. Radiofrequency catheter ablation as a cure for idiopathic tachycardia of both left and right ventricular origin. J Am Coll Cardiol. 1994;23:1333-41.
4. Daoud E, Morady F. Catheter ablation of ventricular tachycardia. Curr Opin Cardiol. 1995;10:21-5.
5. Ito S, Tada H, Naito S, Kurosaki K, Ueda M, Hoshizaki H, Miyamori I, Oshima S, Taniguchi K, Nogami A. Development and validation of an ECG algorithm for identifying the optimal ablation site for idiopathic ventricular outflow tract tachycardia. J Cardiovasc Electrophysiol. 2003;14:1280-6.
6. Callans DJ, Menz V, Schwartzman D, Gottlieb CD, Marchlinski FE. Repetitive monomorphic tachycardia from the left ventricular outflow tract: Electrocardiographic patterns consistent with a left ventricular site of origin. J Am Coll Cardiol. 1997;29:1023-7.
7. Kanagaratnam L, Tomassoni G, Schweikert R, Pavia S, Bash D, Beheiry S, Neibauer M, Saliba W, Chung M, Tchou P, Natale A. Ventricular tachycardias arising from the aortic sinus of Valsalva: An under-recognized variant of left outflow tract ventricular tachycardia. J Am Coll Cardiol. 2001;37: 1408-14.
8. Ouyang F, Fotuhi P, Ho SY, Hebe J, Volkmer M, Goya M, Burns M, Antz M, Ernst S, Cappato R, Kuck KH. Repetitive monomorphic ventricular tachycardia originating from the aortic sinus cusp: electrocardiographic characterization for guiding catheter ablation. J Am Coll Cardiol. 2002;39:500-8.
9. Zipes DP, Foster PR, Troup PJ, Pedersen DH. Atrial induction of ventricular tachycardia: reentry versus triggered automaticity. Am J Cardiol. 1979;44:1-8.
10. Belhassen B, Rotmensch HH, Laniado S. Response of recurrent sustained ventricular tachycardia to verapamil. Br Heart J. 1981;46:679-82.
11. Ohe T, Shimomura K, Aihara N, Kamakura S, Matsuhisa M, Sato I, Nakagawa H, Shimizu A. Idiopathic sustained left ventricular tachycardia: clinical and electrophysiological characteristics. Circulation. 1988;77:560-8.
12. Nogami A, Idiopathic left ventricular tachycardia: assessment and treatment. Card Electrophysiol Rev. 2002;6:448-57.
13. Gallagher JJ, Selle JG, Svenson RH, Fedor JM, Zimmern SH, Sealy WC, Robicsek FR. Surgical treatment of arrhythmias. Am J Cardiol. 1988;61:27A-44A.
14. Suwa M, Yoneda Y, Nagao H, Sakai Y, Nakayama Y, Hirota Y, Kawamura K, Iwa T. Surgical correction of idiopathic paroxysmal ventricular tachycardia possibly related to left ventricular false tendon. Am J Cardiol. 1989;64:1217-20.
15. Thakur RK, Klein GJ, Sivaram CA, Zardini M, Schleinkofer DE, Nakagawa H, Yee R, Jackman WM. Anatomic substrate for idiopathic left ventricular tachycardia. Circulation. 1996;93: 497-501.
16. Maruyama M, Terada T, Miyamoto S, Ino T. Demonstration of the reentrant circuit of verapamil-sensitive idiopathic left ventricular tachycardia: direct evidence for macroreentry as the underlying mechanism. J Cardiovasc Electrophysiol. 2001; 12:968-72.
17. Lin FC, Wen MS, Wang CC, Yeh SJ, Wu D. Left ventricular fibromuscular band is not a specific substrate for idiopathic left ventricular tachycardia. Circulation. 1996;93:525-7.
18. Nogami A, Naito S, Tada H, Taniguchi K, Okamoto Y, Nishimura S, Yamauchi Y, Aonuma K, Goya M, Iesaka Y, Hiroe M. Demonstration of diastolic and presystolic Purkinje potential as critical potentials on a macroreentry circuit of verapamil-sensitive idiopathic left ventricular tachycardia. J Am Coll Cardiol. 2000;36:811-23.
19. Kuo JY, Tai CT, Chiang CE, Yu WC, Huang JL, Hsieh MH, Hou CJ, Tsai CH, Ding YA, Chen SA. Is the fascicle of left bundle branch involved in the reentrant circuit of verapamil-sensitive idiopathic left ventricular tachycardia? Pacing Clin Electrophysiol. 2003;26:1986-92.
20. Morishima I, Nogami A, Tsuboi H, Sone T. Negative participation of the left posterior fascicle in the reentry circuit of verapamil-sensitive idiopathic left ventricular tachycardia. Heart Rhythm. 2012;23:556-9.
21. Ouyang F, Cappato R, Ernst S, Goya M, Volkmer M, Hebe J, Antz M, Vogtmann T, Schaumann A, Fotuhi P, Hoffmann-Riem M, Kuck KH. Electroanatomic substrate of idiopathic left ventricular tachycardia: Unidirectional block and macroreentry within the Purkinje network. Circulation. 2002;105: 462-9.
22. Nogami A, Naito S, Tada H, Oshima S, Taniguchi K, Aonuma K, Iesaka Y. Verapamil-sensitive left anterior fascicular ventricular tachycardia: Results of radiofrequency ablation in six patients. J Cardiovasc Electrophysiol. 1998;9:1269-78.
23. Nishiuchi S, Nogami A, Naito S. A case with occurrence of antidromic tachycardia after ablation of idiopathic left fascicular tachycardia: Mechanism of left upper septal ventricular tachycardia. J Cardiovasc Electrophysiol. 2013;24:825-7.
24. Nakagawa H, Beckman KJ, McClelland JH, Wang X, Arruda M, Santoro I, Hazlitt HA, Abdalla I, Singh A, Gossinger H, et al. Radiofrequency catheter ablation of idiopathic left ventricular tachycardia guided by a Purkinje potential. Circulation. 1993;88:2607-17.
25. Yeh SJ, Wen MS, Wang CC, Lin FC, Wu D. Adenosine-sensitive ventricular tachycardia from the anterobasal left ventricle. J Am Coll Cardiol. 1997;30:339-45.
26. Crijns HJ, Smeets JL, Rodriguez LM, Meijer A. Cure of interfascicular reentrant ventricular tachycardia by ablation to anterior fascicle of the left bundle branch. J Cardiovasc Electrophysiol. 1995;6:486-92.
27. Tsuchiya T, Okumura K, Honda T, Iwasa A, Yasue H, Tabuchi T. Significance of late diastolic potential preceding Purkinje potential in verapamil-sensitive idiopathic left ventricular tachycardia. Circulation. 1999;99:2408-13.
28. Tada H, Nogami A, Naito S, Tomita T, Oshima S, Taniguchi K, Aonuma K, Iesaka Y. Retrograde Purkinje potential activation during sinus rhythm following catheter ablation of idiopathic left ventricular tachycardia. J Cardiovasc Electrophysiol. 1998; 9:1218-24.
29. Kottkamp H, Chen X, Hindricks G, Willems S, Haverkamp W, Wichter T, Breithardt G, Borggrefe M. Idiopathic left ventricular tachycardia: new insights into electrophysiological characteristics and radiofrequency catheter ablation. Pacing Clin Electrophysiol. 1995;18:1285-97.

30. Lin D, Hsia HH, Gerstenfeld EP, Dixit S, Callans DJ, Nayak H, Russo A, Marchlinski FE. Idiopathic fascicular left ventricular tachycardia: Linear ablation lesion strategy for noninducible or nonsustained tachycardia. Heart Rhythm. 2005;2:934-9.

31. Timmermans C, Manusama R, Alzand B, Rodriguez LM. Catheter-based cryoablation of postinfarction and idiopathic ventricular tachycardia: initial experience in a selected population. J Cardiovasc Electrophysiol. 2010;21:255-61.

EDITORS' SUMMARY

One of the pioneers in drawing attention to the importance of carefully annotating the sensed electrograms with fascicular tachycardia— Professor Nogami—has written for us an incredibly lucid and engaging discourse on this difficult topic. The figures that he has selected largely tell us the entire story from diagnosis to difficulties and success with conduction system-related ventricular tachycardia. He provides an informative yet balanced look at what the signals that we see mean and what does and does not constitute a desirable site for where to target energy delivery.

The reader would be encouraged to carefully analyze the intracardiac electrograms without reading the tracings and then comparing notes with an international expert's (Professor Nogami's) interpretation of these tracings. Episodic review of these tracings and the relevant paragraphs in the chapter prior to beginning an ablation procedure for a patient with suspected fascicular tachycardia would likely prove very useful in maximizing success and maintaining safety with these complex procedures.

CHAPTER 36

Jackson J Liang, Sanjay Dixit

Idiopathic Outflow Tract Ventricular Tachycardia

LIST OF ABBREVIATIONS

AAD	Antiarrhythmic Drug	LVOT	Left Ventricular Outflow Tract
AIV	Anterior Interventricular Vein	MA	Mitral Annulus
AMC	Aortomitral Continuity	NCC	Noncoronary Cusp
AMP	Adenosine Monophosphate	OTVT	Outflow Tract Ventricular Tachycardia
ARVC	Arrhythmogenic Right Ventricular Cardiomyopathy	PA	Pulmonary Artery
ASC	Aortic Sinus Cusps	PVC	Premature Ventricular Contraction
cAMP	Cyclic Adenosine Monophosphate	RBBB	Right Bundle Branch Block
DAD	Delayed Afterdepolarization	RCA	Right Coronary Artery
GCV	Great Cardiac Vein	RCC	Right Coronary Cusp
LAD	Left Anterior Descending	RFA	Radiofrequency Ablation
LBBB	Left Bundle Branch Block	RV	Right Ventricle
LCC	Left Coronary Cusp	RVOT	Right Ventricular Outflow Tract
LMCA	Left Main Coronary Artery	SOO	Site of Origin
LV	Left Ventricle	TZI	Transition Zone Index
LVEF	Left Ventricular Ejection Fraction	VT	Ventricular Tachycardia

INTRODUCTION

While ventricular tachycardia (VT) typically occurs in patients with structural heart disease, a minority (10%) of patients with VT have structurally normal hearts.[1] VT in these patients is associated with a more benign prognosis, and has been termed "idiopathic" VT. Idiopathic VT comprises a diverse group of arrhythmias which have been sub-classified based on the underlying mechanisms (triggered activity, abnormal automaticity, or reentry) and/or the clinical presentation. These arrhythmias have been further classified based on the site and/or region of origin as determined by the electrocardiographic characteristics (QRS morphology and axis).

Outflow tract tachycardias (OTVTs) comprise the largest subgroup of idiopathic VTs. As the name suggests, these arrhythmias arise from the outflow tract region (right and left ventricular outflow tracts [RVOT and LVOT]) which also includes the aortic sinus cusps [ASC], pulmonary artery [PA], and left ventricular (LV) summit. Other types of idiopathic VT include fascicular tachycardias, papillary muscle and moderator band VT, etc. This chapter will focus on OTVTs.

We will review the epidemiology, clinical presentation, mechanism, treatment and prognosis of OTVTs. Particular focus will be placed on anatomy of the outflow tract region as well as the electrocardiographic (ECG) characteristics of OTVTs. Understanding these concepts in our opinion, is crucial for optimizing successful catheter ablation of these arrhythmias.

MECHANISM OF ARRHYTHMIA

The mechanism underlying OTVT is accepted to be delayed afterdepolarization mediated triggered activity.[2] Nearly three decades ago, Lerman et al. observed that interventions which reduced the amount of intracellular cyclic adenosine monophosphate (cAMP) could terminate or prevent induction of OTVT, suggesting that the mechanism of the arrhythmia was cAMP-mediated triggered activity.[2] Cyclic AMP (cAMP) facilitates intracellular calcium release (via the calcium channel) which can overwhelm the ability of the sarcoplasmic reticulum to absorb the ion. The resulting transient calcium overload causes afterdepolarizations which result in action potential generation at the end of the repolarization phase, hence the name, delayed afterdepolarization (DAD). Intracellular cAMP levels are regulated by interplay of different receptors. Adenosine A1 receptors and muscarinic cholinergic receptors inhibit adenylate cyclase activity, while beta-adrenergic receptors enhance the activity of this enzyme. Thus, cAMP levels are increased by beta-agonists such as isoproterenol and decreased by beta receptor blockers. Adenosine (via the inhibitory adenosine receptors) as well as acetylcholine and vagal maneuvers (through their effects on the inhibitory muscarinic cholinergic receptors) result in decreased intracellular cAMP.[2,3] Agents that enhance cAMP levels increase OTVTs and those which diminish cAMP inhibit OTVTs. Calcium channel blockers exert their effect through inhibition of the calcium channel which in turn decreases intracellular calcium and thus inhibit OTVT. The differing site of action of calcium channel and beta receptor blockers allows these drugs to have a synergistic effect in suppressing OTVT.[4]

Increase in underlying heart rates (through rapid atrial/ventricular pacing or programmed stimulation) facilitates OTVT.[5] These arrhythmias are also promoted by high catecholamine states, as occurs during or immediately post-exercise. Caffeine can also have a proarrhythmic affect. In women, hormonal influences (i.e. premenstrual, gestational, perimenopausal, oral contraceptive use) have been shown to be stronger triggers for these arrhythmias than exercise.[6]

EPIDEMIOLOGY

While idiopathic OTVTs can manifest at any age and in both genders, the most common age group is during the third to fifth decade of life.[7] RVOT VT is more frequently seen in women, while LVOT VT may be slightly more prevalent in men.[8-10]

CLINICAL PRESENTATION

The most common clinical presentation of OTVT is either isolated premature ventricular contractions (PVCs) or non-sustained repetitive monomorphic VT, and these account for 60 to 90% of cases.[5] Sustained VT is relatively uncommon and may be observed infrequently during stress testing or other catecholaminergic states.[11]

Palpitations are the most common symptom in patients with idiopathic VT, although patients may also experience fatigue, chest pain, or lightheadedness. Syncope is relatively uncommon (10%) in these patients and the underlying mechanism has been speculated to be baroreceptor reflex.[12] Sudden death is extremely rare in patients with true idiopathic VT. However, it is important to rule out other cardiomyopathies in patients with OTVT. This is particularly important in patients manifesting pleomorphic morphologies especially if the left ventricular ejection fraction (LVEF) is not normal and/or there is evidence of right ventricular (RV) dilation or dysfunction.

Differentiating from Arrhythmogenic Right Ventricular Cardiomyopathy (ARVC)

While idiopathic VT has a benign prognosis, in patients manifesting OTVT it is important to exclude early ARVC. Multiple studies have identified electrocardiographic characteristics that can help distinguish idiopathic RVOT VT from ARVC.[13,14] Hoffmayer, et al. found that compared with RVOT VT, the QRS complex during VT in ARVC patients was longer in duration in lead I (150 ± 31 ms vs. 123 ± 34 ms; $p = 0.006$), more frequently exhibited V6 precordial transition (18 vs. 0%, $p = 0.005$), and more frequently had at least one lead with QRS notching (65 vs. 21%; $p = 0.001$).[13] A subsequent scoring algorithm based on ECG characteristics was created using data from a derivation cohort of patients with VT of left bundle branch block (LBBB) morphology with inferior axis which was validated in a prospective cohort.[14] Additionally, modalities such as signal-averaged ECG, cardiac MRI, and electroanatomic mapping to identify occult scar may be helpful to rule out ARVC[15-18] **(Figures 36.1A to C)**.

Tachycardia and PVC-induced Cardiomyopathy

In the past, PVCs were generally considered to be benign, but high PVC burden has been associated with lower LVEF in patients without any other structural heart disease, a disease process known as "PVC-induced cardiomyopathy".[19]

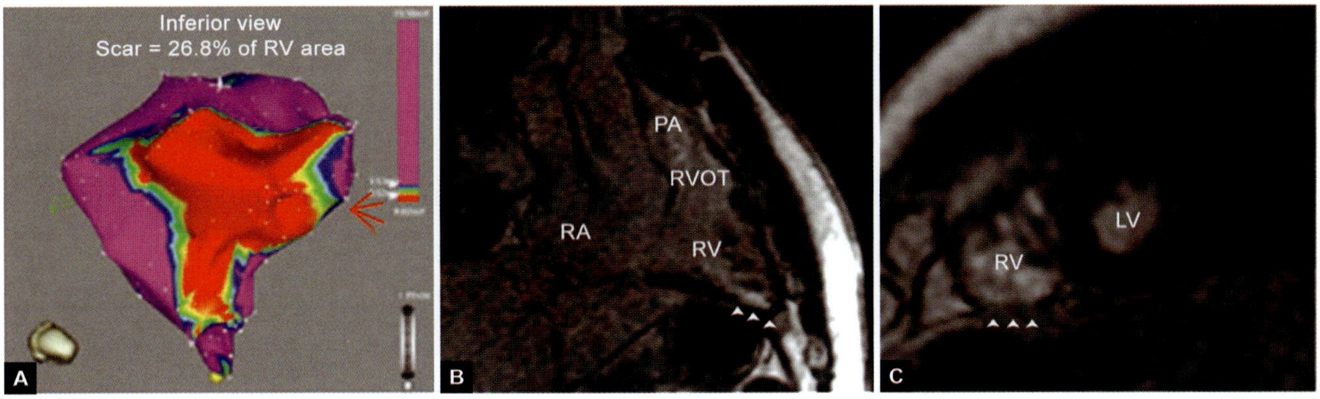

Figures 36.1A to C: Electroanatomic map (A) demonstrating large area of low voltage consistent with scar. Contrast-enhanced cardiac magnetic resonance showing late gadolinium enhancement in the apicoinferior wall as seen in RV long-axis (B, arrowheads) and short-axis planes (C, arrowheads)

Abbreviations: PA, pulmonary artery; LV, left ventricle; RA, right atrium; RV, right ventricle; RVOT, right ventricular outflow tract

From: Santangeli P, Hamilton-Craig C, Dello Russo A, et al. Imaging of scar in patients with ventricular arrhythmias of right ventricular origin: cardiac magnetic resonance versus electroanatomic mapping. J Cardiovasc Electrophysiol. 2011;22:1359-66

In fact, one recent population-based study associated a higher PVC burden with increased rates of systolic dysfunction, incident heart failure, and even increased overall mortality.[20] The mechanisms of PVC-induced cardiomyopathy may be multifactorial.[21] The overall PVC burden necessary for development of LV dysfunction is ≥10%.[22-25] Additional factors that have been implicated in the development of PVC-induced cardiomyopathy include wider QRS duration of PVCs, greater PVC coupling interval dispersion and the sites of origin.[26-29]

In patients with PVC-induced cardiomyopathy, catheter ablation has been shown to be beneficial for both reducing the PVC burden and improving systolic function. The QRS duration during sinus rhythm appears to be an independent predictor of recovery of LV function. We have shown that patients with wider QRS complexes tend to have less recovery of LVEF despite successful PVC ablation. Among those with depressed systolic function (LVEF < 50%) in our cohort, the mean QRS duration among those with >10% improvement in LVEF was 158 ms, compared with 173 ms in those whose LVEF did not improve after ablation ($p < 0.01$).[30] Additionally, the magnitude of recovery appears to be inversely related to residual PVC burden, and we have shown that a >80% reduction in PVC burden has a comparable effect on LVEF recovery as complete abolition of all PVCs.[31]

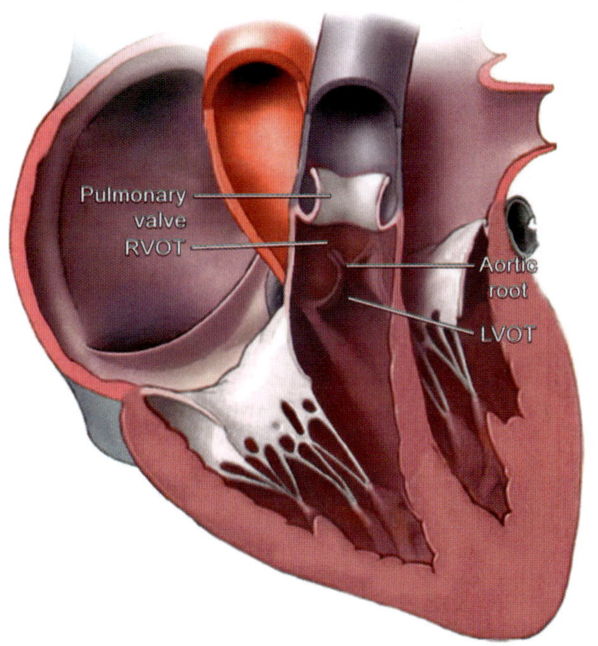

Figure 36.2: Anatomical relationship of the ventricular outflow tracts. The right ventricular outflow tract (RVOT) is anterior to the left ventricular outflow tract (LVOT) and curves leftward as it rises. As such, the distal RVOT and pulmonary artery is actually located leftward of the LVOT and aortic root

From: Hai JJ, Lachman N, Syed FF, et al. The anatomic basis for ventricular arrhythmia in the normal heart: What the student of anatomy needs to know. Clin Anat 2014;27:885-93

ANATOMY OF THE OUTFLOW TRACT REGION

A thorough understanding of the anatomical relationship between the relevant structures is critical for successful localization and ablation of OTVT.[32,33] In-vivo, the heart sits in the thoracic cavity with a leftward rotation and downward apical tilt, such that the RVOT is the most anterior cardiac structure. The LVOT lies posterior to and slightly below the RVOT **(Figure 36.2)**. It is important to recognize the orientation between the RVOT and LVOT. One should think of the RVOT as a tubular structure which twists leftward and crosses the LVOT as it rises superiorly. As such, while the proximal RVOT lies to the right of the LVOT, the distal RVOT and pulmonary artery are actually located to the left of the LVOT and aortic root.

Right Ventricular Outflow Tract

The RVOT is formed by the cone-shaped subpulmonary infundibulum of the RV. It typically extends from the level of the tricuspid valve (entrance) to the pulmonic valve (superior limit). This region is comprised of the free-wall, septum, posterior (rightward) and anterior (leftward) aspect.[34] The septal aspect of the RVOT is directly anterior to the aortic valve and the superior RVOT extends above the aortic cusp region. The left main coronary artery (LMCA) runs near the posterior pulmonic valve cusps, the right coronary artery (RCA) runs near the RVOT and the proximal left anterior descending (LAD) coronary artery runs near the superior anterior septal aspect of the RVOT. The posterior or septal aspect of RVOT is relatively thick and in close proximity to the aortic root.[35] The superior aspect of the RVOT (under the pulmonic valve) has been implicated to be the most common source of arrhythmias arising from this region.[10]

Left Ventricular Outflow Tract

Most foci of idiopathic VT from the LVOT originate in and around the aortic and mitral valves. Both these valves attach to an elliptical structure termed the "LV ostium" which is located at the base of the LV[36] **(Figure 36.3)**. There are certain locations in this region which tend be more common sources of OTVT including the area of the aortomitral continuity (AMC), superior aspect of the mitral valve and the LV summit. The latter is a triangular portion of the LVOT on the epicardium that is located between the bifurcation of the LAD and left circumflex arteries (superiorly), the 1st septal perforator of the LAD (inferiorly) and is bisected by the great cardiac vein (GCV) as it transitions into the anterior interventricular vein (AIV)[37,38] **(Figure 36.4)**. Targeting OTVT in the LV summit can be challenging because of its proximity to major cardiac vessels and the presence of significant amounts of epicardial fat in this distribution.[38]

Semilunar Valves

Myocardial extensions beyond the pulmonary and aortic valves have been implicated to be the source of OTVT from these locations. In general, OTVTs are much more common from the aortic cusp region than the pulmonary artery. The reason for this discrepancy remains unclear. The pulmonic valve lies anterior to and approximately 1–2 cm superior

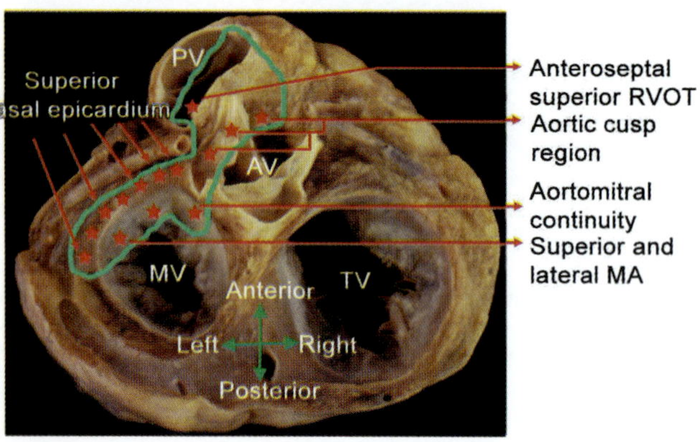

Figure 36.3: Anatomy of the left ventricular ostium (encircled by green line), which houses common sites of origin of outflow tract ventricular tachycardia (red stars)

Abbreviations: AV, aortic valve; MA, mitral annulus; MV, mitral valve; PV, pulmonary valve; RVOT, right ventricular outflow tract; TV, tricuspid valve

(Heart model figure courtesy of Dr. Samuel J. Asirvatham, MD)

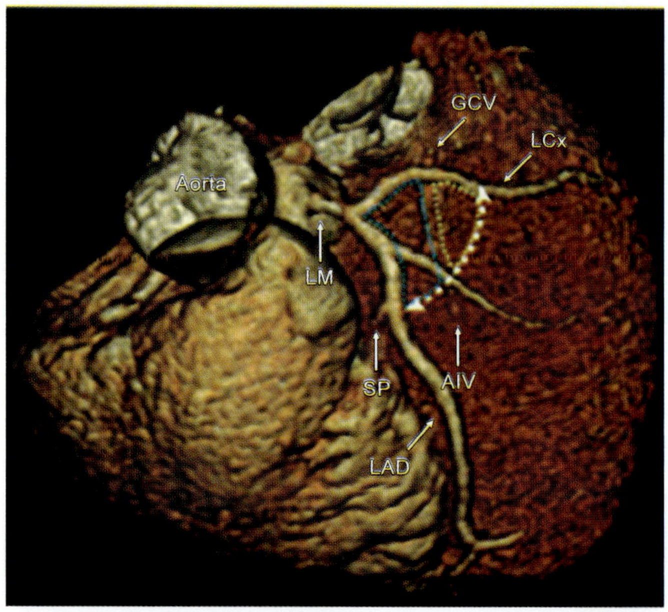

Figure 36.4: Computer tomographic image demonstrating the anatomy of the left ventricular summit (LVS). The LVS is a triangular region of the epicardial LV. The apex of the triangle is formed by the bifurcation of the left main coronary artery into left anterior descending and left circumflex arteries while the base is formed by an arc connecting the origin of the first septal perforator branch with the left circumflex (white dotted line). The great cardiac vein bisects the LVS, separating it into 2 regions (blue and yellow dotted lines). The proximal portion (blue dotted lines) is less accessible for ablation due to proximity of the coronary arteries as well as the presence of thicker layer of epicardial fat

Abbreviations: AIV, anterior interventricular vein; GCV, great cardiac vein; LAD, left anterior descending; LCx, left circumflex; LM, left main; SP, septal perforator

From: Santangeli P, Marchlinski FE, Zado ES, et al. Percutaneous epicardial ablation of ventricular arrhythmias arising from the left ventricular summit: Outcomes and ECG correlates of success. Circ Arrhythm Electrophysiol. 2015;8:337-43

to the aortic valve. The posterior or septal RVOT is in direct continuity with the aortic root (noncoronary and right coronary cusps).

Aortic Root and Cusp Region

The aortic root is centrally located and is in direct contact with multiple critical cardiac structures. The right coronary cusp (RCC) is the most anterior cusp, and sits directly adjacent to the posterior aspect of the RVOT. The left coronary cusp (LCC) is left-posterior and the noncoronary cusp (NCC) is right-posterior to the RCC. The aortic valve is tilted rightward (up to 30–45 degrees) in the horizontal plane and the RCC and NCC tend to be inferior (caudal) to the LCC. The R/LCC commissure sits directly anterior to the superior septal RVOT and the pulmonic valve. The penetrating bundle of His courses through the membranous interventricular septum at the commissure between the RCC and NCC. Analogous to the pulmonic valve, there are frequently muscular sleeves which extend above the aortic valve. However, the distribution of the supra-aortic valve sleeves is quite different from those of the pulmonic valve. In one study, supravalvular myocardial sleeves were most commonly present in the RCC (55%), while they were less frequently seen in the LCC (24%) and extremely rare in the NCC (0.66%).[39] Additionally, the sleeves in the RCC tended to extend a greater distance (2.8 mm) versus those in the LCC (1.5 mm) or NCC (1.3 mm).

DIAGNOSIS: ELECTROCARDIOGRAPHIC LOCALIZATION OF THE ARRHYTHMOGENIC FOCUS

The surface ECG is helpful in localizing the site of origin (SOO) of OTVTs.[40,41] This is important both for preprocedural planning, as well as to counsel the patient on expected outcome and the possible need for additional procedures, since outcomes may differ based on the SOO of the PVC. Success rates are highest in patients with PVCs originating from the RVOT, while PVCs originating from the epicardium or papillary muscles have lower rates of acute procedural success.[42] Due to the anatomically superior location of the OT region, arrhythmias from this location manifest with a QRS that has an inferior axis with positive forces (R-waves) in the inferior leads (II, III, and aVF). Further localization of the arrhythmia focus is facilitated by the QRS morphology in leads I and V1 as well as the precordial QRS transition pattern. The QRS complex may have either a right or left bundle branch block (RBBB and LBBB) pattern, based on whether the complex is predominantly positive or negative in lead V1. RBBB OTVTs originate in the LVOT or lateral basal LV whereas LBBB OTVTs can originate in both the RVOT and the septal aspect of the LVOT.

In order to accurately predict the site of origin based on the 12-lead ECG, one must recognize the importance of appropriate lead placement. Minute aberrations in electrode placement may dramatically alter the QRS morphology and therefore misguide prediction of the VT origin. For example, during electrophysiologic studies and/or VT ablation procedures, the precordial leads V1 and V2 may be misplaced to accommodate precordial defibrillator pads. It has been shown that superior displacement of the precordial leads V1 and V2 reduces R-wave amplitude and decreases the R/S ratio, while inferior displacement of these leads increases R-wave amplitude and R/S ratio.[43] Similarly, during treadmill stress testing, the limb leads are sometimes placed on the anterior chest instead of the arms or shoulders and this can significantly alter the QRS morphology in limb lead I.[43]

Discriminating between RVOT versus LVOT Source

Lead V1

The RV is the anterior—most structure of the heart within the chest and in close proximity to precordial leads V1 and V2. Therefore, VTs originating from the RVOT will have a negative QRS complex in V1 (LBBB pattern) as well as leads V2 and V3. As the arrhythmia site of origin shifts posteriorly and leftward in the heart, the precordial transition pattern becomes earlier. However, predominantly positive R-waves (RBBB) are not seen unless the arrhythmia focus is located in the basal LV at or beyond the AMC region **(Figure 36.5)**.

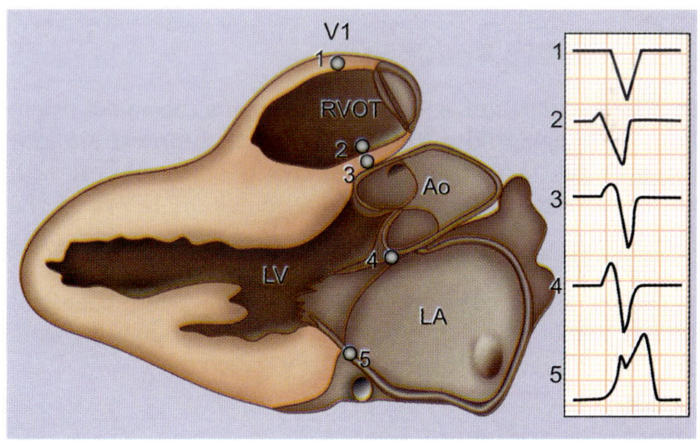

Figure 36.5: Depiction of the electrocardiographic QRS morphology in V1 (inset) based on site of origin. Because lead V1 is an anterior lead, arrhythmias originating in the anterior RVOT (1) result in typical left bundle branch block morphology. As the site of origin moves more posteriorly (2—posterior RVOT; 3—anterior right coronary cusp), the R-wave in V1 begins to increase in size. At the region of the left coronary cusp and aortomitral continuity (4), there is a distinct R-wave. Finally, at the posterior mitral annulus (5), there is right bundle branch block morphology

Abbreviations: Ao, aorta; LA, left atrium; LV, left ventricle; RVOT, right ventricular outflow tract

From: Asirvatham SJ. Correlative anatomy for the invasive electrophysiologist: outflow tract and supravalvular arrhythmia. J Cardiovasc Electrophysiol. 2009;20:955-69

The cusp region is interesting because of its proximity to different aspects of the RVOT. In particular, the RCC is adjacent to septal RVOT so arrhythmias in this location exhibit a LBBB appearance (negative QS in V1) as well but the transition is earlier than that in the RVOT locations. Arrhythmias originating from the LCC usually manifest biphasic complexes in lead V1. Beyond this location, in the LVOT the complexes have predominantly and/or exclusively positive forces in lead V1 (RBBB—appearance). The AMC location is a "water-shed" site and arrhythmias originating in this location typically manifest a qR pattern in V1.

Leads aVR, aVL, II, and III

Leads aVR and aVL are located at the right and left shoulders, respectively, and typically OTVTs have negative (QS) complexes in both these leads. In fact, the QRS complexes in leads aVR and aVL are almost mirror images of QRS complexes in leads II and III. The aVR:aVL ratio of QRS complexes is helpful in distinguishing leftward versus rightward and also inferior versus superior origin within the outflow tract. For example, when the VT focus is from the low RVOT (anatomically inferior and rightward origin, near the His bundle), QRS complexes in lead aVL can be biphasic or even positive whereas they remain predominantly negative in lead aVR. On the other hand, when the VT originates from a superior and leftward location such as the pulmonary artery, QRS complexes in lead aVL will be more negative than in lead aVR.

Precordial QRS Transition

Precordial transition is helpful in localizing the site of origin in the OT region. The RVOT free wall is the most anterior structure and arrhythmias from this region manifest with LBBB morphology with late QRS transition (≥V4) in the precordium. Compared to RVOT free wall, arrhythmias originating from septal RVOT manifest earlier precordial transition (≤V3). Arrhythmias originating from the RCC usually transition at V2 or V3 whereas those originating from the LV summit usually transition at V1-V3.[37]

Importance of Lead V3 for Precordial Transition

A V3 precordial transition is common in patients with OTVT and approximately half of these may be successfully ablated from the RVOT. However, certain locations in the cusp region can also manifest precordial transition by lead V3 and these may not always be successfully targeted from the RVOT. To help better distinguish cusp from RVOT site of origin, Betensky et al. have developed a V2 precordial transition ratio which compares the precordial transition in VT versus sinus rhythm. **(Figure 36.6)**. The V2 transition ratio is defined as [R/(R+S) during VT]/[R/(R+S) in sinus rhythm].[44] Typically, a ratio ≥ 0.6 predicts LVOT origin with

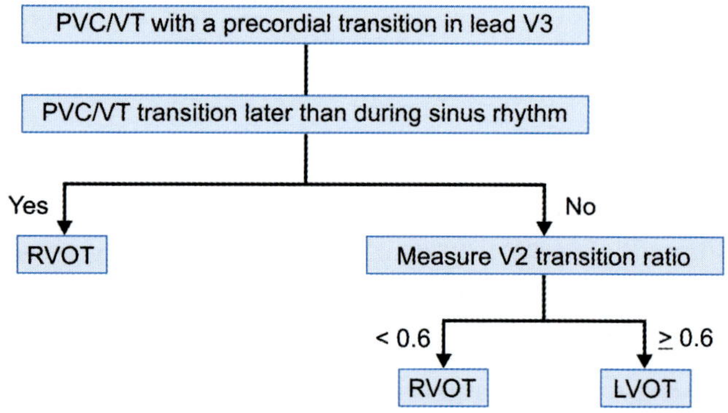

Figure 36.6: Diagnostic algorithm for outflow tract ventricular tachycardia in patients with a V3 transition of the PVC or VT
Abbreviations: LVOT, left ventricular outflow tract; PVC, premature ventricular contraction; RVOT, right ventricular outflow tract; VT, ventricular tachycardia
From: Betensky BP, Park RE, Marchlinski FE, et al. The V(2) transition ratio: a new electrocardiographic criterion for distinguishing left from right ventricular outflow tract tachycardia origin. J Am Coll Cardiol. 2011;57:2255-62

>90% accuracy. Additionally, when the PVC/VT precordial transition occurred later than during sinus rhythm, it essentially excluded an LVOT origin with 100% accuracy.[44]

Other studies have offered additional criteria to predict whether VT originates from the RVOT or LVOT in patients with V3 transition. Cheng et al. found that the presence of a V3 R-wave deflection interval >80 ms combined with V1 R-wave amplitude index >0.3 predicted an LVOT origin with 91.7% accuracy.[45] Yoshida et al. subsequently proposed the V2S/V3R index ([S-wave amplitude in V2]/[R-wave amplitude in V3]) as a criteria, demonstrating smaller V2S/V3R index in patients with LVOT versus RVOT origin (a cutoff of ≤1.5 predicted LVOT origin with 89% sensitivity and 94% specificity).[46]

Localizing within RVOT

Through pace-mapping at different locations in the RVOT, we have developed ECG criteria that can be helpful for accurately localizing the SOO of arrhythmias in this region.[47,48] We have used a numbering system to classify the RVOT septal and free wall regions into nine anatomic sites (1 to 9) **(Figure 36.7)**. Sites 1 to 3 are the most superior sites just inferior to the pulmonic valve, in a posterior to anterior orientation. In our experience, this area is the source of the vast majority of RVOT VTs. Below this location are additional sites 4 to 6 and 7 to 9. The latter are the most inferior and in close proximity to the RV inflow region.

We have compared pace-maps from superior RVOT sites in order to identify unique QRS morphology patterns that can help distinguish septal from free wall locations **(Figure 36.8)**. Typically, RVOT septal sites manifest taller and narrower R-waves in the inferior leads with earlier precordial transition (≤V4). Meanwhile, RVOT free wall sites more

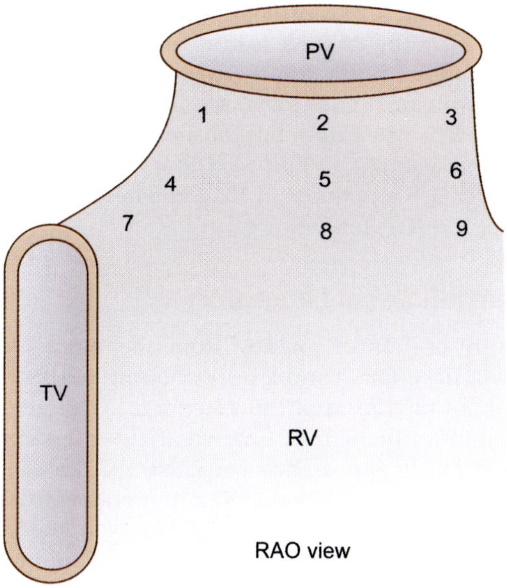

Figure 36.7: Representation of the RVOT septum (as viewed in a 30-degree right anterior oblique projection). The RVOT is divided into 9 sites. Sites 1, 4, and 7 are the posterior sites and 3, 6, and 9 are the anterior sites
Abbreviations: PV, pulmonic valve; RV, right ventricle; TV, tricuspid valve; RAO, right anterior oblique

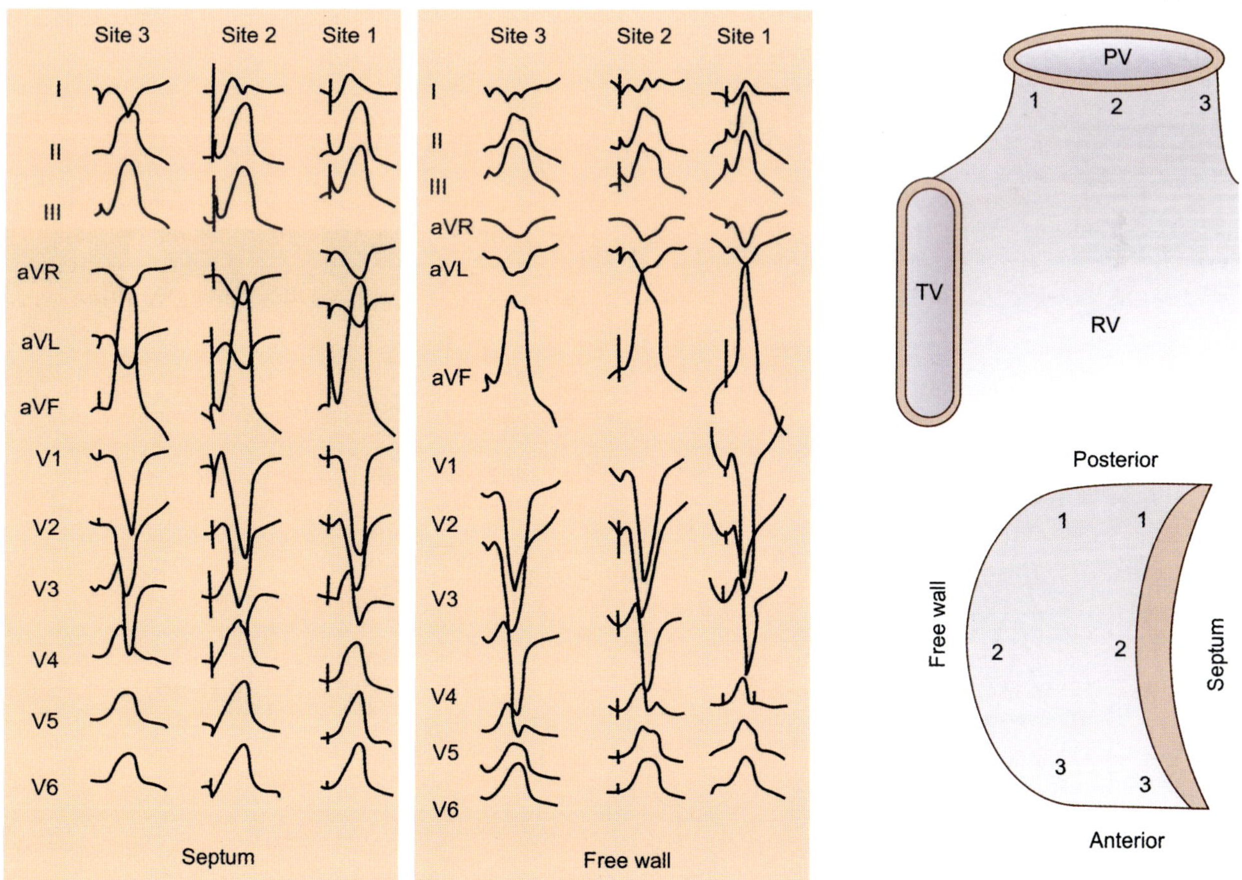

Figure 36.8: Twelve-lead electrocardiogram pace-maps from sites 1 to 3 along the septum and free wall of the right ventricular outflow tract
Abbreviations: PV, pulmonic valve; RV, right ventricle; TV, tricuspid valve

frequently exhibited "notching" of the R-waves in the inferior leads and demonstrate late precordial transition (≥V4).[34]

Limb lead I may be helpful to further localize VT from the superior RVOT. VT originating from site 1 (which is posterior and rightward) usually manifests a positive complex in this lead whereas VT originating from site 3 (which is anterior and leftward) manifests a negative complex. These differences are likely because of the leftward axis of lead I.

Yamauchi et al. further compared ECG characteristics of VT originating from the parahisian (RV inflow) region from the RVOT. They found that a parahisian origin was associated with monophasic tall R in lead I, narrower QRS complexes with relatively small R-waves in the inferior leads (with R-amplitude in II>III), presence of R-wave in aVL, QS pattern in lead V1, early precordial transition (V2-V3), and relatively tall R in V5 and V6. [49]

Identification of Focus from within the Pulmonary Artery

As mentioned earlier, myocardial sleeves may extend above the pulmonic valve into the pulmonary artery.[50] As such, RVOT VT may have a source above the pulmonary valve (in the PA) in 4–6% of patients.[34,51] The focus usually lies 1–2 cm above the pulmonic valve, mostly along the septum.[52] PVCs or VT originating from the PA have features similar to other locations in the superior septal RVOT. However, in some of these cases, the precordial QRS transition is earlier (V2-3). Other features of PVCs or VT from this location include ratio of QS complexes in lead aVL:aVR of >1, QS or rS pattern in lead I, and a larger R/S amplitude in V2 compared with VT from the superior RVOTregion.[52]

Localizing within Basal LV Region

The vast majority of VTs originating from the basal LV endocardium will have QRS complexes exhibiting a RBBB-appearance with an inferior axis. The exception to this rule is VT originating from the high left interventricular septum which manifests LBBB appearance (negative QS in V1), but very early precordial transition (≤V2). The endocardial basal LV includes the septum, anterior, inferior, and lateral walls surrounding the mitral valve. Using pace-mapping, we have developed ECG criteria that can help localize the SOO of VT from various locations in this region such as the septal para-Hisian area, AMC region, superior, lateral, and superolateral mitral annular (MA) locations **(Figure 36.9)**.[9] Septal para-Hisian sites manifest narrower QRS complexes

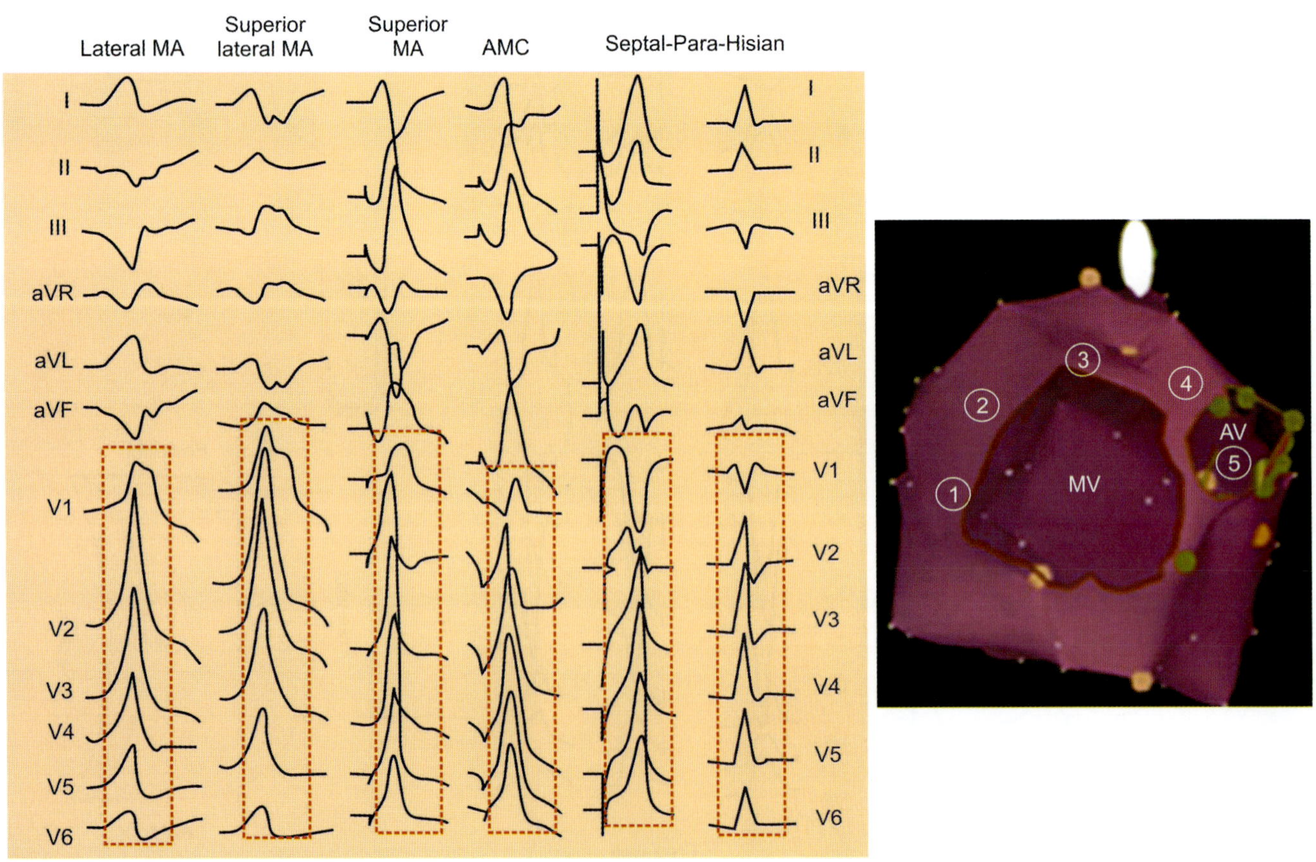

Figure 36.9: Twelve-lead electrocardiogram pace-maps from the following sites in the basal left ventricular outflow tract: Lateral mitral annulus (MA), superior lateral MA, superior MA, aortomitral continuity (AMC), and septal Para-Hisian. MV is mitral valve

(134 ms), initial negative deflections (QS or rS) in lead V1, early precordial transition (≤V2), and predominantly positive forces in lead I. The AMC region manifests qR pattern in V1 and predominantly positive complexes in lead I. All other locations in this region (superior, superolateral and lateral MA) manifest monophasic R waves in lead V1 with either no precordial transition or very late appearance of S-wave (≥V5). Additionally, superolateral and lateral MA locations manifest rS or QS complexes in lead I.[9]

Aortic Sinus Cusps

The aortic sinus cusps have been increasingly recognized to harbor foci of OTVT. ECG characteristics of OTVTs originating from the cusps have been elucidated by our group using pace mapping. QRS complex morphology in lead V1 is useful to localize the site of origin in this region. Arrhythmias and/or pacemaps from the LCC manifest multiphasic, predominantly positive QRS complexes with "M" or "W" patterns in V1 **(Figure 36.10)** with early precordial transition (≤V2).[53] In comparison, pacemaps and/or arrhythmias originating from the RCC usually manifest a LBBB pattern in lead V1 and a later precordial transition (by lead V3). The NCC is in direct contact with the interatrial septum as well as both atria, and in our experience this cusp is not a site for OTVT. In fact pacing from this location typically results in atrial and sometimes His bundle capture.[53]

An interesting site of arrhythmia origin in this region is the RCC/LCC commissure. Arrhythmias from this location manifest unique ECG characteristics in lead V1 which include a QS morphology with prominent notching on the downward deflection[54] **(Figure 36.11).**

As we have pointed out earlier, ECG features (in particular precordial transition) can be helpful in distinguishing RVOT from cusp VTs. Yoshida et al. proposed a "transition zone index" (TZI), accounting for cardiac rotation.[55] They defined the transition zone as "the position of precordial leads in which R/S amplitudes are equal" and the TZI as the "transition zone score during PVC/VT minus the transition zone score during normal sinus rhythm". In their study, the TZI was lower when VT originated from the ASC compared to the RVOT, and a cutoff value of TZI < 0 strongly predicted ASC origin.[55]

It is important to recognize that significant age-related changes in the orientation of the ventricle and aortic root can affect the QRS morphologies of arrhythmias originating from the cusp region. Typically in older patients (compared to younger patients), the RCC is lower and so arrhythmias (and pacemaps) in these subjects have less positive forces in inferior leads.[56]

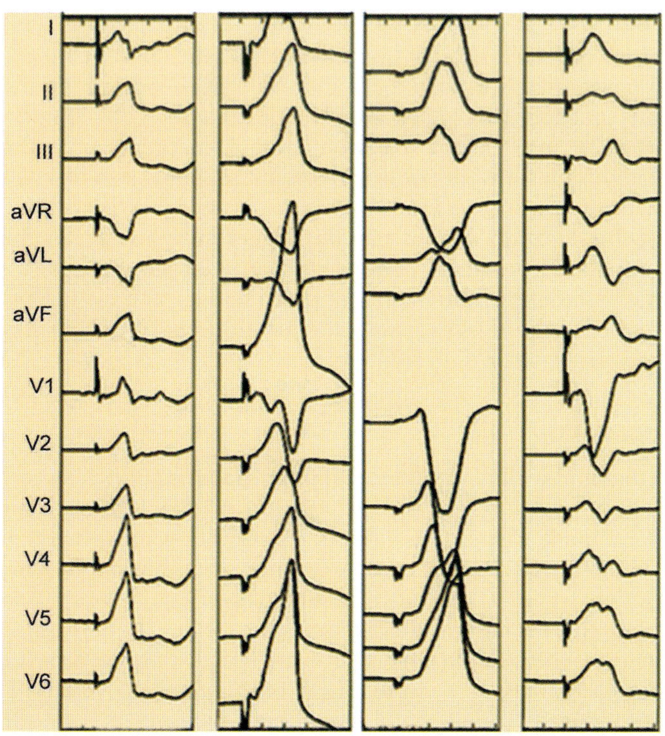

Figure 36.10: Twelve-lead electrocardiogram pace-maps from the right and left coronary cusps

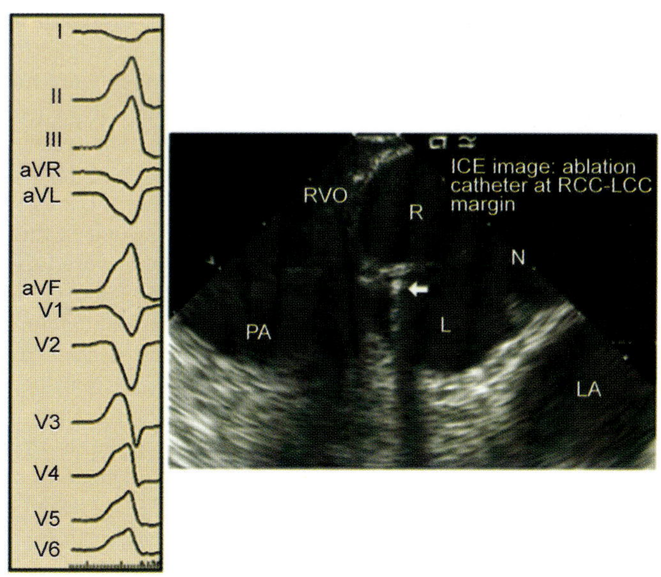

Figure 36.11: Twelve-lead electrocardiogram pace-map from the commissure between the right and left coronary cusps. Intracardiac echocardiographic image demonstrating location of the ablation catheter at the commissure between the right and left coronary cusps (arrow)

Abbreviations: R, right coronary cusp; L, left coronary cusp; N, non-coronary cusp; LA, left atrium; PA, pulmonary artery; RVO, right ventricular outflow; ICE, intracardiac echocardiography

LV Summit

The LV summit has also been recognized to be a source of OTVTs. LV summit is an epicardial triangular area which is defined fluoroscopically as the region bounded superiorly by the bifurcation of LAD and the left circumflex artery and inferiorly by the 1st septal perforator artery. The great cardiac vein (GCV) and anterior interventricular vein (AIV) transect the LV summit dividing it into two parts: superomedial and inferolateral regions. ECG criteria that suggest a SOO from the LV summit include Q-wave in lead I, QRS amplitude ratio in lead III and II of >1.25 and QS ratio in leads aVL and aVR of >1.75.[37] We have recently identified ECG findings that are predictors of successful ablation of VT arising from this region using an epicardial approach. In our experience, arrhythmias arising from inferolateral part of the LV summit are better suited for epicardial ablation and features that can help identify this location within the LV summit include aVL to aVR Q-wave ratio of >1.85, V1 R/S ratio >2, and absence of Q-waves in V1.[38]

TREATMENT OF IDIOPATHIC OUTFLOW TRACT VENTRICULAR TACHYCARDIA

Pharmacologic Therapies

Treatment of OTVT is primarily focused on relief of symptoms. Additionally, suppression of ventricular ectopy may reverse systolic dysfunction in some patients with PVC-induced cardiomyopathy. As mentioned previously, the mechanism underlying these arrhythmias is DAD-mediated triggered activity which involves increased intracellular calcium. Therefore, a number of medications have been shown to suppress these arrhythmias through mechanistic effects at different stages involved in the release of intracellular calcium ion. Beta blockers, through their inhibition of the release of stimulatory G protein, reduce cAMP which in turn decreases triggered activity. These drugs are considered the first-line pharmacologic therapy for suppression of idiopathic VT. Calcium channel blockers inhibit the release of calcium ions through a direct effect on the calcium channel and can be used synergistically with beta-blockers in the treatment of OTVTs. The overall efficacy of beta and calcium channel blockers remains modest (25–50%),[4,5] and in patients that opt for long-term medical management of this condition, membrane stabilizing antiarrhythmic drugs (AADs) may be necessary. Both sodium channel blockers (class I agents),[57] and potassium channel blockers (class III agents) have been used effectively in the treatment of OTVT. However, concerns about the proarrhythmic and noncardiac side effects often prohibit long-term use of these agents, particularly in younger patients. Intravenous lidocaine and adenosine have both been shown to be effective for acute treatment of these arrhythmias. The effectiveness of the latter has resulted in these arrhythmias being labeled as "adenosine sensitive".

Catheter Ablation

Since the first clinical report of successful ablation of OTVT was published in 1990,[58] technological advances over the past two decades have improved both safety and efficacy of ablation, resulting in its widespread acceptance as first-line therapy in the management of these arrhythmias. The overall success rates of catheter ablation for OTVT are high and the occurrence of serious complications remains quite low. One recent large multicenter retrospective study examining safety and efficacy of PVC ablation in over 1,000 patients reported an acute procedural success rate of 84% with a major complication rate of 2.9%.[42]

Catheter ablation has been shown to be superior to AADs with regards to PVC suppression in both retrospective and prospective studies. One single-center retrospective study examined 510 patients with frequent PVCs and demonstrated that catheter ablation resulted in greater PVC reduction and improvement in LVEF compared with antiarrhythmic drugs.[59] Similarly, a prospective randomized controlled trial by Ling et al. randomized 330 patients with frequent RVOT PVCs to radiofrequency ablation (RFA) vs. AADs and confirmed that RFA was more effective in suppressing PVCs.[60]

Activation Mapping

Since triggered activity underlies OTVT, the source of these tachycardias is usually focal and electrical depolarization at this location usually precedes the onset of the QRS complex by ~20 ms. During electroanatomic mapping of these arrhythmias, the site of origin should manifest as a discrete zone of early electrical activity and the distal tip of the catheter at this location should manifest a QS morphology on the unipolar electrogram. When activation mapping results in a nondiscrete or diffuse area of early activity, the likely SOO may be in the adjacent chamber and additional mapping may be warranted prior to ablation.

Pace-Mapping

Together with activation mapping, pace mapping is very helpful in mapping and ablation of OTVTs- although by itself, pace mapping is inferior to activation mapping,[61] in localizing the SOO of OTVTs, it may sometimes be the only option when VT is too infrequent for adequate activation mapping. For best results, pace mapping should be performed at threshold output and at a cycle length that mimics the coupling interval or cycle length of the clinical PVC or VT, respectively. If performed using these parameters from the SOO, the match of the paced QRS complexes to the clinical arrhythmia should be 12/12. When assessing the match, particular attention should be paid to the "notches" and other subtle morphological variations observed in the QRS complexes of the clinical arrhythmia across multiple leads, which should be mimicked on the paced QRS complexes. It is important to note that ablation at sites without perfect pace-matches are less likely to succeed.[62] Innovations such as the PASO™ module (CARTO, Biosense Webster, Diamond Bar, CA) have resulted in the ability to perform automated matching of paced and clinical arrhythmias and provide quantitative estimates (percentage) of the level of match. In our experience, the accuracy of pace mapping is excellent within the RVOT, while the accuracy is lower within the aortic root, where pacing at high outputs may be necessary to achieve capture.

Mapping of Outflow Tract Ventricular Tachycardias

In order to maximize the inducibility of the VT at the time of ablation, medications including beta blockers, calcium channel blockers, and antiarrhythmic medications should be withdrawn several days before the planned procedure. Due to its long half-life, amiodarone is ideally discontinued several weeks in advance. Because of the catecholamine-sensitivity of OTVTs, it is our standard practice to limit the use of propofol and benzodiazepines as sedative agents during the procedure. Instead, remifentanil can be utilized since it is ultra-short acting and has fewer antiarrhythmic properties.[63] When VT is infrequent, isoproterenol, aminophylline, phenylephrine, or burst pacing may be used to induce these arrhythmias.

For LBBB VT/PVCs with precordial transition ≥V3 and/or precordial transition later than that during sinus rhythm, we begin mapping in the RVOT. For LBBB VT/PVCs that manifest precordial transition ≥V2 and/or earlier that during sinus rhythm, we will usually start mapping in the aortic cusps. Additionally, for both LBBB VT/PVCs as well as RBBB PVCs that manifest ECG features suggestive of epicardial origin (i.e., pseudodelta wave ≥34 ms, delayed intrinsicoid deflection ≥85 ms, delayed maximum deflection index, etc.),[64,65] we will also map the GCV/AIV. Determining a site of origin within the RVOT versus the ASC prior to the ablation may be difficult, but is important for preprocedural planning. Yamada et al. have previously showed that 25% of patients with ASC VT had a closer pace-match from the RVOT than from within the aortic cusp region, and that an ASC origin may preferentially conduct to a breakout site within the RVOT.[66] Other ECG features may also be helpful in distinguishing RVOT from cusp arrhythmias. Ouyang et al. found that VT originating from the aortic cusps had longer R-wave duration in leads V1 and V2, and smaller R/S amplitude compared with VT from the RVOT.[67]

Radiofrequency Settings and Ablation Techniques

Since OTVT due to triggered activity originates from a focal area, we typically use 4-mm catheters in either temperature or power-controlled mode (maximum temperature and power 55C and 50W, respectively). More recently, we have found that by varying flow rates and limiting maximum power delivery, we are able to use the 3.5 mm open irrigated tip ablation catheter at all locations in the outflow tract region. Typical RF applications are for a maximum duration of 60–90 seconds targeting an impedance drop of 10–12 ohms. Failure to suppress VT early into the ablation (≤15 seconds) and/or recurrence of VT after late suppression implies origin from a location that is at a distance from the ablation site. In these instances further mapping is advised. Occasionally, the site of ablation manifests late suppression after extensive mapping, and in these instances longer lesions (2–5 minutes) may be required. This is particular true for OTVTs that have been localized to the LV summit, where longer lesions from adjacent areas (cusp region, AMC and/or the septal anterior RVOT) are often required to achieve successful suppression.

When ablating in the aortic cusps, imaging with intracardiac echocardiography is particularly helpful in facilitating real-time visualization of the catheter location as well as identifying the location of the ostium of the LMCA as well as the course of the LMCA and LAD. Additionally, coronary angiography may be necessary to locate the course of the coronary arteries especially when ablating from the GCV-AIV location. This location is in close proximity to the left circumflex artery and its branches. The LMCA originates from the LCC and courses immediately posterior to the RVOT, near the pulmonic valve before it bifurcates giving off the left circumflex and the LAD arteries. The possibility of damage to the LMCA should be considered when ablating OTVTs originating from the pulmonary artery due to its close proximity (<3 mm in one study).[68] In general, ablation within 5 mm of the coronary artery should be avoided. Although case reports have suggested safety and feasibility of catheter ablation of OTVT in close proximity to coronary arteries using adjunctive imaging,[69] the risks versus benefits of such an undertaking must be seriously considered. If ablation is carried out in close proximity to the coronary artery, a post-ablation coronary angiogram should be performed to identify acute damage. It is important to recognize that the absence of acute coronary damage does not guarantee lack of long-term consequences: we have observed at least one scenario where a patient was found to have high-grade stenosis of an obtuse marginal vessel following ablation in the LV epicardium which was incidentally detected during coronary angiography during a subsequent procedure, despite the immediate post-ablation angiogram after the initial procedure showing patent vessels (**Figures 36.12A and B**).

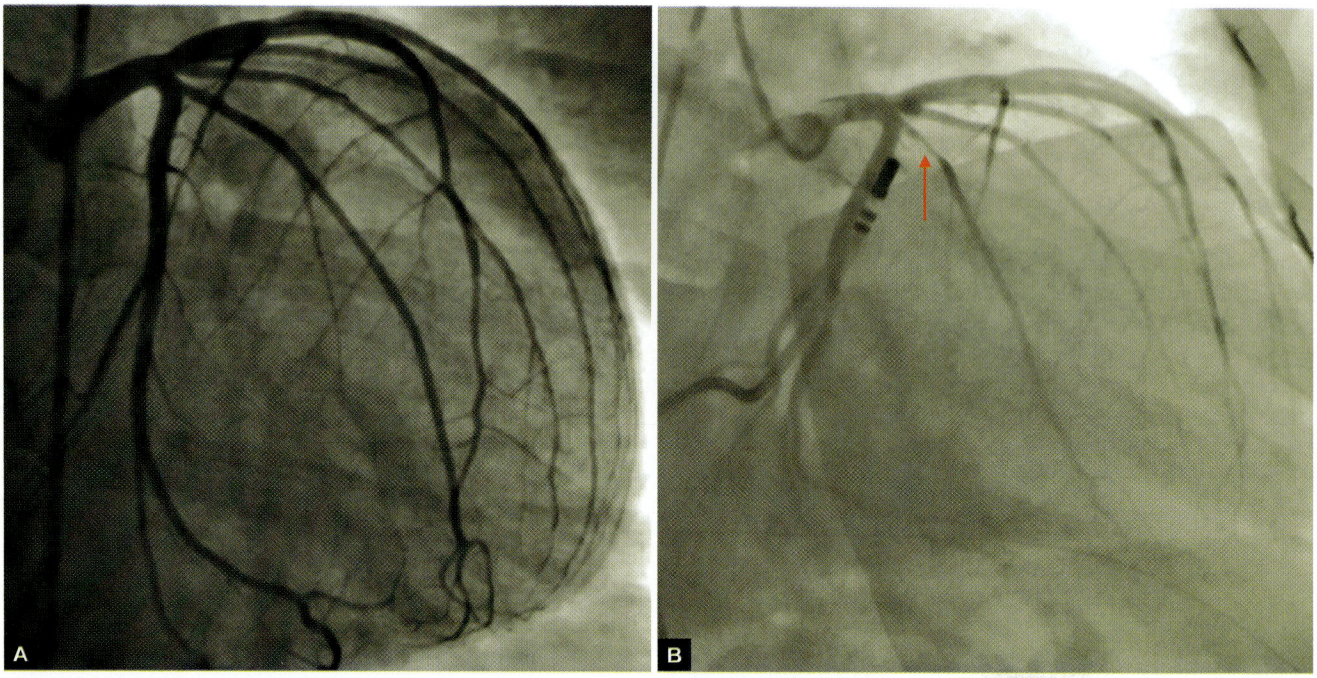

Figures 36.12A and B: Coronary angiogram (A; right anterior oblique view) of a patient both before and immediately after epicardial PVC ablation in the LV summit region demonstrated no evidence of coronary artery disease. The patient returned three months later for repeat PVC ablation and coronary angiogram (B; right anterior oblique view) prior to ablation demonstrated a high-grade stenosis of the obtuse marginal branch (arrow), near the area where epicardial radiofrequency lesions were applied during the prior procedure

CONCLUSION

Idiopathic OTVTs are focal arrhythmias resulting from triggered activity. Although these arrhythmias occur in patients with structurally normal hearts and portend a benign prognosis, they can result in troublesome symptoms and may even lead to cardiomyopathy if left untreated. Medical therapy may be effective in the short-term but is not ideal for long-term management of these arrhythmias. Catheter ablation is a safe and effective treatment option and has become first line therapy in the management of OTVTs now-a-days. The key to successful ablation of OTVTs is accurately localizing the arrhythmia focus. This can be achieved using a combination of 12-lead ECG coupled with activation and pace mapping facilitated by electroanatomic mapping as well as adjunctive imaging with intracardiac echocardiography.

REFERENCES

1. Brooks R, Burgess JH. Idiopathic ventricular tachycardia. A review. Medicine (Baltimore). 1988;67:271-94.
2. Lerman BB, Belardinelli L, West GA, Berne RM, DiMarco JP. Adenosine-sensitive ventricular tachycardia: evidence suggesting cyclic AMP-mediated triggered activity. Circulation. 1986;74:270-80.
3. Lerman BB. Response of nonreentrant catecholamine-mediated ventricular tachycardia to endogenous adenosine and acetylcholine. Evidence for myocardial receptor-mediated effects. Circulation. 1993;87:382-90.
4. Gill JS, Blaszyk K, Ward DE, Camm AJ. Verapamil for the suppression of idiopathic ventricular tachycardia of left bundle branch block-like morphology. Am Heart J. 1993;126:1126-33.
5. Issa ZF, Miller JM, Zipes DP. CHAPTER 19 - Idiopathic Ventricular Tachycardia. In: Zipes ZFIMMP, (Ed). Clinical Arrhythmology and Electrophysiology (1). Philadelphia: W.B. Saunders; 2009. pp. 440-61.
6. Marchlinski FE, Deely MP, Zado ES. Sex-specific triggers for right ventricular outflow tract tachycardia. Am Heart J. 2000;139:1009-13.
7. Lerman BB, Stein KM, Markowitz SM. Idiopathic right ventricular outflow tract tachycardia: a clinical approach. Pacing Clin Electrophysiol. 1996;19:2120-37.
8. Nakagawa M, Takahashi N, Nobe S, Ichinose M, Ooie T, Yufu F, Shigematsu S, Hara M, Yonemochi H, Saikawa T. Gender differences in various types of idiopathic ventricular tachycardia. J Cardiovasc Electrophysiol. 2002;13:633-8.
9. Dixit S, Gerstenfeld EP, Lin D, Callans DJ, Hsia HH, Nayak HM, Zado E, Marchlinski FE. Identification of distinct electrocardiographic patterns from the basal left ventricle: distinguishing medial and lateral sites of origin in patients with idiopathic ventricular tachycardia. Heart Rhythm. 2005;2:485-91.
10. Callans DJ, Menz V, Schwartzman D, Gottlieb CD, Marchlinski FE. Repetitive monomorphic tachycardia from the left ventricular outflow tract: electrocardiographic patterns consistent with a left ventricular site of origin. J Am Coll Cardiol. 1997;29:1023-7.

11. Lerman BB, Stein KM, Markowitz SM. Adenosine-sensitive ventricular tachycardia: a conceptual approach. J Cardiovasc Electrophysiol. 1996;7:559-69.
12. Anter E, Dixit S. Ablation of Ventricular Outflow Tract Tachycardias. In: Huang SKS, Miller JM (Eds). Catheter Ablation of Cardiac Arrhythmias. 3rd edn. Philadelphia, PA: Elsevier Saunders; 2015. pp. 519-39.
13. Hoffmayer KS, Machado ON, Marcus GM, Yang Y, Johnson CJ, Ermakov S, Vittinghoff E, Pandurangi U, Calkins H, Cannom D, Gear KC, Tichnell C, Park Y, Zareba W, Marcus FI, Scheinman MM. Electrocardiographic comparison of ventricular arrhythmias in patients with arrhythmogenic right ventricular cardiomyopathy and right ventricular outflow tract tachycardia. J Am Coll Cardiol. 2011;58:831-8.
14. Hoffmayer KS, Bhave PD, Marcus GM, James CA, Tichnell C, Chopra N, Moxey L, Krahn AD, Dixit S, Stevenson W, Calkins H, Badhwar N, Gerstenfeld EP, Scheinman MM. An electrocardiographic scoring system for distinguishing right ventricular outflow tract arrhythmias in patients with arrhythmogenic right ventricular cardiomyopathy from idiopathic ventricular tachycardia. Heart Rhythm. 2013;10:477-82.
15. Santangeli P, Pieroni M, Dello Russo A, Casella M, Pelargonio G, Macchione A, Camporeale A, Smaldone C, Bartoletti S, Di Biase L, Bellocci F, Natale A. Noninvasive diagnosis of electroanatomic abnormalities in arrhythmogenic right ventricular cardiomyopathy. Circ Arrhythm Electrophysiol. 2010;3:632-8.
16. Santangeli P, Hamilton-Craig C, Dello Russo A, Pieroni M, Casella M, Pelargonio G, Di Biase L, Smaldone C, Bartoletti S, Narducci ML, Tondo C, Bellocci F, Natale A. Imaging of scar in patients with ventricular arrhythmias of right ventricular origin: cardiac magnetic resonance versus electroanatomic mapping. J Cardiovasc Electrophysiol. 2011;22:1359-66.
17. Santangeli P, Pieroni M, Dello Russo A, Casella M, Pelargonio G, Di Biase L, Macchione A, Burkhardt JD, Bellocci F, Santarelli P, Tondo C, Natale A. Correlation between signal-averaged ECG and the histologic evaluation of the myocardial substrate in right ventricular outflow tract arrhythmias. Circ Arrhythm Electrophysiol. 2012;5:475-83.
18. Corrado D, Basso C, Leoni L, Tokajuk B, Turrini P, Bauce B, Migliore F, Pavei A, Tarantini G, Napodano M, Ramondo A, Buja G, Iliceto S, Thiene G. Three-dimensional electroanatomical voltage mapping and histologic evaluation of myocardial substrate in right ventricular outflow tract tachycardia. J Am Coll Cardiol. 2008;51:731-9.
19. Lee YH, Zhong L, Roger VL, Asirvatham SJ, Shen WK, Slusser JP, Hodge DO, Cha YM. Frequency, origin, and outcome of ventricular premature complexes in patients with or without heart diseases. Am J Cardiol. 2014;114:1373-8.
20. Dukes JW, Dewland TA, Vittinghoff E, Mandyam MC, Heckbert SR, Siscovick DS, Stein PK, Psaty BM, Sotoodehnia N, Gottdiener JS, Marcus GM. Ventricular ectopy as a predictor of heart failure and death. J Am Coll of Cardiol. 2015;66:101-9.
21. Lee GK, Klarich KW, Grogan M, Cha Y-M. Premature ventricular contraction-induced cardiomyopathy: a treatable condition. Circ Arrhythm Electrophysiol. 2012;5:229-36.
22. Yarlagadda RK, Iwai S, Stein KM, Markowitz SM, Shah BK, Cheung JW, Tan V, Lerman BB, Mittal S. Reversal of cardiomyopathy in patients with repetitive monomorphic ventricular ectopy originating from the right ventricular outflow tract. Circulation. 2005;112:1092-7.
23. Takemoto M, Yoshimura H, Ohba Y, Matsumoto Y, Yamamoto U, Mohri M, Yamamoto H, Origuchi H. Radiofrequency catheter ablation of premature ventricular complexes from right ventricular outflow tract improves left ventricular dilation and clinical status in patients without structural heart disease. J Am Coll Cardiol. 2005;45:1259-65.
24. Baman TS, Lange DC, Ilg KJ, Gupta SK, Liu T-Y, Alguire C, Armstrong W, Good E, Chugh A, Jongnarangsin K, Pelosi Jr F, Crawford T, Ebinger M, Oral H, Morady F, Bogun F. Relationship between burden of premature ventricular complexes and left ventricular function. Heart Rhythm. 2010;7:865-9.
25. Ban JE, Park HC, Park JS, Nagamoto Y, Choi JI, Lim HE, Park SW, Kim YH. Electrocardiographic and electrophysiological characteristics of premature ventricular complexes associated with left ventricular dysfunction in patients without structural heart disease. Europace. 2013;15:735-41.
26. Del Carpio Munoz F, Syed FF, Noheria A, Cha Y-M, Friedman PA, Hammill SC, Munger TM, Venkatachalam KL, Shen W-K, Packer DL, Asirvatham SJ. Characteristics of premature ventricular complexes as correlates of reduced left ventricular systolic function: study of the burden, duration, coupling interval, morphology and site of origin of PVCs. J Cardiovasc Electrophysiol. 2011;22:791-8.
27. Yokokawa M, Kim HM, Good E, Crawford T, Chugh A, Pelosi Jr F, Jongnarangsin K, Latchamsetty R, Armstrong W, Alguire C, Oral H, Morady F, Bogun F. Impact of QRS duration of frequent premature ventricular complexes on the development of cardiomyopathy. Heart Rhythm. 2012;9:1460-4.
28. Carballeira Pol L, Deyell MW, Frankel DS, Benhayon D, Squara F, Chik W, Kohari M, Deo R, Marchlinski FE. Ventricular premature depolarization QRS duration as a new marker of risk for the development of ventricular premature depolarization-induced cardiomyopathy. Heart Rhythm. 2014;11:299-306.
29. Kawamura M, Badhwar N, Vedantham V, Tseng ZH, Lee BK, Lee RJ, Marcus GM, Olgin JE, Gerstenfeld EP, Scheinman MM. Coupling interval dispersion and body mass index are independent predictors of idiopathic premature ventricular complex-induced cardiomyopathy. J Cardiovasc Electrophysiol. 2014;25:756-62.
30. Deyell MW, Park K-M, Han Y, Frankel DS, Dixit S, Cooper JM, Hutchinson MD, Lin D, Garcia F, Bala R, Riley MP, Gerstenfeld E, Callans DJ, Marchlinski FE. Predictors of recovery of left ventricular dysfunction after ablation of frequent ventricular premature depolarizations. Heart Rhythm. 2012;9:1465-72.
31. Mountantonakis SE, Frankel DS, Gerstenfeld EP, Dixit S, Lin D, Hutchinson MD, Riley M, Bala R, Cooper J, Callans D, Garcia F, Zado ES, Marchlinski FE. Reversal of outflow tract ventricular premature depolarization-induced cardiomyopathy with ablation: effect of residual arrhythmia burden and preexisting cardiomyopathy on outcome. Heart Rhythm. 2011;8:1608-14.
32. Liang JJ, Desimone CV, Lachman N, Noheria A, Nanda S, Asirvatham SJ. Cardiac Anatomy for Catheter Mapping and Ablation of Arrhythmias. In: Huang SKS, Miller JM (Eds). Catheter Ablation of Cardiac Arrhythmias. 3rd edn. Philadelphia, PA: Elsevier Saunders; 2015. pp. 85-105.
33. Asirvatham SJ. Correlative anatomy for the invasive electrophysiologist: outflow tract and supravalvar arrhythmia. J Cardiovasc Electrophysiol. 2009;20:955-68.
34. Dixit S, Gerstenfeld EP, Callans DJ, Marchlinski FE. Electrocardiographic patterns of superior right ventricular

outflow tract tachycardias: distinguishing septal and free-wall sites of origin. J Cardiovasc Electrophysiol. 2003;14:1-7.
35. Suleiman M, Asirvatham SJ. Ablation above the semilunar valves: when, why, and how? Part I. Heart Rhythm. 2008;5:1485-92.
36. Yamada T, Litovsky SH, Kay GN. The left ventricular ostium: an anatomic concept relevant to idiopathic ventricular arrhythmias. Circ Arrhythm Electrophysiol. 2008;1:396-404.
37. Yamada T, McElderry HT, Doppalapudi H, Okada T, Murakami Y, Yoshida Y, Yoshida N, Inden Y, Murohara T, Plumb VJ, Kay GN. Idiopathic ventricular arrhythmias originating from the left ventricular summit: anatomic concepts relevant to ablation. Circ Arrhythm Electrophysiol. 2010;3:616-23.
38. Santangeli P, Marchlinski FE, Zado ES, Benhayon D, Hutchinson MD, Lin D, Frankel DS, Riley MP, Supple GE, Garcia FC, Bala R, Desjardins B, Callans DJ, Dixit S. Percutaneous Epicardial Ablation of Ventricular Arrhythmias Arising from the Left Ventricular Summit: Outcomes and ECG Correlates of Success. Circ Arrhythm Electrophysiol. 2015;8:337-43.
39. Gami AS, Noheria A, Lachman N, Edwards WD, Friedman PA, Talreja D, Hammill SC, Munger TM, Packer DL, Asirvatham SJ. Anatomical correlates relevant to ablation above the semilunar valves for the cardiac electrophysiologist: a study of 603 hearts. J Interv Card Electrophysiol. 2011;30:5-15.
40. Liang JJ, Han Y, Frankel DS. Ablation of outflow tract ventricular tachycardia. Curr Treat Options Cardiovasc Med. 2015;17:1-10.
41. Mehrotra A, Dixit S. Electrocardiogram characteristics of outflow tract ventricular tachycardia. Card Electrophysiol Clin. 2014;6:553-65.
42. Latchamsetty R, Yokokawa M, Morady F, Kim HM, Mathew S, Tilz R, Kuck K-H, Nagashima K, Tedrow U, Stevenson WG, Yu R, Tung R, Shivkumar K, Sarrazin J-F, Arya A, Hindricks G, Vunnam R, Dickfeld T, Daoud EG, Oza NM, Bogun F. Multicenter outcomes for catheter ablation of idiopathic premature ventricular complexes. JACC Clin Electrophysiol. 2015;1:116-23.
43. Anter E, Frankel DS, Marchlinski FE, Dixit S. Effect of electrocardiographic lead placement on localization of outflow tract tachycardias. Heart Rhythm. 2012;9:697-703.
44. Betensky BP, Park RE, Marchlinski FE, Hutchinson MD, Garcia FC, Dixit S, Callans DJ, Cooper JM, Bala R, Lin D, Riley MP, Gerstenfeld EP. The V(2) transition ratio: a new electrocardiographic criterion for distinguishing left from right ventricular outflow tract tachycardia origin. J Am Coll Cardiol. 2011;57:2255-62.
45. Cheng Z, Cheng K, Deng H, Chen T, Gao P, Zhu K, Fang Q. The R-wave deflection interval in lead V3 combining with R-wave amplitude index in lead V1: a new surface ECG algorithm for distinguishing left from right ventricular outflow tract tachycardia origin in patients with transitional lead at V3. Int J Cardiol. 2013;168:1342-8.
46. Yoshida N, Yamada T, McElderry HT, Inden Y, Shimano M, Murohara T, Kumar V, Doppalapudi H, Plumb VJ, Kay GN. A novel electrocardiographic criterion for differentiating a left from right ventricular outflow tract tachycardia origin: the V2S/V3R index. J Cardiovasc Electrophysiol. 2014;25:747-53.
47. Jadonath RL, Schwartzman DS, Preminger MW, Gottlieb CD, Marchlinski FE. Utility of the 12-lead electrocardiogram in localizing the origin of right ventricular outflow tract tachycardia. Am Heart J. 1995;130:1107-13.
48. Movsowitz C, Schwartzman D, Callans DJ, Preminger M, Zado E, Gottlieb CD, Marchlinski FE. Idiopathic right ventricular outflow tract tachycardia: Narrowing the anatomic location for successful ablation. Am Heart J. 1996;131:930-6.
49. Yamauchi Y, Aonuma K, Takahashi A, Sekiguchi Y, Hachiya H, Yokoyama Y, Kumagai K, Nogami A, Iesaka Y, Isobe M. Electrocardiographic characteristics of repetitive monomorphic right ventricular tachycardia originating near the His-bundle. J Cardiovasc Electrophysiol. 2005;16:1041-8.
50. Hasdemir CAN, Aktas S, Govsa F, Aktas EO, Kocak A, Bozkaya YT, Demirbas MI, Ulucan CEM, Ozdogan O, Kayikcioglu M, Can LH, Payzin S. Demonstration of ventricular myocardial extensions into the pulmonary artery and aorta beyond the ventriculo-arterial junction. Pacing Clin Electrophysiol. 2007;30:534-9.
51. Tada H, Tadokoro K, Miyaji K, Ito S, Kurosaki K, Kaseno K, Naito S, Nogami A, Oshima S, Taniguchi K. Idiopathic ventricular arrhythmias arising from the pulmonary artery: prevalence, characteristics, and topography of the arrhythmia origin. Heart Rhythm. 2008;5:419-26.
52. Sekiguchi Y, Aonuma K, Takahashi A, Yamauchi Y, Hachiya H, Yokoyama Y, Iesaka Y, Isobe M. Electrocardiographic and electrophysiologic characteristics of ventricular tachycardia originating within the pulmonary artery. J Am Coll Cardiol. 2005;45:887-95.
53. Lin D, Ilkhanoff L, Gerstenfeld E, Dixit S, Beldner S, Bala R, Garcia F, Callans D, Marchlinski FE. Twelve-lead electrocardiographic characteristics of the aortic cusp region guided by intracardiac echocardiography and electroanatomic mapping. Heart Rhythm. 2008;5:663-9.
54. Bala R, Marchlinski FE. Electrocardiographic recognition and ablation of outflow tract ventricular tachycardia. Heart Rhythm. 2007;4:366-70.
55. Yoshida N, Inden Y, Uchikawa T, Kamiya H, Kitamura K, Shimano M, Tsuji Y, Hirai M, Murohara T. Novel transitional zone index allows more accurate differentiation between idiopathic right ventricular outflow tract and aortic sinus cusp ventricular arrhythmias. Heart Rhythm. 2011;8:349-56.
56. Maeda S, Chik WW, Han Y, Liang JJ, Squara F, Arkles JS, Sadek MM, Santangeli P, Frankel DS, Zado ES, Takebayashi S, Dixit S, Callans DJ, Marchlinski FE, Lin D. Effects of age-related aortic root anatomic changes on left ventricular outflow tract pace-mapping morphologies: a cardiac magnetic resonance imaging validation study. J Cardiovasc Electrophysiol 2015 (EPub Ahead of Print).
57. Stec S, Sikorska A, Zaborska B, Krynski T, Szymot J, Kulakowski P. Benign symptomatic premature ventricular complexes: short- and long-term efficacy of antiarrhythmic drugs and radiofrequency ablation. Kardiol Pol. 2012;70:351-8.
58. Stevenson WG, Nademanee K, Weiss JN, Wiener I. Treatment of catecholamine-sensitive right ventricular tachycardia by endocardial catheter ablation. J Am Coll Cardiol. 1990;16:752-5.
59. Zhong L, Lee YH, Huang XM, Asirvatham SJ, Shen WK, Friedman PA, Hodge DO, Slusser JP, Song ZY, Packer DL, Cha YM. Relative efficacy of catheter ablation vs antiarrhythmic drugs in treating premature ventricular contractions: a single-center retrospective study. Heart Rhythm. 2014;11:187-93.

60. Ling Z, Liu Z, Su L, Zipunnikov V, Wu J, Du H, Woo K, Chen S, Zhong B, Lan X, Fan J, Xu Y, Chen W, Yin Y, Nazarian S, Zrenner B. Radiofrequency ablation versus antiarrhythmic medication for treatment of ventricular premature beats from the right ventricular outflow tract: prospective randomized study. Circ Arrhythm Electrophysiol. 2014;7:237-43.
61. Chung FP, Chong E, Lin YJ, Chang SL, Lo LW, Hu YF, Tuan TC, Chao TF, Liao JN, Huang YC, Chi PC, Chan CS, Yun-Yu C, Huang HK, Chen SA. Different characteristics and electrophysiological properties between early and late recurrences after acute successful catheter ablation of idiopathic right ventricular outflow tract arrhythmias during long-term follow-up. Heart Rhythm. 2014;11:1760-9.
62. Gerstenfeld EP, Dixit S, Callans DJ, Rajawat Y, Rho R, Marchlinski FE. Quantitative comparison of spontaneous and paced 12-lead electrocardiogram during right ventricular outflow tract ventricular tachycardia. J Am Coll Cardiol. 2003;41:2046-53.
63. Mandel JE, Hutchinson MD, Marchlinski FE. Remifentanil-midazolam sedation provides hemodynamic stability and comfort during epicardial ablation of ventricular tachycardia. J Cardiovasc Electrophysiol. 2011;22:464-6.
64. Berruezo A, Mont L, Nava S, Chueca E, Bartholomay E, Brugada J. Electrocardiographic recognition of the epicardial origin of ventricular tachycardias. Circulation. 2004;109:1842-7.
65. Daniels DV, Lu YY, Morton JB, Santucci PA, Akar JG, Green A, Wilber DJ. Idiopathic epicardial left ventricular tachycardia originating remote from the sinus of Valsalva: electrophysiological characteristics, catheter ablation, and identification from the 12-lead electrocardiogram. Circulation. 2006;113:1659-66.
66. Yamada T, Murakami Y, Yoshida N, Okada T, Shimizu T, Toyama J, Yoshida Y, Tsuboi N, Muto M, Inden Y, Hirai M, Murohara T, McElderry HT, Epstein AE, Plumb VJ, Kay GN. Preferential conduction across the ventricular outflow septum in ventricular arrhythmias originating from the aortic sinus cusp. J Am Coll Cardiol. 2007;50:884-91.
67. Ouyang F, Fotuhi P, Ho SY, Hebe J, Volkmer M, Goya M, Burns M, Antz M, Ernst S, Cappato R, Kuck KH. Repetitive monomorphic ventricular tachycardia originating from the aortic sinus cusp: electrocardiographic characterization for guiding catheter ablation. J Am Coll Cardiol. 2002;39:500-8.
68. Walsh KA, Fahy GJ. Anatomy of the left main coronary artery of particular relevance to ablation of left atrial and outflow tract arrhythmias. Heart Rhythm. 2014;11:2231-8.
69. Vaidya V, Syed F, Desimone C, Bdeir S, Munoz FDC, Packer DL, Asirvatham SJ. Outflow tract ventricular tachycardia mapped to the coronary arteries: anatomical correlates and management strategies. J Cardiovasc Electrophysiol. 2013;24:1416-22.

EDITORS' SUMMARY

Professor Dixit and Dr Liang outline in this chapter an essential "what you need to know", informative approach to mapping and ablating outflow tract tachycardias. The difficult areas of distinguishing benign outflow tract tachycardia from arrhythmogenic right ventricular cardiomyopathy and the topic of outflow tract arrhythmia giving rise to cardiomyopathy are covered with a practical and useful approach. This chapter is best used in conjunction with Chapter 37 from Professor Yamada on nonoutflow tract idiopathic VT and the chapter 6 on anatomic correlations for electrophysiology.

CHAPTER 37

Takumi Yamada

Idiopathic Ventricular Tachycardia from the Mitral Annulus, Papillary Muscles and Other Sites

LIST OF ABBREVIATIONS

AIV	Anterior Interventricular Vein	MB	Moderator Band
CS	Coronary Sinus	PAM	Papillary Muscles
GCV	Great Cardiac Vein	PVC	Premature Ventricular Contraction
ICE	Intracardiac Echocardiography	RF	Radiofrequency
LAD	Left Anterior Descending	RV	Right Ventricle
LCx	Left Circumflex	RVOT	Right Ventricular Outflow Tract
LV	Left Ventricle	VA	Ventricular Arrhythmia
MA	Mitral Annulus	VT	Ventricular Tachycardia

INTRODUCTION

Idiopathic ventricular arrhythmias (VAs) are not related to scarring, and occur in patients with and without structural heart disease.[1,2] In the past decade, advances in procedural techniques, and an improved understanding of electrophysiological mechanisms, have allowed catheter ablation to cure most idiopathic VAs arising from the endocardium and epicardium. As a result, the major sites of origin of idiopathic VAs have been revealed **(Table 37.1)**.[3-27] The ventricular outflow tracts are the most common and the left ventricular fascicles are the second most common sites of origins of idiopathic VAs.[1,2] In this chapter, idiopathic VAs originating from the other sites including the papillary muscles (PAMs), atrioventricular annuli, moderator band, and epicardium, are described.

PAPILLARY MUSCLE VENTRICULAR ARRHYTHMIAS

VAs originating from the PAMs account for approximately 7% of patients with idiopathic VAs.[23] PAM VAs are most often idiopathic, but can be complicated with structural heart diseases.[19-24] These VAs are often exercise-induced or require intravenous isoproterenol or epinephrine for induction. They usually occur as premature ventricular contractions (PVCs) rather than ventricular tachycardias (VTs). Anatomically, the PAMs of the heart are the thickest myocardial structure and conical projections into the ventricular myocardium covered by endocardium **(Figures 37.1A and B)**. The basal end of the PAMs is attached to the mitral or tricuspid leaflets by multiple tendons. The left ventricular anterolateral or posteromedial papillary

Table 37.1: Major sites of origin of idiopathic ventricular arrhythmias

	RV	*LV*
Outflow tract region		
Supravalvular	PA	Aorta
Endocardial	RVOT	LVOT (AMC)
Epicardial		LV summit (GCV, AIVV)
Annuli	TA (Peri-Hisian)	MA
Fascicles		LPF>>LAF Upper septum
Intracavital	PAM Moderator band	PPAM>>APAM
Epicardium		Crux (MCV)

(LV ostium: Aorta, LVOT (AMC), LV summit (GCV, AIVV), MA)

Abbreviations: AIVV, anterior interventricular vein; AMC, aortomitral continuity; APAM, anterolateral papillary muscle; GCV, great cardiac vein; LAF, left anterior fascicle; LPF, left posterior fascicle; LV, left ventricle; LVOT, LV outflow tract; MA, mitral annulus; MCV, middle cardiac vein; PA, pulmonary artery; PAM, papillary muscle; PPAM, posteromedial papillary muscle; RV, right ventricle; RVOT, RV outflow tract; TA, tricuspid annulus

muscles originate from the middle to apical site of the anterior or inferior wall of the left ventricle (LV), respectively. VAs originating from the LV PAMs are known to arise more commonly from the posteromedial PAM than anterolateral PAM.[19-23] The sites of the origin of PAM VAs are limited to the base of the PAMs. VAs can rarely originate from the PMs in the right ventricle (RV).[24] It has been reported that VAs can arise from all 3 PAMs in the RV, and half of them arise from the septal PAM.[24]

Electrocardiographic Characteristics

VAs originating from the anterolateral and posteromedial PAMs in the LV exhibit right bundle branch block morphology and right inferior and left or right superior axis of the QRS, respectively.[19-23] RV PAM VAs originating from the posterior or anterior RV PAMs more often exhibit a superior axis with late precordial transition (> lead V4) as compared with septal RV PAM VAs, which more often exhibit an inferior axis with an earlier precordial transition (≤ lead V4).[24] PAM VAs often exhibit multiple QRS morphologies at baseline, which may be caused by a single origin with

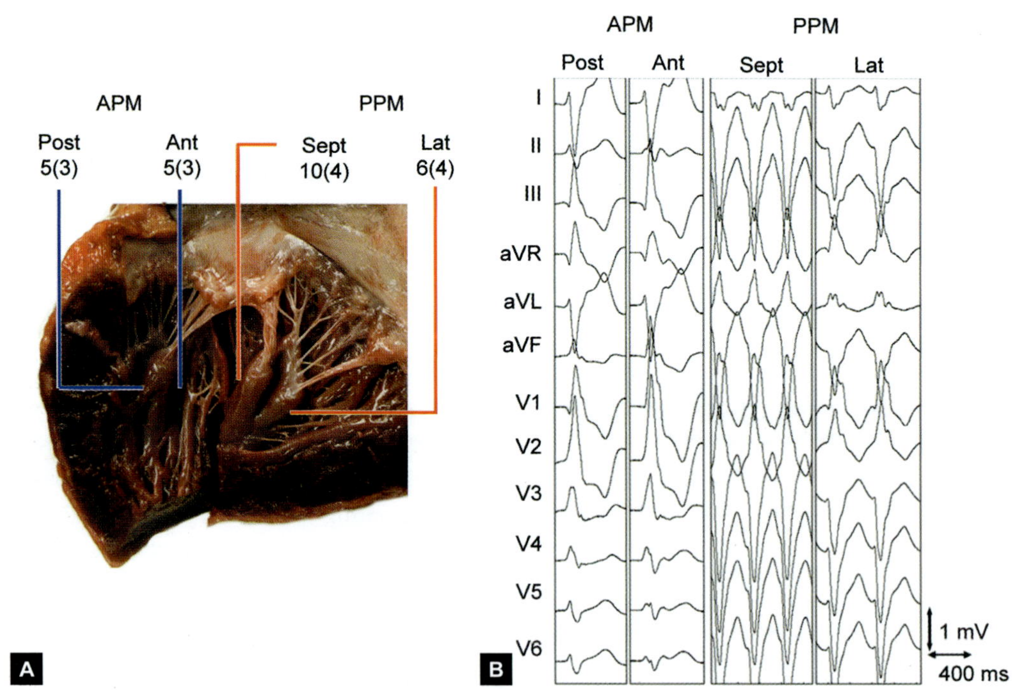

Figures 37.1A and B: The human autopsy heart exhibiting the distribution of the successful ablation sites (A) and representative 12-lead electrocardiograms exhibiting the differences in the QRS morphology of the ventricular arrhythmias successfully ablated between both sides of the papillary muscles in the same patients (B). The number in (A) indicates the number of the patients and the number in the parentheses, the number of the patients with radiofrequency lesions on both sides of the papillary muscle

Abbreviations: Ant, anterior side; APM, anterolateral papillary muscle; Lat, lateral side; Post, posterior side; PPM, posteromedial papillary muscle; Sept, septal side

From: Yamada T, Doppalapudi H, McElderry HT, et al. Electrocardiographic and electrophysiological characteristics in idiopathic ventricular arrhythmias originating from the papillary muscles in the left ventricle: relevance for catheter ablation. Circ Arrhythm Electrophysiol. 2010;3: 24-331. With permission

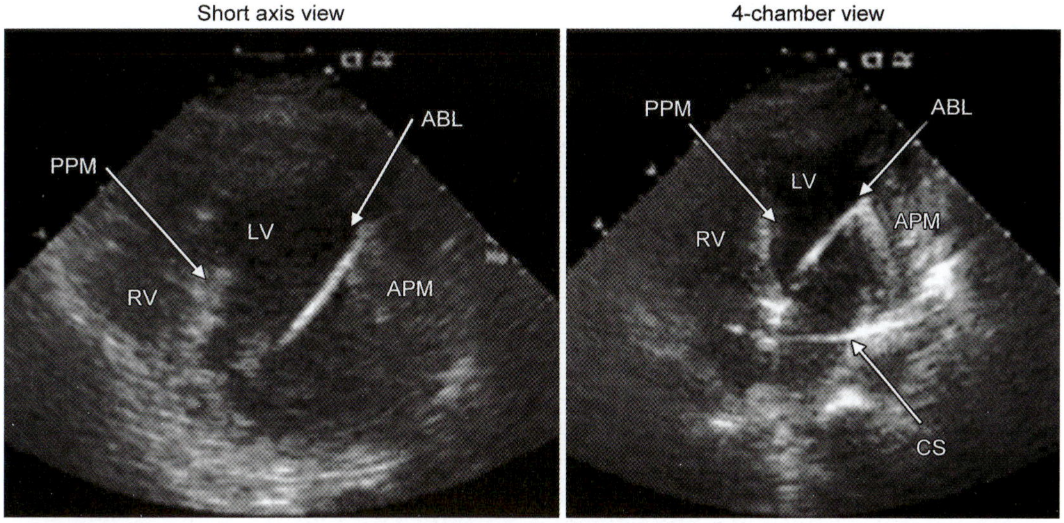

Figure 37.6: Two-dimensional transthoracic echocardiographic images exhibiting a parasternal short-axis view at the level of the papillary muscles and an apical 4-chamber view obtained during the procedure, with the ablation catheter positioned at the site of the successful ablation. The ablation catheter located at the anterior and middle portion of the APM is clearly seen

Abrreviation: RV, right ventricle. The other abbreviations are as in the previous figures

From: Yamada T, McElderry HT, Okada T, et al. Idiopathic focal ventricular arrhythmias originating from the anterior papillary muscle in the left ventricle. J Cardiovasc Electrophysiol 2009;20:866-72. With permission

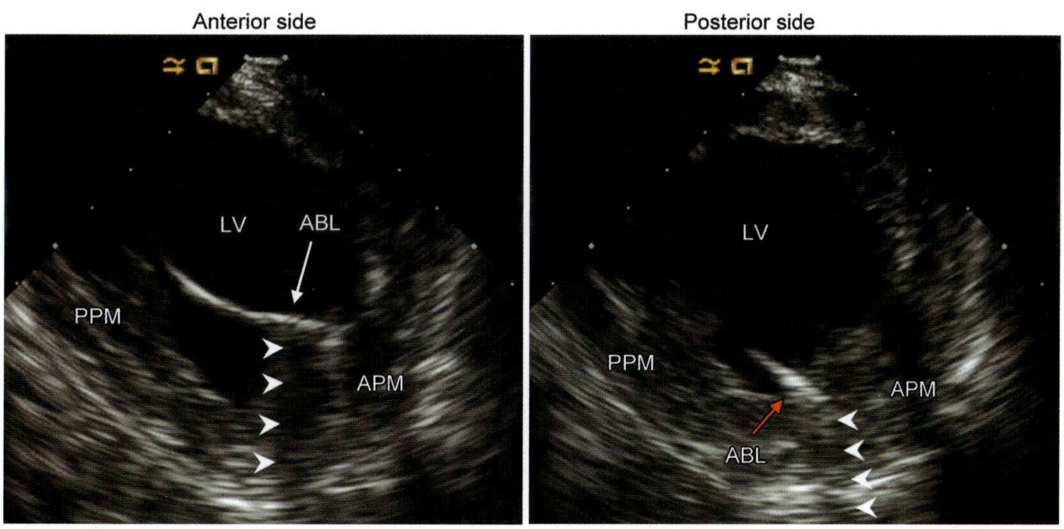

Figure 37.7: The intracardiac echocardiographic images of the successful ablation site. Two-dimensional intracardiac echocardiographic short-axis images at the level of the papillary muscles demonstrate that the ablation catheter (ABL) was positioned on the anterior and posterior sides of the APM. The arrowheads indicate the acoustic shadow from the ablation catheter. Abbreviations are as in the previous figures

From: Yamada T, Doppalapudi H, McElderry HT, et al. Electrocardiographic and electrophysiological characteristics in idiopathic ventricular arrhythmias originating from the papillary muscles in the left ventricle: relevance for catheter ablation. Circ Arrhythm Electrophysiol. 2010;3: 324-31. With permission

ostium that is known as one of the major sites of idiopathic VA origins (*see* **Table 37.1**).[13] The idiopathic VAs originating from the MA account for 5% of all idiopathic VAs. There is no gender difference or a slight male dominance in the incidence of MA VAs.[11,12,32,33] MA VAs most often occur in middle to old age. MA VAs can originate from any of the regions along the MA, but the anterolateral and posteroseptal aspects of the MA are the most and second-most common sites of MA VA origins, respectively.[11,12] MA VAs occur as PVCs rather than VTs.

The anteromedial aspect of the MA, which is termed the aortomitral continuity, may be included in sites of MA VA origins.[33]

Electrocardiographic Characteristics

All MA VAs exhibit a right bundle branch block pattern and monophasic R or Rs in leads V2 to V6 **(Figures 37.11A to C)**.[11,12,32,33] Because the origins of all MA VAs are located in the posterior portion of the LV, distant from the precordial electrodes, the activation from the MA VA origins propagates toward these electrodes, resulting in an early precordial transition and concordant positive QRS pattern in leads V2 to V4 during MA VAs. The electrocardiographic characteristics are very helpful for predicting sites of MA VA origins.[11,12,33] The polarity of the QRS complex in the inferior leads and lateral leads (I and aVL) is useful for distinguishing the anterolateral MA VAs from the posterior and posterolateral MA VAs. The polarity of the QRS complex in the inferior and lateral leads is positive and negative, respectively in the anterolateral MA VAs while that is negative and positive in the posterior and posterolateral MA VAs, respectively. MA VAs originating from the free wall of MA are characterized by a longer QRS duration sometimes with pseudodelta waves and notching in the late phase of the R- or Q-wave in the inferior leads, which may result from phased excitation from the LV free wall to the RV **(Figure 37.12)**. These ECG characteristics are not observed in the posteroseptal, anterior, and anteromedial MA VAs. Posterior MA VAs exhibit a dominant R-wave in lead V1, whereas posteroseptal MA VAs exhibit a negative QRS component in lead V1 (qR, qr, rs, rS, or QS). This is because the activation from the posteroseptal MA VA origin propagates toward the left and away from the electrode of lead V1 which is positioned horizontally to the ventricular septum. The Q-wave amplitude ratio of leads III to II is greater for posteroseptal MA VAs than posterior MA VAs because the activation from the posteroseptal MA VA origins propagates more toward the left than that from the posterior MA VA origins.

Electrophysiological Characteristics

MA VAs occur with a focal (nonreentrant) mechanism which may be triggered activity based on the response to adenosine, verapamil, and pacing maneuvers.[11,12] It has been proposed that a remnant of the atrioventricular conduction system close to the aortomitral continuity, such as a dead-end tract,[34] might be important in the genesis of a nonreentrant mechanism for the MA VAs.[11]

Mapping and Catheter Ablation

During the electrophysiological study, a multipolar mapping catheter should be placed in the coronary sinus (CS) in order to record the earliest ventricular activation during MA VAs. The earliest ventricular activation within the CS is usually presystolic during the MA VAs **(Figure 37.12)**. Mapping should be performed underneath the mitral valve around the electrode of the CS catheter recording the earliest ventricular

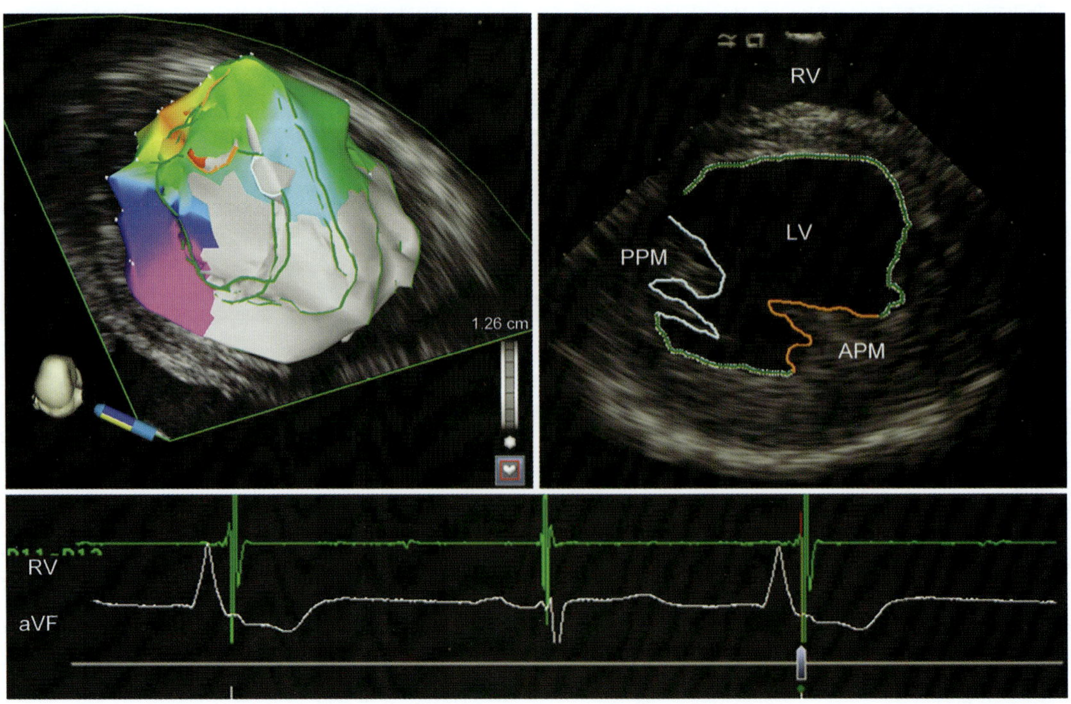

Figure 37.8A

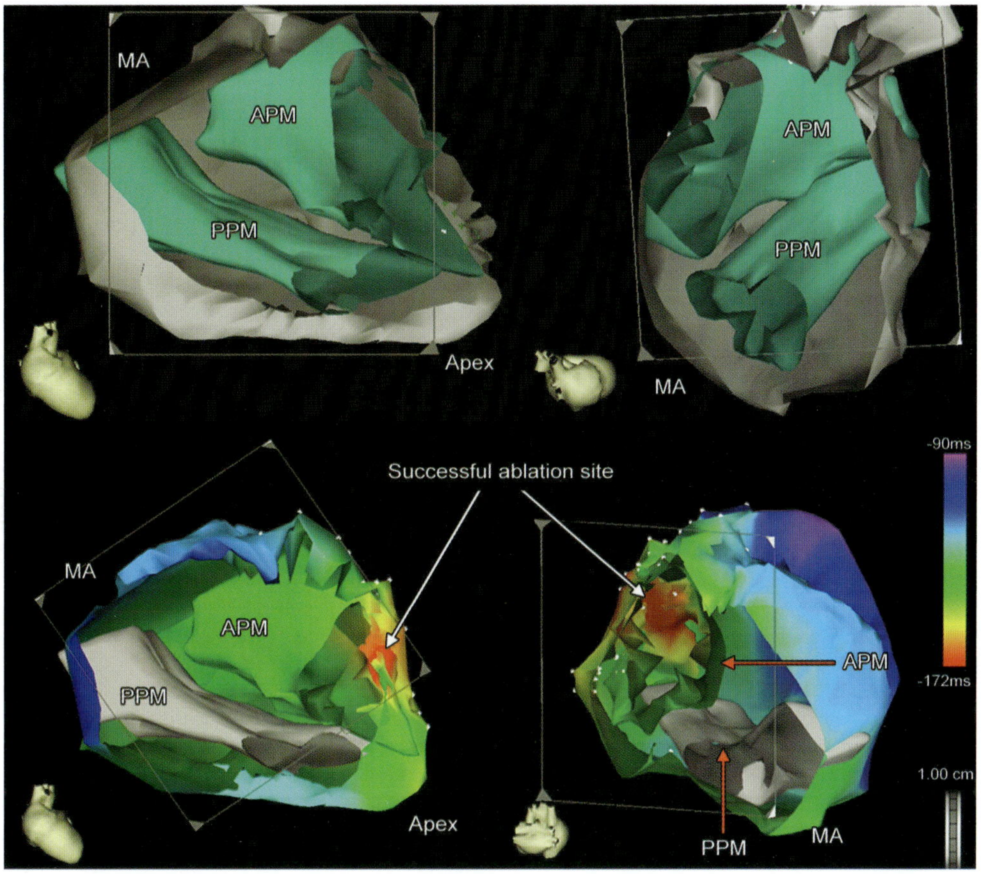

Figure 37.8B

Figures 37.8A and B: (A) Real-time integration of the intracardiac echocardiography (ICE) and three-dimensional (3D) electroanatomic mapping. The left panel exhibits the CARTO map of the LV with the ultrasound "fan" projecting from the tip of the ICE probe to generate the ICE image exhibited in the right panel. A two-dimensional ICE image was registered as part of the CARTO shell of the LV. The green (LV), orange (APM), and light blue (PPM) lines on the 3D reconstruction of the LV (left panel) represent the individual registered contours traced on the ICE images synchronized to the RV electrogram during the PVCs originating from the APM (lower panel); (B) Three-dimensional LV anatomical shells (upper panel) and activation maps during the PVCs originating from the APM (lower panel). The left figure on each panel exhibits the image seen through the LV septum and the right figure on each panel exhibits the image seen from the mitral annulus (MA). Abbreviations are as in the previous figures

From: Yamada T, McElderry HT, Doppalapudi H, et al. Real-time integration of intracardiac echocardiography and electroanatomic mapping in PVCs arising from the LV anterior papillary muscle. Pacing Clin Electrophysiol. 2009;32:1240-3. With permission

activation with an ablation catheter through a retrograde transaortic approach. However, a transseptal approach may sometimes be required for better mapping in the posterior to posteroseptal aspects of the MA. In order to identify the site of an MA VA origin, activation mapping is the most reliable, but pacemapping from the CS and ablation catheter is helpful when MA VAs are infrequent. At the successful ablation site of MA VAs, an atrial electrogram is usually recorded, and the ratio of the local atrial and ventricular electrograms should be less than one **(Figure 37.12)**. RF energy is usually used for catheter ablation of MA VAs. Epicardial catheter ablation within the CS is rarely required for elimination of MA VAs when endocardial catheter ablation is unsuccessful.

Ablation Outcome and Complications

Catheter ablation of MA VAs is highly successful and its complications are very unlikely although there is a potential risk of mitral insufficiency.

TRICUSPID ANNULAR VENTRICULAR ARRHYTHMIAS

Idiopathic VAs also can originate from the tricuspid annulus (TA). These VAs account for 8% of all idiopathic VAs.[14] TA VAs more often occur in males (twice as often as in females) and in old age.[14] TA VAs can originate from any regions along

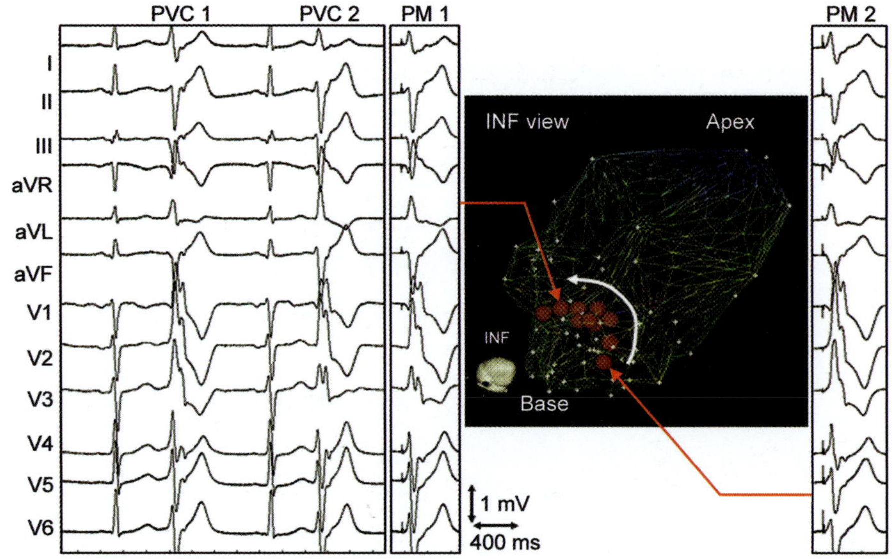

Figure 37.9: The 12-lead electrocardiograms of the PVCs originating from the LV PPM and excellent pace maps (PMs) and an electroanatomic map exhibiting the radiofrequency ablation sites. At baseline, there were 2 main PVCs with differences in the QRS morphology (PVC 1 and PVC 2) and a fused form of them. The depth of the S-waves in the inferior leads was smaller, the R-wave amplitude in lead aVL was smaller, and the QRS duration was longer during PVC 1 than during PVC 2. Excellent pace maps of PVC 1 and PVC 2 were reproduced by pacing from the lateral and septal sides of the PPM, respectively, before the ablation. Radiofrequency ablation at the lateral side of the PPM never interrupted the PVCs. Because the QRS morphology of PVC 1 slightly changed and the earliest activation site gradually moved to the septal side of the PPM after every radiofrequency application, radiofrequency lesions targeting the earliest ventricular activation sites were created on approximately half the circumference of the PPM. Finally, radiofrequency ablation at the septal side completely eliminated all the PVCs. PM 1 and PM 2 correspond to the pace maps for PVC 1 and PVC 2, respectively. The arrow on the electroanatomic map indicates the direction of the creation of the radiofrequency lesions

Abbreviations: PVC, premature ventricular contraction; INF, inferior

From: Yamada T, Doppalapudi H, McElderry HT, et al. Electrocardiographic and electrophysiological characteristics in idiopathic ventricular arrhythmias originating from the papillary muscles in the left ventricle: relevance for catheter ablation. Circ Arrhythm Electrophysiol. 2010;3: 324-31. With permission

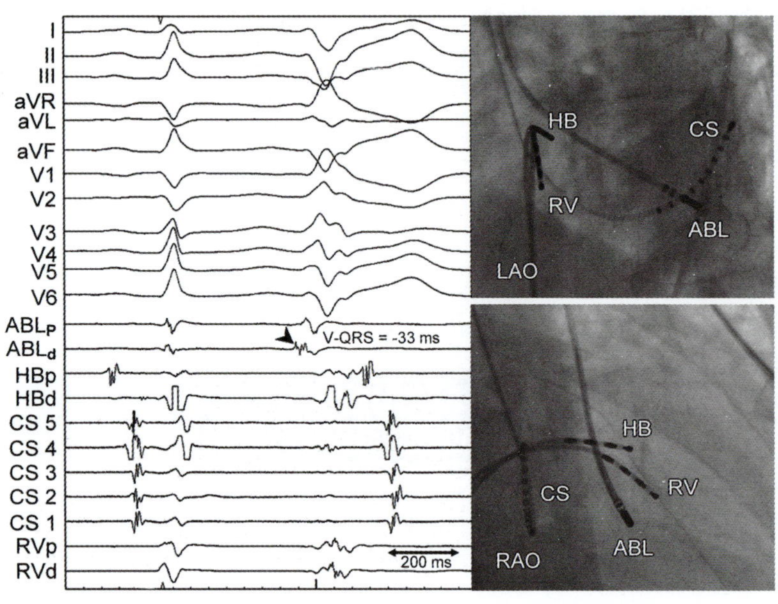

Figure 37.10: Cardiac tracings (left panel) and fluoroscopic images (right panels) exhibiting the successful ablation site of the PVCs originating from the LV PPM. The first beat is a sinus beat and the second one is a PVC. Note that at the successful ablation site, no Purkinje potentials were observed during sinus rhythm and a spiky prepotential (arrowhead) was observed in the local ventricular activity during the PVC

Abrreviations: ABL, HB, RV d(p), the distal (proximal) electrode pair of the ablation, His bundle, right ventricular catheter, respectively; CS 1 to 5, the first to fifth electrode pair of the coronary sinus catheter; V-QRS, the local ventricular activation time relative to the QRS onset. The other abbreviations are as in the previous figures

From: Yamada T, Doppalapudi H, McElderry HT, et al. Electrocardiographic and electrophysiological characteristics in idiopathic ventricular arrhythmias originating from the papillary muscles in the left ventricle: relevance for catheter ablation. Circ Arrhythm Electrophysiol. 2010;3: 324-31. With permission

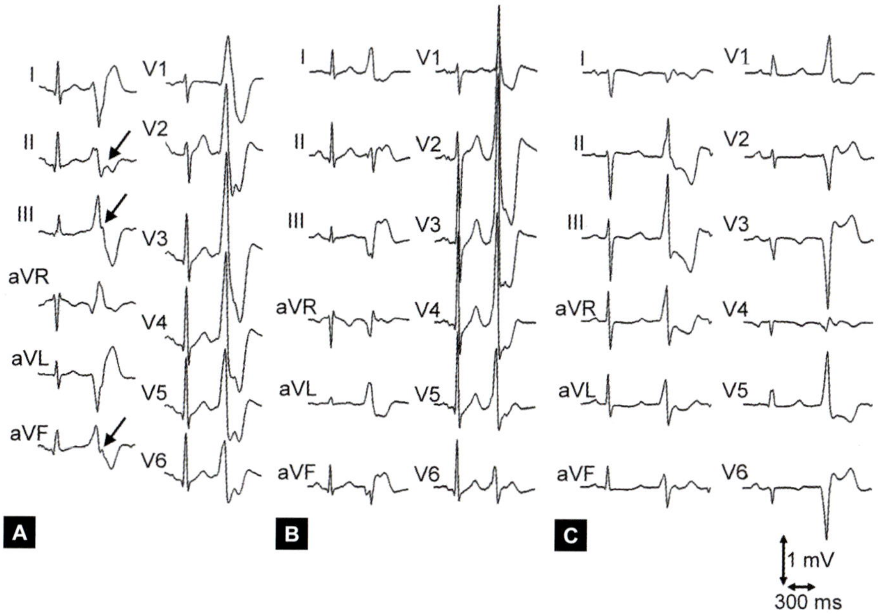

Figures 37.11A to C: The representative 12-lead electrocardiograms of the PVCs originating from the anterolateral (A), posterior (B), and posteroseptal (C) aspects of the mitral annulus. The arrows indicate "notching" of the late phase of the QRS complex in the inferior leads

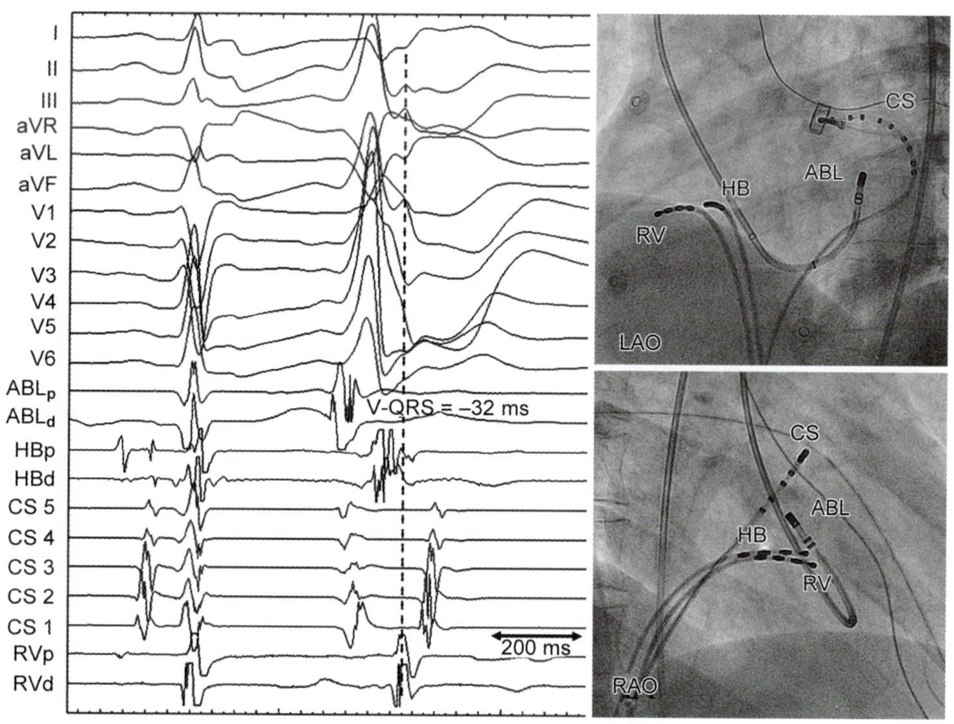

Figure 37.12: Cardiac tracings (left panel) and fluoroscopic images (right panels) exhibiting the successful ablation site of the PVCs originating from the lateral aspect of the mitral annulus. During the PVC, the timing of the second peak of the "notched" R-wave corresponds precisely with that of the activation of the right ventricular free wall (dotted line), which was recorded from the catheter at the anterolateral aspect of the tricuspid annulus. The abbreviations are as in the previous figures

the TA, but more often originate from the septal aspect, especially in the anteroseptal or para-Hisian region than the free wall of the TA.[14] VAs originating from the free wall of the TA more often occur in males than in females while VAs originating from the septum of the TA are distributed almost equally between males and females.[35]

Electrocardiographic Characteristics

All TA VAs exhibit a left bundle branch block QRS morphology and positive QRS polarity in leads I, V5, and V6 **(Figures 37.13A to C)**.[14,33] No negative component of the QRS complex is found in lead I because the TA VA origins are located on the right anterior side of the heart. Because the TA sits at the base of the RV, the activation propagating from the TA VA origins toward the apex generates a positive QRS polarity in leads V5 and V6. The R-wave in lead I is usually taller during TA VAs than during VAs originating from the RV outflow tract (RVOT), which is the most common site of idiopathic VAs because the TA is located more rightward and inferior to the RVOT. For the same reason, a positive QRS polarity in all of the inferior leads is rare in TA VAs although that is common in all RVOT VAs. TA VAs exhibits an rS or QS pattern in lead aVR like RVOT VAs. However, in lead aVL, a QS or rS pattern is rare, and the QRS polarity in lead aVL is positive in almost all TA VAs, which is not the case for RVOT VAs.

Among all TA VAs, the QRS duration and Q-wave amplitude in each of the leads V1 to V3 are greater in TA VAs originating from the free wall of the TA as compared with those from the septal wall of the TA.[14,33] The septal TA VAs exhibit an earlier precordial transition (lead V3), narrower QRS, and QS in lead V1 with the absence of notching in the inferior leads while the free-wall TA VAs are associated with a late precordial transition (> lead V3), wider QRS, absence of Q-waves in lead V1, and notching in the inferior leads (the timing of the second peak of the notched QRS complex in the inferior leads corresponds precisely with the LV free wall activation) **(Figure 37.14)**. These ECG characteristics are helpful for distinguishing between TA VAs originating from the free wall and septal wall of the TA. The negative QRS polarity in the inferior leads predicts VA origins in the posterior aspect of the TA, and otherwise, VA origins in the mid to anterior aspects of the TA are suggested.

Electrophysiological Characteristics

TA VAs often occur spontaneously or can be induced by an isoproterenol infusion. TA VAs most likely have a focal (nonreentrant) mechanism, and can rarely be induced or terminated by programmed ventricular stimulation.

Mapping and Catheter Ablation

In order to identify the site of the TA VA origin, activation mapping is the most reliable, but pace-mapping is helpful when TA VAs are infrequent. At the successful ablation sites of TA VAs, an atrial electrogram is usually recorded, and a

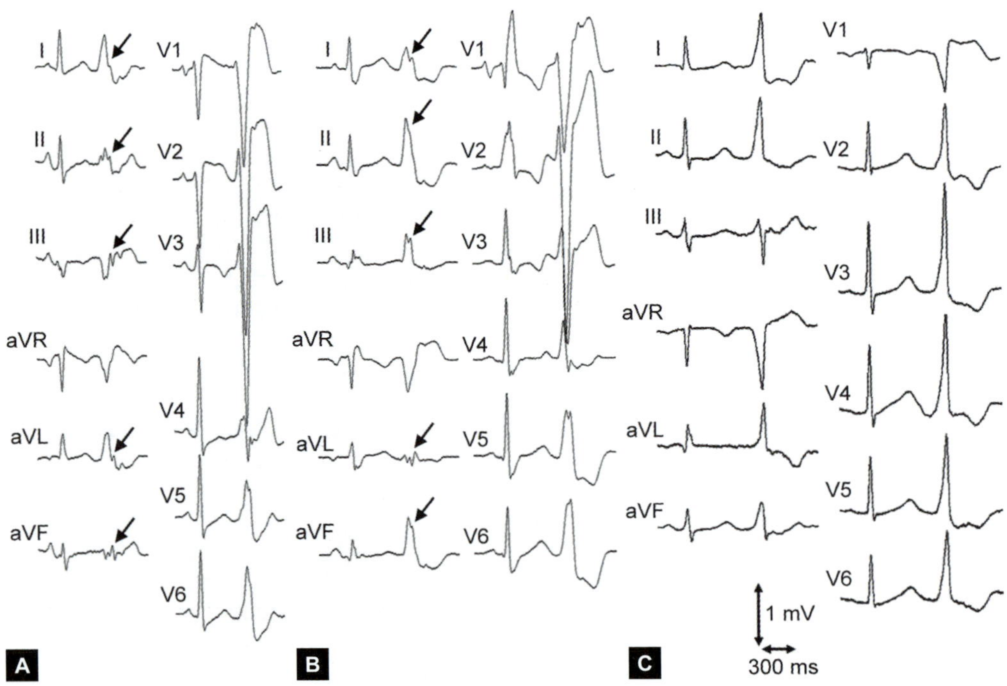

Figures 37.13A to C: The representative 12-lead electrocardiograms of the PVCs originating from the posterolateral (A), anterior (B), and anteroseptal (C) aspects of the triscuspid annulus. The arrows indicate "notching" of the late phase of the QRS complex in the limb leads

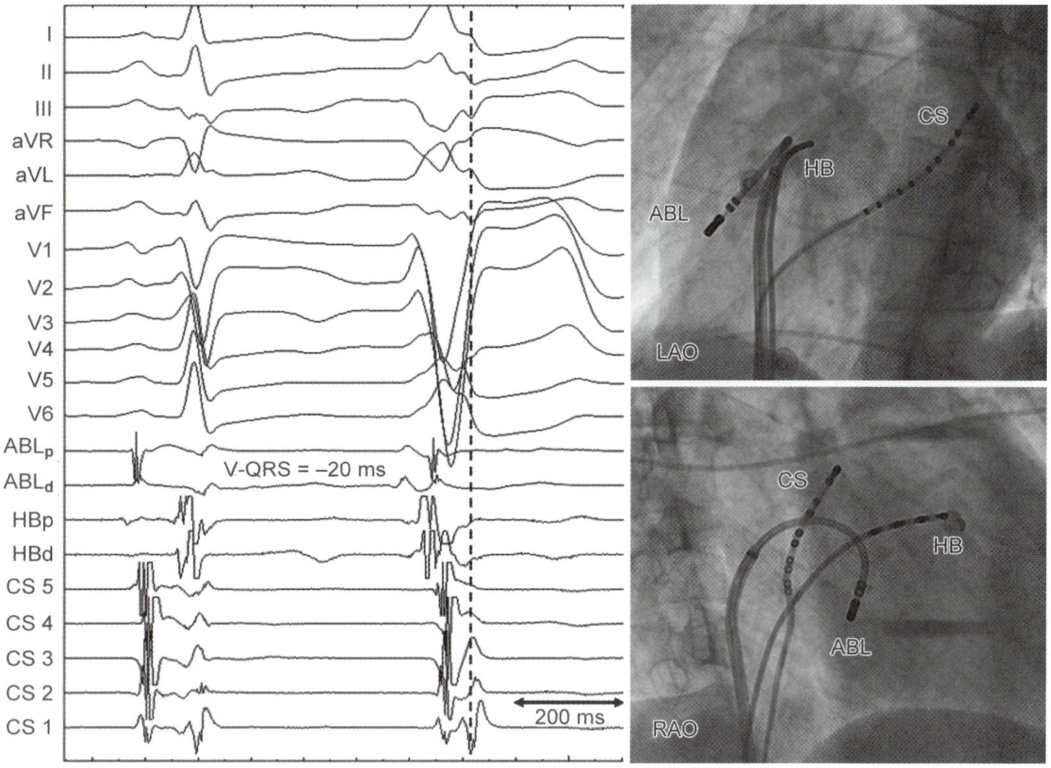

Figure 37.14: Cardiac tracings (left panel) and fluoroscopic images (right panels) exhibiting the successful ablation site of the PVCs originating from the lateral aspect of the tricuspid annulus. During the PVC, the timing of the peak of the late "notched" R-wave corresponded precisely with that of the activation of the left ventricular free wall (dotted line), which was recorded from the catheter at the posterolateral aspect of the mitral annulus. The abbreviations are as in the previous figures

ratio of the local atrial and ventricular electrograms should be less than one **(Figure 37.14)**. RF energy is usually used for catheter ablation of TA VAs.

It is needless to say that the three-dimensional electroanatomic mapping systems are most helpful for mapping TA VAs. However, mapping along the TA with a duodecapolar Halo catheter and His bundle catheter may also be helpful for identifying an area of interest quickly **(Figure 37.15)**.[36] Because the mapping catheter approaches the TA from the right atrium, the TA is usually mapped on the tricuspid valve. Therefore, it is often challenging to achieve adequate contact and stability of the mapping catheter on the TA. In order to overcome such challenges, the use of long guiding sheaths may be recommended for mapping TA VAs **(Figures 37.14 and 37.15)**. The use of high RF power settings delivered from an irrigated or nonirrigated 8 mm tip ablation catheter may also be recommended in the catheter ablation of TA VAs in order to create an effective RF lesion underneath the tricuspid valve. When catheter ablation on the tricuspid valve is unsuccessful, a catheter inversion technique should be attempted for mapping and catheter ablation underneath the tricuspid valve **(Figure 37.16)**.

RF catheter ablation may be abandoned when a TA VA origin is located close to the atrioventricular conduction system. VAs originating from the RV near the His bundle exhibit ECG end electrophysiological characteristics similar to those of VAs originating from the right and noncoronary sinuses of Valsalva and near the membranous septum underneath those coronary cusps.[17,18] Therefore, when RV mapping reveals the earliest ventricular activation near the His bundle region, mapping in the right coronary and noncoronary cusps and the LV underneath those cusps should be added to identify the VA origin and reduce the risk of damage to the atrioventricular conduction system. When it is assured that a VA origin is located close to the His bundle in the RV, cryothermal ablation may be a viable alternative.[14]

Ablation Outcome and Complications

RF catheter ablation is often unsuccessful for VAs originating from the septal aspect of the TA.[14] Junctional rhythm or mild impairment of the atrioventricular conduction can occur during RF energy applications delivered to this region, resulting in an inadequate RF lesion formation. Considering

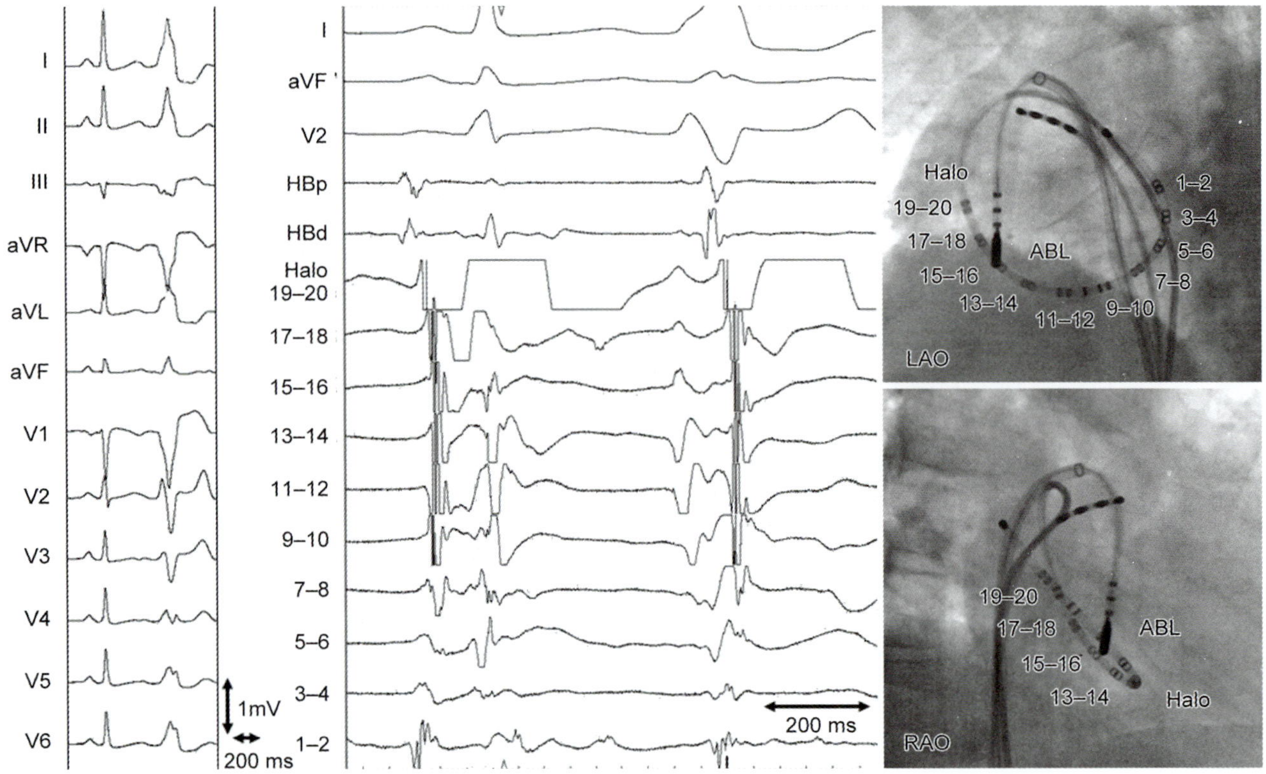

Figure 37.15: Twelve-lead electrocardiogram (left panel), cardiac tracings (middle panel), and successful ablation site (right panel) of the PVCs originating from the posterolateral aspect of the tricuspid annulus. The first beats are sinus beats and the second beats are premature ventricular contractions in the left and middle panels. The abbreviations are as in the previous figures

From: Yamada T, Allison JS, McElderry HT, et al. Successful catheter ablation of premature ventricular contractions originating from the tricuspid annulus using a Halo-type catheter. Europace. 2008;10:1228-9. With permission

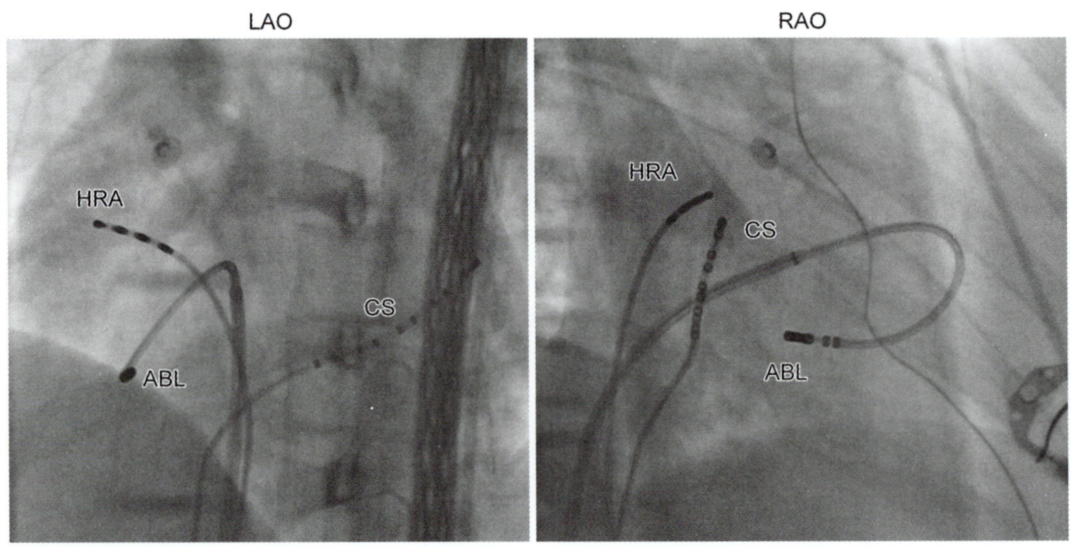

Figure 37.16: Fluoroscopic images exhibiting the successful ablation site at the posterolateral aspect of the tricuspid annulus by using the catheter inversion technique

Abrreviation: HRA, high right atrium. The other abbreviations are as in the previous figures that VAs are idiopathic, most care should be taken to prevent the incidence of atrioventricular conduction block. On the other hand, RF catheter ablation of VAs originating from the free-wall aspect of the TA is usually successful without any significant complications.

MODERATOR BAND VENTRICULAR ARRHYTHMIAS

It has been recently reported that the moderator band (MB) can be a source of VAs including PVCs, VTs, and ventricular fibrillation.[27] PVCs from the MB can be particularly prone to induce ventricular fibrillation. There is a significant male gender (90%) preponderance in the occurrence of MB VAs.

Anatomically, the MB is considered to be a part of the septomarginal trabeculation, crossing from the septum to the RV free wall and supporting the anterior PAM of the tricuspid valve **(Figure 37.17)**.[27] There is a wide variation in the morphology and insertion sites of the MB. In addition, the peripheral Purkinje network extends to the surface of the MB. These anatomical backgrounds should contribute to the electrocardiographic and electrophysiological characteristics of the MB VAs and affect the outcome of catheter ablation treatment of the MB VAs.

Electrocardiographic Characteristics

VAs arising from the MB have a distinctive ECG morphology. They exhibit a left bundle branch block and left superior frontal plane axis QRS morphology, sharp downstroke of the QRS in the precordial leads, and relatively narrow QRS duration **(Figures 37.18A and B)**.[27] MB VAs not only have a late precordial transition pattern, typically after lead V4, but also the transition is always later than that of the sinus rhythm QRS. Among the idiopathic right VAs, the late precordial transition and superiorly directed nature are helpful for distinguishing MB VAs from VAs originating in the RV base or septum.[27] Although the precordial transition is later during MB VAs than VAs originating from the septal RV PAM, there are no ECG features that clearly distinguish MB VAs from septal RV PAM VAs likely because of the similar insertion on the RV free wall and highly variable anatomy.

It is also noted that MB VAs exhibit varied ECG morphologies because of the altitudinal orientation of the heart, and the variation in the origin and insertion of the MB as well.

Electrophysiological Characteristics

During the electrophysiological study, PVCs originating from the MB often occur spontaneously.[27] When PVCs are infrequent, MB VAs can be induced by burst pacing from the RV on or off an isoproterenol infusion.

Mapping and Catheter Ablation

Because MB VAs originate from a specific anatomical structure, the guide of real-time imaging with ICE and three-dimensional electroanatomic mapping is necessary for an effective and safe mapping and catheter ablation of MB VAs **(Figures 37.19A and B)**. Given the heterogeneous morphology of the MB, ICE imaging during the procedure is important to allow accurate MB mapping and ensure catheter contact during the ablation.

The successful anatomic ablation sites along the MB are varied, including the septal insertion, body of the MB, and free-wall insertion.[27] In the challenging cases, changes in the

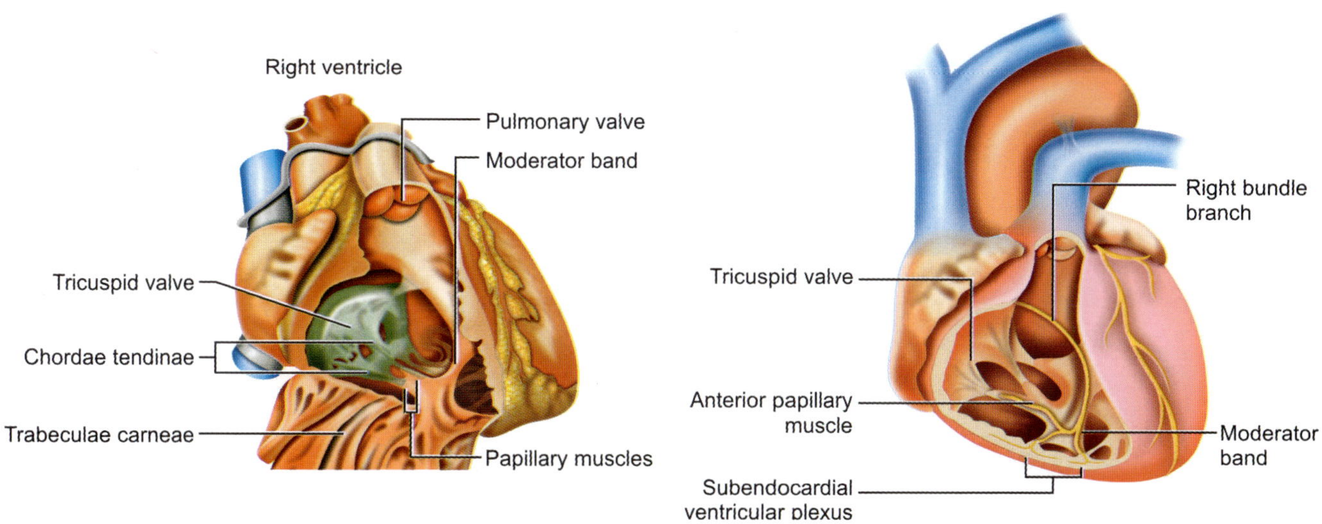

Figure 37.17: The schema exhibiting the moderator band crossing from the septum to the free wall of the right ventricle and supporting the anterior papillary muscle of the tricuspid valve

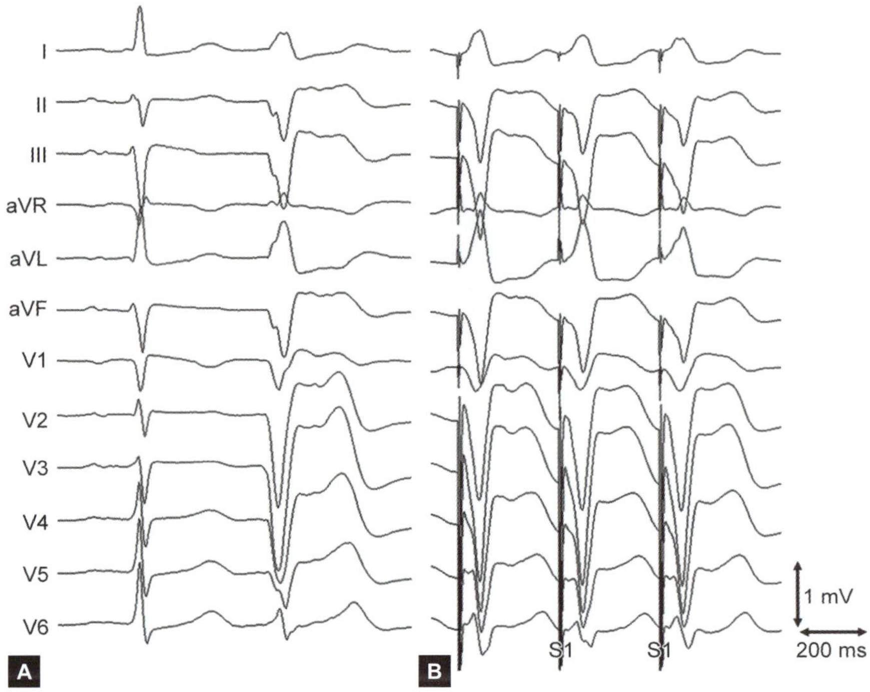

Figures 37.18A and B: Twelve-lead electrocardiograms exhibiting a PVC originating from the moderator band (A) and an excellent pace map (B)

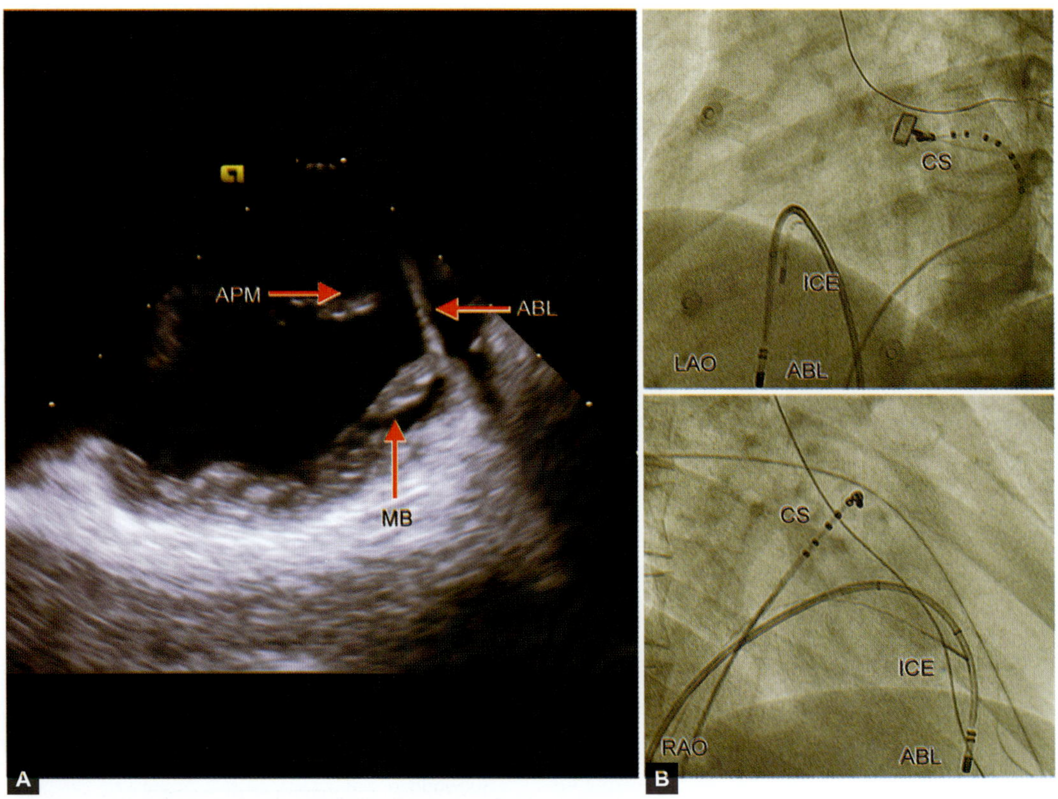

Figures 37.19A and B: The ICE images (A) and fluoroscopic images (B) exhibiting the successful ablation site of the PVCs originating from the moderator band (MB)

Abbreviation: ICE, intracardiac echocardiography catheter. The other abbreviations are as in the previous figures

QRS morphology can occur during the RF ablation, suggesting a change in the exit site, with eventual PVC elimination after extensive ablation, particularly on the free-wall insertion (subendocardial ventricular plexus). This might be explained by a deep origin within the MB with lateral exits that are modified progressively until all exits are eliminated. PVC termination can rarely be achievable with ablation of the right bundle branch. Whether the optimal approach for ablation of MB VAs involves targeting ablation at the site of the earliest activation, an extensive MB ablation including the free-wall insertion, or ablation of the right bundle branch remains to be elucidated.

Ablation Outcome and Complications

RF catheter ablation of MB VAs can be performed safely although it is challenging. Although long-term outcomes of the catheter ablation are generally excellent, a repeat procedure is often required likely due to challenging catheter contact and stability leading to a low power delivery to the thick intracavitary structure, despite adequate visualization with ICE.[27]

IDIOPATHIC EPICARDIAL VENTRICULAR ARRHYTHMIAS

Idiopathic VAs can arise from the epicardial sites. Although endocardial RF catheter ablation is highly successful for idiopathic RV VAs,[3] epicardial RF catheter ablation is sometimes required to cure LV VAs because the LV myocardial wall is thicker than that of the RV.[1,2,25,26,37] There are two major sites of origin of idiopathic epicardial VAs such as the crux of the heart[25] and LV summit.[26]

CRUX VENTRICULAR ARRHYTHMIAS

Anatomically, the crux of the heart is formed by the junction of the atrioventricular groove and the posterior interventricular groove and corresponds roughly to the junction of the middle cardiac vein and CS, near the origin of the posterior descending coronary artery.[25] Crux VAs are very rare (1% of all idiopathic VAs). They are usually exercise-induced and most often occur as a sustained VT, which is associated with syncope or presyncope.[25]

Electrocardiographic Characteristics

VAs arising from the crux of the heart exhibit a left superior axis QRS morphology with deeply negative deltoid waves (QS pattern) in the inferior leads and an early precordial transition (a prominent R-wave in lead V2) which may be associated with a polarity reversal between leads V1 and V2 **(Figure 37.20)**. It is noted that a QS or large S-wave is possible in lead V6 although crux VAs arise from the LV base. These ECG characteristics are similar to those associated with maximally preexcited posteroseptal accessory pathways because the latter insert into the same area of the LV as the origins of crux VAs. The maximum deflection index (calculated by dividing the shortest time from the QRS onset to the maximum deflection in any of the precordial leads by the total QRS duration)[37] is always greater than 0.55.

Electrophysiological Characteristics

Crux VAs occur with a focal (nonreentrant) mechanism.[25] They can be induced by pacing, and require isoproterenol

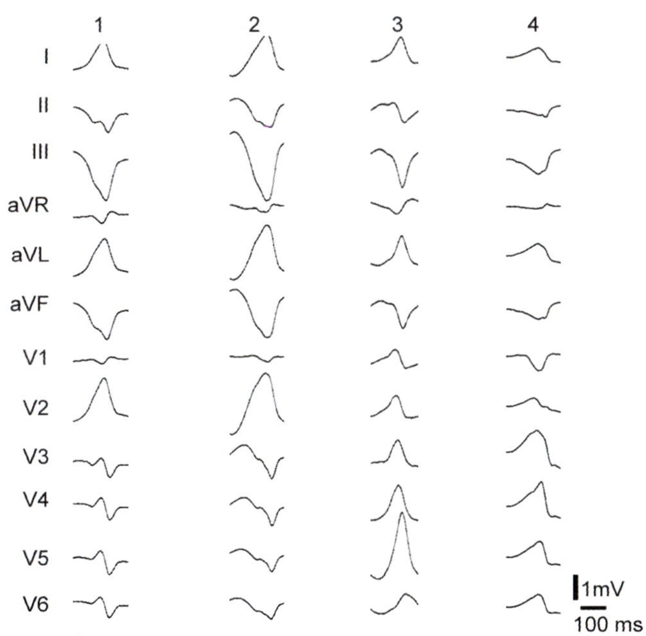

Figure 37.20: Twelve-lead electrocardiograms exhibiting QRS complexes of the VAs originating from the crux of the heart
From: Doppalapudi H, Yamada T, Ramaswamy K, et al. Idiopathic focal epicardial ventricular tachycardia originating from the crux of the heart. Heart Rhythm. 2009;6:44-50. With permission

(catecholamine sensitive) for induction. However, pacing during VT fails to demonstrate any criterion for transient entrainment, suggesting a nonreentrant mechanism, and likely triggered activity.

Mapping and Catheter Ablation

During endocardial mapping, the earliest ventricular activation is recorded within the middle cardiac vein or proximal CS **(Figure 37.21)**.[25] If the local ventricular activation precedes the QRS onset by greater than 20 ms and/or an excellent pace map is recorded at that site, irrigated RF catheter ablation may be attempted in power-control mode, starting at 20 W and titrated up to 30 W with an irrigation flow rate of 30 mL/min. If it is unsuccessful, epicardial mapping via a subxiphoid pericardial approach should be performed. A prior coronary angiography is strongly recommended to determine a safer area for the epicardial RF ablation **(Figure 37.22)**. It may be important to maintain a distance of more than 5 mm between the coronary artery and distal electrode of the ablation catheter at any point of the cardiac cycle in order to reduce the risk of damage to the coronary artery during the epicardial RF ablation. For an epicardial catheter ablation, irrigated RF current should be delivered in a power-controlled mode, starting at 30 W and titrated up to 50 W with an irrigation flow rate of 30 mL/min.

Ablation Outcome and Complications

RF catheter ablation of crux VAs appears to be effective and safe despite the limited data.[25] There is a potential risk of perforation of the CS or damage of the coronary artery (posterior descending artery) when catheter ablation is performed within the CS or middle cardiac vein or on the epicardial surface.

LEFT VENTRICLE SUMMIT VENTRICULAR ARRHYTHMIAS

Anatomically, a region of the LV epicardial surface bounded by the left anterior descending (LAD) coronary artery and

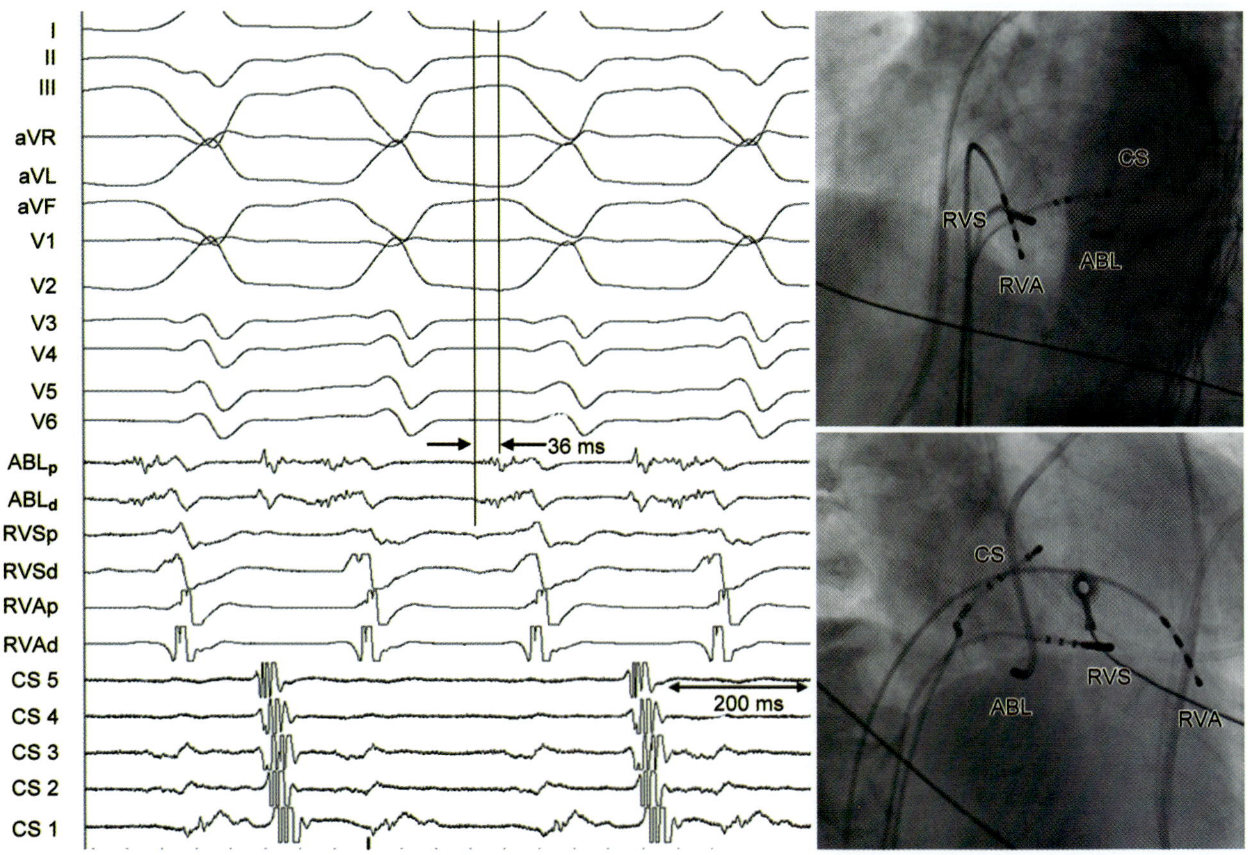

Figure 37.21: Cardiac tracings (left panel) and fluoroscopic images (right panels) exhibiting the successful ablation site of the ventricular tachycardia originating from the crux of the heart

Abbreviations: RVA, right ventricular apex; RVS, right ventricular septum. The other abbreviations are as in the previous figures

From: Doppalapudi H, Yamada T, Ramaswamy K, et al. Idiopathic focal epicardial ventricular tachycardia originating from the crux of the heart. Heart Rhythm. 2009;6:44-50. With permission

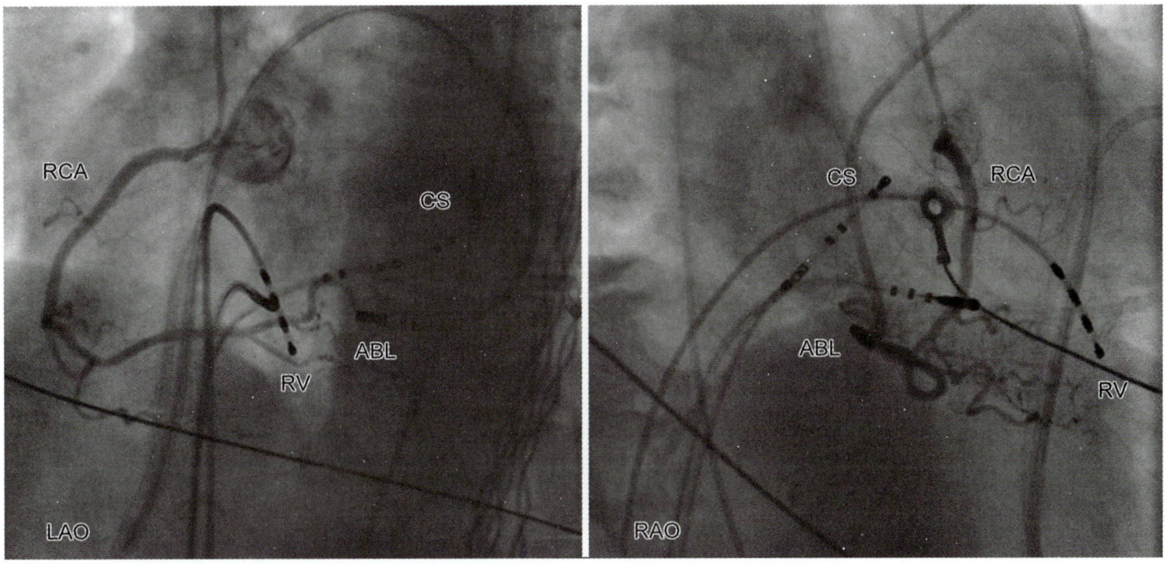

Figure 37.22: Fluoroscopic images exhibiting the relationship between the successful ablation site of ventricular tachycardia originating from the crux of the heart and the right coronary artery (RCA). The other abbreviations are as in the previous figures
From: Doppalapudi H, Yamada T, Ramaswamy K, et al. Idiopathic focal epicardial ventricular tachycardia originating from the crux of the heart. Heart Rhythm. 2009;6:44-50. With permission

left circumflex (LCx) coronary artery that lies superior to the aortic portion of the LV ostium occupies the most superior portion of the LV and has been termed the LV summit by McAlpine **(Figure 37.23)**.[38] This region near where the great cardiac vein (GCV) ends and the anterior interventricular vein (AIV) begins is one of the major sources of epicardial idiopathic VAs. The LV summit is bisected by the GCV into an area lateral to this structure which is accessible to epicardial catheter ablation (the *accessible area*) and a superior region that is inaccessible to catheter ablation due to the close proximity of the coronary arteries and the thick layer of epicardial fat that overlies the proximal portion of these vessels (the *inaccessible area*) **(Figure 37.23)**.[26]

The prevalence of LV summit VAs has been reported to account for 12% of idiopathic LV VAs. They most often occur as PVCs or nonsustained VT[26] and very unlikely to result in syncope. There is no significant difference in the gender in patients with LV summit VAs.[26]

Electrocardiographic Characteristics

The common ECG characteristics of the LV summit VAs are a right inferior axis QRS morphology, wider QRS, and larger maximum deflection index than the other idiopathic LV outflow tract VAs.[26] There are different ECG characteristics of the LV summit VAs among the 3 areas of the LV summit that are reasonably understood in consideration of the anatomical relationships among the 3 areas. First, the maximal amplitude of the R-wave in the inferior leads is highest for VAs with a presumed origin in the inaccessible area, lowest in those with an origin in the accessible area and in-between in those with an origin in the GCV and AIV. Second, a right bundle branch block pattern of the VAs is always observed in VAs with an origin in the accessible area and is dominant in those with an origin in the GCV and AIV but rare in those with an origin in the inaccessible area. Third, a very early precordial transition of the VAs (earlier than in lead V1) is dominant in VAs with an origin in the accessible area and GCV and AIV, whereas it is never observed in those with an origin in the inaccessible area. Fourth, the ratio of the Q-wave amplitude in leads aVL to aVR (aVL/aVR) and that of the R-wave amplitude in leads III to II (III/II) are significantly higher in the VAs with an origin in the accessible area than in those with an origin in the GCV and AIV and the inaccessible area. When VAs are considered to originate from the LV summit, a right bundle branch block pattern, transition zone earlier than lead V1, aVL/aVR amplitude ratio >1.1, and presence of S-waves in lead V5 or V6 suggest with a high accuracy that a VA origin is likely to be ablated within the GCV, AIV, and accessible area. When VAs are considered to originate from the GCV and AIV and the accessible area, both a III/II amplitude ratio >1.25 and aVL/aVR amplitude ratio >1.75 suggest the necessity of a epicardial approach with a high accuracy.

Electrophysiological Characteristics

LV summit VAs occur with a focal (nonreentrant) mechanism.[26] They may be induced by pacing, and an isoproterenol infusion may be helpful for their induction.

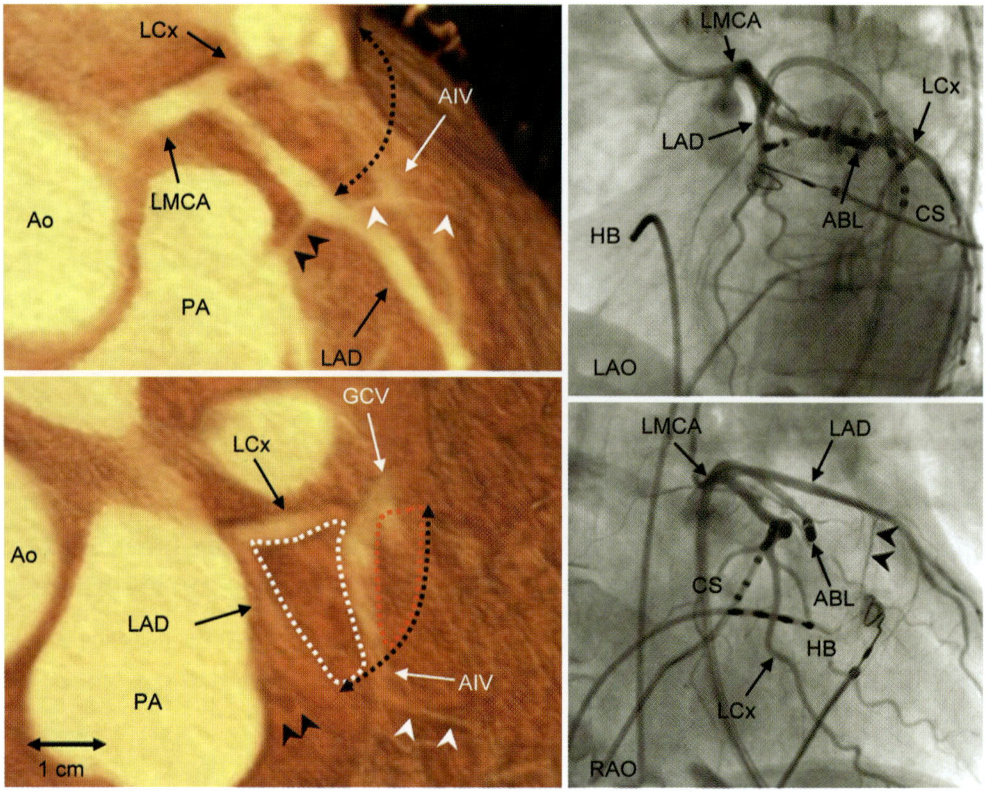

Figure 37.23: Computed tomographic (CT) (left panels) and fluoroscopic (right panels) images exhibiting the summit of the left ventricle. The LV summit was defined as the region on the LV epicardial surface near the bifurcation of the left main coronary artery (LMCA) that is bounded by an arc (black dotted line) from the left anterior descending (LAD) coronary artery superior to the first septal perforating branch (black arrowheads) extending anteriorly to the left circumflex (LCx) coronary artery laterally. The great cardiac vein (GCV) bisects the LV summit into a superior portion surrounded by the white dotted line (the *inaccessible area*) and an inferior portion surrounded by red dotted line (the *accessible area*). The white arrowheads indicate the first diagonal branch of the LAD. The ablation catheter (ABL) was positioned at the successful ablation site in the *accessible* area

Abbreviations: AIV, anterior interventricular cardiac vein; Ao, aorta; PA, pulmonary artery. The other abbreviations are as in the previous figures

From: Yamada T, McElderry HT, Doppalapudi H, et al. Idiopathic ventricular arrhythmias originating from the left ventricular summit: anatomic concets relevant to ablation. Circ Arrhythm Electrophysiol. 2010;3:616-23. With permission

Mapping and Catheter Ablation

Because the LV summit is bounded by the LAD and LCx coronary arteries and the inaccessible area is separated from the accessible area by the GCV and AIV, a catheter within these veins is essential for mapping LV summit VAs. During the electrophysiological study, mapping in the GCV and AIV with a 6 or 7-French decapolar catheter is very helpful for making a diagnosis of LV summit VAs **(Figure 37.23)**. This mapping catheter should be advanced until the electrode pair 3–4 records earlier ventricular activation than the most distal electrode pair 1–2 during the VAs. Pacing from the electrode pair recording the earliest ventricular activation within the GCV or AIV should be attempted, and the pace map should be compared with the VAs especially with respect to the bundle branch block pattern, maximum deflection index, and R-wave amplitude in the inferior leads **(Figure 37.24)**. When the maximum deflection index in the VA is similar to that in the pace map from the GCV or AIV, the VA is likely to be epicardial. When the R-wave amplitude in the inferior leads is taller in the VAs than that in the pace map from the GCV or AIV, the VAs are likely to arise from an inaccessible area of the LV summit.

Comprehensive mapping within the GCV and AIV should be performed first for LV summit VAs. Venography with an angiographic catheter or irrigated ablation catheter will be helpful for a guide of mapping within these venous structures **(Figure 37.25)**.[39] When the local ventricular activation during the VAs is earlier in the GCV or AIV (usually earlier than –20 ms relative to the QRS onset) than for any endocardial site, epicardial catheter ablation using transvenous or transpericardial approaches should be considered.

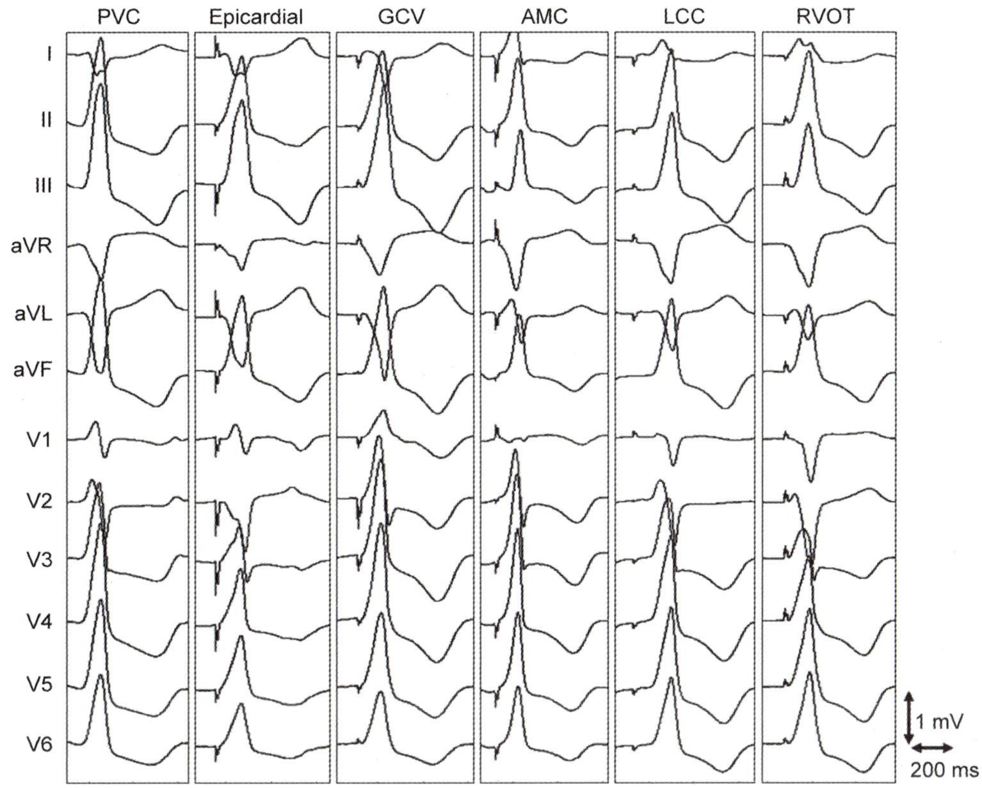

Figure 37.24: Comparison of the 12-lead electrocardiograms between the PVCs arising from the inaccessible area and pace maps. Note that pacing from any endocardial or epicardial site never produced an excellent pace map especially with a higher amplitude of the R-waves in the inferior leads

Abbreviations: AMC, aortomitral continuity; LCC, left coronary cusp; RVOT; right ventricular outflow tract. The other abbreviations are as in the previous figures

From: Yamada T, McElderry HT, Doppalapudi H, et al. Idiopathic ventricular arrhythmias originating from the left ventricular summit: anatomic concepts relevant to ablation. Circ Arrhythm Electrophysiol. 2010;3:616-23. With permission

When the local ventricular activation within the GCV or AIV precedes the QRS onset by more than 20 ms and pacing from the site of the earliest ventricular activation within the GCV or AIV produces an excellent match to the QRS complex of the VAs, catheter ablation within the GCV or AIV may be attempted. Otherwise or when the RF ablation within the GCV or AIV fails to eliminate the VAs, epicardial mapping and ablation via a subxiphoid approach should be performed **(Figure 37.23)**. Irrigated RF current should be used in the power-control mode starting at 20 W in the GCV and AIV and 30 W on the epicardial surface with an irrigation flow rate of 30 mL/min. The RF power was titrated to as high as 30 W and 40 W, respectively, with the goal being to achieve a decrease in the impedance of 8 to 10 Ω and with care taken to limit the temperature to less than 40°C. During the epicardial catheter ablation using transvenous and transpericardial approaches, left coronary angiography should be performed to ensure the location of the ablation catheter relative to the left coronary arteries and to minimize the risk of thermal injury to that vessel **(Figure 37.23)**. An RF application should never be delivered within 5 mm of a coronary artery.

Ablation Outcome and Complications

The prevalence of LV summit VA origin is much higher within the GCV and AIV (70%) than on the epicardial surface of either side of these veins (15% for each side). Catheter ablation of the LV summit VAs within the distal GCV or AIV may be challenging because of the inability to position the tip of an ablation catheter and high impedance and temperature within these veins. Cryothermal ablation may be a viable alternative when RF current delivery is limited by high impedance and temperature.[40] Although an LV summit VA origin lateral to the GCV (in the accessible area) is usually amenable to ablation using an intrapericardial approach, catheter ablation of a VA origin superior to this structure (in the inaccessible area) is unlikely to be successful because of a thick layer of epicardial fat overlying the proximal coronary arteries and may be potentially hazardous to these vessels although anatomic variations in some patients may allow catheter ablation even in this region **(Figures 37.26A and B)**. Although this area may be ablated with surgical approaches allowing dissection of the epicardial fat and

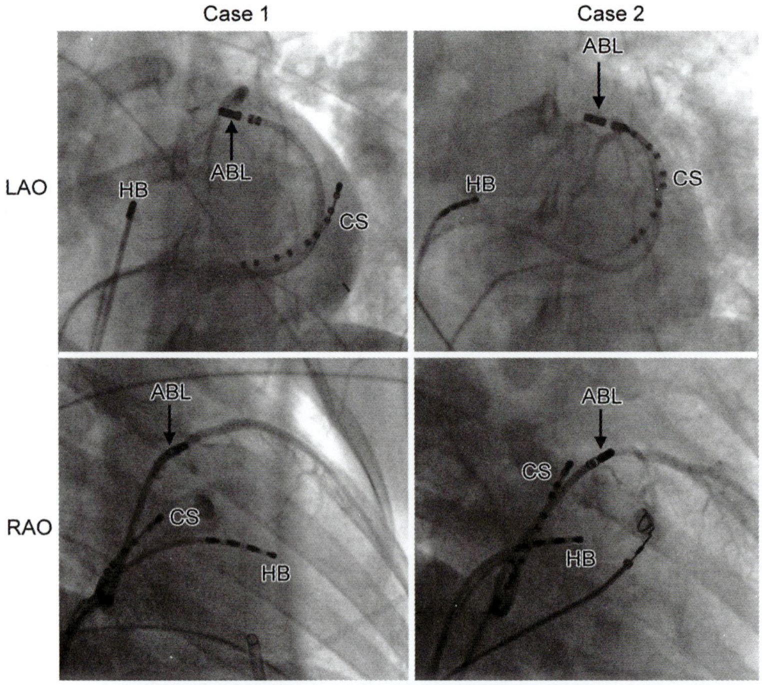

Figure 37.25: Fluoroscopic images exhibiting the great cardiac venograms during a contrast injection through an external irrigation catheter. In Case 1, the tip of the ablation catheter was positioned in the main trunk of the GCV whereas in Case 2, it was in a small branch of the GCV. In both cases, the contrast filled even the peripheral branches and clear venograms were obtained

Abbreviation: ABL, the externally irrigated ablation catheter. The other abbreviations are as in the previous figures

From: Yamada T, McElderry HT, Doppalapudi H, et al. Great cardiac venography by contrast injection through an external irrigation catheter. Heart Rhythm. 2012;9:156-7. With permission

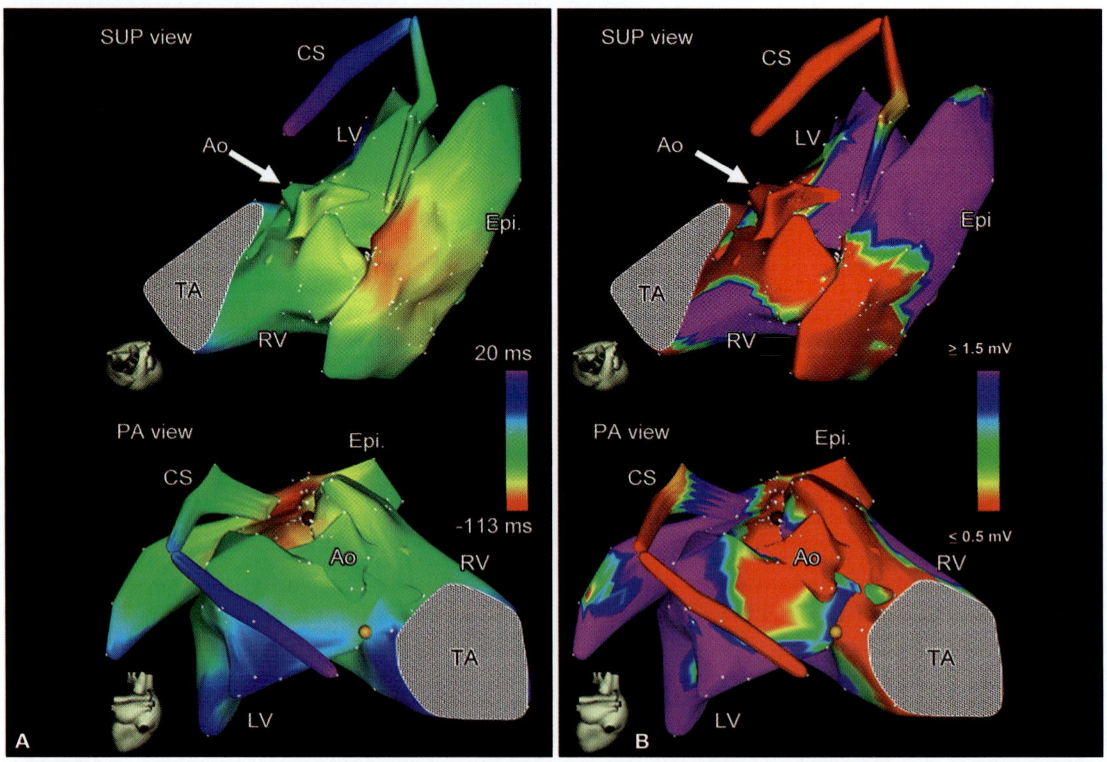

Figures 37.26A and B: Activation (A) and voltage (B) maps in a patient with ventricular arrhythmias (VAs) arising from the inaccessible area in the LV summit. Note that the earliest ventricular activation during the VAs was observed in the inaccessible area with a low voltage of the local ventricular electrogram. The red tag indicates the ablation site in the right ventricular outflow tract

Abbreviations: EPI, epicardial surface; PA, posteroanterior; RV, right ventricle; SUP, superior; TA, tricuspid annulus. The other abbreviations are as in the previous figures

From: Yamada T, McElderry HT, Doppalapudi H, et al. Idiopathic ventricular arrhythmias originating from the left ventricular summit: anatomic concepts relevant to ablation. Circ Arrhythm Electrophysiol. 2010;3:616-23. With permission direct application of ablative energy to this region, the safety of this approach is uncertain.

Because catheter ablation of LV summit VAs is challenging for the reasons mentioned above, appropriate decision-making about the necessity of a pericardial approach and abandonment of the ablation may save procedural and fluoroscopic time and avoid some complications.

REFERENCES

1. Stevenson WG, Soejima K. Catheter ablation for ventricular tachycardia. Circulation. 2007;115:2750-60.
2. Yamada T, Kay GN. Optimal ablation strategies for different types of ventricular tachycardias. Nat Rev Cardiol. 2012;9: 512-25.
3. Coggins DL, Lee RJ, Sweeney J, Chein WW, Van Hare G, Epstein L, Gonzalez R, Griffin JC, Lesh MD, Scheinman MM. Radiofrequency catheter ablation as a cure for idiopathic tachycardia of both left and right ventricular origin. J Am Coll Cardiol. 1994;23:1333-41.
4. Tsuchiya T, Okumura K, Honda T, Honda T, Iwasa A, Yasue H, Tabuchi T. Significance of late diastolic potential preceding Purkinje potential in verapamil-sensitive idiopathic left ventricular tachycardia. Circulation. 1999;99:2408-13.
5. Nogami A, Naito S, Tada H, Taniguchi K, Okamoto Y, Nishimura S, Yamauchi Y, Aonuma K, Goya M, Iesaka Y, Hiroe M. Demonstration of diastolic and presystolic Purkinje potentials as critical potentials in a macroreentry circuit of verapamil-sensitive idiopathic left ventricular tachycardia. J Am Coll Cardiol. 2000;36:811-23.
6. Kanagaratnam L, Tomassoni G, Schweikert R, Pavia S, Bash D, Beheiry S, Neibauer M, Saliba W, Chung M, Tchou P, Natale A. Ventricular tachycardias arising from the aortic sinus of valsalva: an under-recognized variant of left outflow tract ventricular tachycardia. J Am Coll Cardiol. 2001;37:1408-14.
7. Ouyang F, Fotuhi P, Ho SY, Hebe J, Volkmer M, Goya M, Burns M, Antz M, Ernst S, Cappato R, Kuck KH. Repetitive monomorphic ventricular tachycardia originating from the aortic sinus cusp: electrocardiographic characterization for guiding catheter ablation. J Am Coll Cardiol. 2002;39:500-8.
8. Yamada T, Yoshida N, Murakami Y, Okada T, Muto M, Murohara T, McElderry HT, Kay GN. Electrocardiographic characteristics of ventricular arrhythmias originating from the junction of the left and right coronary sinuses of Valsalva in the aorta: the activation pattern as a rationale for the electrocardiographic characteristics. Heart Rhythm. 2008;5:184-92.
9. Yamada T, McElderry HT, Doppalapudi H, Murakami Y, Yoshida Y, Yoshida N, Okada T, Tsuboi N, Inden Y, Murohara T, Epstein AE, Plumb VJ, Singh SP, Kay GN. Idiopathic ventricular arrhythmias originating from the aortic root: prevalence, electrocardiographic and electrophysiological characteristics, and results of the radiofrequency catheter ablation. J Am Coll Cardiol. 2008;52:139-47.
10. Yamada T, Lau YR, Litovsky SH, Thomas McElderry H, Doppalapudi H, Osorio J, Plumb VJ, Neal Kay G. Prevalence and clinical, electrocardiographic, and electrophysiologic characteristics of ventricular arrhythmias originating from the noncoronary sinus of Valsalva. Heart Rhythm. 2013;10: 1605-12.
11. Tada H, Ito S, Naito S, Kurosaki K, Kubota S, Sugiyasu A, Tsuchiya T, Miyaji K, Yamada M, Kutsumi Y, Oshima S, Nogami A, Taniguchi K. Idiopathic ventricular arrhythmia arising from the mitral annulus: a distinct subgroup of idiopathic ventricular arrhythmias. J Am Coll Cardiol. 2005;45:877-86.
12. Kumagai K, Yamauchi Y, Takahashi A, Yokoyama Y, Sekiguchi Y, Watanabe J, Iesaka Y, Shirato K, Aonuma K. Idiopathic left ventricular tachycardia originating from the mitral annulus. J Cardiovasc Electrophysiol. 2005;16:1029-36.
13. Yamada T, Litovsky SH, Kay GN. The left ventricular ostium: an anatomic concept relevant to idiopathic ventricular arrhythmias. Circ Arrhythmia Electrophysiol. 2008;1:396-404.
14. Tada H, Tadokoro K, Ito S, Naito S, Hashimoto T, Kaseno K, Miyaji K, Sugiyasu A, Tsuchiya T, Kutsumi Y, Nogami A, Oshima S, Taniguchi K. Idiopathic ventricular arrhythmias originating from the tricuspid annulus: Prevalence, electrocardiographic characteristics, and results of radiofrequency catheter ablation. Heart Rhythm. 2007;4:7-16.
15. Sekiguchi Y, Aonuma K, Takahashi A, Yamauchi Y, Hachiya H, Yokoyama Y, Iesaka Y, Isobe M. Electrocardiographic and electrophysiologic characteristics of ventricular tachycardia originating within the pulmonary artery. J Am Coll Cardiol. 2005;45:887-95.
16. Yamauchi Y, Aonuma K, Takahashi A, Sekiguchi Y, Hachiya H, Yokoyama Y, Kumagai K, Nogami A, Iesaka Y, Isobe M. Electrocardiographic characteristics of repetitive monomorphic right ventricular tachycardia originating near the His-bundle. J Cardiovasc Electrophysiol. 2005;16:1041-8.
17. Yamada T, McElderry HT, Doppalapudi H, Kay GN. Catheter ablation of ventricular arrhythmias originating in the vicinity of the His bundle: significance of mapping the aortic sinus cusp. Heart Rhythm. 2008;5:37-42.
18. Yamada T, Plumb VJ, McElderry HT, Doppalapudi H, Epstein AE, Kay GN. Focal ventricular arrhythmias originating from the left ventricle adjacent to the membranous septum. Europace. 2010;12:1467-74.
19. Doppalapudi H, Yamada T, McElderry HT, Plumb VJ, Epstein AE, Kay GN. Ventricular tachycardia originating from the posterior papillary muscle in the left ventricle: a distinct clinical syndrome. Circ Arrhythm Electrophysiol. 2008;1: 23-9.
20. Yamada T, McElderry HT, Okada T, Murakami Y, Doppalapudi H, Yoshida N, Allred JD, Murohara T, Kay GN. Idiopathic focal ventricular arrhythmias originating from the anterior papillary muscle in the left ventricle. J Cardiovasc Electrophysiol. 2009;20:866-72.
21. Yamada T, Doppalapudi H, McElderry HT, Okada T, Murakami Y, Inden Y, Yoshida Y, Yoshida N, Murohara T, Epstein AE, Plumb VJ, Litovsky SH, Kay GN. Electrocardiographic and electrophysiological characteristics in idiopathic ventricular arrhythmias originating from the papillary muscles in the left ventricle: relevance for catheter ablation. Circ Arrhythm Electrophysiol. 2010;3:324-31.
22. Yamada T, Doppalapudi H, McElderry HT, Okada T, Murakami Y, Inden Y, Yoshida Y, Kaneko S, Yoshida N, Murohara T, Epstein AE, Plumb VJ, Kay GN. Idiopathic ventricular arrhythmias originating from the papillary muscles in the left ventricle: prevalence, electrocardiographic and electrophysiological characteristics, and results of the radiofrequency catheter ablation. J Cardiovasc Electrophysiol. 2010;21:62-9.

23. Good E, Desjardins B, Jongnarangsin K, Oral H, Chugh A, Ebinger M, Pelosi F, Morady F, Bogun F. Ventricular arrhythmias originating from a papillary muscle in patients without prior infarction: a comparison with fascicular arrhythmias. Heart Rhythm. 2008;5:1530-7.
24. Crawford T, Mueller G, Good E, Jongnarangsin K, Chugh A, Pelosi F Jr, Ebinger M, Oral H, Morady F, Bogun F. Ventricular arrhythmias originating from papillary muscles in the right ventricle. Heart Rhythm. 2010;7:725-30.
25. Doppalapudi H, Yamada T, Ramaswamy K, Ahn J, Kay GN. Idiopathic focal epicardial ventricular tachycardia originating from the crux of the heart. Heart Rhythm. 2009;6:44-50.
26. Yamada T, McElderry HT, Doppalapudi H, Okada T, Murakami Y, Yoshida Y, Yoshida N, Inden Y, Murohara T, Plumb VJ, Kay GN. Idiopathic ventricular arrhythmias originating from the left ventricular summit: anatomic concepts relevant to ablation. Circ Arrhythm Electrophysiol. 2010;3:616-23.
27. Sadek MM, Benhayon D, Sureddi R, Chik W, Santangeli P, Supple GE, Hutchinson MD, Bala R, Carballeira L, Zado ES, Patel VV, Callans DJ, Marchlinski FE, Garcia FC. Idiopathic ventricular arrhythmias originating from the moderator band: Electrocardiographic characteristics and treatment by catheter ablation. Heart Rhythm. 2015;12:67-75.
28. Seiler J, Lee JC, Roberts-Thomson KC, Stevenson WG. Intracardiac echocardiography guided catheter ablation of incessant ventricular tachycardia from the posterior papillary muscle causing tachycardia--mediated cardiomyopathy. Heart Rhythm. 2009;6:389-92.
29. Yamada T, McElderry HT, Doppalapudi H, Kay GN. Real-time integration of intracardiac echocardiography and electroanatomic mapping in PVCs arising from the LV anterior papillary muscle. Pacing Clin Electrophysiol. 2009;32:1240-3.
30. Liu XK, Barrett R, Packer DL, Asirvatham SJ. Successful management of recurrent ventricular tachycardia by electrical isolation of anterolateral papillary muscle. Heart Rhythm. 2008;5:479-82.
31. Yamada T, McElderry HT, Allred JD, Doppalapudi H, Kay GN. Ventricular fibrillation induced by a radiofrequency energy delivery for idiopathic premature ventricular contractions arising from the left ventricular anterior papillary muscle. Europace. 2009;11:1115-7.
32. Wasmer K, Köbe J, Dechering DG, Bittner A, Pott C, Mönnig G, Milberg P, Frommeyer G, Zellerhoff S, Kochhäuser S, Eckardt L. Ventricular arrhythmias from the mitral annulus: patient characteristics, electrophysiological findings, ablation, and prognosis. Heart Rhythm. 2013;10:783-8.
33. Nogami A, Tada H. Ablation of idiopathic left and right ventricular and fascicular tachycardias. In: Shoei K, Stephen Huang, John M Miller (Eds). Catheter ablation of cardiac catheter ablation of cardiac arrhythmias, 3rd edn. Saunders; 2015. pp. 540-78.
34. Kurosawa H, Becker AE. Dead-end tract of the conduction axis. Int J Cardiol. 1985;7:13-20.
35. Tanaka Y, Tada H, Ito S, Naito S, Higuchi K, Kumagai K, Hachiya H, Hirao K, Oshima S, Taniguchi K, Aonuma K, Isobe M. Gender and age differences in candidates for radiofrequency catheter ablation of idiopathic ventricular arrhythmias. Circ J. 2011;75:1585-91.
36. Yamada T, Allison JS, McElderry HT, Doppalapudi H, Epstein AE, Plumb VJ, Kay GN. Successful catheter ablation of premature ventricular contractions originating from the tricuspid annulus using a Halo-type catheter. Europace. 2008; 10:1228-9.
37. Daniels DV, Lu YY, Morton JB, Santucci PA, Akar JG, Green A, Wilber DJ. Idiopathic epicardial left ventricular tachycardia originating remote from the sinus of Valsalva: electrophysiological characteristics, catheter ablation, and identification from the 12-lead electrocardiogram. Circulation. 2006;113:1659-66.
38. McAlpine WA. Heart and Coronary Arteries. New York: Springer-Verlag; 1975.
39. Yamada T, McElderry HT, Doppalapudi H, Kay GN. Great cardiac venography by contrast injection through an external irrigation catheter. Heart Rhythm. 2012;9:156-7.
40. Obel OA, d'Avila A, Neuzil P, Saad EB, Ruskin JN, Reddy VY. Ablation of left ventricular epicardial outflow tract tachycardia from the distal great cardiac vein. J Am Coll Cardiol. 2006;48:1813-7.

EDITORS' SUMMARY

Professor Yamada has provided in this chapter a veritable treatise on idiopathic ventricular tachycardias arising from sites less frequently than those from the ventricular outflow tracts. An outstanding anatomic/electrogram/ECG correlation is presented that the reader will greatly benefit from with careful study. This chapter right along with Chapter 6 on anatomy and Professor Dixit's chapter on outflow tract tachycardia (Chapter 36) will form a comprehensive unit for approaching ventricular arrhythmia in a patient with a normal heart.

The reader will do well to study the figures in isolation from the chapter and writing to appreciate the anatomy and themselves attempt correlation with possible electrocardiographic findings as well as specific challenges with ablating at those sites. Professor Yamada brings into focus the common sites and their relationship to the coronary vascular and conduction systems.

CHAPTER 38

Zalmen Blanck, Anwer Dhala, Masood Akhtar

Bundle Branch Reentry: Mechanisms, Diagnosis and Management

LIST OF ABBREVIATIONS

AV	Atrioventricular	LBBB	Left Bundle Branch Block
BBR	Bundle Branch Reentry	LV	Left Ventricle
EGM	Electrogram	RBB	Right Bundle Branch
EP	Electrophysiology	RBBB	Right Bundle Branch Block
HB	His-Bundle	RV	Right Ventricle
HPS	His-Purkinje System	SMVT	Sustained Monomorphic Ventricular Tachycardia
IF-VT	Interfascicular Ventricular Tachycardia	SR	Sinus Rhythm
LBB	Left Bundle Branch	VT	Ventricular Tachycardia

INTRODUCTION

The most common mechanism of sustained monomorphic ventricular tachycardia (SMVT) is reentry related to scar tissue, usually in patients with ischemic or nonischemic cardiomyopathies. However, reentry in the His-Purkinje system (HPS), also called bundle branch reentry (BBR), accounts for approximately 6% of SMVT in patients with structural heart disease.[1] This is a unique type of VT because the reentry circuit is well defined: the His-bundle (HB), the bundle branches and transseptal myocardial conduction are the components of the reentry circuit.[2-4] Although relatively uncommon, this type of VT may be more frequent than generally suspected for the following reasons:

- Syncope or sudden death are the most common manifestations of this arrhythmia,[1,5] and 12-lead electrocardiographic (ECG) documentation usually is not available.
- Induction of this mechanism of VT in the electrophysiology (EP) laboratory may be difficult or not reproducible, and a variety of electric stimulation techniques or pharmacologic maneuvers that might not be used routinely in EP laboratories may be required.
- An HB recording during VT is necessary for the diagnosis of this arrhythmia,[5-8] and may not be obtained during EP studies performed solely for VT.
- In the United States and in many parts of the world, defibrillator implantation is usually performed without EP evaluation, even in patients implanted for secondary prevention of life-threatening ventricular arrhythmias.

It is important to recognize BBR as the mechanism of VT because catheter ablation of the right bundle branch

(RBB), a procedure that can be easily performed in most patients and has a high success rate,[1,5,9-12] is curative of this type of VT.

MECHANISMS OF BUNDLE BRANCH REENTRY

Isolated BBR beats can be found in up to 50% of patients with normal intraventricular conduction undergoing EP studies; it is a finding without any prognostic significance.[2-4] The QRS morphology in these beats, or when sustained tachycardia is induced, will depend upon which bundle branch is used for antegrade propagation of the electric impulse: the QRS will exhibit a left (L), or right bundle branch block (RBBB) morphology, if the impulse propagates down the RBB or the LBB, respectively. The induction of isolated BBR beats or sustained BBR tachycardia share a common mechanism, as follows **(Figure 38.1)**.

During right ventricular (RV) programmed stimulation using a constant basic drive, a premature beat (S2) with a long coupling period is introduced and retrograde conduction to the HB occurs via the RBB, resulting in short V2-H2 intervals **(Figure 38.1A)**. As the S2 coupling periods are shortened, progressive delay in the retrograde RBB conduction is encountered (longer V2-H2), while propagation of the impulse proceeds transseptally into the LBB (which has shorter refractoriness than the RBB). Additional shortening of the coupling periods reach the effective refractory of the RBB, resulting in retrograde conduction block **(Figures 38.1B and C)**. Propagation of the stimulus continues transseptally, and via the LBB to the HB. A retrograde HB potential, inscribed after the local ventricular electrogram (EGM), becomes apparent. Further conduction delay in the LBB allows recovery of the initial site of the block in the RBB, allowing the impulse to propagate antegradely and activate the RV. This results in a wide QRS complex with a left bundle branch block (LBBB) pattern, the so-called V3 phenomenon, BBR beat, or a macro-reentrant beat. It should be noted that there is an inverse relationship between the retrograde conduction delay in the LBB (V2-H2), and the degree of recovery of the antegrade conduction in the RBB (H2-V3). Longer conduction times in the LBB (longer V2-H2), facilitate the antegrade recovery of the RBB, resulting in shorter H2-V3 intervals. On the other hand, insufficient delay in V2-H2 (i.e., longer coupling periods) may result in a longer H2-V3.[2-4]

It has been shown that reentry in the HPS is more likely to occur when premature beats are introduced during basic drives that incorporate short-long sequences, in contrast to constant basic drives. This is due to the cycle length dependency of the HPS refractoriness.[13-15] It has been suggested that an abrupt change in cycle length (short-to-long) may result in conduction block at a more distal site in the muscle-Purkinje-RBB axis, which will allow sufficient recovery of excitability in the RBB-Purkinje-muscle to allow antegrade conduction and reentry. This also will result in a shorter H2-V3 interval.

Although the most common type of BBR has an LBBB pattern, BBR with an RBBB pattern also may occur during RV stimulation. During this type of reentry, there is a retrograde LBBB and the impulse retrogradely propagates to the HB via the RBB. This can only occur when the LBB refractoriness is longer than that of the RBB or when retrograde RBB conduction resumes after a bilateral HPS block (gap phenomenon). This type of reentry also may be seen during left ventricular (LV) stimulation, as retrograde LBBB may be easier to accomplish given the proximity of the LBB to the stimulation site.

In patients with normal intraventricular conduction, BBR is a limited phenomenon, and if short-to-long pacing sequences are used, up to 3 BBR beats may be seen.[3,13-15] In most cases, the reentry terminates in the retrograde limb of the circuit, in the muscle-Purkinje-LBB axis.[16] Rarely, the reentry will terminate in the antegrade limb. The maintenance of this phenomenon is critically dependent upon the relationship between the conduction velocity and the recovery of excitability in front of the reentrant impulse. The presence of conduction abnormalities (i.e., intraventricular conduction delay) facilitates the development of clinically relevant sustained reentry.

Another, much less common, type of HPS reentry with a narrow QRS complex has been described in the presence of normal intraventricular conduction during RV stimulation.[17] This occurs when there is retrograde conduction via the LBB, followed by antegrade propagation via the RBB and one of the LBB fascicles, resulting in a narrow QRS with variable axis, depending upon which fascicle is used for antegrade conduction.

CLINICAL CHARACTERISTICS OF PATIENTS WITH BBR-VT

Sustained BBR-VT usually occurs in patients with significant structural heart disease: LV dysfunction with low ejection fraction and congestive heart failure are typical findings. Although nonischemic cardiomyopathy is the underlying substrate in about 45% of these patients,[1,5-7,9] this type of VT can also be seen in ischemic and valvular cardiomyopathies,[18] and also has been reported in patients with Ebstein's anomaly,[19] hypertrophic cardiomyopathy,[11] and any other type of structural heart disease associated with abnormal intraventricular conduction.[16] Myotonic dystrophy and other types of dystrophies also can be a substrate for this VT given the involvement of the HPS in these conditions.[20] Rarely, patients with isolated HPS disease, without other evidence of cardiac disease, have been reported to develop sustained BBR.[16,21] In some patients, valvular replacement surgery (aortic or mitral) predisposes them to develop

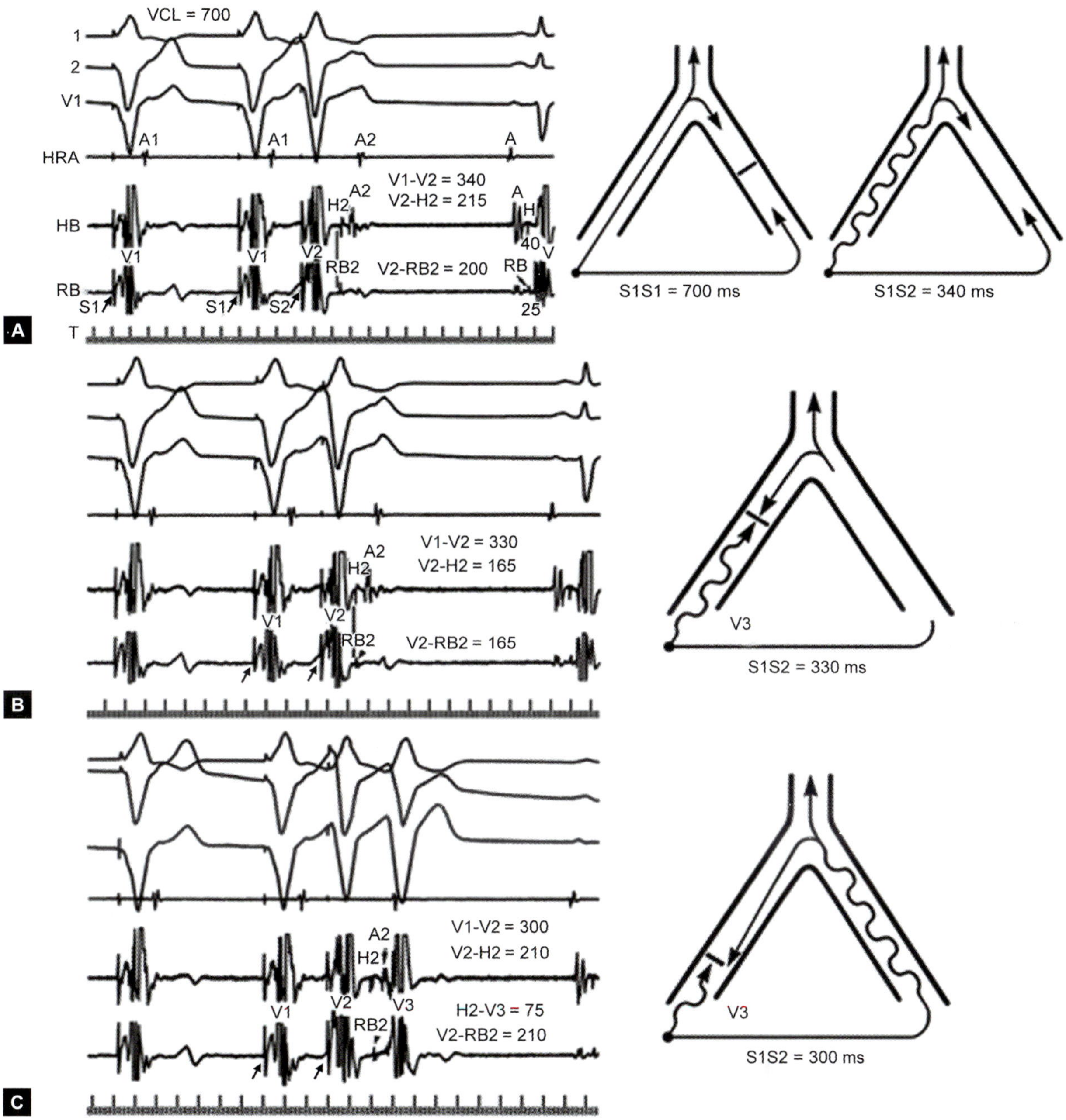

Figures 38.1A to C: In Panels A, B, and C, the tracings displayed are, from top to bottom, surface ECG leads 1, 2 and V1, and intracardiac recordings from the high right atrium (HRA), His-bundle (HB), right bundle branch (RB), and time lines (T). The three panels show the effect of premature ventricular beats introduced with progressively shorter coupling periods to a constant basic drive in the retrograde conduction in the His-Purkinje system. During the constant ventricular drive (700 ms), retrograde conduction is by way of the right bundle branch; this impulse collides with the transeptally conducted impulse in the left bundle branch (see diagram). A premature ventricular beat (coupling period 340 ms) results in slowing of the retrograde right bundle branch conduction, with subsequent emergence of the right bundle branch and HB potentials after the local ventricular electrogram. Note that the right bundle branch potential precedes the HB potential (V2 – RB2 = 200 ms versus V2 – HB2 = 215 ms) as expected with retrograde conduction proceeding via the right bundle branch. In Panel B, the introduction of a premature beat with a shorter coupling period (S2 330 ms) results in (proximal) retrograde block in the right bundle branch, which allows the transeptally conducted impulse to reach the HB via the left bundle branch. Note the change in the sequence of HB activation compared to Panel A (V2 – RB2 = 165 ms versus V2 – H2 = 165 ms). The HB and the right bundle branch are simultaneously activated, as expected during retrograde conduction via the LBB. In Panel C, the coupling period of S2 is further shortened to 300 ms, which results in retrograde block in the distal right bundle branch. This shift in the site of right bundle branch block, and the slower transeptal (not shown) and left bundle branch retrograde conduction, allow recovery of the site of block and activation of the right ventricle via the RBB (see diagram), resulting in a bundle branch reentrant beat with a left bundle branch block morphology, also called V3 phenomenon, or macro-reentrant beat

sustained BBR in the immediate postoperative period.[18] This group of patients who developed BBR postoperatively had better preserved cardiac function and left ventricular ejection fraction than the typical patient with cardiomyopathy and BBR (LVEF 44%). Of course, the most important determinant of long-term survival in these patients is the degree of cardiac dysfunction.[1,5,16,18,21]

Clinical Presentation

Sustained BBR is usually a fast tachycardia, and given the association with significant cardiac disease, it results in significant hemodynamic compromise: syncope or sudden death are the clinical presentation in up to 70% of these patients.[1,5] Twelve-lead ECG documentation of the VT is rarely available, so the relative incidence of spontaneous VT with LBBB or RBBB morphology is unknown.

ECG Findings

The most common abnormalities include mild PR interval prolongation in sinus rhythm (SR) (average 256 ms)[1,5] About 25% of patients have atrial fibrillation as the intrinsic rhythm. Most patients have an intraventricular conduction delay with an LBBB pattern. Rarely, an RBBB pattern is seen, a finding that does not exclude BBR as the mechanism of the VT, because the RBBB pattern may reflect antegrade conduction delay, rather than complete antegrade block, in the RBB. In the same context, a complete LBBB pattern may also be a manifestation of antegrade conduction delay, rather than complete conduction block. Even in the presence of a complete antegrade conduction block, the bundle branch may still be able to exhibit retrograde conduction, a necessary requirement for BBR to occur.[16]

In our experience, atrioventricular (AV) dissociation was present in nearly 100% of patients with sustained BBR.[1,5] This may be due to the fast cycle lengths of BBR and the presence of drugs that may depress AV conduction (e.g., beta-blockers, digoxin).

ELECTROPHYSIOLOGIC CHARACTERISTICS OF PATIENTS WITH BBR-VT

The presence of conduction disease in the HPS, manifested as prolongation of the His-ventricle (HV) interval, is a cardinal finding in this patient population, regardless of the type of underlying structural substrate.[1,5,6-12] In our experience, the HV interval ranged from 60 ms to 110 ms (average 80 ms).[5]

BBR is most commonly induced by RV stimulation. This can be accomplished by the introduction of premature ventricular stimuli to a constant basic drive, or more commonly, by the introduction of premature stimuli to a drive incorporating a pause before introducing the premature beat(s), so-called short-long-short.[13-15] We routinely use a 600 ms pause during a 400 ms drive prior to introducing premature beats. As the electric properties of the HPS may vary between patients, the use of protocols incorporating different short-long sequences may be necessary (i.e. 350–650, 400–700, etc.).[13-15] Induction of BBR with an RBBB may also require LV stimulation.

In some instances, the use of class 1A anti-arrhythmic drugs (e.g., procainamide) may facilitate induction of sustained BBR when the VT is not induced in the baseline state. Procainamide prolongs the antegrade and retrograde conduction times of the HPS, and by prolonging the HV and VH intervals, allows the penetration by the reentrant impulse into a better recovered RBB or LBB, respectively.[22] It should be noted that induction of BBR should be attempted during the slow administration of these drugs, as they may also abolish this type of reentry. Sometimes, isoproterenol may also be useful to induce this type of VT. However, the use of these drugs has not been systematically studied in patients with sustained BBR.

In contrast to other types of VT, BBR-VT can almost always be terminated by overdrive ventricular stimulation, regardless of the VT cycle length (unless, of course, ventricular fibrillation is induced). The rationale for this is the relative large size of the reentrant circuit, the presence of an "excitable conduction gap," and the proximity of the RV stimulation site to the reentrant circuit. All these factors facilitate the penetration of the circuit by the propagated stimulated impulses.

Diagnostic Criteria for BBR-VT

The EP criteria diagnostic of BBR are shown in **Table 38.1**. The diagnosis of BBR-VT requires intracardiac recordings during the induced VT (i.e., HB and/or bundle branch potentials). In some cases, it may be difficult to obtain an HB recording during the VT, in which case, an RBB potential may be more stable and easier to record, and may facilitate the diagnosis.[8]

Table 38.1: Diagnostic criteria for BBR-VT

1. The VT exhibits QRS morphology that is typical of an LBBB or RBBB, consistent with ventricular depolarization via the His-Purkinje system.
2. The onset of ventricular activation is preceded by a His-bundle potential and bundle branch potentials, with an appropriate sequence of activation to the corresponding QRS morphology, and with stable HV, RB-V, or LB-V intervals.
3. Spontaneous variations in V-V intervals are preceded by similar variations in H-H intervals.
4. Induction of tachycardia is consistently dependent upon achieving a critical delay in the His-Purkinje system.
5. The VT cannot be induced after successful catheter ablation of the RBB.

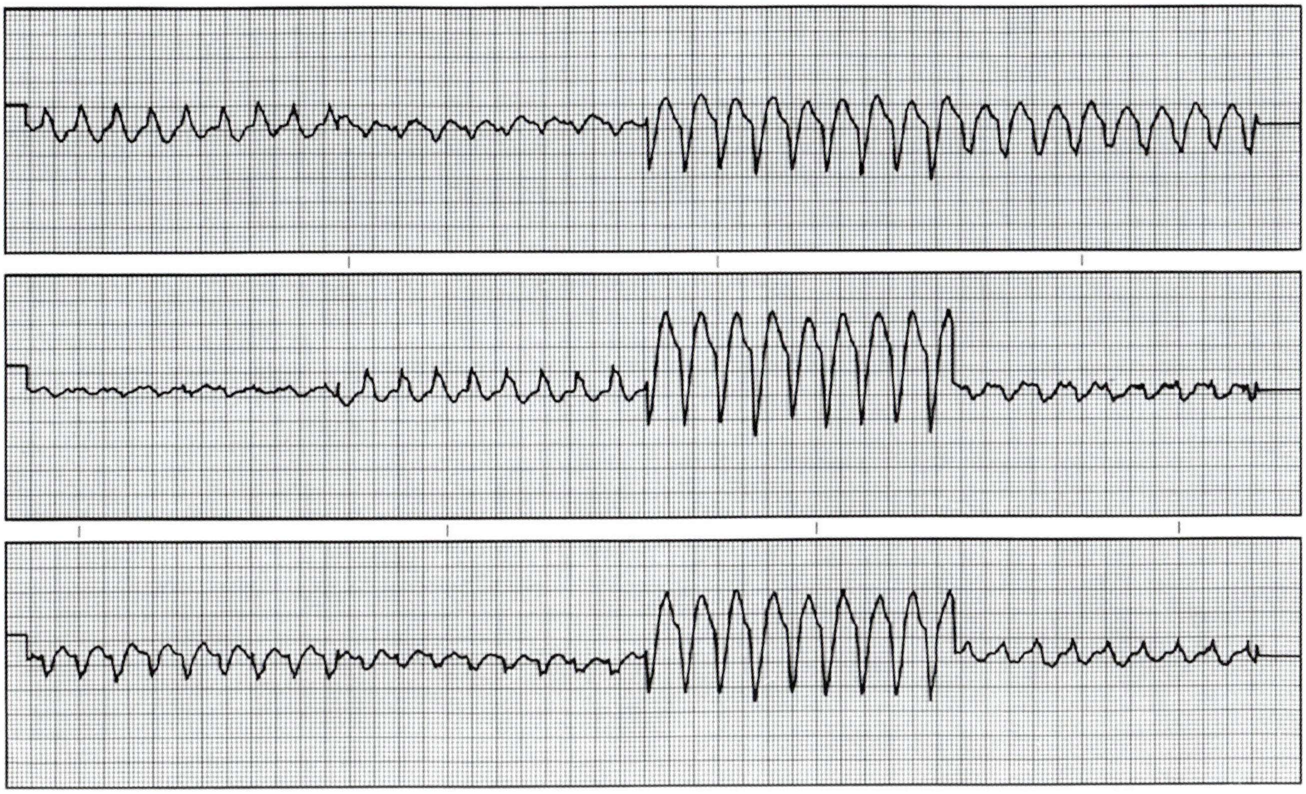

Figure 38.2: Twelve-lead surface electrocardiogram of spontaneous bundle branch reentrant tachycardia with left bundle branch QRS pattern and left-axis deviation at a rate of 215 bpm (not labeled). Because ventricular activation occurs by way of the right bundle branch, the QRS configuration is suggestive of intraventricular aberrant conduction. (Used with permission from Elsevier from Zipes DP, Jalife J. Cardiac Electrophysiology: From Cell to Bedside, 2nd edn. (2005) Saunders, Philadelphia, Penn. p. 881).

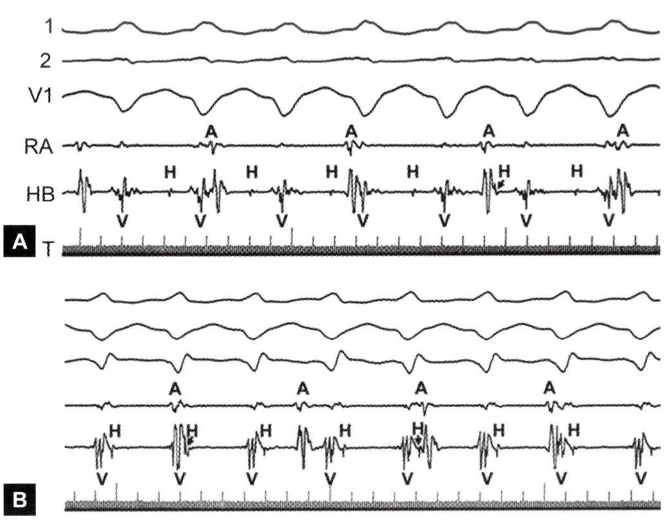

Figures 38.3A and B: Bundle branch reentry with left (A) and right (B) bundle branch block morphology. Tracings, from top to bottom in each panel, include surface ECG leads 1, 2 and V1, and intracardiac recordings from the right atrium (RA), His-bundle (HB), and time lines (T). In Panel A, bundle branch reentry tachycardia with a left bundle branch block morphology is displayed. Note the relatively slow cycle length, unusual in this type of tachycardia. The HV interval of 90 ms was identical to the one in sinus rhythm. In contrast, during tachycardia with a right bundle branch block, the HV interval is much longer, 250 ms. Antegrade activation in each tachycardia is dependent upon the RBB and the LBB, respectively, resulting in significantly different HV intervals

During BBR-VT with an LBBB pattern **(Figure 38.2)**, the most common type of induced BBR-VT, the HV interval is similar to, or slightly longer than, the HV interval in SR **(Figure 38.3A)**.[1,5,6-12] Rarely, if a very proximal HB recording is obtained, a slightly shorter HV interval may be obtained during the VT as the HB and the RBB may be simultaneously activated via the LBB.

In contrast, the induction of BBR with an RBBB pattern may result in an HV interval that is significantly different than in sinus rhythm **(Figure 38.3B)**. In patients with BBR, the HV interval during SR is generally determined by the conduction properties of the RBB. However, during VT with an RBBB pattern, the HV interval is determined by the conduction properties of the LBB. Different antegrade conduction properties of the RBB and the LBB may account for different HV intervals during intrinsic rhythm versus tachycardia.

Recording the HB potential and the bundle branch potentials can document the sequence of activation of the HPS during the VT, an important diagnostic criteria for BBR **(Table 38.1, Figures 38.4, 38.5 and 38.6A)**. During VT with an LBBB pattern, activation of the LBB is followed by activation of the HB, which in turn is followed by activation of the RBB. The opposite sequence of activation occurs during BBR-VT with an RBBB pattern.

As ventricular activation is dependent upon the propagation of the impulse in the HPS, irregularities in the H-H cycle lengths during BBR (typically seen at the onset of the tachycardia), will precede similar irregularities in the corresponding V-V cycle lengths **(Figure 38.6B)**. This is an important criterion to distinguish VT due to BBR from scar-related VT with incidental (retrograde) activation of the HPS.

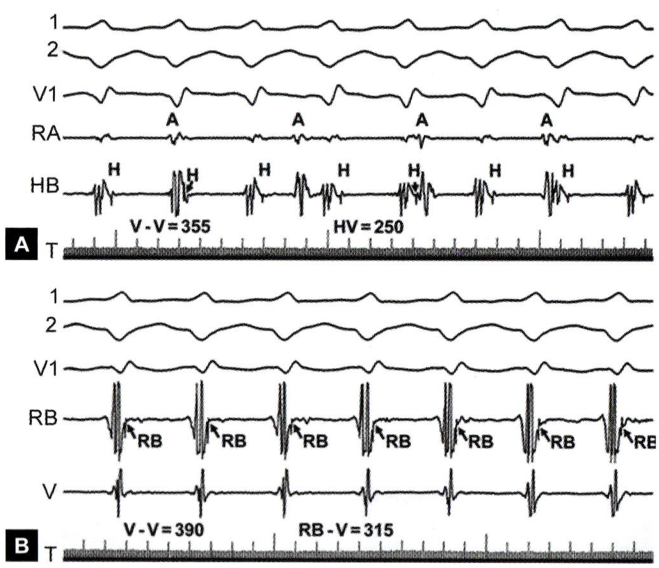

Figures 38.4A and B: Bundle branch reentry (BBR) with right bundle branch block (RBBB) morphology. Panel A shows, from top to bottom, surface ECG leads 1, 2 and V1, and intracardiac recordings from the right atrium (RA), His-bundle, and time lines (T). Panel B shows the same surface ECG leads, and intracardiac recordings from the right bundle branch (RB), right ventricle (RV), and time lines (T). During BBR with RBBB morphology (Panel A), the HV is determined by the conduction properties of the left bundle branch, in this case, 250 ms. In contrast, during sinus rhythm, the HV interval, determined primarily by the right bundle branch, was 90 ms (not shown). In Panel B, the right bundle branch potential is shown. Note the appropriate sequence of activation: the RBB potential is recorded before the His-bundle potential, as expected in this type of BBR reentry

Merino et al.[23] described another diagnostic criterion for BBR. Given the close proximity between the BBR reentry circuit (i.e., distal RBB) and the RV apex, the post-pace interval was equal or <30 ms when RV stimulation was performed during BBR with an LBBB (compared to >100 ms for myocardial VT) **(Figure 38.7)**. This may be particularly useful when an HB or RBB potential cannot be recorded.

BBR-VT with LBBB Pattern

As previously mentioned, this is, by far, the most common type of HPS-related VT,[1,5,6-12] perhaps because programmed stimulation is routinely performed from the RV. In our experience,[1,5] induction of this VT required LV stimulation in 2 of 59 patients. The QRS morphology is suggestive of aberrant conduction **(Figure 38.2)** because myocardial activation is by way of the HPS, in this case the RBB. In the absence of anti-arrhythmic drugs, the cycle length of this VT is fast, ranging from 200 ms to 300 ms. The QRS axis is usually normal or leftward. Rightward axis is rare, unless the QRS in SR also is rightward. The HV interval ranges from 55 ms to 160 ms.

BBR-VT with RBBB Pattern

In this type of VT, activation of the HB is by the RBB, followed by antegrade conduction via the LBB **(Figures 38.4A and B)**. We induced this VT in 6 of 59 patients. In 2 of the 6 patients, it was the only type of VT inducible. This type of VT, in contrast to the one with LBBB pattern, more often required LV or atrial stimulation. A functional proximal RBBB may occur during atrial pacing (or atrial fibrillation);[24] slow antegrade propagation over the LBB may allow recovery of the RBB, facilitating BBR. This type of VT may be less common than BBR with an LBBB pattern because LV stimulation is not routinely performed, but also due to the shorter retrograde refractoriness of the LBB (compared to the RBB), in which case, retrograde block may be more difficult to accomplish during RV pacing. The QRS axis in this type of VT may be normal, leftward, or rightward, depending upon which fascicle is used for antegrade propagation. In our experience, the cycle length of this tachycardia has ranged from 220 ms to 360 ms, and the HV interval between 65 ms and 250 ms.[1,5,18] Although rare, this type of VT was more commonly seen in the immediate postoperative period after valvular replacement surgery, compared to patients with nonischemic cardiomyopathy.[18]

Interfascicular (IF)–VT

In this type of VT,[25-27] the reentry circuit involves the distal LBB, the left-sided fascicles, and myocardial conduction **(Figure 38.8)**. The RBB is not part of the reentry circuit and is activated incidentally; therefore, catheter ablation of the RBB will not eliminate this type of VT. This mechanism of VT needs to be excluded from BBR with an RBBB pattern because in both cases the QRS morphology is RBBB pattern.

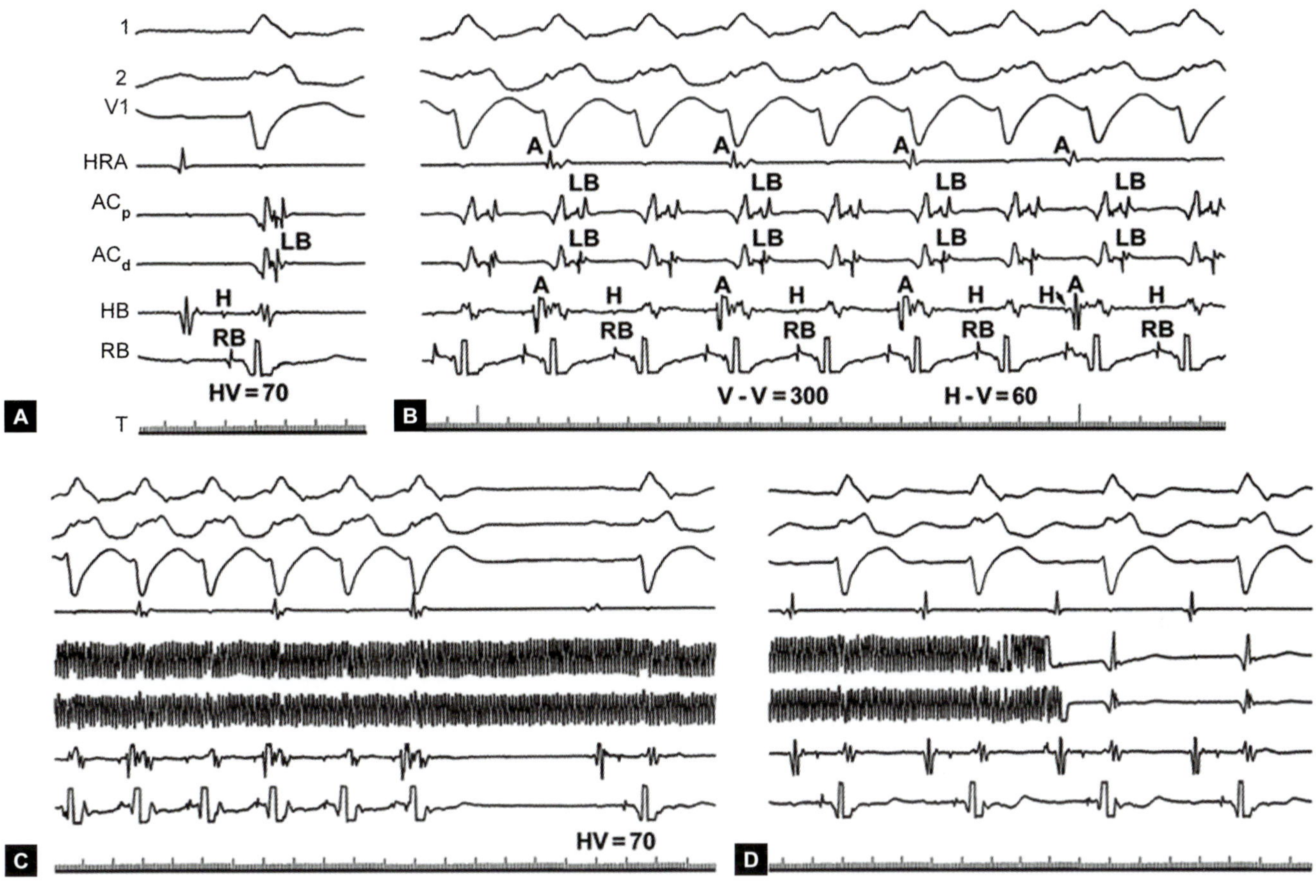

Figures 38.5A to D: Catheter ablation of the left bundle branch for bundle branch reentrant tachycardia. The four panels in this figure display, from top to bottom, surface ECG leads 1, 2 and V1 and intracardiac recordings from the high right atrium (HRA), proximal and distal ablation catheter (AC_p and AC_d), His-bundle (HB), right bundle branch (RB), and time lines (T). Panel A shows sinus rhythm with His and right bundle branch potentials. The ablation catheter is positioned in the left side of the interventricular septum and is recording a left bundle branch potential (LB) after the local ventricular electrogram. This is a retrograde (transeptally conducted impulse) potential given the complete antegrade left bundle branch block. During bundle branch reentrant tachycardia (Panel B), the same sequence of activation is displayed as in sinus rhythm, with a slightly shorter HV interval. Panel C displays delivery of radiofrequency current to the left bundle branch during bundle branch reentry, which results in termination of the tachycardia. The first escape beat has the same HV interval as before the ablation and there is no change in the QRS morphology. Note in Panel D that the LB potential is no longer recorded. (From Blanck Z, Deshpande S, Jazayeri MR, Akhtar M. Catheter ablation of the left bundle branch for the treatment of sustained bundle branch reentrant ventricular tachycardia. J Cardiovasc Electrophysiol 1995; 6:40-3. Used with permission from John Wiley and Sons)

The sequence of activation of the HPS, being different in these two tachycardias, may be helpful in differentiating them. During BBR with RBBB (i.e., retrograde conduction via the RBB), the RBB is activated before the HB is activated. In contrast, during IF-VT, the RBB is expected to be activated after the HB activation. Patients with IF-VT usually have concomitant BBR.[25,26] We recently noted that an RBBB may be a prerequisite for IF reentry (spontaneous or inducible).[25] The RBBB may be pre-existing or occur after catheter ablation for BBR-VT. The HV interval during IF-VT is usually shorter than in SR, as the "turnaround" between the fascicles is distal to the HB. Depending on the fascicle used for antegrade conduction, the QRS during IF-VT will be rightward or leftward. Ablation of the LBB, or one of its fascicles, is necessary to eliminate this type of VT and has been performed successfully.[25-27]

DIFFERENTIAL DIAGNOSIS OF BBR-VT

BBR-VT should be suspected in the presence of a wide QRS complex tachycardia with AV dissociation, where HB potentials precede ventricular activation. The diagnosis of BBR-VT requires careful analysis of the sequence of HPS activation and the relationship between changes in H-H and V-V cycle lengths. Otherwise, this mechanism may go unrecognized and be attributed to the common variety of

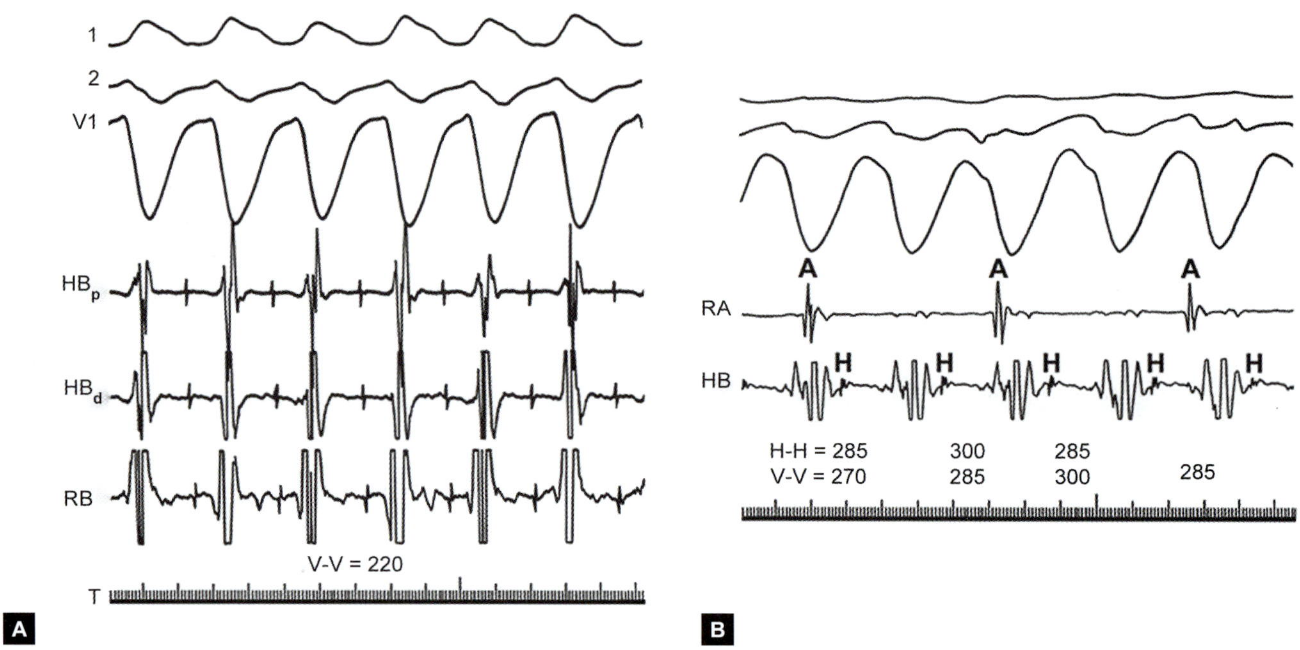

Figures 38.6A and B: Diagnosis of bundle branch reentry. Panel A, from top to bottom, shows surface ECG leads 1, 2 and V1, and intracardiac recordings from proximal and distal His-bundle (HB_p and HB_d), right bundle branch (RB), and time lines (T). Intracardiac recordings during bundle branch reentrant tachycardia show the His and bundle branch potentials to precede the onset of the surface ECG, the appropriate sequence of His-Purkinje system activation during tachycardia with a left bundle branch pattern (i.e., from proximal to distal), and a very short cycle length, typical of this type of reentry. Panel B, from top to bottom, shows surface ECG leads 1, 2 and V1, and intracardiac recordings from the right atrium (RA), His-bundle (HB), and time lines (T). This figure shows an important criteria for bundle branch reentrant tachycardia: during irregular cycle lengths, H-H changes will precede and dictate the corresponding V-V changes

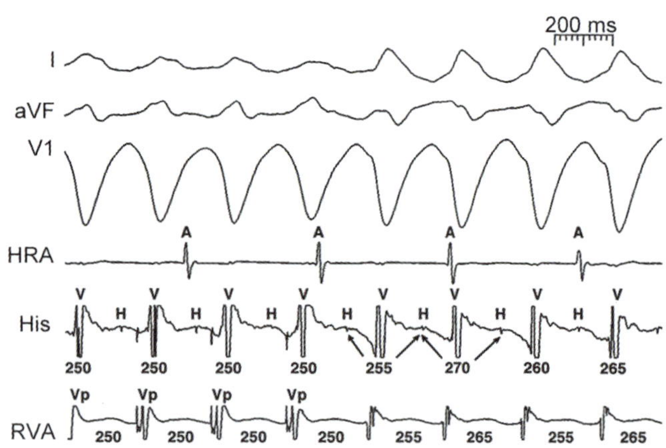

Figure 38.7: Post-pace interval during bundle branch reentry. Tracings, from top to bottom, include surface ECG leads 1, 2 and V1, and intracardiac recordings from the right atrium (RA), His-bundle (His), and right ventricular apex (RVA). This figure shows a post-pace interval (PPI) of 250 ms after a train of ventricular pacing from the RV apex (first four beats of the figure). A similar PPI from this pacing site as the cycle length of tachycardia is consistent with bundle branch reentry

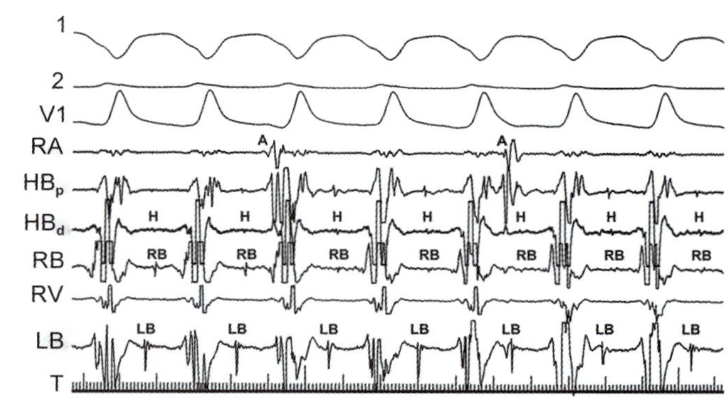

Figure 38.8: Interfascicular reentrant tachycardia. Displayed from top to bottom are surface ECG leads 1, 2 and V1 and intracardiac recordings from the right atrium (RA), proximal and distal His-bundle (HB_p and HB_d), right ventricle (RV), left bundle branch (LB), and time lines (T). Intracardiac recordings during interfascicular tachycardia show the appropriate sequence of His-Purkinje system activation: the left bundle branch is activated first, followed by simultaneous activation of the HB and the RB. The HV interval (not labeled) is 25 ms shorter than in sinus rhythm, a finding consistent with this mechanism of tachycardia. The QRS morphology is right bundle branch block (RBBB). In bundle branch reentry with the same QRS pattern (e.g., RBBB), the opposite sequence of activation would be expected (e.g., RB, followed by HB, followed by LB)

scar-related VT. Perhaps, the most important factor in the diagnosis of BBR-VT is to suspect it in the appropriate clinical setting.

Myocardial Scar-related VT

This type of VT, with retrograde activation of the HPS, is the most important consideration and should always be differentiated from BBR-VT. In most scar-related VTs, the HB activation is "obscured" by the local ventricular EGM, and it is not usually seen. However, in some VTs, the HB potential may be recorded before the local ventricular EGM but after the onset of the QRS in the 12-lead ECG, which rules out BBR. In other VTs, an HB or BB potential may appear to precede the onset of the surface QRS, a finding similar to BBR-VT **(Figure 38.9)**. In these cases, and in contrast to BBR, changes in V-V intervals will precede subsequent changes in H-H intervals. In addition, given the same QRS morphology (i.e., RBBB), analysis of the sequence of HPS activation may be helpful as it may differ between myocardial VT, where the HB may be activated retrogradely by the LBB, and BBR-VT, where the HB also is activated retrogradely, but by the RBB. Finally, if myocardial VT is suspected, RV pacing during SR at the same cycle length as the VT may be helpful to demonstrate retrograde HPS activation **(Figures 38.10A and B)**, a finding that would support a myocardial VT.

Supraventricular Tachycardia with Aberrant Conduction

Patients with BBR almost never exhibit 1:1 AV conduction during tachycardia. In addition, the sequence of activation

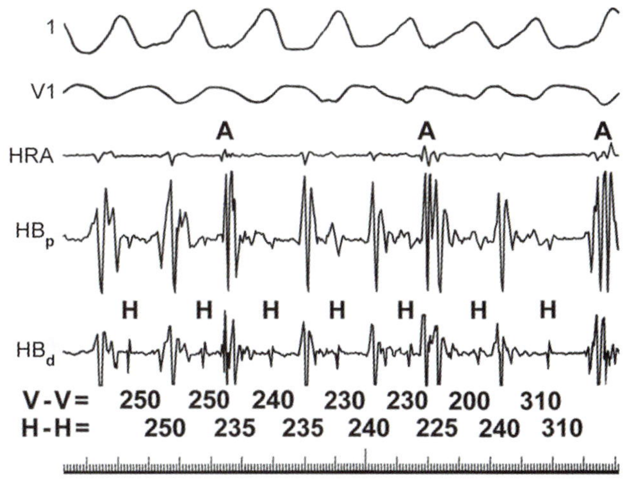

Figure 38.9: Incidental activation of the His-bundle during myocardial ventricular tachycardia initiated after catheter ablation of the right bundle branch. Tracings, from top to bottom, are surface ECG leads I and V1; high right atrium (HRA) and proximal and distal His-bundle recordings (HB$_p$ and HB$_d$); and time lines (T). All intervals are in milliseconds. During induced sustained ventricular tachycardia with a left bundle branch block QRS configuration, each ventricular electrogram is preceded by a His-bundle potential. However, retrograde activation of the His-Purkinje system is coincidental, and changes in V-V intervals precede or are unrelated to changes in H-H intervals, as expected during myocardial ventricular tachycardia. In this case, activation of the His-bundle is retrograde through the left bundle branch, the conduction of which was severely impaired. (From Blanck Z, et al. Bundle Branch Reentrant Ventricular Tachycardia: Cummulative Experience in 48 Patients. J Cardiovasc Electrophysiol 1993;4:253-63. Used with permission from John Wiley and Sons)

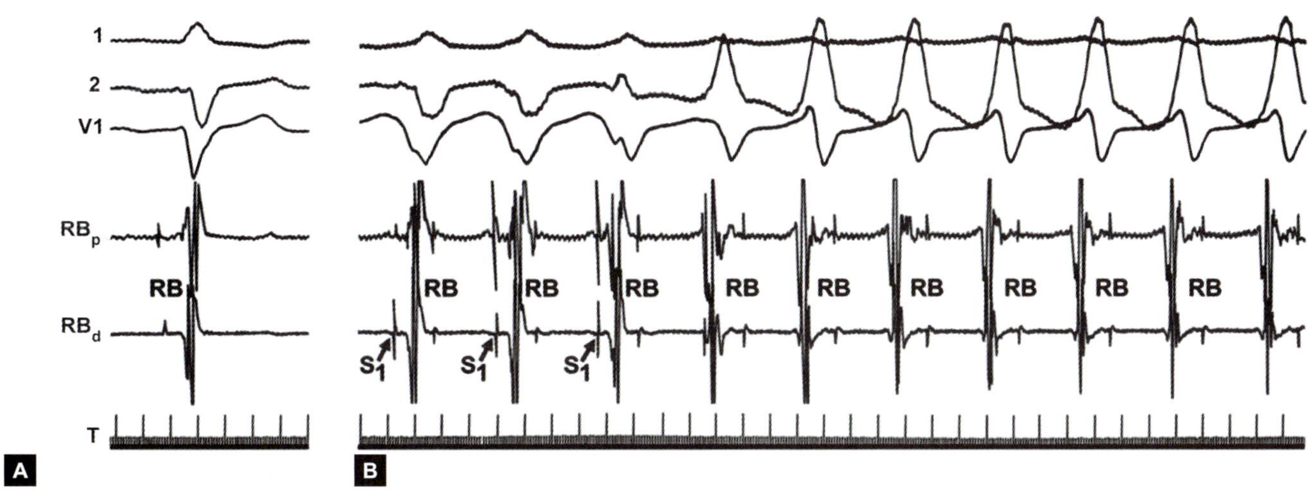

Figures 38.10A and B: Tracings, from top to bottom, show surface ECG leads 1, 2 and V1, and intracardiac recordings from proximal and distal right bundle branch (RB$_p$ and RB$_d$) and time lines (T). Panel A shows the RB potentials in sinus rhythm. Panel B displays the end of a ventricular pacing drive (first 4 beats) followed by ongoing ventricular tachycardia (VT). Note that the RB is captured during ventricular pacing, with a similar sequence as during VT, a finding consistent with myocardial, scar-related VT

of the HPS is different: in supraventricular tachycardia, the HPS is activated antegradely, with a similar sequence as in sinus rhythm. In contrast, during BBR, the HPS sequence of activation is retrograde usually via the LBB.

Atriofascicular Reentry

In this tachycardia, ventricular activation also is by way of the RBB,[28] and the HB is activated retrogradely, as in BBR. However, the sequence of HPS activation is different in both tachycardias: in BBR with an LBBB pattern, the HB is activated before the RBB, and the opposite sequence is seen in atriofascicular reentry. Also, the atrium is part of the atriofascicular reentry circuit, and most patients with atriofascicular reentry do not have structural heart disease. Atrial pacing in patients with atriofascicular reentry may show pre-excitation.

BBR-VT should always be suspected in patients with nonischemic cardiomyopathy presenting with syncope or sudden death. It also should be suspected in patients with inducible SMVT and conduction abnormalities, or when the VT has an LBBB pattern.

TREATMENT OF BBR-VT

Radiofrequency catheter ablation of the RBB is the treatment of choice for BBR-VT[8] **(Figures 38.11A to C)**. This procedure will eliminate both types of BBR (LBBB and RBBB) by creating complete conduction block in the RBB.[1,5,9-12] In this ablation, a catheter is placed in the septum until an RBB potential is recorded. The nature of this potential is confirmed by the absence of an atrial EGM and an H-RB interval of at least 20 ms.[9,10] Inadvertent ablation of the HB will result in complete AV block and persistent inducibility

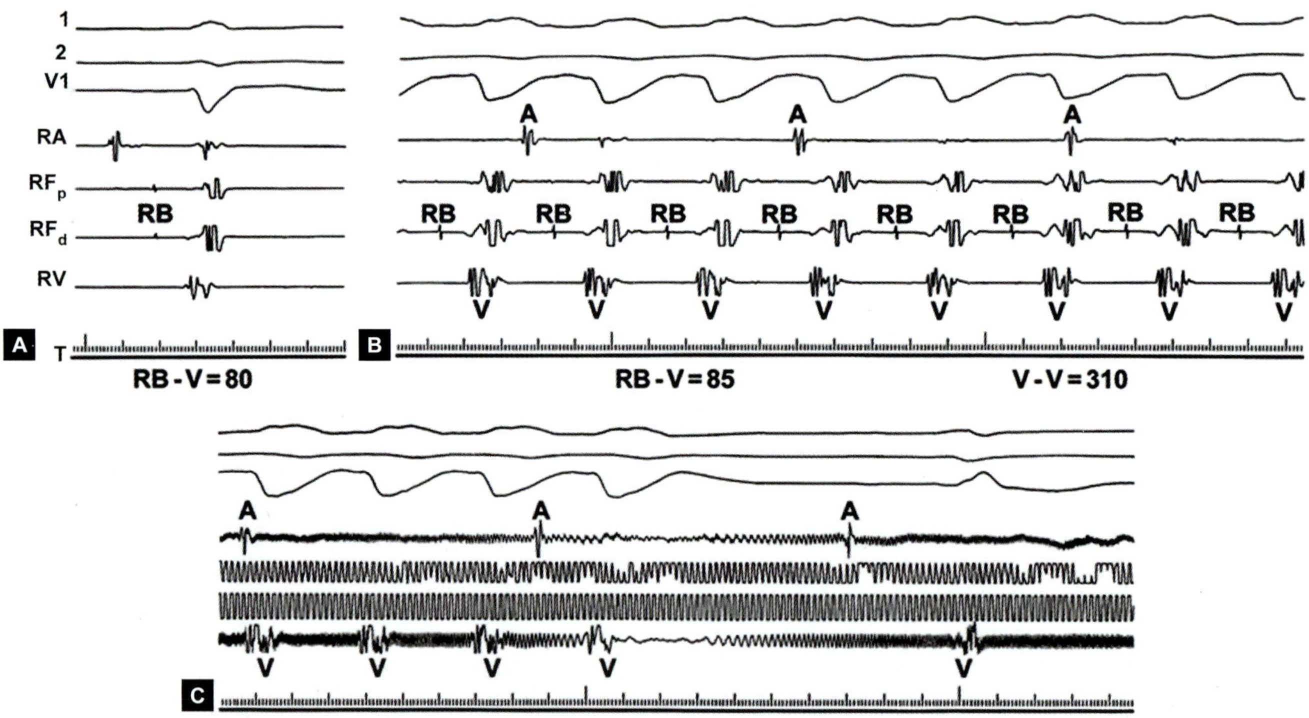

Figures 38.11A to C: Termination of sustained bundle branch reentrant tachycardia during catheter ablation of the right bundle branch using radiofrequency current. Displayed from top to bottom are ECG leads 1, 2, and V1; intracardiac recordings from the right atrium (RA), proximal and distal ablating catheter (RF_p, RF_a), and right ventricle electrogram (RV); and time lines (T). All intervals are in milliseconds. In Panel A, activation of the right bundle branch is recorded in the distal bipole of the ablating catheter during sinus rhythm. Panel B shows bundle branch reentrant ventricular tachycardia with a left bundle branch block pattern and a cycle length of 310 ms. Activation of the right bundle branch is recorded in the ablating catheter. In Panel C, ablation of the right bundle branch and termination of the tachycardia occur within 6 seconds of energy application. Note the expected complete right bundle branch block QRS morphology in the first sinus beat after terminating the tachycardia. (From Blanck Z, et al. Bundle Branch Reentrant Ventricular Tachycardia: Cumulative Experience in 48 Patients. J Cardiovasc Electrophysiol 1993;4:253-63. Used with permission from John Wiley and Sons)

of BBR. Given the anatomic features of the RBB (relatively thin and superficially located in the sub-endocardium) this procedure is easily performed and successful in the majority of patients.[29]

Although catheter ablation of the LBB is technically more challenging than RBB ablation, it can be attempted in select patients with BBR or in patients with IF-VT, as described previously **(Figure 38.5)**.[16,24,26,27,30] Patients with complete antegrade LBBB (i.e., QRS duration >140 ms) may benefit more from LBB ablation as this will eliminate retrograde conduction in the LBB, eliminate induction of BBR, and prevent complete AV block, a likely complication of RBB ablation in the presence of a complete LBBB.[16]

After RBB ablation, prophylactic pacemaker implantation was carried out only if the HV interval prolonged significantly (>90–100 ms), or infra-His block could be documented during atrial stimulation.[5] However, with the advent of biventricular pacing, the role of prophylactic pacing and defibrillator implantation has changed over the years, and the presence of LV dysfunction and congestive heart failure are additional considerations for prophylactic device implantation in these patients. Of note, in 25% of our patients with BBR, a concomitant scar-related SMVT also was induced,[1,5] another factor when considering device implantation post-ablation.

REFERENCES

1. Caceres J, Jazayeri M, McKinnie J, Avitall B, Denker ST, Tchou P, Akhtar M. Sustained bundle branch reentry as a mechanism of clinical tachycardia. Circulation. 1989;79:256-70.
2. Akhtar M, Damato AN, Batsford WP, Ruskin JN, Ogunkelu JB, Vargas G. Demonstration of re-entry within the His-Purkinje system in man. Circulation. 1974;50:1150-62.
3. Akhtar M, Denker S, Lehmann MH, Mahmud R. Macro-reentry within the His Purkinje system. Pacing Clin Electrophysiol. 1983;6:1010-28.
4. Akhtar M, Gilbert C, Wolf FG, Schmidt DH. Reentry within the His-Purkinje system. Elucidation of reentrant circuit using right bundle branch and His bundle recordings. Circulation. 1978;58:295-304.
5. Blanck Z, Dhala A, Deshpande S, Sra J, Jazayeri M, Akhtar M. Bundle branch reentrant ventricular tachycardia: cumulative experience in 48 patients. J Cardiovasc Electrophysiol. 1993;4:253-62.
6. Welch WJ, Strasberg B, Coelho A, Rosen KM. Sustained macroreentrant ventricular tachycardia. Am Heart J. 1982;104:166-9.
7. Reddy CP, Slack JD. Recurrent sustained ventricular tachycardia: report of a case with His-bundle branches reentry as the mechanism. Eur J Cardiol. 1980;11:23-31.
8. Chien WW, Scheinman MM, Cohen TJ, Lesh MD. Importance of recording the right bundle branch deflection in the diagnosis of His-Purkinje reentrant tachycardia. Pacing Clin Electrophysiol. 1992;15:1015-24.
9. Tchou P, Jazayeri M, Denker S, Dongas J, Caceres J, Akhtar M. Transcatheter electrical ablation of right bundle branch. A method of treating macroreentrant ventricular tachycardia attributed to bundle branch reentry. Circulation. 1988;78:246-57.
10. Touboul P, Kirkorian G, Atallah G, Lavaud P, Moleur P, Lamaud M, Mathieu MP. Bundle branch reentrant tachycardia treated by electrical ablation of the right bundle branch. J Am Coll Cardiol. 1986;7:1404-9.
11. Cohen TJ, Chien WW, Lurie KG, Young C, Goldberg HR, Wang YS, Langberg JJ, Lesh MD, Lee MA, Griffin JC, et al. Radiofrequency catheter ablation for treatment of bundle branch reentrant ventricular tachycardia: results and long-term follow-up. J Am Coll Cardiol. 1991;18:1767-73.
12. Langberg JJ, Desai J, Dullet N, Scheinman MM. Treatment of macroreentrant ventricular tachycardia with radiofrequency ablation of the right bundle branch. Am J Cardiol. 1989;63:1010-3.
13. Denker S, Shenasa M, Gilbert CJ, Akhtar M. Effects of abrupt changes in cycle length on refractoriness of the His-Purkinje system in man. Circulation. 1983;67:60-8.
14. Denker S, Lehmann MH, Mahmud R, Gilbert C, Akhtar M. Facilitation of macroreentry within the His-Purkinje system with abrupt changes in cycle length. Circulation. 1984;69:26-32.
15. Denker S, Lehmann M, Mahmud R, Gilbert C, Akhtar M. Effects of alternating cycle lengths on refractoriness of the His-Purkinje system. J Clin Invest. 1984;74:559-70.
16. Schmidt B, Tang M, Chun KR, Antz M, Tilz RR, Metzner A, Koektuerk B, Xie P, Kuck KH, Ouyang F. Left bundle branch-Purkinje system in patients with bundle branch reentrant tachycardia: lessons from catheter ablation and electroanatomic mapping. Heart Rhythm. 2009;6:51-8.
17. Reddy CP, Khorasanchian A. Intraventricular reentry with narrow QRS complex. Circulation. 1980;61:641-7.
18. Narasimhan C, Jazayeri MR, Sra J, Dhala A, Deshpande S, Biehl M, Akhtar M, Blanck Z. Ventricular tachycardia in valvular heart disease: facilitation of sustained bundle-branch reentry by valve surgery. Circulation. 1997;96:4307-13.
19. Andress JD, Vander Salm TJ, Huang SK. Bidirectional bundle branch reentry tachycardia associated with Ebstein's anomaly: cured by extensive cryoablation of the right bundle branch. Pacing Clin Electrophysiol. 1991;14:1639-47.
20. Merino JL, Carmona JR, Fernandez-Lozano I, Peinado R, Basterra N, Sobrino JA. Mechanisms of sustained ventricular tachycardia in myotonic dystrophy: implications for catheter ablation. Circulation. 1998;98:541-6.
21. Blanck Z, Jazayeri M, Dhala A, Deshpande S, Sra J, Akhtar M. Bundle branch reentry: a mechanism of ventricular tachycardia in the absence of myocardial or valvular dysfunction. J Am Coll Cardiol. 1993;22:1718-22.
22. Reddy CP, Damato AN, Akhtar M, Dhatt MS, Gomes JA, Calon AH. Effect of procainamide on reentry within the His-Purkinje system in man. Am J Cardiol. 1977;40:957-64.
23. Merino JL, Peinado R, Fernandez-Lozano I, Lopez-Gil M, Arribas F, Ramirez LJ, Echeverria IJ, Sobrino JA. Bundle-branch reentry and the postpacing interval after entrainment by right ventricular apex stimulation: a new approach to elucidate the mechanism of wide-QRS-complex tachycardia with atrioventricular dissociation. Circulation. 2001;103:1102-8.
24. Blanck Z, Jazayeri M, Akhtar M. Facilitation of sustained bundle branch reentry by atrial fibrillation. J Cardiovasc Electrophysiol. 1996;7:348-52.

25. Blanck Z, Sra J, Akhtar M. Incessant interfascicular reentrant ventricular tachycardia as a result of catheter ablation of the right bundle branch: case report and review of the literature. J Cardiovasc Electrophysiol. 2009;20:1279-83.
26. Berger RD, Orias D, Kasper EK, Calkins H. Catheter ablation of coexistent bundle branch and interfascicular reentrant ventricular tachycardias. J Cardiovasc Electrophysiol. 1996;7:341-7.
27. Crijns HJ, Smeets JL, Rodriguez LM, Meijer A, Wellens HJ. Cure of interfascicular reentrant ventricular tachycardia by ablation of the anterior fascicle of the left bundle branch. J Cardiovasc Electrophysiol. 1995;6:486-92.
28. Tchou P, Lehmann MH, Jazayeri M, Akhtar M. Atriofascicular connection or a nodoventricular Mahaim fiber? Electrophysiologic elucidation of the pathway and associated reentrant circuit. Circulation. 1988;77:837-48.
29. Massing GK, James TN. Anatomical configuration of the His bundle and bundle branches in the human heart. Circulation. 1976;53:609-21.
30. Blanck Z, Deshpande S, Jazayeri MR, Akhtar M. Catheter ablation of the left bundle branch for the treatment of sustained bundle branch reentrant ventricular tachycardia. J Cardiovasc Electrophysiol. 1995;6:40-3.

EDITORS' SUMMARY

The authors who have taught the electrophysiology community about this unique and fascinating arrhythmia —bundle-branch reentrant tachycardia—provide a well-referenced and well-illustrated summary that is enjoyable to read. Although not a common arrhythmia, bundle-branch reentry is imminently treatable and is a veritable microcosm of all invasive arrhythmia diagnosis. The principles of reset, attempting to find what is in and not in a circuit of a reentrant tachycardia, identifying the driver or the critical link, and the concept of pseudo intervals (the HV during tachycardia and proximal His-V during bundle-branch reentry) are all represented and clearly discussed in this chapter. The early student of invasive electrophysiology would do well to read this chapter along with those on AV node reentry (Chapter 17) and diagnostic maneuvers both for SVT (Chapters 15 and 16) and entrainment (Chapter 43) for a comprehensive foray into the art and science of diagnostic maneuvers for arrhythmia diagnosis.

CHAPTER 39

Charles Antzelevitch, Bence Patocskai

J Wave Syndromes

LIST OF ABBREVIATIONS

AP	Action Potential	LV	Left Ventricle
ARI	Activation Recovery Intervals	MAP	Monophasic Action Potential
ARVC	Arrhythmogenic Right Ventricular Cardiomyopathy	MRI	Magnetic Resonance Imaging
BrS	Brugada Syndrome	P2R	Phase 2 Reentry
CT	Computed Tomography	PDE	Phosphodiesterase
DS	Desmosomal	PES	Programmed Electrical Stimulation
ECGI	Electrocardiographic Imaging	RBBB	Right Bundle Branch Block
EG	Electrogram	RF	Radiofrequency
ER	Early Repolarization	RFA	Radiofrequency Ablation
ERP	Early Repolarization Pattern	RV	Right Ventricle
ERS	Early Repolarization Syndrome	RVOT	Right Ventricular Outflow Tract
GWAS	Genome Wide Association Studies	SCD	Sudden Cardiac Death
ICD	Implantable Cardioverter-Defibrillator	SIDS	Sudden Infant Death Syndrome
iPSC-CM	Induced Pluripotent Stem Cell-derived Cardiac Myocytes	TRPM4	Transient Receptor Potential Melastatin Protein 4
IVCD	Intraventricular Conduction Defect	VF	Ventricular Fibrillation
LP	Late Potential	VT	Ventricular Tachycardia

INTRODUCTION

The J wave syndromes are so named because they involve accentuation of the electrocardiographic J wave.[1] The J wave is thought to be inscribed as a consequence of transmural differences in the manifestation of the action potential (AP) notch between epicardium and endocardium secondary to heterogeneous transmural distribution of the transient outward current (I_{to}).[2] The appearance of prominent electrocardiographic J waves has long been associated with hypothermia[3-5] and hypercalcemia,[6,7] and more recently with life-threatening ventricular arrhythmias.[1] Two principal inherited cardiac arrhythmia syndromes, Brugada (BrS) and early repolarization syndromes (ERS), comprise the J wave syndromes. Pedro and Josep Brugada provided the initial delineation of BrS as a clinical entity in 1992.[8] The clinical impact of ERS was not fully realized until 2008, when publication of the now classical studies of Haïssaguerre and coworkers,[9] Nam and coworkers[10] and Rosso et al.[11] appeared. The genetic basis for BrS and ERS has progressed, but the Mendelian nature of their inheritance has recently been questioned. The cellular mechanisms underlying the J wave syndromes have also been the subject of some debate. This chapter provides a review of the genetic, ionic and cellular mechanisms underlying the J wave syndromes.

J WAVE SYNDROMES: DEFINITIONS AND DESCRIPTIONS

The J wave, when associated with life-threatening ventricular arrhythmias,[1] may be so tall and broad as to appear as an ST segment elevation, as in cases of Brugada syndrome (BrS). The normal J wave in humans commonly appears as a J point elevation, with a good part of the J wave buried inside the QRS. An early repolarization (ER) pattern in the ECG, characterized by a distinct J wave, J point elevation, a notch or slur of the terminal part of the QRS with and without an ST segment elevation was long considered as benign.[12,13] In 2000, Gussak and Antzelevitch[14] challenged this view on the basis of experimental data showing that this ECG manifestation predisposes to the development of polymorphic ventricular tachycardia and fibrillation (VT/VF) in coronary-perfused wedge preparations.[1,14-16] Validation of this hypothesis came years later with the seminal work of Haïssaguerre et al.,[9] Nam et al.[10] and Rosso et al.[11] These studies were followed by a wave of case control and population-based studies, providing clinical evidence for an increased risk for development of life-threatening arrhythmic events and sudden cardiac death (SCD) among patients presenting with an ER pattern, particularly in inferior and inferolateral leads. In order to avoid the many inconsistencies in the terminology of ER appearing in early reports,[17-19] MacFarlane and coworkers provided and expert consensus statement with recommendations for the measurement and reporting of ER and J waves. The task force recommends that peak of an end QRS notch and/or the onset of an end QRS slur be designated as J_p and that J_p should exceed 0.1 mV in ≥2 contiguous inferior and/or lateral leads of a standard 12-lead ECG for early repolarization to be present.[20] It was further recommended that the start of the end QRS notch or J wave be designated as J_o and the termination as J_t.

BrS, and more recently ERS, have been associated with a risk of development of polymorphic VT and VF leading to SCD[1,8-10] in young adults and occasionally of sudden infant death syndrome (SIDS).[21-23] The region of the heart most affected in ERS, is generally the inferior region of the left ventricle, whereas in BrS, it is the anterior right ventricular outflow tract (RVOT).[9,11,24-28] BrS is characterized by the appearance of accentuated J waves, often appearing as a coved-type ST segment elevation in the right precordial leads, V1-V3, whereas ERS is characterized by the appearance of J waves, J_o elevation, notch or slur of the terminal part of the QRS and ST-segment or J_t elevation in the lateral (type I), inferolateral (type II) or in inferolateral + anterior or right ventricular leads (type III).[1]

An early repolarization pattern (ERP) is commonly encountered in healthy individuals, particularly in young, black individuals and athletes. ERP is also observed in acquired conditions, including hypothermia and ischemia.[1,29,30] When associated with VT or VF, ERP is referred to as early repolarization syndrome (ERS).

The prevalence of type 1 BrS ECG varies widely among different international regions. It is traditionally higher in Asian countries, such as Japan (0.15–0.27%),[31,32] the Philippines (0.18%),[33] and among Japanese-Americans in North America (0.15%)[34] than in Western countries, including Europe (0–0.017%)[35-37] or North America (0.005–0.1%).[38,39] In contrast, the prevalence of an ERP in the inferior and/or lateral leads with a J_o elevation of ≥ 0.1 mV ranges between 1% and 24% and for J_o of ≥ 0.2 mV, it ranges between 0.6% to 6.4%.[40-42] An ERP is significantly more common in blacks than in Caucasians and appears to be more common in Aboriginal Australians than in Caucasian Australians.[43]

DIAGNOSIS OF BrS

According to the first two consensus statements,[44,45] BrS is diagnosed with the appearance of a Type 1 ECG displaying a coved-type ST-segment elevation of 2 mm (0.2 mV) or more followed by a negative T wave in more than one right precordial leads (V1 to V3) in the presence or absence of a sodium channel-blocking agent, and in conjunction with one of the following: documented VF, polymorphic VT, a family history of SCD at ≤45 years old, coved-type ECGs in family members, inducibility of VT with programmed electrical stimulation, syncope, or nocturnal agonal respiration. This was modified in the 2013 consensus statement on inherited cardiac arrhythmias[46] and 2015 Guidelines for the management of patients with ventricular arrhythmias and prevention of sudden cardiac death.[47]: According to the new criteria, BrS is to be diagnosed in patients with ST-segment elevation with type 1 morphology ≥2 mm in ≥1 lead among the right precordial leads V1, V2, positioned in the 2nd, 3rd or 4th intercostal space occurring either spontaneously or after provocative drug test with intravenous administration of Class I antiarrhythmic drugs. BrS is diagnosed in patients with type 2 or type 3 ST-segment elevation in ≥1 lead among the right precordial leads V1, V2 positioned in the 2nd, 3rd or 4th intercostal space when a provocative drug test with intravenous administration of Class I antiarrhythmic drugs induces a type I ECG morphology." There was no longer a requirement for manifestation of any symptoms. This modification has raised a concern that this could result in an over-diagnosis of BrS, particularly in patients displaying a Type 1 ECG only after a drug challenge, an issue that is being addressed by an expert consensus statement currently under development.

All consensus documents agree that a Type 2 (saddleback type) or Type 3 ST segment elevation cannot substitute for a Type 1 unless converted to Type 1 with fever or sodium channel blocking drug challenge. A drug challenge-induced type 1 can be used to diagnose BrS only if accompanied by one of the criteria specified above. Type 2 is characterized by ST segment elevation of ≥0.5 mm (generally ≥2 mm in V2) in ≥1 right precordial lead (V1-V3), followed by a convex ST. The ST segment is followed by a positive T wave in V2 and variable morphology V1. Type 3 is characterized by either a saddleback or coved appearance with an ST-segment elevation of <1 mm. The placement of the right precordial leads in more cranial positions (in the 3rd or 2nd intercostal space) in a 12 lead resting ECG or 12 lead Holter ECG increases the sensitivity of ECG.[48-50] Veltman et al. showed that RVOT localization using MRI correlates with type 1 ST segment elevation in BrS and that lead positioning according to RVOT location improves the diagnosis of Brugada syndrome.

Diagnostic Aids

When a patient presents with a clinical suspicion of BrS (Type 2 or 3 ST segment elevation, syncope or family history), a pharmacological challenge using a sodium channel blocker is recommended. These tests include use of ajmaline (1 mg/kg over 10 minutes, IV), flecainide (2 mg/kg over 10 minutes, IV or 200-300 mg, orally); procainamide (2 mg/kg over 10 minutes IV or 200-300 mg, orally); or pilsicainide (1 mg/kg over 10 minutes, IV). The test is considered positive only if a type 1 ECG pattern is achieved and it should be discontinued in case of frequent ventricular extrasystoles or other arrhythmias, or widening of the QRS >130% over the baseline value.[44] Alternatively, the "full stomach test" has been proposed for diagnosing BrS.[51] In this case, ECGs are performed before and after a large meal. The use of "high-electrodes" increases the sensitivity for recognizing spontaneous type 1 ST segment elevation at night or after heavy meals.[52] A type 1 ST segment elevation recorded using a Holter is a spontaneous type 1.

Drug challenge is generally not indicated in asymptomatic patients displaying the type 1 ECG under baseline conditions because of the lack of the additional diagnostic value. These provocative drug tests are also not recommended in cases in which fever has been documented to induce a Type 1 ECG, other than for research purposes. Much debate has centered around the definition of a false positive sodium channel block challenge.[53] It is difficult to define a false positive because of the lack of a gold standard. The development of a Type 1 ST segment elevation in response to sodium block challenge should be considered as probabilistic, rather than binary, in nature.

It is generally agreed that asymptomatic patients with a family history of BrS or SCD should be informed of the availability of a sodium channel blocker challenge test to provide a more definitive diagnosis of BrS. However, patients should be advised that no therapy may be recommended regardless of the outcome because the long-term risk of patients with BrS diagnosed by this test is significantly lower than the risk of patients with spontaneous type 1. The decision as to whether to undergo the drug challenge ultimately should be left up to the well informed patient, who should be informed as to the risk of the test and about the emotional consequences of having a positive test not followed by definitive therapy.

Performing a sodium block challenge in children is problematic because the test appears to be less sensitive in children than in adults[54] and because the test is associated with greater risk than in adults.[54,55] Caution needs to be exercised when performing a sodium blocker challenge in adults with a known pathogenic sodium channel mutation or in patients with prolonged PR intervals, pointing to a carrier of such a mutation.[56]

Table 39.1 presents other causes of ST segment elevation that must be excluded before establishing the diagnosis of BrS. A Type 1 Brugada-like ECG is encountered in a variety of circumstances including right bundle branch block (RBBB), pectus excavatum, arrhythmogenic right ventricular cardiomyopathy (ARVC), as well as occlusion of the left anterior descending artery or the conus branch of the right coronary artery, which supplies the RVOT. Distinguishing between BrS and ARVC can be especially challenging. Although debate continues as to the extent to which structural abnormalities contribute to BrS, most investigators consider BrS to be a channelopathy. Concealed structural abnormalities, such as histologic myocardial fibrosis of the RVOT, which may not become evident using conventional imaging techniques have been proposed to account for or

Table 39.1: Differential diagnosis of Brugada syndrome

- Atypical right bundle branch block
- Ventricular hypertrophy
- Early repolarization (especially in athletes)
- Acute pericarditis/myocarditis
- Acute myocardial ischemia or infarction (especially of the right ventricle)
- Pulmonary thromboembolism
- Prinzmetal angina
- Dissecting aortic aneurysm
- Central and autonomic nervous systems abnormalities
- Duchenne's muscular dystrophy
- Friedreich's ataxia
- Spinobulbar muscular atrophy
- Myotonic dystrophy
- Arrhythmogenic right ventricular cardiomyopathy
- Mechanical compression of the right ventricular outflow tract (for instance, *Pectus excavatum*, mediastinal tumor, hemopericardium etc.)
- Hypothermia
- Post-defibrillation ECG

contribute to delayed conduction and ventricular arrhythmias in BrS. MRI and electron beam computed tomography (CT) studies of BrS patients consistently show subtle abnormalities, including wall motion abnormalities and reduced contractile function of the right ventricle (RV) and to a lesser extent of the left ventricle (LV), and dilatation of the RVOT.[57-60] Cardiac dilatation and reduced contractility in all of these studies have been attributed to structural changes (fibrosis, fatty degeneration), despite the fact that virtually no signs of fibrosis or fatty degeneration could be detected.[61] Antzelevitch and co-workers have long argued for an alternative explanation.[27,62,63] They suggested that loss of the action potential dome, which has been shown to create the arrhythmogenic substrate in BrS leads to contractile changes that could explain the wall motion abnormalities. The all-or-none repolarization at the end of phase 1 of the epicardial AP responsible for loss of the dome causes the calcium channels to inactivate very soon after they activate, thus dramatically reducing calcium channel current. Cells become depleted of calcium and contractile function ceases. This is expected to lead to wall motion abnormalities and dilatation, particularly in the RVOT, and reduced ejection fraction observed in patients with BrS. They also proposed that loss of the AP dome, because it creates a hibernation-like state, may over long periods of time lead to mild structural changes, including intracellular lipid accumulation, vacuolization and connexin 43 redistribution. These structural changes may in turn contribute to the arrhythmogenic substrate of the Brugada syndrome, although they are very different from those encountered in ARVC.[27,35,64,65]

In marked contrast, imaging techniques in ARVC clearly reveal morphological and functional changes (e.g., dilatation and wall motion abnormalities). ARVC is an inherited cardiomyopathy caused by genetically defective desmosomal (DS) proteins.[66,67] The syndrome is characterized by fibro-fatty myocardial replacement predisposing to scar-related ventricular arrhythmias which may lead to SCD, mostly in young people and athletes.[68] Interestingly, life-threatening ventricular arrhythmias have been reported during the "concealed phase" of the disease, prior to overt structural changes.[66,67,69] A recent series of studies by the Delmar group have demonstrated that loss of expression of DS proteins can induce electrical ventricular instability by causing sodium channel dysfunction and current reduction, as a consequence of the cross-talk between these molecules at the intercalated discs, which predisposes to sodium current-dependent lethal arrhythmias, similar to those leading to SCD in patients with J-wave/BrS.[69-73] These findings support the concept that Desmosomal-gene mutations involved in the pathogenesis of ARVC can lead to a reduction in sodium channel current and manifest as BrS, at least in the early stages of the disease, even before major structural changes are evident. In the more advanced stages of the disease, the ECG displays a constant T-wave inversion, epsilon waves, and monomorphic VT with left bundle branch block morphology[74] whereas BrS is associated with a dynamically changing ST segment elevation and polymorphic VT occurring predominantly during sleep or rest.[75] A positive ajmaline challenge is reported in 16% of patients with ARVC.[76,77]

Acquired Brugada Pattern and Syndrome

The J waves associated with BrS are often concealed and can be unmasked with a wide variety of drugs and conditions, including a febrile state, vagotonic agents and maneuvers, β adrenergic blockers, α adrenergic agonists, tricyclic or tetracyclic antidepressants, hypokalemia, hyperkalemia, hypercalcemia, as well as by alcohol and cocaine toxicity.[78-88] Chiale and co-workers were the first to demonstrate that pre-excitation of RV can unmask the BrS ECG in cases of RBBB.[89] An up to date list of agents to avoid in BrS can be found at www.brugadadrugs.org.[90]

DIAGNOSIS OF ERS

The ERS is diagnosed in patients displaying ER in the inferior and/or lateral leads and presenting with aborted cardiac arrest, documented VF or polymorphic VT. Consistent with the recent Consensus Report on ER pattern,[20] early repolarization is recognized if when there is an end QRS notch (J wave) or slur on the downslope of a prominent R wave with and without an ST segment elevation; the peak of the notch or J wave (Jp) $\geq$ 0.1 mV in two or more contiguous leads of the 12 lead ECG, excluding leads V1-V3. and QRS duration (measured in leads in which a notch or slur is absent) <120 ms.

SIMILARITIES AND DIFFERENCES BETWEEN BrS AND ERS

BrS and ERS display several phenotypic similarities, once again suggesting similar pathophysiological mechanisms.[2,15,17,91,92] In both syndromes (1) males strongly predominate;[93,94] (2) patients may be totally asymptomatic until presenting with sudden cardiac arrest; (3) appearance of accentuated J waves and ST segment elevation are generally associated with bradycardia or pauses,[95,96] explaining why VF in both syndromes often occurs during sleep or at a low level of physical activity;[97,98] (4) the highest incidence of VF or SCD occurs in the third decade of life, perhaps tied to testosterone levels in males;[99] (5) Phenotype is associated with mutations or rare variants in the same genes; (6) Electrical storms and associated J wave manifestations can be suppressed using β-adrenergic agonists;[100-103] and (7) Chronic oral pharmacological therapy using quinidine,[104,105] cilostazol,[100,102,106-110] denopamine,[100,106] and bepridil[102] suppress the development of VT/VF secondary to inhibition of I_{to}, augmentation of I_{Ca}, I_{Na} or both.[10,107,111]

The principal differences between the two syndromes include: (1) the region of the heart most affected (RVOT vs. inferior LV); (2) greater incidence of late potentials in signal-averaged ECGs in BrS (60%) vs. ERS (7%);[98] (3) greater inducibility of VF during electrophysiological study in BrS than in ERS; (4) greater elevation of J_O, J_P or J_t (ST segment elevation) in response to sodium channel blockers in BrS vs. ERS and (5) higher prevalence of atrial fibrillation in BrS vs. ERS.[112]

Initial studies of the effect of sodium channel blockers on ER, suggested different pathophysiological basis for ERS and BrS based on the observation that the sodium channel blockers unmask or accentuate J wave manifestation in BrS, but reduce the amplitude in ERS.[98] A recent study by Nakagawa et al., however, provided a different perspective. They showed that J waves recorded using unipolar LV epicardial leads introduced into the left lateral coronary vein in ERS patients are indeed augmented, even though J waves recorded in the lateral precordial leads are diminished. The latter were diminished due to engulfment of the surface J wave by the widened QRS.[25,98] Also in support of the thesis that these ECG patterns and syndromes are closely related are reports of cases in which ERS transitions into ERS plus BrS.[92,113]

GENETICS OF THE J WAVE SYNDROMES

Candidate gene, Next Generation, whole exome and whole genome sequencing as well as genome wide association studies (GWAS) have identified variants in 18 different genes cases of BrS and 7 different genes cases of ERS. **Table 39.2** lists the genes uncovered and the effect of mutations or rare variants in these genes on ion channel currents. Available data suggests that the presence of a prominent I_{to} determines whether loss of function mutations resulting in a reduction in I_{Na} will manifest as BrS/ERS or as conduction disease.[114-117]

Recent studies have identified two new susceptibility genes, which await confirmation: Transient Receptor Potential Melastatin Protein 4 gene (*TRPM4*)[118] and the *KCND2* gene. A *KCND2* variant has been identified in a single patient and shown to cause a gain of function in I_{to} when heterologously expressed.[119] Variants in *KCNH2, KCNE5, SEMA3A* although not causative, have been identified as capable of modulating the substrate for the development of BrS.[120-123] Loss-of-function mutations in *HCN4* causing a reduction in pacemaker current, I_f, can unmask BrS by reducing heart rate.[124]

Interpretation of the genetic tests has become a challenging problem. Very few variants in the genes associated with BrS, ERS and other syndromes have been evaluated using functional expression studies to ascertain causality and to establish pathogenicity. Very few have been studied in genetically engineered animal models, native cardiac cells or in induced pluripotent stem cell-derived cardiac myocytes (iPSC-CM) isolated from ERS and BrS patients. *In silico* tools developed to predict the functional consequences of mutations are helpful, but have not been rigorously tested. The lack of functional validation remains a severe limitation of genetic test interpretation.[125] Recent technological advances have resulted in expansion of disease specific databases,[126] which have challenged our understanding of the extent of background genetic variation within cardiac channelopathy-susceptibility genes.[127-129] These issues are transitioning us to consider the results of genetic tests as

Table 39.2: Genetics of Brugada and early repolarization syndromes

		Locus	Ion channel	Gene/Protein
BrS	BrS1	3p21	↓ I_{Na}	*SCN5A*, $Na_V1.5$
	BrS2	3p24	↓ I_{Na}	*GPD1L*
	BrS3	12p13.3	↓ I_{Ca}	*CACNA1C*,$Ca_V1.2$
	BrS4	10p12.33	↓ I_{Ca}	*CACNB2b*, $Ca_V\beta2b$
	BrS5	19q13.1	↓ I_{Na}	*SCN1B*, $Na_V\beta1$
	BrS6	11q13-q14	↓ I_{Ca}	*KCNE3*. MiRP2
	BrS7	11q23.3	↓ I_{Na}	*SCN3B*, Navb3
	BrS8	12p11.23	↑ $I_{K\text{-}ATP}$	*KCNJ8*, Kir6.1
	BrS9	7q21.11	↓ I_{Ca}	*CACNA2D1*, $Ca_V\alpha2\delta1$
	BrS10	1p13.2	↑ I_{to}	*KCND3*, $K_V4.3$
	BrS11	17p13.1	↓ I_{Na}	*RANGRF*, MOG1
	BrS12	3p21.2-p14.3	↓ I_{Na}	*SLMAP*
	BrS13	12p12.1	↑ $I_{K\text{-}ATP}$	*ABCC9*, SUR2A
	BrS14	11q23	↓ I_{Na}	*SCN2B*, $Na_V\beta2$
	BrS15	12p11	↓ I_{Na}	*PKP2*, Plakophilin2
	BrS16	3q28	↓ I_{Na}	*FGF12*, FHAF1
	BrS17	3p22.2	↓ I_{Na}	*SCN10A*, $Na_V1.8$
	BrS18	6q	↑ I_{Na}	*HEY2 (transcriptional factor)*
ERS	ERS1	12p11.23	↑ $I_{K\text{-}ATP}$	*KCNJ8*, Kir6.1
	ERS2	12p13.3	↓ I_{Ca}	*CACNA1C*, $Ca_V1.2$
	ERS3	10p12.33	↓ I_{Ca}	*CACNB2b*, $Ca_V\beta2b$
	ERS4	7q21.11	↓ I_{Ca}	*CACNA2D1*, $Ca_V\alpha2\delta1$
	ERS5	12p12.1	↑ $I_{K\text{-}ATP}$	*ABCC9*, SUR2A
	ERS6	3p21	↓ I_{Na}	*SCN5A*, $Na_V1.5$
	ERS7	3p22.2	↓ I_{Na}	*SCN10A*, $Na_V1.8$

Listed in chronological order of discovery.
Abbreviations: BrS, Brugada syndrome; ERS, Early repolarization syndrome.

probabilistic, rather than binary or deterministic. Additional evidence obtained from co-segregation, studies,[130] *in silico* prediction tools[131-134] and variant frequency in cases and control databases are helpful in determining causality.[127] Despite these aids, a large number of variants remain in "genetic purgatory". Kapplinger et al. recently reported the synergistic use of up to seven *in silico* tools to help promote or demote a variant's pathogenic status and alter its relegation to genetic purgatory.[135]

Available data suggest that in individual cases, BrS and the susceptibility to SCD may not be due to a single mutation, but rather to oligogenic inheritance of multiple BrS-susceptibility variants.[136] The multifactorial nature of the genetics, can be further confounded by the fact that expressivity of the syndrome may be multifactorial in that the phenotype can be modulated by hormonal (testosterone, thyroxine) and other environmental factors.

CELLULAR MECHANISMS UNDERLYING BrS AND ERS

The J wave syndromes are characterized by accentuation of the electrocardiographic J wave leading in some cases to the development of malignant arrhythmias.[1] The electrocardiographic J wave is believed to be inscribed as a consequence of transmural differences in the manifestation of the AP notch between epicardium and endocardium secondary to heterogeneous transmural distribution of the transient outward current (I_{to}).[2]

The available data suggests that an outward shift in the balance of currents active during phases 1 and 2 of the right ventricular epicardial action potential via either a reduction of inward current (I_{Na} or I_{Ca}) or increase in outward current (I_{to}, I_{Kr} or $I_{K\text{-}ATP}$), allows the intrinsically prominent I_{to} to accentuate phase 1 repolarization **(Figures 39.1 and 39.2)**. When phase-1 repolarizes to a voltage below that needed to activate the L-type Ca^{+2} channels, the Ca^{+2} channels fail to activate, resulting in loss of the action potential plateau, predominantly in the right ventricular subepicardial cells where I_{to} is most prominent.

Loss of the AP dome is usually heterogeneous so that loss of the AP dome at some epicardial sites but not in others creates both an epicardial and transmural dispersion of repolarization. Conduction of the AP dome from epicardial sites at which it is maintained to sites at which it is lost results in the development of a very closely coupled extrasystole, a phenomenon termed phase 2 reentry.[27] Interestingly, these repolarization abnormalities give rise to low voltage fractionated electrogram activity **(Figure 39.3)** and high frequency late potentials when a bipolar electrogram is recorded in the region of the RVOT **(Figure 39.4)**.[116] The low voltage fractionated electrogram activity is due to dysynchrony in the appearance of the epicardial action potential dome secondary to accentuation of the action potential notch and the high frequency late potentials are due to concealed phase 2 reentry.

The propensity for the right ventricular AP to lose its dome, particularly under conditions of sodium or calcium channel block, giving rise to phase 2 reentry and other characteristics of the Brugada syndrome were identified in the early 1990's and evolved in parallel with the clinical syndrome.[137-140]

The development of prominent J waves, appearing as ST segment elevation, in the right precordial leads of BrS patients is thought to be due to accentuation of the right ventricular epicardial AP notch secondary to the rebalancing of the currents active at the end of phase 1.[141] A spike and dome morphology due to a prominent transient outward current (I_{to}), or notch, in ventricular epicardium, but not endocardium, generates a transmural voltage gradient that inscribes the electrocardiographic J wave in larger mammals and in man. The ST segment is usually isoelectric because of the absence of transmural voltage gradients at the level of the action potential plateau. Under pathophysiologic conditions such as those associated with BrS, accentuation of the right ventricular action potential notch leads to exaggeration of transmural voltage gradients and thus to exaggeration of the J wave, often referred to as an ST segment elevation.[141] A delay in epicardial activation and repolarization time leads to progressive inversion of the T wave.

Accentuation of the AP notch in the RVOT can give rise to the typical Brugada ECG without creating an arrhythmogenic substrate, as illustrated in **Figure 39.1B**. The arrhythmogenic substrate gradually arises with a further shift in the balance of currents causing loss of the AP dome at some epicardial sites but not others. Disappearance of the action potential dome in epicardium but not endocardium results in marked transmural dispersion of repolarization and refractoriness, thus creating a vulnerable window, as illustrated in **Figure 39.1C**. Because loss of the epicardial AP dome is usually heterogeneous, a marked dispersion of repolarization develops in epicardium and between epicardium and endocardium. Propagation of the AP potential dome from RVOT sites at which it is maintained to sites at which it is lost can cause local re-excitation via a phase 2 reentry mechanism (P2R). The phase 2 reentrant extrasystole is often concealed because it is surrounded by refractory tissue. These concealed P2Rs are responsible for the appearance of high frequency late potentials **(Figures 39.3 and 39.4)** in epicardial electrograms recorded over these epicardial sites in patients with BrS.[116] When the P2R succeeds in propagating out of its protected focus and capturing the vulnerable window, it can trigger a circus movement reentry, usually manifest as polymorphic VT/VF **(Figure 39.1F)**.[15,142,143] The phase 2 reentrant beat fuses with the negative T wave of the basic response. Support for these hypotheses derives in part from experiments involving arterially perfused right ventricular wedge preparations as well as from studies such as those of Kurita et al. **(Figure 39.5)** who obtained monophasic action potential (MAP) recordings form the epicardial

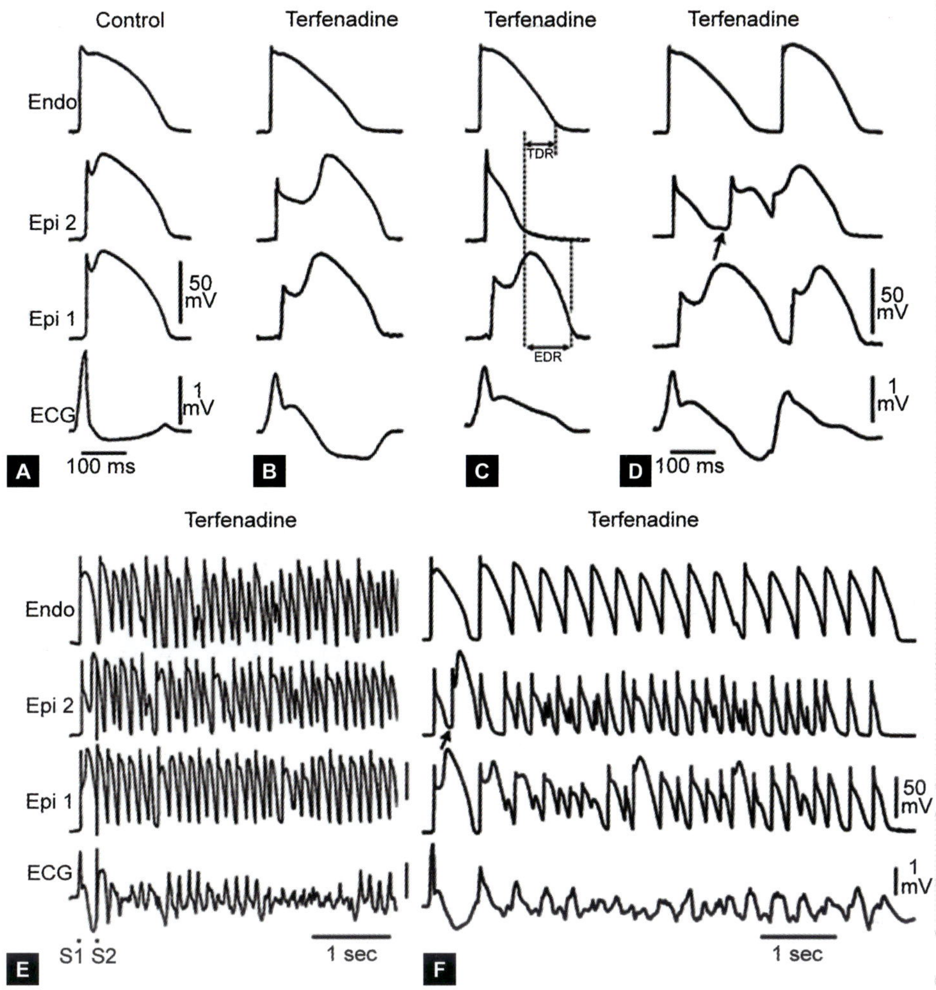

Figures 39.1A to F: Cellular basis for electrocardiographic and arrhythmic manifestation of BrS. Each panel shows transmembrane action potentials from one endocardial (top) and two epicardial sites together with a transmural ECG recorded from a canine coronary-perfused right ventricular wedge preparation. (A) Control [Basic cycle length (BCL) 400 ms]; (B) Combined sodium and calcium channel block with terfenadine (5 µM) accentuates the epicardial action potential notch creating a transmural voltage gradient that manifests as an ST segment elevation or exaggerated J wave in the ECG; (C) Continued exposure to terfenadine results in all-or-none repolarization at the end of phase 1 at some epicardial sites but not others, creating a local epicardial dispersion of repolarization (EDR) as well as a transmural dispersion of repolarization (TDR); (D) Phase 2 reentry occurs when the epicardial action potential dome propagates from a site where it is maintained to regions where it has been lost giving rise to a closely coupled extrasystole; (E) Extrastimulus (S1-S2 = 250 ms) applied to epicardium triggers a polymorphic VT; (F) Phase 2 reentrant extrasystole triggers a brief episode of polymorphic VT. (Modified from reference 143 with permission)

and endocardial surfaces of the RVOT of patients with the Brugada syndrome.[139,144] **Figure 39.1E** illustrates an example of programmed electrical stimulation-induced VT/VF under similar conditions.

Although an abundance of data point to the repolarization defects of the type illustrated above as the basis for the electrocardiographic and arrhythmic manifestations of BrS, the ionic and cellular mechanisms underlying BrS have long been a matter of debate.[145,146] The two principal hypotheses advanced to explain BrS are: (1) The *repolarization hypothesis*, which maintains that an outward shift in the balance of currents in right ventricular epicardium leads to repolarization abnormalities that give rise to phase 2 reentry and the generation of closely-coupled premature beats capable of precipitating VT/VF; and (2) The *depolarization hypothesis*, which suggests that slow conduction in the RVOT and other regions of RV, secondary to structural defects including fibrosis and reduced Cx43, leading to discontinuities in conduction, play a key role in the development of the electrocardiographic and arrhythmic manifestations of the syndrome. While quite distinct, these theories are not mutually exclusive and may indeed be synergistic.

The most apparently persuasive evidence in support of the depolarization hypothesis derives from the study of Nademanee et al.[147] showing that radiofrequency (RF)

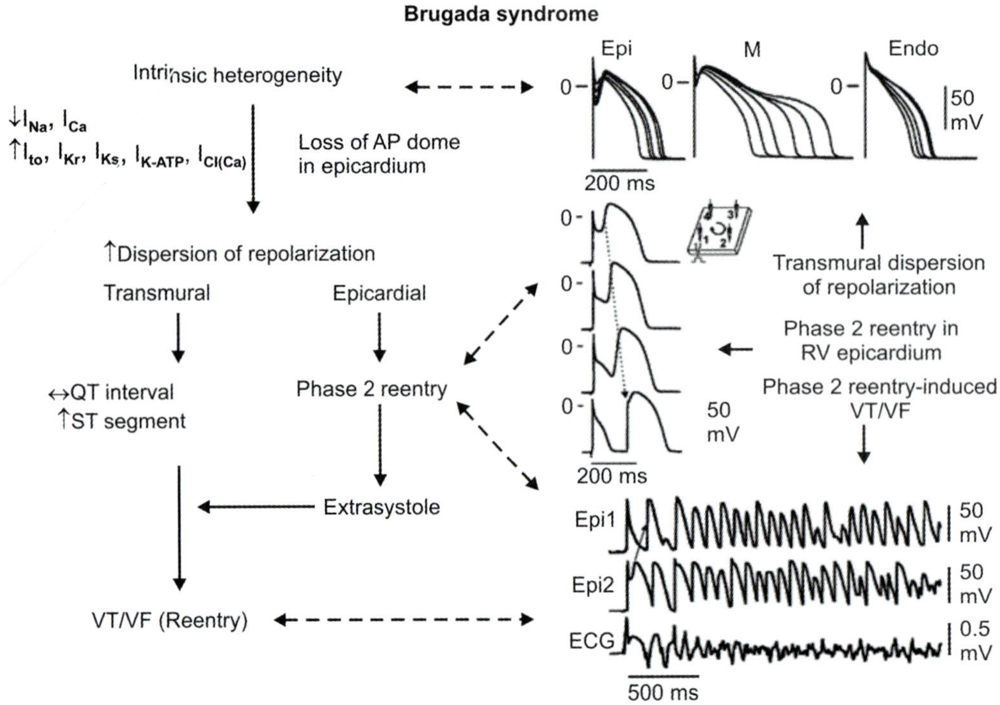

Figure 39.2: Proposed mechanism for the Brugada syndrome. An outward shift in the balance of currents serves to amplify existing heterogeneities by causing loss of the action potential dome at some epicardial, but not endocardial sites. A vulnerable window develops as a result of the dispersion of repolarization and refractoriness within epicardium as well as across the wall. Epicardial dispersion leads to the development of phase 2 reentry, which provides the extrasystole that captures the vulnerable window and initiates VT/VF via a circus movement reentry mechanism. (Modified from reference 225 with permission)

ablation of epicardial sites displaying fractionated bipolar electrograms (EGs) and late potentials in the RVOT of patients with BrS reduces the ECG and arrhythmic manifestations of the syndrome. Similar results have been reported by Brugada et al.[148] and in a case report published by Sacher and co-workers.[149] Based largely on traditional beliefs, these authors concluded that the late potential (LP) and fractionated electrogram activity are due to conduction delays within the RVOT and that ablation of the sites of slow conduction is the basis for the ameliorative effect of ablation therapy.[147-149] In a direct test of this hypothesis, Szél and co-workers[116] provided evidence for an alternative mechanism. Using an experimental model of BrS, they showed that low-voltage fractionated electrogram activity similar to that observed by Nademaneee et al. in the RVOT of BrS patients develops due to desynchronization in the appearance of the second action potential upstroke, secondary to accentuation of the epicardial AP notch and not to slow or delayed conduction **(Figure 39.3)**. They also demonstrated that high frequency late potentials develop in RV epicardium due to concealed phase 2 reentry. Slow or delayed conduction of the primary beat was never observed in a wide variety of BrS models created by exposing canine right ventricular wedge preparations to drugs mimicking the different genetic defects that have been associated with BrS.[116] These findings produced a paradigm shift in our interpretation of fractionated electrograms and late potentials from a mechanism involving delayed conduction, usually secondary to structural remodeling of ventricular myocardium, to a mechanism in which conduction disturbances played little or no role and in which repolarization defects dominated.

If the low voltage fractionated electrograms and late potentials recorded from the RVOT were not attributable to conduction disturbances, then why is it that ablation of these sites was effective in diminishing the ECG and arrhythmic manifestations of BrS? Patocskai et al. went on to test the hypothesis that ablation ameliorates the BrS phenotype by destroying sites of abnormal conduction. They ablated the epicardial regions displaying fractionated electrograms and LPs in the experimental models of BrS. Once again, they found that these manifestations were not due to slow or delayed conduction but rather to repolarization abnormalities and concealed phase 2 reentry. Ablation of the RV epicardium reduced the manifestation of J waves and ST segment elevation and abolished all arrhythmic activity, a result identical to that obtained by the clinical investigators **(Figure 39.4)**. These observations provided direct evidence that ablation can exert an ameliorative effect by destroying

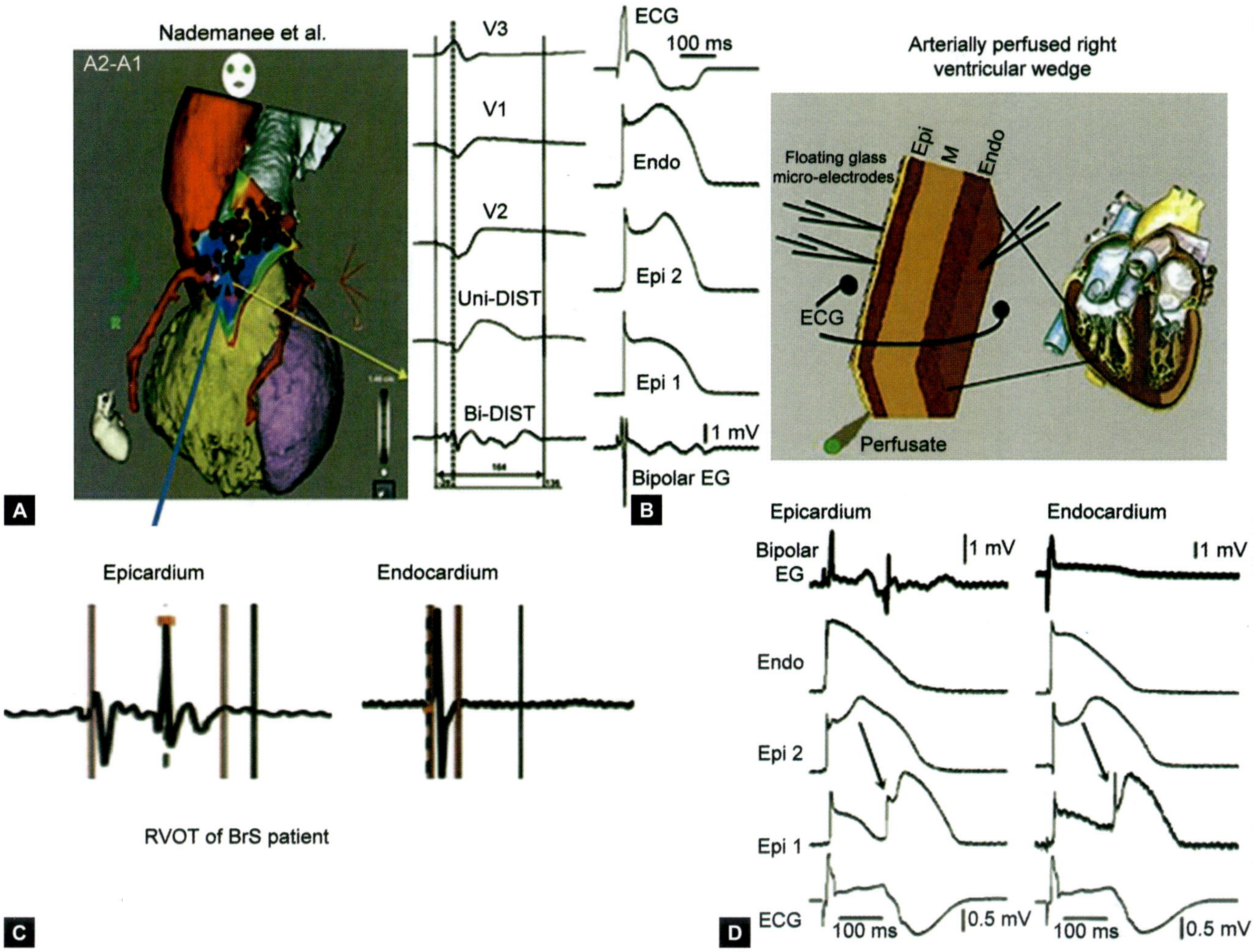

Figures 39.3A to D: New interpretation of fractionated electrogram activity and late potentials. Desynchrony in the appearance of the epicardial action potential second upstroke gives rise to fractionated epicardial electrogram (EG) activity and concealed phase 2 reentry gives rise to high frequency late potentials in the setting of Brugada syndrome (BrS). (A) Shown are right precordial lead recordings, unipolar and bipolar EGs from the right ventricular outflow tract of a BrS patient; (B) ECG, action potentials from endocardium (Endo) and two epicardial (Epi) sites, and a bipolar epicardial EG (Bipolar EG) all simultaneously recorded from a coronary-perfused right ventricular wedge preparation treated with the I_{to} agonist NS5806 (5 μM) and the calcium channel blocker verapamil (2 μM) to induce the Brugada phenotype. Basic cycle length = 1000 ms; (C) Bipolar EGs recorded from the epicardial and endocardial surfaces of the RVOT in a patient with BrS. The epicardial EG displays fractionated electrogram activity as well as a high frequency late potential late potential (130 ms delay); (D) Bipolar electrograms recorded from the epicardium and endocardium of a coronary-perfused wedge model of BrS, together with AP recordings from an endocardial and two epicardial sites and a transmural ECG. Slow or delayed conduction was never observed. The clinical data are modified from Nademanee et al.[147] and the experimental data are from Szel and co-workers,[116] with permission)

the cells with the most prominent action potential notch, thus eliminating the cells responsible for the repolarization abnormalities that give rise to phase 2 reentry and VT/VF.[1,150]

The only experimental models of BrS currently available are those involving the canine RV wedge models, originally developed by Yan and Antzelevitch.[2,15] The need for whole heart or whole animal model of BrS has long been recognized. In an attempt to create an *in vivo* model of BrS, Park et al. genetically engineered Yucatan minipigs to heterozygously express a nonsense mutation in SCN5A (E558X) originally identified in a child with Brugada syndrome.[114] Atrial myocytes isolated from the $SCN5A^{E558X/+}$ pigs showed a marked reduction in I_{Na}. Consistent with the loss of function of sodium channel activity, the minipigs displayed conduction abnormalities consisting of prolongation of the P wave, QRS complex and PR interval. Interstingly, a BrS phenotype was never observed, nor could it be provoked by the administration of flecainide. These observations

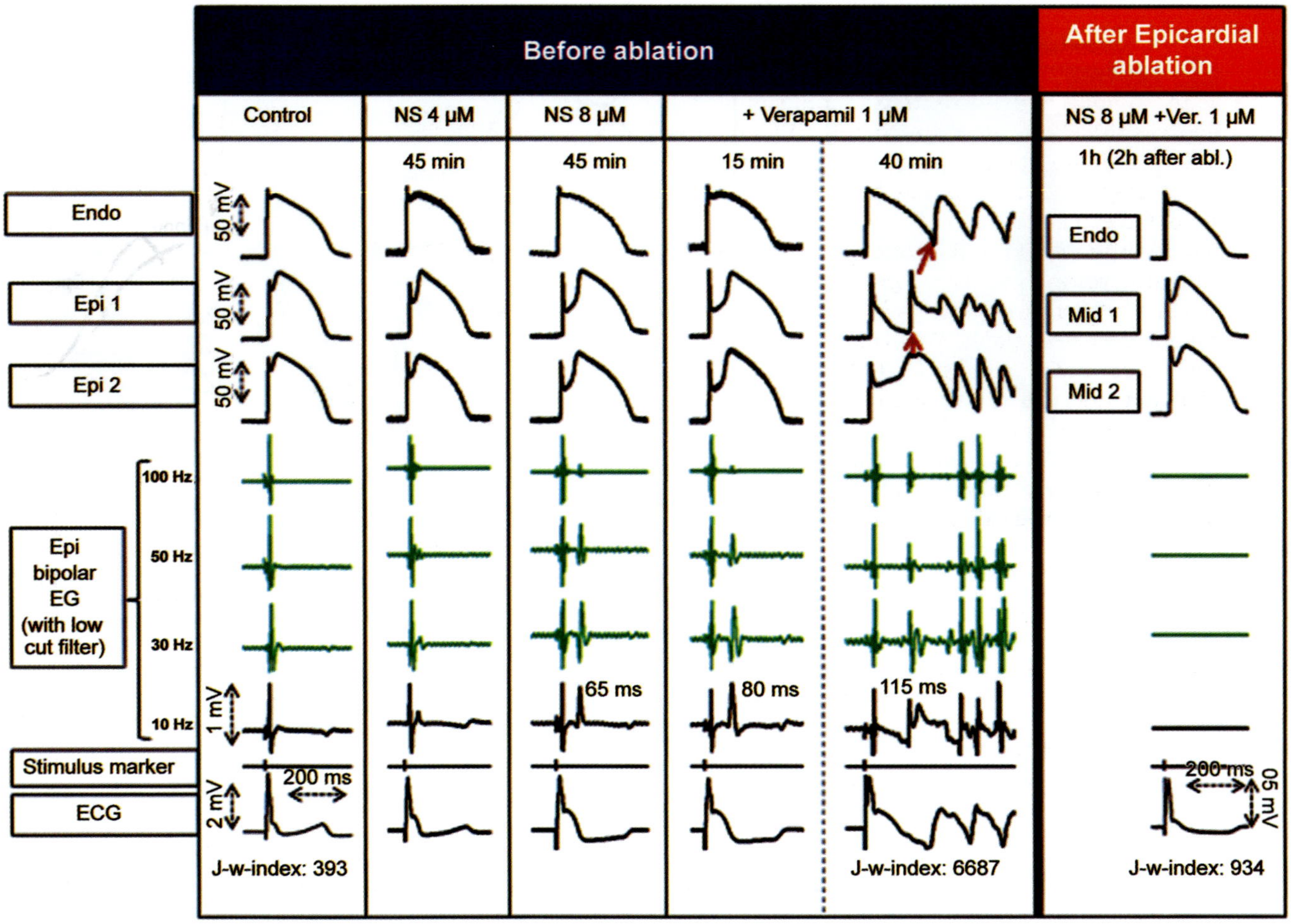

Figure 39.4: Radiofrequency ablation of the epicardial surface abolishes the BrS ECG and suppresses arrhythmogenesis in coronary-perfused canine right ventricular wedge model of BrS. Transmembrane action potentials (AP) were simultaneously recorded from one endocardial (Endo) and two epicardial (Epi) sites together with epicardial bipolar electrograms (EG) and a transmural pseudo-ECG. The epicardial bipolar EGs were recorded at 10–1000 Hz bandwidth (black trace), and were simultaneously band-pass filtered at 30–200 Hz, 50–200 Hz and 100–200 Hz (green traces). *Column 1*: Control. *Column 2*: Recorded 45 min after the addition of the I_{to}-agonist NS5806 (4 μM) to the coronary perfusate. *Column 3*: Recorded 45 min after the concentration of NS5806 was raised to 8 μM. High and low frequency late potentials (LP) are apparent in the EG recordings resulting from progressive delay in the appearance of the second upstroke of the Epi AP secondary to accentuation of the AP notch. *Column 4*: Recorded 15 min after the addition of the I_{Ca}-blocker verapamil (1 μM) to the coronary perfusate. *Column 5*: Recorded after 40 min of exposure to verapamil (1 μM). Loss of the AP dome at Epi 1 but not Epi 2 gives rise to a phase 2 reentrant beat, which precipitates polymorphic VT. *Column 6*: Recorded 2 h after radiofrequency ablation of the epicardial surface, and 1 h after reintroduction of the provocative agents to the perfusate (in the same concentration as before ablation). APs are now recorded from the deep subepicardium-midmyocardium (Mid 1, Mid 2) instead of the epicardial surface. Ablation markedly suppressed the BrS phenotype and abolished all arrhythmic activity by destroying the cells exhibiting the pronounced repolarization abnormalities. Slow or delayed conduction was not observed at any phase. (Modified from reference 150 with permission)

are expected owing to the lack of I_{to} in the pig, which is a prerequisite for the development of the repolarization abnormalities associated with BrS. These findings provide strong evidence against the depolarization hypothesis and for the repolarization hypothesis.

These experiments also provide the first test in a large mammal of the hypothesis that a slowly conducting embryonic phenotype is maintained in the adult RVOT and is unmasked with a loss of function of sodium channel activity.[151] The hypothesis is not supported since conduction in the RVOT of the $SCN5A^{E558X/+}$ pigs was no different from conduction in the rest of RV. Both were equally depressed by the loss of function of sodium channel activity.[114]

Additional evidence in support of the repolarization hypothesis derives from the observation of Kurita and coworkers that MAPs recorded from the endocardial and epicardial surfaces of the RVOT of a patient with BrS are nearly identical to transmembrane APs recorded from the endocardial and epicardial surfaces of the wedge model of BrS.[139,144] In both cases, the AP displays a prominent accentuation of the notch in epicardium, but not endocardium without any major transmural conduction delays **(Figure 39.5)**. It is noteworthy that these differences were not observed in an isolated heart explanted from a BrS patient after transplantation of a new heart. However, the epicardium of the explanted heart was extremely depressed, perhaps as a result of the 129 shocks delivered by the implantable cardioverter-defibrillator (ICD) in an attempt to control the cascade of electrical storms.[28]

Rudy's group, recently studied 25 BrS and 6 RBBB patients using noninvasive ECG imaging (ECGI).[152] The authors concluded that both slow discontinuous conduction and steep dispersion of repolarization are present in the RVOT of patients with BrS. ECGI was able to differentiate between BrS and RBBB. Unlike BrS, RBBB showed delayed activation in the entire right ventricle, without ST-segment elevation, fractionation, or repolarization abnormalities on the electrograms. Importantly, in 6 BrS patients they evaluated the response to an increase in rate and found that the increase in rate increased fractionation of the electrogram but reduced ST-segment elevation, indicating that the conduction impairment was not the principal cause of the BrS ECG.

The strong similarity between BrS and ERS with respect to clinical manifestations and response to treatment modalities lend further support for the repolarization hypothesis. Koncz et al.,[26] using an experimental model of ERS, provided evidence in support of the hypothesis that, similar to the mechanism operative in BrS, an accentuation of transmural gradients in the LV wall is responsible for the repolarization abnormalities underlying ERS. The transmural voltage gradients gave rise to J point elevation, distinct J waves, or slurring of the terminal part of the QRS. The repolarization defect was accentuated by cholinergic agonists and reduced by quinidine, isoproterenol, cilostazol and milrinone, accounting for the ability of these agents to reverse the repolarization abnormalities responsible for ERS.[26,153] These authors went on to show that greater intrinsic levels of I_{to} in the inferior LV underlie the greater vulnerability of the inferior LV wall to VT/VF.[26] Using ECGI, Rudy and co-workers provided additional evidence in support of the repolarization abnormalities by identifying abnormally short activation-recovery intervals (ARI) in the inferior and lateral regions of LV and a marked dispersion of repolarization.[154] Recent ECGI mapping studies performed in an ERS patient during VF demonstrated VF rotors anchored in the inferior-lateral left ventricular wall.[18]

Is it Possible to Distinguish between a Depolarization and a Repolarization Defect?

When notches appear in the rising phase of the electrocardiographic R wave, it is generally accepted that these are due to conduction defects within the ventricular myocardium. When the notch occurs at the terminal portion of the QRS, resembling a J wave, it may be due either to a conduction or repolarization defect.[17,155] We and others have suggested that the response to prematurity or to an increase in rate may be helpful in differentiating between the two mechanisms.[115] Delayed conduction invariably becomes more exaggerated at faster rates or during premature beats, thus leading to accentuation of the QRS notch, whereas repolarization defects are usually moderated at faster rates resulting in a diminution of the J wave. Although typical J waves are usually accentuated with bradycardia or long pauses, the opposite has also been described.[156,157] J waves are often seen in young males with no apparent structural heart diseases, whereas intra-ventricular conduction delay is often observed in older individuals or in cases of post-myocardial infarction or cardiomyopathy.[155,156] The prognostic value of a fragmented QRS has been demonstrated in BrS,[158,159] although fragmentation of the QRS is not associated with increased risk in the absence of cardiac disease.[160] It is also noteworthy that unlike IVCD-mediated syndromes, the appearance of J waves is strongly male predominant.

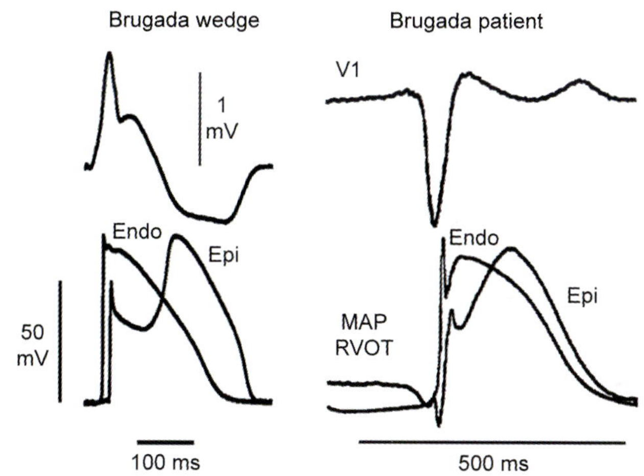

Figure 39.5: Comparison of transmembrane and monophasic action potentials and ECGs recorded from a wedge model of BrS and a patient diagnosed with BrS. Left panel shows a pseudo-ECG and transmembrane action potentials recorded from the epicardium and endocardium of a right ventricular wedge preparation in which the Brugada phenotype was elicited using 5 μM terfenadine to block I_{Na} and I_{Ca}, thus mimicking the genetic variants associated with BrS. Right panel shows lead V1 and monophasic action potentials recorded from epicardium and endocardium of the RVOT of a patient with BrS. Note that the apparent notch in the endocardial MAP is an "intrinsic potential" and not a true notch. Modified from[139,144]

THERAPY FOR THE J WAVE SYNDROMES

The only proven effective therapy for the prevention of SCD in high risk BrS and ERS patients is an implantable cardioverter defibrillator (ICD).[161,162] The decision to implant an ICD must be approached with great care since ICDs are associated with complications, especially in young active individuals that comprise this cohort.[163,164] Subcutaneous ICDs are thought to represent the future for this indication in that they are expected to be associated with fewer complications over a life-time.[165]

ICD is first line therapy for J wave syndrome patients who present with aborted SCD or documented VT/VF with or without syncope (Class I recommendation).[161,166] ICDs can be useful (Class IIa) in symptomatic BrS patients with Type 1 pattern, in whom syncope was likely caused by VT/VF. The HRS/EHRA/APHRS Expert Consensus statement indicates that ICD may be considered (Class IIb) in asymptomatic patients with inducible VF during programmed electrical stimulation (PES).[46] Some studies suggest that the predictive value of EP studies may be improved by limiting the PES protocol to 2 extrastimuli[167] but that observation is not supported by other studies.[168,169]

Arrhythmic events and sudden cardiac death in both BrS and ERS generally occur during sleep or at rest and are associated with slow heart rates. These observations notwithstanding, a potential therapeutic role for cardiac pacing remains largely unexplored.[170-172]

Nademanee et al.[147] was the first to show the benefit of radiofrequency ablation (RFA) of the RVOT *epicardium*. Additional evidence in support of the effectiveness of epicardial ablation was provided by several other prominent investigative groups.[148,149,173,174] Ablation therapy can be life-saving in otherwise uncontrollable cases. RF ablation is a *Class IIa* recommendation in BrS-patient with frequent appropriate ICD-shocks due to recurrent electrical storms.[175] There are no clinical reports of ablation of the LV substrate in patients with ERS.

Pharmacologic Approach to Therapy

Approach to Therapy of BrS

The pharmacologic approach to therapy is geared to reversing the substrate responsible for the repolarization abnormalities that underlie the ECG and arrhythmic manifestations of BrS as well as ERS. Because the repolarization abnormalities are caused by an outward shift in the balance of current in the early phases of the epicardial action potential in the RVOT, the approach to therapy involves creation of an inward shift of the balance of current. This can be accomplished by increasing inward currents such as I_{Ca} or reducing outward currents such as I_{to}. The inward shift in the balance of current results in a diminution in the magnitude of the action potential notch and restoration of action potential dome, thus restoring homogeneity within epicardium as well as across the ventricular wall. Because the presence of a prominent I_{to} is a prerequisite for the development of both BrS and ERS, partial inhibition of this current appears to be effective regardless of the genetic or ionic basis for the disease. Regrettably, cardioselective and I_{to}-specific blockers are at present not available.

Quinidine is the only agent available with significant I_{to} blocking properties.[15,62] Experimental studies stemming back to 1999 have shown that quinidine is effective in restoring the epicardial action potential dome, thus normalizing the ST segment and preventing phase 2 reentry and polymorphic VT in a variety of different experimental models of Brugada syndrome.[15,116,176-178] A recent experimental study suggests that quinidine, owing to its effect to block I_{to}, can also exert a protective effect against hypothermia-induced VT/VF in a J wave syndrome model.[179] Historically, quinidine was used to prevent ventricular fibrillation in patients who required hypothermia for surgical procedures.[178]

Quinidine's effectiveness to normalize the ST segment elevation and or prevent arrhythmic events in patients with BrS has been reported in numerous studies and case reports.[102,104,105,109,180-193] Belhassen and co-workers[194] reported a 90% efficacy in prevention of VF induction with quinidine despite the use of very aggressive extrastimulation protocols. Importantly, there were no arrhythmic events among BrS patients treated with quinidine during a mean follow-up period of 10 years. A prospective registry of empiric quinidine for asymptomatic Brugada syndrome has been established. The study appears at the National Institutes of Health website (ClinicalTrials.gov: http://clinicaltrials.gov/ct2/show/NCT00789165?term_brugada&rank_2.) Doses between 600 and 900 mg were recommended, if tolerated.[184]

Agents that augment I_{Ca}, such as β adrenergic agents like isoproterenol, denopamine or orciprenaline, are useful as well.[15,102,106,141,189,195] Isoproterenol, at times in combination with quinidine, has been utilized successfully to quiet VF storms and normalize ST elevation particularly in children.[81,100,101-103,181,182,187,193,196-204] Adminisitration of isoprotereonol is a Class IIa recommendation for BrS patients presenting with electrical storms.[175]

Another promising pharmacologic approach for BrS is phosphodiesterase III (PDE3) inhibition using cilostazol,[102,106,108] which has been shown to normalize the ST segment, by augmenting I_{Ca} as well as by reducing I_{to} secondary to an increase in cAMP and heart rate.[205] Other effects of cilostazol may contribute as well. (e.g.: adenosine, NO, mitochondrial I_{KATP}).[206] Its efficacy in combination with bepridil in preventing VF-episodes was recently reported by Shinohara et al.[110] The failure of cilostazol in the treatment of BrS has been described in a single case report.[207] Another PDE3 inhibitor, milrinone, was recently identified as a more potent alternative to cilostazol in suppressing ST elevation and arrhythmogenesis in an experimental model of BrS.[116,208] No clinical reports have appeared as yet. The greater potency of milrinone is consistent with the results of previous studies reporting that milrinone produces a greater increase in cytosolic cAMP than cilostazol,[209,210] possibly due to the fact that milrinone blocks both PDE-3 and PDE4.[210]

A traditional Chinese medicine, Wenxin Keli, has recently been reported to inhibit I_{to} and thus to suppress polymorphic VT in experimental models of BrS when combined with low concentrations of quinidine (5 μM).[177]

Agents that augment peak and late I_{Na}, including bepridil and dimethyl lithospermate B (dmLSB), have been suggested to be of value in BrS. Bepridil reportedly suppresses VT/VF in patients with BrS.[102,211-213] The drug's actions are thought to be mediated by: (1) inhibition of I_{to}; (2) augmentation of I_{Na} via upregulation of the sodium channels;[214] and (3) prolongation of QT interval at slow rates thus increasing the QT/RR slope.[211,213] Finally, dimethyl lithospermate B, an extract of Danshen, another traditional Chinese medicine, has been reported to slow inactivation of I_{Na}, thus increasing I_{Na} during the early phases of the AP and suppressing arrhythmogenesis in experimental models of BrS.[215]

Participation in sports has long been a concern. Because life-threatening ventricular arrhythmias are infrequent in asymptomatic patients with BrS[216] or ER pattern[40] and usually unrelated to physical activity, these patterns do not contraindicate participation in sports.

Approach to Therapy of ERS

It is of no surprise that the approach to therapy of ERS is similar to that of BrS, since the mechanisms underlying the two syndromes are similar. Quinidine, isoproterenol and PDE3 inhibitors have all been reported to exert an ameliorative effect in preventing or quieting arrhythmias associated with ERS. Isoproterenol is effective in quieting electrical storms developing in patients with either BrS[102,196] or ERS.[217] Isoproterenol acts by reversing the repolarization abnormalities responsible for the disease phenotype secondary to restoration of the epicardial action potential dome in experimental models of both BrS[15,176] and ERS.[26] This action of the beta-adrenergic agonist is expected due to its actions to potently increase I_{Ca} and reduced I_{to}.

Cilostazol, a PDE3 inhibitor, has been reported to reduce the ECG and arrhythmic manifestations of ERS.[107] PDE inhibitors are known to activate I_{Ca} and reduce I_{to} secondary to an increase in cAMP.[106,205,218-222] These actions prevent arrhythmias associated with the J wave syndromes by reversing the repolarization defects and restoring electrical homogeneity across the ventricular wall secondary to restoration of the epicardial action potential dome in both BrS[208] and ERS.[179] The effectiveness of bepridil in ERS has been reported in a single patient thus far.[223]

The effectiveness of RF ablation in the setting of ERS has not been evaluated, despite the fact that low voltage fractionated electrogram activity and high frequency late potentials are observed in the LV in patients with ERS[224] and in experimental models of ERS (Yoon and Antzelevitch, unpublished observation). Nakagawa et al.[224] reported the results of a study in which they recorded epicardial electrograms directly from the left ventricle of patients diagnosed with ERS by introducing a multipolar catheter into the left lateral (marginal) coronary vein, anterior interventricular vein, and middle cardiac vein via the coronary sinus. The authors reported late potentials in the bipolar electrograms recorded from the LV epicardium of the ERS patients similar to what has been reported in the RVOT of patients with BrS.[225]

REFERENCES

1. Antzelevitch C, Yan GX. J wave syndromes. Heart Rhythm. 2010;7:549-58.
2. Yan GX, Antzelevitch C. Cellular basis for the electrocardiographic J wave. Circulation. 1996;93:372-9.
3. Clements SD, Hurst JW. Diagnostic value of ECG abnormalities observed in subjects accidentally exposed to cold. Am J Cardiol. 1972;29:729-34.
4. Thompson R, Rich J, Chmelik F, Nelson WL. Evolutionary changes in the electrocardiogram of severe progressive hypothermia. J Electrocardiol. 1977;10:67-70.
5. Eagle K. Images in clinical medicine. Osborn waves of hypothermia. N Engl J Med. 1994;10:680.
6. Kraus F. Ueber die wirkung des kalziums auf den kreislauf. Dtsch Med Wochenschr. 1920;46:201-3.
7. Sridharan MR, Horan LG. Electrocardiographic J wave of hypercalcemia. Am J Cardiol. 1984;54:672-3.
8. Brugada P, Brugada J. Right bundle branch block, persistent ST segment elevation and sudden cardiac death: a distinct clinical and electrocardiographic syndrome: a multicenter report. J Am Coll Cardiol. 1992;20:1391-6.
9. Haissaguerre M, Derval N, Sacher F, Jesel L, Deisenhofer I, De Roy L, Pasquie JL, Nogami A, Babuty D, Yli-Mayry S, De Chillou C, Scanu P, Mabo P, Matsuo S, Probst V, Le Scouarnec S, Defaye P, Schlaepfer J, Rostock T, Lacroix D, Lamaison D, Lavergne T, Aizawa Y, Englund A, Anselme F, O'Neill M, Hocini M, Lim KT, Knecht S, Veenhuyzen GD, Bordachar P, Chauvin M, Jais P, Coureau G, Chene G, Klein GJ, Clementy J. Sudden cardiac arrest associated with early repolarization. N Engl J Med. 2008;358:2016-23.
10. Nam GB, Kim YH, Antzelevitch C. Augmentation of J waves and electrical storms in patients with early repolarization. N Engl J Med. 2008;358:2078-9.
11. Rosso R, Kogan E, Belhassen B, Rozovski U, Scheinman MM, Zeltser D, Halkin A, Steinvil A, Heller K, Glikson M, Katz A, Viskin S. J-point elevation in survivors of primary ventricular fibrillation and matched control subjects: incidence and clinical significance. J Am Coll Cardiol. 2008;52:1231-8.
12. Wasserburger RH, Alt WJ. The normal RS-T segment elevation variant. Am J Cardiol. 1961;8:184-92.
13. Mehta MC, Jain AC. Early repolarization on scalar electrocardiogram. Am J Med Sci. 1995;309:305-11.
14. Gussak I, Antzelevitch C. Early repolarization syndrome: clinical characteristics and possible cellular and ionic mechanisms. J Electrocardiol. 2000;33:299-309.
15. Yan GX, Antzelevitch C. Cellular basis for the Brugada syndrome and other mechanisms of arrhythmogenesis associated with ST segment elevation. Circulation. 1999;100:1660-6.
16. Shu J, Zhu T, Yang L, Cui C, Yan GX. ST-segment elevation in the early repolarization syndrome, idiopathic ventricular fibrillation, and the Brugada syndrome: cellular and clinical linkage. J Electrocardiol. 2005;38:26-32.

17. Antzelevitch C. J wave syndromes: molecular and cellular mechanisms. J Electrocardiol. 2013;46:510-8.
18. Mahida S, Derval N, Sacher F, Berte B, Yamashita S, Hooks DA, Denis A, Lim H, Amraoui S, Aljefairi N, Hocini M, Jais P, Haissaguerre M. History and clinical significance of early repolarization syndrome. Heart Rhythm. 2015;12:242-9.
19. Wellens HJ, Schwartz PJ, Lindemans FW, Buxton AE, Goldberger JJ, Hohnloser SH, Huikuri HV, Kaab S, La Rovere MT, Malik M, Myerburg RJ, Simoons ML, Swedberg K, Tijssen J, Voors AA, Wilde AA. Risk stratification for sudden cardiac death: current status and challenges for the futuredagger. Eur Heart J. 2014;35:1642-51.
20. Macfarlane PW, Antzelevitch C, Haissaguerre M, Huikuri HV, Potse M, Rosso R, Sacher F, Tikkanen JT, Wellens H, Yan GX. The Early Repolarization Pattern: A Consensus Paper. J Am Coll Cardiol. 2015;66:470-7.
21. Kanter RJ, Pfeiffer R, Hu D, Barajas-Martinez H, Carboni MP, Antzelevitch C. Brugada-like syndrome in infancy presenting with rapid ventricular tachycardia and intraventricular conduction delay. Circulation. 2012;125:14-22.
22. Antzelevitch C. Molecular biology and cellular mechanisms of Brugada and long QT syndromes in infants and young children. J Electrocardiol. 2001;34:177-81.
23. Wedekind H, Smits JP, Schulze-Bahr E, Arnold R, Veldkamp MW, Bajanowski T, Borggrefe M, Brinkmann B, Warnecke I, Funke H, Bhuiyan ZA, Wilde AA, Breithardt G, Haverkamp W. De novo mutation in the *SCN5A* gene associated with early onset of sudden infant death. Circulation. 2001;104: 1158-64.
24. Nagase S, Kusano KF, Morita H, Fujimoto Y, Kakishita M, Nakamura K, Emori T, Matsubara H, Ohe T. Epicardial electrogram of the right ventricular outflow tract in patients with the Brugada syndrome: using the epicardial lead. J Am Coll Cardiol. 2002;39:1992-5.
25. Nakagawa K, Nagase S, Morita H, Ito H. Left ventricular epicardial electrogram recordings in idiopathic ventricular fibrillation with inferior and lateral early repolarization. Heart Rhythm. 2014;11:314-7.
26. Koncz I, Gurabi Z, Patocskai B, Panama BK, Szel T, Hu D, Barajas-Martinez H, Antzelevitch C. Mechanisms underlying the development of the electrocardiographic and arrhythmic manifestations of early repolarization syndrome. J Mol Cell Cardiol. 2014;68C:20-8.
27. Antzelevitch C. Brugada syndrome. Pacing Clin Electrophysiol. 2006;29:1130-59.
28. Coronel R, Casini S, Koopmann TT, Wilms-Schopman FJ, Verkerk AO, de Groot JR, Bhuiyan Z, Bezzina CR, Veldkamp MW, Linnenbank AC, van der Wal AC, Tan HL, Brugada P, Wilde AA, de Bakker JM. Right ventricular fibrosis and conduction delay in a patient with clinical signs of Brugada syndrome: a combined electrophysiological, genetic, histopathologic, and computational study. Circulation. 2005;112:2769-77.
29. Bastiaenen R, Hedley PL, Christiansen M, Behr ER. Therapeutic hypothermia and ventricular fibrillation storm in early repolarization syndrome. Heart Rhythm. 2010;7:832-4.
30. Federman NJ, Mechulan A, Klein GJ, Krahn AD. Ventricular fibrillation induced by spontaneous hypothermia in a patient with early repolarization syndrome. J Cardiovasc Electrophysiol. 2013;24:586-8.
31. Sakabe M, Fujiki A, Tani M, Nishida K, Mizumaki K, Inoue H. Proportion and prognosis of healthy people with coved or saddle-back type ST segment elevation in the right precordial leads during 10 years follow-up. Eur Heart J. 2003;24: 1488-93.
32. Tsuji H, Sato T, Morisaki K, Iwasaka T. Prognosis of subjects with Brugada-type electrocardiogram in a population of middle-aged Japanese diagnosed during a health examination. Am J Cardiol. 2008;102:584-7.
33. Gervacio-Domingo G, Isidro J, Tirona J, Gabriel E, David G, Amarillo ML, Morales D, Dans A. The Brugada type 1 electrocardiographic pattern is common among Filipinos. J Clin Epidemiol. 2008;61:1067-72.
34. Ito H, Yano K, Chen R, He Q, Curb JD. The prevalence and prognosis of a Brugada-type electrocardiogram in a population of middle-aged Japanese-American men with follow-up of three decades. Am J Med Sci. 2006;331:25-9.
35. Letsas KP, Weber R, Astheimer K, Kalusche D, Arentz T. Tpeak-Tend interval and Tpeak-Tend/QT ratio as markers of ventricular tachycardia inducibility in subjects with Brugada ECG phenotype. Europace. 2010;12:271-4.
36. Gallagher MM, Forleo GB, Behr ER, Magliano G, De LL, Morgia V, De LF, Romeo F. Prevalence and significance of Brugada-type ECG in 12,012 apparently healthy European subjects. Int J Cardiol. 2008;130:44-8.
37. Pecini R, Cedergreen P, Theilade S, Haunso S, Theilade J, Jensen GB. The prevalence and relevance of the Brugada-type electrocardiogram in the Danish general population: data from the Copenhagen City Heart Study. Europace. 2010;12: 982-6.
38. Patel SS, Anees SS, Ferrick KJ. Prevalence of a Brugada pattern electrocardiogram in an urban population in the United States. Pacing Clin Electrophysiol. 2009;32:704-8.
39. Lee C, Soni A, Tate RB, Cuddy TE. The incidence and prognosis of Brugada electrocardiographic pattern in the Manitoba Follow-Up Study. Can J Cardiol. 2005;21:1286-90.
40. Tikkanen JT, Anttonen O, Junttila MJ, Aro AL, Kerola T, Rissanen HA, Reunanen A, Huikuri HV. Long-term outcome associated with early repolarization on electrocardiography. N Engl J Med. 2009;361:2529-37.
41. Sinner MF, Reinhard W, Muller M, Beckmann BM, Martens E, Perz S, Pfeufer A, Winogradow J, Stark K, Meisinger C, Wichmann HE, Peters A, Riegger GA, Steinbeck G, Hengstenberg C, Kaab S. Association of early repolarization pattern on ecg with risk of cardiac and all-cause mortality: a population-based prospective cohort study (MONICA/KORA). PLoS Med. 2010;7:e1000314.
42. Haruta D, Matsuo K, Tsuneto A, Ichimaru S, Hida A, Sera N, Imaizumi M, Nakashima E, Maemura K, Akahoshi M. Incidence and prognostic value of early repolarization pattern in the 12-lead electrocardiogram. Circulation. 2011;123: 2931-7.
43. Brosnan MJ, Kumar S, LaGerche A, Brown A, Stewart S, Kalman JM, Prior DL. Early repolarization patterns associated with increased arrhythmic risk are common in young non-Caucasian Australian males and not influenced by athletic status. Heart Rhythm. 2015;12:1576-83.
44. Antzelevitch C, Brugada P, Borggrefe M, Brugada J, Brugada R, Corrado D, Gussak I, LeMarec H, Nademanee K, Perez Riera AR, Shimizu W, Schulze-Bahr E, Tan H, Wilde A. Brugada syndrome: report of the second consensus conference: endorsed by the Heart Rhythm Society and the European Heart Rhythm Association. Circulation. 2005;111:659-70.

45. Wilde AA, Antzelevitch C, Borggrefe M, Brugada J, Brugada R, Brugada P, Corrado D, Hauer RN, Kass RS, Nademanee K, Priori SG, Towbin JA. Proposed diagnostic criteria for the Brugada syndrome: consensus report. Circulation. 2002;106:2514-9.
46. Priori SG, Wilde AA, Horie M, Cho Y, Behr ER, Berul C, Blom N, Brugada J, Chiang CE, Huikuri H, Kannankeril P, Krahn A, Leenhardt A, Moss A, Schwartz PJ, Shimizu W, Tomaselli G, Tracy C. HRS/EHRA/APHRS expert consensus statement on the diagnosis and management of patients with inherited primary arrhythmia syndromes: document endorsed by HRS, EHRA, and APHRS in May 2013 and by ACCF, AHA, PACES, and AEPC in June 2013. Heart Rhythm. 2013;10:1932-63.
47. Priori SG, Blomstrom-Lundqvist C, Mazzanti A, Blom N, Borggrefe M, Camm J, Elliott PM, Fitzsimons D, Hatala R, Hindricks G, Kirchhof P, Kjeldsen K, Kuck KH, Hernandez-Madrid A, Nikolaou N, Norekval TM, Spaulding C, Van Veldhuisen DJ. 2015 ESC Guidelines for the management of patients with ventricular arrhythmias and the prevention of sudden cardiac death: The Task Force for the Management of Patients with Ventricular Arrhythmias and the Prevention of Sudden Cardiac Death of the European Society of Cardiology (ESC) Endorsed by: Association for European Paediatric and Congenital Cardiology (AEPC). Eur Heart J. 2015;36:2793-867.
48. Sangwatanaroj S, Prechawat S, Sunsaneewitayakul B, Sitthisook S, Tosukhowong P, Tungsanga K. Right ventricular electrocardiographic leads for detection of Brugada syndrome in sudden unexplained death syndrome survivors and their relatives. Clin Cardiol. 2001;24:776-81.
49. Miyamoto K, Yokokawa M, Tanaka K, Nagai T, Okamura H, Noda T, Satomi K, Suyama K, Kurita T, Aihara N, Kamakura S, Shimizu W. Diagnostic and prognostic value of a type 1 Brugada electrocardiogram at higher (third or second) V1 to V2 recording in men with Brugada syndrome. Am J Cardiol. 2007;99:53-7.
50. Nagase S, Hiramatsu S, Morita H, Nishii N, Murakami M, Nakamura K, Kusano KF, Ito H, Ohe T. Electroanatomical correlation of repolarization abnormalities in Brugada syndrome: detection of type 1 electrocardiogram in the right ventricular outflow tract. J Am Coll Cardiol. 2010;56:2143-5.
51. Ikeda T, Abe A, Yusa S, Nakamura K, Ishiguro H, Mera H, Yotsukura M, Yoshino H. The full stomach test as a novel diagnostic technique for identifying patients at risk for Brugada Syndrome. J Cardiovasc Electrophysiol. 2006;17:602-7.
52. Shimeno K, Takagi M, Maeda K, Tatsumi H, Doi A, Yoshiyama M. Usefulness of multichannel Holter ECG recording in the third intercostal space for detecting type 1 Brugada ECG: comparison with repeated 12-lead ECGs. J Cardiovasc Electrophysiol. 2009;20:1026-31.
53. Viskin S, Rosso R, Friedensohn L, Havakuk O, Wilde AA. Everybody has Brugada syndrome until proven otherwise? Heart Rhythm. 2015;12:1595-8.
54. Conte G, de Asmundis C, Ciconte G, Julia J, Sieira J, Chierchia GB, Brugada P. Follow-up from childhood to adulthood of individuals with family history of Brugada syndrome and normal electrocardiograms. JAMA. 2014;312:2039-41.
55. Conte G, Dewals W, Sieira J, De Asmundis C, Ciconte G, Chierchia GB, Di Giovanni G, Baltogiannis G, Saitoh Y, Levinstein M, La Meir M, Wellens F, Pappaert G, Brugada P. Drug-induced Brugada syndrome in children: clinical features, device-based management and long-term follow-up. J Am Coll Cardiol. 2014;63:2272-9.
56. Gandjbakhch E, Fressart V, Duthoit G, Marquie C, Deharo JC, Pousset F, Hebert JL, Simon F, Himbert C, Klug D, Charron P, Hidden-Lucet F. Malignant response to ajmaline challenge in SCN5A mutation carriers: experience from a large familial study. Int J Cardiol. 2014;172:256-8.
57. Papavassiliu T, Wolpert C, Fluchter S, Schimpf R, Neff W, Haase KK, Duber C, Borggrefe M. Magnetic resonance imaging findings in patients with Brugada syndrome. J Cardiovasc Electrophysiol. 2004;15:1133-8.
58. Papavassiliu T, Veltmann C, Doesch C, Haghi D, Germans T, Schoenberg SO, van Rossum AC, Schimpf R, Brade J, Wolpert C, Borggrefe M. Spontaneous type 1 electrocardiographic pattern is associated with cardiovascular magnetic resonance imaging changes in Brugada syndrome. Heart Rhythm. 2010;7:1790-6.
59. Takagi M, Aihara N, Kuribayashi S, Taguchi A, Kurita T, Suyama K, Kamakura S, Takamiya M. Abnormal response to sodium channel blockers in patients with Brugada syndrome: augmented localised wall motion abnormalities in the right ventricular outflow tract region detected by electron beam computed tomography. Heart. 2003;89:169-74.
60. Catalano O, Antonaci S, Moro G, Mussida M, Frascaroli M, Baldi M, Cobelli F, Baiardi P, Nastoli J, Bloise R, Monteforte N, Napolitano C, Priori SG. Magnetic resonance investigations in Brugada syndrome reveal unexpectedly high rate of structural abnormalities. Eur Heart J. 2009;30:2241-8.
61. van Hoorn F, Campian ME, Spijkerboer A, Blom MT, Planken RN, van Rossum AC, de Bakker JM, Wilde AA, Groenink M, Tan HL. SCN5A mutations in Brugada syndrome are associated with increased cardiac dimensions and reduced contractility. PLoS One. 2012;7:e42037.
62. Antzelevitch C, Brugada P, Brugada J, Brugada R, Nademanee K, Towbin JA. Clinical approaches to tachyarrhythmias. The Brugada syndrome. Armonk, NY: Futura Publishing Company, Inc.; 1999.
63. Antzelevitch C. Brugada syndrome: historical perspectives and observations. Eur Heart J. 2002;23:676-8.
64. Slezak J, Tribulova N, Okruhlicova L, Dhingra R, Bajaj A, Freed D, Singal P. Hibernating myocardium: pathophysiology, diagnosis, and treatment. Can J Physiol Pharmacol. 2009;87:252-65.
65. Nademanee K, Raju H, de Noronha SV, Papadakis M, Robinson L, Rothery S, Makita N, Kowase S, Boonmee N, Vitayakritsirikul V, Ratanarapee S, Sharma S, van der Wal AC, Christiansen M, Tan HL, Wilde AA, Nogami A, Sheppard MN, Veerakul G, Behr ER. Fibrosis, Connexin-43, and Conduction Abnormalities in the Brugada Syndrome. J Am Coll Cardiol. 2015;66:1976-86.
66. Corrado D, Thiene G. Arrhythmogenic right ventricular cardiomyopathy/dysplasia: clinical impact of molecular genetic studies. Circulation. 2006;113:1634-7.
67. Corrado D, Basso C, Pilichou K, Thiene G. Molecular biology and clinical management of arrhythmogenic right ventricular cardiomyopathy/dysplasia. Heart. 2011;97:530-9.
68. Thiene G, Nava A, Corrado D, Rossi L, Pennelli N. Right ventricular cardiomyopathy and sudden death in young people. N Engl J Med. 1988;318:129-33.
69. Delmar M, McKenna WJ. The cardiac desmosome and arrhythmogenic cardiomyopathies: from gene to disease. Circ Res. 2010;107:700-14.
70. Delmar M, Makita N. Cardiac connexins, mutations and arrhythmias. Curr Opin Cardiol. 2012;27:236-41.

71. Cerrone M, Noorman M, Lin X, Chkourko H, Liang FX, van der Nagel R, Hund T, Birchmeier W, Mohler P, van Veen TA, van Rijen HV, Delmar M. Sodium current deficit and arrhythmogenesis in a murine model of plakophilin-2 haploinsufficiency. Cardiovasc Res. 2012;95:460-8.
72. Corrado D, Basso C, Buja G, Nava A, Rossi L, Thiene G. Right bundle branch block, right precordial ST-segment elevation, and sudden death in young people. Circulation. 2001;103: 710-7.
73. Cerrone M, Lin X, Zhang M, Agullo-Pascual E, Pfenniger A, Chkourko Gusky H, Novelli V, Kim C, Tirasawadichai T, Judge DP, Rothenberg E, Chen HS, Napolitano C, Priori SG, Delmar M. Missense mutations in plakophilin-2 cause sodium current deficit and associate with a Brugada syndrome phenotype. Circulation. 2014;129:1092-103.
74. Corrado D, Leoni L, Link MS, Della Bella P, Gaita F, Curnis A, Salerno JU, Igidbashian D, Raviele A, Disertori M, Zanotto G, Verlato R, Vergara G, Delise P, Turrini P, Basso C, Naccarella F, Maddalena F, Estes NA, 3rd, Buja G, Thiene G. Implantable cardioverter-defibrillator therapy for prevention of sudden death in patients with arrhythmogenic right ventricular cardiomyopathy/dysplasia. Circulation. 2003;108:3084-91.
75. Matsuo K, Kurita T, Inagaki M, Kakishita M, Aihara N, Shimizu W, Taguchi A, Suyama K, Kamakura S, Shimomura K. The circadian pattern of the development of ventricular fibrillation in patients with Brugada syndrome. Eur Heart J. 1999;20: 465-70.
76. Peters S, Trummel M, Denecke S, Koehler B. Results of ajmaline testing in patients with arrhythmogenic right ventricular dysplasia-cardiomyopathy. Int J Cardiol. 2004;95:207-10.
77. Peters S, Trummel M, Koehler B. QRS fragmentation in standard ECG as a diagnostic marker of arrhythmogenic right ventricular dysplasia-cardiomyopathy. Heart Rhythm. 2008;5:1417-21.
78. Shimizu W. Acquired forms of the Brugada syndrome. J Electrocardiol. 2005;38 Suppl:22-5.
79. Brugada P, Brugada J, Brugada R. Arrhythmia induction by antiarrhythmic drugs. Pacing Clin Electrophysiol. 2000;23: 291-2.
80. Brugada R, Brugada J, Antzelevitch C, Kirsch GE, Potenza D, Towbin JA, Brugada P. Sodium channel blockers identify risk for sudden death in patients with ST-segment elevation and right bundle branch block but structurally normal hearts. Circulation. 2000;101:510-5.
81. Miyazaki T, Mitamura H, Miyoshi S, Soejima K, Aizawa Y, Ogawa S. Autonomic and antiarrhythmic drug modulation of ST segment elevation in patients with Brugada syndrome. J Am Coll Cardiol. 1996;27:1061-70.
82. Babaliaros VC, Hurst JW. Tricyclic antidepressants and the Brugada syndrome: an example of Brugada waves appearing after the administration of desipramine. Clin Cardiol. 2002; 25:395-8.
83. Goldgran-Toledano D, Sideris G, Kevorkian JP. Overdose of cyclic antidepressants and the Brugada syndrome. N Engl J Med. 2002;346:1591-2.
84. Tada H, Sticherling C, Oral H, Morady F. Brugada syndrome mimicked by tricyclic antidepressant overdose. J Cardiovasc Electrophysiol. 2001;12:275-.
85. Ortega-Carnicer J, Bertos-Polo J, Gutierrez-Tirado C. Aborted sudden death, transient Brugada pattern, and wide QRS dysrrhythmias after massive cocaine ingestion. J Electrocardiol. 2001;34:345-9.
86. Nogami A, Nakao M, Kubota S, Sugiyasu A, Doi H, Yokoyama K, Yumoto K, Tamaki T, Kato K, Hosokawa N, Sagai H, Nakamura H, Nitta J, Yamauchi Y, Aonuma K. Enhancement of J-ST-segment elevation by the glucose and insulin test in Brugada syndrome. Pacing Clin Electrophysiol. 2003;26:332-7.
87. Araki T, Konno T, Itoh H, Ino H, Shimizu M. Brugada syndrome with ventricular tachycardia and fibrillation related to hypokalemia. Circ J. 2003;67:93-5.
88. Pastor A, Nunez A, Cantale C, Cosio FG. Asymptomatic Brugada syndrome case unmasked during dimenhydrinate infusion. J Cardiovasc Electrophysiol. 2001;12:1192-4.
89. Chiale PA, Garro HA, Fernandez PA, Elizari MV. High-degree right bundle branch block obscuring the diagnosis of Brugada electrocardiographic pattern. Heart Rhythm. 2012;9:974-6.
90. Postema PG, Wolpert C, Amin AS, Probst V, Borggrefe M, Roden DM, Priori SG, Tan HL, Hiraoka M, Brugada J, Wilde AA. Drugs and Brugada syndrome patients: review of the literature, recommendations, and an up-to-date website (www.brugadadrugs.org). Heart Rhythm. 2009;6:1335-41.
91. Nam GB. Idiopathic ventricular fibrillation, early repolarization and other J wave-related ventricular fibrillation syndromes. Circ J. 2012;76:2723-31.
92. McIntyre WF, Perez-Riera AR, Femenia F, Baranchuk A. Coexisting early repolarization pattern and Brugada syndrome: recognition of potentially overlapping entities. J Electrocardiol. 2012;45:195-8.
93. Benito B, Sarkozy A, Mont L, Henkens S, Berruezo A, Tamborero D, Arzamendi D, Berne P, Brugada R, Brugada P, Brugada J. Gender differences in clinical manifestations of Brugada syndrome. J Am Coll Cardiol. 2008;52:1567-73.
94. Kamakura T, Kawata H, Nakajima I, Yamada Y, Miyamoto K, Okamura H, Noda T, Satomi K, Aiba T, Takaki H, Aihara N, Kamakura S, Kimura T, Shimizu W. Significance of non-type 1 anterior early repolarization in patients with inferolateral early repolarization syndrome. J Am Coll Cardiol. 2013;62:1610-8.
95. Kalla H, Yan GX, Marinchak R. Ventricular fibrillation in a patient with prominent J (Osborn) waves and ST segment elevation in the inferior electrocardiographic leads: a Brugada syndrome variant? J Cardiovasc Electrophysiol. 2000;11:95-8.
96. Aizawa Y, Sato A, Watanabe H, Chinushi M, Furushima H, Horie M, Kaneko Y, Imaizumi T, Okubo K, Watanabe I, Shinozaki T, Aizawa Y, Fukuda K, Joo K, Haissaguerre M. Dynamicity of the J-wave in idiopathic ventricular fibrillation with a special reference to pause-dependent augmentation of the J-wave. J Am Coll Cardiol. 2012;59:1948-53.
97. Nademanee K. Sudden unexplained death syndrome in southeast Asia. Am J Cardiol. 1997;79(6A):10-1.
98. Kawata H, Noda T, Yamada Y, Okamura H, Satomi K, Aiba T, Takaki H, Aihara N, Isobe M, Kamakura S, Shimizu W. Effect of sodium-channel blockade on early repolarization in inferior/lateral leads in patients with idiopathic ventricular fibrillation and Brugada syndrome. Heart Rhythm. 2012;9:77-83.
99. Matsumoto AM. Fundamental aspects of hypogonadism in the aging male. Rev Urol. 2003;5(Suppl 1):S3-10.
100. Shimizu W, Kamakura S. Catecholamines in children with congenital long QT syndrome and Brugada syndrome. J Electrocardiol. 2001;34 Suppl:173-5.
101. Suzuki H, Torigoe K, Numata O, Yazaki S. Infant case with a malignant form of Brugada syndrome. J Cardiovasc Electrophysiol. 2000;11:1277-80.
102. Ohgo T, Okamura H, Noda T, Satomi K, Suyama K, Kurita T, Aihara N, Kamakura S, Ohe T, Shimizu W. Acute and chronic

management in patients with Brugada syndrome associated with electrical storm of ventricular fibrillation. Heart Rhythm. 2007;4:695-700.

103. Watanabe A, Fukushima KK, Morita H, Miura D, Sumida W, Hiramatsu S, Banba K, Nishii N, Nagase S, Nakamura K, Sakuragi S, Ohe T. Low-dose isoproterenol for repetitive ventricular arrhythmia in patients with Brugada syndrome. Eur Heart J. 2006;27:1579-83.
104. Hermida JS, Denjoy I, Clerc J, Extramiana F, Jarry G, Milliez P, Guicheney P, Di Fusco S, Rey JL, Cauchemez B, Leenhardt A. Hydroquinidine therapy in Brugada syndrome. J Am Coll Cardiol. 2004;43:1853-60.
105. Belhassen B, Glick A, Viskin S. Efficacy of quinidine in high-risk patients with Brugada syndrome. Circulation. 2004;110:1731-7.
106. Tsuchiya T, Ashikaga K, Honda T, Arita M. Prevention of ventricular fibrillation by cilostazol, an oral phosphodiesterase inhibitor, in a patient with Brugada syndrome. J Cardiovasc Electrophysiol. 2002;13:698-701.
107. Iguchi K, Noda T, Kamakura S, Shimizu W. Beneficial effects of cilostazol in a patient with recurrent ventricular fibrillation associated with early repolarization syndrome. Heart Rhythm. 2013;10:604-6.
108. Agac MT, Erkan H, Korkmaz L. Conversion of Brugada type I to type III and successful control of recurrent ventricular arrhythmia with cilostazol. Arch Cardiovasc Dis. 2013.
109. Hasegawa K, Ashihara T, Kimura H, Jo H, Itoh H, Yamamoto T, Aizawa Y, Horie M. Long-term pharmacological therapy of Brugada syndrome: is J-wave attenuation a marker of drug efficacy? Intern Med. 2014;53:1523-6.
110. Shinohara T, Ebata Y, Ayabe R, Fukui A, Okada N, Yufu K, Nakagawa M, Takahashi N. Combination therapy of cilostazol and bepridil suppresses recurrent ventricular fibrillation related to J-wave syndromes. Heart Rhythm. 2014;11:1441-5.
111. Haissaguerre M, Sacher F, Nogami A, Komiya N, Bernard A, Probst V, Yli-Mayry S, Defaye P, Aizawa Y, Frank R, Mantovan R, Cappato R, Wolpert C, Leenhardt A, De Roy L, Heidbuchel H, Deisenhofer I, Arentz T, Pasquie JL, Weerasooriya R, Hocini M, Jais P, Derval N, Bordachar P, Clementy J. Characteristics of recurrent ventricular fibrillation associated with inferolateral early repolarization role of drug therapy. J Am Coll Cardiol. 2009;53:612-9.
112. Junttila MJ, Tikkanen JT, Kentta T, Anttonen O, Aro AL, Porthan K, Kerola T, Rissanen HA, Knekt P, Huikuri HV. Early repolarization as a predictor of arrhythmic and nonarrhythmic cardiac events in middle-aged subjects. Heart Rhythm. 2014;11:1701-6.
113. Nam GB, Ko KH, Kim J, Park KM, Rhee KS, Choi KJ, Kim YH, Antzelevitch C. Mode of onset of ventricular fibrillation in patients with early repolarization pattern vs. Brugada syndrome. Eur Heart J. 2010;31:330-9.
114. Park DS, Cerrone M, Morley G, Vasquez C, Fowler S, Liu N, Bernstein SA, Liu FY, Zhang J, Rogers CS, Priori SG, Chinitz LA, Fishman GI. Genetically engineered SCN5A mutant pig hearts exhibit conduction defects and arrhythmias. J Clin Invest. 2015;125:403-12.
115. Antzelevitch C, Yan GX. J-wave syndromes: Brugada and early repolarization syndromes. Heart Rhythm. 2015;12:1852-66.
116. Szel T, Antzelevitch C. Abnormal repolarization as the basis for late potentials and fractionated electrograms recorded from epicardium in experimental models of brugada syndrome. J Am Coll Cardiol. 2014;63:2037-45.
117. Patocskai B, Szel T, Yoon N, Antzelevitch C. Cellular mechanisms underlying the fractionated and late potentials on epicardial electrograms and the ameliorative effect of epicardial radiofrequency ablation in an experimental model of Brugada syndrome. In: Program and abstracts of the 24th Annual Upstate New York Cardiac Electrophysiology Society Meeting, November 3, 2014, Buffalo, NY 2014:Abstact 006.
118. Liu H, Chatel S, Simard C, Syam N, Salle L, Probst V, Morel J, Millat G, Lopez M, Abriel H, Schott JJ, Guinamard R, Bouvagnet P. Molecular genetics and functional anomalies in a series of 248 Brugada cases with 11 mutations in the TRPM4 channel. PLoS One. 2013;8:e54131.
119. Perrin MJ, Adler A, Green S, Al-Zoughool F, Doroshenko P, Orr N, Uppal S, Healey JS, Birnie D, Sanatani S, Gardner M, Champagne J, Simpson C, Ahmad K, van Den Berg MP, Chauhan V, Backx PH, Van Tintelen JP, Krahn AD, Gollob MH. Evaluation of genes encoding for the transient outward current (Ito) identifies the *KCND2* gene as a cause of J wave syndrome associated with sudden cardiac death. Circ Cardiovasc Genet. 2014;7:782-9.
120. Verkerk AO, Wilders R, Schulze-Bahr E, Beekman L, Bhuiyan ZA, Bertrand J, Eckardt L, Lin D, Borggrefe M, Breithardt G, Mannens MM, Tan HL, Wilde AA, Bezzina CR. Role of sequence variations in the human *ether-a-go-go*-related gene (HERG, KCNH2) in the Brugada syndrome. Cardiovasc Res. 2005;68:441-53.
121. Wilders R, Verkerk AO. Role of the R1135H *KCNH2* mutation in Brugada syndrome. Int J Cardiol. 2010;144:149-51.
122. Ohno S, Zankov DP, Ding WG, Itoh H, Makiyama T, Doi T, Shizuta S, Hattori T, Miyamoto A, Naiki N, Hancox JC, Matsuura H, Horie M. KCNE5 (KCNE1L) variants are novel modulators of Brugada syndrome and idiopathic ventricular fibrillation. Circ Arrhythm Electrophysiol. 2011;4:352-61.
123. Boczek NJ, Ye D, Johnson EK, Wang W, Crotti L, Tester DJ, Dagradi F, Mizusawa Y, Torchio M, Alders M, Giudicessi JR, Wilde AA, Schwartz PJ, Nerbonne JM, Ackerman MJ. Characterization of SEMA3A-encoded semaphorin as a naturally occurring Kv4.3 protein inhibitor and its contribution to Brugada syndrome. Circ Res. 2014;115:460-9.
124. Ueda K, Nakamura K, Hayashi T, Inagaki N, Takahashi M, Arimura T, Morita H, Higashiuesato Y, Hirano Y, Yasunami M, Takishita S, Yamashina A, Ohe T, Sunamori M, Hiraoka M, Kimura A. Functional characterization of a trafficking-defective *HCN4* mutation, D553N, associated with cardiac arrhythmia. J Biol Chem. 2004;279:27194-8.
125. Schwartz PJ, Ackerman MJ, George AL, Jr., Wilde AA. Impact of genetics on the clinical management of channelopathies. J Am Coll Cardiol. 2013;62:169-80.
126. Raffan E, Semple RK. Next generation sequencing--implications for clinical practice. rBr Med Bull. 2011;99:53-71.
127. Refsgaard L, Holst AG, Sadjadieh G, Haunso S, Nielsen JB, Olesen MS. High prevalence of genetic variants previously associated with LQT syndrome in new exome data. European journal of human genetics: Eur J Hum Genet. 2012;20:905-8.
128. Kapa S, Tester DJ, Salisbury BA, Harris-Kerr C, Pungliya MS, Alders M, Wilde AA, Ackerman MJ. Genetic testing for long-QT syndrome: distinguishing pathogenic mutations from benign variants. Circulation. 2009;120:1752-60.
129. Andreasen C, Refsgaard L, Nielsen JB, Sajadieh A, Winkel BG, Tfelt-Hansen J, Haunso S, Holst AG, Svendsen JH, Olesen MS. Mutations in genes encoding cardiac ion channels previously

associated with sudden infant death syndrome (SIDS) are present with high frequency in new exome data. Can J Cardiol. 2013;29:1104-9.
130. Song W, Shou W. Cardiac sodium channel Nav1.5 mutations and cardiac arrhythmia. Pediatr Cardiol. 2012;33: 943-9.
131. Ruklisa D, Ware JS, Walsh R, Balding DJ, Cook SA. Bayesian models for syndrome- and gene-specific probabilities of novel variant pathogenicity. Genome Med. 2015;7:5.
132. Juang JM, Lu TP, Lai LC, Hsueh CH, Liu YB, Tsai CT, Lin LY, Yu CC, Hwang JJ, Chiang FT, Yeh SS, Chen WP, Chuang EY, Lai LP, Lin JL. Utilizing multiple in silico analyses to identify putative causal SCN5A variants in Brugada syndrome. Sci Rep. 2014;4:3850.
133. Walsh R, Peters NS, Cook SA, Ware JS. Paralogue annotation identifies novel pathogenic variants in patients with Brugada syndrome and catecholaminergic polymorphic ventricular tachycardia. J Med Genet. 2014;51:35-44.
134. Kapplinger JD, Giudicessi JR, Tester DJ, Callis TE, Ackerman MJ. Enhanced classification of non-synonymous single nucleotide variants in the SCN5A-Encoded Nav1.5 cardiac sodium channel. Heart Rhythm. 2012;9:1912.
135. Kapplinger JD, Giudicessi JR, Ye D, Tester DJ, Callis TE, Valdivia CR, Makielski JC, Wilde AA, Ackerman MJ. Enhanced Classification of Brugada syndrome-associated and long-QT syndrome-associated genetic variants in the SCN5A-Encoded Nav1.5 cardiac sodium channel. Circ Cardiovasc Genet. 2015;8:582-95.
136. Bezzina CR, Barc J, Mizusawa Y, Remme CA, Gourraud JB, Simonet F, Verkerk AO, Schwartz PJ, Crotti L, Dagradi F, Guicheney P, Fressart V, Leenhardt A, Antzelevitch C, Bartkowiak S, Schulze-Bahr E, Zumhagen S, Behr ER, Bastiaenen R, Tfelt-Hansen J, Olesen MS, Kaab S, Beckmann BM, Weeke P, Watanabe H, Endo N, Minamino T, Horie M, Ohno S, Hasegawa K, Makita N, Nogami A, Shimizu W, Aiba T, Froguel P, Balkau B, Lantieri O, Torchio M, Wiese C, Weber D, Wolswinkel R, Coronel R, Boukens BJ, Bezieau S, Charpentier E, Chatel S, Despres A, Gros F, Kyndt F, Lecointe S, Lindenbaum P, Portero V, Violleau J, Gessler M, Tan HL, Roden DM, Christoffels VM, Le MH, Wilde AA, Probst V, Schott JJ, Dina C, Redon R. Common variants at *SCN5A-SCN10A* and *HEY2* are associated with Brugada syndrome, a rare disease with high risk of sudden cardiac death. Nat Genet. 2013;45:1044-9.
137. Antzelevitch C, Sicouri S, Litovsky SH, Lukas A, Krishnan SC, Di Diego JM, Gintant GA, Liu DW. Heterogeneity within the ventricular wall. Electrophysiology and pharmacology of epicardial, endocardial, and M cells. Circ Res. 1991;69:1427-49.
138. Krishnan SC, Antzelevitch C. Sodium channel block produces opposite electrophysiological effects in canine ventricular epicardium and endocardium. Circ Res. 1991;69:277-91.
139. Antzelevitch C, Brugada P, Brugada J, Brugada R, Shimizu W, Gussak I, Perez Riera AR. Brugada syndrome: a decade of progress. Circ Res. 2002;91:1114-9.
140. Krishnan SC, Antzelevitch C. Flecainide-induced arrhythmia in canine ventricular epicardium. Phase 2 reentry? Circulation. 1993;87:562-72.
141. Antzelevitch C. The Brugada syndrome: ionic basis and arrhythmia mechanisms. J Cardiovasc Electrophysiol. 2001; 12:268-72.
142. Lukas A, Antzelevitch C. Phase 2 reentry as a mechanism of initiation of circus movement reentry in canine epicardium exposed to simulated ischemia. Cardiovasc Res. 1996;32: 593-603.
143. Fish JM, Antzelevitch C. Role of sodium and calcium channel block in unmasking the Brugada syndrome. Heart Rhythm. 2004;1:210-7.
144. Kurita T, Shimizu W, Inagaki M, Suyama K, Taguchi A, Satomi K, Aihara N, Kamakura S, Kobayashi J, Kosakai Y. The electrophysiologic mechanism of ST-segment elevation in Brugada syndrome. J Am Coll Cardiol. 2002;40:330-4.
145. Wilde AA, Postema PG, Di Diego JM, Viskin S, Morita H, Fish JM, Antzelevitch C. The pathophysiological mechanism underlying Brugada syndrome: depolarization versus repolarization. J Mol Cell Cardiol. 2010;49:543-53.
146. Morita H, Zipes DP, Wu J. Brugada syndrome: insights of ST elevation, arrhythmogenicity, and risk stratification from experimental observations. Heart Rhythm. 2009;6:S34-S43.
147. Nademanee K, Veerakul G, Chandanamattha P, Chaothawee L, Ariyachaipanich A, Jirasirirojanakorn K, Likittanasombat K, Bhuripanyo K, Ngarmukos T. Prevention of ventricular fibrillation episodes in Brugada syndrome by catheter ablation over the anterior right ventricular outflow tract epicardium. Circulation. 2011;123:1270-9.
148. Brugada J, Pappone C, Berruezo A, Vicedomini G, Manguso F, Ciconte G, Giannelli L, Santinelli V. Brugada syndrome phenotype elimination by epicardial substrate ablation. Circ Arrhythm Electrophysiol. 2015;8:1373-81.
149. Sacher F, Jesel L, Jais P, Haissaguerre M. Insight into the mechanism of Brugada syndrome: epicardial substrate and modification during ajmaline testing. Heart Rhythm. 2014;11:732-4.
150. Patocskai B, Antzelevitch C. Novel therapeutic strategies for the management of ventricular arrhythmias associated with the Brugada syndrome. Expert Opin Orphan Drugs. 2015;3: 633-51.
151. Boukens BJ, Sylva M, de Gier-de VC, Remme CA, Bezzina C, Christoffels VM, Coronel R. Reduced sodium channel function unmasks residual embryonic slow conduction in the adult right ventricular outflow tract. Circ Res. 2013;113:137-41.
152. Zhang J, Sacher F, Hoffmayer K, O'Hara T, Strom M, Cuculich P, Silva J, Cooper D, Faddis M, Hocini M, Haissaguerre M, Scheinman M, Rudy Y. Cardiac electrophysiological substrate underlying the ECG phenotype and electrogram abnormalities in Brugada syndrome patients. Circulation. 2015;131:1950-9.
153. Gurabi Z, Koncz I, Patocskai B, Nesterenko VV, Antzelevitch C. Cellular mechanism underlying hypothermia-induced ventricular tachycardia/ventricular fibrillation in the setting of early repolarization and the protective effect of quinidine, cilostazol, and milrinone. Circ Arrhythm Electrophysiol. 2014;7:134-42.
154. Ghosh S, Cooper DH, Vijayakumar R, Zhang J, Pollak S, Haissaguerre M, Rudy Y. Early repolarization associated with sudden death: insights from noninvasive electrocardiographic imaging. Heart Rhythm. 2010;7:534-7.
155. Huikuri HV. Separation of Benign from Malignant J waves. Heart Rhythm. 2015;12:384-5.
156. Aizawa Y, Sato M, Kitazawa H, Aizawa Y, Takatsuki S, Oda E, Okabe M, Fukuda K. Tachycardia-dependent augmentation of "notched J waves" in a general patient population without ventricular fibrillation or cardiac arrest: Not a repolarization but a depolarization abnormality? Heart Rhythm. 2015;12: 376-83.

157. Badri M, Patel A, Yan G. Cellular and ionic basis of J-wave syndromes. Trends Cardiovasc Med. 2015;25:12-21.
158. Morita H, Kusano KF, Miura D, Nagase S, Nakamura K, Morita ST, Ohe T, Zipes DP, Wu J. Fragmented QRS as a marker of conduction abnormality and a predictor of prognosis of Brugada syndrome. Circulation. 2008;118:1697-704.
159. Priori SG, Gasparini M, Napolitano C, Della BP, Ottonelli AG, Sassone B, Giordano U, Pappone C, Mascioli G, Rossetti G, De NR, Colombo M. Risk stratification in Brugada syndrome: results of the PRELUDE (PRogrammed ELectrical stimUlation preDictive valuE) registry. J Am Coll Cardiol. 2012;59: 37-45.
160. Terho HK, Tikkanen JT, Junttila JM, Anttonen O, Kentta TV, Aro AL, Kerola T, Rissanen HA, Reunanen A, Huikuri HV. Prevalence and prognostic significance of fragmented QRS complex in middle-aged subjects with and without clinical or electrocardiographic evidence of cardiac disease. Am J Cardiol. 2014;114:141-7.
161. Brugada J, Brugada R, Brugada P. Pharmacological and device approach to therapy of inherited cardiac diseases associated with cardiac arrhythmias and sudden death. J Electrocardiol. 2000;33 Suppl:41-7.
162. Nademanee K, Veerakul G, Mower M, Likittanasombat K, Krittayapong R, Bhuripanyo K, Sitthisook S, Chaothawee L, Lai MY, Azen SP. Defibrillator Versus beta-Blockers for Unexplained Death in Thailand (DEBUT): a randomized clinical trial. Circulation. 2003;107:2221-6.
163. Sacher F, Probst V, Maury P, Babuty D, Mansourati J, Komatsu Y, Marquie C, Rosa A, Diallo A, Cassagneau R, Loizeau C, Martins R, Field ME, Derval N, Miyazaki S, Denis A, Nogami A, Ritter P, Gourraud JB, Ploux S, Rollin A, Zemmoura A, Lamaison D, Bordachar P, Pierre B, Jais P, Pasquie JL, Hocini M, Legal F, Defaye P, Boveda S, Iesaka Y, Mabo P, Haissaguerre M. Outcome after Implantation of Cardioverter-Defibrillator in Patients with Brugada Syndrome: A Multicenter Study - Part 2. Circulation. 2013;128:1739-47.
164. Conte G, Sieira J, Ciconte G, de Asmundis C, Chierchia GB, Baltogiannis G, Di Giovanni G, La Meir M, Wellens F, Czapla J, Wauters K, Levinstein M, Saitoh Y, Irfan G, Julia J, Pappaert G, Brugada P. Implantable cardioverter-defibrillator therapy in brugada syndrome: a 20-year single-center experience. J Am Coll Cardiol. 2015;65:879-88.
165. De Maria E, Olaru A, Cappelli S. The entirely subcutaneous defibrillator (s-icd): state of the art and selection of the ideal candidate. Curr Cardiol Rev. 2015;11:180-6.
166. Brugada P, Brugada R, Brugada J, Geelen P. Use of the prophylactic implantable cardioverter defibrillator for patients with normal hearts. Am J Cardiol. 1999;83:98D-100D.
167. Makimoto H, Kamakura S, Aihara N, Noda T, Nakajima I, Yokoyama T, Doi A, Kawata H, Yamada Y, Okamura H, Satomi K, Aiba T, Shimizu W. Clinical impact of the number of extrastimuli in programmed electrical stimulation in patients with Brugada type 1 electrocardiogram. Heart Rhythm. 2012;9:242-8.
168. Takagi M, Tatsumi H, Yoshiyama M. Approach to the asymptomatic patients with Brugada syndrome. Indian Pacing Electrophysiol J. 2007;7:73-6.
169. Priori SG, Gasparini M, Napolitano C, Della Bella P, Ottonelli AG, Sassone B, Giordano U, Pappone C, Mascioli G, Rossetti G, De Nardis R, Colombo M. Risk stratification in Brugada syndrome: results of the PRELUDE (PRogrammed ELectrical stimUlation preDictive valuE) registry. J Am Coll Cardiol. 2012;59:37-45.
170. van Den Berg MP, Wilde AA, Viersma TJW, Brouwer J, Haaksma J, van der Hout AH, Stolte-Dijkstra I, Bezzina TCR, Van Langen IM, Beaufort-Krol GC, Cornel JH, Crijns HJ. Possible bradycardic mode of death and successful pacemaker treatment in a large family with features of long QT syndrome type 3 and Brugada syndrome. J Cardiovasc Electrophysiol. 2001;12:630-6.
171. Bertomeu-Gonzalez V, Ruiz-Granell R, Garcia-Civera R, Morell-Cabedo S, Ferrero A. Syncopal monomorphic ventricular tachycardia with pleomorphism, sensitive to antitachycardia pacing in a patient with Brugada syndrome. Europace. 2006;8:1048-50.
172. Lee KL, Lau C, Tse H, Wan S, Fan K. Prevention of ventricular fibrillation by pacing in a man with Brugada syndrome. J Cardiovasc Electrophysiol. 2000;11:935-7.
173. Shah AJ, Hocini M, Lamaison D, Sacher F, Derval N, Haissaguerre M. Regional substrate ablation abolishes Brugada syndrome. J Cardiovasc Electrophysiol. 2011;22:1290-1.
174. Cortez-Dias N, Placido R, Marta L, Bernardes A, Sobral S, Carpinteiro L, de SJ. Epicardial ablation for prevention of ventricular fibrillation in a patient with Brugada syndrome. Rev Port Cardiol. 2014;33:305.
175. Priori SG, Wilde AA, Horie M, Cho Y, Behr ER, Berul C, Blom N, Brugada J, Chiang CE, Huikuri H, Kannankeril P, Krahn A, Leenhardt A, Moss A, Schwartz PJ, Shimizu W, Tomaselli G, Tracy C. Executive Summary: HRS/EHRA/APHRS Expert Consensus Statement on the Diagnosis and Management of Patients with Inherited Primary Arrhythmia Syndromes. Heart Rhythm. 2013;15:1389-406.
176. Minoura Y, Di Diego JM, Barajas-Martinez H, Zygmunt AC, Hu D, Sicouri S, Antzelevitch C. Ionic and cellular mechanisms underlying the development of acquired Brugada syndrome in patients treated with antidepressants. J Cardiovasc Electrophysiol. 2012;23:423-32.
177. Minoura Y, Panama BK, Nesterenko VV, Betzenhauser M, Barajas-Martinez H, Hu D, Di Diego JM, Antzelevitch C. Effect of Wenxin Keli and quinidine to suppress arrhythmogenesis in an experimental model of Brugada syndrome. Heart Rhythm. 2013;10:1054-62.
178. Johnson P, Lesage A, Floyd Wl, Young Wg, Jr., Sealy WC. Prevention of ventricular fibrillation during profound hypothermia by quinidine. Ann Surg. 1960;151:490-5.
179. Gurabi Z, Koncz I, Patocskai B, Nesterenko VV, Antzelevitch C. Cellular mechanism underlying hypothermia-induced VT/VF in the setting of early repolarization and the protective effect of quinidine, cilostazol and milrinone. Circ Arrhythm Electrophysiol. 2014;7:134-42.
180. Belhassen B, Shapira I, Shoshani D, Paredes A, Miller H, Laniado S. Idiopathic ventricular fibrillation: inducibility and beneficial effects of class I antiarrhythmic agents. Circulation. 1987;75:809-16.
181. Belhassen B, Viskin S, Antzelevitch C. The Brugada syndrome: is an implantable cardioverter defibrillator the only therapeutic option? Pacing Clin Electrophysiol. 2002;25: 1634-40.
182. Alings M, Dekker L, Sadee A, Wilde A. Quinidine induced electrocardiographic normalization in two patients with Brugada syndrome. Pacing Clin Electrophysiol. 2001;24: 1420-2.

183. Belhassen B, Viskin S. Pharmacologic approach to therapy of Brugada syndrome: quinidine as an alternative to ICD therapy? In: Antzelevitch C, Brugada P, Brugada J, Brugada R, (Eds). The Brugada Syndrome: From Bench to Bedside. Oxford: Blackwell Futura; 2004:202-11.
184. Viskin S, Wilde AA, Tan HL, Antzelevitch C, Shimizu W, Belhassen B. Empiric quinidine therapy for asymptomatic Brugada syndrome: time for a prospective registry. Heart Rhythm. 2009;6:401-4.
185. Belhassen B, Glick A, Viskin S. Excellent long-term reproducibility of the electrophysiologic efficacy of quinidine in patients with idiopathic ventricular fibrillation and Brugada syndrome. Pacing Clin Electrophysiol. 2009;32:294-301.
186. Marquez MF, Bonny A, Hernandez-Castillo E, De SA, Gomez-Flores J, Nava S, Hidden-Lucet F, Iturralde P, Cardenas M, Tonet J. Long-term efficacy of low doses of quinidine on malignant arrhythmias in Brugada syndrome with an implantable cardioverter-defibrillator: A case series and literature review. Heart Rhythm. 2013;9:1995-2000.
187. Pellegrino PL, Di BM, Brunetti ND. Quinidine for the management of electrical storm in an old patient with Brugada syndrome and syncope. Acta Cardiol. 2013;68:201-3.
188. Probst V, Evain S, Gournay V, Marie A, Schott JJ, Boisseau P, H LEM. Monomorphic ventricular tachycardia due to Brugada syndrome successfully treated by hydroquinidine therapy in a 3-year-old child. J Cardiovasc Electrophysiol. 2006;17:97-100.
189. Schweizer PA, Becker R, Katus HA, Thomas D. Successful acute and long-term management of electrical storm in Brugada syndrome using orciprenaline and quinine/quinidine. Clin Res Cardiol. 2010;99:467-70.
190. Marquez MF, Rivera J, Hermosillo AG, Iturralde P, Colin L, Moragrega JL, Cardenas M. Arrhythmic storm responsive to quinidine in a patient with Brugada syndrome and vasovagal syncope. Pacing ClinElectrophysiol. 2005;28:870-3.
191. Viskin S, Antzelevitch C, Marquez MF, Belhassen B. Quinidine: a valuable medication joins the list of 'endangered species'. Europace. 2007;12:1105-6.
192. Rosso R, Glick A, Glikson M, Wagshal A, Swissa M, Rosenhek S, Shetboun I, Khalamizer V, Fuchs T, Boulos M, Geist M, Strasberg B, Ilan M, Belhassen B. Outcome after implantation of cardioverter defribrillator in patients with Brugada syndrome: a multicenter Israeli study (ISRABRU). Isr Med AssocJ. 2008;10:435-9.
193. Mok NS, Chan NY, Chi-Suen CA. Successful use of quinidine in treatment of electrical storm in Brugada syndrome. Pacing Clin Electrophysiol. 2004;27:821-3.
194. Belhassen B, Rahkovich M, Michowitz Y, Glick A, Viskin S. Management of Brugada syndrome: a 33-year experience using electrophysiologically-guided therapy with class 1A antiarrhythmic drugs. Circ Arrhythm Electrophysiol 2015.
195. Kyriazis K, Bahlmann E, van der SH, Kuck KH. Electrical storm in Brugada syndrome successfully treated with orciprenaline; effect of low-dose quinidine on the electrocardiogram. Europace. 2009;11:665-6.
196. Maury P, Couderc P, Delay M, Boveda S, Brugada J. Electrical storm in Brugada syndrome successfully treated using isoprenaline. Europace. 2004;6:130-3.
197. Maury P, Hocini M, Haissaguerre M. Electrical storms in Brugada syndrome: review of pharmacologic and ablative therapeutic options. Indian Pacing Electrophysiol J. 2005;5: 25-34.
198. Jongman JK, Jepkes-Bruin N, Ramdat Misier AR, Beukema WP, Delnoy PP, Oude LH, Dambrink JH, Hoorntje JC, Elvan A. Electrical storms in Brugada syndrome successfully treated with isoproterenol infusion and quinidine orally. Neth Heart J. 2007;15:151-5.
199. Furniss G. Isoprenaline and quinidine to calm Brugada VF storm. BMJ Case Rep 2012.
200. Shimizu W, Matsuo K, Takagi M, Tanabe Y, Aiba T, Taguchi A, Suyama K, Kurita T, Aihara N, Kamakura S. Body surface distribution and response to drugs of ST segment elevation in Brugada syndrome: clinical implication of eighty-seven-lead body surface potential mapping and its application to twelve-lead electrocardiograms. J Cardiovasc Electrophysiol. 2000;11:396-404.
201. Tanaka H, Kinoshita O, Uchikawa S, Kasai H, Nakamura M, Izawa A, Yokoseki O, Kitabayashi H, Takahashi W, Yazaki Y, Watanabe N, Imamura H, Kubo K. Successful prevention of recurrent ventricular fibrillation by intravenous isoproterenol in a patient with Brugada syndrome. Pacing Clin Electrophysiol. 2001;24:1293-4.
202. Sharif-Kazemi MB, Emkanjoo Z, Tavoosi A, Kafi M, Kheirkhah J, Alizadeh A, Sadr-Ameli MA. Electrical storm in Brugada syndrome during pregnancy. Pacing Clin Electrophysiol. 2011;34:e18-e21.
203. Roten L, Derval N, Sacher F, Pascale P, Scherr D, Komatsu Y, Ramoul K, Daly M, Denis A, Shah AJ, Hocini M, Jais P, Haissaguerre M. Heterogeneous response of J wave syndromes to beta-adrenergic stimulation. Heart Rhythm. 2012;9:1970-6.
204. Kaneko Y, Horie M, Niwano S, Kusano K, Takatsuki S, Kurita T, Mitsuhashi T, Nakajima T, Irie T, Hasegawa K, Noda T, Kamakura S, Aizawa Y, Yasuoka R, Torigoe K, Suzuki H, Ohe T, Shimizu A, Fukuda K, Kurabayashi M, Aizawa Y. Electrical storm in patients with Brugada syndrome is associated with early repolarization. Circ Arrhythm Electrophysiol 2014.
205. Kanlop N, Chattipakorn S, Chattipakorn N. Effects of cilostazol in the heart. J Cardiovasc Med (Hagerstown). 2011;12:88-95.
206. Bai Y, Muqier, Murakami H, Iwasa M, Sumi S, Yamada Y, Ushikoshi H, Aoyama T, Nishigaki K, Takemura G, Uno B, Minatoguchi S. Cilostazol protects the heart against ischaemia reperfusion injury in a rabbit model of myocardial infarction: focus on adenosine, nitric oxide and mitochondrial ATP-sensitive potassium channels. Clin Exp Pharmacol Physiol. 2011;38:658-65.
207. Abud A, Bagattin D, Goyeneche R, Becker C. Failure of cilostazol in the prevention of ventricular fibrillation in a patient with Brugada syndrome. J Cardiovasc Electrophysiol. 2006;17: 210-2.
208. Szel T, Koncz I, Antzelevitch C. Cellular mechanisms underlying the effects of milrinone and cilostazol to supress arrhythmogenesis associated with Brugada syndrome. Heart Rhythm. 2013;10:1720-7.
209. Cone J, Wang S, Tandon N, Fong M, Sun B, Sakurai K, Yoshitake M, Kambayashi J, Liu Y. Comparison of the effects of cilostazol and milrinone on intracellular cAMP levels and cellular function in platelets and cardiac cells. J Cardiovasc Pharmacol. 1999;34:497-504.
210. Shakur Y, Fong M, Hensley J, Cone J, Movsesian MA, Kambayashi J, Yoshitake M, Liu Y. Comparison of the effects of cilostazol and milrinone on cAMP-PDE activity, intracellular cAMP and calcium in the heart. Cardiovasc Drugs Ther. 2002;16:417-27.

211. Sugao M, Fujiki A, Nishida K, Sakabe M, Tsuneda T, Iwamoto J, Mizumaki K, Inoue H. Repolarization dynamics in patients with idiopathic ventricular fibrillation: pharmacological therapy with bepridil and disopyramide. J Cardiovasc Pharmacol. 2005;45:545-9.
212. Murakami M, Nakamura K, Kusano KF, Morita H, Nakagawa K, Tanaka M, Tada T, Toh N, Nishii N, Nagase S, Hata Y, Kohno K, Miura D, Ohe T, Ito H. Efficacy of low-dose bepridil for prevention of ventricular fibrillation in patients with Brugada syndrome with and without SCN5A mutation. J Cardiovasc Pharmacol. 2010;56:389-95.
213. Aizawa Y, Yamakawa H, Takatsuki S, Katsumata Y, Nishiyama T, Kimura T, Nishiyama N, Fukumoto K, Tanimoto Y, Tanimoto K, Mitamura H, Ogawa S, Fukuda K. Efficacy and safety of bepridil for prevention of ICD shocks in patients with Brugada syndrome and idiopathic ventricular fibrillation. Int J Cardiol. 2013;168:5083-5.
214. Kang L, Zheng MQ, Morishima M, Wang Y, Kaku T, Ono K. Bepridil up-regulates cardiac Na+ channels as a long-term effect by blunting proteasome signals through inhibition of calmodulin activity. Br J Pharmacol. 2009;157:404-14.
215. Fish JM, Welchons DR, Kim YS, Lee SH, Ho WK, Antzelevitch C. Dimethyl lithospermate B, an extract of danshen, suppresses arrhythmogenesis associated with the Brugada syndrome. Circulation. 2006;113:1393-400.
216. Probst V, Veltmann C, Eckardt L, Meregalli PG, Gaita F, Tan HL, Babuty D, Sacher F, Giustetto C, Schulze-Bahr E, Borggrefe M, Haissaguerre M, Mabo P, Le Marec H, Wolpert C, Wilde AA. Long-term prognosis of patients diagnosed with Brugada syndrome: Results from the FINGER Brugada Syndrome Registry. Circulation. 2010;121:635-43.
217. Haissaguerre M, Chatel S, Sacher F, Weerasooriya R, Probst V, Loussouarn G, Horlitz M, Liersch R, Schulze-Bahr E, Wilde A, Kaab S, Koster J, Rudy Y, Le MH, Schott JJ. Ventricular fibrillation with prominent early repolarization associated with a rare variant of KCNJ8/K_{ATP} channel. J Cardiovasc Electrophysiol. 2009;20:93-8.
218. Kanlop N, Shinlapawittayatorn K, Sungnoon R, Weerateer-angkul P, Chattipakorn S, Chattipakorn N. Cilostazol attenuates ventricular arrhythmia induction and improves defibrillation efficacy in swine. Can J Physiol Pharmacol. 2010;88:422-8.
219. Endoh M, Yanagisawa T, Taira N, Blinks JR. Effects of new inotropic agents on cyclic nucleotide metabolism and calcium transients in canine ventricular muscle. Circulation. 1986;73:III117-33.
220. Rapundalo ST, Grupp I, Grupp G, Abdul Matlib M, Solaro RJ, Schwartz A. Myocardial actions of milrinone: characterization of its mechanism of action. Circulation. 1986;73:III134-44.
221. Atarashi H, Endoh Y, Saitoh H, Kishida H, Hayakawa H. Chronotropic effects of cilostazol, a new antithrombotic agent, in patients with bradyarrhythmias. J Cardiovasc Pharmacol. 1998;31:534-9.
222. Matsui K, Kiyosue T, Wang JC, Dohi K, Arita M. Effects of pimobendan on the L-type Ca^{2+} current and developed tension in guinea-pig ventricular myocytes and papillary muscle: comparison with IBMX, milrinone, and cilostazol. Cardiovasc Drugs Ther. 1999;13:105-13.
223. Aizawa Y, Chinushi M, Hasegawa K, Naiki N, Horie M, Kaneko Y, Kurabayashi M, Ito S, Imaizumi T, Aizawa Y, Takatsuki S, Joo K, Sato M, Ebe K, Hosaka Y, Haissaguerre M, Fukuda K. Electrical storm in idiopathic ventricular fibrillation is associated with early repolarization. J Am Coll Cardiol. 2013;62:1015-9.
224. Nakagawa K, Nagase S, Morita H, Ito H. Left ventricular epicardial electrogram recordings in idiopathic ventricular fibrillation with inferior and lateral early repolarization. Heart Rhythm. 2013;11:314-7.
225. Antzelevitch C. The Brugada syndrome: diagnostic criteria and cellular mechanisms. Eur Heart J. 2001;22:356-63.

EDITORS' SUMMARY

A pioneer and recognized world leader in the understanding of basic arrhythmogenesis, Dr Antzelevitch has provided for the readers of this textbook an outstanding overview of J wave syndromes that is exhaustively referenced.

While the details of the clinical epidemiology and evaluation specific to early repolarization is discussed elsewhere (Chapter 40), here, the reader can make quick comparisons between all the J wave syndromes, and this comparative understanding will aid in the differential diagnosis when confronted with an abnormal pattern of late depolarization/early repolarization.

A hallmark of the approach taken in this chapter is the repeated correlation between cellular electrophysiology, the findings on the wedge preparation, the electrocardiogram, and the clinical impact of these findings.

CHAPTER 40

Peter A Noseworthy

Early Repolarization Syndrome and Risk of Sudden Cardiac Death

LIST OF ABBREVIATIONS

APL	Action Potential	SCD	Sudden Cardiac Death
ER	Early Repolarization	VF	Ventricular Fibrillation
PVC	Premature Ventricular Contraction	VT	Ventricular Tachycardia

INTRODUCTION

The electrocardiographic early repolarization (ER) pattern has long been felt to be a normal variant. However, over the past decade, emerging evidence has identified the pattern as a potential marker of increased risk of ventricular arrhythmias. Although, case reports of ventricular arrhythmia occurring in the context of early repolarization patterns on ECG have percolated the literature for years,[1] it was not until a landmark paper by Haissaguerre in 2008 demonstrated a high prevalence of the pattern among survivors of resuscitated sudden death,[2] that there has been renewed interest in defining this phenomenon. We now understand early repolarization syndrome as a cause of sudden death among individuals with structurally normal hearts. Although the syndrome has clinical and electrophysiologic similarities to the Brugada syndrome, the electrophysiologic, genetic underpinning and clinical management are less well established.

There is considerable confusion and controversy about the syndrome, its definitions, and its clinical implications.[3] This is in part due to the fact that the early repolarization pattern is quite prevalent and is commonly seen in young, healthy individuals who are likely at low risk of sudden cardiac death. The distinction between early repolarization syndrome (a definition that requires a history of resuscitated sudden death) and the early repolarization pattern on ECG (a highly prevalent finding) is the key. The manifestations of early repolarization exist on a spectrum **(Figure 40.1)** with common, relatively benign manifestations at one end, and rare, potentially dangerous manifestations at the other. Generally, as the prevalence of the particular feature increases, the incremental risk to the individual is less. Those at highest risk represent only a 'tip of the iceberg' of all patients along this spectrum.

This chapter will primarily focus on the early repolarization syndrome that is known to increase the risk of sudden cardiac death and is of particular concern to the electrophysiologist.

DEFINITIONS AND NOMENCLATURE

It is important for electrophysiologists to understand the various terms commonly used in the medical literature to describe patterns of early repolarization. The electrocardiographic early repolarization pattern requires the presence of J-point elevation ≥1 mm in ≥2 contiguous inferior and/or lateral leads of a standard 12-lead ECG. In general, the right precordial leads are excluded from the diagnosis to

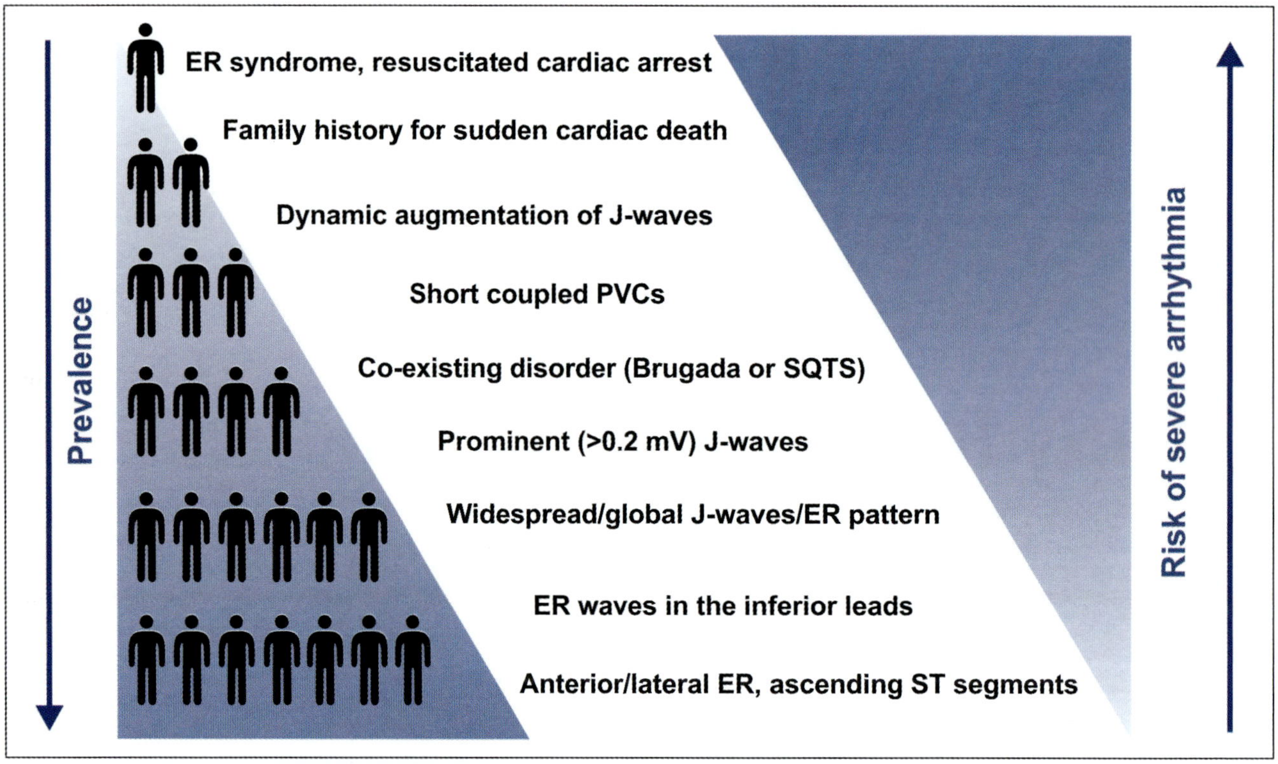

Figure 40.1: The prevalence and risk associated with various electrocardiographic findings in early repolarization pattern. Modified from Tikkanen JT et al.[32]

Abbreviations: ER, early repolarization; PVC, premature ventricular contraction; SQTS, short QT syndrome

Table 40.1: Diagnostic criteria for the early repolarization syndrome

Early repolarization (ER) expert consensus recommendations on early repolarization diagnosis	
1.	ER *syndrome is diagnosed* in the presence of J-point elevation ≥1 mm in ≥2 contiguous inferior and/or lateral leads of a standard 12-lead ECG in a patient resuscitated from otherwise unexplained VF/polymorphic VT
2.	ER syndrome *can be diagnosed* in an SCD victim with a negative autopsy and medical chart review with a previous ECG demonstrating J-point elevation ≥1 mm in ≥2 contiguous inferior and/or lateral leads of a standard 12-lead ECG
3.	ER pattern *can be diagnosed* in the presence of J-point elevation ≥1 mm in ≥2 contiguous inferior and/or lateral leads of a standard 12-lead ECG

Abbreviations: ER, early repolarization; SCD, sudden cardiac death; VF, ventricular fibrillation; VT, ventricular tachycardia
Modified with permission from Priori et al.[31]

avoid confusion with the Brugada syndrome and because right precordial ER pattern is particularly common in young, healthy athletes and has no negative prognostic implications. Early repolarization syndrome can be diagnosed only in patients resuscitated from otherwise unexplained ventricular fibrillation (VF) or polymorphic ventricular tachycardia (VT) who meet criteria for the ER pattern on ECG.

The term J-wave syndromes (also *see* chapter 39) are often used interchangeably with 'early repolarization,' but they are not truly synonymous. J-waves are often present, but are not required, for the diagnosis of ER pattern. Rather, J-waves syndromes reflect a range of clinical entities in which there is prominent elevation of the J-point on ECG. This pattern was first described as occurring during extreme hypothermia, the so-called 'Osborne wave',[4] but is now recognized to include inherited and acquired early repolarization (when there is notching or slurring of the J-wave) and the Brugada syndrome in which there are marked right precordial J-waves. It is felt that prominent J-waves may be a particular marker of arrhythmic risk (in comparison to smooth, ascending elevation of the ST segment), and some care has been taken to describe various J-wave abnormalities in the early repolarization pattern.[5]

Because ER pattern is relatively common, the current HRS/EHRA/APHRS guidelines recommend a strict definition of the condition **(Table 40.1)**. At present, family members of ER syndrome patients are not considered to have the syndrome based only on the presence of the ECG pattern because the genetic underpinnings and risk stratification of the syndrome are not well established.

EPIDEMIOLOGY OF EARLY REPOLARIZATION

The early repolarization pattern is common. Depending on the population studied and precise definition of the trait used, prevalence estimates range from 1 to 15%.[6-8] It is the most common in young males,[9] particularly those of African[10] or Southeast Asian[11] descent. Among young athletes the prevalence can approach 50% in some studies.[12] However, in this population, the pattern does not portend a poor prognosis.[13]

The trait appears to be at least partially heritable,[8] but also dynamic, decreasing with age,[14] increased heart rate,[15] and, in athletes, in periods of relative inactivity.[9] There appears to be an effect of vagal tone (the pattern is accentuated by bradycardia) as well as metabolic effects such as hypothermia and hypocalcemia. The mere observation that the pattern is so common, and that unexplained sudden death is so rare, underscores the fact that the pattern alone is not a marker of significantly increased absolute risk at the individual level.

There also appears to be some overlap between ER and the Brugada and short QT syndromes. ER pattern is common among patients with Brugada syndrome (11–15%),[16] and many individuals with the ER syndrome have a relatively short QT interval.[17]

GENETIC UNDERPINNINGS

Although, the ER pattern has been shown to be partially heritable,[8] its genetic causes are not well established. Since the trait is so prevalent and varies with clinical factors and over time, it is unlikely to be a monogenetic disorder. However, mutations in KCNJ8,[18] L-type calcium channel genes (*CACNA1C, CACNB2B*, and *CACNA2D1*),[19] and *SCN5A*[20] have been identified in some isolated cases. Genome-wide association studies have identified several single nucleotide polymorphisms (one of which was located at the *KCND*3 gene),[6] but these data have not been widely replicated. Despite some recent inroads, the genetic architecture of the syndrome remains relatively unknown.

ASSOCIATION TO VENTRICULAR ARRHYTHMIAS AND SUDDEN DEATH

At the population level, there are data to suggest a slightly increased risk of sudden cardiac death (SCD) with the early repolarization pattern. The first major study to establish an association between ER and sudden death was a case-control study by Haissaguerre and colleagues in 2008 that demonstrated ER prevalence of 31% among SCD survivors compared to 5% in controls.[2] This study was followed by several confirmatory case-control studies,[21-23] and, ultimately prospective and community-based studies that demonstrated an incremental increased relative risk at the population level. The first major retrospective community-based study demonstrated a relative risk of 1.4 for inferior ER of >1 mm and 2.9 for ER >2 mm.[7] Subsequent retrospective community-based studies have demonstrated similar relative risks ranging from 1.4 to 2.5[11,24-26] with one study demonstrating no increased risk.[14] The preponderance of evidence suggests that the pattern confers some increased risk of arrhythmogenic sudden death, but it is important to understand that these relative risks do not translate to a high absolute risk to an individual. More important to the practicing electrophysiologist is the fact that individuals who have suffered an unexplained cardiac arrest and have ER pattern on ECG are at heightened risk of recurrent events.

MOLECULAR MECHANISMS OF THE J-WAVE, ST ELEVATION, AND VF

The J-wave occurs during phase 1 of the action potential (APL). During this phase, transient outward potassium current (so called I_{to}) results in a negative deflection just prior to the calcium-mediated plateau phase (phase 2), leading to a characteristic 'spike and dome' curvature of the APL. There is heterogeneity of the density of this current, such that the 'spike and dome' pattern prominent in the epicardium may be absent from the endocardium. The gradient between endo- and epicardial layers results in the generation of a prominent J-point on the surface ECG **(Figure 40.2)**.

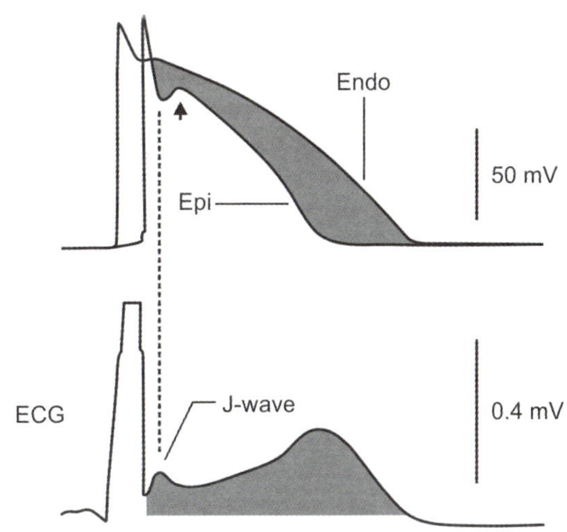

Figure 40.2: Simultaneous recordings of epicardial (Epi) and endocardial (Endo) action potentials (APLs) and a simulated ECG resulting from the gradient between these two layers. The ECG demonstrates a J-wave which reflects a prominent epicardial but not endocardial APL notch. Relative loss of the epicardial APL dome results in a epi-endo gradient which manifests as ST-segment elevation during the plateau phase. Modified from Yan and Antzelevitch[33]

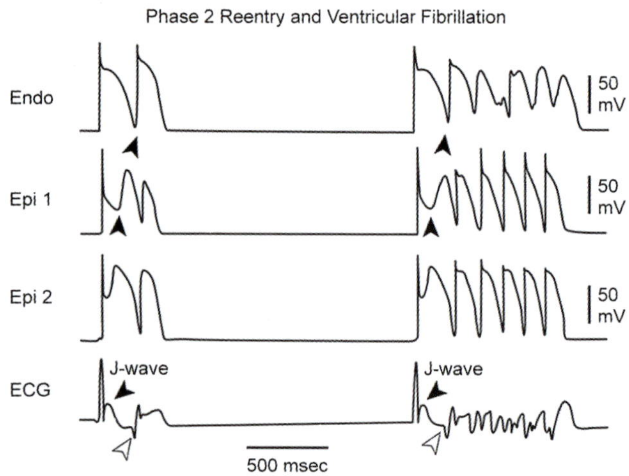

Figure 40.3: Phase 2 reentry resulting in ventricular fibrillation (VF). Loss of action potential (APL) dome in Epi 1 but not in Epi 2 caused propagation of an APL from Epi 2 to Epi 1 (phase 2 reentry, solid arrows). Phase 2 reentry can result in a short-coupled PVC (open arrows) capable of triggering VF. Modified from Yan and Antzelevitch[33]

Because I_{to} is slow to recover from the inactive state, the J-wave may be accentuated by bradycardia or after a pause. The dynamic nature of the J-wave is useful in distinguishing them from abnormalities of depolarization (QRS notching or delay).[27]

A prominent J-wave is often associated with ST-segment elevation. Accentuation of the notch in the action potential (increase in I_{to}) may result in sensitivity to repolarization currents during phase 2 and a reduction in the APL 'dome.' This can cause a continuous gradient during the plateau phase, which is inscribed as ST-segment elevation on the surface ECG.

When the I_{to} current is marked, it may result in inactivation of L-type calcium current and complete loss of the APL 'dome' and marked shortening of the APL. This local APL shortening induces marked repolarization heterogeneity and the opportunity for phase 2 reentry. An APL may propagate from the adjacent depolarized tissue to this repolarized tissue, resulting in a short-coupled premature ventricular contraction (PVC) and the potential for VF **(Figure 40.3)**.

RISK STRATIFICATION

Various electrocardiographic features have been associated with risk. For instance, the degree of J-point elevation appears to increase risk, with those with >2 mm at highest risk.[7] Further, the extent of the pattern (number of territories affected)[28] and the slope of the ST segment (**Figure 40.4**, horizontal or descending ST segment at higher risk than ascending)[25] are important considerations. Notching or slurring of the J-point (rather than a smooth J-point and ST segment) may also be a marker of risk.[29] Occasionally, pause-dependent accentuation of J-point elevation can be a harbinger of impending VF **(Figures 40.5A and B)**.[30] In general, ER found in healthy athletes tends to have an ascending ST segment, whereas ER associated with adverse outcomes in the general population tends to have a horizontal ST segment **(Figure 40.6)**.

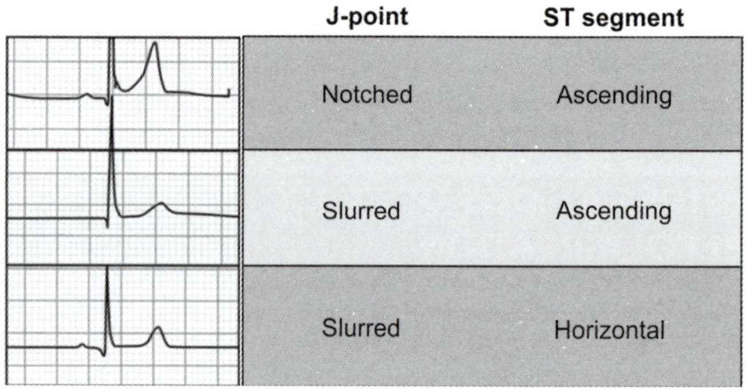

Figure 40.4: Early repolarization pattern, morphological classifications based on J-point and ST segment. Modified from Tanguturi VK et al.[10]

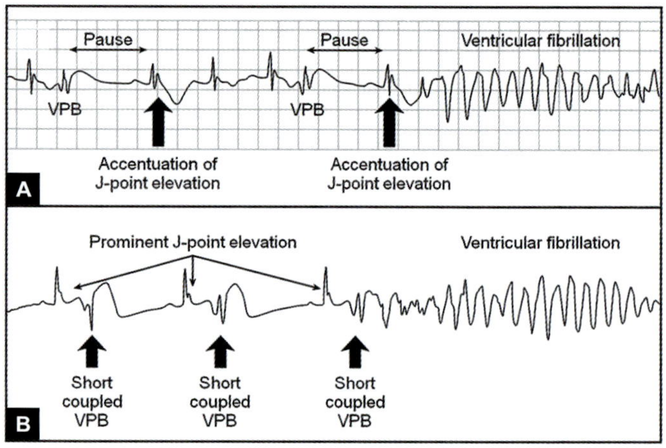

Figures 40.5A and B: (A) Pause-induced augmentation of the J-wave in a patient with ventricular fibrillation (VF) and the onset of VF. The pause was produced by a ventricular premature beat (VPB). Modified from Shinohara T et al.[34] (B) Short-coupled ventricular bigeminy in a middle-aged patient with prominent J-waves before the initiation of ventricular fibrillation. Modified from Aizawa Y et al.[30]

MANAGEMENT

Current HRS/EHRA/APHRS expert consensus recommendations on therapy for ER syndrome are outlined in **Table 40.2**. For patients with no symptoms, the implications of the ER pattern are uncertain, and no further diagnostic testing or intervention is warranted. Among patients at higher risk, the option for implantable cardioverter-defibrillator (ICD) implantation or medical therapy remains. According to the current guidelines, secondary prevention ICD implantation is warranted for those with ER syndrome.

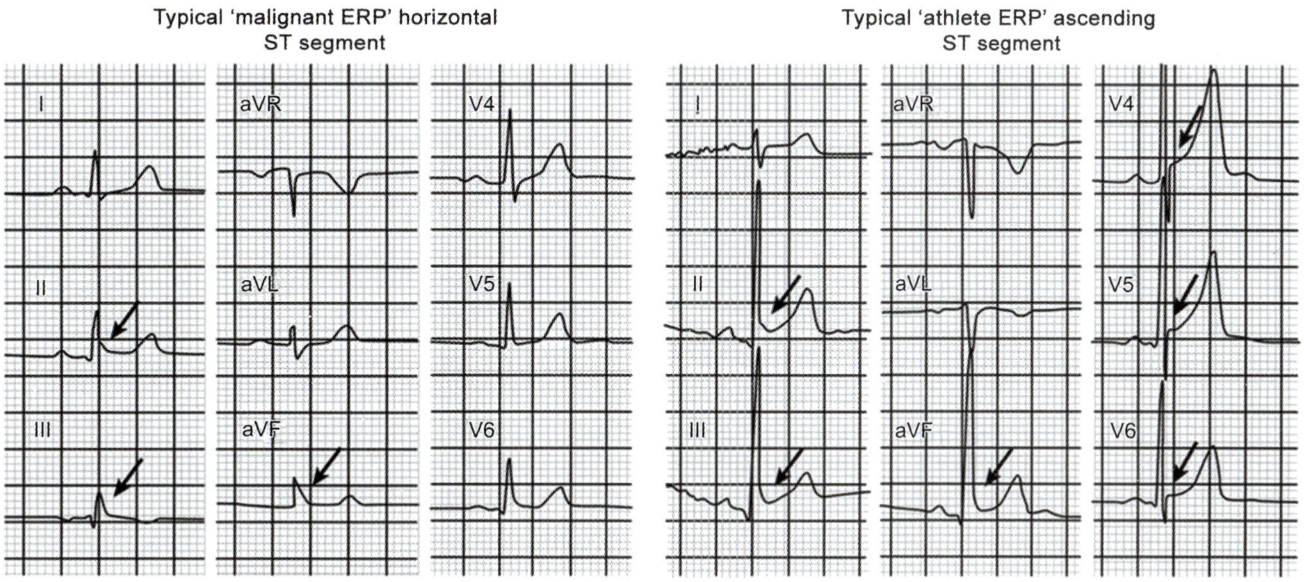

Figure 40.6: The typical early repolarization patterns seen in athletes and the pattern associated with adverse events in the general population. Modified from Tanguturi VK et al.[10]

Table 40.2: Recommendations on the management of early repolarization syndrome

Class	Recommendation
Class I	• ICD implantation is recommended in patients with a diagnosis of ER syndrome who have survived a cardiac arrest
Class IIa	• Isoproterenol infusion can be useful in suppressing electrical storms in patients with a diagnosis of ER syndrome • Quinidine in addition to an ICD can be useful for secondary prevention of VF in patients with a diagnosis of ER syndrome
Class IIb	• ICD implantation may be considered in symptomatic family members of ER syndrome patients with a history of syncope in the presence of ST-segment elevation >1 mm in 2 or more inferior or lateral leads • ICD implantation may be considered in asymptomatic individuals who demonstrate a high-risk ER ECG pattern (high J-wave amplitude, horizontal/descending ST segment) in the presence of a strong family history of juvenile unexplained sudden death with or without a pathogenic mutation
Class III	• ICD implantation is not recommended in asymptomatic individuals with isolated ER ECG pattern

Abbreviations: ER, early repolarization; ICD, implantable cardioverter-defibrillator; VF, ventricular fibrillation
Modified with permission from Priori et al.[31]

ICD implantation may be considered in some high risk family members of ER syndrome patients such as those with a history of syncope in the presence of a high risk ECG pattern (marked or horizontal/downsloping ST-segment elevation). Medical therapy may include isoproterenol infusion for acute management during electrical storm. Quinidine may be considered (as in Brugada syndrome) to prevent recurrent ICD therapies in high risk secondary prevention ER syndrome patients, though data on this approach are lacking.

REFERENCES

1. Otto CM, Tauxe RV, Cobb LA, Greene HL, Gross BW, Werner JA, Burroughs RW, Samson WE, Weaver WD, Trobaugh GB. Ventricular fibrillation causes sudden death in Southeast Asian immigrants. Ann Intern Med. 1984;101:45-7.
2. Haissaguerre M, Derval N, Sacher F, Jesel L, Deisenhofer I, de Roy L, Pasquie JL, Nogami A, Babuty D, Yli-Mayry S, De Chillou C, Scanu P, Mabo P, Matsuo S, Probst V, Le Scouarnec S, Defaye P, Schlaepfer J, Rostock T, Lacroix D, Lamaison D, Lavergne T, Aizawa Y, Englund A, Anselme F, O'Neill M, Hocini M, Lim KT, Knecht S, Veenhuyzen GD, Bordachar P, Chauvin M, Jais P, Coureau G, Chene G, Klein GJ, Clementy J. Sudden cardiac arrest associated with early repolarization. N Engl J Med. 2008;358:2016-23.
3. Surawicz B, Macfarlane PW. Inappropriate and confusing electrocardiographic terms: J-wave syndromes and early repolarization. J Am Coll Cardiol. 2011;57:1584-6.
4. Osborn JJ. Experimental hypothermia; respiratory and blood pH changes in relation to cardiac function. Am J Physiol. 1953;175:389-98.

5. Merchant FM, Noseworthy PA, Weiner RB, Singh SM, Ruskin JN, Reddy VY. Ability of terminal QRS notching to distinguish benign from malignant electrocardiographic forms of early repolarization. Am J Cardiol. 2009;104:1402-6.
6. Sinner MF, Porthan K, Noseworthy PA, Havulinna AS, Tikkanen JT, Muller-Nurasyid M, Peloso G, Ulivi S, Beckmann BM, Brockhaus AC, Cooper RR, Gasparini P, Hengstenberg C, Hwang SJ, Iorio A, Junttila MJ, Klopp N, Kahonen M, Laaksonen MA, Lehtimaki T, Lichtner P, Lyytikainen LP, Martens E, Meisinger C, Meitinger T, Merchant FM, Nieminen MS, Peters A, Pietila A, Perz S, Oikarinen L, Raitakari O, Reinhard W, Silander K, Thorand B, Wichmann HE, Sinagra G, Viikari J, O'Donnell CJ, Ellinor PT, Huikuri HV, Kaab S, Newton-Cheh C, Salomaa V. A meta-analysis of genome-wide association studies of the electrocardiographic early repolarization pattern. Heart Rhythm. 2012;9:1627-34.
7. Tikkanen JT, Anttonen O, Junttila MJ, Aro AL, Kerola T, Rissanen HA, Reunanen A, Huikuri HV. Long-term outcome associated with early repolarization on electrocardiography. N Engl J Med. 2009;361:2529-37.
8. Noseworthy PA, Tikkanen JT, Porthan K, Oikarinen L, Pietila A, Harald K, Peloso GM, Merchant FM, Jula A, Vaananen H, Hwang SJ, O'Donnell CJ, Salomaa V, Newton-Cheh C, Huikuri HV. The early repolarization pattern in the general population: clinical correlates and heritability. J Am Coll Cardiol. 2011;57:2284-9.
9. Noseworthy PA, Weiner R, Kim J, Keelara V, Wang F, Berkstresser B, Wood MJ, Wang TJ, Picard MH, Hutter AM, Jr., Newton-Cheh C, Baggish AL. Early repolarization pattern in competitive athletes: clinical correlates and the effects of exercise training. Circ Arrhythm Electrophysiol. 2011;4:432-40.
10. Tanguturi VK, Noseworthy PA, Newton-Cheh C, Baggish AL. The electrocardiographic early repolarization pattern in athletes: normal variant or sudden death risk factor? Sports Med. 2012;42:359-66.
11. Haruta D, Matsuo K, Tsuneto A, Ichimaru S, Hida A, Sera N, Imaizumi M, Nakashima E, Maemura K, Akahoshi M. Incidence and prognostic value of early repolarization pattern in the 12-lead electrocardiogram. Circulation. 2011;123: 2931-7.
12. Peidro RM, Brion GB, Bruzzese M, Castiello G. [Early repolarization in soccer players' ECG. Prevalence, characteristics and evolution]. Medicina (B Aires). 2014;74:443-7.
13. Quattrini FM, Pelliccia A, Assorgi R, DiPaolo FM, Squeo MR, Culasso F, Castelli V, Link MS, Maron BJ. Benign clinical significance of J-wave pattern (early repolarization) in highly trained athletes. Heart Rhythm. 2014;11:1974-82.
14. Uberoi A, Jain NA, Perez M, Weinkopff A, Ashley E, Hadley D, Turakhia MP, Froelicher V. Early repolarization in an ambulatory clinical population. Circulation. 2011;124: 2208-14.
15. Yan GX, Antzelevitch C. Cellular basis for the electrocardiographic J wave. Circulation. 1996;93:372-9.
16. Sarkozy A, Chierchia GB, Paparella G, Boussy T, De Asmundis C, Roos M, Henkens S, Kaufman L, Buyl R, Brugada R, Brugada J, Brugada P. Inferior and lateral electrocardiographic repolarization abnormalities in Brugada syndrome. Circ Arrhythm Electrophysiol. 2009;2:154-61.
17. Panicker GK, Manohar D, Karnad DR, Salvi V, Kothari S, Lokhandwala Y. Early repolarization and short QT interval in healthy subjects. Heart Rhythm. 2012;9:1265-71.
18. Haissaguerre M, Chatel S, Sacher F, Weerasooriya R, Probst V, Loussouarn G, Horlitz M, Liersch R, Schulze-Bahr E, Wilde A, Kaab S, Koster J, Rudy Y, Le Marec H, Schott JJ. Ventricular fibrillation with prominent early repolarization associated with a rare variant of KCNJ8/KATP channel. J Cardiovasc Electrophysiol. 2009;20:93-8.
19. Burashnikov E, Pfeiffer R, Barajas-Martinez H, Delpon E, Hu D, Desai M, Borggrefe M, Haissaguerre M, Kanter R, Pollevick GD, Guerchicoff A, Laino R, Marieb M, Nademanee K, Nam GB, Robles R, Schimpf R, Stapleton DD, Viskin S, Winters S, Wolpert C, Zimmern S, Veltmann C, Antzelevitch C. Mutations in the cardiac L-type calcium channel associated with inherited J-wave syndromes and sudden cardiac death. Heart Rhythm. 2010;7:1872-82.
20. Watanabe H, Nogami A, Ohkubo K, Kawata H, Hayashi Y, Ishikawa T, Makiyama T, Nagao S, Yagihara N, Takehara N, Kawamura Y, Sato A, Okamura K, Hosaka Y, Sato M, Fukae S, Chinushi M, Oda H, Okabe M, Kimura A, Maemura K, Watanabe I, Kamakura S, Horie M, Aizawa Y, Shimizu W, Makita N. Electrocardiographic characteristics and SCN5A mutations in idiopathic ventricular fibrillation associated with early repolarization. Circ Arrhythm Electrophysiol. 2011;4: 874-81.
21. Rosso R, Kogan E, Belhassen B, Rozovski U, Scheinman MM, Zeltser D, Halkin A, Steinvil A, Heller K, Glikson M, Katz A, Viskin S. J-point elevation in survivors of primary ventricular fibrillation and matched control subjects: incidence and clinical significance. J Am Coll Cardiol. 2008;52:1231-8.
22. Nam GB, Kim YH, Antzelevitch C. Augmentation of J waves and electrical storms in patients with early repolarization. N Engl J Med. 2008;358:2078-9.
23. Rosso R, Glikson E, Belhassen B, Katz A, Halkin A, Steinvil A, Viskin S. Distinguishing "benign" from "malignant early repolarization": the value of the ST-segment morphology. Heart Rhythm. 2012;9:225-9.
24. Sinner MF, Reinhard W, Muller M, Beckmann BM, Martens E, Perz S, Pfeufer A, Winogradow J, Stark K, Meisinger C, Wichmann HE, Peters A, Riegger GA, Steinbeck G, Hengstenberg C, Kaab S. Association of early repolarization pattern on ECG with risk of cardiac and all-cause mortality: a population-based prospective cohort study (MONICA/KORA). PLoS Med. 2010;7:e1000314.
25. Tikkanen JT, Junttila MJ, Anttonen O, Aro AL, Luttinen S, Kerola T, Sager SJ, Rissanen HA, Myerburg RJ, Reunanen A, Huikuri HV. Early repolarization: electrocardiographic phenotypes associated with favorable long-term outcome. Circulation. 2011;123:2666-73.
26. Olson KA, Viera AJ, Soliman EZ, Crow RS, Rosamond WD. Long-term prognosis associated with J-point elevation in a large middle-aged biracial cohort: the ARIC study. Eur Heart J. 2011;32:3098-106.
27. Aizawa Y, Sato M, Kitazawa H, Takatsuki S, Oda E, Okabe M, Fukuda K. Tachycardia-dependent augmentation of "notched J waves" in a general patient population without ventricular fibrillation or cardiac arrest: Not a repolarization but a depolarization abnormality? Heart Rhythm. 2015;12:376-83.
28. Derval N, Simpson CS, Birnie DH, Healey JS, Chauhan V, Champagne J, Gardner M, Sanatani S, Yee R, Skanes AC, Gula LJ, Leong-Sit P, Ahmad K, Gollob MH, Haissaguerre M, Klein GJ, Krahn AD. Prevalence and characteristics of early repolarization in the CASPER registry: cardiac arrest survivors

with preserved ejection fraction registry. J Am Coll Cardiol. 2011;58:722-8.
29. Merchant FM, Noseworthy PA, Weiner RB, Singh SM, Ruskin JN, Reddy VY. Ability of terminal QRS notching to distinguish benign from malignant electrocardiographic forms of early repolarization. Am J Cardiol. 2009;104:1402-6.
30. Aizawa Y, Sato A, Watanabe H, Chinushi M, Furushima H, Horie M, Kaneko Y, Imaizumi T, Okubo K, Watanabe I, Shinozaki T, Fukuda K, Joo K, Haissaguerre M. Dynamicity of the J-wave in idiopathic ventricular fibrillation with a special reference to pause-dependent augmentation of the J-wave. J Am Coll Cardiol. 2012;59:1948-53.
31. Priori SG, Wilde AA, Horie M, Cho Y, Behr ER, Berul C, Blom N, Brugada J, Chiang CE, Huikuri H, Kannankeril P, Krahn A, Leenhardt A, Moss A, Schwartz PJ, Shimizu W, Tomaselli G, Tracy C. HRS/EHRA/APHRS expert consensus statement on the diagnosis and management of patients with inherited primary arrhythmia syndromes: document endorsed by HRS, EHRA, and APHRS in May 2013 and by ACCF, AHA, PACES, and AEPC in June 2013. Heart Rhythm. 2013;10:1932-63.
32. Tikkanen JT, Huikuri HV. Characteristics of "malignant" vs. "benign" electrocardiographic patterns of early repolarization. J Electrocardiol. 2015;48:390-4.
33. Yan GX, Antzelevitch C. Cellular basis for the Brugada syndrome and other mechanisms of arrhythmogenesis associated with ST-segment elevation. Circulation. 1999;100:1660-6.
34. Shinohara T, Takahashi N, Saikawa T, Yoshimatsu H. Characterization of J wave in a patient with idiopathic ventricular fibrillation. Heart Rhythm. 2006;3:1082-4.

EDITORS' SUMMARY

Among the most vexing situations that we as electrophysiologists need to think about and advise patients on occurs when a pattern of early repolarization is noted on an electrocardiogram. The whole spectrum of a benign incidental finding that requires no further evaluation all the way to diagnosing the culprit for a sudden cardiac death event is evoked. Dr Noseworthy provides an outstanding summary of our current knowledge in a straightforward and practical manner. A thorough reading of this chapter will serve as a foundation not only on what we know about the syndrome but what remains undefined. A comparison between the specific early repolarization syndrome and other J-wave syndromes is discussed in depth elsewhere (Chapter 39), and these two chapters read in conjunction with others that discuss cellular arrhythmogenesis and arrhythmia mechanism would serve the student of electrophysiology with a cornerstone upon which our clinical decision making and invasive diagnostic and ablative therapy are based.

CHAPTER 41

Arnon Adler, Raphael Rosso, Sami Viskin

Idiopathic Ventricular Fibrillation: Mechanisms and Management Strategies

LIST OF ABBREVIATIONS

ACTN-2	Alpha Actinin-2
ARVC	Arrhythmogenic Right Ventricular Cardiomyopathy
AV	Atrioventricular
BrS	Brugada Syndrome
CA	Cardiac Arrest
CASPER	Cardiac Arrest Survivors with Preserved Ejection Fraction Registry
CPVT	Catecholaminergic Polymorphic Ventricular Tachycardia
DPP-6	Dipeptidyl Aminopeptidase-like Protein-6
EPS	Electrophysiology Study
ERS	Early Repolarization Syndrome
HCM	Hypertrophic Cardiomyopathy
ICD	Implantable Cardioverter-Defibrillator
LQTS	Long QT Syndrome
PVC	Premature Ventricular Contraction
RVOT	Right Ventricular Outflow Tract
RYR2	Ryanodine Receptor 2
SCD	Sudden Cardiac Death
SEMA3A	Semaphorin 3A
SQTS	Short QT Syndrome
VF	Ventricular Fibrillation
VT	Ventricular Tachycardia
WPW	Wolff-Parkinson-White

INTRODUCTION

Idiopathic ventricular fibrillation (VF) is a rare but lethal disease that typically strikes without warning and at a young age.[1] Many of those who survive the first event suffer from recurrent arrhythmias and, therefore, are at considerable risk of sudden cardiac death (SCD).[2] Consequently, despite being rare, idiopathic VF has a significant impact on morbidity and mortality.

As the term implies, idiopathic VF is a diagnosis of exclusion; only after all possible causes of cardiac arrest (CA) are ruled-out can the diagnosis be made. As a result, patients with idiopathic VF are probably a heterogeneous group comprised of patients with different, yet unidentified, medical conditions. Indeed, in the past two and a half decades the identification of Brugada syndrome (BrS),[3] short QT syndrome (SQTS)[4] and, recently, early repolarization syndrome (ERS)[2] has shifted patients' diagnosis from idiopathic VF to these "new" syndromes. Nevertheless, typical patients with idiopathic VF share several clinical characteristics that may differentiate them from other CA survivors and enable us to reach a diagnosis based on inclusion criteria as well. In this chapter, we will focus on these patients and discuss the approach to their diagnosis and management.

WHAT IS IDIOPATHIC VENTRICULAR FIBRILLATION?

In a recent expert consensus statement endorsed by major heart rhythm societies[5] an idiopathic VF patient was defined as "....a resuscitated cardiac arrest victim, preferably with documentation of VF, in whom known cardiac, respiratory, metabolic and toxicological etiologies have been excluded through clinical evaluation." Importantly, VF documentation is not actually required for clinching the diagnosis according to this definition. Nevertheless, documentation of VF and, especially, its mode of initiation, are important for identification of the "classic" idiopathic VF patient as will be discussed below.

EPIDEMIOLOGY

The exact prevalence of idiopathic VF is unknown, yet some insight may be gained from the incidence of unexplained SCD which is estimated to be between 0.76 and 1.34 per 100,000.[6-8] As the difference between "unexplained CA" and "unexplained SCD" may be merely a few minutes in delay of the emergency medical services, it may be assumed that the incidence of idiopathic VF is generally similar (i.e. very rare). It is important to remember, however, that unexplained SCD and idiopathic VF are not synonymous. Not only may there be confounding factors other than time to emergency medical service contact, the postmortem evaluation is very different from the work-up of a survivor of CA, making exclusion of many syndromes difficult in the deceased. Indeed, one study showed that familial evaluation of unexplained CA patients yielded a diagnosis in 62% but only in 18% of families of SCD victims was a diagnosis made.[9]

CLINICAL CHARACTERISTICS

Based on published data from idiopathic VF series[1,2] the majority of patients (54–73%) are male. The mean age at presentation in these series was 36–37, with 73% of patients being younger than 45 years.[1]

The presenting symptoms are, as expected, syncope or CA. However, unlike in other syndromes presenting with polymorphic ventricular arrhythmias, [e.g. long QT syndrome (LQTS), catecholaminergic polymorphic ventricular tachycardia (CPVT)] the majority of idiopathic VF patients present with CA rather than syncope.[10] In fact, about 25% present with arrhythmic storms (clusters of recurrent VF occurring within 24–48 hours).[1,11,12] Another distinction between idiopathic VF and many of the other primary arrhythmia syndromes is the lack of specific triggers- only 4% were found to suffer CA during sleep and 13% during physical effort.[2]

THE ELECTROCARDIOGRAM

As a rule, the ECG of patients with idiopathic VF is normal. As exclusion of all other causes of CA is obligatory, this is not surprising. The only positive finding in these patients is a *relatively* short QT interval. Patients with idiopathic VF (particularly males) have been found to have shorter QT intervals than age-matched controls (often in 360–370 ms range) and have insufficient QT prolongation during slow heart rates.[13,14] Based on these findings it was proposed that some of the idiopathic VF patients actually have "SQTS with not so-short QT intervals".[15] The fact that around half of LQTS patients are now known to have borderline or frankly normal corrected QT intervals[16] serves as precedence to this hypothesis. Further support comes from SQTS mutation-carriers with corrected QT intervals in the low-normal range demonstrating that "concealed SQTS" is possible.[17,18]

The typical ventricular arrhythmia in idiopathic VF is polymorphic ventricular tachycardia (VT) or VF triggered by a short-coupled premature ventricular contraction (PVC) **(Figures 41.1A to C)**. In several series, the mean coupling interval was 300 ms with a confidence interval of about ±40 ms.[19-22] Because of the short coupling interval, the PVCs fall on the summit or on the descending limb of the T-wave. In the series from our center,[19] all VF episodes were started by PVCs falling within 40 ms (with the vast majority falling within 20 ms) of the peak of the T-wave. Furthermore, there appears to be an inverse relationship between the coupling interval of the PVC and the risk for malignant arrhythmias with longer bursts of polymorphic VT triggered by PVCs with shorter coupling intervals.[20] Although one publication suggest that idiopathic VF often has a pause dependent initiation,[22] other publications and many illustrations suggest otherwise.[1,2,11,12,21]

In early reports showing the onset of idiopathic VF,[1,11,23] a similar ECG pattern of the first short-coupled ventricular PVC was observed, namely left bundle branch block pattern and left axis. However, later reports,[20,24] showed that initiating PVCs with other patterns also exist, suggesting various possible sites of origin. Interestingly, when multiple episodes of polymorphic VTs are recorded with 12-lead recordings, the morphology of the initiating beats of all these episodes is similar. This applies not only to the first complex, but to the second and third complexes of the polymorphic arrhythmias as well **(Figure 41.2)**. The last observation supports the notion that idiopathic VF has a focal origin (see "possible mechanisms" below).[20,24]

ELECTROPHYSIOLOGICAL DATA

Like with the electrocardiogram, the electrophysiologic study in patients with idiopathic VF is generally normal. The A-H

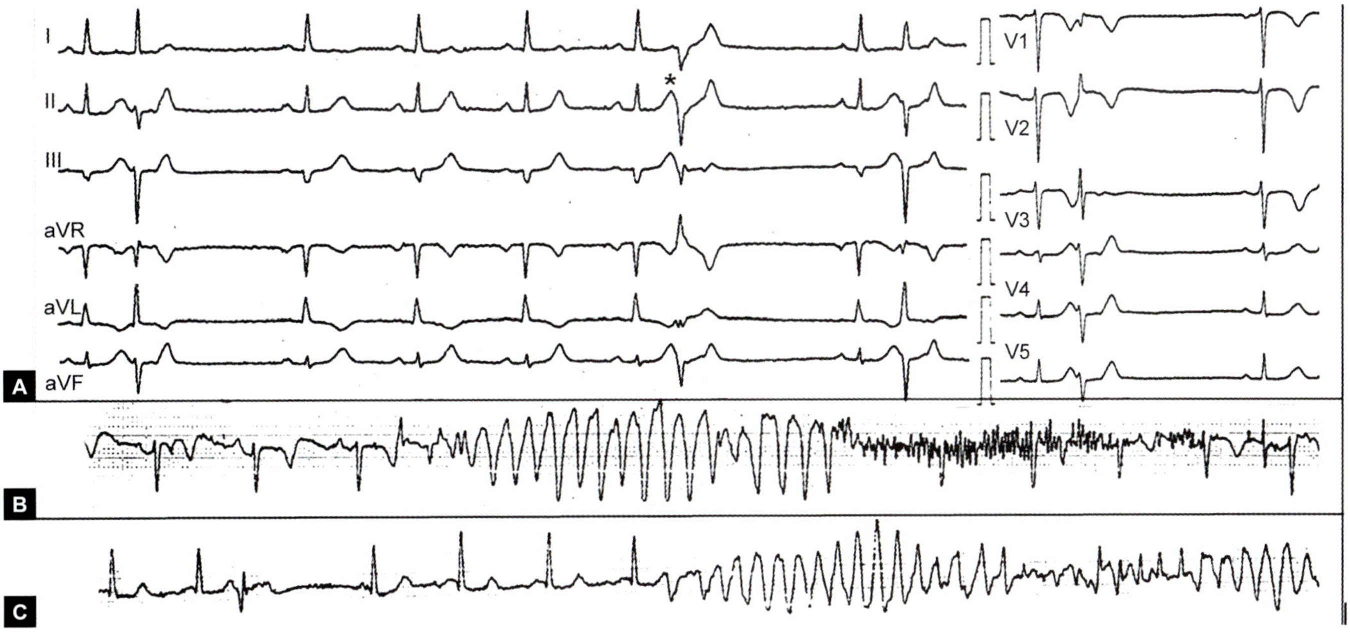

Figures 41.1A to C: Typical example of idiopathic VF. This 54-year-old female was referred for neurological consultation because of "recurrent seizures." Her baseline electrocardiogram shows sinus rhythm with normal PR, QRS and QT intervals (A). However, there are several ventricular extrasystoles with varying coupling intervals, including short-coupled extrasystoles falling on the peak of the preceding T-wave (*). Because of the short-coupled extrasystoles the patient was admitted to the Cardiology Department (instead of the Neurology Department). Soon thereafter a self-terminating episode of rapid polymorphic ventricular tachycardia was recorded during one of her "seizures" (B). Ventricular fibrillation requiring defibrillation was also recorded shortly thereafter (C). The patient was diagnosed with "idiopathic ventricular fibrillation" and has been free of ventricular arrhythmias during treatment with quinidine for more than 10 years

and H-V intervals and the ventricular refractory periods are unremarkable.[25,26] This is in contrast to patients with BrS, who often have prolonged H-V interval[3] and patients with SQTS, who have short refractory periods in the atrium and the ventricle.[27,28]

The ventricular arrhythmias induced by programmed ventricular stimulation are invariably of polymorphic morphology, namely polymorphic VT or VF. Induction of monomorphic VT makes the diagnosis of idiopathic VF highly unlikely. This is at variance with patients with Brugada syndrome who, although usually present with polymorphic VT/VF, [29] may rarely have monomorphic VT.[30-34]

As the inducibility rate is a function of the protocol used during programmed ventricular stimulation, many electrophysiologists are reluctant to shorten the coupling interval of the delivered ventricular extrastimuli beyond a "nominal" value of 200 ms. This is because the risk of "accidentally" inducing VF in healthy individuals also increases as the coupling interval of the second and third extrastimuli is shortened below 200 ms.[35-37] Indeed, in small studies performed 20 years ago, 9% of healthy individuals without documented or suspected spontaneous ventricular arrhythmias had inducible VF when the coupling intervals were limited only by ventricular refractoriness.[35-37] Moreover, an additional 40% of these healthy subjects had inducible nonsustained polymorphic VT that lead to premature discontinuation of the pacing protocol. Therefore, one must recognize that *at least* 9% of healthy individuals will have inducible VF if aggressive protocols with double and triple extrastimulation and coupling intervals shorter than 200 ms are used.[38] In patients with idiopathic VF, it is our experience that as many as 80% have inducible VF with such aggressive protocols at two right ventricular pacing sites and using repetition of extrastimulation at the shortest coupling interval that captures the ventricle.[23,25,26] One study reported much lower percentage of VF induction but detailed extrastimulation protocols were not published making direct comparison difficult.[20]

Haissaguerre et al. performed endocardial recordings in patients with idiopathic VF at a time when they had frequent spontaneous PVCs and/or bursts of polymorphic VT.[20,24] The investigators were able to locate the site of origin of these ventricular arrhythmias in 27 patients. Successful localization was guided by very early endocardial recordings and confirmed by abolition of these ventricular arrhythmias following radiofrequency ablation of the firing focus. Purkinje potentials were recorded at the site of origin of ventricular arrhythmias in 23 (85%) out of these 27 patients

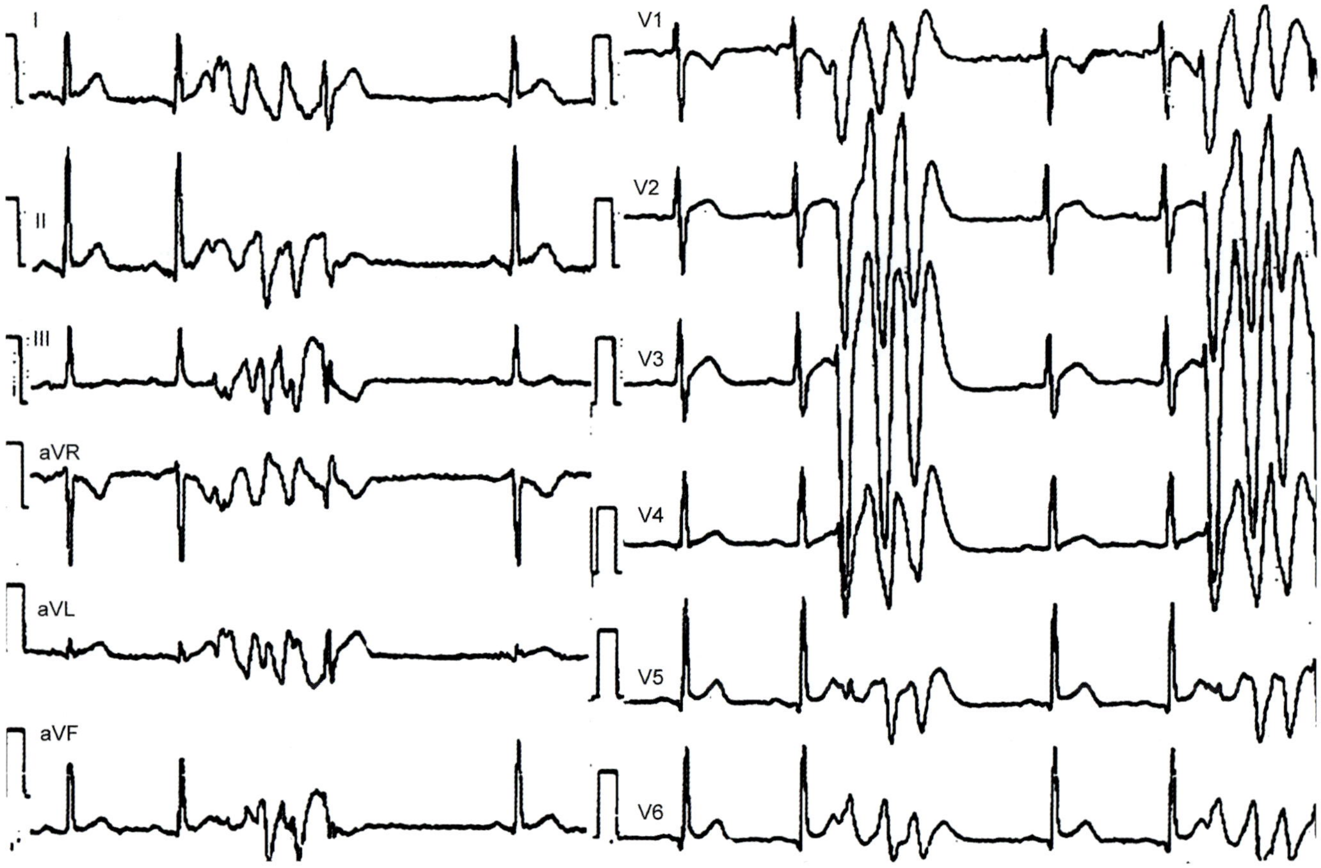

Figure 41.2: Typical mode of onset of idiopathic VF. Note the very short coupling interval of the extrasystoles initiating the polymorphic ventricular tachycardia. Also, note that despite the polymorphic morphology of the arrhythmia, when more than one VT episode is recorded (like in the precordial leads), the first, second and third complexes of the tachycardias are remarkably similar

(in the left ventricular septum in 10 patients, the anterior right ventricle in 9 patients and in both locations in 4). The Purkinje potentials preceded the local myocardial activation by 11 ± 5 ms during sinus rhythm and by 38 ± 28 ms during spontaneous ventricular ectopy.[20,24] These endocardial recordings, like the electrocardiographic findings described above, suggest that idiopathic VF has a focal origin and that the triggering focus is within the Purkinje fibers in the majority of patients. Of note, the firing focus was not within the Purkinje network in only 4 (15%) patients and in all these patients the arrhythmias originated in the right ventricular outflow tract (RVOT). It is possible that idiopathic VF originating from the RVOT, the "short-coupled variant of RVOT" described by our group,[39] and the "malignant idiopathic RVOT-VT described by Noda[40] represent the same entity.

POSSIBLE MECHANISMS

As alluded to in the introduction, patients with BrS, SQTS or ERS have been previously regarded as idiopathic VF patients. Though these syndromes and idiopathic VF are now regarded as separate entities, they share some common clinical characteristics: (1) the majority of patients are young adult males,[1,2,41-43] (2) the arrhythmias are not exercise- or stress-related,[1,2,4,44] (3) the arrhythmias are polymorphic by nature [2,3,45] and (4) there is a favorable response to quinidine.[12,25,42,46] It is, therefore, plausible that similarities in the pathophysiology of these 4 conditions also exist. The fact that patients with idiopathic VF and ERS have been demonstrated to have relatively short QT intervals[2,15] further supports this hypothesis.

In the case of BrS and ERS there is an accumulating body of evidence suggesting that both syndromes share repolarization abnormalities.[47] Specifically, an outward shift of early repolarization currents has been implicated. Such a shift may be due to decrease in calcium or sodium currents or increase in potassium currents (I_{to}, $T_{K\text{-}ATP}$ or I_{ACh}).[47] Similarly, in SQTS abbreviation of the action potential is thought to result from abnormal augmentation of one of the potassium currents (I_{Kr}, I_{Ks} or I_{K1}) or reduction in calcium currents.[48] In all these cases, differences in the degree of abbreviation of the action potential between different myocardial layers (endo-, mid- and epicardium) is thought to result in transmural dispersion of repolarization setting the stage for initiation and maintenance of reentry arrhythmias.[47,48] Data connecting to a possibly similar pathophysiology in idiopathic VF was found in large Dutch kindred with idiopathic VF and a risk haplotype spanning the dipeptidyl aminopeptidase-like protein-6 (*DPP6*) gene.[49] The risk haplotype was associated with over-expression of DPP6. Although this protein is not an ionic channel, it has been shown to influence trafficking and kinetics of the I_{to} channel.[50,51] Interestingly, a recent in-vitro study demonstrated that DPP6 is highly expressed in Purkinje fibers but to a lesser extent in ventricular myocardium.[52] Furthermore, over-expression of DPP6 augmented I_{to} in canine Purkinje cells but not in ventricular myocytes. Therefore, it was suggested that a local gradient of repolarization between Purkinje fibers and adjacent myocardium is responsible for arrhythmogenesis in these patients. The relatively small mass of Purkinje fibers relative to ventricular myocardium may explain why in patients with the Dutch risk haplotype the ECG is normal while in other I_{to}-related syndromes (e.g. BrS) it is not.[52]

Further evidence implicating Purkinje fibers in idiopathic VF pathophysiology comes from a recent study on a family with multiple idiopathic VF cases presenting during childhood or adolescence.[53] Exome sequencing identified a mutation in the *CALM1* gene encoding for calmodulin. This mutation was subsequently shown to reduce protein stability, Ca^{2+} binding affinity and interaction with the ryanodine receptor.[54] Importantly, *CALM1* mRNA was found in greater abundance in Purkinje fibers than in atrial or ventricular myocardium.[55] The greater expression of these genes in Purkinje fibers is of special interest due to the prior observations by Haissaguerre linking these fibers to the origin of PVCs in idiopathic VF patients.[24]

Role of Genetics

In rare cases, a clear family history of SCD may be obtained from patients with CA of unknown etiology. In few such cases, genetic studies have been able to isolate specific mutations and segregate them with disease. The most robust data linking a specific mutation with idiopathic VF comes from Dutch kindred carrying the *DPP6* risk halpotype (see previous section).[49] Although no mutations were found in the coding region of the *DPP6* gene, a variant (c.1-340C>T) thought to effect gene regulation resulting in overexpression of DPP6, was discovered. In symptomatic patients, "typical" idiopathic VF arrhythmias (i.e. polymorphic VT triggered by short-coupled PVCs) were documented. In fact, this haplotype was found to be so malignant (50% of affected patients dying or suffering CA before the age of 60) that asymptomatic mutation carriers between the ages of 20 and 50 were recommended to undergo implantable cardioverter-defibrillator (ICD) implantation for *primary* prevention.[56] Importantly, such a recommendation is specific to carriers of this risk haplotype and not generally advised for other idiopathic VF patients' family members.

The second gene to be associated with idiopathic VF is *CALM1* encoding for calmodulin.[53] A missense mutation (p.F90L) was found in 3 siblings suffering CA or SCD during childhood and adolescence. In one of the patients, ICD recordings demonstrated episodes of VF which were neither pause-dependent nor initiated by short-coupled PVC. Although mutations in genes encoding for calmodulin have been previously associated with LQTS and CPVT,[57,58] the patients studied did not have exercise-induced arrhythmias or significant QT-prolongation. It was speculated that calmodulin mutations result in different phenotypes with different mechanism depending on the mutation's effect on protein and calcium binding sites.[53]

Recently, a mutation in the alpha-actinin-2 (*ACTN2*) gene was segregated with disease in 2 families.[59] Typical short-coupled PVCs initiating polymorphic VT were documented in some affected family members without evidence of structural heart disease. However, the phenotype was highly variable with some mutation-carriers having hypertrophic cardiomyopathy (HCM) and others left-ventricular non-compaction. Therefore, the exact role of this gene in "pure" idiopathic VF remains to be resolved.

Mutations in the ryanodine receptor-2 (*RYR2*) gene, typically associated with CPVT, were found in some CA patients without exercise-induced arrhythmias.[60-62] Whether these patients should be regarded as idiopathic VF patients or atypical CPVT patients is unclear. Finally, a polymorphism in the Semaphorin 3A (*SEMA3A*) gene affecting sympathetic innervation has been associated with unexplained CA.[63] However, more research is required in order to substantiate its role in idiopathic VF.

DIAGNOSIS

By definition, diagnosis of idiopathic VF is based on the exclusion of all other etiologies of CA. A detailed discussion on all possible causes of CA/SCD is beyond the scope of this chapter; however, some general principles should be kept in mind. First and foremost, there is no alternative to a detailed and systematic diagnostic evaluation at the time of presentation. The treating cardiologist may sometimes forget that, although sudden unexplained CA is frequently the result of a cardiac disease, it is not invariably so. This is especially true in cases in which loss of consciousness is unwitnessed and VF is not documented. Furthermore, detailed electrocardiographic documentation in the initial time period after presentation is crucial for subsequent diagnosis. An effort should be made to record 12-lead ECGs, monitor strips and, especially, initiation of sustained and nonsustained arrhythmias. Unfortunately, this is easier said

Table 41.1: Diagnostic tests for evaluation of patients with undiagnosed cardiac arrest

Diagnostic test	*Conditions in which test may be positive*
ECG-based tests	
ECG with elevated leads	BrS[75]
SAECG	All cardiomyopathies,[106,107] BrS,[108-110] sarcoidosis[111]
Holter	ARVC,[107] LQTS,[112] BrS,[113,114] SQTS,[115] ERS,[80] coronary vasospasm,[116] "M-RVOT-VT"[39,40]
Imaging	
Echocardiogram	All cardiomyopathies, myocarditis, valvular heart disease
Coronary angiography	Coronary artery disease/vasospasm#
Cardiac MRI	All cardiomyopathies†, myocarditis, sarcoidosis[117]
Cardiac PET CT*	Sarcoidosis[118]
Provocation tests	
Quick standing test	LQTS[119,120]
Exercise test	LQTS,[121] CPVT,[122] ARVC,[123] BrS[124]‡
Epinephrine tests*	LQTS,[125,126] CPVT,[122] ARVC[127]
Sodium-channel blockers	BrS[75]
Adenosine test	Preexcitation,[128] LQTS[129]
*EP Study**	Preexcitation,[84] ARVC,[130] SQTS[27,42]

Order of tests depends on clinical findings.
*Provisional tests
#If provocative tests are used
†Especially useful in ARVC and subtle forms of other cardiomyopathies
‡Brugada pattern during recovery
Abbreviations: ARVC, arrhythmogenic right ventricular cardiomyopathy; BrS, Brugada syndrome; CPVT, catecholaminergic polymorphic ventricular tachycardia; EP, electrophysiology; ERS, early repolarization syndrome; HCM, hypertrophic cardiomyopathy; LQTS, long QT syndrome; MRI, magnetic resonance imaging; M-RVOT-VT, malignant right ventricular outflow tract VT; PET-CT, positron emission tomography-computed tomography; SAECG, signal averaged ECG; SQTS, short QT syndrome

than done and lack of such information frequently impedes diagnostic work-up at a later time.

A tiered approach for evaluation of CA survivors was implemented in the Cardiac Arrest Survivors With Preserved Ejection Fraction Registry (CASPER).[64] Such an approach was demonstrated to result in a diagnosis in more than half of the unexplained CA cases (i.e. with normal echocardiogram, coronary angiogram and ECG). **Table 41.1** lists suggested diagnostic tests for the evaluation of CA patients.

Genetic testing for evaluation of patients with unexplained cardiac arrest should be limited to those cases in which a specific condition is suspected.[5] Genetic testing of a wide panel of genes in cases without such suspicion should be avoided. In idiopathic VF patients with a strong family history of CA/SCD there may be a place for genetic testing. Nevertheless, the data to date regarding possible genes to be tested is scarce and, therefore, such evaluation should be limited to research or highly specialized centers.

Differential Diagnosis

Subtle Forms of Structural Heart Disease

In most cases an echocardiogram suffices for the diagnosis or exclusion of structural heart disease. However, in some cases CA may occur in cardiomyopathies without significant abnormalities demonstrated by echocardiogram. Such cases include certain types of HCM,[65,66] arrhythmogenic right ventricular cardiomyopathy (ARVC),[67] granulomatous myocarditis and certain other mild forms of myocarditis. Therefore, cardiac MRI with gadolinium injection, which is more sensitive for wall motion abnormalities and may also demonstrate edema and fibrosis, should be an integral part of any unexplained CA evaluation. Cardiac MRI may also be of benefit in the exclusion of sarcoidosis which is a rare cause of CA even in the absence of extracardiac manifestations.[68]

At the same time it is important to remember that signs of severe left ventricular dysfunction after resuscitation should not necessarily be used to exclude the diagnosis of idiopathic VF because prolonged resuscitation may result in transient electrocardiographic and echocardiographic abnormalities that are indistinguishable from those seen in patients with dilated cardiomyopathy.[69,70] If such abnormalities resolve, the diagnosis of idiopathic VF should obviously be considered.

"Forme Fruste" of Other Primary Arrhythmia Syndromes

Although the majority of primary arrhythmias will be readily diagnosed based on personal and family history and ECG, some forms of these disorders may be missed if a high level of suspicion is not maintained. For instance, in LQTS 12% of patients have corrected QT intervals in the normal range (<440 ms)[71,72] and in BrS only a third of patients have persistent Brugada pattern on recurrent ECGs.[73] It is, therefore, important to utilize appropriate tests (see **Table 1**) in order to rule out these disorders. SQTS requires special attention, as a clear QT interval cut-off for diagnosis is a matter of debate.[5] A corrected QT interval of 330 ms is usually used for strict criteria, however, it is reasonable to suspect that subtle forms of SQTS with "not so short QT" exist (see "the electrocardiogram" section above).[72] In this regard holter testing for evaluation of appropriate QT prolongation during bradycardia may be of value in patients with QT intervals in the low-normal range.[74]

Similar to the precautions with structural heart disease, some findings immediately after CA may erroneously be regarded as diagnostic of primary arrhythmia syndromes. ST segment elevation in right precordial leads after cardioversion of CA does not necessarily indicate BrS.[75] Likewise, QT prolongation or J-point elevation are frequently found during hypothermia and should not be used as proof of LQTS or ERS.

Early Repolarization Syndrome

ERS is the "youngest" of all primary arrhythmia syndromes, described only in the past few years. In a consensus statement endorsed by major heart rhythm societies, patients with ERS are basically defined as idiopathic VF patients with J-point elevation of at least 1 mm on 2 contiguous non-right precordial leads.[5] Nevertheless, the high prevalence of J-point elevation in the general population, estimated to be 3–13%,[76-79] makes it possible that at least some of these patients have idiopathic VF with J-point elevation being an innocent bystander (i.e. early repolarization does not play a role in arrhythmogenesis in these patients). Practically speaking, this has little impact on the patients themselves as management of patients with idiopathic VF and ERS is currently very similar,[80] however, this may have significance for family screening in some cases. A detailed discussion regarding ERS may be found in Chapters 39 and 40 and in several contemporary reviews.[81-83]

Preexcitation

Patients with atrioventricular accessory pathways may have minimal or no ventricular preexcitation (i.e. may have narrow QRS complexes) if they also have fast conduction along the AV node or if their accessory pathways is located on the left lateral wall (far away from the sinus node). Yet, these pathways may have short refractory periods. Such patients may develop atrial fibrillation with rapid ventricular rates that may deteriorate to VF. If the preexcited atrial fibrillation is not recorded and the patient is found in VF, the near-normal electrocardiogram during sinus rhythm may lead to an erroneous diagnosis of "idiopathic VF" because all imaging tests will be normal. The diagnosis of idiopathic VF may erroneously gain further support from electrophysiologic studies if *atrial* stimulation is not performed prior to ventricular pacing because programmed ventricular stimulation is likely to induce VF in patients with Wolff-Parkinson-White (WPW) syndrome.[84] Therefore, excluding accessory pathways–either with adenosine injection as a bedside test or with atrial pacing during electrophysiologic studies is a mandatory step in the work-up of VF survivors even when the electrocardiogram is judged to be "normal." Of note, rare cases of cardiac arrest caused by very rapid supraventricular tachyarrhythmias in patients without preexcitation have also been described.[85]

Short-coupled Variant of Right Ventricular Outflow Tachycardia

The RVOT is the site of origin of the most common type of VT occurring in patients *without* organic heart disease.[11] This RVOT-VT has a distinctive morphology (QRS complexes with left bundle branch block pattern and tall R-waves in the inferior leads) and, in general, does not lead to hemodynamic decompensation. Therefore, RVOT-VT is considered a benign arrhythmia.[11] However, our group[39] and the group of Noda and Shimizu[40] have described patients with otherwise typical "benign RVOT ectopy" who went on to develop spontaneous VF or polymorphic VT. It is not clear if patients with idiopathic VF and patients with this form of "polymorphic VT from the RVOT" represent different aspects of one disease or two distinct disorders.[86] However, several characteristics differ between both groups: (1) patients with malignant polymorphic RVOT-VT usually also have *monomorphic* RVOT-VT,[39,40] however monomorphic arrhythmias are never seen in idiopathic VF, (2) Only 5% of patients with "malignant polymorphic RVOT-VT"[39,40] but the majority of idiopathic VF patients[11,23] have inducible VF by programmed ventricular stimulation, (3) the coupling interval of the ventricular PVCs initiating the malignant ventricular arrhythmias is invariably very short in idiopathic VF[1,19] but is longer, varying from "relatively short"[39] to "normal"[40] in the "polymorphic RVOT-VT".[87] The last observation is consistent with the results of intracardiac mapping performed by Haissaguerre et al.[20] In that series, idiopathic VF originated from Purkinje fibers in 85% of the patients and from the RVOT in the remaining 15%. Again, the coupling interval of the PVCs initiating VF was *longer* for arrhythmias originating in the RVOT than for arrhythmias triggered by Purkinje fibers (355 ± 30 ms vs 280 ± 26 ms, $p<0.01$).[20]

Coronary Vasospasm

Coronary vasospasm should be suspected in any case of CA preceded by chest pain in the absence of significant coronary stenosis. Furthermore, asymptomatic episodes triggering arrhythmias have been described making this diagnosis possible in patients without angina as well.[88,89] Diagnosis, however, remains a challenge due to the transient nature of findings (e.g. ST-segment elevation) and lack of clear guidelines.[90]

Ambulatory ECG monitoring demonstrating transient ST-elevation may be useful for diagnosis in patients with recurrent events.[89] Diagnostic provocation tests (e.g. ergonovine, acetylcholine) have been shown to be effective, however they are not always utilized.[90] In the CASPER registry, for instance, coronary spasm was diagnosed in 11% of patients with CA of unknown etiology-based solely on transient ST-segment elevation and lack of significant coronary stenosis.[64] Provocation tests were not used.

Heat Stroke

A recent study suggests that heat stroke is an under-diagnosed cause of SCD and CA during endurance racing[91] As heat stroke may be easily missed if timely *rectal* temperature is not measured, a high level of suspicion is required in any CA case occurring during prolonged high endurance activity in high (or relatively high) ambient temperatures.

MANAGEMENT

Several studies reported the outcomes of patients with idiopathic VF followed for several years (mean- 42 to 76 months). In all these studies, the recurrence rate of major arrhythmic episodes, majority of which were appropriate ICD shocks, was high (23–46%).[2,21,92,93] One study reported the time to first recurrence to be between 1 and 27 months.[21] In our experience, patients suffered cardiac events up to 8 years after the first episode indicating that even a long period with the absence of symptoms cannot be regarded as a sign of low risk. Fortunately, effective therapy for both prevention and treatment of arrhythmic episodes in idiopathic VF is available. These treatments include ICD implantation, quinidine and ablation.

Implantable Cardioverter-Defibrillator

ICD implantation is the only treatment option for idiopathic VF patients that has a Class I recommendation.[5] Although there is no doubt that ICDs are very effective in treatment of VF, they also have a significant rate of complications. This is especially true in a young patient population. For instance, in patients with BrS undergoing ICD implantation, the complication rate was found to be 28%.[94] It is, therefore, important to remember that pharmacological treatment with quinidine has also been demonstrated to be effective (see below).

Drug Therapy with Quinidine

The very first patients with idiopathic VF described in the literature, back in 1929[95] and 1949,[96] were treated with quinidine after multiple documented episodes of spontaneous polymorphic VT and VF. Both patients had an excellent response. In fact, a second publication reporting the long-term follow-up of the patient initially reported in 1949, established that this patient eventually died of cancer at old age, without ever experiencing arrhythmia recurrence while on quinidine therapy for 40 years.[97] In 1987, Belhassen pioneered the therapy of idiopathic VF with electrophysiology study (EPS) guided quinidine after observing that VF is easily inducible at the baseline state but no longer inducible after quinidine therapy.[25] Of note, one of the patients included in that original report,[23] has completed >25 uneventful years of EPS-guided therapy with amiodarone and quinidine after experiencing arrhythmic storms of VF in the absence of therapy and recurrent arrhythmic syncope on amiodarone alone.[98]

In 1990, we found that the recurrence rate of cardiac arrest was high during therapy with other antiarrhythmic drugs (including amiodarone, beta-blockers or verapamil).[1] The high-rate of arrhythmia recurrence with verapamil is worth noting because that drug was empirically proposed by Leenhardt and Coumel to treat the "short-coupled variant of torsade de pointes",[99] an entity that probably represents idiopathic VF. In contrast, we found that the recurrence rate with quinidine was nil.[1] By the time the ICD became commercially available, *we continued to recommend quinidine as the sole therapy for appropriately selected patients with idiopathic VF, including patients resuscitated from spontaneous cardiac arrest.*[100] Our criteria for quinidine therapy in VF survivors includes *all the following*: 1) diagnosis of idiopathic VF with or without Brugada syndrome; 2) inducible VF in the absence of drugs with programmed ventricular stimulation; 3) no inducible arrhythmias during oral quinidine therapy despite a very aggressive protocol of ventricular stimulation;[25,46,101] 4) informed consent by a patient who is well informed of the risk and benefits of ICD and quinidine therapy for this disease;[100] 5) repeated assertion of drug compliance during long-term follow-up (compliance is assessed with quinidine serum levels and quinidine-effect on the QT interval). Our results using this approach were published in 1999.[26] These results may be summarized as follows: Of 34 patients with idiopathic VF (all after resuscitation from cardiac arrest),[26] (80%) had inducible VF at baseline electrophysiologic study and all but one of them were rendered noninducible with quinidine. Side effects from quinidine led to discontinuation of the drug in 14% of our patients. Nevertheless, 23 patients (2/3 of the patients from the original cohort of cardiac arrest survivors) remained on quinidine therapy without ICD back-up and all are alive and completely free of arrhythmic symptoms during a follow-up period that now exceeds 10 years.[102] Relatively early in our experience, three patients who had negative electrophysiologic studies in the absence of drugs received empiric quinidine. All these patients died 4–8 years after the original VF episode. These 3 patients discontinued follow-up long before they died. Therefore, we do not know if the fatalities were due to poor compliance or due to drug failure and weather such failure was related to the fact that quinidine therapy for these particular patients was empiric and not guided by electrophysiologic studies (since these 3 patients were noninducible at baseline). Nevertheless, we no longer recommend empiric use of quinidine for noninducible patients after spontaneous cardiac arrest. However, we have successfully used quinidine to control arrhythmic storms in patients who originally received an ICD either because of noninducibility in the baseline EPS or because of the extremely rare persistence of inducibility while on quinidine therapy.

Ablation

The fact that the PVC initiating polymorphic VT/VF in idiopathic VF patients is frequently of the same morphology raised the possibility of ablation as an effective treatment for idiopathic VF. This form of therapy has been used primarily to treat patients with implanted ICDs who are receiving multiple ICD shocks because of arrhythmic storms. The first successful ablation was reported by Aizawa in 1992.[103] Subsequently, relatively large series have been reported by Haissaguerre[104] and by Noda and Shimizu.[40] The series of Haissaguerre and Noda differ in the site of origin of the targeted arrhythmias. Noda targeted polymorphic VT originating from the right ventricular outflow tract.[40] In contrast, 87% of the polymorphic ventricular arrhythmias ablated by Haissaguerre's group were mapped to the Purkinje system in the right or left ventricle while the site of origin of the VF was in the right ventricular outflow tract in only 11% of patients.[104] The risk of recurrent spontaneous VF during long-term follow-up (mean of 63 months) was 18% with repeated ablation resulting in abolition of arrhythmias during an additional follow-up period of 28 months. Nevertheless, the recurrence of arrhythmias in a significant minority of patients should be kept in mind and ablation is not regarded as "curative" or as an alternative to ICD implantation.

Family Screening

As idiopathic VF is a diagnosis primarily based on exclusion and there is no diagnostic test which is 100% sensitive, there's always a possibility of missing a subtle underlying condition. Therefore, basic screening of first degree family members is reasonable in order to rule out other possible familial diagnoses.[5] An ECG, echocardiogram and exercise test may be considered for such screening, however data on the yield of this approach is lacking. The use of genetic testing for cascade screening is limited to the very rare cases in which a genetic substrate (e.g. the Dutch risk haplotype)[49] is found in the proband.

LIMITATIONS OF KNOWLEDGE

As VF is the final common pathway of any hemodynamically unstable arrhythmia, its documentation does not rule out other conditions that may present initially with monomorphic ventricular tachycardia (VT), bradyarrhythmias or even supraventricular tachycardia. The work-up required for exclusion of all other etiologies is not strictly defined and, obviously, has changed considerably during the years. Therefore, cohorts and series of idiopathic VF patients may include slightly different patients depending on the exclusion protocol used. Furthermore, although "positive" findings of short-coupled PVCs initiating polymorphic VT/VF makes the diagnosis of idiopathic VF more certain, this kind of documentation is possible only in patients with arrhythmic storms. Thus, any study focusing solely on these "classic" idiopathic VF patients would have to exclude patients without storms that may have a different (better?) prognosis. The result of the abovementioned points is that our current knowledge of idiopathic VF is probably tainted by heterogeneous cohorts. Indeed, follow-up of patients with undiagnosed CA in the CASPER registry demonstrated that a change of diagnosis from idiopathic VF to a specific cardiomyopathy or primary arrhythmia syndrome is not rare.[105] Further studies are necessary in order to define more clearly this patient population.

REFERENCES

1. Viskin S, Belhassen B. Idiopathic ventricular fibrillation. Am Heart J. 1990;120:661-71.
2. Haissaguerre M, Derval N, Sacher F, Jesel L, Deisenhofer I, de Roy L, Pasquie JL, Nogami A, Babuty D, Yli-Mayry S, De Chillou C, Scanu P, Mabo P, Matsuo S, Probst V, Le Scouarnec S, Defaye P, Schlaepfer J, Rostock T, Lacroix D, Lamaison D, Lavergne T, Aizawa Y, Englund A, Anselme F, O'Neill M, Hocini M, Lim KT, Knecht S, Veenhuyzen GD, Bordachar P, Chauvin M, Jais P, Coureau G, Chene G, Klein GJ, Clementy J. Sudden cardiac arrest associated with early repolarization. N Engl J Med. 2008;358:2016-23.
3. Brugada P, Brugada J. Right bundle branch block, persistent ST segment elevation and sudden cardiac death: a distinct clinical and electrocardiographic syndrome. A multicenter report. J Am Coll Cardiol. 1992;20:1391-6.
4. Gussak I, Brugada P, Brugada J, Wright RS, Kopecky SL, Chaitman BR, Bjerregaard P. Idiopathic short QT interval: a new clinical syndrome? Cardiology. 2000;94: 99-102.

5. Priori SG, Wilde AA, Horie M, Cho Y, Behr ER, Berul C, Blom N, Brugada J, Chiang CE, Huikuri H, Kannankeril P, Krahn A, Leenhardt A, Moss A, Schwartz PJ, Shimizu W, Tomaselli G, Tracy C. HRS/EHRA/APHRS expert consensus statement on the diagnosis and management of patients with inherited primary arrhythmia syndromes: document endorsed by HRS, EHRA, and APHRS in May 2013 and by ACCF, AHA, PACES, and AEPC in June 2013. Heart Rhythm. 2013;10:1932-63.
6. Behr ER, Casey A, Sheppard M, Wright M, Bowker TJ, Davies MJ, McKenna WJ, Wood DA. Sudden arrhythmic death syndrome: a national survey of sudden unexplained cardiac death. Heart 2007;93:601-5.
7. Bowker TJ, Wood DA, Davies MJ, Sheppard MN, Cary NR, Burton JD, Chambers DR, Dawling S, Hobson HL, Pyke SD, Riemersma RA, Thompson SG. Sudden, unexpected cardiac or unexplained death in England: a national survey. QJM. 2003;96:269-79.
8. Winkel BG, Holst AG, Theilade J, Kristensen IB, Thomsen JL, Ottesen GL, Bundgaard H, Svendsen JH, Haunso S, Tfelt-Hansen J. Nationwide study of sudden cardiac death in persons aged 1-35 years. Eur Heart J. 2011;32:983-90.
9. Kumar S, Peters S, Thompson T, Morgan N, Maccicoca I, Trainer A, Zentner D, Kalman JM, Winship I, Vohra JK. Familial cardiological and targeted genetic evaluation: low yield in sudden unexplained death and high yield in unexplained cardiac arrest syndromes. Heart Rhythm. 2013;10:1653-60.
10. Viskin S, Belhassen B. Polymorphic ventricular tachyarrhythmias in the absence of organic heart disease: classification, differential diagnosis, and implications for therapy. Prog Cardiovasc Dis. 1998;41:17-34.
11. Belhassen B, Viskin S. Idiopathic ventricular tachycardia and fibrillation. J Cardiovasc Electrophysiol. 1993;4:356-68.
12. Haissaguerre M, Sacher F, Nogami A, Komiya N, Bernard A, Probst V, Yli-Mayry S, Defaye P, Aizawa Y, Frank R, Mantovan R, Cappato R, Wolpert C, Leenhardt A, de Roy L, Heidbuchel H, Deisenhofer I, Arentz T, Pasquie JL, Weerasooriya R, Hocini M, Jais P, Derval N, Bordachar P, Clementy J. Characteristics of recurrent ventricular fibrillation associated with inferolateral early repolarization role of drug therapy. J Am Coll Cardiol. 2009;53:612-9.
13. Fujiki A, Sugao M, Nishida K, Sakabe M, Tsuneda T, Mizumaki K, Inoue H. Repolarization abnormality in idiopathic ventricular fibrillation: assessment using 24-hour QT-RR and QaT-RR relationships. J Cardiovasc Electrophysiol. 2004;15:59-63.
14. Sugao M, Fujiki A, Sakabe M, Nishida K, Tsuneda T, Iwamoto J, Mizumaki K, Inoue H. New quantitative methods for evaluation of dynamic changes in QT interval on 24 hour Holter ECG recordings: QT interval in idiopathic ventricular fibrillation and long QT syndrome. Heart. 2006;92:201-7.
15. Viskin S, Zeltser D, Ish-Shalom M, Katz A, Glikson M, Justo D, Tekes-Manova D, Belhassen B. Is idiopathic ventricular fibrillation a short QT syndrome? Comparison of QT intervals of patients with idiopathic ventricular fibrillation and healthy controls. Heart Rhythm. 2004;1:587-91.
16. Taggart NW, Haglund CM, Tester DJ, Ackerman MJ. Diagnostic miscues in congenital long-QT syndrome. Circulation. 2007;115:2613-20.
17. Templin C, Ghadri JR, Rougier JS, Baumer A, Kaplan V, Albesa M, Sticht H, Rauch A, Puleo C, Hu D, Barajas-Martinez H, Antzelevitch C, Luscher TF, Abriel H, Duru F. Identification of a novel loss-of-function calcium channel gene mutation in short QT syndrome (SQTS6). Eur Heart J. 2011;32:1077-88.
18. Redpath CJ, Green MS, Birnie DH, Gollob MH. Rapid genetic testing facilitating the diagnosis of short QT syndrome. Can J Cardiol. 2009;25:e133-5.
19. Viskin S, Lesh MD, Eldar M, Fish R, Setbon I, Laniado S, Belhassen B. Mode of onset of malignant ventricular arrhythmias in idiopathic ventricular fibrillation. J Cardiovasc Electrophysiol. 1997;8:1115-20.
20. Haissaguerre M, Shoda M, Jais P, Nogami A, Shah DC, Kautzner J, Arentz T, Kalushe D, Lamaison D, Griffith M, Cruz F, de Paola A, Gaita F, Hocini M, Garrigue S, Macle L, Weerasooriya R, Clementy J. Mapping and ablation of idiopathic ventricular fibrillation. Circulation. 2002;106:962-7.
21. Champagne J, Geelen P, Philippon F, Brugada P. Recurrent cardiac events in patients with idiopathic ventricular fibrillation, excluding patients with the Brugada syndrome. BMC Med. 2005;3:1.
22. Nam GB, Ko KH, Kim J, Park KM, Rhee KS, Choi KJ, Kim YH, Antzelevitch C. Mode of onset of ventricular fibrillation in patients with early repolarization pattern vs. Brugada syndrome. Eur Heart J. 2010;31:330-9.
23. Belhassen B, Pelleg A, Miller HI, Laniado S. Serial electrophysiological studies in a young patient with recurrent ventricular fibrillation. Pacing Clin Electrophysiol. 1981;4:92-9.
24. Haissaguerre M, Shah DC, Jais P, Shoda M, Kautzner J, Arentz T, Kalushe D, Kadish A, Griffith M, Gaita F, Yamane T, Garrigue S, Hocini M, Clementy J. Role of Purkinje conducting system in triggering of idiopathic ventricular fibrillation. Lancet. 2002;359:677-8.
25. Belhassen B, Shapira I, Shoshani D, Paredes A, Miller H, Laniado S. Idiopathic ventricular fibrillation: inducibility and beneficial effects of class I antiarrhythmic agents. Circulation. 1987;75:809-16.
26. Belhassen B, Viskin S, Fish R, Glick A, Setbon I, Eldar M. Effects of electrophysiologic-guided therapy with Class IA antiarrhythmic drugs on the long-term outcome of patients with idiopathic ventricular fibrillation with or without the Brugada syndrome. J Cardiovasc Electrophysiol. 1999;10: 1301-12.
27. Gussak I, Bjerregaard P. Short QT syndrome--5 years of progress. J Electrocardiol. 2005;38:375-7.
28. Gaita F, Giustetto C, Bianchi F, Schimpf R, Haissaguerre M, Calo L, Brugada R, Antzelevitch C, Borggrefe M, Wolpert C. Short QT syndrome: pharmacological treatment. J Am Coll Cardiol. 2004;43:1494-9.
29. Brugada P, Geelen P, Brugada R, Mont L, Brugada J. Prognostic value of electrophysiologic investigations in Brugada syndrome. J Cardiovasc Electrophysiol. 2001;12:1004-7.
30. Shimada M, Miyazaki T, Miyoshi S, Soejima K, Hori S, Mitamura H, Ogawa S. Sustained monomorphic ventricular tachycardia in a patient with Brugada syndrome. Jpn Circ J. 1996;60:364-70.
31. Viskin S, Belhassen B. Clinical problem-solving. When you only live twice. N Engl J Med. 1995;332:1221-5.
32. Boersma LV, Jaarsma W, Jessurun ER, Van Hemel NH, Wever EF. Brugada syndrome: a case report of monomorphic ventricular tachycardia. Pacing Clin Electrophysiol. 2001;24:112-5.
33. Dinckal MH, Davutoglu V, Akdemir I, Soydinc S, Kirilmaz A, Aksoy M. Incessant monomorphic ventricular tachycardia during febrile illness in a patient with Brugada syndrome: fatal electrical storm. Europace. 2003;5:257-61.
34. Mok NS, Chan NY, Chiu AC. Successful use of quinidine in treatment of electrical storm in Brugada syndrome. Pacing Clin Electrophysiol. 2004;27:821-3.

35. Brugada P, Green M, Abdollah H, Wellens HJ. Significance of ventricular arrhythmias initiated by programmed ventricular stimulation: the importance of the type of ventricular arrhythmia induced and the number of premature stimuli required. Circulation. 1984;69:87-92.
36. Morady F, DiCarlo LA, Jr., Baerman JM, de Buitleir M. Comparison of coupling intervals that induce clinical and nonclinical forms of ventricular tachycardia during programmed stimulation. Am J Cardiol. 1986;57:1269-73.
37. Stevenson WG, Brugada P, Waldecker B, Zehender M, Wellens HJ. Can potentially significant polymorphic ventricular arrhythmias initiated by programmed stimulation be distinguished from those that are nonspecific? Am Heart J. 1986;111:1073-80.
38. Viskin S, Rogowski O. Asymptomatic Brugada syndrome: a cardiac ticking time-bomb? Europace. 2007;9:707-10.
39. Viskin S, Rosso R, Rogowski O, Belhassen B. The "short-coupled" variant of right ventricular outflow ventricular tachycardia: a not-so-benign form of benign ventricular tachycardia? J Cardiovasc Electrophysiol. 2005;16:912-6.
40. Noda T, Shimizu W, Taguchi A, Aiba T, Satomi K, Suyama K, Kurita T, Aihara N, Kamakura S. Malignant entity of idiopathic ventricular fibrillation and polymorphic ventricular tachycardia initiated by premature extrasystoles originating from the right ventricular outflow tract. J Am Coll Cardiol. 2005;46:1288-94.
41. Probst V, Veltmann C, Eckardt L, Meregalli PG, Gaita F, Tan HL, Babuty D, Sacher F, Giustetto C, Schulze-Bahr E, Borggrefe M, Haissaguerre M, Mabo P, Le Marec H, Wolpert C, Wilde AA. Long-term prognosis of patients diagnosed with Brugada syndrome: Results from the FINGER Brugada Syndrome Registry. Circulation. 2010;121:635-43.
42. Giustetto C, Schimpf R, Mazzanti A, Scrocco C, Maury P, Anttonen O, Probst V, Blanc JJ, Sbragia P, Dalmasso P, Borggrefe M, Gaita F. Long-term follow-up of patients with short QT syndrome. J Am Coll Cardiol. 2011;58:587-95.
43. Mazzanti A, Kanthan A, Monteforte N, Memmi M, Bloise R, Novelli V, Miceli C, O'Rourke S, Borio G, Zienciuk-Krajka A, Curcio A, Surducan AE, Colombo M, Napolitano C, Priori SG. Novel insight into the natural history of short QT syndrome. J Am Coll Cardiol. 2014;63:1300-8.
44. Mizumaki K, Fujiki A, Tsuneda T, Sakabe M, Nishida K, Sugao M, Inoue H. Vagal activity modulates spontaneous augmentation of ST elevation in the daily life of patients with Brugada syndrome. J Cardiovasc Electrophysiol. 2004;15:667-73.
45. Schimpf R, Wolpert C, Gaita F, Giustetto C, Borggrefe M. Short QT syndrome. Cardiovasc Res. 2005;67:357-66.
46. Belhassen B, Glick A, Viskin S. Efficacy of quinidine in high-risk patients with Brugada syndrome. Circulation. 2004;110:1731-7.
47. Antzelevitch C, Yan GX. J wave syndromes. Heart Rhythm. 2010;7:549-58.
48. Patel C, Yan GX, Antzelevitch C. Short QT syndrome: from bench to bedside. Circ Arrhythm Electrophysiol. 2010;3:401-8.
49. Alders M, Koopmann TT, Christiaans I, Postema PG, Beekman L, Tanck MW, Zeppenfeld K, Loh P, Koch KT, Demolombe S, Mannens MM, Bezzina CR, Wilde AA. Haplotype-sharing analysis implicates chromosome 7q36 harboring DPP6 in familial idiopathic ventricular fibrillation. Am J Hum Genet. 2009;84:468-76.
50. Radicke S, Cotella D, Graf EM, Ravens U, Wettwer E. Expression and function of dipeptidyl-aminopeptidase-like protein 6 as a putative beta-subunit of human cardiac transient outward current encoded by Kv4.3. J Physiol. 2005;565:751-6.
51. Colinas O, Perez-Carretero FD, Lopez-Lopez JR, Perez-Garcia MT. A role for DPPX modulating external TEA sensitivity of Kv4 channels. J Gen Physiol. 2008;131:455-71.
52. Xiao L, Koopmann TT, Ordog B, Postema PG, Verkerk AO, Iyer V, Sampson KJ, Boink GJ, Mamarbachi MA, Varro A, Jordaens L, Res J, Kass RS, Wilde AA, Bezzina CR, Nattel S. Unique cardiac Purkinje fiber transient outward current beta-subunit composition: a potential molecular link to idiopathic ventricular fibrillation. Circ Res. 2013;112:1310-22.
53. Marsman RF, Barc J, Beekman L, Alders M, Dooijes D, van den Wijngaard A, Ratbi I, Sefiani A, Bhuiyan ZA, Wilde AA, Bezzina CR. A mutation in CALM1 encoding calmodulin in familial idiopathic ventricular fibrillation in childhood and adolescence. J Am Coll Cardiol. 2014;63:259-66.
54. Nomikos M, Thanassoulas A, Beck K, Vassilakopoulou V, Hu H, Calver BL, Theodoridou M, Kashir J, Blayney L, Livaniou E, Rizkallah P, Nounesis G, Lai FA. Altered RyR2 regulation by the calmodulin F90L mutation associated with idiopathic ventricular fibrillation and early sudden cardiac death. FEBS Lett. 2014;588:2898-902.
55. Gaborit N, Le Bouter S, Szuts V, Varro A, Escande D, Nattel S, Demolombe S. Regional and tissue specific transcript signatures of ion channel genes in the non-diseased human heart. J Physiol. 2007;582:675-93.
56. Postema PG, Christiaans I, Hofman N, Alders M, Koopmann TT, Bezzina CR, Loh P, Zeppenfeld K, Volders PG, Wilde AA. Founder mutations in the Netherlands: familial idiopathic ventricular fibrillation and DPP6. Neth Heart J. 2011;19:290-6.
57. Nyegaard M, Overgaard MT, Sondergaard MT, Vranas M, Behr ER, Hildebrandt LL, Lund J, Hedley PL, Camm AJ, Wettrell G, Fosdal I, Christiansen M, Borglum AD. Mutations in calmodulin cause ventricular tachycardia and sudden cardiac death. Am J Hum Genet. 2012;91:703-12.
58. Crotti L, Johnson CN, Graf E, De Ferrari GM, Cuneo BF, Ovadia M, Papagiannis J, Feldkamp MD, Rathi SG, Kunic JD, Pedrazzini M, Wieland T, Lichtner P, Beckmann BM, Clark T, Shaffer C, Benson DW, Kaab S, Meitinger T, Strom TM, Chazin WJ, Schwartz PJ, George AL, Jr. Calmodulin mutations associated with recurrent cardiac arrest in infants. Circulation. 2013;127:1009-17.
59. Bagnall RD, Molloy LK, Kalman JM, Semsarian C. Exome sequencing identifies a mutation in the ACTN2 gene in a family with idiopathic ventricular fibrillation, left ventricular noncompaction, and sudden death. BMC Med Genet. 2014;15:99.
60. Priori SG, Chen SR. Inherited dysfunction of sarcoplasmic reticulum Ca2+ handling and arrhythmogenesis. Circ Res. 2011;108:871-83.
61. Paech C, Gebauer RA, Karstedt J, Marschall C, Bollmann A, Husser D. Ryanodine receptor mutations presenting as idiopathic ventricular fibrillation: A report on two novel familial compound mutations, c.6224T>C and c.13781A>G, with the clinical presentation of idiopathic ventricular Fibrillation. Pediatr Cardiol. 2014;35:1437-41.
62. Cheung JW, Meli AC, Xie W, Mittal S, Reiken S, Wronska A, Xu L, Steinberg JS, Markowitz SM, Iwai S, Lacampagne A, Lerman BB, Marks AR. Short-coupled polymorphic ventricular tachycardia at rest linked to a novel ryanodine receptor (RyR2)

cardiac sarcoidosis: a systematic review and metaanalysis including the Ontario experience. J Nucl Med. 2012;53:241-8.

119. Viskin S, Postema PG, Bhuiyan ZA, Rosso R, Kalman JM, Vohra JK, Guevara-Valdivia ME, Marquez MF, Kogan E, Belhassen B, Glikson M, Strasberg B, Antzelevitch C, Wilde AA. The response of the QT interval to the brief tachycardia provoked by standing: a bedside test for diagnosing long QT syndrome. J Am Coll Cardiol. 2010;55:1955-61.

120. Adler A, van der Werf C, Postema PG, Rosso R, Bhuiyan ZA, Kalman JM, Vohra JK, Guevara-Valdivia ME, Marquez MF, Halkin A, Benhorin J, Antzelevitch C, Wilde AA, Viskin S. The phenomenon of "QT stunning": the abnormal QT prolongation provoked by standing persists even as the heart rate returns to normal in patients with long QT syndrome. Heart Rhythm. 2012;9:901-8.

121. Sy RW, van der Werf C, Chattha IS, Chockalingam P, Adler A, Healey JS, Perrin M, Gollob MH, Skanes AC, Yee R, Gula LJ, Leong-Sit P, Viskin S, Klein GJ, Wilde AA, Krahn AD. Derivation and validation of a simple exercise-based algorithm for prediction of genetic testing in relatives of LQTS probands. Circulation. 2011;124:2187-94.

122. Leenhardt A, Lucet V, Denjoy I, Grau F, Ngoc DD, Coumel P. Catecholaminergic polymorphic ventricular tachycardia in children. A 7-year follow-up of 21 patients. Circulation. 1995; 91:1512-9.

123. Perrin MJ, Angaran P, Laksman Z, Zhang H, Porepa LF, Rutberg J, James C, Krahn AD, Judge DP, Calkins H, Gollob MH. Exercise testing in asymptomatic gene carriers exposes a latent electrical substrate of arrhythmogenic right ventricular cardiomyopathy. J Am Coll Cardiol. 2013;62: 1772-9.

124. Makimoto H, Nakagawa E, Takaki H, Yamada Y, Okamura H, Noda T, Satomi K, Suyama K, Aihara N, Kurita T, Kamakura S, Shimizu W. Augmented ST-segment elevation during recovery from exercise predicts cardiac events in patients with Brugada syndrome. J Am Coll Cardiol. 2010;56:1576-84.

125. Ackerman MJ, Khositseth A, Tester DJ, Hejlik JB, Shen WK, Porter CB. Epinephrine-induced QT interval prolongation: a gene-specific paradoxical response in congenital long QT syndrome. Mayo Clin Proc. 2002;77:413-21.

126. Shimizu W, Noda T, Takaki H, Nagaya N, Satomi K, Kurita T, Suyama K, Aihara N, Sunagawa K, Echigo S, Miyamoto Y, Yoshimasa Y, Nakamura K, Ohe T, Towbin JA, Priori SG, Kamakura S. Diagnostic value of epinephrine test for genotyping LQT1, LQT2, and LQT3 forms of congenital long QT syndrome. Heart Rhythm. 2004;1:276-83.

127. Denis A, Sacher F, Derval N, Lim HS, Cochet H, Shah AJ, Daly M, Pillois X, Ramoul K, Komatsu Y, Zemmoura A, Amraoui S, Ritter P, Ploux S, Bordachar P, Hocini M, Jais P, Haissaguerre M. Diagnostic value of isoproterenol testing in arrhythmogenic right ventricular cardiomyopathy. Circ Arrhythm Electrophysiol. 2014;7:590-7.

128. Garratt CJ, Antoniou A, Griffith MJ, Ward DE, Camm AJ. Use of intravenous adenosine in sinus rhythm as a diagnostic test for latent preexcitation. Am J Cardiol. 1990;65:868-73.

129. Viskin S, Rosso R, Rogowski O, Belhassen B, Levitas A, Wagshal A, Katz A, Fourey D, Zeltser D, Oliva A, Pollevick GD, Antzelevitch C, Rozovski U. Provocation of sudden heart rate oscillation with adenosine exposes abnormal QT responses in patients with long QT syndrome: a bedside test for diagnosing long QT syndrome. Eur Heart J. 2006;27:469-75.

130. Marra MP, Leoni L, Bauce B, Corbetti F, Zorzi A, Migliore F, Silvano M, Rigato I, Tona F, Tarantini G, Cacciavillani L, Basso C, Buja G, Thiene G, Iliceto S, Corrado D. Imaging study of ventricular scar in arrhythmogenic right ventricular cardiomyopathy: comparison of 3D standard electroanatomical voltage mapping and contrast-enhanced cardiac magnetic resonance. Circ Arrhythm Electrophysiol. 2012;5:91-100.

EDITORS' SUMMARY

Professor Viskin and colleagues have provided for us an insightful and comprehensive yet streamlined summary of idiopathic ventricular fibrillation. This condition and closely-related syndromes are among the most difficult for clinical and invasive electrophysiologists to understand and guide patients appropriately. The reader will find the information provided invaluable in developing an overall understanding of the subject while providing a platform for more in depth study.

The approach taken by the authors is clinical with multiple pearls related to the cardiac region of abnormality, coupling interval of PVC's, the somewhat short QT interval found in some survivors of idiopathic ventricular fibrillation, and a practical differential diagnostic approach that they have outlined. Importantly, this internationally leading group in this area has given us the highpoints on the potential genetic basis including a succinct summary of recent advances in this area. They highlight both from the genetic perspective and clinical mapping, the regional importance of the Purkinje network and the outflow tract. Both areas of considerable present research interest, that those who have read this chapter will be better equipped to comprehend, analyze, and assimilate appropriately into their practice. The chapter will provide an excellent overview along with the chapters that deal with repolarization syndromes (Chapters 39 and 40), specifically the early repolarization syndrome (Chapter 40), and Purkinje-related arrhythmias (Chapter 35).

CHAPTER 42

SP Abhilash, Narayanan Namboodiri

Ventricular Arrhythmia Storm: Etiology, Mechanisms and Management

LIST OF ABBREVIATIONS

ACLS	Advanced Cardiac Life Support	LV	Left Ventricle
ATP	Antitachycardia Pacing	MI	Myocardial Infarction
BLS	Basic Life Support	RF	Radiofrequency
CRT	Cardiac Resynchronization Therapy	SVT	Supraventricular Tachycardia
ES	Electrical Storm	VF	Ventricular Fibrillation
IABP	Intra-aortic Balloon Pump	VPC	Ventricular Premature Contraction
ICD	Implantable Cardioverter-Defibrillator	VT	Ventricular Tachycardia

INTRODUCTION

Ventricular arrhythmia storm, or electrical storm (ES) as commonly known, is a potentially lethal clinical situation characterized by recurrent episodes of ventricular arrhythmias. It is defined as 3 or more sustained episodes of ventricular tachycardia (VT), ventricular fibrillation (VF), or appropriate implantable cardioverter-defibrillator (ICD) shocks during a 24-hour period.[1] Sustained VT lasts at least 30 seconds, can result in hemodynamic compromise, and may require medical intervention to terminate the episode. Electrical storm can manifest during the acute phase of a myocardial infarction and in the presence of structural heart disease, advanced heart failure or an inherited arrhythmia syndrome. Among patients with ICDs, electrical storm has been reported in 10–20% of patients in whom the indication was secondary prevention,[2] but has a lower incidence in patients with primary prevention indication.[3] The major symptoms are recurrent palpitations, presyncope and syncope. A significant number of patients may present with worsening heart failure. Since many such patients already have advanced cardiac illness, hemodynamic deterioration is common. The clinical presentation might be dramatic and can involve cardiac arrest or multiple episodes of potentially fatal ventricular arrhythmias.

Management of ES is challenging and requires a systematic approach. Every effort has to be made to identify the underlying cause. Patients who have an ICD can present with recurrent shocks which is an agonizing experience for the patient physically as well as mentally. Effective management of electrical storm requires not only knowledge of arrhythmia mechanisms and therapeutic options, but also expertise in ICD programming.

ETIOLOGY AND MECHANISMS

ES develops when a vulnerable anatomic substrate [such as structural heart disease or scarring after an myocardial infarction (MI)] is affected by a triggering event, such as ventricular premature contractions (VPCs) or electrolyte imbalance.[4] Potential triggering factors include modification of or noncompliance to drug therapy, worsening of heart failure, early postoperative period, emotional stress and anger, alcohol excess, electrolyte abnormalities like hypokalemia and hypocalcemia, hyperthyroidism, fever, renal failure and myocardial ischemia. However, most cases of ES occur without any apparent cause.[5-8] Determining the cause of electrical storm is crucial, because treatment must target the underlying mechanism. The underlying arrhythmia that result in storm is predominantly (more than 80%) monomorphic VT.[9,10] However, ES can also occur due to polymorphic VT or VF, especially in the context of myocardial ischemia and in long QT syndrome. Multiple ICD shocks lead to elevations in cardiac troponin levels, which are indicative of minor degrees of myocardial injury,[11,12] and pathological studies have demonstrated fibrosis and acute cellular injury in the hearts of patients who had received recent shocks.[13,14] Recurrent episodes of VF are also associated with increased intracellular myocardial calcium levels,[15] which in turn have been linked to progressive left ventricular dysfunction,[16] cardiac apoptosis,[17] and arrhythmia facilitation. In addition, myocardial injury can lead to adrenergic neurohormonal stimulation and can lead to worsening heart failure and further propagation of electrical storm.

Flow chart 42.1: Approach to electrical storm

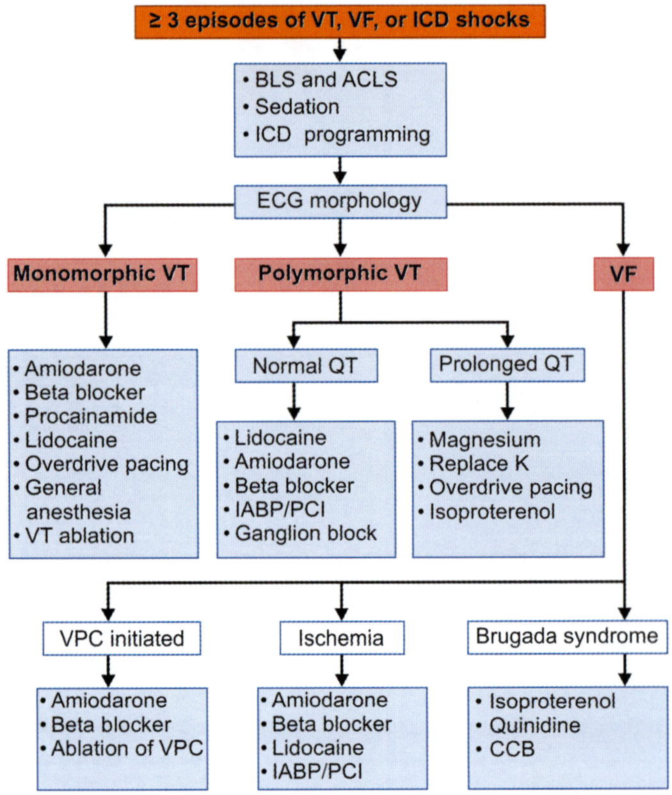

Abbreviations: ACLS, advanced cardiac life support; BLS, basic life support; CCB, calcium channel blockers; IABP, intra-aortic balloon counterpulsation; ICD, implantable cardioverter-defibrillator; K, potassium; PCI, percutaneous coronary intervention; VF, ventricular fibrillation; VPC, ventricular premature contraction; VT, ventricular tachycardia

APPROACH TO A PATIENT PRESENTING WITH ELECTRICAL STORM

Management of patients with electrical storm begins by accurately recognizing the clinical arrhythmia **(Flow chart 42.1)**. A brief history should be obtained while the patient is being evaluated for hemodynamic stability. Vitals are recorded first and if unstable; basic life support (BLS) and advanced cardiac life support (ACLS) algorithms initiated. Once the patient is stabilized, a detailed history regarding structural heart disease, hereditary syndromes, previous interventions and other precipitating factors should be sought. Special attention should be given to drug history, compliance to drugs, and metabolic disturbances like hypokalemia and hypomagnesemia. Every patient should be screened for evidence of myocardial ischemia and worsening heart failure. Endocrine evaluation to rule out hyperthyroidism and diabetic ketoacidosis can be crucial. Hyperthyroidism presenting as electrical storm is not rare in patients who are on chronic amiodarone therapy. Also, issues like acute infection, worsening renal failure or emotional stress, all of which can initiate and sustain an electrical storm, should be looked into. The patients often have severe anxiety and raised catecholamine levels, which can amplify the severity and perpetuate an electrical storm.

In patients who have preexisting bundle branch block, ventricular preexcitation, or a rate-related aberrancy, supraventricular tachycardia (SVT) can resemble VT. The differentiation of VT from SVT with aberrant conduction is very important in deciding further course of action. An SVT, resulting in inappropriate shock is not an uncommon clinical scenario in patients with ICD. **(Flow chart 42.2)** Such inappropriate shocks may be more common in patients who have a single chamber ICD and in old generation ICDs where SVT discrimination algorithms were not fully evolved. A simple step of checking for regularity of rhythm during tachycardia helps to distinguish atrial fibrillation from other more complex arrhythmias.

It needs to be strongly emphasized that the patient's hemodynamic status may misguide us in the distinction between SVT and VT. VT may result in minimal symptoms that may lead to the erroneous diagnosis of SVT with aberrant conduction. On the contrary, an SVT with fast rate in a patient with left ventricular (LV) dysfunction can easily result in heart failure and/or hemodynamic collapse. For this reason, an ambiguous wide-complex tachycardia should be considered as VT, especially in patients who have structural

Flow chart 42.2: Approach to electrical storm in a patient with ICD

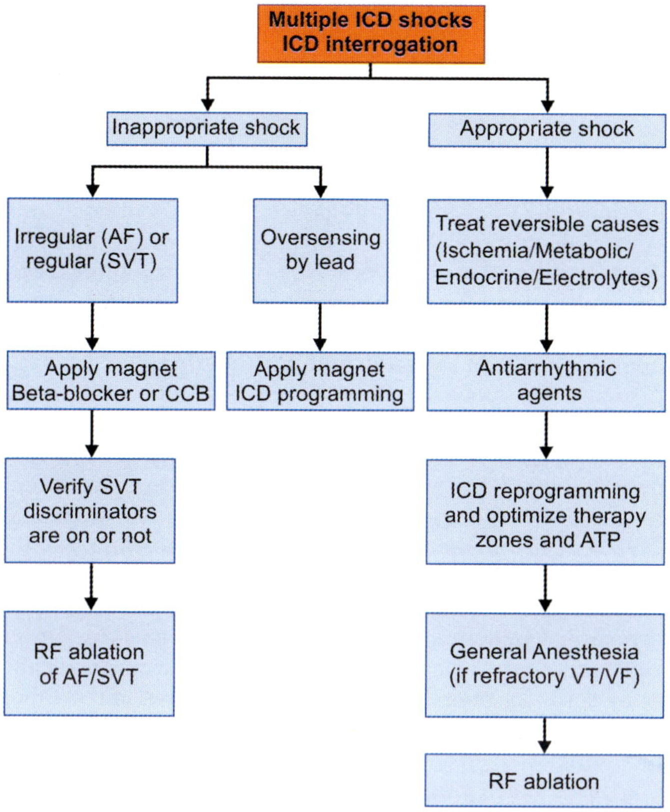

Abbreviations: AF, atrial fibrillation; ATP, antitachycardia pacing; CCB, calcium channel blocker; ICD, implantable cardioverter-defibrillator; RF, radiofrequency; SVT, supraventricular tachycardia; VF, ventricular fibrillation; VT, ventricular tachycardia

heart disease. If this rule is followed, the diagnosis of electrical storm will be accurate in 80% of all patients with tachycardia and in 95% of those who have had a previous MI.[18] Moreover, in general, treatment aimed at converting VT usually treats SVTs as well. However, the reverse may not be true and at times risky. A typical example would be treating VT in a patient with LV dysfunction using calcium channel blockers and thereby resulting in cardiac arrest.

Intravenous analgesics and sedatives should be given early and aggressively to patients who experience electrical storm especially those with multiple ICD shocks.[19] Not only are the shocks extremely painful and distressing to patients, but repeated shocks can cause depression and posttraumatic stress syndrome, and many patients report phantom shocks subsequently.[20]

Recurrent ICD shocks may result from appropriate therapy (cardioversion or defibrillation for VT or VF) or inappropriate therapy (shocks for supraventricular arrhythmias or for overdetection in the absence of any arrhythmia). Interrogation of the device and analysis of stored electrograms by a trained person can help to distinguish appropriate

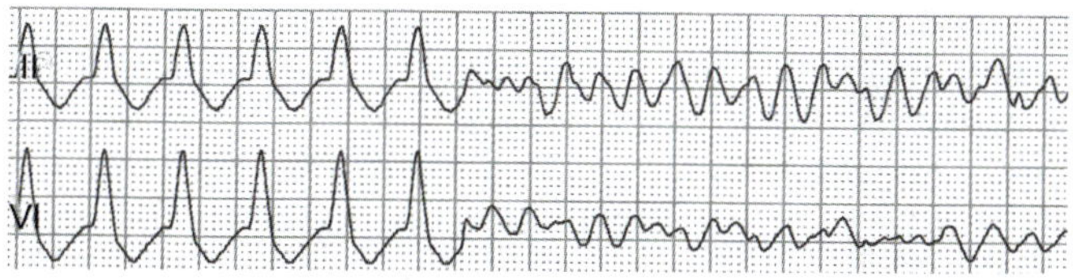

Figure 42.1: Monomorphic ventricular tachycardia degenerating into ventricular fibrillation

from inappropriate therapy. If the device reveals appropriate therapies for VT or VF, patient should be evaluated for triggering factors like ischemia, electrolyte imbalance, worsening heart failure, and others. Shocks without evidence of an arrhythmia may indicate device malfunction, such as the oversensing of myopotentials or electrical noise due to a fractured lead. In addition, as already discussed, SVT or atrial fibrillation can result in inappropriate shocks. In such cases, a magnet can be placed over the ICD to inhibit sensing to prevent further shocks until device reprogramming is done. Keeping magnet over the device will not hamper its pacing function and will also help to prevent further battery depletion in addition to preventing further unnecessary shocks. It goes without saying that the patient should be constantly monitored in such a scenario and external shock delivered or magnet removed if there is any hemodynamic instability. Optimal device programming can not only help in preventing inappropriate shocks due to oversensing or supraventricular arrhythmias but can also reduce appropriate but unnecessary shocks (for e.g., for fast VT amenable to antitachycardia pacing).

ELECTRICAL STORM: CLINICAL TYPES

Electrical storm can be classified on the basis of underlying arrhythmia as diagnosed with surface ECG into three clinical types: monomorphic VT, polymorphic VT or VF **(Flow chart 42.1)**.

Monomorphic VT

This is the most common variety and constitutes 85–90% of all patients with electrical storm **(Figure 42.1)**. Monomorphic VT occurs when the QRS complex morphology remains the same in all complexes and is usually due to reentry around a fixed anatomical barrier such as post-myocardial infarct scar tissue or perivalvular structure. Monomorphic VT due to wavefront reentry implies presence of underlying substrate and does not indicate active myocardial ischemia. It interesting to know that monomorphic VT is quite uncommon in patients with first acute MI, due to absence of scar tissue. Instead ongoing ischemia during acute MI or acute coronary syndrome can result in polymorphic VT or VF.

In ischemic as well as nonischemic cardiomyopathy, the substrate for reentry lies within heterogeneous areas of scarred myocardium. After an acute MI, or as nonischemic cardiomyopathy progresses, structural changes like fibrosis and scar formation occur in the myocardium. Fibrosis and scar tissue creates areas of slow conduction or block that along with areas of normal electrical conduction result in formation of reentrant circuits. The bundles of surviving myofibrils particularly around the border of a scar can lead to heterogeneous electrical conduction resulting in electrically stable reentry. Then, an otherwise harmless trigger, such as a VPC, is all that is required to initiate and sustain monomorphic VT.

Monomorphic VT can be totally asymptomatic or can present with hemodynamic collapse or cardiac arrest with varying severity of symptoms between the two extreme presentations. The degree of hemodynamic compromise depends upon the ventricular rate, LV function, and the presence of clinical heart failure. In addition, loss of atrioventricular synchrony, and the pattern of ventricular activation may determine the tolerance to monomorphic VT in particular patient.[21] The management of monomorphic VT is immediate cardioversion if hemodynamically unstable whereas stable VTs can be initially managed with drugs. Amiodarone and β-blockers are the preferred drugs for pharmacologic management of monomorphic VT **(Flow chart 42.1)**.

Polymorphic VT

Polymorphic VT (2–8% of electrical storm) is said to present when the QRS morphology varies from beat to beat during tachycardia **(Figures 42.2A to C)**. Polymorphic VT is due to multiple wave fronts propagating throughout the heart or appearing simultaneously in several parts of the heart.[22] Polymorphic VT can be associated with a normal or a prolonged QT interval in sinus rhythm and the management of both situations differ remarkably **(Flow chart 42.1)**.

Polymorphic VT with Normal QT Interval

Polymorphic VT is commonly associated with acute ischemic syndromes, but can also occur in the absence of organic heart disease. Patients with myocarditis or hypertrophic cardiomyopathy may also present with episodes of polymorphic VT. Therapy for polymorphic VT and VF varies, depending upon the mode of initiation and the underlying QT interval. In acute MI, polymorphic VT can be due to ischemia, altered membrane potential, or triggered activity. Ischemia may result in transmural dispersion of electrical refractory periods between the endocardium and epicardium, resulting in reentry.[23] In addition, ischemia increases Purkinje cell automaticity, that can result in polymorphic VT or VF.

The most effective treatment for polymorphic VT due to myocardial ischemia is to reverse the ischemia with emergency coronary revascularization either pharmacologically or by coronary intervention. Adequate sedation and sympathetic blockade using beta-blockers are crucial in preventing perpetuation of electrical storm. Amiodarone and lignocaine are the antiarrhythmic drugs found to be most useful in this situation **(Flow chart 42.1)**. It is interesting to note that magnesium therapy is not effective in treatment of polymorphic VT that is associated with normal QT intervals.

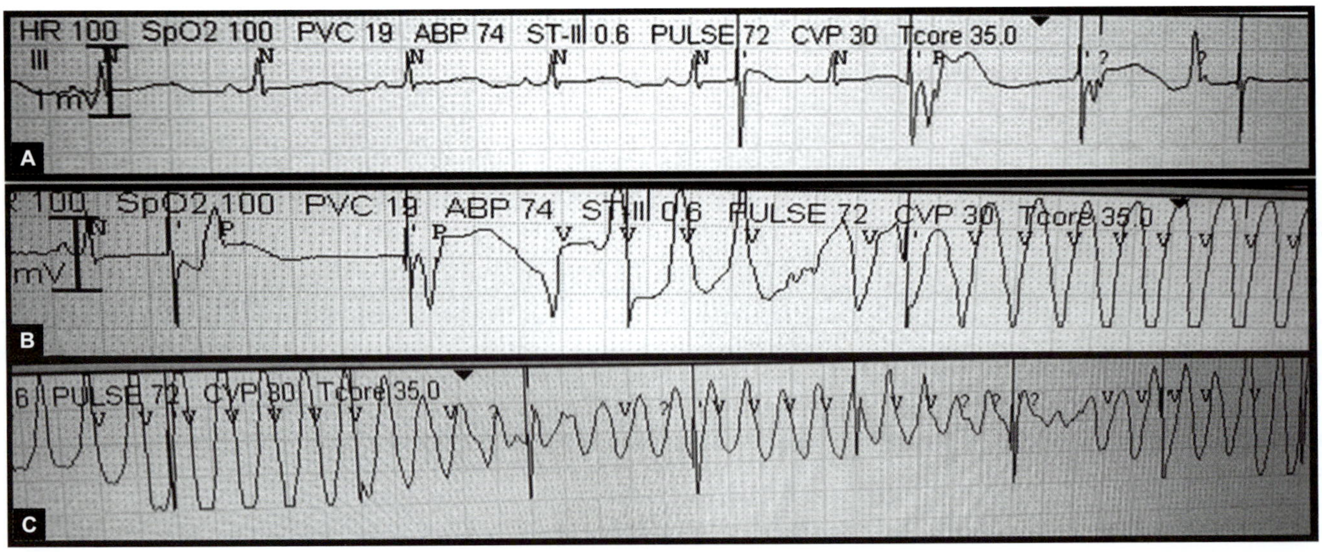

Figures 42.2A to C: Telemetry ECG of a patient with recent aortic valve replacement on temporary ventricular pacing through epicardial wire. The patient has diuretic induced hypokalemia. (A) Prolonged QT and ventricular undersensing by the temporary pacemaker; (B) VT triggered probably by pacing stimulus delivered on the T wave; (C) Polymorphic VT with temporary pacing spikes. He had recurrent polymorphic VT that settled after correction of hypokalemia and turning off pacemaker

Polymorphic VT with Prolonged QT Interval

Patients with recurrent polymorphic VT should have their baseline ECG carefully evaluated for a prolonged QT interval. "Torsades de pointes" is a type of pause-dependent polymorphic VT (name derived from QRS morphology "twisting around an axis" on surface ECG) occurring in patients with a long QT interval at baseline. It typically occurs when patients have bradycardia in addition to QT prolongation. QT prolongation can occur due to congenital or acquired causes. Inherited long QT syndromes usually present with syncope or sudden cardiac death, and presentation as electrical storm is rare.[24] Use of catecholamines, including isoproterenol, should be avoided in these patients.

Acquired causes for prolonged QT interval include electrolyte imbalances (hypokalemia, hypocalcemia, or hypomagnesemia), hypothyroidism, and the use of medications that are known to prolong the QT interval. Commonly used drugs which can prolong QT interval includes tricyclic antidepressants like amitriptyline, antipsychotics like haloperidol, and antibiotics such as clarithromycin, levofloxacin and erythromycin. Class Ia and class III antiarrhythmic drugs are well known to prolong the QT. Apart from correction of acquired causes, intravenous magnesium administration is the therapy of choice for patients with polymorphic VT and a long QT interval **(Flow chart 42.1)**. In all cases, keeping serum potassium level above 4.5 mEq/L is recommended. In patient with bradycardia or heart block, torsades de pointes should be managed with isoproterenol therapy or temporary pacing. In such cases, implantation of a permanent pacemaker is to be considered if VT is refractory.[1] Occasionally a VPC or a ventricular pacing stimulus that falls on the T wave in a patient with prolonged QT can result in polymorphic VT/VF **(Figures 42.2A to C)**. Correction of prolonged QT, avoiding ventricular pacing on T wave and correction of predisposing conditions for both prolonged QT and VPC like hypokalemia, are the mainstays of treatment.

Ventricular Fibrillation

Ventricular fibrillation (1–20% of electrical storm) manifests as chaotic ventricular activation on surface ECG, and is usually fatal if not treated promptly. Monomorphic or polymorphic VT can degenerate to ventricular fibrillation as well **(Figure 42.1)**. Even after successful defibrillation, VF may recur repeatedly and present as electrical storm. When VF occurs as electrical storm, mortality rates are extremely high at more than 90%.[25] The most common etiology of VF storm is myocardial ischemia and emergency coronary revascularization is the sole hope for survival in such cases.

Patients who have structurally normal heart and normal QT, may develop a VF storm that is triggered by closely coupled monomorphic VPCs.[26] Electrical storm presenting as VF initiated by VPCs has been reported late after myocardial infarction as well.[27] The triggering VPC often originates in the distal Purkinje system. Radiofrequency (RF) catheter ablation at these sites can eliminate these VPCs and prevent recurrence of VF.

Brugada syndrome, caused by a defective cardiac sodium channel gene, can also manifest as recurrent VF.[28] The prevalence of fatal arrhythmia ranges from 5% in patients without previous arrhythmias to 40% in those with a prior history of cardiac arrest. Fever, hypokalemia, high vagal tone and bradycardia are considered predisposing factors for occurrence of VF in Brugada syndrome. In one study, continuous isoproterenol infusion could normalize ST-segment elevation in V1-V3 and suppressed electrical storm in patients with Brugada syndrome.[29] Oral antiarrhythmic therapy may be required, because attempts to wean patients from isoproterenol can result in recurrent VF. Antiarrhythmic drug, quinidine has been shown to prevent ventricular arrhythmias in these patients by blocking the transient outward potassium channel that is responsible for phase 1 of the action potential. Quinidine is recommended therapy for refractory cases of electrical storm caused by Brugada syndrome and once electrical storm is settled; an ICD implantation is strongly indicated.

PRINCIPLES OF MANAGEMENT OF ELECTRICAL STORM

Role of Anesthesia in Electrical Storm

The physical and emotional stress, that patients experience during electrical storm with multiple electrical cardioversions are tremendous and this stress itself can lead to further perpetuation of arrhythmias by activation of the adrenergic system. Post-MI patients with electrical storm have significantly increased sympathetic activity, which plays a major role in the pathophysiology of ventricular arrhythmogenesis. It is reported that MI and myocardial ischemia result in denervation of sympathetic-parasympathetic fibers, which enhances sympathetic activity, thereby increasing the propensity for ventricular tachyarrhythmias.[30] All patients with electrical storm should be sedated. Short-acting anesthetics such as propofol, benzodiazepines, and some general anesthetic agents have been associated with suppression of electrical storm.[31] Left stellate ganglion blockade and thoracic epidural anesthesia have also reportedly suppressed electrical storms that were refractory to multiple antiarrhythmic agents and β blockade.[32]

Nonpharmacological Management of VT Storm

Radiofrequency ablation aims at modifying the myocardial substrate for reentry apart from eliminating the focal triggering discharges as described already for VPCs. Patients with advanced structural heart disease have VTs of multiple morphologies. Mapping and ablating multiple and frequently hemodynamically unstable VTs is challenging, and usually requires 3-D electroanatomic mapping. Timely performance of this procedure can often be life saving and in one prospective study, emergency RF ablation was successful in completely suppressing drug-refractory electrical storm in all of the 95 patients studied.[33] Use of percutaneous LV assist devices and intraaortic balloon pump (IABP) can provide hemodynamic support and enable the mapping and ablation of hemodynamically unstable VTs in these usually sick patients.[34] The Heart Rhythm Society and the European Heart Rhythm Association support the use of ablation early in the management of recurrent VT and electrical storm.[35]

Progressive heart failure has been a predictor of electrical storm, in several studies[3,36] and cardiac resynchronization therapy (CRT) in selected patients may reduce its incidence.[37] CRT-related reverse remodeling is sustained over the long term in patients with ischemic and nonischemic cardiomyopathy.[38] In one of the largest trials of CRT, the CARE-HF study CRT recipients had a reduction in all-cause death by 40%, heart-failure death by 45%, and sudden death by 46% compared to medical therapy alone.[39] The reduction in electrical storm might indicate a CRT-induced improvement in the underlying cardiac gene expression, myocardial substrate, and hemodynamic characteristics.[40]

Special Considerations in Patients with ICD Presenting as Electrical Storm

ICDs are used in patients who are at high risk of sudden cardiac death. However, these devices do not prevent the occurrence of arrhythmias, and many of these patients will require antiarrhythmic medications to reduce arrhythmic burden. When a patient with an ICD presents with recurrent shocks, device interrogation and reprogramming as discussed earlier are crucial for the diagnosis as well as guiding further management **(Flow chart 42.2)**. Programming ICDs to deliver antitachycardia pacing (ATP) for fast VTs can reduce the incidence of shocks in these patients. ATP has been shown to terminate fast VTs in a significant number of patients.[41]

RF ablation of VT can reduce appropriate ICD shocks in patients who present with multiple episodes of VTs.[42] Such patients may have multiple morphologies of VTs that are often hemodynamically unstable and a substrate based ablation approach is usually more useful rather than targeting and ablating the induced VT. The QRS morphology and cycle length of the clinical VT on surface ECG as well as location of prior MI and scar on imaging studies greatly help in localization the target region for mapping and RF ablation.

Recently, reports suggest that prophylactic RF ablation at the time of ICD implantation is beneficial to reduce future ICD shocks [43,44] in patients with high risk of recurrent VT.

Long-term Management

The risk of cardiac death is maximum within first three months of an electrical storm.[3,6] An electrical storm generally lasts less than 36–48 hours and aggressive efforts need to be made to stabilize the patient and prevent its future occurrence. Once and electrical storm has been taken care of, prompt implementation or augmentation of therapies demonstrated to be efficacious in preventing cardiovascular mortality is warranted. ACE inhibitors improve outcome in patients with left ventricular dysfunction,[45] primarily via a reduction in heart failure progression and should be titrated to most optimal doses. Beta blockers further reduce mortality in these patients[46, 47] through reductions in sudden death and heart failure progression. Spironolactone has also been demonstrated to reduce mortality in patients with advanced heart failure.[48] Coronary artery revascularization is very important in patients with ischemic left ventricular dysfunction, both in terms of reducing the risk of future arrhythmias[49] and in optimizing ventricular function. It is needless to say that optimal ICD programming to reduce unnecessary shocks in future is essential in all these patients.

CONCLUSION

Patients with electrical storm have a poor outcome and electrical storm might be an independent risk factor for cardiac death.[3,6] The presence or absence of structural heart disease and the ECG morphology during sinus rhythm and during arrhythmia, provide important diagnostic clues to the mechanism of electrical storm. Initial management involves hemodynamic stabilization followed by identifying and correcting the precipitating factors like ischemia, heart failure, electrolyte imbalances, or other inciting factors. Most patients present with monomorphic VT and amiodarone and β-blockers form the cornerstone of antiarrhythmic drug therapy. Patients who have ICDs can present with multiple shocks and may require device reprogramming in addition to drug therapy. Nonpharmacologic treatment, including RF catheter ablation may be implemented in drug-refractory patients to improve their clinical outcome.

REFERENCES

1. Zipes DP, Camm AJ, Borggrefe M, Buxton AE, Chaitman B, Fromer M, Gregoratos G, Klein G, Moss AJ, Myerburg RJ, Priori SG, Quinones MA, Roden DM, Silka MJ, Tracy C, Smith SC, Jacobs AK, Adams CD, Antman EM, Anderson JL, Hunt SA, Halperin JL, Nishimura R, Ornato JP, Page RL, Riegel B, Blanc JJ, Budaj A, Dean V, Deckers JW, Despres C, Dickstein K, Lekakis J, McGregor K, Metra M, Morais J, Osterspey A, Tamargo JL, Zamorano JL. ACC/AHA/ESC 2006 guidelines for management of patients with ventricular arrhythmias and the prevention of sudden cardiac death: a report of the American College of Cardiology/American Heart Association Task Force and the European Society of Cardiology Committee for Practice Guidelines (Writing Committee to Develop

Guidelines for Management of Patients With Ventricular Arrhythmias and the Prevention of Sudden Cardiac Death). J Am Coll Cardiol. 2006;48:e247-346.
2. Emkanjoo Z, Alihasani N, Alizadeh A, Tayyebi M, Bonakdar H, Barakpour H, Sadr-Ameli MA. Electrical storm in patients with implantable cardioverter-defibrillators: can it be forecast? Tex Heart Inst J. 2009;36:563-7.
3. Sesselberg HW, Moss AJ, McNitt S, Zareba W, Daubert JP, Andrews ML, Hall WJ, McClinitic B, Huang DT. Ventricular arrhythmia storms in postinfarction patients with implantable defibrillators for primary prevention indications: a MADIT-II substudy. Heart Rhythm. 2007;4:1395-402.
4. Eifling M, Razavi M, Massumi A. The evaluation and management of electrical storm. Tex Heart Inst J. 2011;38: 111-21.
5. Credner SC, Klingenheben T, Mauss O, Sticherling C, Hohnloser SH. Electrical storm in patients with transvenous implantable cardioverter-defibrillators: incidence, management and prognostic implications. J Am Coll Cardiol. 1998;32:1909-15.
6. Exner DV, Pinski SL, Wyse DG, Renfroe EG, Follmann D, Gold M, Beckman KJ, Coromilas J, Lancaster S, Hallstrom AP. Electrical storm presages nonsudden death: the antiarrhythmics versus implantable defibrillators (AVID) trial. Circulation. 2001;103:2066-71.
7. Brigadeau F, Kouakam C, Klug D, Marquie C, Duhamel A, Mizon-Gerard F, Lacroix D, Kacet S. Clinical predictors and prognostic significance of electrical storm in patients with implantable cardioverter defibrillators. Eur Heart J. 2006;27:700-7.
8. Hohnloser SH, Al-Khalidi HR, Pratt CM, Brum JM, Tatla DS, Tchou P, Dorian P. Electrical storm in patients with an implantable defibrillator: incidence, features, and preventive therapy: insights from a randomized trial. Eur Heart J. 2006;27:3027-32.
9. Verma A, Kilicaslan F, Marrouche NF, Minor S, Khan M, Wazni O, Burkhardt JD, Belden WA, Cummings JE, Abdul-Karim A, Saliba W, Schweikert RA, Tchou PJ, Martin DO, Natale A. Prevalence, predictors, and mortality significance of the causative arrhythmia in patients with electrical storm. J Cardiovasc Electrophysiol. 2004;15:1265-70.
10. Huang DT, Traub D. Recurrent ventricular arrhythmia storms in the age of implantable cardioverter defibrillator therapy: a comprehensive review. Prog Cardiovasc Dis. 2008;51: 229-36.
11. Hurst TM, Hinrichs M, Breidenbach C, Katz N, Waldecker B. Detection of myocardial injury during transvenous implantation of automatic cardioverter-defibrillators. J Am Coll Cardiol. 1999;34:402-8.
12. Joglar JA, Kessler DJ, Welch PJ, Keffer JH, Jessen ME, Hamdan MH, Page RL. Effects of repeated electrical defibrillations on cardiac troponin I levels. Am J Cardiol. 1999;83:270-2, A6.
13. Singer I, Hutchins GM, Mirowski M, Mower MM, Veltri EP, Guarnieri T, Griffith LS, Watkins L, Juanteguy J, Fisher S, et al. Pathologic findings related to the lead system and repeated defibrillations in patients with the automatic implantable cardioverter-defibrillator. J Am Coll Cardiol. 1987;10: 382-8.
14. Epstein AE, Kay GN, Plumb VJ, Dailey SM, Anderson PG. Gross and microscopic pathological changes associated with nonthoracotomy implantable defibrillator leads. Circulation. 1998;98:1517-24.
15. Jones DL, Narayanan N. Defibrillation depresses heart sarcoplasmic reticulum calcium pump: a mechanism of postshock dysfunction. Am J Physiol. 1998;274:H98-105.
16. Swynghedauw B. Molecular mechanisms of myocardial remodeling. Physiol Rev. 1999;79:215-62.
17. Marks AR. Intracellular calcium-release channels: regulators of cell life and death. Am J Physiol. 1997;272:H597-605.
18. Baerman JM, Morady F, DiCarlo LA, de Buitleir M. Differentiation of ventricular tachycardia from supraventricular tachycardia with aberration: value of the clinical history. Ann Emerg Med. 1987;16:40-3.
19. Dijkman B, den Dulk K, Wellens HJ. Management of electrical instability after ICD implantation. Pacing Clin Electrophysiol. 1995;18:148-51.
20. Sears SF, Todaro JF, Urizar G, Lewis TS, Sirois B, Wallace R, Sotile W, Curtis AB, Conti JB. Assessing the psychosocial impact of the ICD: a national survey of implantable cardioverter defibrillator health care providers. Pacing Clin Electrophysiol. 2000;23:939-45.
21. Saksena S, Ciccone JM, Craelius W, Pantopoulos D, Rothbart ST, Werres R. Studies on left ventricular function during sustained ventricular tachycardia. J Am Coll Cardiol. 1984;4:501-8.
22. Recurrent ventricular tachycardia. In: Josephson ME, (Ed). Clinical cardiac electrophysiology: techniques and interpretation. 3rd edn. Philadelphia: Lippincott Williams & Wilkins; 2002. p. 528.
23. Bigger JT, Dresdale FJ, Heissenbuttel RH, Weld FM, Wit AL. Ventricular arrhythmias in ischemic heart disease: mechanism, prevalence, significance, and management. Prog Cardiovasc Dis. 1977;19:255-300.
24. Roden DM. Clinical practice. Long-QT syndrome. N Engl J Med. 2008;358:169-76.
25. Herlitz J, Bang A, Holmberg M, Axelsson A, Lindkvist J, Holmberg S. Rhythm changes during resuscitation from ventricular fibrillation in relation to delay until defibrillation, number of shocks delivered and survival. Resuscitation. 1997;34:17-22.
26. Haissaguerre M, Shoda M, Jais P, Nogami A, Shah DC, Kautzner J, Arentz T, Kalushe D, Lamaison D, Griffith M, Cruz F, de Paola A, Gaita F, Hocini M, Garrigue S, Macle L, Weerasooriya R, Clementy J. Mapping and ablation of idiopathic ventricular fibrillation. Circulation. 2002;106:962-7.
27. Bansch D, Oyang F, Antz M, Arentz T, Weber R, Val-Mejias JE, Ernst S, Kuck KH. Successful catheter ablation of electrical storm after myocardial infarction. Circulation. 2003;108: 3011-6.
28. Maury P, Hocini M, Haissaguerre M. Electrical storms in Brugada syndrome: review of pharmacologic and ablative therapeutic options. Indian Pacing Electrophysiol J. 2005;5: 25-34.
29. Ohgo T, Okamura H, Noda T, Satomi K, Suyama K, Kurita T, Aihara N, Kamakura S, Ohe T, Shimizu W. Acute and chronic management in patients with Brugada syndrome associated with electrical storm of ventricular fibrillation. Heart Rhythm. 2007;4:695-700.
30. Zipes DP. Influence of myocardial ischemia and infarction on autonomic innervation of heart. Circulation. 1990;82: 1095-105.
31. Burjorjee JE, Milne B. Propofol for electrical storm; a case report of cardioversion and suppression of ventricular tachycardia by propofol. Can J Anaesth. 2002;49:973-7.

32. Mahajan A, Moore J, Cesario DA, Shivkumar K. Use of thoracic epidural anesthesia for management of electrical storm: a case report. Heart Rhythm. 2005;2:1359-62.
33. Carbucicchio C, Santamaria M, Trevisi N, Maccabelli G, Giraldi F, Fassini G, Riva S, Moltrasio M, Cireddu M, Veglia F, Della Bella P. Catheter ablation for the treatment of electrical storm in patients with implantable cardioverter-defibrillators: short- and long-term outcomes in a prospective single-center study. Circulation. 2008;117:462-9.
34. Zanobini M, Rossi F, Bertera A, Sandano S, Costa C, Fabrizi R, Viola S, Annoni A, Alamanni F, Biglioli P. Cardiopulmonary support during electrophysiological procedures for ventricular tachycardias not haemodynamically tolerated. Perfusion. 2003;18:79-82.
35. Aliot EM, Stevenson WG, Almendral-Garrote JM, Bogun F, Calkins CH, Delacretaz E, Della Bella P, Hindricks G, Jais P, Josephson ME, Kautzner J, Kay GN, Kuck KH, Lerman BB, Marchlinski F, Reddy V, Schalij MJ, Schilling R, Soejima K, Wilber D. EHRA/HRS Expert Consensus on Catheter Ablation of Ventricular Arrhythmias: developed in a partnership with the European Heart Rhythm Association (EHRA), a Registered Branch of the European Society of Cardiology (ESC), and the Heart Rhythm Society (HRS); in collaboration with the American College of Cardiology (ACC) and the American Heart Association (AHA). Heart Rhythm. 2009;6:886-933.
36. Pacifico A, Ferlic LL, Cedillo-Salazar FR, Nasir N, Doyle TK, Henry PD. Shocks as predictors of survival in patients with implantable cardioverter-defibrillators. J Am Coll Cardiol. 1999;34:204-10.
37. Nordbeck P, Seidl B, Fey B, Bauer WR, Ritter O. Effect of cardiac resynchronization therapy on the incidence of electrical storm. Int J Cardiol. 2010;143:330-6.
38. Bristow MR, Saxon LA, Boehmer J, Krueger S, Kass DA, De Marco T, Carson P, DiCarlo L, DeMets D, White BG, DeVries DW, Feldman AM. Cardiac-resynchronization therapy with or without an implantable defibrillator in advanced chronic heart failure. N Engl J Med. 2004;350:2140-50.
39. Cleland JG, Daubert JC, Erdmann E, Freemantle N, Gras D, Kappenberger L, Tavazzi L. The effect of cardiac resynchronization on morbidity and mortality in heart failure. N Engl J Med. 2005;352:1539-49.
40. Vanderheyden M, Mullens W, Delrue L, Goethals M, de Bruyne B, Wijns W, Geelen P, Verstreken S, Wellens F, Bartunek J. Myocardial gene expression in heart failure patients treated with cardiac resynchronization therapy responders versus nonresponders. J Am Coll Cardiol. 2008;51:129-36.
41. Wathen MS, DeGroot PJ, Sweeney MO, Stark AJ, Otterness MF, Adkisson WO, Canby RC, Khalighi K, Machado C, Rubenstein DS, Volosin KJ. Prospective randomized multi-center trial of empirical antitachycardia pacing versus shocks for spontaneous rapid ventricular tachycardia in patients with implantable cardioverter-defibrillators: Pacing Fast Ventricular Tachycardia Reduces Shock Therapies (PainFREE Rx II) trial results. Circulation. 2004;110:2591-6.
42. Stevenson WG, Wilber DJ, Natale A, Jackman WM, Marchlinski FE, Talbert T, Gonzalez MD, Worley SJ, Daoud EG, Hwang C, Schuger C, Bump TE, Jazayeri M, Tomassoni GF, Kopelman HA, Soejima K, Nakagawa H. Irrigated radiofrequency catheter ablation guided by electroanatomic mapping for recurrent ventricular tachycardia after myocardial infarction: the multicenter thermocool ventricular tachycardia ablation trial. Circulation. 2008;118:2773-82.
43. Reddy VY, Reynolds MR, Neuzil P, Richardson AW, Taborsky M, Jongnarangsin K, Kralovec S, Sediva L, Ruskin JN, Josephson ME. Prophylactic catheter ablation for the prevention of defibrillator therapy. N Engl J Med. 2007;357:2657-65.
44. Kuck KH, Schaumann A, Eckardt L, Willems S, Ventura R, Delacretaz E, Pitschner HF, Kautzner J, Schumacher B, Hansen PS. Catheter ablation of stable ventricular tachycardia before defibrillator implantation in patients with coronary heart disease (VTACH): a multicentre randomised controlled trial. Lancet. 2010;375:31-40.
45. Effect of enalapril on survival in patients with reduced left ventricular ejection fractions and congestive heart failure. The SOLVD Investigators. N Engl J Med. 1991;325: 293-302.
46. Effect of metoprolol CR/XL in chronic heart failure: Metoprolol CR/XL Randomised Intervention Trial in Congestive Heart Failure (MERIT-HF). Lancet. 1999;353:2001-7.
47. The Cardiac Insufficiency Bisoprolol Study II (CIBIS-II): a randomised trial. Lancet. 1999;353:9-13.
48. Pitt B, Zannad F, Remme WJ, Cody R, Castaigne A, Perez A, Palensky J, Wittes J. The effect of spironolactone on morbidity and mortality in patients with severe heart failure. Randomized Aldactone Evaluation Study Investigators. N Engl J Med. 1999;341:709-17.
49. O'Rourke RA. Role of myocardial revascularization in sudden cardiac death. Circulation. 1992;85:I112-7.

EDITORS' SUMMARY

All electrophysiologists and indeed critical care physicians and general cardiologists need to be completely conversant with the causes and management approaches for patients with a ventricular arrhythmia storm. Dr Namboodiri and colleagues review our present understanding in this area and provide some practical approaches for management. The mainstay for therapy remains beta-blockade along with sedation (with associated sympatholysis) and expeditiously identifying and treating provocative factors including ongoing ischemia. The additional role of antiarrhythmic therapy, percutaneous and surgical sympathetic blockade, and radiofrequency ablation are also outlined and referenced.

SECTION F

Miscellaneous

CHAPTER 43

Ivan Cakulev, Albert L Waldo

Entrainment: Principles and Clinical Applications

LIST OF ABBREVIATIONS

AEGM	Atrial Electrogram	EGM	Electrogram
AFL	Atrial Flutter	HRA	High Right Atrium
AP	Accessory Pathway	ms	milliseconds
AV	Atrioventricular	PCL	Pacing Cycle Length
AVNRT	Atrioventricular Nodal Reentrant Tachycardia	PPI	Post Pacing Interval
AVRT	Atrioventricular Reentrant Tachycardia	RA	Right Atrium
bpm	Beats per minute	TCL	Tachycardia Cycle Length
CL	Cycle Length	VEGM	Ventricular Electrogram
CS	Coronary Sinus	VT	Ventricular Tachycardia
ECG	Electrocardiogram		

INTRODUCTION

The concept of entrainment evolved from a clinical question: was it possible to terminate atrial flutter (AFL) with atrial pacing? But also important was the discovery of triggered rhythms,[1] and the technological revolution in pacing the human heart, particularly to initiate and terminate reentrant arrhythmias. Until the late 1960s and early 1970s, it was generally thought that tachycardias were either due to an automatic mechanism or a reentrant mechanism. Nevertheless, apart from the early and classic experiments of Mayer[2] on reentry in the Medusa ring, and subsequent studies by Mines[3] on ring preparations cut from dogfish auricles or from canine right ventricles, it was only with the publications of the in vitro studies of depressed bundles in loops of canine Purkinje fibers in 1972 by Wit et al.[4,5] that the occurrence of reentry actually was documented. Before the latter studies, although reentrant mechanisms were postulated as being the cause of most arrhythmias, this was based primarily on indirect evidence. Moreover, for in vivo rhythms, it had long been thought that one could distinguish reentrant arrhythmias from automatic rhythms by a few key characteristics. Simply stated, it was generally accepted that if an arrhythmia could be either induced or terminated by premature beats or rapid pacing, the arrhythmia was due to a reentrant mechanism.[6]

Also, the best proof of reentry had long been thought to be mapping the sequence of activation of the heart during the tachycardia, thereby demonstrating the reentrant circuit. Even so, the admonition of Mines[3] that "... the chief error to be guarded against is that of mistaking a series of automatic beats originating in one point of a ring [substitute apparent reentrant circuit] and traveling around it in one direction only owing to a complete block close to the point of origin of the rhythm on one side of this point" must be remembered. The point, of course, is that even sequence of activation mapping may not provide proof of reentry per se, even though it appears to be just that. Mines suggested that severing the ring [again, substitute reentrant circuit] or the like, and then demonstrating that no further reentrant excitation could occur was required for proof of reentry. Nevertheless, although it became possible to perform sequence of activation mapping of the human heart in vivo, simple pacing techniques were far easier to use in clinical and most animal studies, during which investigators relied on the above responses to cardiac pacing to establish the presence or absence of reentry. With the discovery of triggered rhythms, we learned that they, too, could be induced and terminated with premature beats or rapid pacing[1,7] Thus, no longer was pacing induction or termination of a rhythm the *sine qua non* for identifying whether the rhythm was due to reentry. Clearly, new pacing criteria were needed to demonstrate the presence of reentry. This was the perspective when we confronted the management of AFL in patients following open heart surgery.

DISCOVERING ENTRAINMENT

The discovery of entrainment begins with studies in patients with AFL. In the early 1970s, the mechanism of AFL was not very well understood. There were two schools, one thought that AFL was due to a single focus firing rapidly, and the other that it was due to a reentrant mechanism.[8] During that time, attempts to terminate AFL in patients using rapid atrial pacing techniques, introduction of premature atrial beats, or both were reported.[9] These studies were not performed systematically, and their results were quite variable. Some reported limited success, and some reported overt failure.[9] In short, whether one could reliably terminate AFL with cardiac pacing was seriously questioned.

One day in the fall of 1972, at The University of Alabama at Birmingham (UAB) Medical Center, a cardiologist was about to perform DC cardioversion of AFL in a post-open heart surgical patient. Since a pair of temporary wire electrodes had been placed on the right atrial epicardium at the time of surgery, and aware of "recent" reports that AFL could be terminated by rapid atrial pacing, he asked us to try to pace terminate the patient's the AFL, and, thereby, restore sinus rhythm. Using overdrive pacing at rates chosen arbitrarily, but all faster than the intrinsic rate of the AFL, we were unable to terminate the AFL. We then began systematic atrial pacing studies in patients with AFL following open heart surgery using the temporary epicardial wire electrodes placed in the high right atrium (near the sinus node) at the time of surgery.[9]

Entrainment of Atrial Flutter

During these studies, we soon found that to terminate AFL, pacing had to be performed at a critically rapid overdrive pacing rate, and for a critically long duration. When the pacing rate was faster than the AFL rate but insufficiently rapid or of insufficient duration, although the pacing captured the atria, with abrupt cessation of pacing or slowing of the pacing rate below the intrinsic AFL rate, the AFL was still present **(Figures 43.1A to D)**.[9] Also, during such pacing, the AFL complexes in ECG leads II, III, and aVF changed little, and the positive atrial complexes in the ECG expected when pacing from the high right atrium were not seen **(Figure 43.1)**. But when the atria were paced at a sufficiently rapid rate for a critically long duration, upon cessation of pacing the AFL had terminated **(Figures 43.2A to C)**. However, we didn't understand why both a critically rapid rate and duration of pacing were required. Also, as demonstrated in **Figures 43.2A to C**, termination of AFL was associated with the appearance of a positive P wave in ECG leads II, II, and aVF, the expected morphology when pacing from the high right atrium. However, the explanation for the abrupt change in the atrial complex morphology in the ECG **(Figures 43.2A to C)** initially was not apparent. Additionally, the abrupt change in atrial morphology in the ECG was associated with a decrease (mean of 100 ms) in activation time from the high right atrial pacing site to a posterior-inferior left atrial electrode recording site despite the fact that the pacing site, the pacing rate, and the recording site had not changed.[9] This, too, was initially not understood except as a marker of successful AFL termination.

Based on our initial series of overdrive atrial pacing studies in patients with AFL, we coined the term "transient entrainment of a tachycardia." It was initially defined as an increase in the rate of a tachycardia to the faster pacing rate, with resumption of the tachycardia either upon abrupt

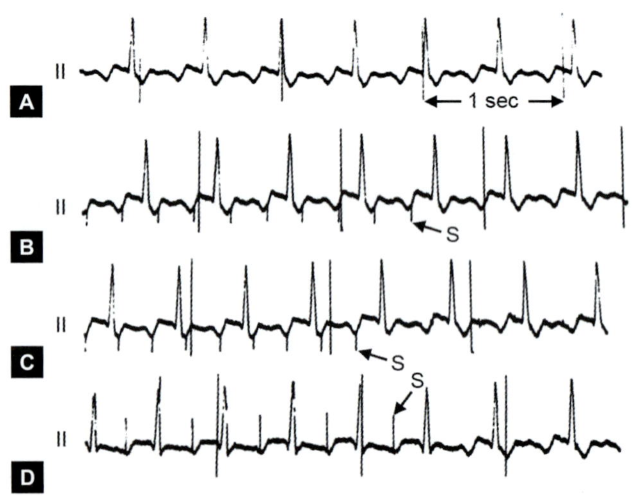

Figures 43.1A to D: (A) ECG lead II recorded from a patient during AFL (atrial CL = 264 ms); and at the end of 30 s of rapid atrial pacing from a high right atrial site at CLs of 254 ms (B), 242 ms (C), and 232 ms (D). The atrial flutter was entrained, but not terminated at each pacing CL. Timelines are at 1 s intervals. See text for discussion. (Modified from reference #11)

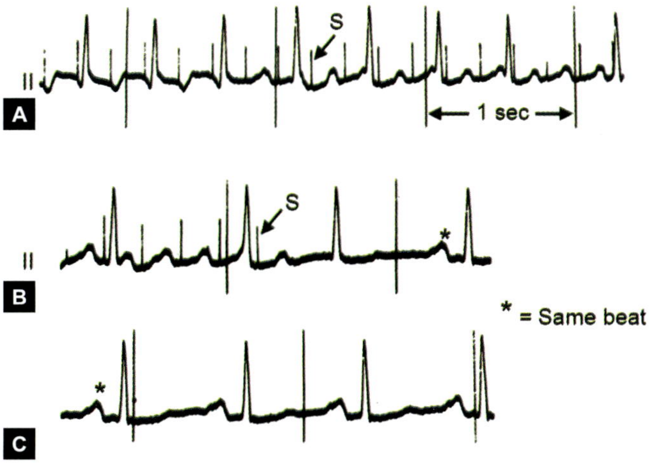

Figures 43.2A to C: (A) ECG lead II recorded from the same patient as in Figure 43.1 during high right atrial pacing from the same site, but now at a CL of 224 ms. With the 7th beat in this tracing, and after 22 s of atrial pacing at a constant rate, the atrial complexes suddenly became positive; (B) ECG lead II recorded from the same patient immediately before and after cessation of pacing at a CL of 224 ms. Note that sinus rhythm is present; (C) Continued sinus rhythm. The asterisk identifies the same beat at the end of (B) and beginning of (C). See text for discussion. (Modified from reference #11)

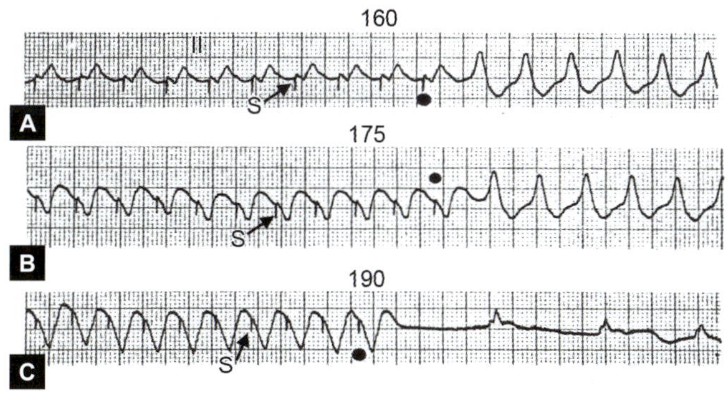

Figures 43.3A to C: ECG lead II recorded from a patient with ventricular tachycardia (VT) at a rate of 150 bpm. (A) Cessation of ventricular pacing (dot) at a rate of 160 bpm, with prompt return of VT; (B) Cessation of pacing (dot) at a rate of 175 bpm, with prompt return of VT; (C) Termination of pacing at a rate of 190 bpm, with successful termination of the VT. See text for discussion. (Modified from reference #11)

cessation of pacing or slowing of the pacing rate below the intrinsic rate of the tachycardia. This was a descriptive definition because we did not yet understand the mechanism of entrainment sufficiently.

Entrainment of Ventricular Tachycardia

We then started to examine overdrive pacing of other tachyarrhythmias. During entrainment of ventricular tachycardia, we again demonstrated that when pacing at a rate faster than the tachycardia rate, a critical pacing rate and duration of pacing were required to terminate the tachycardia[10] **(Figure 43.3C)**. What was new during entrainment of VT was the clear recognition of progressive fusion of the QRS complexes in the ECG during pacing at two or more constant rates, each of which were faster than the rate of the tachycardia, but each of which failed to terminate the tachycardia[10] **(Figures 43.3A and B)**.

The critical insight that led to our understanding the mechanism (physiology) of entrainment resulted from analysis of a single case of entrainment and termination of VT.[11] What we finally understood about entrainment and termination of reentrant VT turned out to be true for every ordered reentrant tachyarrhythmia (AFL,[9,11-14] VT,[10,11,15-17] atrioventricular reentrant tachycardia [AVRT],[14,18] AV nodal reentrant tachycardia [AVNRT,[14,19] and intra-atrial reentrant tachycardia[14,20]) we have studied. Moreover, the phenomena observed during entrainment and termination of a tachycardia identify the tachycardia mechanism as reentrant.

ENTRAINMENT: A PACING TECHNIQUE TO IDENTIFY REENTRANT ARRHYTHMIAS

On the basis of a series of studies during overdrive pacing of AFL,[9,11-14] VT,[10,11,15-17] AVRT,[11,18] AVNRT,[14,19] and intra-atrial reentrant tachycardia,[14,20] we demonstrated that entrainment of a tachycardia is an increase in the rate of all tissues responsible for sustaining the tachycardia to the faster pacing rate, with resumption of the intrinsic rate of the tachycardia on either abrupt cessation of pacing or slowing of the pacing rate below the intrinsic rate of the tachycardia.[8] On the basis of studies during the above rhythms in patients, and in an experimental model of AFL,[21] we demonstrated that entrainment is best explained by pacing capture of a reentrant circuit from two directions. Thus, during entrainment of a tachycardia, the wavefront from each pacing impulse enters into the excitable gap of the reentrant circuit, and travels in two directions, antidromically, i.e. in the opposite direction of the circulating wavefront of the spontaneous tachycardia, where it collides with the orthodromic wavefront of the previous beat, and orthodromically, i.e. in the same direction as the circulating wavefront of the spontaneous tachycardia. The latter wavefront continues the tachycardia, resetting it to the pacing rate. On the basis of those and subsequent studies, we demonstrated that entrainment of a tachycardia indicates that the tachycardia is due to a reentrant mechanism, with an excitable gap being present in the reentrant circuit.

THE BREAKTHROUGH CASE IN UNDERSTANDING ENTRAINMENT, AND DEVELOPMENT OF THE FIRST THREE ENTRAINMENT CRITERIA

The "Eureka!" case was one of postoperative VT with 1:1 retrograde atrial activation during the VT.[11] Because of the latter, and especially because this VT was relatively slow (141 bpm) and well-tolerated, we thought we could pace the atria to terminate the VT. **Figure 43.4** shows the first of a series of diagrams to represent the reentrant VT circuit using a figure-of-eight model of reentry with a central isthmus. At the time, we thought that the isthmus represented an area of slow conduction. But as we now know from the work of Wit et al.,[8] the area of slow conduction in the model is probably on either side of the isthmus. For purposes of simplicity, and as originally reported, we chose to continue to use the figure-of-eight reentrant circuit to illustrate what occurs during entrainment and termination of VT. However, an example of entrainment of a single loop reentrant VT circuit with an excitable gap would work as well.

In **Figure 43.4**, the top left panel illustrates the spontaneous VT wavefronts traveling around the reentrant circuit at a cycle length (CL) of 425 ms (141 bpm). With the onset of atrial pacing (**Figure 43.4**, top middle panel) at a CL of 400 ms (150 bpm), a rate faster than the spontaneous VT rate, the ventricular wavefront from the pacing impulse is able to enter the excitable gap of the reentrant circuit, whereupon it travels both antidromically and orthodromically. Antidromically, it collides with the orthodromic wavefront of the previous beat, creating a fusion beat morphology in the ECG. Orthodromically, it enters the reentrant circuit early, so that it captures the reentrant circuit at the pacing CL, and resets it to the pacing rate (CL). Because this orthodromic wavefront isn't blocked, it travels around the reentrant circuit until it collides with the antidromic wavefront of the next paced beat (**Figure 43.4**, top right panel). Thus, during pacing, there is a constant fusion of the QRS complex morphology in the ECG, as the ventricles are activated simultaneously by wavefronts from two different directions, and from two different paced beats; and b) there is continuous resetting of the tachycardia to the pacing rate (CL) by the orthodromic wave from each pacing impulse. This, in fact, is the mechanistic definition of entrainment: Entrainment of a tachycardia occurs during pacing at a rate faster than the tachycardia rate when each orthodromic wavefront from the pacing impulse resets the tachycardia to the pacing rate, and each antidromic wavefront from the pacing impulse either collides with the orthodromic wavefront of the previous beat or is otherwise blocked. An example of the latter occurs when entraining AVRT during atrial pacing in the presence of an accessory AV connection or an accessory pathway (AP) capable only of unidirectional retrograde conduction (a concealed AV bypass pathway).

The ECG and ventricular electrogram (VEGM) recordings during atrial pacing at 150 bpm with 1:1 capture of the ventricles are shown in the bottom panel of **Figure 43.4**. Note that during pacing, the QRS complexes a) have changed in morphology compared to those during the spontaneous VT, and b) are narrower in duration (120 ms) compared to those during the spontaneous VT (148 ms), but the VEGM morphology was the same during pacing as during the spontaneous VT, indicating that the direction of activation at this recording site was the same in both the instances.

The top panel of **Figure 43.5** diagrammatically illustrates what happened with cessation of pacing. The top left panel shows the last paced beat, and, as expected, its antidromic wavefront collided with the orthodromic wavefront of the previous beat, creating a fusion QRS complex beat in the ECG (i.e., the ventricles are activated simultaneously by wavefronts from two different beats). The orthodromic wavefront of the last paced beat again resets the tachycardia to the pacing rate (CL), but this time, this orthodromic wavefront, which travels around the reentrant circuit at the pacing cycle length, is unopposed because there is no subsequent pacing impulse. Therefore, this last captured beat is entrained, but there is no QRS complex fusion in the ECG. The bottom panel of **Figure 43.5** shows the ECG and VEGM recordings. The last pacing impulse captured the ventricles at the 400 ms pacing CL, but while the last captured ventricular beat was entrained (asterisk), the QRS complex was not a result of fusion. Rather, because the orthodromic wavefront from the last pacing impulse was unopposed by a subsequent antidromic pacing wavefront, this beat had the QRS complex morphology of the spontaneous VT. These observations illustrate the first entrainment criterion: during a tachycardia, when pacing at a constant rate that is faster than the rate of tachycardia, and which fails to terminate the tachycardia, there is the demonstration of constant fusion beats in the ECG except for the last captured beat, which is entrained but not fused.[8]

Then with atrial pacing at 155 bpm (CL 387 ms), the same events occurred. The VT reentrant circuit was captured at the pacing rate CL, the morphology of the QRS complexes (fusion beats) changed even more, as did the QRS duration, which narrowed to 91 ms **(Figure 43.6)**. Also, as before, the VEGM morphology was unchanged from that during the spontaneous VT. And as before, the last pacing impulse captured the ventricles at the pacing rate CL, but the morphology of the last entrained beat was not fused. Because the pacing CL was shorter, the antidromic wavefront from each pacing impulse entered the excitable gap of the reentrant circuit earlier, resulting in greater antidromic penetration of the reentrant circuit, and, therefore, resulting in collision with the orthodromic wavefront of the previous beat at a different place **(Figure 43.6)**. This created constant fusion QRS complexes in the ECG which were different from when seen pacing at 150 bpm **(Figures 43.4 and 43.5)**. And then when pacing the atria at 160 bpm (375 ms CL),

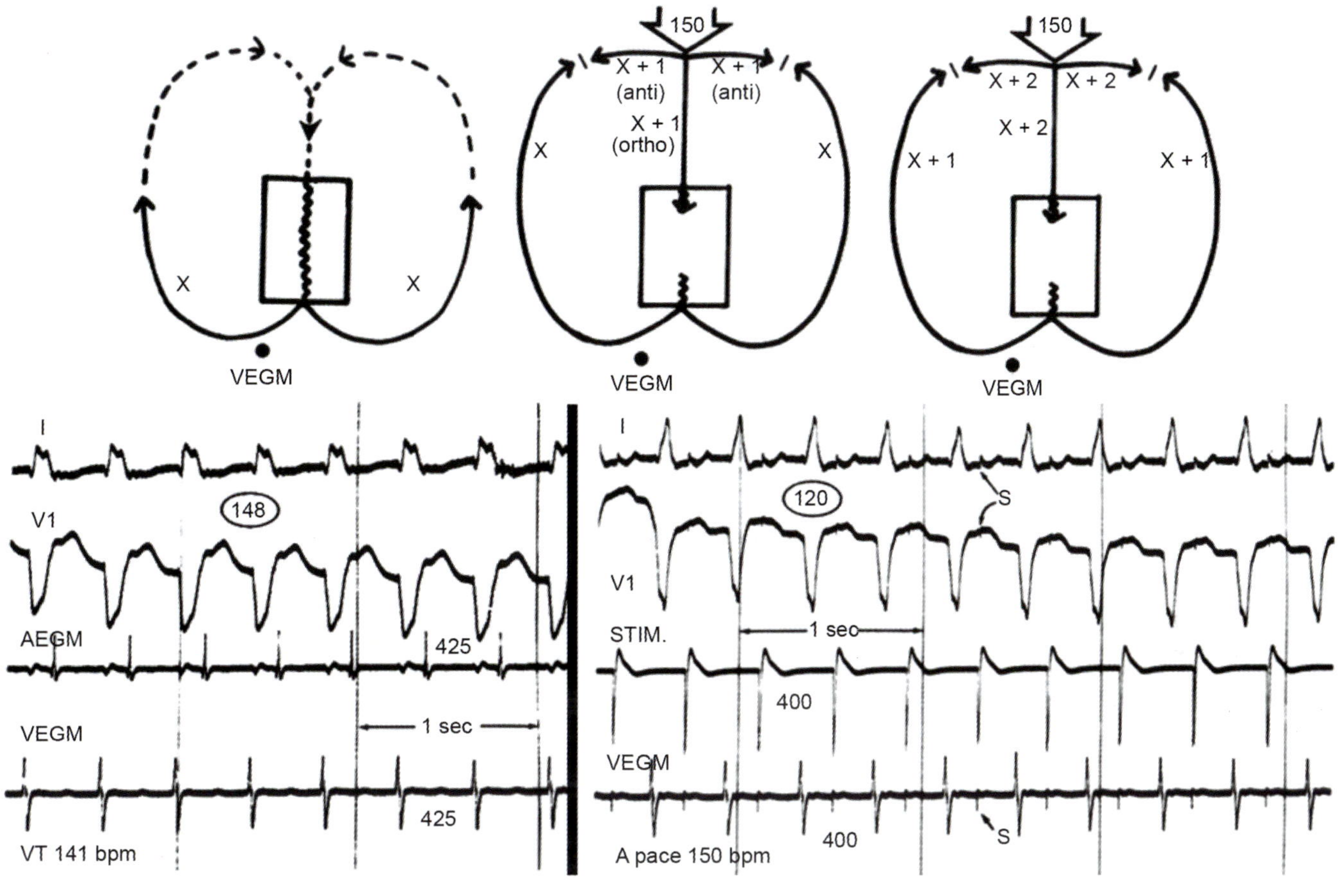

Figure 43.4: Top panel: Diagrammatic representation of entrainment, in this case, of ventricular tachycardia (VT) during atrial pacing. In this and subsequent diagrams, arrows indicate the direction of activation in the reentrant circuit, the box represents an isthmus in the reentrant circuit, the serpentine line indicates slow conduction, the dashed line indicates the excitable gap in the reentrant circuit, the black dot represents a right ventricular electrogram (VEGM) recording site, and the large arrow (middle and right panels) indicates wavefronts from the pacing impulse entering the excitable gap of the VT reentrant circuit, where they are conducted orthodromically (ortho) and antidromically (anti).

Top left panel: Diagram of the reentrant circuit (figure-of-eight model) during VT at a rate of 141 bpm. *X* = orthodromic wavefronts of the reentrant rhythm.

Top middle panel: Introduction of the first pacing impulse (*X* + 1) during atrial pacing at a rate of 150 bpm during the VT. The antidromic wavefronts (*X* + 1) collide with the orthodromic wavefronts of the previous spontaneous beat (X), resulting in a fusion ventricular beat, which, in effect, terminates the VT. However, the orthodromic wavefront from the pacing impulse continues the tachycardia, resetting it to the pacing rate.

Top right panel: Introduction of the second pacing impulse (*X* + 2) during atrial pacing at 150 bpm. The antidromic wavefronts (*X* + 2) collide with the orthodromic wavefronts (*X* + 1) of the previous paced beat, again resulting in ventricular fusion, which, again, in effect, terminates the VT. But again, the orthodromic wavefronts from the pacing impulse (*X* + 2) continue the VT, resetting it to the pacing rate. During the period of pacing, the VEGM site is always activated by an orthodromic wavefront.

Bottom left panel: ECG leads I and VI recorded simultaneously with a bipolar atrial electrogram (AEGM) and a unipolar ventricular electrogram (VEGM) during VT at a rate of 141 bpm (425 ms CL). In this and Figure 43.5, the circled number indicates the duration (ms) of each QRS complex.

Bottom right panel: ECG leads I and V1, recorded simultaneously with the atrial pacing (A Pace) stimulus (S) artifact (STIM) and the unipolar ventricular electrogram (VEGM) during atrial pacing at 150 bpm (400 ms CL). Timelines are at 1 second intervals. See text for discussion. (Modified from reference #11)

there was a still different QRS complex morphology, and the QRS complex duration was now only 80 ms **(Figure 43.6)**, but the ventricular electrode recording site was still activated from the same direction during pacing as during the spontaneous tachycardia, and the last entrained beat was not fused. Because this pacing CL was shorter still, the antidromic wavefront of each pacing impulse was able to penetrate further into the reentrant circuit **(Figure 43.6)**, explaining the yet again different QRS complex morphology of the fusion beats in the ECG leads. The different degree of fusion in the ECG leads at each pacing rate (CL) which entrains but fails to terminate the tachycardia is called progressive fusion

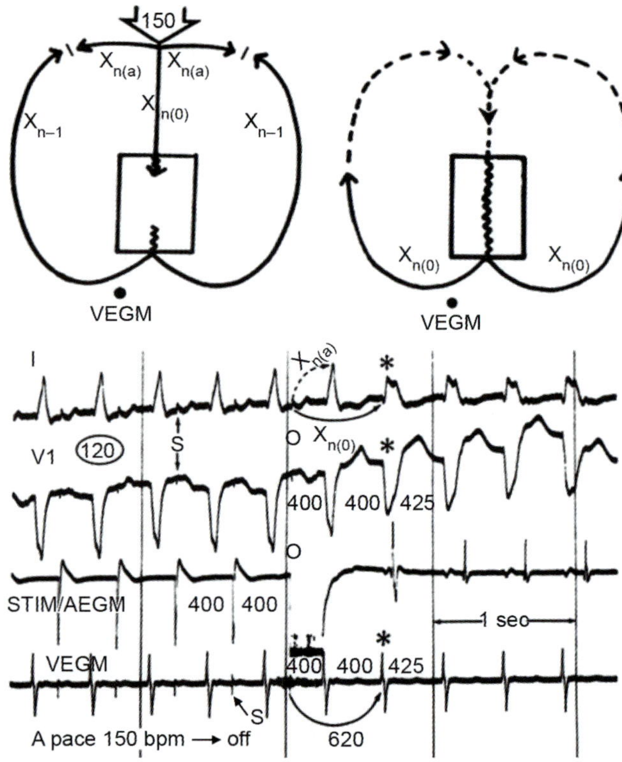

Figure 43.5: Diagrammatic representation and tracings of the cessation of atrial pacing at 150 bpm, illustrating the first entrainment criterion.

Top left panel: The wavefront from the last pacing impulse (rate 150 bpm) enters the excitable gap of the VT reentrant circuit, where it is conducted orthodromically and antidromically. The antidromic wavefronts $X_{n(a)}$ collide with the orthodromic wavefronts X_{n-1}, resulting in a fusion beat. The orthodromic wavefront $X_{n(o)}$ from the last pacing impulse continues the tachycardia, resetting it to the pacing rate.

Top right panel: The orthodromic wavefronts from the last pacing impulse are now unopposed by antidromic wavefronts because there is no subsequent pacing impulse, so that no fusion of ventricular activation occurs despite the presence of entrainment. This last entrained beat continues the tachycardia (dashed lines), which then resumes at its previous spontaneous rate.

Bottom panel: ECG leads I and V1 recorded simultaneously with the atrial pacing (A Pace) stimulus (S) artifact (STIM) or atrial electrogram (AEGM), and the unipolar ventricular electrogram (VEGM) at the cessation of atrial pacing at a rate of 150 bpm (400 ms CL). In this and subsequent figures, the open circle denotes the last stimulus, the asterisk denotes the last entrained beat, the arrow from the stimulus in the VEGM points to the resulting VEGM (with the stimulus-to-VEGM interval indicated in ms); the dashed arrow in lead I represents the last antidromic wavefronts $X_{n(a)}$; and the solid arrow represents the last orthodromic wavefronts, $X_{n(o)}$ from the last pacing impulse. See text for discussion. (Modified from reference #11)

(Figure 43.6). These observations illustrate the second entrainment criterion: during a tachycardia: when pacing at two or more constant rates that are each faster than the rate of the tachycardia, but which fail to terminate the tachycardia, there is the demonstration of constant fusion beats in the ECG at each different pacing rate, but different degrees of constant fusion at each pacing rate (CL).[8]

Then with atrial pacing at a rate of 165 bpm (364 ms CL), still with 1:1 conduction to the ventricles (**Figure 43.7**, top panel), initially there is further progressive fusion of the QRS complexes in the ECGs. Then, denoted by the asterisks, there was an abrupt change in morphology of both the recorded VEGMs and the QRS complexes in the ECG leads. Immediately before the change in morphology of both the QRS complexes and of the VEGMs, the stimulus-to-VEGM interval was 640 ms (recall that this includes conduction time from the atrial pacing site through the AV node and His-Purkinje system, and then entry into the excitable gap of the ventricular reentrant circuit). Then, there was localized conduction block to the VEGM recording site for one beat (i.e., the impulse from the next stimulus captured most of the ventricles, but never activated this ventricular recording site), after which, the impulse from the next stimulus was conducted to that VEGM site with a stimulus-to-VEGM interval of only 305 ms. The localized conduction block for one beat was associated with a one cycle prolongation of the beat-to-beat interval at the VEGM recording site (from a pacing CL of 364 ms, to 425 ms, and then back to the pacing CL of 364 ms). There was no similar prolongation of the QRS complex CLs. In the ECG lead I tracing, the dashed arrows represent the antidromic wavefronts, and the solid arrows represent the orthodromic wavefronts from the fifth and sixth pacing impulses shown in the figure. After the block of both the antidromic and orthodromic wavefronts in the VT reentrant circuit during the sixth pacing impulse, the ventricles were activated by the seventh pacing impulse as expected during overdrive atrial pacing of a sinus rhythm because the VT had been terminated, and the reentrant circuit was no longer present. This explains the change in morphology of both the QRS complexes and the VEGMs. The QRS complexes returned to their usual morphology during activation as in sinus rhythm (actually now an atrial paced rhythm, but in the absence of VT). The VEGM morphology also changed to that seen during sinus rhythm, as the VEGM electrode site was now being activated as during sinus rhythm, different from that during the VT. Finally, had the pacing been stopped prior to achieving block of both the antidromic and orthodromic wavefronts of the same pacing impulse during the same beat, the tachycardia would not have been terminated, emphasizing the critical duration of pacing at the critical pacing rate required for termination of the tachycardia.

Termination of the tachycardia is shown diagrammatically (**Figure 43.7**, bottom panel). When pacing the atria at 165 bpm (364 ms CL), the antidromic wavefront of the pacing impulse collided, as usual, with the orthodromic wavefront of the previous beat. But now the orthodromic wavefront of that same pacing impulse also blocked, presumably in an area of slow conduction in the reentrant circuit.[8] Therefore, an area of the ventricles was never activated by this paced beat.

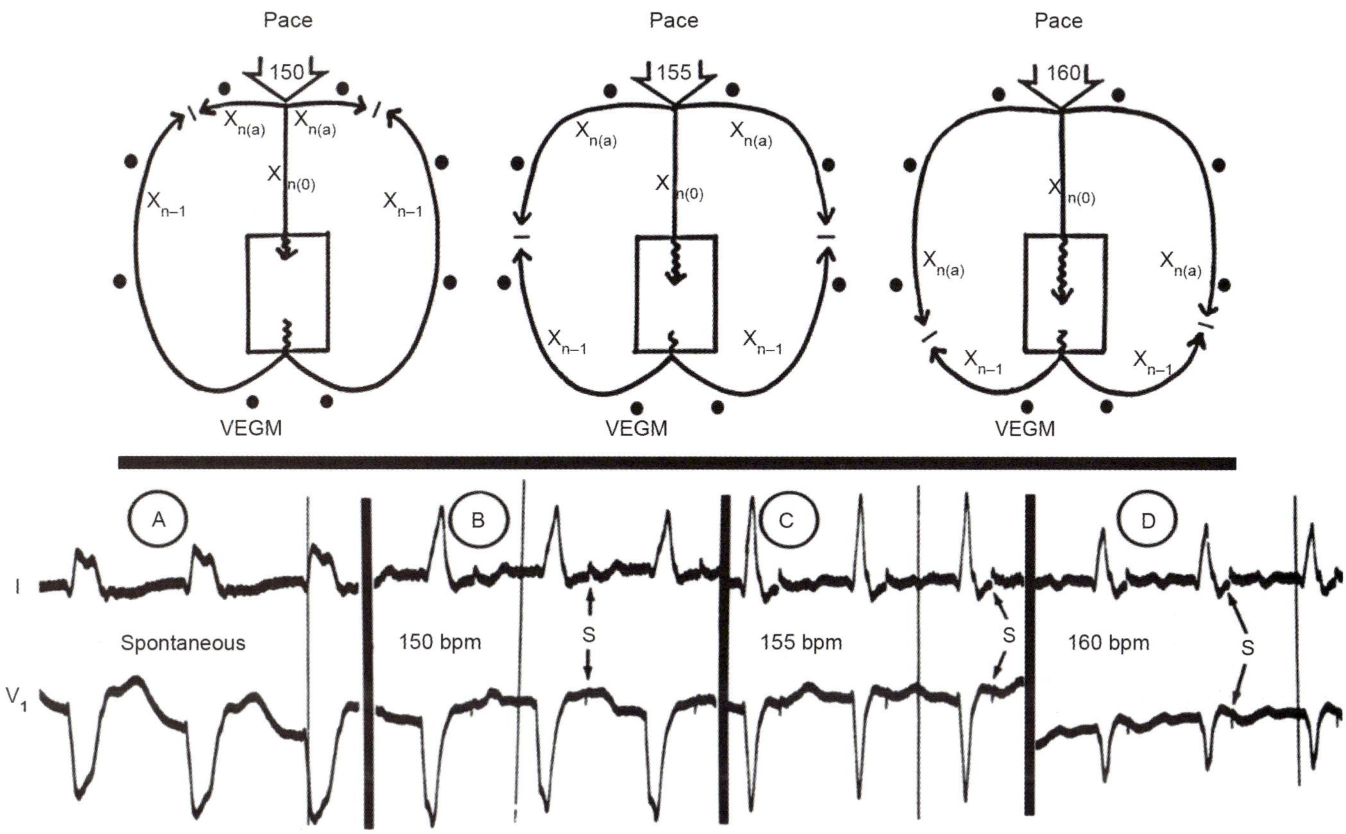

Figure 43.6: Illustration of the second entrainment criterion.
Top panel: Diagrammatic representation of entrainment of the VT illustrated in Figure 43.4 during pacing at 150 bpm, 155 bpm, and 160 bpm. In each example, the antidromic wavefronts from each pacing impulse, $X_{n(a)}$, collide with the orthodromic wavefront of the previous beat, X_{n-1}. However, in each case, the orthodromic wavefront from each pacing impulse, $X_{n(0)}$, entrains the VT by resetting it to the pacing rate. Because the pacing CL progressively decreases as the pacing rate increases, the antidromic wavefronts from each pacing impulse at each faster rate penetrate the reentrant circuit to a greater degree. Therefore, although ventricular fusion occurs in each instance, the degree of fusion is different. This results in progressive fusion in the ECGs (see bottom panel).
Bottom panel: ECG leads I and V_1 recorded simultaneously during VT at a rate of 141 bpm (A), and during atrial pacing which entrains the VT at 150 bpm (B), 155 bpm (C), and 160 bpm (D). S = stimulus artifact. See text for discussion. (Modified from reference #11)

This is localized conduction block. With block of both the antidromic and orthodromic wavefronts of the atrial pacing impulse during the same beat, the tachycardia was terminated, and the functionally determined components of the reentrant circuit disappeared. Thus, with the next atrial pacing impulse at the same 165 bpm rate (364 ms CL), the site at which localized conduction block had just occurred now is activated from a different direction and with a shorter conduction time. These observations demonstrate the third entrainment criterion: during a tachycardia, when pacing at a constant rate that is faster than the rate of tachycardia and which terminates the tachycardia, there is the demonstration of localized conduction block to a site or sites for one beat followed by activation of that site or those sites by the next paced beat from a different direction and with a shorter conduction time.[8]

From the above, we can understand what happened in **Figure 43.2** during overdrive pacing of AFL. Recall that after the 22 seconds of high right atrial pacing at a constant rate of 373 bpm, suddenly there was the appearance of positive P waves in ECG lead II, and with the cessation of pacing, the AFL had been terminated, with return of sinus rhythm. This was the demonstration of the third entrainment criterion, in this case, during overdrive pacing of AFL. Thus, during entrainment, the antidromic wavefront of each atrial pacing impulse collided with the orthodromic wavefront of the previous beat, and each orthodromic wavefront reset the tachycardia to the pacing rate. But when the antidromic and orthodromic wavefronts of the same pacing impulse were blocked during the same beat, the tachycardia was terminated. Therefore, the next pacing impulse captured the atria as if overdriving sinus rhythm. Since pacing was being performed from the

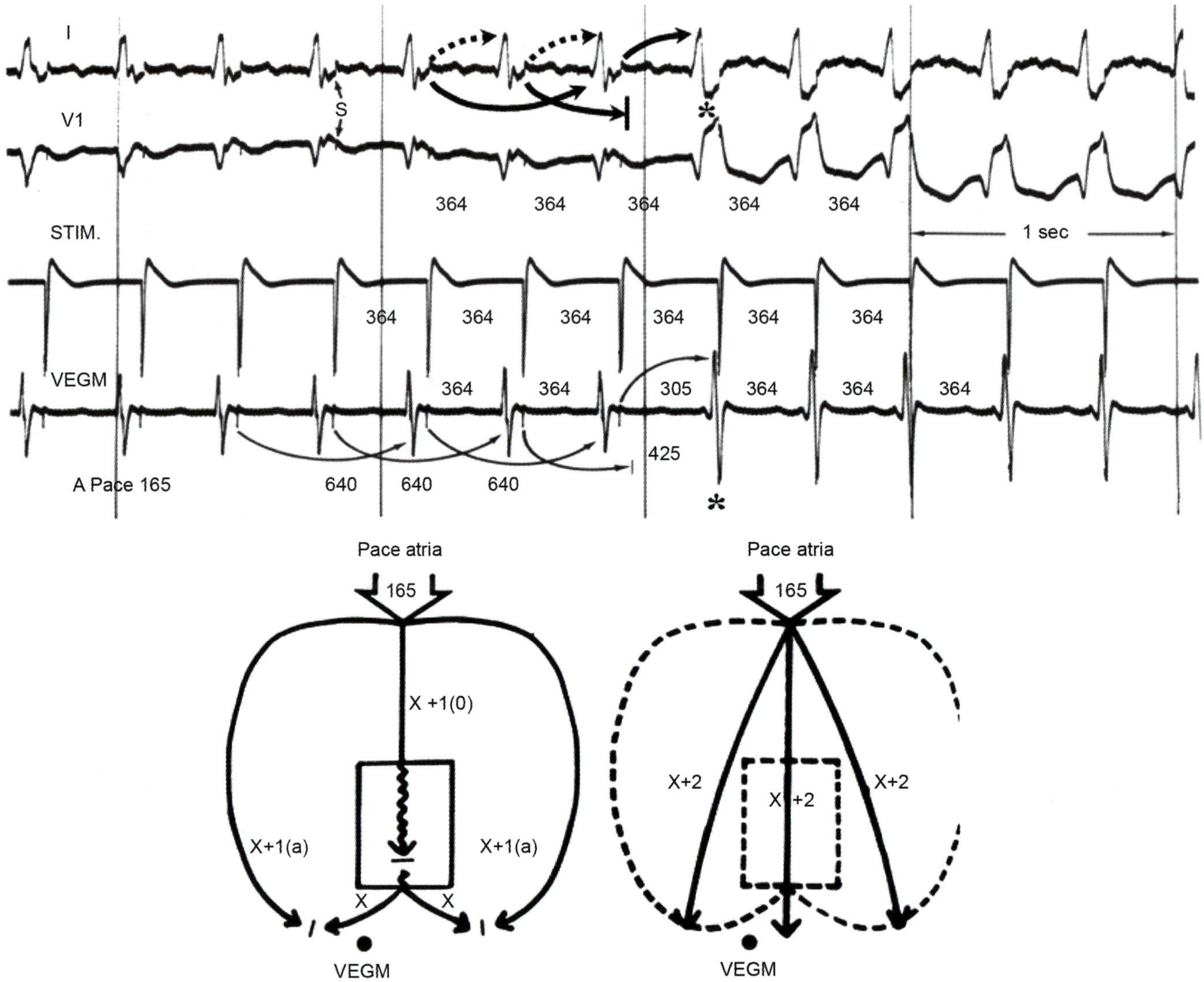

Figure 43.7: Illustration of the third entrainment criterion.

Top panel: ECG leads I and V_1 recorded simultaneously with the atrial pacing stimulus (s) artifact (STIM), and the unipolar ventricular electrogram (VEGM) during atrial pacing at 165 bpm (364 ms CL) which terminates the VT. The asterisks denote an abrupt change in configuration of the recorded QRS complexes in both ECG leads and VEGM. Before the change in configuration of the QRS complexes and the VEGM, the atrial stimulus-to-VEGM interval is 640 ms. Then, after the localized block to the VEGM recording site, this interval becomes 305 ms. Note also that this localized conduction block is associated with a one-cycle increase in the beat-to-beat CL localized to the VEGM recording site (from 364 to 425 ms, and then back again to 364 ms). S = stimulus artifact.

The **bottom panel** is a diagrammatic representation of events recorded in the top panel during the termination of the VT with pacing at 165 bpm.

Bottom left panel: The wavefront from the pacing impulse enters the excitable gap of the VT reentrant circuit, where it is conducted antidromically, X + 1(a), and orthodromically, X + 1(o). The antidromic wavefronts collide with the orthodromic wavefronts of the previous beat (*X*) resulting in a fusion beat. Note that this collision is at a site still different from that illustrated in Figure 43.6. However, this time, the orthodromic wavefront is also blocked during the same cycle. Note that sites immediately orthodromically distal to the site of block of X +1(0), although activated by the orthodromic wavefront (X) of the previous beat, are not activated by X + 1.

Bottom right panel: The next pacing impulse at the same 165 bpm rate (X + 2) now activates the ventricles. But because the VT was terminated by the previous (X + 1) paced beat, the sequence of ventricular activation during X + 2 is as expected during atrial overdrive pacing of sinus rhythm. Thus the sites which had just demonstrated localized conduction block for one beat, including the VEGM site, are now activated from a different direction and with a shorter conduction time. This is because there no longer is a VT reentrant circuit to direct activation to these latter sites. See text for discussion. (Modified from reference #11) high right atrium, a positive P wave appeared in ECG lead II **(Figure 43.2)**. Thus, we finally understood what happened during entrainment and termination of classical AFL when pacing from the high right atrium. With the pacing termination of atrial flutter, because there was no longer a re-entrant circuit to engage, including orthodromic conduction through an area of slow conduction, conduction time from the pacing site to the postero-inferior left atrial recording site was as if overdriving sinus rhythm, so that conduction from the high right atrial pacing site became considerably shorter. This is now diagrammed in **Figure 43.8**.

THE FOURTH ENTRAINMENT CRITERION

During these entrainment studies, it was recognized that it is sometimes difficult to see or demonstrate some or all of the first three entrainment criteria, particularly fusion in the ECG when pacing from the atria during AFL or a reentrant supraventricular tachycardia. From that evolved the fourth entrainment criterion: during a tachycardia, when pacing at two constant rates, both of which are faster than the rate of tachycardia, but which fail to terminate the tachycardia, there is the demonstration of a change in conduction time to and EGM morphology at an electrode recording site.[8,9,11,14] This is the EGM equivalent of the second entrainment criterion.

Figures 43.9A and B well illustrates the fourth entrainment criterion in a patient during atrial pacing from the high right atrium (HRA) during an AVRT (CL 339 ms). Shown in both panels is ECG lead II recorded simultaneously with EGMs from the proximal pair of electrodes of a catheter placed in the HRA and the coronary sinus (CS) during termination of pacing at CLs of 308 ms **(Figure 43.9A)**, and 292 ms **(Figure 43.9B)**. In the recordings from the coronary sinus (CS), the arrows from each stimulus artifact (S) indicate the EGMs that resulted from that stimulus. Note that the AEGMs at the CS site in panel A were identical to those during the spontaneous rhythm, and that conduction time during pacing was long (390 ms). However, with pacing at a shorter CL (292 ms) in panel B, the AEGM morphology changed at the CS site during entrainment, indicating that this site was now activated from a different direction associated with a shorter conduction time (90 ms). Note also that the tachycardia was not terminated by pacing at either rate. This fulfilled the fourth criterion for the demonstration of entrainment. As diagrammatically illustrated in the bottom half of panels A and B in **Figure 43.9**, the CS site was activated orthodromically during pacing at a CL of 308 ms, but antidromically during pacing at a CL of 292 ms. Actually, in **Figure 43.9A**, the disappearance of a positive P wave in the ECG with the last captured beat that was entrained but not fused is apparent, also fulfilling the first entrainment criterion. Finally, note also in **Figure 43.9B**, that with the last paced beat, the CS site was first activated antidromically and then orthodromically by the same beat because the orthodromic wavefront from the last paced beat was not blocked.

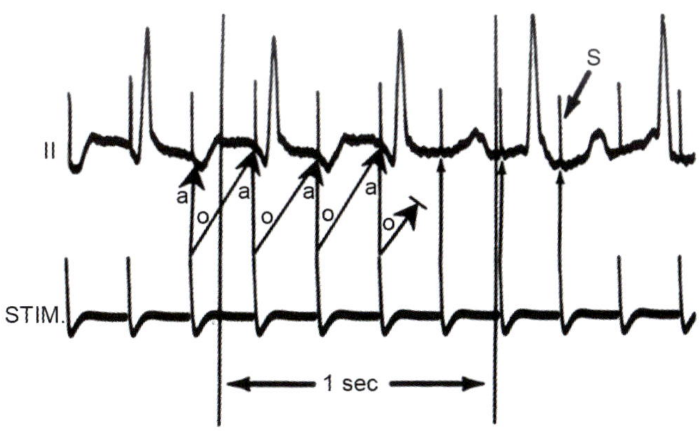

Figure 43.8: ECG lead II previously shown in Figure 43.2 is now shown recorded simultaneously with the stimulus artifact (STIM) from the high right atrial pacing site. Arrows from each stimulus artifact represent the antidromic (a) and orthodromic (o) wavefronts from each pacing impulse in association with each atrial complex in the ECG. Note that the appearance of the positive atrial complex in the ECG lead is associated with block of both the antidromic and orthodromic wavefronts of the same pacing impulse during the same pacing cycle. The antidromic wavefront blocks because it collides with the orthodromic wavefront of the previous beat, as usual. When the orthodromic wavefront of the same beat blocks during the same cycle, the AFL is terminated, and continued atrial pacing activates the atria from the high right atrial pacing site as expected during overdrive pacing of sinus rhythm. (Modified from reference #11)

CONCEALED ENTRAINMENT

A tachycardia may be entrained and even terminated during rapid pacing without being able to demonstrate any of the entrainment criteria, i.e. there may be concealed entrainment.[8,15-17] When this occurs, to prove the presence of entrainment, pacing must be performed from a site demonstrating manifest entrainment. This almost always means pacing from a site orthodromically proximal to an area of slow conduction in the reentrant circuit.

There are two types of concealed entrainment described. **Figure 43.10** illustrates and explains one form of concealed entrainment in a figure-of-eight reentrant VT circuit. During pacing from an isthmus in the circuit, with pacing at a rate faster than the spontaneous rate, but which doesn't terminate the tachycardia, the orthodromic wavefront from each pacing impulse captures the reentrant circuit, and resets it to the pacing rate, but each antidromic wavefront blocks in an area of slow conduction (here diagrammed as being in the isthmus, although in double loop reentry, it is probably not that simple[22]), so that the antidromic wavefront never exits the isthmus. Key to this is that the antidromic impulse is blocked in the isthmus at all pacing rates faster than the tachycardia rate which fail to interrupt the tachycardia. Therefore, a fusion morphology is not present in the ECG because, except for a very small area activated antidromically,

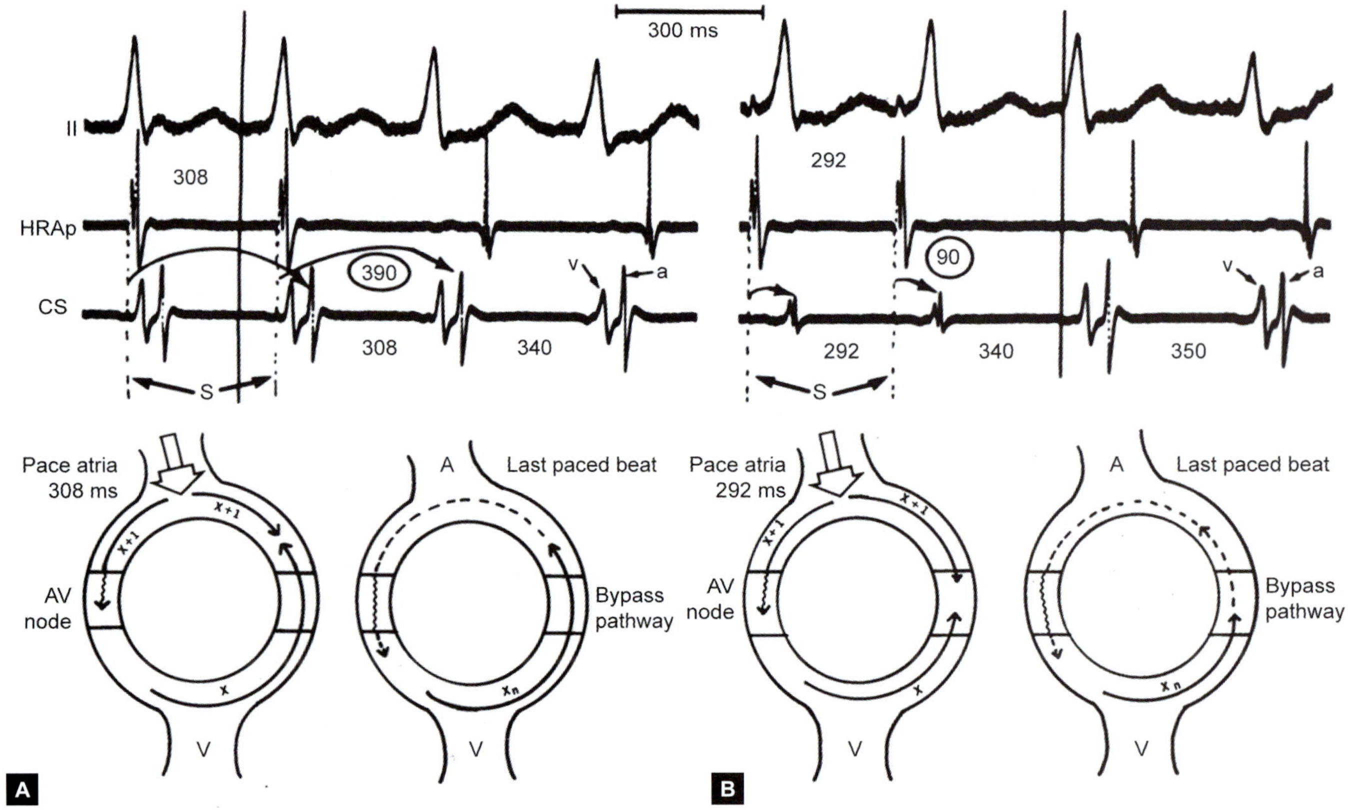

Figures 43.9A and B: Illustration of the fourth criterion of entrainment during atrial pacing from the high right atrium (HRA) during an atrioventricular reentrant tachycardia (AVRT) at a CL of 339 ms. In the upper part of both panels A and B, ECG lead II is recorded simultaneously with bipolar EGMs from the proximal pair of catheter electrodes in the HRA_p and the coronary sinus (CS) before and following cessation of pacing at a CL of 308 ms **(A)** and 292 ms **(B)**. In the CS recordings, the arrows from each stimulus (s) indicate the atrial complexes that result from that stimulus; a = atrial complex; v = ventricular complex. The last arrow in each panel goes to the last entrained beat. S = stimulus artifact.

The bottom diagrams in each panel represent the recorded events during pacing at each CL. The left panel of each diagram indicates the pacing impulse (X + 1) from the distal HRA electrode pair entering into the reentrant circuit, where upon it is conducted antidromically and orthodromically. The antidromic wavefront collides in the atria with the orthodromic wavefront (X) of the previous beat in panel A, but in the AV bypass pathway in panel B. However, in each case, the orthodromic wavefront, which is not blocked during that beat, resets the tachycardia to the pacing rate, continuing the tachycardia. Thus, with the last paced beat, the unopposed orthodromic wavefront from the last paced beat continues the tachycardia. In panel B, note that with resumption of the AVRT, the CS will again be activated orthodromically (it had been activated antidromically during pacing at 292 ms CL). The serpentine line represents slow conduction in the AV node. See text for discussion. (Modified from reference #11)

all sites are activated the same way during pacing as during the tachycardia. Although the tachycardia is entrained, there is no proof of that in the ECG. Therefore, the entrainment is concealed. And with pacing at a still faster rate that fails to terminate the tachycardia, because the activation sequence is the same, there is no progressive fusion. What happens with the last paced beat is that the orthodromic wavefront from the pacing impulse goes around the reentrant circuit, and the tachycardia resumes **(Figures 43.10A to C)**. With termination of the tachycardia, there is no demonstration of the third entrainment criterion. Thus, when pacing is fast enough to terminate the tachycardia, the presence of any localized conduction block for one beat rarely, if ever, is demonstrable. Understanding this form of concealed entrainment has become very useful, particularly during ablation of the "AFL isthmus," and during the ablation of VTs with an isthmus, in concert with criteria of Stevenson et al.,[23] which use the post- pacing interval to demonstrate the participation of sites in the reentrant circuit.

There is another form of concealed entrainment that we described,[15,17] but which is not widely appreciated. It occurs when pacing from a site orthodromically distal to an area of slow conduction in the reentrant circuit, but outside the isthmus (if present) or away from the core of the reentrant circuit. Using the same VT shown in **Figures 43.4** to **43.7** as illustrated, if the ventricles are paced at rates of 150, 155, and 160 bpm from a site distal to an area of slow conduction in the reentrant circuit, but away from the reentrant core **(Figure 43.11)**, the tachycardia will be entrained because the pacing impulse will enter the excitable gap and reset the

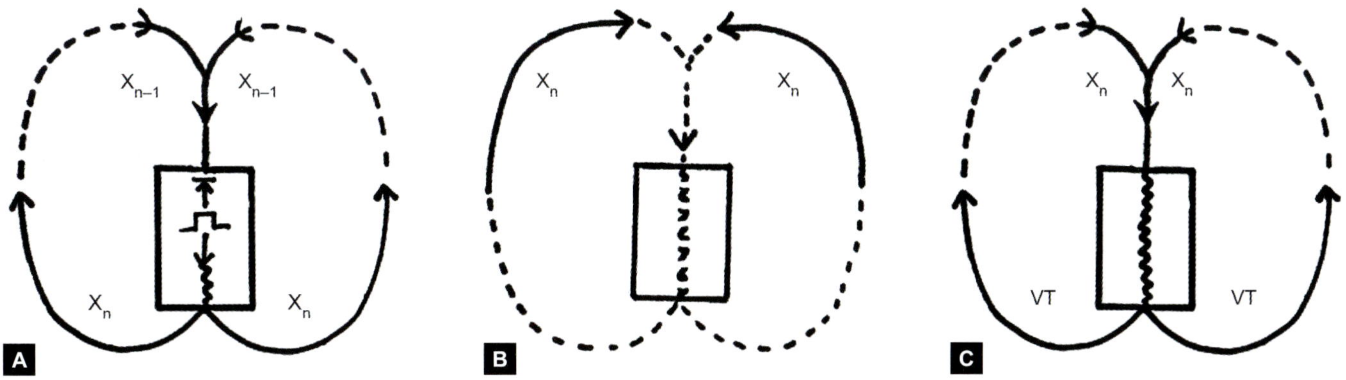

Figures 43.10A to C: Diagrammatic representation of one form of concealed entrainment of VT by pacing from an isthmus in a reentrant circuit. (A) The last paced beat (X_n) during concealed entrainment. The square wave indicates the pacing site. X_{n-1} = an orthodromic wavefront of the next-to-last paced beat. The antidromic wavefront from the last pacing impulse blocks (unidirectional block) within or very close to the isthmus. The orthodromic wavefront from the last pacing impulse activates the ventricles virtually identically as during the spontaneous VT, so that there is no fusion QRS complex morphology in the ECG; (B and C) Following the last paced beat (X_n), the VT resumes at its previous rate. See text for discussion. (Modified from reference #11)

tachycardia to the pacing rate. However, despite the fact that the tachycardia is entrained and subsequently terminated when pacing at 165 bpm, none of the criteria of transient entrainment will be demonstrable. The latter occurs because of the same reasons described above. Thus, when pacing orthodromically distal to the area of slow conduction in the reentrant circuit at 150 bpm (**Figure 43.11**, top panel), each pacing impulse enters the excitable gap of the reentrant circuit. The antidromic wavefront encounters unidirectional block in the area of slow conduction. The orthodromic wavefront of each pacing impulse resets the tachycardia to the pacing rate. With cessation of pacing, the orthodromic wavefront of the last paced beat continues the tachycardia. Since the last captured beat has the same morphology as that throughout the period of pacing[16], the first criterion of transient entrainment is not met; i.e., there is no constant fusion except for the last entrained beat.

With pacing at 155 or 160 bpm (**Figure 43.11**, bottom panel), because the pacing CL is shorter than pacing at 150 bpm, the wavefront from each pacing impulse enters the reentrant circuit earlier, but block of the antidromic wavefront still occurs at the same place. The orthodromic wavefront continues to activate the ventricles as during pacing at 150 bpm. Thus, the QRS complex during pacing at these faster rates does not change, and progressive fusion, the second entrainment criterion, will not be present. Therefore, the fourth criterion also will not be present. Finally, when pacing at a sufficiently rapid rate (165 bpm), termination of VT occurs because now the orthodromic wavefront blocks independently, presumably in the area of slow conduction (**Figure 43.11**, bottom right panel), along with block of the antidromic wavefront of the same paced beat. However, the only way to know that termination of the tachycardia has occurred is to stop pacing because the third criterion of entrainment is not demonstrable. In some instances, because the reentrant circuit is no longer present, the ECG morphology may change to that which occurs with overdrive pacing from the pacing site during sinus rhythm. In sum, when pacing from a site orthodromically distal to an area of slow conduction in the reentrant circuit, the demonstration of manifest entrainment likely will not be possible.

Figure 43.12 is a representative example of this type of concealed entrainment in a case of AFL during pacing from the coronary sinus. The left panel demonstrates the termination of pacing at a rate (352 bpm) faster than the rate of the AFL. Although the atria are clearly captured at the pacing rate, note the absence of anything to distinguish the last captured atrial beat from the other captured atrial beats or even from the atrial complexes seen during AFL. With cessation of pacing, the AFL resumes at its previous rate. The right panel demonstrates pacing at 365 bpm. Despite pacing at a faster rate, there is again no change in the morphology of the atrial complexes compared with that during pacing at the slower rate. However, this time, with cessation of pacing, the AFL has been terminated. There is no evidence during pacing that the AFL had been terminated. In fact, the only way to know that the AFL has been interrupted was to stop pacing.

CLINICAL APPLICATIONS OF ENTRAINMENT

When approaching tachycardias in the electrophysiology laboratory, the first question that needs to be answered is if the mechanism of the tachycardia is reentrant or focal. This question can be answered by using the four entrainment criteria delineated above. Although it might be

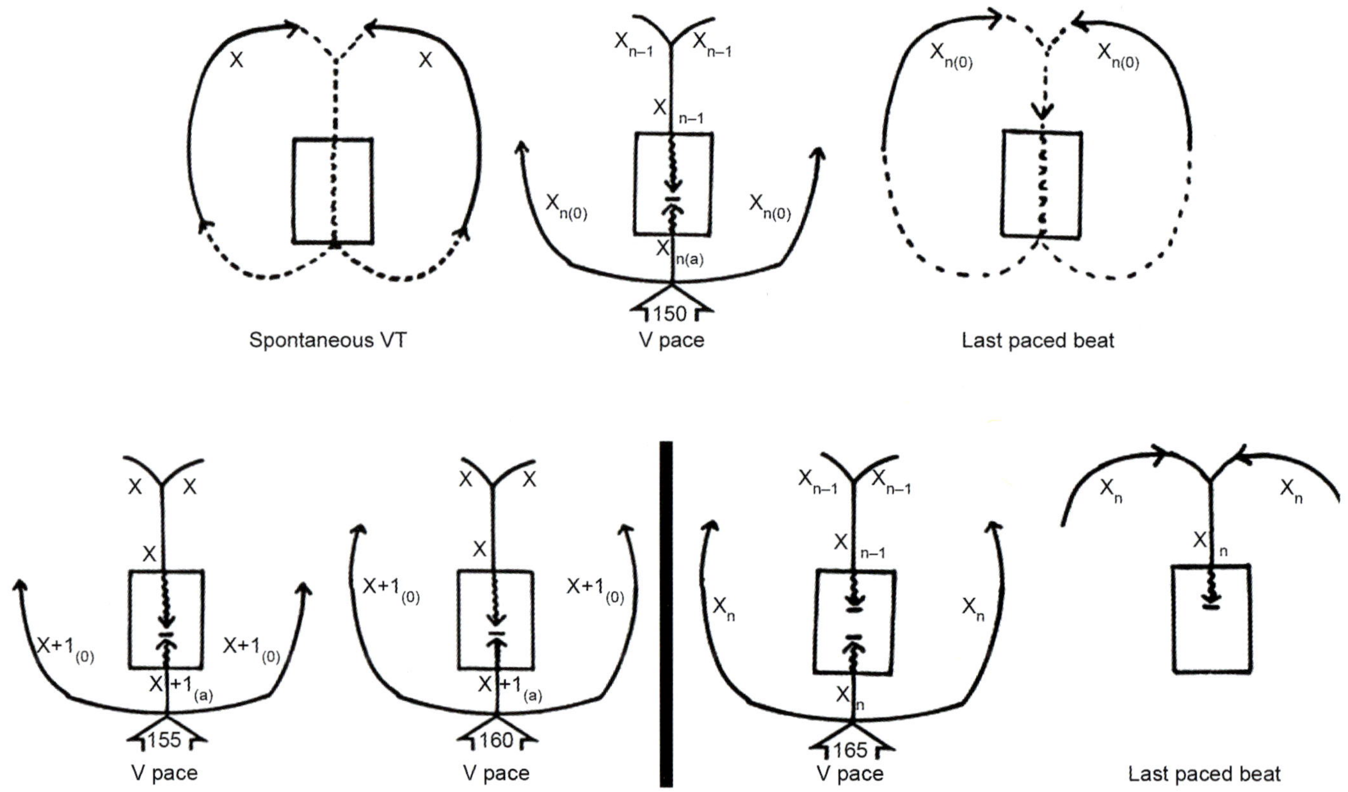

Figure 43.11: Diagrammatic representation of another form of concealed entrainment during ventricular pacing at rates of 150, 155, 160, and 165 bpm from a site distal to an area of slow conduction in the reentrant circuit.

Top left panel: Diagrammatic representation of the same VT as seen in **Figures 43.4 to 43.7**. Dashed lines represent the excitable gap. X_{n-1} = the orthodromic wavefronts of the next-to-last pacing impulse. X = circulating reentrant wavefronts of the VT.

Top middle panel: The large arrow represents the wavefront from the last pacing impulse entering the reentrant circuit, where it is conducted orthodromically, $X_{n(o)}$ and antidromically $X_{n(a)}$. The antidromic wavefront blocks in an area of slow conduction (unidirectional block). The orthodromic wavefronts reset the tachycardia to the pacing rate.

Top right panel: The orthodromic wavefronts from the last pacing impulse continue around the reentrant circuit, so that the VT resumes at its previous rate.

Bottom left two panels: Diagrammatic representations of concealed entrainment during ventricular pacing at rates of 155 bpm and 160 bpm from the same site shown in the top panel. $X + 1_{(o)}$ and $X + 1_{(a)}$ indicate the orthodromic and antidromic wavefronts, respectively, from the pacing impulse. Note the absence of progressive fusion.

Bottom right two panels: Diagrammatic representation of the termination of VT while pacing at 165 bpm from the same pacing site as shown in the upper and two left bottom panels. The wavefront from the last pacing impulse at a rate of 165 bpm enters into the VT reentrant circuit. The antidromic wavefront of the pacing impulse is again blocked (unidirectionally) in the same place as during pacing at 150, 155, and 160 bpm. The orthodromic wavefront from the pacing impulse travels around the reentrant circuit as before, but now it is also blocked, presumably in the area of slow conduction. However, this cannot be appreciated either from the ECG or from standard electrode catheter recording sites. Only with cessation of pacing, can it be appreciated that the VT has been terminated. See text for discussion. (Modified after reference #11)

an over simplification, all four criteria can be summarized briefly as follows: during reentrant tachycardias, overdrive pacing interacts with the reentrant circuit. This interaction becomes apparent in the recorded intracardiac electrograms (EGMs) and surface ECGs. In contrast, overdrive pacing during a focal tachyarrhythmia will "overdrive" the focus, so that the EGM and ECG recordings will be identical as if overdrive pacing during sinus rhythm. This is a starting point to understand the clinical applications of entrainment.

Consider overdrive pacing of the right ventricle during orthodromic AVRT. When overdrive pacing accelerates all the EGMs, the orthodromic wavefront from the pacing impulse will enter the excitable gap of the reentrant circuit, and travel to the atria via the AP. It will then continue to travel to the ventricles via the AV node. If the antidromic wavefront from the pacing impulse collides with the wavefront of the previous spontaneous beat in the ventricles, the ventricles are activated in part by the antidromic wavefront from each

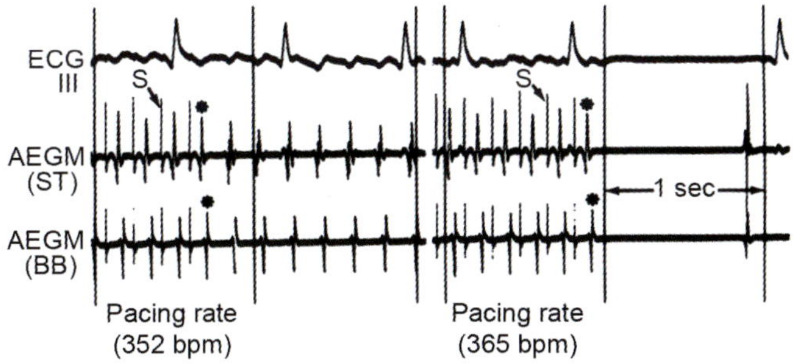

Figure 43.12: Demonstration of concealed entrainment of AFL. ECG lead III is recorded simultaneously with bipolar AEGMs from the sulcus terminalis (ST) and Bachmann's bundle (BB) before and after the cessation of 30 s of rapid atrial pacing (352 bpm – left panel; 365 bpm – right panel) from the postero-inferior left atrium in a patient with AFL (rate of 320 bpm). Comparison of events during rapid atrial pacing and its cessation at each rate fails to manifest any entrainment criteria, even despite termination of the AFL by pacing at 365 bpm. In fact, only when the pacing was stopped was it realized that AFL had been interrupted

Abbreviation: S = stimulus artifact. Asterisk = last captured beat during atrial pacing. Time lines are at 1 s intervals. See text for discussion. (Modified after reference #11)

pacing stimulus, and in part by the orthodromic wavefront of the previous orthodromic AVRT impulse that came through the AV node. This is the first entrainment criterion. If we are unaware that the narrow complex tachycardia is orthodromic AVRT, we still do not know if an antidromic pacing wavefront is colliding with the orthodromic wavefront of the previous beat of the tachycardia (in the case of a reentrant mechanism) or its simply overdriving the atria during the presence of a focal tachycardia or a sinus tachycardia. To see if there is fusion, there are two ways to do that. First, with cessation of pacing, if the last beat is entrained, but not fused, i.e. there is no fusion in the ECG during the last entrained beat, we have identified the presence of entrainment, and, consequently, reentry. Another way is to compare the EGMs during overdrive pacing of the tachycardia with the EGMs during pacing from the same site during sinus rhythm. If pacing is performed during sinus rhythm or, to make it closer to our scenario, if pacing is performed from the same location in the right ventricle during sinus tachycardia at the same CL as that of the orthodromic AVRT, the recorded EGMs and ECGs would be different when compared with the EGMs and ECGs when pacing during orthodromic AVRT that fails to terminate the tachycardia. This is how we can tell the presence of fusion vs. simple overdrive pacing, and if fusion is seen, this establishes the mechanism of the tachycardia as reentry. It is worth mentioning that when pacing during a focal tachycardia, or, as in our example, if pacing is performed from the right ventricle during sinus tachycardia, the initial few pacing wavefronts may collide at different sites with the wavefront emanating from the focal tachycardia. However, once the chamber from which pacing is performed is overridden by the pacing wavefronts, the morphology of the EGMs will not change. In this scenario, with overdrive pacing of a focal tachycardia or a sinus rhythm/sinus tachycardia, pacing at increasingly faster rates that do not terminate the tachycardia will not change the morphology of the either the ECG or the EGMs. But such pacing during a reentrant arrhythmia or, as in our example, an orthodromic AVRT, will result in change of the EGMs. This is because the pacing wavefront penetrates further antidromically at each faster rate, so that now, more of the ventricles is being activated by the pacing wavefront, and the site of fusion occurs more distant from the pacing site. This is the second criterion of entrainment – progressive fusion.

It is precisely this scenario of overdrive pacing from the right ventricle during a narrow QRS complex tachycardia, along with the fusion criteria that have recently been used to differentiate between AVNRT and AVRT.[24] In this report, during right ventricular pacing, if the His bundle was activated anterogradely, a diagnosis of AVRT was certain. This is so because during overdrive pacing from the right ventricle, in order for the AVNRT circuit to be captured and accelerated to the pacing CL, the pacing wavefront has to penetrate the AV node. Therefore, the His bundle has to be, and can only be, activated retrogradely. Anterograde activation of the His bundle during overdrive pacing from the right ventricle when all the EGMs are accelerated to the pacing CL can exist only in AVRT. In this case, the pacing and the orthodromic wavefronts of the tachycardia are colliding below the AV node in the His bundle. Theoretically, if one now starts pacing still faster, part of the His bundle (the distal part) could be activated by a wavefront from the pacing impulse, which will result in retrograde His bundle activation, and part of the His bundle can be activated anterogradely by the wavefront of the previous orthodromic beat. In this scenario, although the His bundle is being activated simultaneously by two different beats, no fusion in the ECG is seen because there is no ECG marker of His bundle activation. Nevertheless, a fusion equivalent is occurring at the level of the His bundle, and if this is seen during faster pacing, it fulfills the 4th entrainment criterion.

Now, if pacing is performed from, let's say, the AV AP itself, and captures only the AV AP orthodromically, the morphology of the EGMs and ECGs would be identical to the ones during orthodromic AVRT. This is an example of concealed entrainment, also known in the literature as concealed fusion.

In summary, one has to look carefully for the evidence of the presence of entrainment. Entrainment is not simply continuous resetting of the tachycardia. It is carefully comparing the EGMs during overdrive pacing of the tachycardia, and, if needed, comparing EGM morphology during overdrive pacing of sinus rhythm. Often, pacing from multiple sites during the tachycardia and during sinus rhythm is necessary to see if entrainment is present. On the other hand, if during overdrive pacing, the morphology of the EGMs and

ECG is identical with that during tachycardia, concealed entrainment is present, and a reentrant arrhythmia is present.

There is a theoretical caveat to be aware of when one is performing overdrive pacing during a focal tachycardia. It is possible that the cardiac activation during overdrive pacing of the focal tachycardia will be different from the one during overdrive pacing in sinus rhythm. This may happen if, associated with the tachycardia, there are areas of refractoriness and preferential pathways of conduction that do not exist in sinus rhythm, and are present only during the tachycardia. To avoid this, pacing should be performed at a site relatively close to the focal source of the tachycardia, and from multiple areas.

Postpacing Interval

During overdrive pacing of a reentrant tachycardia, it was observed that upon cessation of pacing, the time to the first recorded spontaneous beat of the tachycardia at the pacing site can provide some helpful information. The post pacing interval (PPI) can be defined as the time recorded at the pacing electrode site that spans the interval from the last pacing stimulus to the first recorded beat (EGM) of the native tachycardia. It has nothing to do with entrainment criteria, nor does it help to differentiate between a reentrant and focal mechanism of the tachyarrhythmia. But it does tell us how far the pacing site is from the source of the tachycardia or from the reentrant circuit. In the case of a reentrant tachycardia, the PPI is the time it takes from the orthodromic wavefront of the last paced beat to enter the reentrant circuit, travel the reentrant circuit along its path length, and return from the reentrant circuit back to the pacing site. From this, it follows that if the pacing site is within the reentrant circuit, the PPI will equal the tachycardia CL, or the PPI-TCL will be close to zero, as the pacing wavefront travels along the path of the reentrant circuit. In focal tachycardia, the PPI that is closest to the tachycardia CL is closest to the site of the successful ablation.[25]

Pitfalls Regarding the Postpacing Interval

The analysis of the PPI is very important, but one has to be aware of potential pitfalls that exist. If pacing is performed from within the reentrant circuit, the PPI can be (unexpectedly) either shorter or longer than the tachycardia cycle.

Shorter postpacing interval

If the pacing stimulus is strong enough, far field capture of the excitable gap can occur at a distance beyond the site immediately beneath the pacing electrode. The size of the virtual electrode varies with the strength of the pacing stimulus. During overdrive pacing at high or maximum stimulus strength from a site within or close to the reentrant tachycardia circuit, a large area, including quite a distance from the pacing electrode site, can be captured, and the orthodromic wavefront is then advanced from this site.

The second reason why the post pacing interval can be misleadingly short is when delayed activation is present during pacing.

The two scenarios are summarized in **Figures 43.13** and **43.14**.

Another common reason for a misleadingly short PPI is when the analysis of the PPI involves far field EGMs.[26] Recognition of far field EGMs is very important when performing overdrive pacing, especially when abnormal myocardium with a significant amount of scar is present. In an infarct scar, EGMs with low amplitude and multiple deflections are commonly recorded, often referred to as "multiple potentials," "isolated potentials," or "double potentials." These potentials often indicate depolarization of muscle bundles that are separated by areas of fibrosis, and, consequently, are depolarized at different times. Such bundles can lie beneath the recording electrode. Alternatively, some potential can be "far field" signals from depolarization of the tissue remote from the recording electrode. These signals are often timed with larger amplitude than the local EGMs. Pacing from the recording electrode can distinguish the near field or local EGMs that are of interest from the far field EGMs. When pacing is initiated at just or minimally greater than threshold strength, the electrical field of the electrode first depolarizes the tissue beneath itself, and that is the tissue responsible for generating the local EGMs. The potentials that are visible and separate from the stimulus artifact are then far field EGMs. A representative scenario is shown on **Figure 43.15**.

Misleading long postpacing interval

In addition to the misleadingly short PPI, when pacing from within the reentrant circuit, a spuriously long PPI can be observed. This can happen when local pacing latency occurs in the segment activated first by the paced wavefront. The most common mechanism for this is incomplete recovery of excitability of the tissue that is immediately adjacent to the pacing electrodes. In fact, in patients with typical atrial flutter, long PPI minus the tachycardia cycle length (PPI-TCL) values >30 ms after entrainment from the cavotricuspid isthmus were observed in 18% of patients.[27] Pacing significantly faster than the tachycardia CL (>20–40 ms) can result in even misleadingly longer PPIs.[28-31] It is important, then, to pace just slightly faster (10–20 ms) than the tachycardia CL in order to avoid this problem.

Misleadingly long PPIs can also happen when overdrive pacing results in decremental conduction in the reentrant circuit. This is most obvious when the circuit involves decrementally conducting cardiac tissue like the AV node. During overdrive pacing of AVRT and/or AVNRT, decremental conduction through the AV node has to be taken into account, so that the PPI can be accurately adjusted.

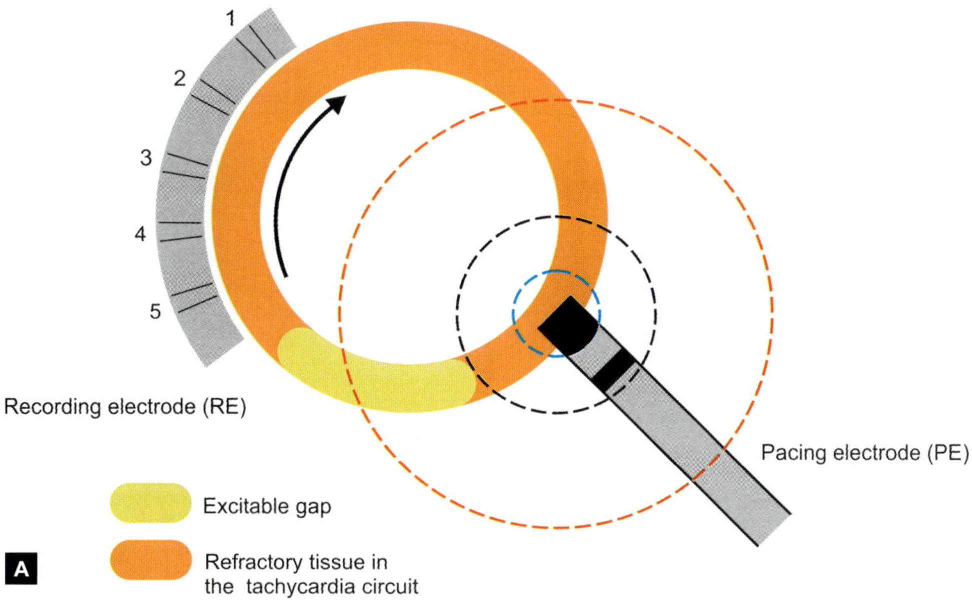

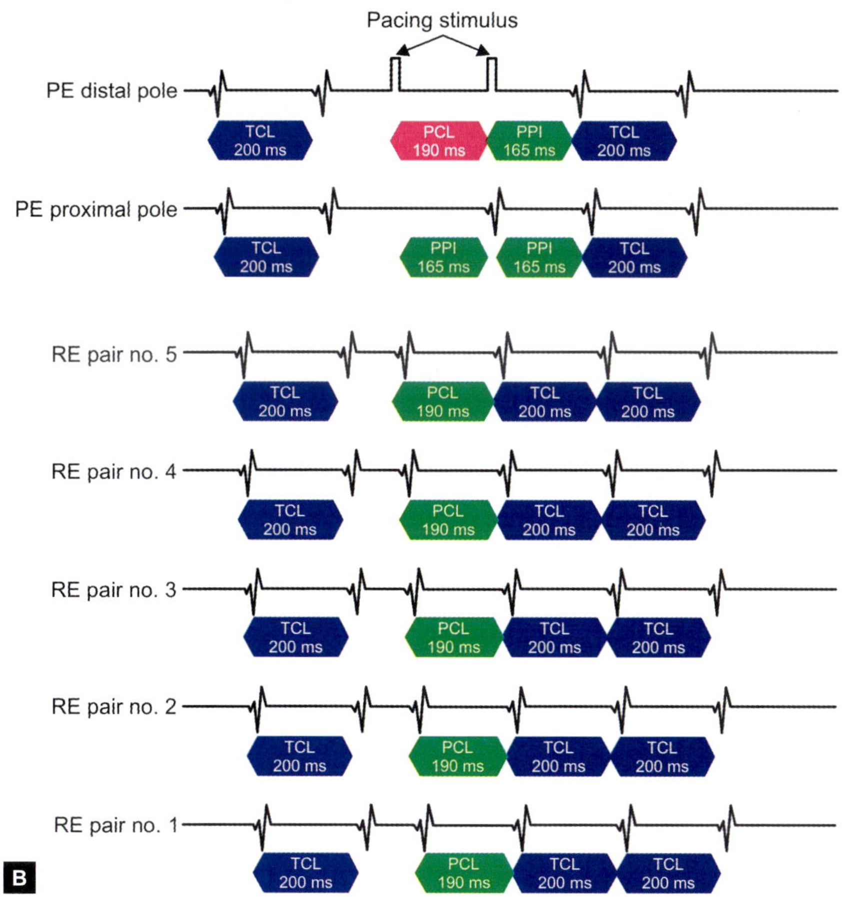

Figures 43.13A and B: (A) Schematic representation of a reentrant circuit with the excitable gap and the refractory area of the reentrant circuit during overdrive pacing. An example of a reentrant tachycardia with a cycle length of 200 ms is shown. Overdrive pacing is initiated from the pacing electrode (PE) at an area that is refractory. The blue, black and the red circles around the pacing site represent pacing with different stimulus strengths. The blue circle is pacing at a threshold stimulus, and the red circle is pacing at the highest stimulus output. The virtual electrode created by pacing at the highest stimulus output captures the excitable gap away from the area of contact between the PE and the refractory tissue. The tachycardia is accelerated from the area where the virtual electrode captures the excitable gap, not from where the pacing electrode is located. A multielectrode catheter is positioned along the course of the reentrant circuit, with electrode pairs labeled from 5 to 1. The black arrow inside the reentrant circuit indicates the direction of travel in the reentrant circuit; (B) EGM recordings from the PE (distal and proximal pole) and the 5 electrode pairs. The native tachycardia cycle length is abbreviated with TCL. Pacing is initiated from the distal pole of the PE. The EGMs recorded from poles 5 to 1 are accelerated to the pacing cycle length (PCL). The EGM on the PE (proximal pole of the PE) is activated last because the activation starts not from the site of the pacing, but from the site where the virtual electrode captures the excitable gap. The postpacing interval (PPI) is shorter because it does not travel the whole path length of the reentrant circuit

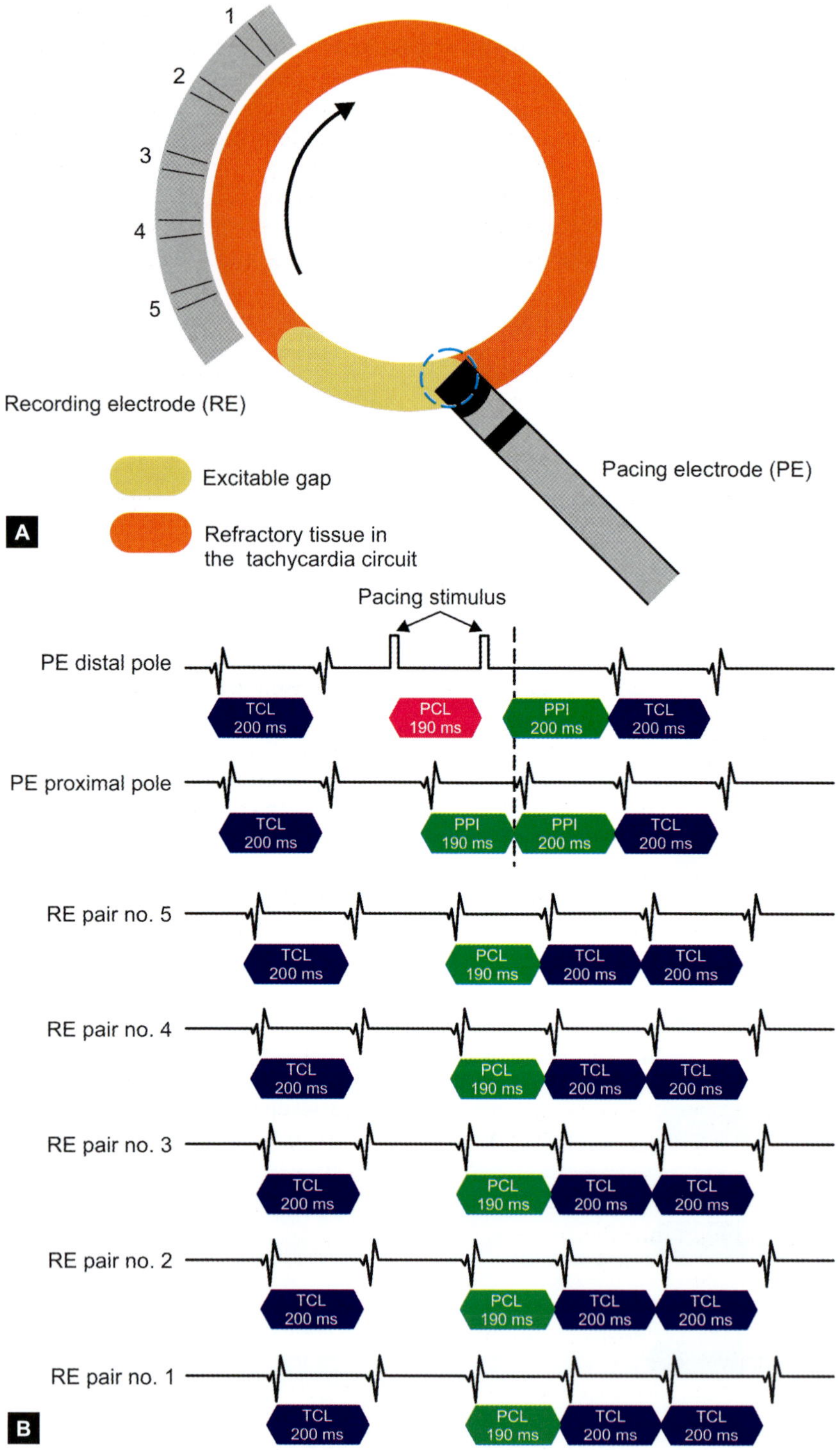

Figures 43.14A and B: (A) Schematic representation of a reentrant circuit with the excitable gap and the refractory area of the reentrant circuit during overdrive pacing. The example of a reentrant tachycardia with a CL of 200 ms is shown. Overdrive pacing is initiated from the pacing electrode (PE) in an area of the excitable gap; (B) EGM recordings from the PE (distal and proximal pole) and the 5 electrode pairs. The EGMs on the poles from 5 to 1 are accelerated to the PCL when pacing is initiated. In this example, the EGM from the proximal pole of the PE is also accelerated to the PCL, and precedes the activation of the other electrodes. However, there is a delay between the stimulus and the EGM on the PE. If one measures the PPI from the pacing stimulus to the next EGM on the PE (the interrupted vertical line) the PPI will be misleadingly short. The true PPI should be measured from the last entrained EGM, which is marked with the vertical interrupted line, to the next EGM of the tachycardia. In this example, the true PPI equals the TCL because pacing is performed from within the reentrant circuit

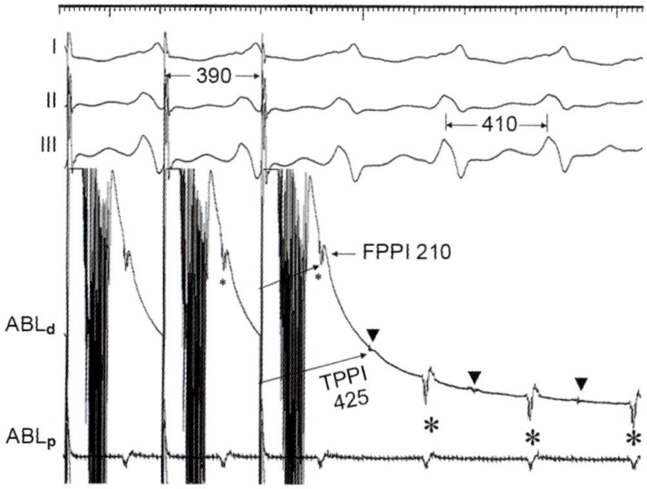

Figure 43.15: Entrainment of ventricular tachycardia (VT) at a site with a double potential is shown. From the top are surface electrocardiogram leads I, II, and III, and bipolar EGMs recorded from the distal (ABL_d) and proximal (ABL_P) electrode pairs of the ablation catheter. VT with a CL of 410 ms is present. Pacing at a CL of 390 ms entrains the tachycardia without altering the QRS complex morphology (concealed entrainment). Recordings at the pacing site show two EGMs marked with an **asterisk** and **arrowhead**, respectively. During entrainment, the EGM marked with the **asterisk** is present and has accelerated to the pacing CL. The tissue generating this EGM is not directly depolarized by the pacing stimulus, and is, therefore, designated as a far-field potential (FFP). The local EGM (indicated by an **arrowhead**) is not discernible during pacing, consistent with direct capture, but reappears after the last stimulus. The true post-pacing interval (PPI) (TPPI), which is measured from the last stimulus to the local EGM, is 425 ms. The false PPI (FPPI), which is measured from the last stimulus to the FFP, is 210 ms, or, if measured to the next FFP EGM one cycle later, would be 620 ms. Radiofrequency ablation at this site abolished the tachycardia. Time lines are 20 ms[26]

Although the PPI has important implications, it is also important to go beyond the simple concept of being "inside" or "outside the reentrant circuit. Note that relying on it to determine if the electrode is in the reentrant circuit or not is not sufficient to ablate the arrhythmia successfully. For instance, the atrial flutter circuit has been mapped with PPIs to clarify the "active" and "passive" part of the circuit by using PPIs that are shorter or longer than 20 ms.[32] Such distinction between passive and active circuit means little given the fact that both the "passive" (with long PPIs) and "active" portions of the reentrant circuit travel together between wide boundaries. What really matters is to identify the critical boundaries that the wavefront is using to pass through.[33] In the case of typical atrial flutter, it is the ablation line across the cavotricuspid isthmus that terminates the tachycardia regardless of the fact that some parts of the isthmus are part of the passive, and some of the active circuit. Studies of patients in ventricular tachycardia have shown that ablating just on the basis of PPIs has not been shown to be clinically useful for identifying successful sites, and ablation at these sites should not be attempted.[34] This is where entrainment especially helps us. Once the tachycardia is determined to be reentrant, the next step would be to define the boundaries through which the wavefront travels or to identify a critically protected area in the reentry circuit through which the wavefront travels. Ablation between the wider boundaries aiming to block the path of the circuit or inside the protected area of the circuit should successfully treat these arrhythmias.

Entrainment in Specific Tachycardia

The principles of entrainment are identical in supraventricular and ventricular tachycardia. Some specifics, however, do exist, and will be discussed.

Supraventricular Tachycardias—Atrioventricular Nodal Reentrant Tachycardia and Atrioventricular Reentrant Tachycardia

During a narrow complex tachycardia with a 1 to 1 relationship between the atria and ventricles, the PPI while pacing from the right ventricle has been used to distinguish between atrioventricular nodal reentrant tachycardia (AVNRT) and atrioventricular reentrant tachycardia (AVRT) (AP mediated tachycardia).[35,36] When pacing from the right ventricle, the PPI is longer in AVNRT because the site of pacing is further away from the AV node. Conversely, since the ventricles are part of the circuit in AVRT, the PPI is shorter. A post pacing interval minus tachycardia CL (PPI-TCL) that is greater than 115 ms is suggestive of AVNRT.[35] Similarly, during right ventricular overdrive pacing of AVNRT, because of the distance from the reentrant circuit, it takes several pacing beats to entrain the tachycardia. Since the ventricles are part of the circuit in AVRT, the first pacing wavefront readily entrains the tachycardia. In a recent study, no case of AVNRT (typical or atypical) demonstrated acceleration of TCL to the pacing CL (PCL) with the first RV pacing beat. On the contrary, every orthodromic AVRT case demonstrated acceleration of TCL to PCL by the first beat of RV pacing, resulting in both positive and negative predictive values of 100% if a cutoff ≤ 1 beat was used.[37]

Atrial Tachycardia

The criteria of entrainment are, of course, also valid for atrial tachycardias. However, it is often challenging or impossible to look for fusion or progressive fusion by comparing the P wave morphologies or the EGMs, the latter being the 4th entrainment criterion. One can rely on the scenario where a PPI that equals the tachycardia CL (TCL) from 2 or more sites distant from each other strongly suggests a reentrant tachycardia. Recently, another technique utilizing the principles of entrainment was used to identify a reentrant atrial tachycardia.[38] In this study, a single pacing maneuver during tachycardia was analyzed. Pacing was performed from a multielectrode catheter. When the multielectrode catheter was within or near a reentrant circuit, as judged by a PPI–TCL < 40 milliseconds, the neighboring electrodes were activated sequentially (from the earliest to the latest pair of the electrode). Overdrive pacing from an electrode that had a later local activation time when compared with its neighbor electrodes resulted in a long stimulus-to-EGM interval from the pacing site, with later activation to a neighboring electrode that was at least 75% of the TCL. This happens because the electrode is with earlier activation time is activated by the orthodromic wavefront of the tachycardia. In focal tachycardia, one can expect short activation time from the pacing electrode to its neighboring electrodes because the wavefront proceeds directly from the pacing electrode to the neighboring electrodes. For instance, in clockwise perimitral atrial flutter with distal-to-proximal sequential coronary sinus activation, overdrive pacing from the proximal coronary sinus electrode will result in a long pacing stimulus to the distal coronary sinus electrode interval.

Multiple mapping strategies have been suggested to efficiently diagnose common atrial arrhythmias arising during or after catheter ablation. This becomes especially important when diagnosing atrial tachycardia after atrial fibrillation ablation. Entrainment mapping for rapid distinction of left and right atrial tachycardia has been published, and relies on overdrive pacing from the high RA, proximal coronary sinus (CS), and distal CS sites. At these sites, the PPI-TCL is calculated, as it is an indicator of how close the pacing electrode is to the reentrant circuit. Based on the value of PPI-TCL, the location of the atrial tachycardia is determined according to an algorithm prospectively confirmed by mapping and successfully ablating the atrial tachycardia[39] **(Figure 43.16)**.

Ventricular Tachycardia

We already mentioned that successful ablation of a tachycardia requires identification of its mechanism, and in the case of reentrant tachycardias, defining the boundaries and intersecting possible pathways of potential conduction for the reentrant circuit. In reentrant atrial tachycardias, usually an ablation that intersects two anatomical boundaries suffices in eliminating the tachycardia. Ventricular tachycardia due to a reentrant mechanism can also be ablated applying similar principles, but some specifics do exists. For instance, finding protected pathways of slow conduction is much less common in reentrant atrial tachycardias, but it is a standard approach when ablating reentrant ventricular tachycardia.

Finding a protected pathway of slow conduction when ablating reentrant VT has origins from the initial observations that VT can be ablated with a single radiofrequency application. Successful ablation of ventricular tachycardia in patients with coronary artery disease was achieved with a single radiofrequency application when all the following mapping criteria were met: (1) an exact QRS complex match in the 12-lead ECG during entrainment; (2) a return CL </=10 ms of the VT CL; (3) presystolic potentials (<70% of VT CL) with an activation time-to-QRS complex within 10 ms of the stimulus-to-QRS complex.[40] Previously, ablating from a site within the reentrant circuit demonstrating concealed entrainment was shown not to be a predictably successful strategy.[41] In order to understand why successful ablation requires the ablation catheter to be in the reentrant circuit and also to have the stimulus-to-QRS complex activation time equal to the ventricular electrogram (presystolic or midiastolic potential)-to-QRS complex interval to be <70% of the VT CL, it is important to understand the anatomy and functions of

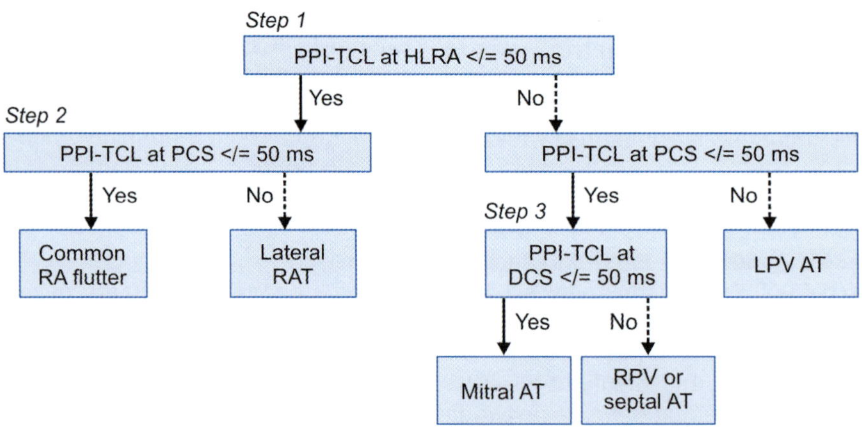

Figure 43.16: Stepwise algorithm for determining the location of atrial tachycardia (AT) reentrant circuits. See text for discussion
Abbreviations: DCS, distal coronary sinus; HLRA, high lateral right atrium; Lateral RAT, AT involving the lateral region in the RA; LPV, left pulmonary vein; PCS, proximal coronary sinus; PPI-TCL, difference between the postpacing interval and the tachycardia cycle length; RA, right atrium; RPV, right pulmonary vein[39]

different regions within the reentrant VT circuit. Consider an example of reentrant VT with a cycle length of 400 ms and the duration of the QRS complex during the tachycardia of 100 ms. On the ECG, 300 ms of diastole are "silent," but since this is a reentrant tachycardia, the reentrant circuit must be continuing during these 300 ms. The reason for this "silence" is thought to be that the reentrant circuit is depolarizing very small amount of myocytes, and is traveling through a protected area called an isthmus. In addition, because the reentrant circuit is traveling, in our example, at 300 ms through the ventricle, it is assumed that the conduction is slow during this period of the cardiac cycle. Most VT reentrant circuits are found to have evidence of an isthmus, also referred to as a channel.[42] The isthmus as studied in humans is a region of abnormal conduction in the scarred area. The approach in the electrophysiology laboratory is to find this area with the ablation catheter by detecting EGMs during this ECG silent period (diastole). EGMs recorded from the isthmus are often of low amplitude, and fractionated EGMs are common. This is understandable given the fact that, as we mentioned already, conduction is slow and abnormal in this area. The QRS complex in the ECG most often only begins when the VT wavefront emerges from the exit of the isthmus to activate the rest of the ventricles. This wavefront then returns to the entrance of the isthmus. If pacing is performed from the isthmus, a short stimulus-to-QRS complex interval will be present in the areas of the isthmus closer to its exit site, and, conversely, a long stimulus-to-QRS complex interval suggests that pacing is being performed from an area closer to the entrance of the isthmus. It has been demonstrated that when the stimulus-to-QRS complex interval is greater than 70% of the tachycardia CL, the pacing electrode is located outside of the critical isthmus.[17]

The conduction time between the pacing site and the reentrant circuit exit indicated by the stimulus-QRS complex interval (S-QRS) can be used to classify the pacing site position as at the exit (S-QRS < 30% of the VT CL), central (30–70% of the VT CL), or inner loop (> 70% of the VT CL). Ablation should target the central part of the isthmus.

So, the approach when ablating ventricular tachycardia first involves finding the reentrant circuit during "silent diastole" in the ECG by detecting the low amplitude, fractionated EGMs. These EGMs may or may not be part of the circuit. Demonstrating concealed entrainment from these sites is the next step. Concealed entrainment tells us that we are in the reentrant circuit, and that the recorded EGMs are part of it. Additional analyses of the PPI or S-QRS intervals and EGM-to-QRS interval are then used to determine if the site is in an isthmus in the reentrant circuit, and pacing from that site results in concealed entrainment. During overdrive pacing that result in concealed entrainment, the S-QRS interval indicates the time required for the paced wavefront to propagate from the pacing site to the reentrant circuit exit. Similarly, the interval from recorded EGMs at the pacing site to the QRS complex onset describes the same activation time. Thus, if these two intervals match for sites with concealed entrainment, they are in the reentrant circuit.

Sites with concealed entrainment but that result in a difference in the S-QRS interval compared to the EGM-QRS intervals at the pacing site are not sites where successful ablation has been demonstrated. This is so because these EGMs, although part of the reentrant circuit, are not in the critically important part of the isthmus.

CONCLUSION

Despite recent technological advancements in mapping of atrial and ventricular tachycardias, an understanding of the mechanism of the tachycardia is critically important to successfully ablate the tachycardia in the invasive electrophysiology laboratory. Entrainment is the first, and often the only, technique that is used during ablation of abnormal tachycardias. Thorough understanding of its principles is necessary to be able to accurately apply it in different situations. It is beyond the scope of this chapter to describe every possible scenario in every possible tachycardia, but with enough practice, one can become sufficiently proficient in looking for and finding the four criteria of entrainment. Again, to re-emphasize, one has to remember that entrainment is an interaction of the pacing wavefront with the tachycardia. This interaction simply does not exist in focal arrhythmias, and can be compared to overdrive pacing during sinus rhythm. This should be the starting point upon which experience should be built.

REFERENCES

1. Cranefield PF, Aronson RS. Triggered activity sustained by delayed after-depolarizations (Chapter 8). In: Cardiac Arrhythmias: The Role of Triggered Activity and Other Mechanisms. Vol illustrated edition. Mount Kisco, NY: Futura Pub Co; 1988.
2. Mayer AG. Rhythmical pulsation in Scyphomedusae: II. Papers from the Tortugas Laboratory of the Carnegie Institution of Washington. Washington, DC: Carnegie Institution of Washington. 1908;1:113.
3. Mines GR. On circulating excitations in heart muscles and their possible relation to tachycardia and fibrillation. Trans R Soc Can. 1914;IV:43-52.
4. Wit AL, Hoffman BF, Cranefield PF. Slow conduction and reentry in the ventricular conducting system. I. Return extrasystole in canine Purkinje fibers. Circ Res. 1972;30:1-10.
5. Wit AL, Cranefield PF, Hoffman BF. Slow conduction and reentry in the ventricular conducting system. II. Single and sustained circus movement in networks of canine and bovine Purkinje fibers. Circ Res. 1972;30:11-22.
6. Wellens HJ. Value and limitations of programmed electrical stimulation of the heart in the study and treatment of tachycardias. Circulation. 1978;57:845-53.
7. Waldo AL, Wit AL. Mechanisms of cardiac arrhythmias. Lancet Lond Engl. 1993;341:1189-93.

8. Waldo AL, Witt AL. Mechanism of cardiac arrhythmias and conduction disturbances. In: Fuster V, Alexander RW, O'Rourke RA, Roberts R, King SB, Wellens HJJ (Eds). Hurst's The Heart. New York: McGraw-Hill Companies. 2001;10:751-96.
9. Waldo AL, MacLean WA, Karp RB, Kouchoukos NT, James TN. Entrainment and interruption of atrial flutter with atrial pacing: studies in man following open heart surgery. Circulation. 1977;56:737-45.
10. MacLean WAH, Plumb VJ, Waldo AL. Transient entrainment and interruption of ventricular tachycardia. Pacing Clin Electrophysiol. 1981;4:358-66.
11. Waldo AL, Henthorn RW, Plumb VJ, MacLean WA. Demonstration of the mechanism of transient entrainment and interruption of ventricular tachycardia with rapid atrial pacing. J Am Coll Cardiol. 1984;3:422-30.
12. Waldo AL, Plumb VJ, Henthorn RW. Observations on the mechanism of atrial flutter. In: Tachycardia. Edited by B Surawicz. The Hague, Martinus Nijhoff; 1981. pp. 213-29.
13. Olshansky B, Okumura K, Henthorn RW, Waldo AL. Entrainment of human atrial flutter localizes the area of slow conduction in the inferior right atrium. J Am Coll Cardiol. 1990;15:833-41.
14. Henthorn RW, Okumura K, Olshansky B, Plumb VJ, Hess PG, Waldo AL. A fourth criterion for transient entrainment: the electrogram equivalent of progressive fusion. Circulation. 1988;77:1003-12.
15. Waldo AL, Henthorn RW. Use of transient entrainment during ventricular tachycardia to localize a critical area in the reentry circuit for ablation. Pacing Clin Electrophysiol. 1989;12:231-44.
16. Okumura K, Olshansky B, Henthorn RW, Epstein AE, Plumb VJ, Waldo AL. Demonstration of the presence of slow conduction during sustained ventricular tachycardia in man: use of transient entrainment of the tachycardia. Circulation. 1987;75:369-78.
17. Okumura K, Henthorn RW, Epstein AE, Plumb VJ, Waldo AL. Further observations on transient entrainment: importance of pacing site and properties of the components of the reentry circuit. Circulation. 1985;72:1293-307.
18. Waldo AL, Plumb VJ, Arciniegas JG, MacLean WA, Cooper TB, Priest MF, James TN. Transient entrainment and interruption of A-V bypass pathway type paroxysmal atrial tachycardia. A model for understanding and identifying re-entrant arrhythmias in man. Circulation. 1982;67:73-83.
19. Brugada P, Waldo AL, Wellens HJ. Transient entrainment and interruption of atrioventricular nodal tachycardia. J Am Coll Cardiol. 1987;9:769-75.
20. Henthorn RW, Plumb VJ, Arciniegas JG, Waldo AL. Entrainment of "ectopic atrial tachycardia:" Evidence for reentry. Am J Cardiol. 1984;53:1750-6.
21. Waldo AL. The canine sterile pericarditis model of atrial flutter. In: Waldo AL, Touboul P (Eds). Atrial Flutter: Advances in Mechanisms and Management. Vol Armonk, NY: Futura Publishing Co., Inc.; 1966. pp. 173-92.
22. Dillon SM, Allessie MA, Ursell PC, Wit AL. Influences of anisotropic tissue structure on re-entrant circuits in the epicardial border zone of subacute canine infarcts. Circ Res. 1988;63:182-206.
23. Stevenson WG, Khan H, Sager P, Saxon LA, Middlekauff HR, Natterson PD, Wiener I. Identification of reentry circuit sites during catheter mapping and radiofrequency ablation of ventricular tachycardia late after myocardial infarction. Circulation. 1993;88:1647-70.
24. Nagashima K, Kumar S, Stevenson WG. Epstein LM, John RM, Tedrow UB, Koplan BA, Michaud GF. Anterograde conduction to the His bundle during right ventricular overdrive pacing distinguishes septal pathway atrioventricular reentry from atypical atrioventricular nodal re-entrant tachycardia. Heart Rhythm. 2015;12:735-43.
25. Mohamed U, Skanes AC, Gula LJ, Leong-Sit P, Krahn AD, Yee R, Subbiah R, Klein GJ. A novel pacing maneuver to localize focal atrial tachycardia. J Cardiovasc Electrophysiol. 2007;18: 1-6.
26. Tung S, Soejima K, Maisel WH, Suzuki M, Epstein L, Stevenson WG. Recognition of far-field electrograms during entrainment mapping of ventricular tachycardia. J Am Coll Cardiol. 2003;42:110-5.
27. Vollmann D, Stevenson WG, Lüthje L, Sohns C, John RM, Zabel M, Michaud GF. Misleading long post-pacing interval after entrainment of typical atrial flutter from the cavotricuspid isthmus. J Am Coll Cardiol. 2012;59:819-24.
28. Cosío FG, López Gil M, Arribas F, Palacios J, Goicolea A, Núñez A. Mechanisms of entrainment of human common flutter studied with multiple endocardial recordings. Circulation. 1994;89:2117-25.
29. Stevenson WG, Sager PT, Friedman PL. Entrainment techniques for mapping atrial and ventricular tachycardias. J Cardiovasc Electrophysiol. 1995;6:201-16.
30. Fatemi M, Mansourati J, Rosu R, Blanc J-J. Value of entrainment mapping in determining the isthmus-dependent nature of atrial flutter in the presence of amiodarone. J Cardiovasc Electrophysiol. 2004;15:1409-15.
31. Deo R, Berger R. The clinical utility of entrainment pacing. J Cardiovasc Electrophysiol. 2009;20:466-70.
32. Santucci PA, Varma N, Cytron J, Akar JG, Wilber DJ, Al Chekakie MO, Brysiewicz N. Electroanatomic mapping of postpacing intervals clarifies the complete active circuit and variants in atrial flutter. Heart Rhythm. 2009;6:1586-95.
33. Sahadevan J, Waldo AL. Actively rethinking the re-entrant circuit. Heart Rhythm. 2009;6:1596-7.
34. Bogun F, Knight B, Goyal R, Strickberger SA, Hohnloser SH, Morady F. Clinical value of the postpacing interval for mapping of ventricular tachycardia in patients with prior myocardial infarction. J Cardiovasc Electrophysiol. 1999;10:43-51.
35. Michaud GF, Tada H, Chough S, Baker R, Wasmer K, Sticherling C, Oral H, Pelosi F Jr, Knight BP, Strickberger SA, Morady F. Differentiation of atypical atrioventricular node re-entrant tachycardia from orthodromic reciprocating tachycardia using a septal accessory pathway by the response to ventricular pacing. J Am Coll Cardiol. 2001;38:1163-7.
36. Gonzalez-Torrecilla E, Arenal A, Atienza F, Osca J, Garcia-Fernandez J, Puchol A, Sanchez A, Almendral J. First postpacing interval after tachycardia entrainment with correction for atrioventricular node delay: a simple maneuver for differential diagnosis of atrioventricular nodal re-entrant tachycardias versus orthodromic reciprocating tachycardias. Heart Rhythm. 2006;3:674-9.
37. Dandamudi G, Mokabberi R, Assal C, Das MK, Oren J, Storm R, Vijayaraman P, Miller JM. A novel approach to differentiating orthodromic reciprocating tachycardia from atrioventricular nodal re-entrant tachycardia. Heart Rhythm. 2010;7:1326-9.

38. Barbhaiya CR, Kumar S, Ng J, Tedrow U, Koplan B, John R, Epstein LM, Stevenson WG, Michaud GF. Overdrive pacing from downstream sites on multielectrode catheters to rapidly detect fusion and to diagnose macroreentrant atrial arrhythmias. Circulation. 2014;129:2503-10.
39. Miyazaki H, Stevenson WG, Stephenson K, Soejima K, Epstein LM. Entrainment mapping for rapid distinction of left and right atrial tachycardias. Heart Rhythm. 2006;3: 516-23.
40. El-Shalakany A, Hadjis T, Papageorgiou P, Monahan K, Epstein L, Josephson ME. Entrainment/mapping criteria for the prediction of termination of ventricular tachycardia by single radiofrequency lesion in patients with coronary artery disease. Circulation. 1999;99:2283-9.
41. Bogun F, Bahu M, Knight BP,. Weiss R, Paladino W, Harvey M, Goyal R, Daoud E, Man KC, Strickberger SA, Morady F. Comparison of effective and ineffective target sites that demonstrate concealed entrainment in patients with coronary artery disease undergoing radiofrequency ablation of ventricular tachycardia. Circulation. 1997;95:183-90.
42. Stevenson WG, Friedman PL, Sager PT, Saxon LA, Kocovic D, Harada T, Wiener I, Khan H. Exploring postinfarction re-entrant ventricular tachycardia with entrainment mapping. J Am Coll Cardiol. 1997;29:1180-9.

EDITORS' SUMMARY

Drs Cakulev and Waldo provide this chapter for our textbook what will undoubtedly be a cornerstone contribution that is comprehensive yet an outstanding practical reference for electrophysioloigists of all levels of training and experience. Dr Waldo, a pioneer for the description and understanding of entrainment mapping not only has outlined the principles with clear illustrations but has discussed in detail the major pitfalls in a manner that's organized and cannot be gleaned easily from the existing literature.

When used in conjunction with the detailed explanations elsewhere on the correct technique for activation and substrate mapping, the student of electrophysiology will be excellently equipped to apply his or her knowledge and skills for even the most complex of arrhythmias in patients in our practice.

Normal QRS, besides being less than 100 ms in duration, also has a certain orientation in frontal and horizontal planes and should not be confused with narrow QRS, which may not be normal. As an example, a narrow QRS may be associated with a Q-wave myocardial infarction.

In essence, therefore, a wide QRS implies that there is sequential rather than simultaneous depolarization of the two ventricles, such as in:

1. Bundle-branch block (BBB)
2. Preexcitation via anomalous or accessory pathway (AP)
3. Ventricular origin of the impulse. Additional mechanisms of wide QRS include
4. Nonspecific intraventricular conduction defect (NSIVCD), which is caused by extensive scarring, Class I antiarrhythmic drugs, particularly 1C, electrolyte abnormalities, that is hyperkalemia, metabolic derangements, etc.
5. Ventricular pacing where the stimulus artifact may not be identifiable.
6. Mechanical irritation from temporary catheters and sometimes by permanent pacemaker or implantable cardioverter-defibrillator (ICD) leads. While the contribution of anisotropic conduction during inscription of normal QRS, if any, is not clear, it does contribute in several forms of wide QRS tachycardias, particularly in patients with NSIVCD, and/or during trans-septal conduction. The extent of its role is not completely understood.

In this chapter, only the monomorphic (MM) forms of wide QRS tachycardia are addressed, particularly of the sustained variety. Excluded are irregular and polymorphic tachycardias.

At the outset, some aspects of wide QRS complex tachycardia are important to point out.

1. The description of morphologic features in the text is what is recorded on a 12-lead surface ECG, rather than a single lead rhythm strip.
2. Width of QRS on a 12-lead ECG is used in a given patient from the earliest to latest QRS recording and one or more leads may be used to achieve this goal. It is assumed that the initial ECG is taken in a non-medicated state.
3. The rhythm strip alone may be insufficient in some instances, unless the width and morphology of QRS are not in question and the cycle length (CL) change is the only focus.
4. Ventricular tachycardias in outpatient settings could present in many forms, but the three main forms of presentation are cardiac arrest, unexplained syncope and hemodynamically-tolerated tachycardia. It is only the latter of the three that lends itself to this type of analysis, that is, a differential diagnosis of a wide QRS tachycardia on a 12-lead surface ECG. It goes without saying that a thorough history of the patient's symptoms, current medications, cardiovascular disease, if any and family history are also important to achieve an accurate diagnosis.

NARROW VERSUS WIDE QRS TACHYCARDIA: ECG DISTINCTION

The vast majority of wide QRS tachycardias are ventricular and, to a much lesser extent, supraventricular with aberrant conduction.[1] With that in mind, this distinction will be dealt with first.

Initially suggested ECG criteria for distinction between ventricular tachycardia (VT) and supraventricular tachycardia (SVT) with aberrant conduction, that is, BBB with or without fascicular block, was done with five ECG leads, i.e. I, II, III, V_1 and V_6. The criteria favoring VT were:[2]

1. QRS of duration ≥ 140 ms
2. Left axis deviation
3. Certain QRS configurations
4. Atrioventricular (AV) dissociation.

While collectively these criteria would reliably diagnose VT, the individual criteria have significantly changed, except AV dissociation or ventriculoatrial (VA) block. The VA block was seen infrequently in the initial description but is easier to identify than AV dissociation when present. A key point to keep in mind is that the quoted study above compared an almost equal number of laboratory-induced tachycardias to define the surface ECG criteria.[2] This gave some readers the unintended impression that VT and SVT with aberrant conduction are equally common. However, when consecutive patients with regular uniform wide QRS tachycardia presenting on a 12-lead ECG were studied, the vast majority (81%) turned out to be VT.[1] Aberrant conduction was noted in only 14% and preexcitation was seen in 5%. The perception of equal frequency of VT and SVT with aberrant conduction is not observed in any population of consecutive patients presenting with spontaneous wide QRS tachycardia. At the time of referral only 32% were labeled VT and almost the same percentage, that is 35 and 33 were labeled aberrant conduction and preexcitation, respectively.[1] This reflects gross underestimation of VT among the referred patients. A similar experience has been noted by other investigators.[3-5] The general reason for this mistake is related to the fact that most physicians have difficulty accepting that a patient with VT can have stable hemodynamics.[5]

The surface ECG criteria, even collectively, do not lead to a 100% accuracy of distinction between VT and aberrant conduction. This is unfortunate, because one is comparing a relatively benign SVT to a potentially malignant, in other words life-threatening, VT. In the practice of medicine, no one is satisfied until a malignant tumor is either diagnosed or excluded with 100% certainty. What makes accurate distinction between VT and SVT even more important is that many patients with VT may die in a relatively short time after a missed diagnosis. Furthermore, these deaths are preventable; which is not the case with most malignant tumors.

Distinction between myocardial VT and aberrant conduction, in essence, is based upon the manner in which the ventricles are depolarized. In other words, via the His-Purkinje system (HPS) or by muscle-to-muscle spread. Since ventricular preexcitation also begins with muscle-to-muscle spread, it is dealt with separately in this communication because it closely mimics myocardial VT on the ECG.

Current Status of ECG Criteria for VT versus Aberrant Conduction Distinction

Atrioventricular (AV) Dissociation or VA Block (2:1, 3:1, etc.) (Figures 44.1 and 44.2)

This is perhaps the most diagnostic of subjunctional rhythms, including all forms of VT.[1-5] Automatic junctional tachycardia arising from the His bundle (HB) associated with aberrant conduction and dissociated from the atrium due to retrograde AV nodal block, and intra-HB re-entry with aberrant conduction will be the only SVTs that could be confused with VT. Fasciculoventricular pathways do not cause SVT, but can be a source of confusion during regular wide QRS tachycardia.

While AV dissociation is fairly diagnostic of VT **(Figure 44.1)**, it is recognizable in only one-third of the patients. This is primarily because the P-waves cannot be identified during a wide QRS tachycardia, particularly when the tachycardia rate is more than 170 per minute or the QRS complex duration ≥ 200 ms.[1-5] **(Figures 44.3A and B)**. The P waves are sometimes identified erroneously, and when studied with the help of intracardiac studies, these turn out to be part of the QRS complex **(Figures 44.4A and B)**. With intracardiac electrograms, AV dissociation can be recognized more often **(Figures 44.5A and B)**.[1,2] However, 1:1 VA conduction is also common during VTs.[1,2] The sensitivity of this criterion from surface ECG alone is, therefore, unacceptably low, and sole reliance on this observation leads to frequent misdiagnosis.

There are no convincing examples of AV nodal reentry (AVNRT) with aberrant conduction and AV dissociation.

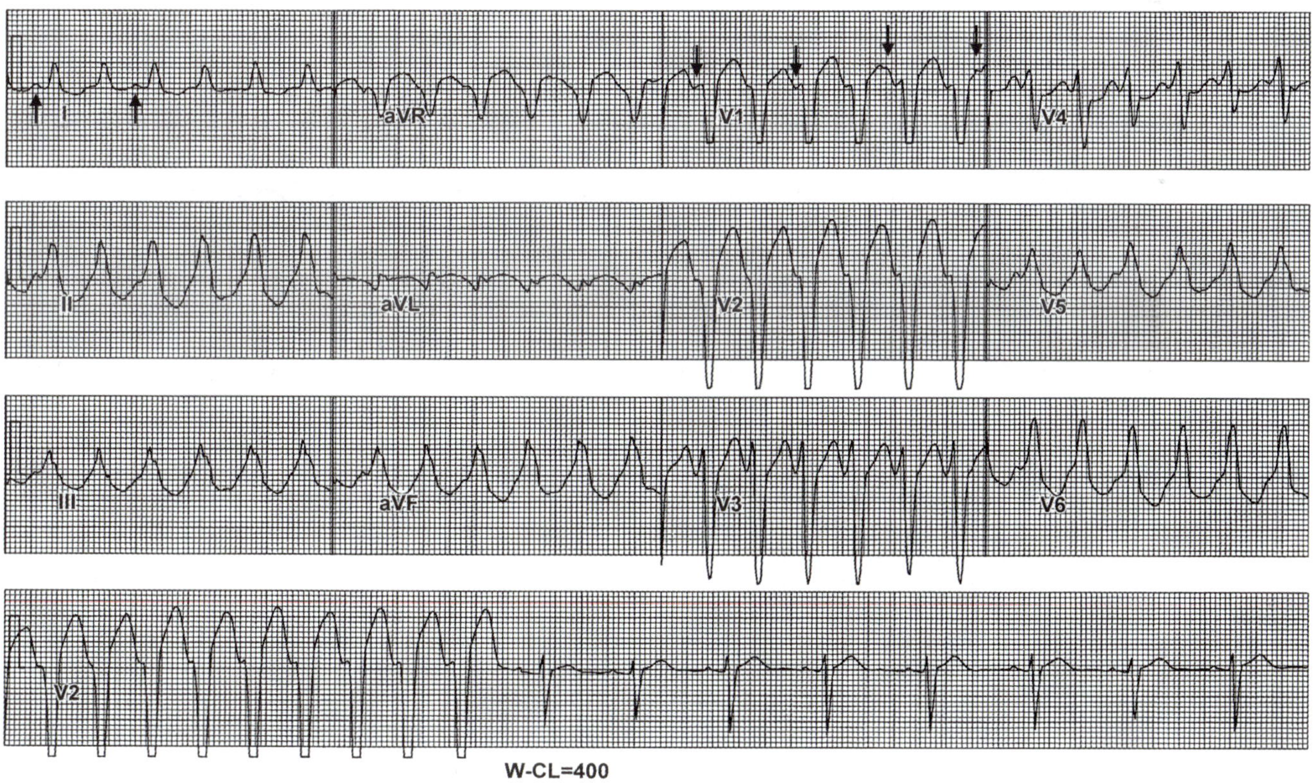

Figure 44.1: AV dissociation during wide QRS tachycardia (myocardial VT). The ECG shows a wide QRS tachycardia (QRS duration 180 ms best appreciated in leads III and aVL) with LBBB and normal axis pattern. Marching of the dissociated P-waves is easily recognizable and depicted by arrows. The initial part of this QRS shows slurring best seen in lead aVL. It is also noticeable that the maximum width of QRS complex is not appreciated in lead I and V6. The bottom trace (lead V2 in this case, but in other instances may be lead II, V1 or both) shows spontaneous termination into sinus rhythm. The lead organization from top to bottom and then left to right are surface ECGs I, II and III, aVR, aVL, aVF, V1 to V3, and lastly V4 to V6. The same orientation is recorded in other Figures unless indicated otherwise

Abbreviation: W-CL, wide QRS tachycardia cycle length

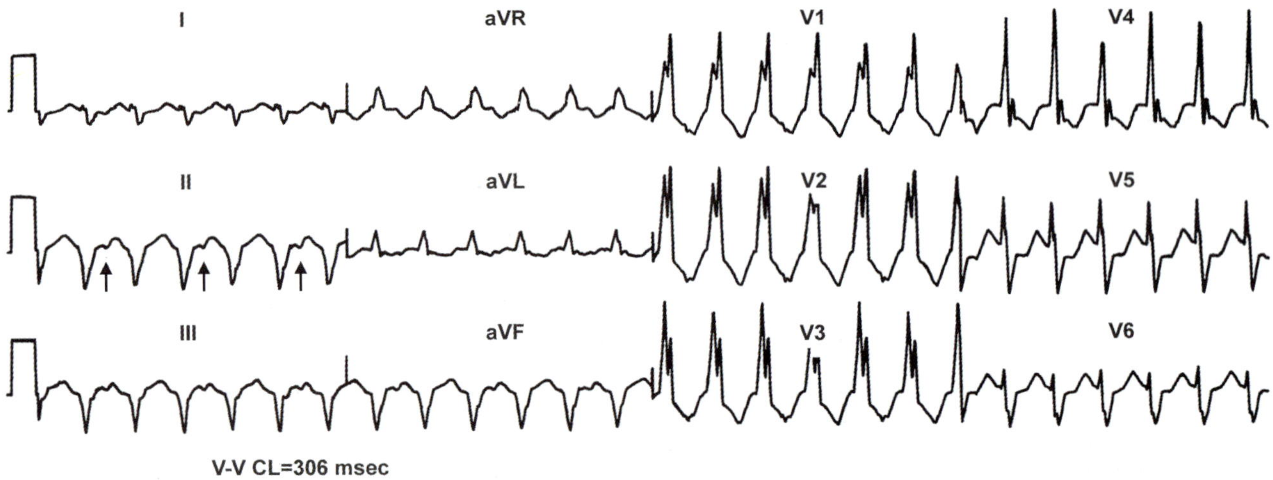

Figure 44.2: VA block during a wide QRS tachycardia (myocardial VT). The leads are organized the same way as in Figure 44.1. The morphology of QRS is that of RBBB pattern with a QRS axis of -100° (northwest quadrant). A 2 : 1 VA block can be recognized following every other QRS complex shown by arrows. QRS duration is 140 ms but appears narrower in lead aVL and I

Abbreviation: V-V CL, ventricular tachycardia cycle length

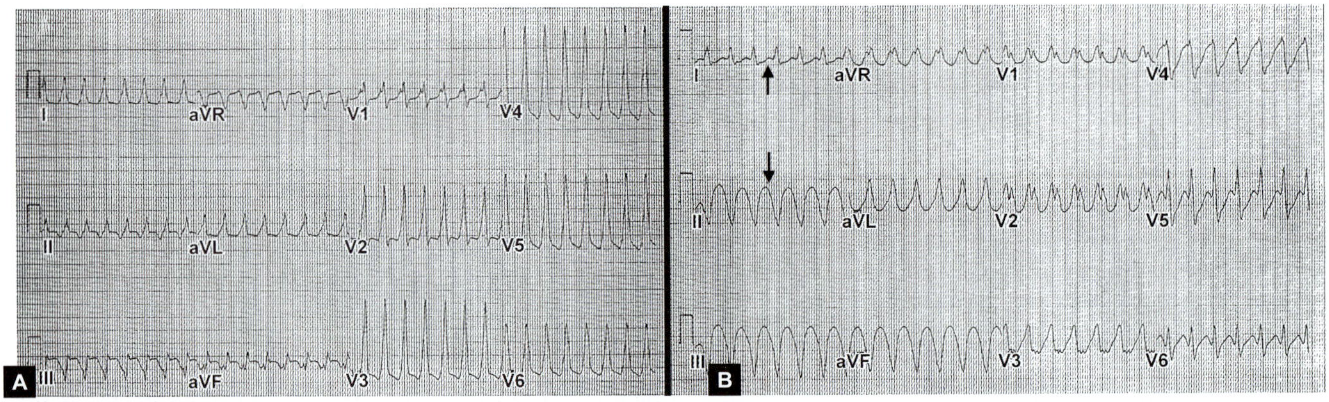

Figures 44.3A and B: The role of rate and width of QRS and P-wave identification. Both Figures (A and B) are examples of myocardial VT. RBBB pattern is seen in both panels. The VT cycle length in Figure A is 320 ms and in Figure B is 360 ms. The QRS duration is 200 ms and 280 ms respectively. Several points can be observed in the two ECGs. 1. In both examples, the diagnosis of myocardial VT (versus aberrant conduction) are made with the usual ECG criteria, i.e. the width of QRS, initial slurring, and QRS morphology in V1. 2. Due to the rate in Figure A and the width of the QRS in both figures, P-wave recognition is difficult. 3. Apparent P-waves at the onset of QRS in lead II and aVF in Figure A and the end of QRS in lead V3 in Figure B are actually part of the QRS. 4. The width of the QRS is underestimated in lead I and aVR in Figure A and in some of the leads (lead I and V6) in Figure B where the QRS duration is literally half compared to the other leads. Not recognized often enough but a relatively common observation in patients with VT and a RBBB pattern is the evidence of prior Q-wave myocardial infarction. In both figures, inferior wall infarction is detectable. When looked for and observed not only does it help the diagnosis of myocardial VT but also the underlying pathology

A 2:1 VA block is occasionally seen during AVNRT (i.e. HA block) in the EP laboratory, and when also accompanied by aberrant conduction can cause confusion, but this type of HA block during AVNRT seldom lasts longer than a few cycles, and in essence therefore, a 2:1 VA block is diagnostic of VT or subjunctional rhythm **(Figure 44.2)**.[6] In this context, it seems appropriate to make a comment about the polarity of P wave during wide QRS tachycardia. Aside from extensive experience, the statement regarding the polarity is seldom accompanied by more convincing evidence, i.e. concomitant atrial recording (intra-atrial or esophageal) **(Figures 44.6A and B)**. We have examined this during ventricular pacing and progressively shorter coupling intervals of extrastimuli where the observed P-wave polarity changes depending upon which part of the ST-T segment it coincides with. The same P-wave polarity can be interpreted as negative to positive or vice versa depending on the location in the ST-T segment even in atrial tachycardias, and particularly in the presence of a wide QRS

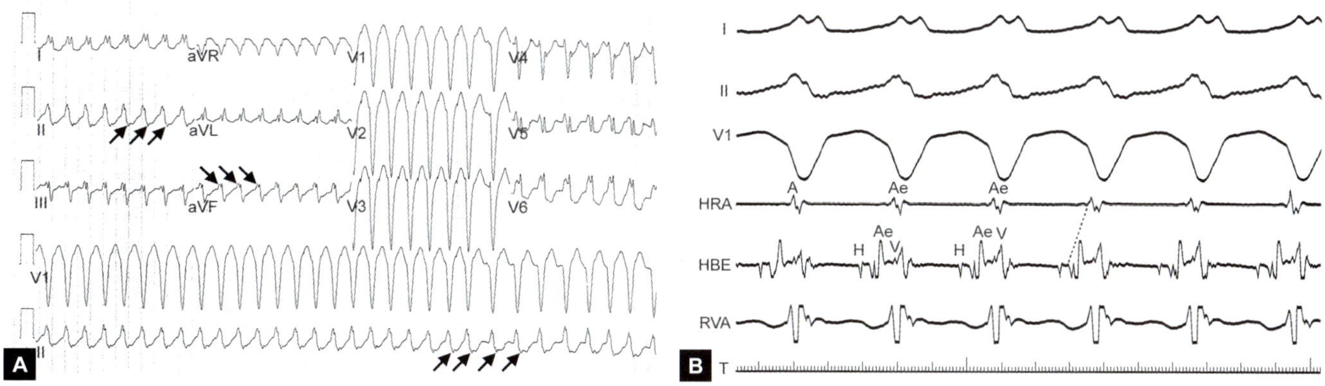

Figures 44.4A and B: Retrograde P-wave and wide QRS tachycardia. 12-lead ECG and rhythm strip (lead V1 and II) shows a wide QRS tachycardia with a LBBB and normal axis pattern. There is a strong suggestion in lead II of a retrograde P-wave at the end of the QRS, however, Figure B documents the retrograde P-wave location with intracardiac electrograms. The tachycardia is slow-fast AV nodal reentry, the same as Figure A. HB deflection (H) and the retrograde atrial echo beats (Ae) are labeled. Note the location of retrograde P-wave precedes the QRS and does not follow the QRS as suggested by surface ECG in Figure A. A positive deflection is seen at the beginning of the QRS in leads III and aVF of Figure A, which is part of the QRS. On the tracing in Figure B, from top to bottom are surface ECG leads I, II and V1, intracardiac electrograms from the region of the right atrium (HRA), HB (HBE) and right ventricular apex (RVA) and timelines are 10 and 100 ms. Similar labeling is used in all intracardiac electrogram tracings unless specified otherwise

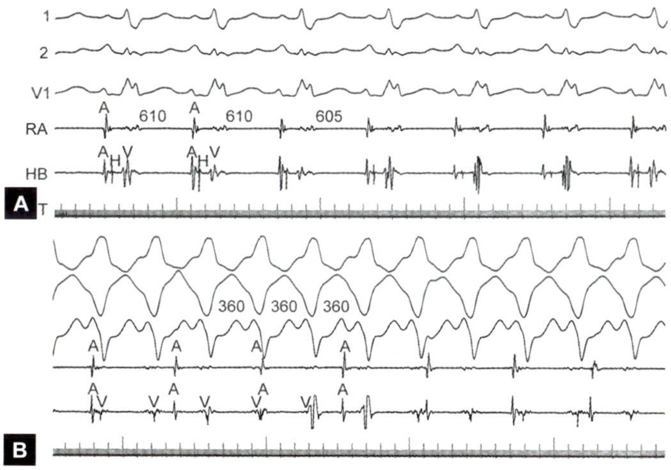

Figures 44.5A and B: AV dissociation with intracardiac signals. Figure A depicts sinus rhythm with 1:1 AV conduction and RBBB. Note that the QRS morphology in V1 is RR, (with taller first R), often quoted as diagnostic configuration for myocardial VT. Figure B depicts myocardial VT with no clearly identifiable P-waves on the surface ECG but clear AV dissociation on the intracardiac tracings. Myocardial nature of VT is suggested from surface ECG, i.e. QRS slurring and on HB electrogram with no H deflection visible

(Figure 44.7). The recognition of the entire P-wave duration is also difficult to measure during a wide QRS tachycardia, and more so at rapid rates and/or wider QRS complexes **(Figures 44.3A and B)**. Occasionally, the P-wave creates changes in the appearance of the ST-T segment; but if it does not march out, it will not be reliable. In patients with wide QRS tachycardia and 1:1 AV/VA relationship, carotid sinus massage and/or adenosine can be used to change the P-QRS relationship which may help P-wave identification. The problem with this approach is that at times, atrial, AV junctional and ventricular tachycardias may all terminate before a definitive diagnosis is made.

QRS Complex Axis

While earlier literature indicated that left or superior axis, that is, –30° to <90° suggests VT, this has not been the experience since.[1,2,5] Some of the reasons for this discrepancy are: (a) The initial series included mostly laboratory-induced tachycardia which did not have consecutive non-selected patients and could not be reproduced in outpatient or ambulatory settings. (b) Left (superior) axis (–30 to < 90°) is common with functional or pre-existing right (R) or left (L) bundle-branch block (RBBB, LBBB, respectively) during sinus rhythm. Therefore, during SVT, the same QRS morphology and axis will be expected, and hence this criterion is unreliable for VT diagnosis. In fact, some forms of VT are characterized by right (inferior) axis (i.e. right ventricular outflow tract VT, **Figure 44.8**) and pulmonic or aortic cusp VT. In our own series, the only axis that was diagnostic of VT was extreme left or so-called northwest axis (–90 to ±180°).[1] Since that publication, we have learned that even the so-called northwest axis has some definitive exceptions for diagnosis of VT for three reasons. Firstly, the part of the normal QRS orientation (–30° to +110°) is due to left ventricular (LV) preponderance or dominance in terms of electrical forces. If that was reversed by virtue of extreme right ventricular hypertrophy, seen sometimes in severe congenital heart disease even in the adult, pulmonary hypertension or chest cage deformity, the axis orientation may be northwest even during sinus rhythm

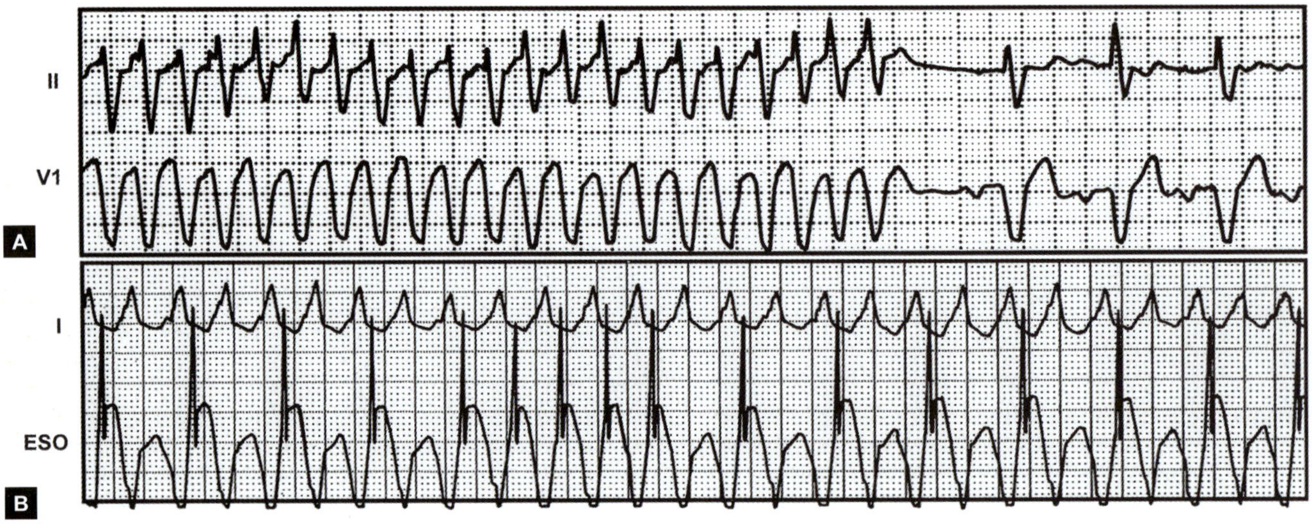

Figures 44.6A and B: P-QRS relationship via esophageal recording. In situations where documentation of AV relationship cannot be ascertained from the surface ECG and it is not practical to get satisfactory atrial electrogram, such as with patients in the Intensive Care Unit, atrial signal can be recorded via esophageal electrogram. The recording from the monitor lead II and V1 during rapid wide QRS tachycardia is shown in the Figure A. Here the surface ECG leads show a similar QRS configuration as sinus rhythm and the nature of tachycardia that is SVT versus VT is difficult to assess. Esophageal recording obtained at the bedside makes it clear (Figure B) that there is 2:1 (in most part) and 1:1 (in the middle part) VA relationship which clarifies the diagnosis. It is worthnoting that in this example of BBR the QRS complex in VT and sinus rhythm are identical

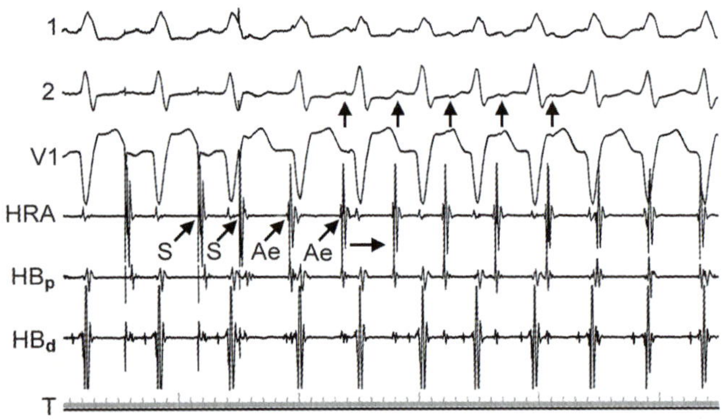

Figure 44.7: P-wave polarity during wide QRS tachycardia. The initiation of atrial tachycardia in a patient with pre-existing rate-related LBBB is shown. Due to the changing relationship between P and QRS, the P-wave timing is changing, which in turn changes the perception of P-wave polarity. This is an important clinical point because the interpretation of P-wave can change from positive to negative polarity (2nd and 3rd arrow, respectively) depending upon where the P-wave coincides with different parts of the ST-T segment. This is even more difficult in patients with wide QRS tachycardia. Since no standard exists at this time, for interpreting P-wave polarity in this setting, the assessment is mostly subjective

and/or SVT. Secondly, on rare occasions, it may occur with left anterolateral pathway-related preexcited tachycardia. Thirdly, LV pacing can result in northwest axis and should be easy to recognize unless the pacing artifact is not visible. Regardless of these limitations, northwest axis during wide QRS tachycardia is more likely in VT than any other cause of wide QRS tachycardia. Its importance almost equals that of AV dissociation because it can be recognized in almost 100% of the cases, unlike AV dissociation plus VA block that is observed in only 24% of the cases of VT. Other investigators have also found little value of axis orientation when it is in the left, normal or right axis category.[5] Since differences exist among investigators regarding the value of other axes, i.e. left, normal, or right axis for diagnosis of VT, it can only be explained on the basis of the differences in the samples.[1,2,5] When one is aiming at reaching accuracy of close to 100%, it seems no axis orientation has value in distinguishing between aberrant conduction and VT.

QRS Complex Duration

One of the simplest criteria, one that is always measureable on surface ECG, is the duration of the QRS complex. It is mentioned by several investigators employing the multiple ECG leads and is ideally determined from the earliest to latest QRS complex inscription using all 12 ECG leads. In a given lead, the QRS duration can be misleadingly narrow **(Figures 44.1, 44.3 and 44.9)**, because part of the QRS complex, particularly the initial part, may be isoelectric. At the very least, two leads perpendicular to each other must be used. In the lab-induced setting used by Wellens et al. five leads, that is, I, II, III, V_1 and V_6 were recorded which may not be sufficient in some patients. This earlier study used 140 ms as a cut-off point for diagnosis of VT[2]. Subsequently, it was modified somewhat so that, during the RBBB pattern,

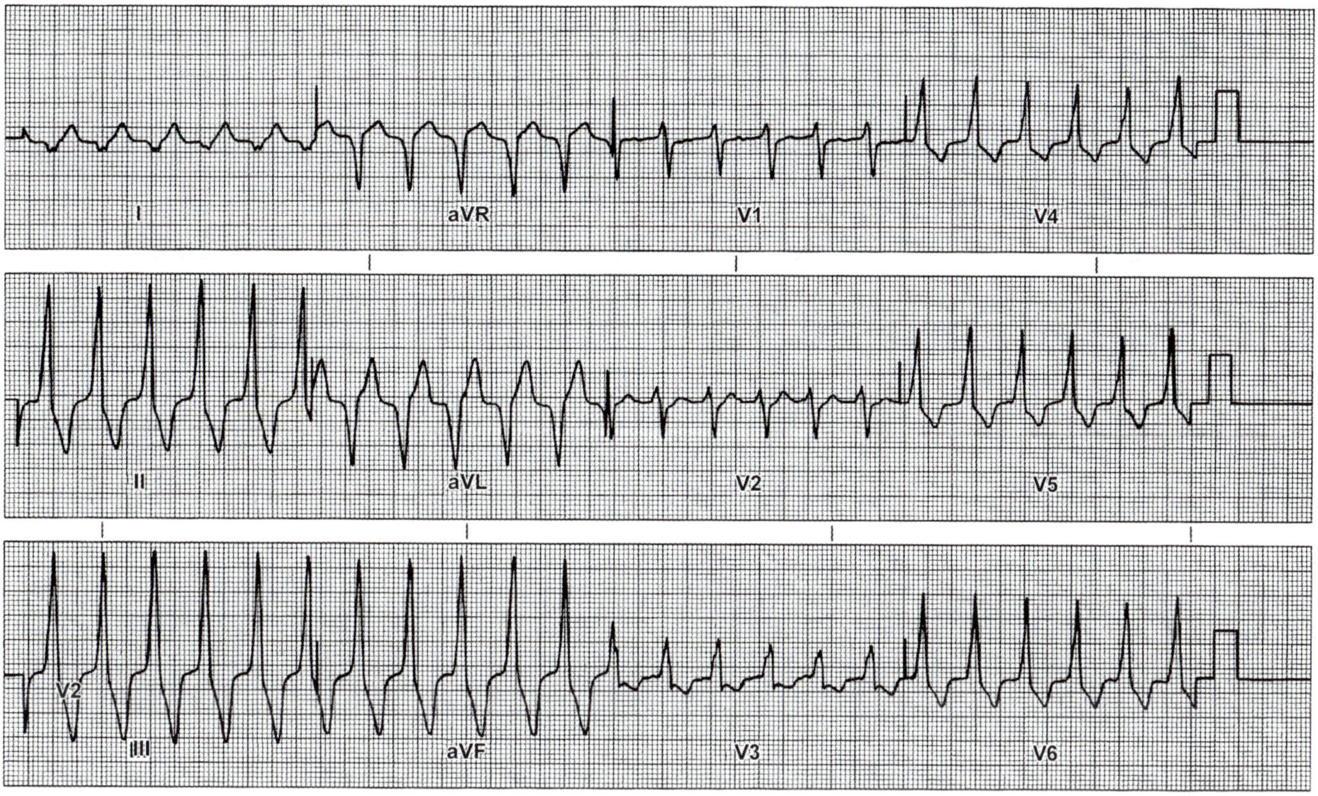

Figure 44.8: Right ventricular (RV) outflow VT. The 12-lead ECG depicts a classic example of RV outflow ventricular tachycardia. There are several locations that have been identified with axes mostly rightward and such ECGs are considered typical of RV outflow VT. This suggests a minimum diagnostic value of left, normal, or rightward axes in distinction of various types of wide QRS tachycardias

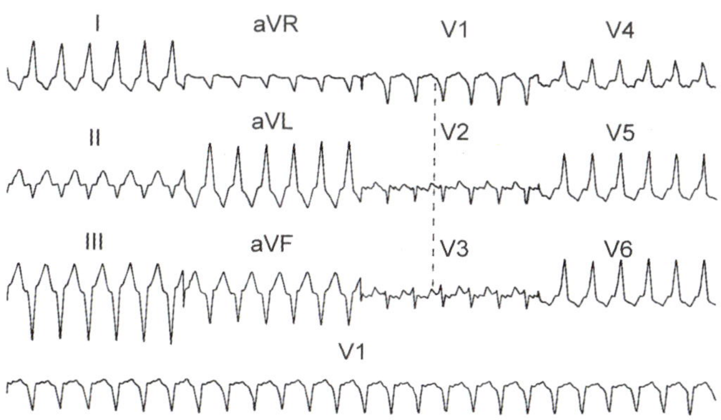

Figure 44.9: QRS duration in multiple leads. A preexcited tachycardia is seen in this Figure. If only lead II, V2 or V3 were recorded the width of the QRS will be grossly underestimated. This finding can also be observed in Figures 44.1 and 44.3

a QRS duration of more than 140 ms was sufficient in distinguishing VT from aberrant conduction. For LBBB configuration, the QRS duration must be at least 160 ms to diagnose VT.[1] A later study suggested that the QRS duration should be more than 160 ms in all types of configurations to label VT as the cause of wide QRS.[5] Another issue that influences this particular aspect is whether the patient is on any cardioactive medications. While the lab-induced tachycardias are usually in an unmedicated state, ambulatory patients may be on several drugs. Class I antiarrhythmic effect (particularly in 1c agents) is the culprit most of the time and Class Ic agents were frequently used many years ago. At this time, Class Ic agents are still prescribed for other arrhythmias such as atrial fibrillation and can broaden the QRS. One form of NSIVCD noted not infrequently in clinical practice is where atrial fibrillation is treated by Class Ic drugs, and the rhythm converts to atrial flutter **(Figures 44.10 and 44.11)**. These agents also cause slowing of the atrial flutter rate, widening of the QRS during 1:1 AV conduction, and further prolongation of the QRS particularly in patients who have preexisting BBB. So in the outpatient setting, QRS duration ≥ 140 ms during a wide QRS tachycardia clearly cannot exclude a diagnosis of SVT. Patients with VT may also show Class I antiarrhythmic drug effect producing further prolongation of QRS complex duration.

It is critical to take a thorough history of the patient's current pharmaceutical use in order to arrive at a correct

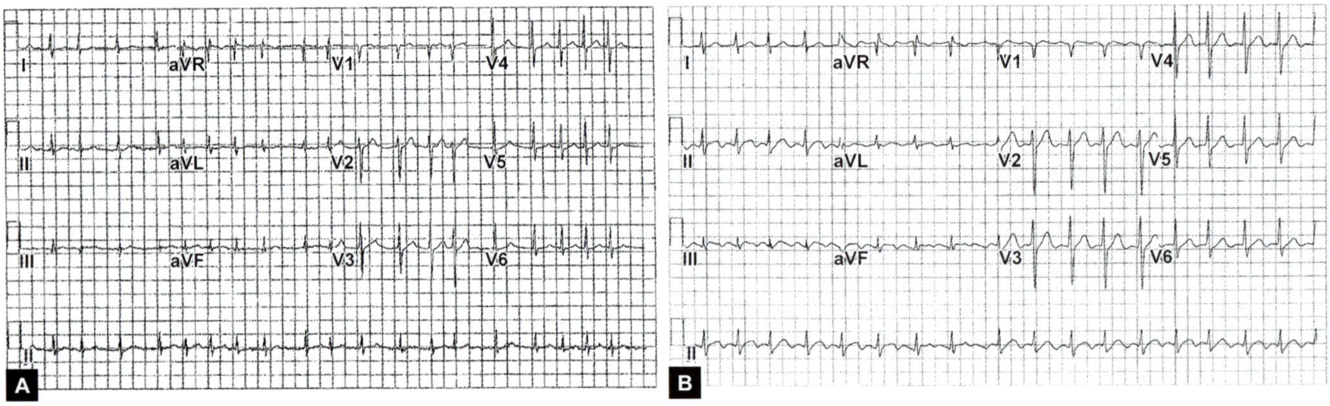

Figures 44.10A and B: Wide QRS and Class I antiarrhythmic agents. Atrial fibrillation with moderate ventricular rate and the QRS duration of 90 ms is seen in Figure A. Following initiation of therapy with flecainide the rhythm converts to atrial flutter with atrial cycle length of 300 ms and variable AV ratio (B). There is also a QRS widening to 105 ms (NSIVCD)

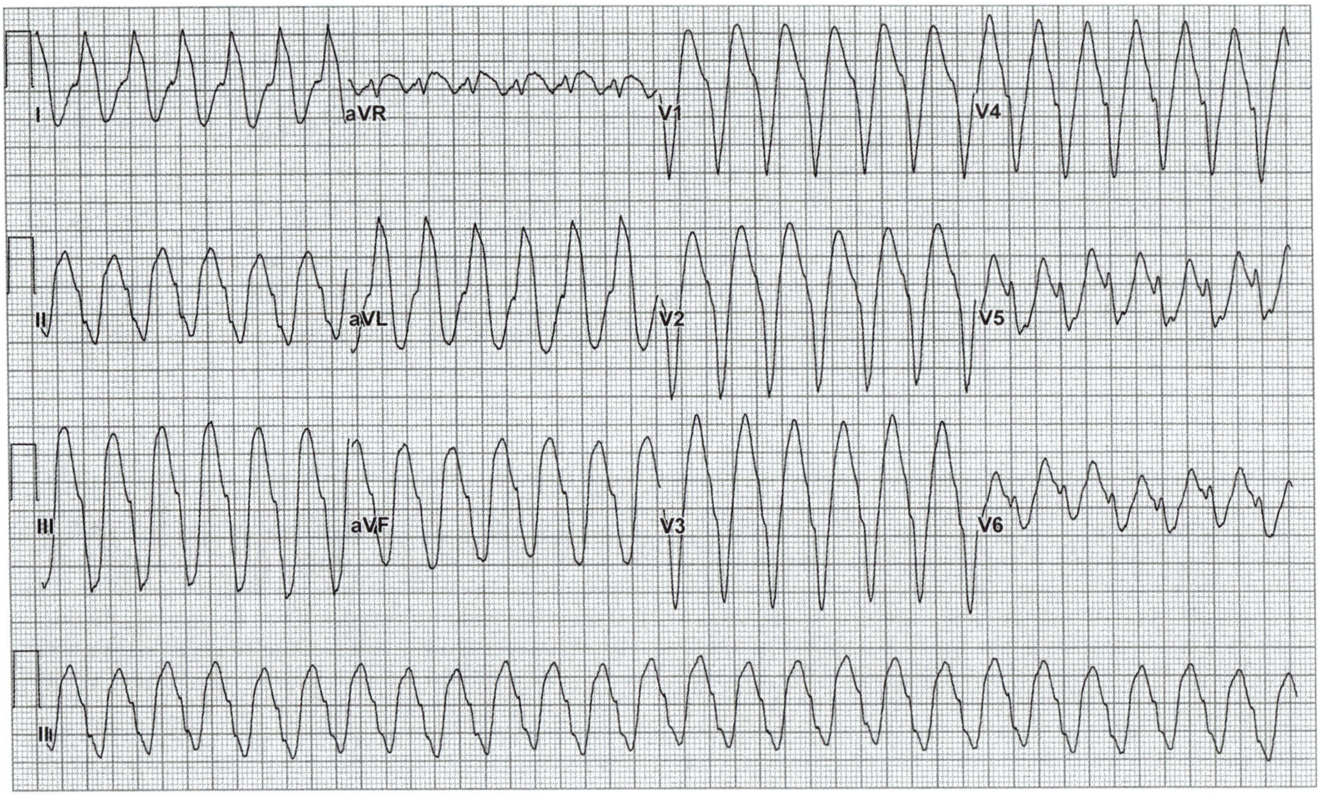

Figure 44.11: Wide QRS and Class Ic agents. Same patient as Figure 44.10. With further slowing of atrial flutter rate to 400 ms, there is 1:1 AV conduction and marked widening of the QRS complex duration to 200 ms with LBBB configuration and left axis deviation. While the general orientation of the QRS in Figures 44.10A and B are similar, there is a marked leftward shift of axis in Figure 44.11 suggesting LBBB in addition to concomitant NSIVCD already present

diagnosis. While Class Ic antiarrhythmic drugs are often the cause of this dilemma, other agents with Class I properties should also be inquired about. Over the counter agents are often not considered by the patient to be drugs and may not be brought to the physician's attention. Other reasons why the QRS duration has limited importance to distinguish VT from aberrant conduction are the following:

a. Many patients have myocardial scarring and NSIVCD and other mechanisms and have a wide QRS complex at the baseline. Even without any specific BBB, one would expect that the width of the QRS will remain the same or further prolong with SVT making a wide QRS even broader if aberrant conduction coexists. This would further reduce the diagnostic value of QRS duration.

b. At the other end of the spectrum, VT can be narrower than the baseline QRS complex. This scenario is more likely when the VT arises in the interventricular septum or is fascicular in nature but not rare in the presence of a pre-existing BBB **(Figure 44.12)**, when the baseline QRS is wider.

c. The role of the HPS participation towards the width of the QRS complex has never been well documented. It is possible that a myocardial impulse can enter the HPS, and then rapidly conduct and create shortening of the QRS duration as compared to no HPS participation. Conversely, if there is extensive fibrosis, the aberrant conduction-related wide QRS tachycardia may even be much broader than otherwise.

QRS Complex Morphology

This is one of the most commonly used since it is readily available and remarkably easy to apply, but there are many aspects that need addressing to put it in proper perspective.

a. RBBB (positive in V1) versus LBBB (negative in V_1) configurations are common in both VT and aberrant conduction (58% versus 42% respectively in VT and 52% versus 48% respectively with aberrant conduction, hence of no value for differentiation.[1]

b. Positive concordance (only R-wave V1 to V6) versus negative (QS in V1-V6) concordance. While in our series positive concordance was only seen in VT (**Figure 44.13A**), negative concordance was also noted in aberrant conduction.[1] Since the publication, some preexcited wide QRS tachycardias with positive concordance have also been shown. (**Figure 44.13B**). In other words, exceptions do exist in both cases, but the pattern heavily favors VT when there is positive concordance. Like many of the other criteria, it is not common to see these patterns (27 out of 122 in VT and 3 out of 21 in aberrant conduction). Hence, these criteria have a low sensitivity and acceptable specificity as was noted in AV dissociation and northwest axis.

c. Specific QRS morphology (mono-, bi- or triphasic QRS complexes) is emphasized by anyone who has examined

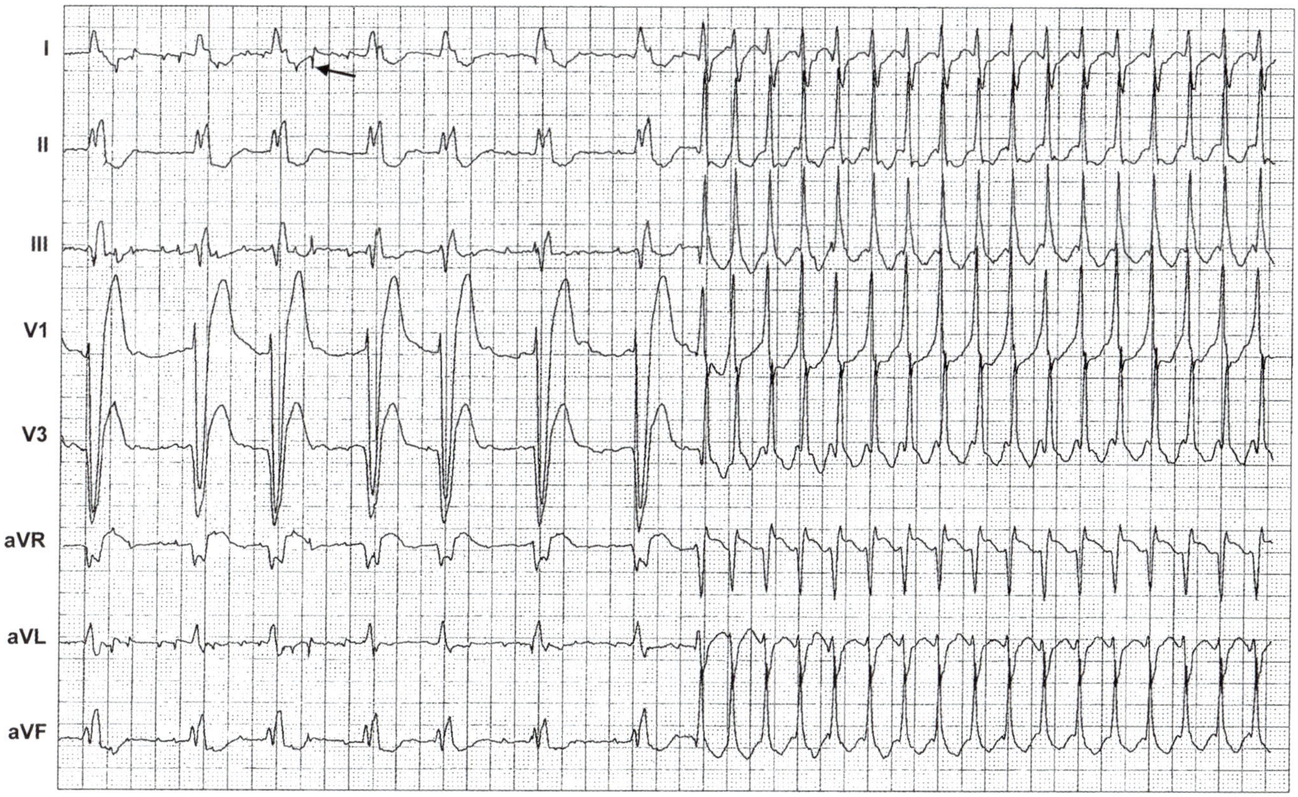

Figure 44.12: Narrower VT QRS compared to baseline (8 leads). The baseline rhythm is atrial fibrillation and the conducted QRS complex shows a LBBB pattern with QRS duration of 160 ms. Sudden onset of regular narrower QRS tachycardia (cycle length 280 ms) is noted. Since the AV node is not capable of conducting at this rate during atrial fibrillation, the tachycardia is subjunctional. The QRS morphology is that of a RBBB plus right axis pattern. In most leads, the onset of QRS is rapid and hence the fascicular nature of the tachycardia cannot be excluded. An alternate possibility is myocardial VT originating from the basal septum and breaking through into the left ventricle. (Arrow is an artifact)

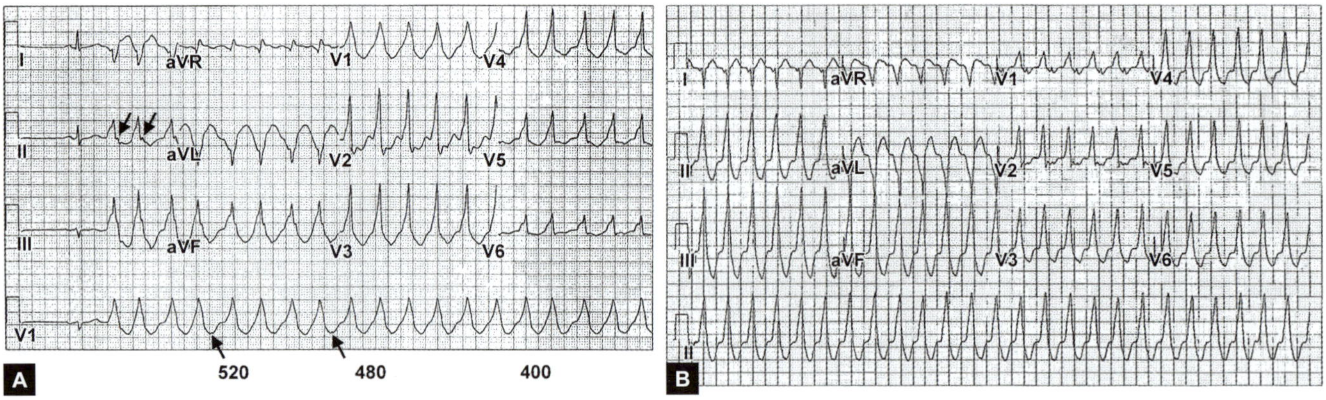

Figures 44.13A and B: Positive concordance and wide QRS tachycardia. A positive QRS concordance, that is positive QRS complex V1 through V6, can be appreciated in both Figures A and B. The tracing in (A) is an example of myocardial VT, whereas the preexcited circus movement tachycardia using a left free wall accessory pathway anterogradely is seen in (B). The two arrows above lead II in (A) are drawing attention to deflections that are part of the QRS and not P-waves mechanisms. Note the RR CL variation in (A) as labeled (520, 480 and 400 ms). Also, there is a hint of P-wave pointed out by the two bottom arrows in the rhythm strip (V1)

this issue closely.[1-5,7] While easiest of all to examine, it is the least helpful and often misleading. **Figure 44.14** shows QRS with RBBB configuration from more than 80 different patients and none of the complexes look identical to any other in the figure. Usually, these shapes are drawn in various publications and do not reflect the true diversity of morphologies. There seems to be less diversity in patients showing a LBBB pattern but nonetheless it exists.

It has been repeatedly stated that monophasic and biphasic complexes in V_1 and RsR pattern where the first R is taller than the second (right versus left rabbit ear) suggest ventricular origin (**Figures 44.14A to K**; 5 examples of first R being taller during sinus rhythm) while the triphasic rsR type of pattern is indicative of aberrant conduction. The irony here is that once you realize that VT is the underlying cause of most wide QRS tachycardias, it is more likely that a triphasic complex, which typically represents aberrant conduction, may in fact be VT in more patients, as was the case in our series.[1] Classic triphasic complex was observed in 9 patients with VT and 7 patients with SVT, even though the higher percentage of patients with aberrant conduction (7 out of 11, or 63%), versus VT (9 out of 70, or 13%) had this pattern. It is obvious that significant overlap exists using this QRS morphology for distinction between VT and aberrant conduction. Interestingly, a triphasic QRS complex in association with wide QRS showing a LBBB configuration which means a notch during the QRS complex in V_1 was only seen in VT. This observation has limited appeal because of its infrequency (occurring in 8 out of 52 patients), and has also been mentioned previously with a somewhat different description.[7] We find that specific QRS morphology as a solo criterion to make a definitive diagnosis of VT versus aberrant conduction not very useful for patient care, albeit a good intellectual exercise. When such inflammatory remarks about any of the so-called "established criteria" are made

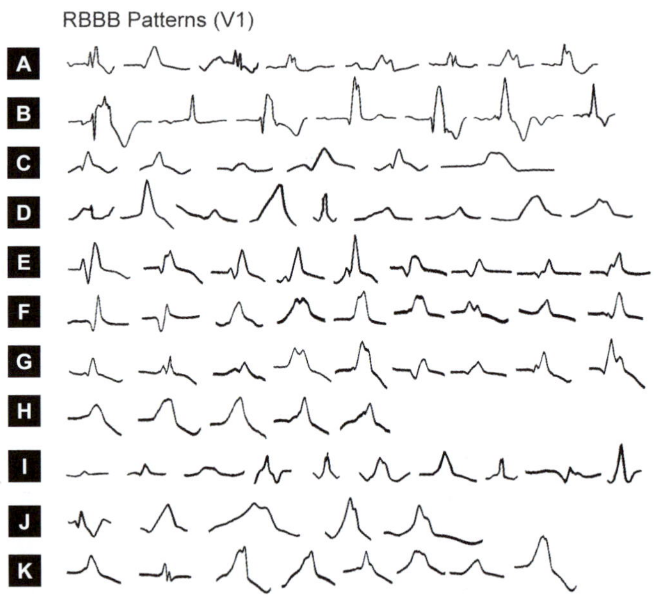

Figures 44.14A to K: Overlap of wide QRS complex configurations (V1) from different etiologies. The Figure depicts RBBB pattern, with wide QRS complexes from various mechanisms in more than 80 patients. Since only lead V1 is being shown some of the QRS complexes may not appear wide but the QRS duration was measured from a combination of leads as was suggested in the text. Figures A and B are sinus rhythm, Figure C shows fascicular tachycardias, Figure D is BBR, Figures E and F are SVT with aberrant conduction, Figures G to I are myocardial VT and finally Figures J and K are preexcited tachycardias. This Figure is an attempt to display some of the QRS configurations, by no means complete. It shows however, that many of the QRS morphologies defy the traditional criteria. In clinical practice, all forms of wide QRS tachycardia are encountered, not just myocardial VT and SVT with aberrant conduction. The diversity of QRS appearances seen in this Figure with actual QRS from patients is far greater than what is usually drawn

in our writing, it should not be forgotten that we are looking for near 100% accuracy, not a 90% sensitivity or specificity. In patients with wide QRS tachycardia and LBBB pattern, several of the previously written criteria apply with a reasonable accuracy, certainly not reaching anywhere close to the desired goal of not missing a single patient with VT. These criteria include:

A. From onset of QRS to nadir measuring 70 ms or more[7]
B. Notching during the S wave in V1
C. rS or QS in V1–V6 measuring ≥ 100 ms. While in some series the rS or QS was only seen in VT, this has not been the case in other published series where negative concordance was also seen in SVT

In the series by Brugada et al., the authors suggested a very high degree of sensitivity and specificity in their approach,[8] but it has not been replicated by others.[9] In their protocol, the first two steps were new whereas the others were previously published. Furthermore, patients with bundle branch reentry (BBR) (6% in our experience) will not be diagnosed as VT using the Brugada algorithm. Additionally, VT with only R wave in V1 to V6 (positive concordance) will also not be appropriate for this approach and will be excluded. These are two categories, i.e. positive concordance and BBR will exclude nearly 15% of the patients, a rather unacceptable number for distinction between VT and aberrant conduction. In about 10% of the cases, the QRS morphology simply defies the surface ECG criteria regardless of who the author is **(Figures 44.15 and 44.16)** and this has been expressed previously.[5]

Value of Pre-existing Bundle-branch Block

Common sense suggests that patients with so-called complete BBB at baseline, which is persistent or permanent, will maintain the same morphology during SVT, and if the QRS is different than the baseline it should be considered VT **(Figures 44.17 and 44.18)**.[10] While some exceptions have been noted, generally it follows the rule.[11] In reference to the latter publication, I would like to make the following comments. None of the ECGs shown in the publication will qualify as identical (though similar) QRS configuration in 12-lead.[11] Also, this criterion requires a 12-lead ECG at baseline, which may not be available until after the conversion of the tachycardia and hence, is only useful for long-term management. So a significant limitation of this feature is that in many patients, the diagnosis cannot be

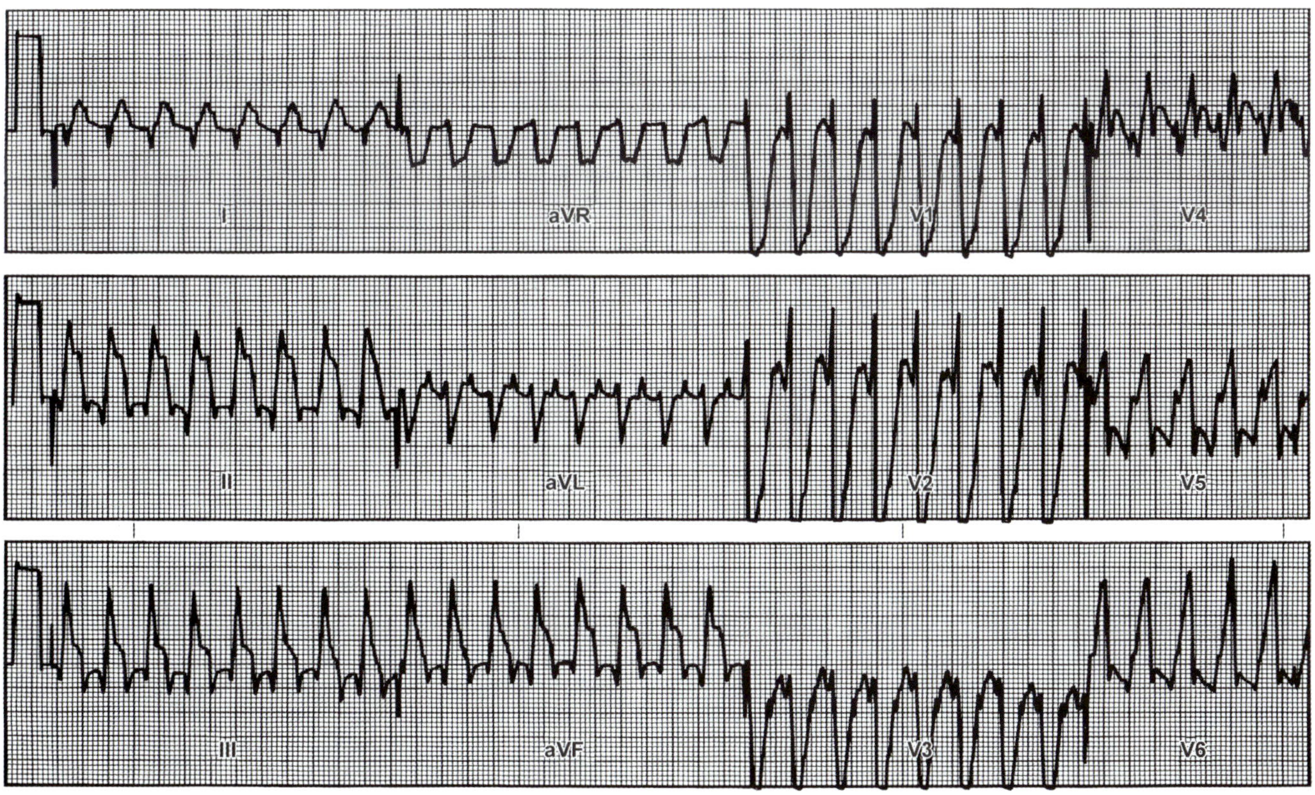

Figure 44.15: Unusual QRS complex during a wide QRS tachycardia. The 12 lead ECG shows a wide QRS tachycardia, duration 200 ms with LBBB and a +100° axis and a rapid initial deflection. Alternating amplitude of initial forces does not represent P-waves (best seen in lead II) and is a part of the QRS as are the positive signals in Lead aVL. What appears to be ST elevation in Leads II, III and aVF is part of the QRS and is not myocardial injury. The example shown here is sustained BBR. The baseline ECG showed a NSIVCD of the LBBB type

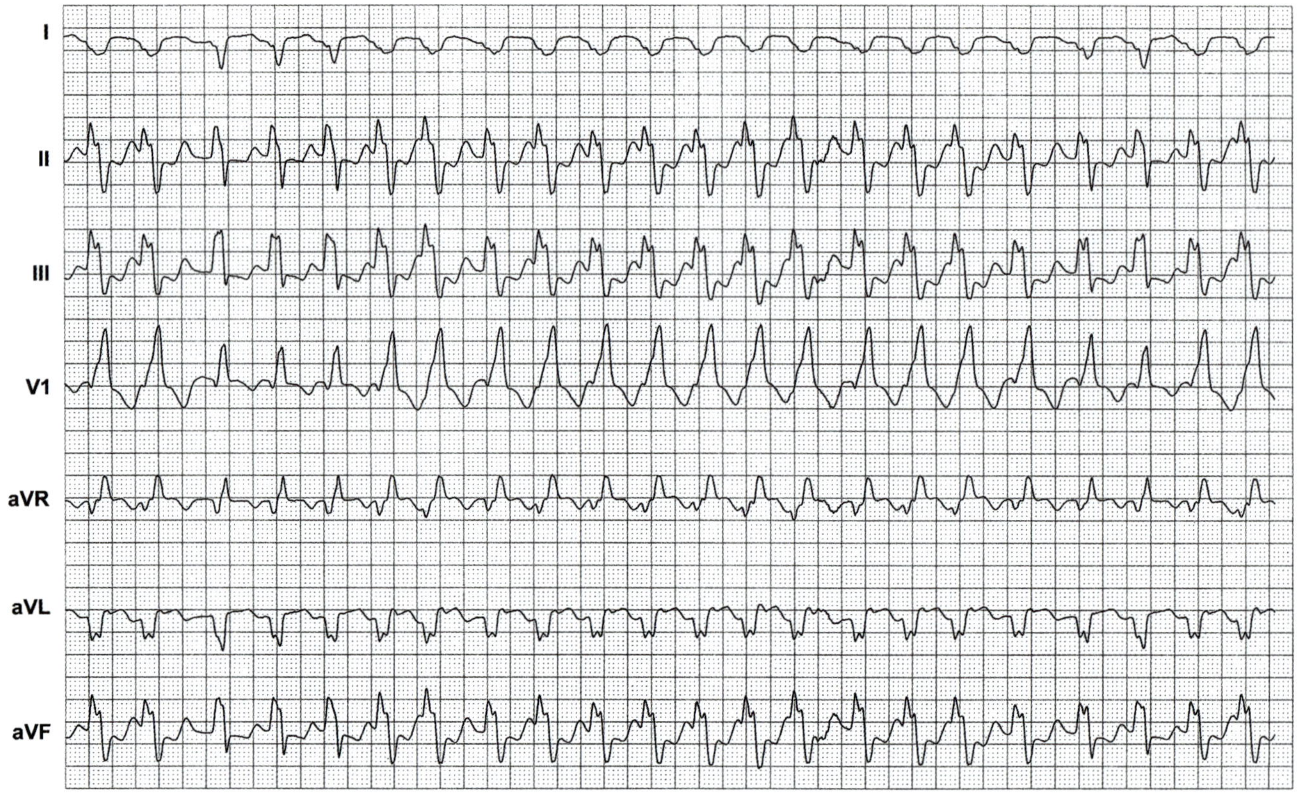

Figure 44.16: Unusual QRS complex configuration. Seven simultaneous leads are available and from top to bottom are Leads I, II, III, V_1 aVR, aVL, and aVF. The QRS morphology is that of a RBBB and right axis with wide QRS complexes measuring 240 ms, and the narrower complexes (3rd to 5th and then 3rd from the end) best seen in lead I or V1 measuring 150 ms. While it fits many of the VT criteria, the rhythm is atrial fibrillation with relatively regular RR and aberrant conduction. The BBB shows some rate relationship and there are three sets of QRS complexes (best appreciated in V1) depending upon whether the T-wave encroaches on the onset of next QRS or does not

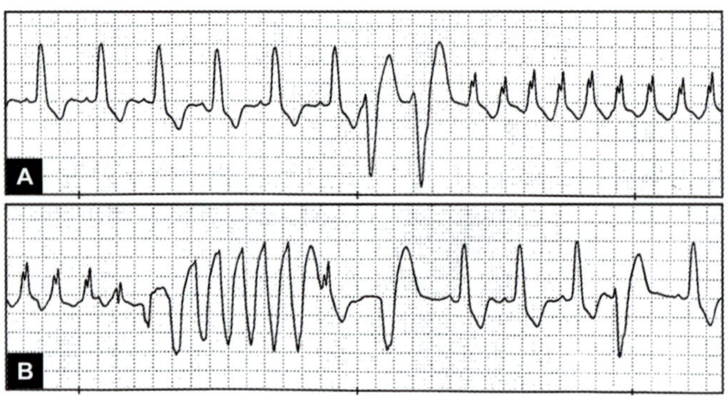

Figures 44.17A and B: Wide QRS tachycardia with pre-existing BBB. Figure A shows LBBB during sinus rhythm and a sudden onset of a wide QRS tachycardia with a different morphology. Although, only one lead is shown, the change in QRS appearance is sufficient to identify differences in QRS morphology during sinus rhythm versus VT. The interruption of VT by another run of spontaneous and rapid nonsustained VT restores sinus rhythm (B)

made at the patient's presentation. Another issue is that the QRS morphology, which may be quite similar to the baseline during the tachycardia, may look slightly different in tachycardias where the rate exceeds 190–200 per minute because the T-wave of prior QRS may alter the appearance at the onset of next QRS in any wide QRS tachycardia (*see* **Figures 44.3A and B**).[5] This will be further complicated if the patient is on agents with Class I antiarrhythmic effect.

It was not previously mentioned strongly enough that BBR VT can and often does have an identical QRS configuration to sinus rhythm **(Figures 44.19 and 44.20)**. Regardless of the QRS morphology, the onset of QRS in BBR is rapid and identical during the first 40 milliseconds. This feature also distinguishes aberrant conduction and BBR from any type of preexcited tachycardia using a rapidly conducting AV-AP or myocardial VT.

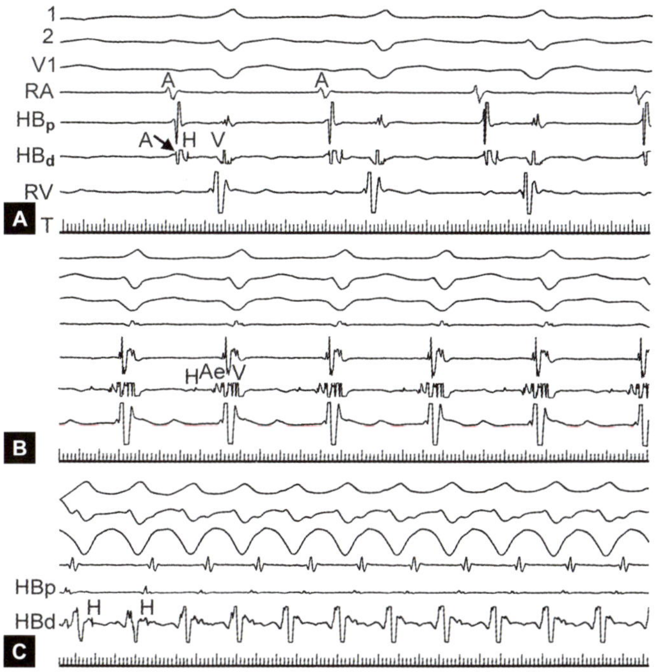

Figures 44.18A to C: Pre-existing BBB and wide QRS tachycardia. Sinus rhythm is seen in Figure A and the HV is prolonged, measuring 105 ms. the same leads are seen in Figure B. An example of AVNRT (slow-fast) is observed in (B) with a cycle length of 500 ms. Note that the QRS configuration on the three ECG leads shown is identical in Figure A. Sustained BBR is depicted in (C). Here the QRS complex is similar but not identical to the Figures A and B already discussed. In BBR, QRS morphologies vary from identical to similar (*see* **Figures 44.19 and 44.20**) and are quite different, if the circuit is reversed

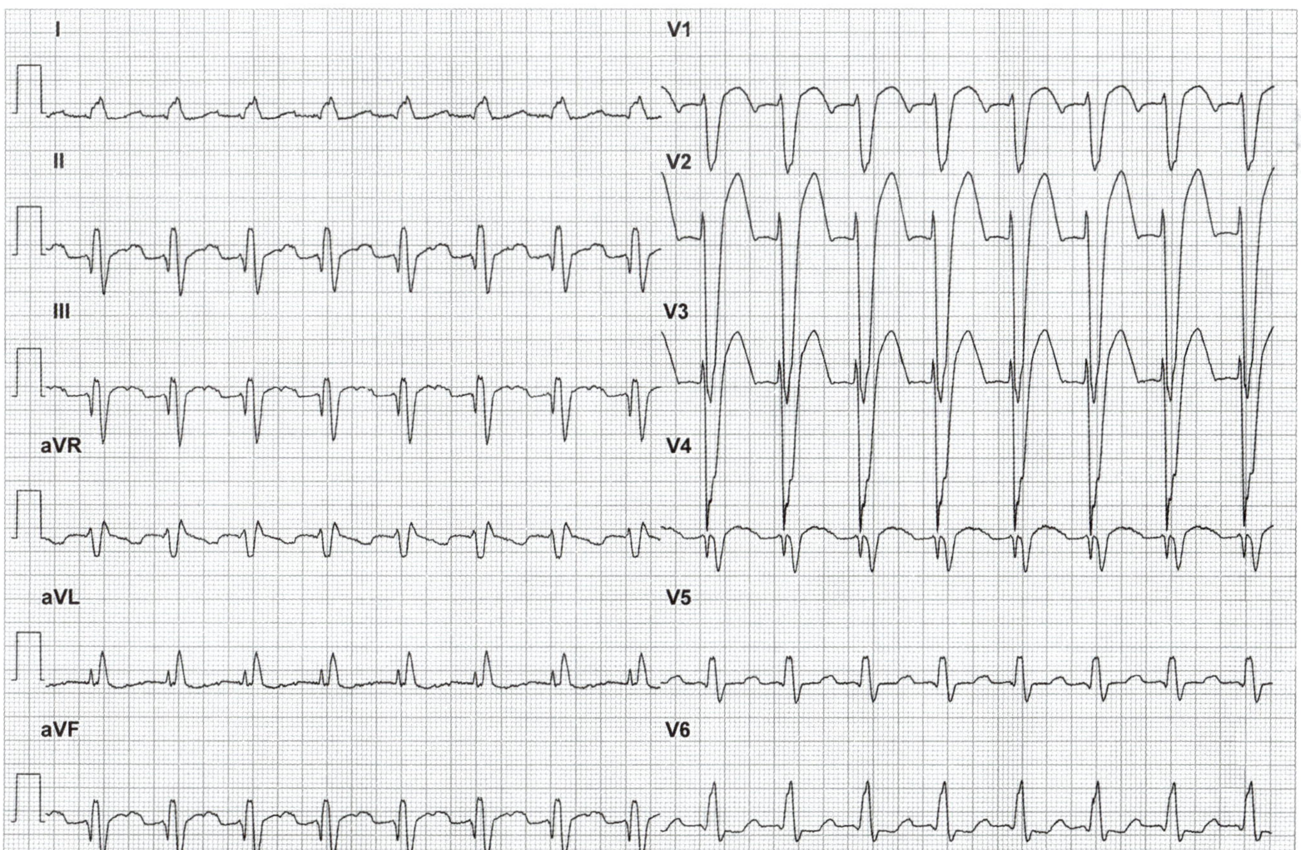

Figure 44.19A

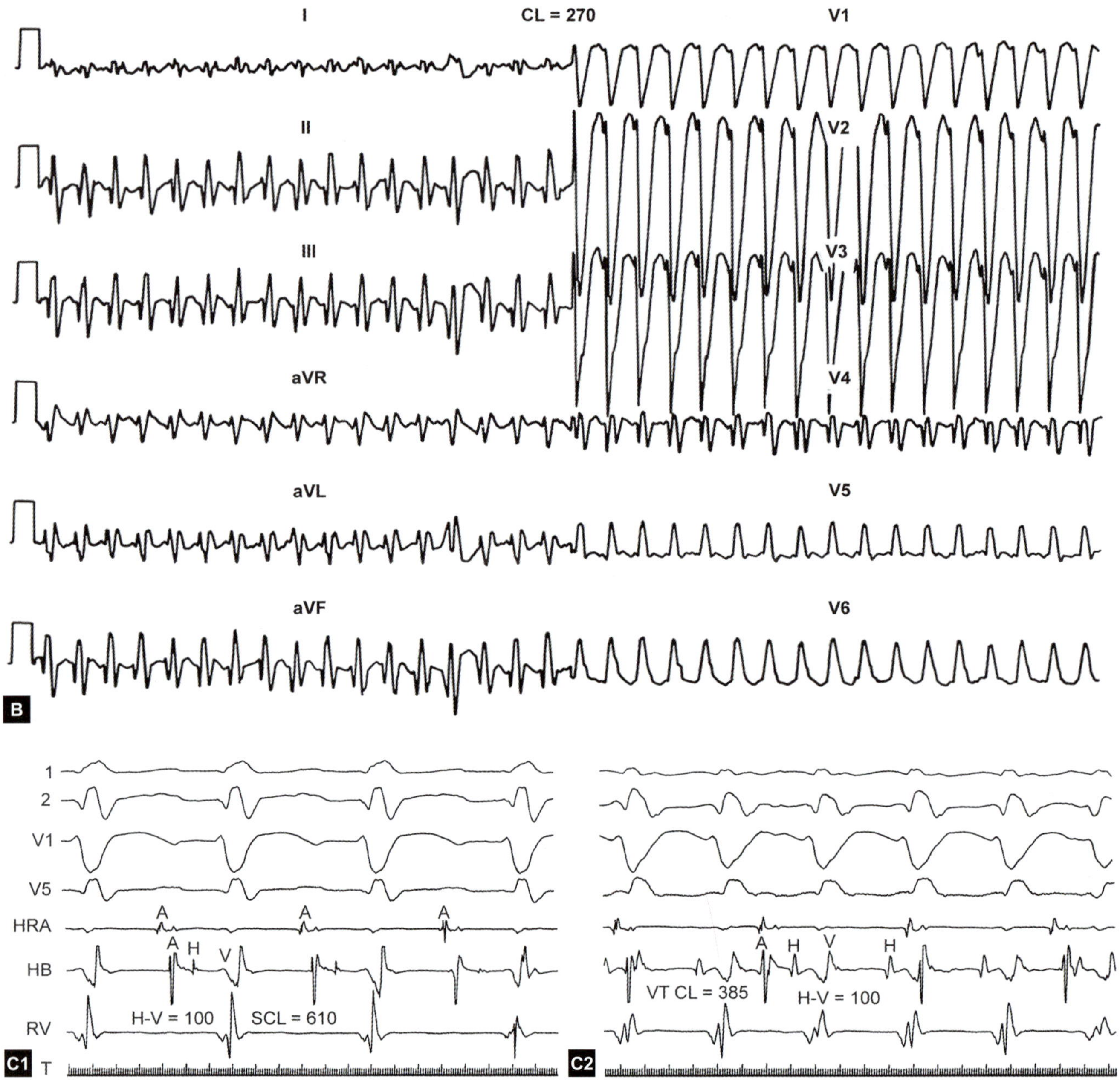

Figures 44.19B and C

Figures 44.19A to C: Pre-existing BBB and BBR. Sinus rhythm is depicted in Figure 44.19A and sustained BBR in Figure 44.19B. The QRS appearance is identical. Sometimes, minor change at the onset of QRS during any rapid wide QRS tachycardia may look different due to the encroachment of T-wave of previous QRS. This is due to the fact that in some leads the vector orientation of the T-wave may be quite different compared with the onset of subsequent QRS. The PR interval measures 300 ms during sinus rhythm (RR 600 ms). The AV node is unlikely to accommodate SVT with CL of 270 ms shown in Figure 44.19B. Another point of emphasis here and has been mentioned before that a so-called complete BBB in these and many other cases is not a complete block which would have cured BBR but simply conduction delay. The latter in either direction, that is anterograde and/or retrograde direction will facilitate BBR as is often the case. Both sinus rhythm and BBR VT with intracardiac tracings are shown in Figures 44.19C1 and 44.19C2 respectively

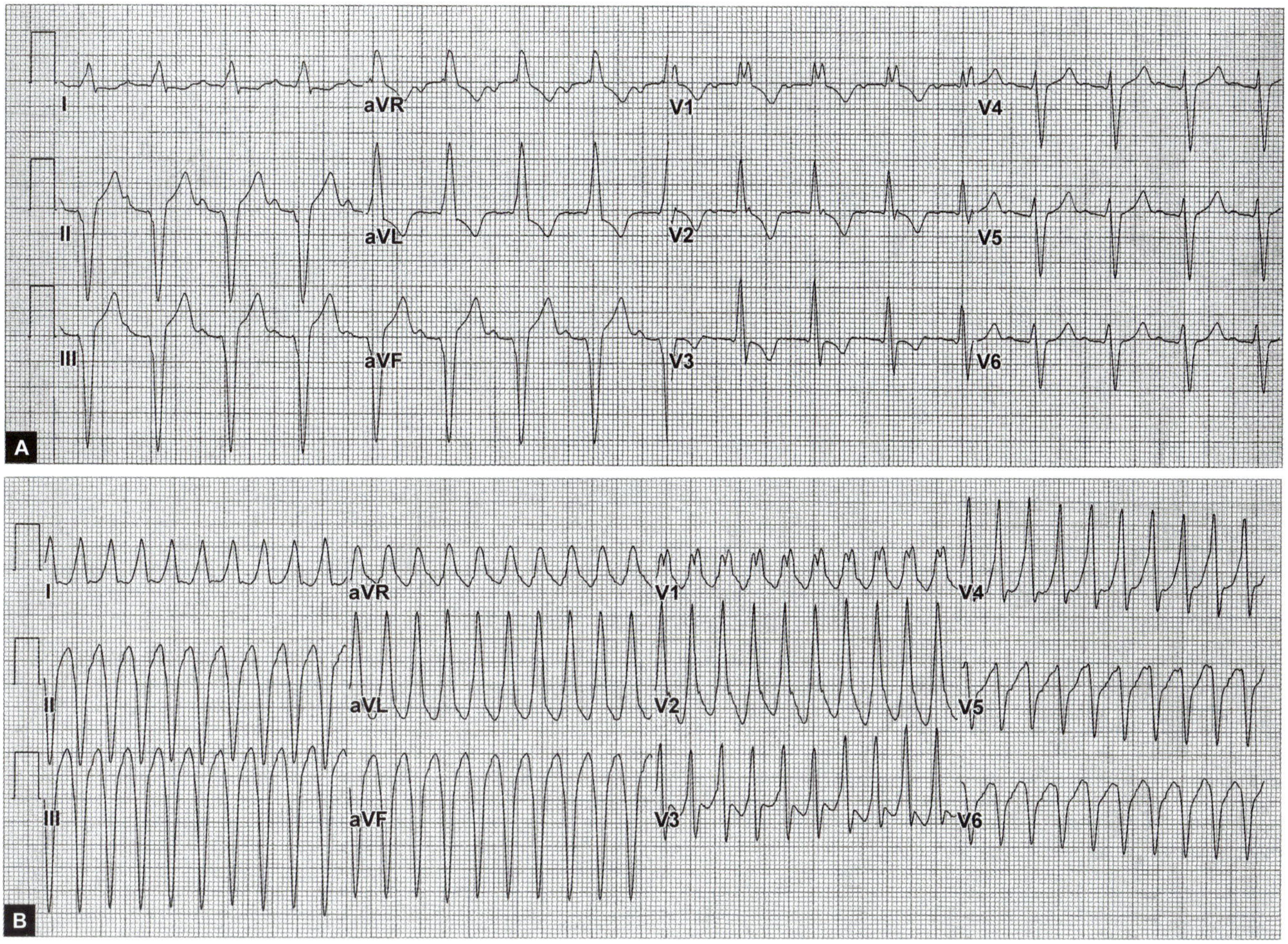

Figures 44.20A and B: Pre-existing BBB and BBR. Sinus rhythm is evident in (A). The sinus complex shows an RBBB and a left axis ventricular pattern. Note the similarity of QRS complex during sinus rhythm and sustained BBR in (B). With rapid VT as seen in Figure (B) the onset of QRS may not look identical in some leads due to superimposition of T-wave from the prior QRS complex

Role of QRS Rate for Distinction Among Wide QRS Tachycardias

Beyond the usual heart rate during wide QRS tachycardia (i.e. 150–180 beats per minute), the rate itself creates difficulty for application of standard ECG criteria. Some aspect of rate can be helpful in making distinction.

1. A change of wide QRS to narrow QRS with the same QRS rate suggests SVT and aberrant conduction **(Figure 44.21)**. It is seldom the case that a narrow complex SVT and wide complex VT have identical rates.
2. A slowing of the heart rate with wide QRS tachycardia and acceleration with conversion to narrow QRS (or vice versa), not only suggests that it is a aberrantly conducted orthodromic tachycardia but also reveals that the AP location is ipsilateral to the BBB **(Figure 44.22)**.[12,13] In right or left free wall APs, there should be a greater than 25 ms change, measurable on most occasions from surface ECG.
3. Ironically, the reverse may happen, where narrow QRS tachycardia emerging from a wide QRS tachycardia shows a slowing of heart rate **(Figure 44.23)**.[14] The reason this happens is that about 10 to 15% of patients with so-called Kent bundle type AP also have AVNRT and dual AV nodal physiology. At the time of conversion from wide to narrow QRS, the ventriculoatrial (VA) interval shortens and hence the corresponding A-A interval **(Figures 44.22 and 44.23)**. This shortening may switch conduction from a fast to a slow pathway of the AV node, prolonging the RR interval and the tachycardia continues with a longer cycle length. The emergent narrow QRS tachycardia may be orthodromic reciprocating tachycardia **(Figure 44.23)** or slow-fast AVNRT.
4. At the onset, some irregularity of RR interval is noted in many patients with MMVT, particularly during non-sustained episodes **(Figures 44.13A and 44.24)**. However, this stabilizes, and marked changes in CL are not common

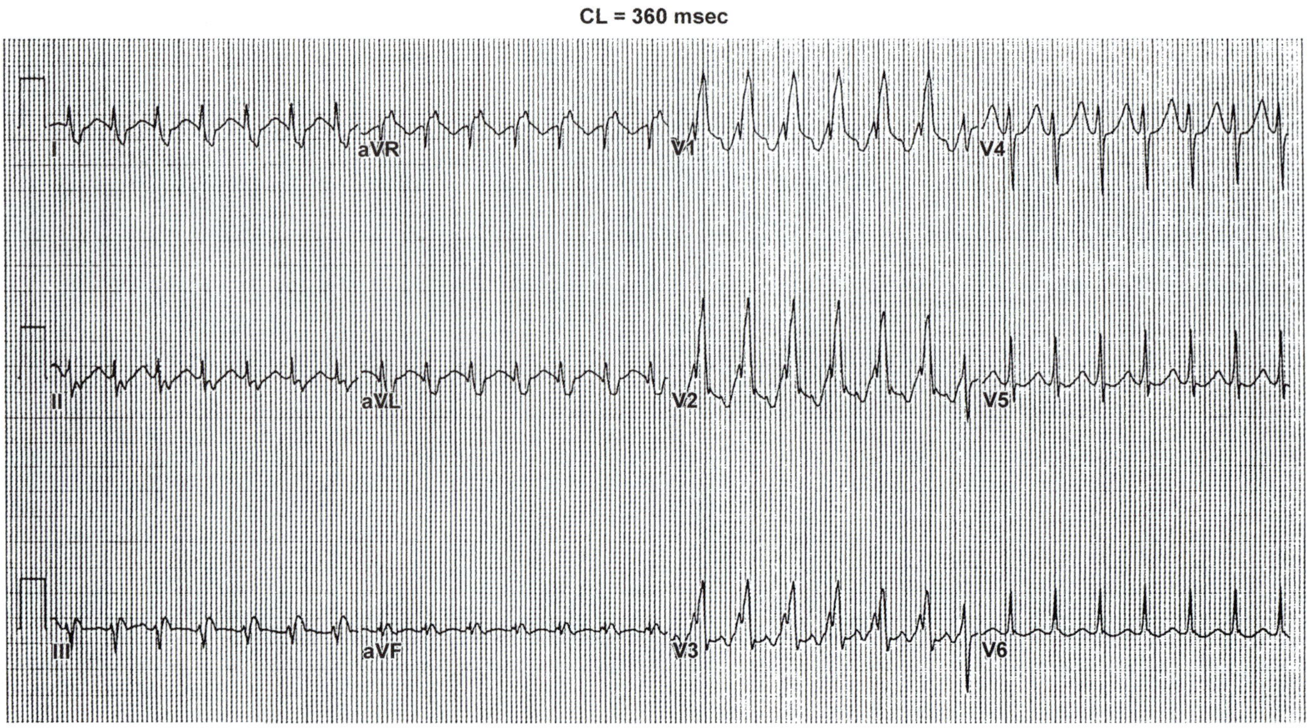

Figure 44.21: Wide to narrow QRS change and the rate of tachycardia. 12 lead ECG of a wide QRS tachycardia with RBBB pattern is seen. Spontaneous change to a narrow QRS occurs in the last three leads (V4 to V6). Note there is no change in the cycle length of the tachycardia and it measures 360 ms throughout. This suggests a diagnosis of SVT with aberrant conduction because the rate of the wide QRS VT and wide QRS SVT are seldom identical. Spontaneous resolution of RBBB is due to forward migration of linking phenomena. A fusion complex is seen at the transition

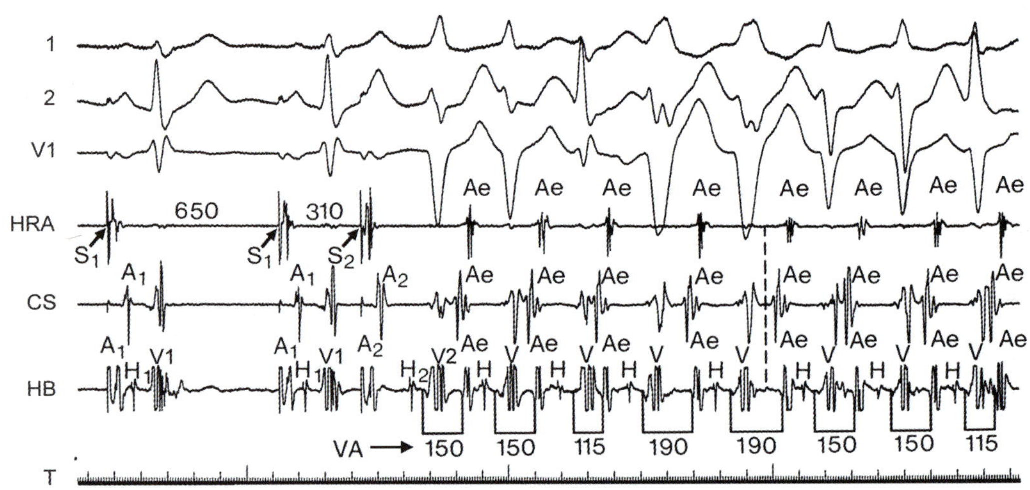

Figure 44.22: The effect of aberrant conduction in AV reentry. The best way to display the effect of various aberrant conduction patterns in a patient with rapidly conducting AV-AP is with intracardiac ECG. The surface ECG-QRS configuration can be appreciated in the top three panels which are labelled. Induction of orthodromic AV reentry is depicted with atrial premature complex (S_2) from HRA at a basic CL of 650 ms. The V2 complex shows a left anterior fascicular block and the VA measures 150 ms. This can be compared with QRS configurations showing the RBBB with right axis in the third tachycardia complex (VA = 115 ms), LBBB plus superior axis (VA = 190 ms 4th and 5th), and with narrow QRS and normal axis (last complex VA = 115 ms). The AP is located in the left free wall. Development of incomplete RBB and left posterior fascicular block has no effect on VA interval (3rd and last VA intervals are identical). The HV interval does not change much during the episode and does not contribute to the VA interval. These changes can also be easily detected on the HRA (for A-A CL) and RR intervals on the surface ECG. These fluctuations in cycle length are a result of fascicular and/or BBB. This phenomenon also occurs in the retrograde direction with His-Purkinje system block which will be shown later in this communication. Reproduced with permission from reference 15

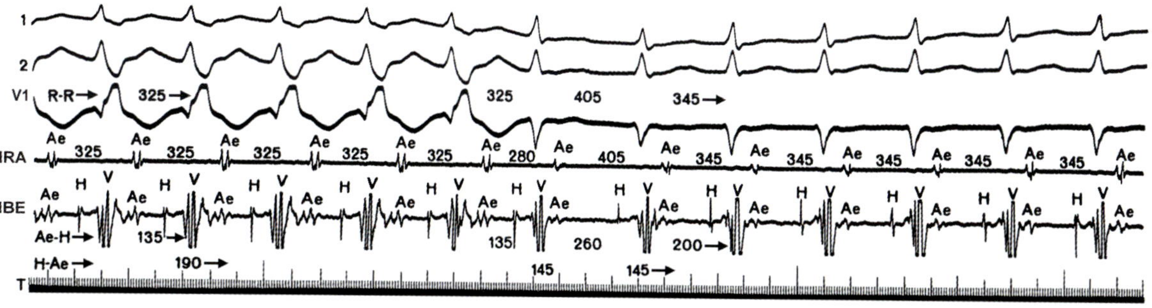

Figure 44.23: Tachycardia cycle length prolongation with abolition of ipsilateral BBB. In patients with right free wall accessory pathway and orthodromic AV re-entry, the abolition of RBBB and a change to narrow QRS shortens the VA interval. In this example, this in return prolongs the anterograde AV nodal conduction time due to engagement of slow AV nodal pathway. This prolongs the AA interval and consequent RR intervals which is opposite of what is expected. Reproduced with permission from reference 14

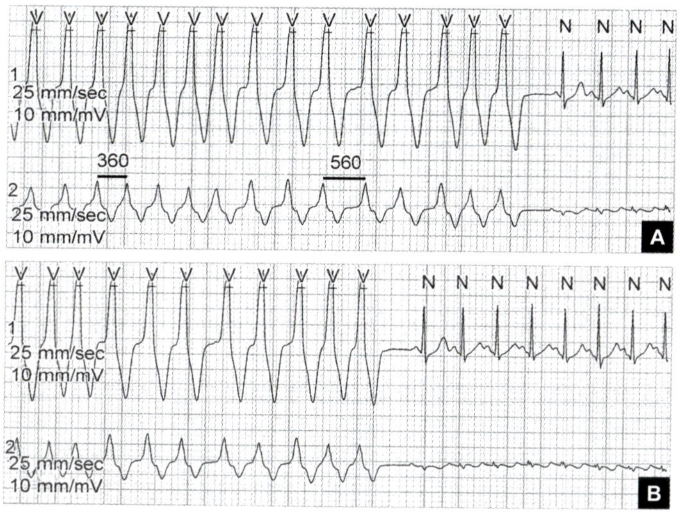

Figure 44.24: Irregular R-R intervals during VT. A non-sustained run of VT is depicted in both panels. There is a marked irregularity of the R-R interval. There is a 200 ms variation during the tachycardia with RR intervals of 360 ms and 560 ms CL shown in (A)

during the rest of the tachycardia but can and do happen in VT.

5. If a short pause is observed or created [carotid sinus massage (CSM), etc.] during a wide complex tachycardia the underlying nature of the arrhythmia may reveal itself and should be looked for very carefully **(Figure 44.25)**.

Multiple Wide QRS VT Morphologies (Pleomorphic VT)

Some patients with a significant area of scarring and diffuse disease may have multiple morphologies of MMVT or a different exit points from the same re-entry circuit. This is uncommon in aberrant conduction or for that matter, pre-excitation or BBR because the aberrant conduction has limited morphologies, that is, right and/or left bundle-branch block with or without superior or inferior axis.[15] Regardless of an individual's experiences, the general patterns of aberrant conduction are commonly known. Similarly, the AP locations are limited, with some exceptions. The most commonly quoted patterns are left and right free wall, posteroseptal, and anteroseptal. So a wide QRS tachycardia which is outside of these patterns should be considered as VT of myocardial origin unless proven otherwise.

Multiple Mechanisms/Causes in Patients with Wide QRS Tachycardia

Several mechanisms may be operative to produce wide QRS tachycardia in the same patient. Some of these scenarios are:

Coexistence of aberrant conduction and myocardial VT: Patients with myocardial VT and with cardiac pathologies such as coronary artery disease, valvular disease, and particularly in conjunction with LV systolic dysfunction may have more than one morphology and mechanism, i.e. several different MMVT (pleomorphism) and if associated with persistent BBB at the baseline, may also have wide QRS tachycardia due to SVT with preexisting BBB. These patients with an LV ejection fraction (LVEF) of less than 40% may be on multiple medications for hypertension, angina or congestive heart failure, etc. and in addition, may have NSIVCD. It is assumed that these patients are not on Class I or Class III agents with some exceptions such as amiodarone. The diagnosis of aberrant conduction related SVT in patients with pre-existing or rate related BBB should be straightforward (i.e. either aberrant conduction or BBR) and a tachycardia with a different QRS would be considered myocardial VT. Otherwise the criteria outlined earlier should be applied. Occasionally, the coexistence of SVT with wide QRS myocardial VT may occur in the absence of myocardial pathology.

Myocardial VT versus BBR: The overall incidence of sustained BBR VT is around 6% of MMVT in our population;

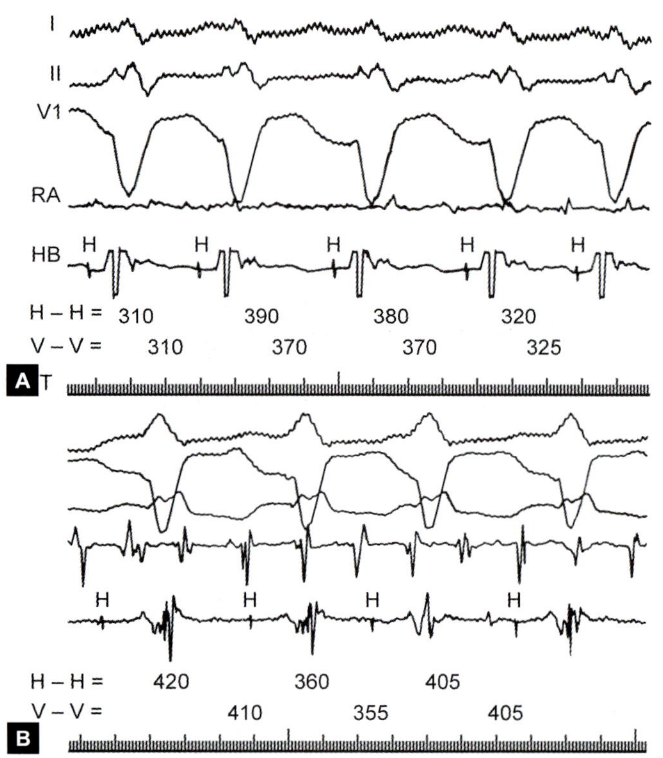

Figures 44.45A and B: H-H and V-V relationship in BBR. In a different patient, two types of BBR are shown with LBBB and normal axis pattern (A) and RBBB plus left axis pattern (B). The underlying atrial rhythm is atrial fibrillation. It can be clearly noted that H-H interval variations drive the subsequent V-V (R-R) CL. The shift of axis (B) is due to exclusive conduction over the LBB (form of complete RBBB pattern) which exposes differential delay in the three fascicles of LBB. This is a common finding following ablation of RBB for BBR

during orthodromic tachycardia regardless of AP location, but is merged within the ventricular electrogram in slow-fast AVNRT and antidromic SVT using AFP. The reason is the AV-AP cannot be engaged in either direction without myocardial activation. Therefore, some intramyocardial conduction time has to be added to VA and then the conduction through the AP before the impulse can reach the atrium. This comparison of VA time must only be done on the HB electrogram because it provides a reliable and reproducible marker. None of the other atrial signals can be used because of two reasons: first, uncertainty of the exact location of other catheters; and second, all of these tachycardia use AV node and the HPS; i.e., the NP which provides a central marker. These distinctions just elaborated can be seen in all the figures in this and other published examples of slow-fast AVNRT, AV re-entry, and AFP related re-entry even though the figures selected here were not chosen to make this point. **Figures 44.55 to 44.57** are also examples of spontaneous or induced termination of wide QRS tachycardias where the atrial impulse does not reach the ventricle and yet terminates the arrhythmia.

Role of Over-under Drive Pacing as a Diagnostic Tool in a Wide QRS Tachycardia

Altering the AV relationship in wide complex tachycardia where there is 1:1 fixed AV/VA interval would clarify the mechanism and the next four figures show some examples of these maneuvers.

a. This patient **(Figure 44.58)** had a concealed left free wall AP and the tachycardia seems to be an orthodromic AVRT, with RBBB, normal axis, and 1:1 VA conduction. The QRS configuration is fairly typical of aberrant conduction, however, there is no detectable HB potential prior to the QRS. Atrial pacing at a CL of 280 ms (tachycardia CL is 350 ms) was attempted. As can be appreciated, the atrial pacing has no impact on the rate of tachycardia. The somewhat different QRS complexes that are seen occasionally in the tracing are due to the paced atrial signal coinciding with various parts of the QRS. Hence, this in essence is a subjunctional tachycardia.
b. **Figures 44.59A and B** displays BBR with CL 240 ms, 1:1 VA conduction, and also had a slow-fast AVNRT with exactly the same morphology (as was the sinus rhythm QRS). In **Figure 44.59A**, the tachycardia starts out with a RBBB and left axis morphology, overdrive pacing from the atrium at 200 ms reverses the circuit, the tachycardia rate accelerates and there is a brief period of entrainment. At the termination of pacing, the tachycardia CL remains same at 200 ms and there is a 2:1 VA block unmasking the ventricular origin. Further evidence is seen in **Figure 44.59B** where deliberate induction of atrial fibrillation has minimal effect on the CL of the tachycardia.
c. During a wide complex tachycardia **(Figure 44.60)** with a RBBB pattern and CL 305 ms (AeAe), overdrive right ventricular pacing at a CL of 230 ms (SS) has no influence on the tachycardia rate. The AV relationship is altered, which can be more clearly noticed at the end of pacing. The atrial activation is high to low, which also suggests the atrial nature of wide QRS tachycardia.
d. A wide QRS complex tachycardia seen **(Figure 44.61A)** at a CL of 320 ms, 1:1 AV relationship, the HB recording was not possible due to access issues. The determination of the tachycardia driver was difficult particularly with a bizarre wide QRS complex (LBBB and Right axis pattern). Ventricular pacing **(Figure 44.61B)** gives the clue. None of the paced ventricular impulses reach the atria during sinus rhythm excluding subjunctional nature of the wide QRS tachycardia which most likely is due to atrial mechanism.
e. Another wide complex tachycardia **(Figure 44.62A)** with a 1:1 AV relationship, CL 250 ms where in the QRS morphology in V_1 hardly suggests VT and aberrant conduction. Atrial pacing at a CL of 280 ms replicates

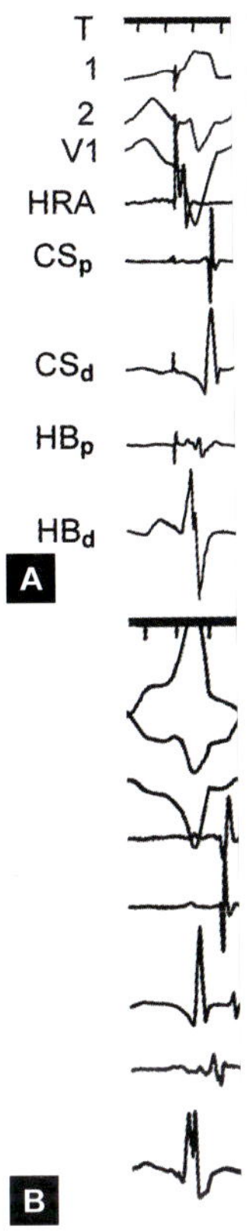

Figures 44.56A to the first three cycl before the QRS wh of wide QRS tachy the tachycardia w anterograde direc AP) interval is bec termination where

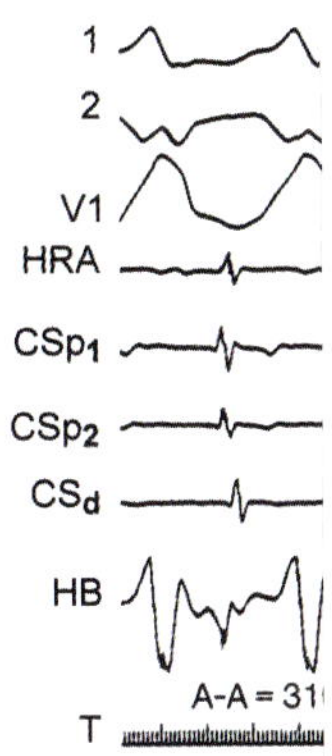

Figure 44.57: Tern tachycardia with 1 before or after the a single atrial prer does not alter the ventricle but term from reference 26

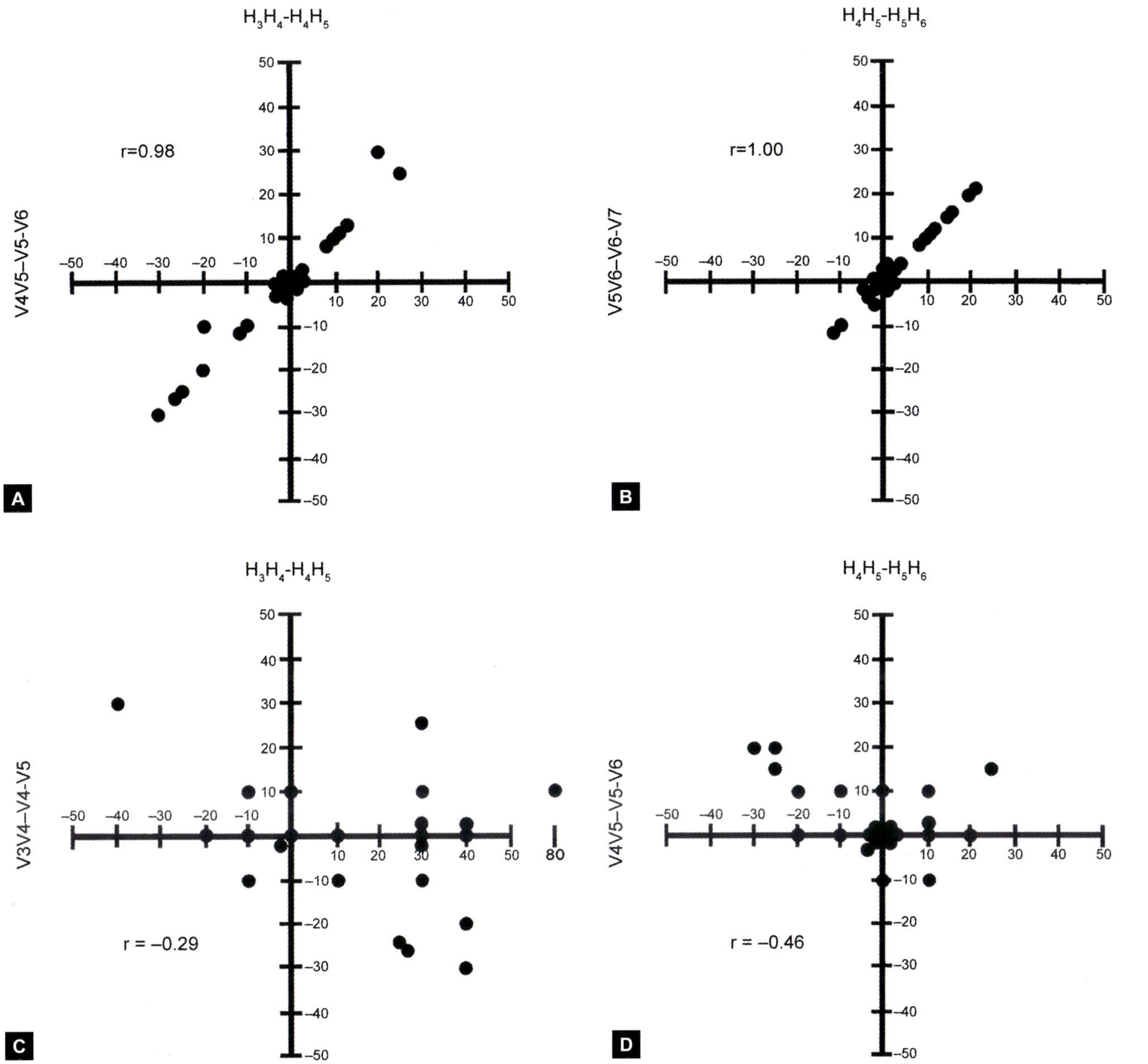

Figures 44.46A to D: Correlation of H-H to next V-V and prior V-V. A plot of H_3-H_4 and H_4-H_5 shows an excellent correlation with subsequent V4-V5 and V5-V6 (A) and a negative correlation with previous V-V interval, i.e. V3-V4 and V4-V5 (C). The same trend is noted with the next HB to V relationship (compare B and D). Reproduced with permission from reference 19

the QRS morphology, suggesting SVT with a rate related BBB, also because the QRS complex narrows during sinus escape seen at the end of the **Figure 44.62B** indicating a retro relationship.

f. Entrainment. While entrainment is not necessary to diagnose a given tachycardia but it is definitely important to establish the mechanism and the reentrant circuit. For effective entrainment, several other phenomena must happen: 1. Intact conduction from the site of pacing to the site of entrainment or for that matter, from one tachycardia entraining another, 2. An excitable gap, 3. Antidromic linking by collision in the reentrant circuit. Effective entrainment of BBR is displayed in **Figure 44.63** showing a RBBB pattern, HV of 90 ms, and AV dissociation (top panel). Ventricular pacing is from the right ventricle at a CL of 270 ms. There is a short period of entrainment with the RV impulse. At the bottom a schema is shown with BBR circuit **(Figure 44.63A)**,

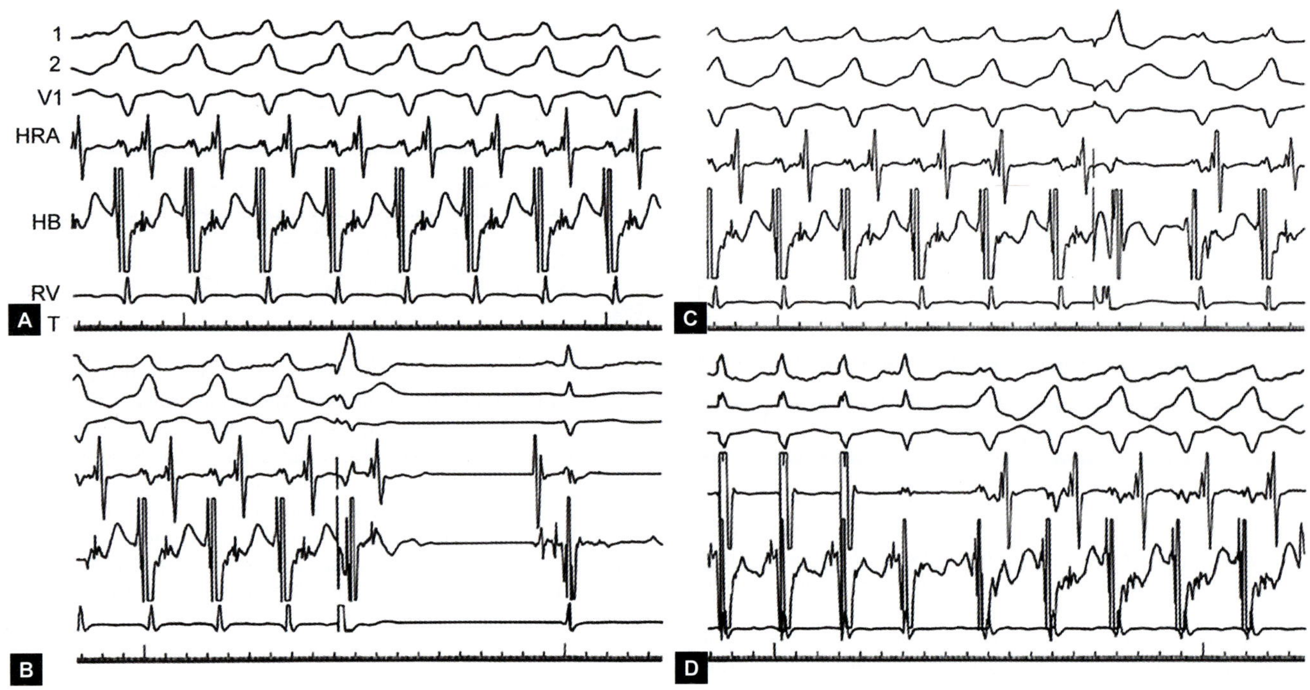

Figures 44.64A to D: Determination of the tachycardia driver in a wide QRS tachycardia. Wide QRS tachycardia with a LBBB and normal axis pattern (A). There is 1:1 AV relationship. The HB is not recognizable during tachycardia but it is well seen during the narrow QRS sinus complex [(B), last complex]. Termination is accomplished in B with a single ventricular extrastimulus. Since the extrastimulus captures the atria earlier than expected, neither myocardial VT nor preexcitation related tachycardia can be excluded. It is clear that HB deflection should have preceded the QRS if it was aberrant conduction. Single ventricular extrastimulus (C) does not influence the tachycardia but the resultant AVVA sequence suggests VT (D). (also see Figure 44.56). A clear driver is seen when the atrial pacing induced normal QRS is followed by an escaped ventricular complex indicating that myocardial VT is the driver

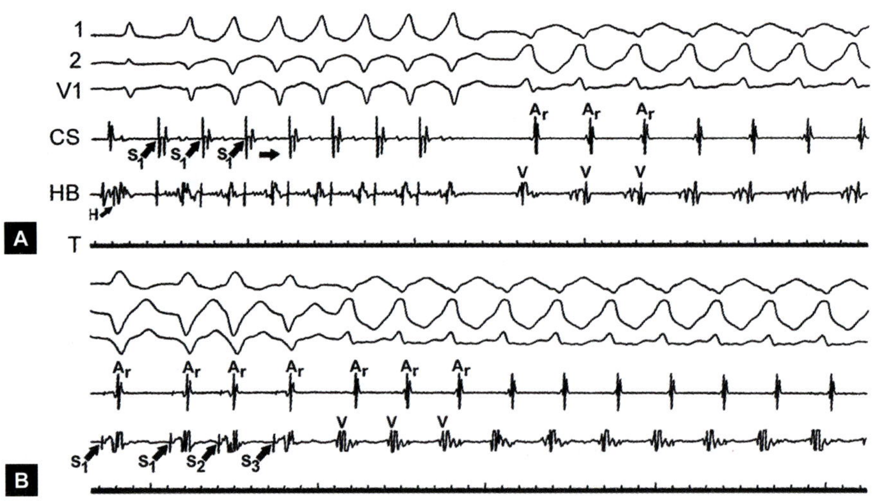

Figures 44.65A and B: Determination of the tachycardia driver. This patient had a history of WPW syndrome and was anticipated to have orthodromic tachycardia. Atrial pacing however is followed by preexcitation from a right posteroseptal accessory pathway, and at the end of pacing there is a clear myocardial VT which is driving the wide QRS. (B) The same arrhythmia is initiated during ventricular pacing. Note the AVVA pattern at the onset of the tachycardia in Figure A, but a VAVA sequence at induction in B. No SVT was induced in this patient. Reproduced with permission from reference 39

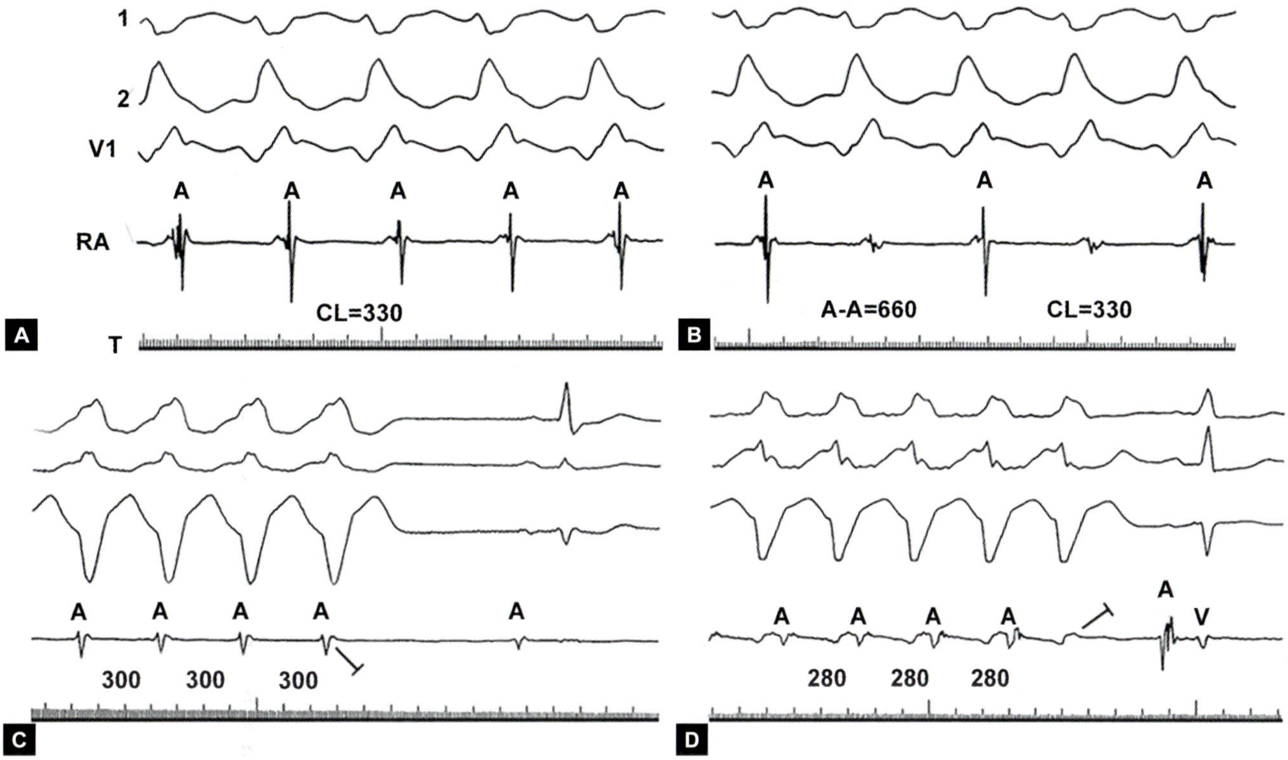

Figures 44.66A to D: Role of adenosine in wide QRS complex tachycardia. (A) A wide QRS tachycardia with 1:1 AV ratio; (B) After adenosine, there is a 2:1 ventriculoatrial block due to the effect of adenosine on the AV node, while the wide QRS tachycardia continues at the same rate (VT CL = 330 ms). This strongly suggests that it is myocardial VT. (C and D) Show termination of AV node dependent reentry tachycardias with adenosine that results in block in antegrade (C) and retrograde (D) limbs of the circuit. Reproduced from reference 39

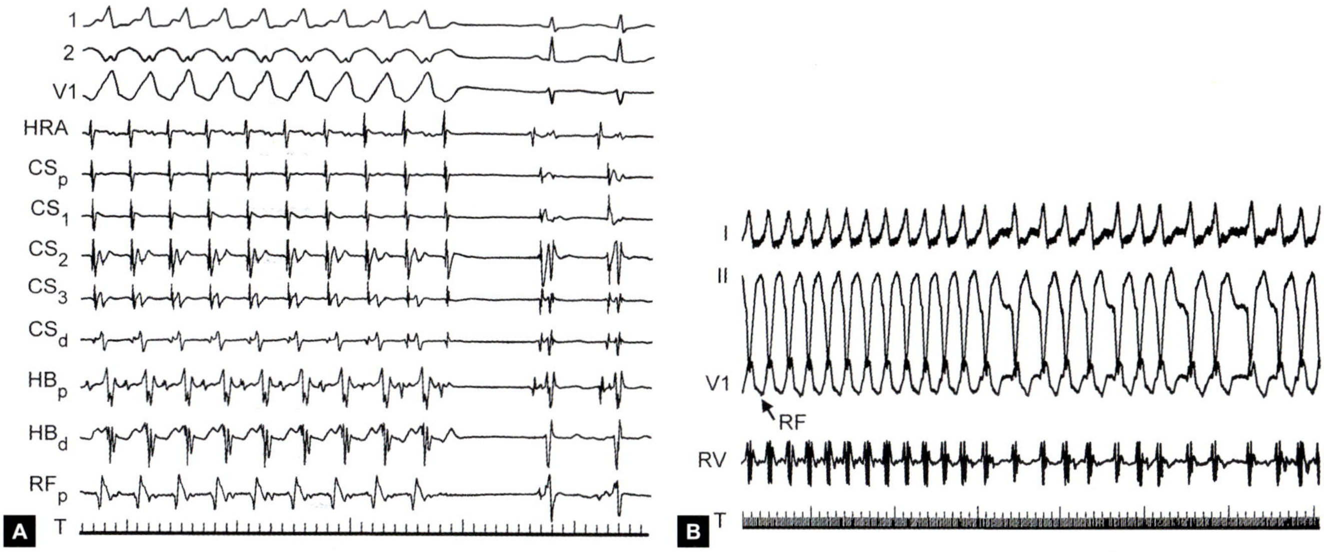

Figures 44.67A and B: Diagnosis of wide QRS tachycardia during RF ablation. (A) A preexcited tachycardia where RF ablation terminates the arrhythmia after the last atrial signal (AV-AP); (B) The ablation of RBB during sustained BBR. Notice the change in CL and irregularity, even though the QRS morphology remains identical (1st[13] QRS complexes compared to the rest). The underlying atrial rhythm was atrial fibrillation. Reproduced with permission from reference 41 (Figure 44.67A) and reference 42 (Figure 44.67B)

Use of Catheter Ablation as a Diagnostic Tool

The next two figures **(Figures 44.67A and B)** depict the examples where ablative maneuvers are applied. This is done after a careful analysis, and if the diagnosis is not certain, a brief RF lesion will clarify the diagnosis. This is shown for the two tachycardias. The first one is preexcited AV reentry **(Figure 44.67A)**.[41] The second is BBR **(Figure 44.67B)** where the underlying rhythm is atrial fibrillation.[42] The morphology of BBR tachycardia and QRS after termination of BBR is identical, but a change in rate and regularity are noticeable (i.e. VT > atrial fibrillation and aberrant conduction).

REFERENCES

1. Akhtar M, Shenasa M, Jazayeri M, Caceres J, Tchou PJ. Wide QRS complex tachycardia. Reappraisal of a common clinical problem. Ann Intern Med. 1988;109:905-12.
2. Wellens HJ, Bar FW, Lie KI. The value of the electrocardiogram in the differential diagnosis of a tachycardia with a widened QRS complex. Am J Med. 1978;64:27-33.
3. Jackman WM, Friday KJ, Naccarelli GV. VT or not VT? An approach to the diagnosis and management of wide QRS complex tachycardia. Clinical Progress in Pacing and Electrophysiology. 1983;1:225-68.
4. Miller J, Das M, Arora R, et al. Differential Diagnosis of Wide QRS Complex Tachycardia. In Cardiac Electrophysiology: From Cell to Bedside, 4th edn. Elsevier; 2004. pp. 747-57.
5. Drew BJ, Scheinman MM. ECG criteria to distinguish between aberrantly conducted supraventricular tachycardia and ventricular tachycardia: practical aspects for the immediate care setting. Pacing Clin Electrophysiol. 1995;18:2194-208.
6. Wellens HJ. Unusual examples of supraventricular re-entrant tachycardias. Circulation. 1975;51:997-1002.
7. Kindwall KE, Brown J, Josephson ME. Electrocardiographic criteria for ventricular tachycardia in wide complex left bundle branch block morphology tachycardias. Am J Cardiol. 1988;61:1279-83.
8. Brugada P, Brugada J, Mont L, Smeets J, Andries EW. A new approach to the differential diagnosis of a regular tachycardia with a wide QRS complex. Circulation. 1991;83:1649-59.
9. Isenhour JL, Craig S, Gibbs M, Littmann L, Rose G, Risch R. Wide-complex tachycardia: continued evaluation of diagnostic criteria. Acad Emerg Med. 2000;7:769-73.
10. Dongas J, Lehmann MH, Mahmud R, Denker S, Soni J, Akhtar M. Value of preexisting bundle branch block in the electrocardiographic differentiation of supraventricular from ventricular origin of wide QRS tachycardia. Am J Cardiol. 1985;55:717-21.
11. Olshansky B. Ventricular tachycardia masquerading as supraventricular tachycardia: a wolf in sheep's clothing. J Electrocardiol. 1988;21:377-84.
12. Jazayeri MR, Sra JJ, Akhtar M. Wide QRS complexes: electrophysiologic basis of a common electrocardiographic diagnosis. J Cardiovasc Electrophysiol. 1992;3:365-93.
13. Coumel P, Attuel P, Flammang D: The role of the conduction system in supraventricular tachycardias. In: Wellens HJJ, Lie H, Janse MJ et al (Eds). The Conduction of the Heart. Lea & Febiger, Philadelphia; 1976. pp. 424-52.
14. Akhtar M, Damato AN, Ruskin JN, Batsford WP, Reddy CP, Ticzon AR, Dhatt MS, Gomes JA, Calon AH. Antegrade and retrograde conduction characteristics in three patterns of paroxysmal atrioventricular junctional reentrant tachycardia. Am Heart J. 1978;95:22-42.
15. Jazayeri MR, Caceres J, Tchou P, Mahmud R, Denker S, Akhtar M. Electrophysiologic characteristics of sudden QRS axis deviation during orthodromic tachycardia. Role of functional fascicular block in localization of accessory pathway. J Clin Invest. 1989;83:952-9.
16. Tchou P, Young P, Mahmud R, Denker S, Jazayeri M, Akhtar M. Useful clinical criteria for the diagnosis of ventricular tachycardia. Am J Med. 1988;84:53-6.
17. Akhtar M, Gilbert C, Al-Nouri M, Denker S. Site of conduction delay during functional block in the His-Purkinje system in man. Circulation. 1980;61:1239-48.
18. Lehmann MH, Denker S, Mahmud R, Addas A, Akhtar M. Linking: a dynamic electrophysiologic phenomenon in macroreentry circuits. Circulation. 1985;71:254-65.
19. Caceres J, Jazayeri M, McKinnie J, Avitall B, Denker ST, Tchou P, Akhtar M. Sustained bundle branch reentry as a mechanism of clinical tachycardia. Circulation. 1989;79:256-70.
20. Blanck Z, Dhala A, Deshpande S, Sra J, Jazayeri M, Akhtar M. Bundle branch reentrant ventricular tachycardia: cumulative experience in 48 patients. J Cardiovasc Electrophysiol. 1993;4: 253-62.
21. Narasimhan C, Jazayeri MR, Sra J, Dhala A, Deshpande S, Biehl M, Akhtar M, Blanck Z. Ventricular tachycardia in valvular heart disease: facilitation of sustained bundle-branch reentry by valve surgery. Circulation. 1997;96:4307-13.
22. Merino JL, Carmona JR, Fernandez-Lozano I, Peinado R, Basterra N, Sobrino JA. Mechanisms of sustained ventricular tachycardia in myotonic dystrophy: implications for catheter ablation. Circulation. 1998;98:541-6.
23. Scherlag BJ, Lau SH, Helfant RH, Berkowitz WD, Stein E, Damato AN. Catheter technique for recording His bundle activity in man. Circulation. 1969;39:13-8.
24. Akhtar M, Gilbert C, Wolf FG, Schmidt DH. Reentry within the His-Purkinje system. Elucidation of reentrant circuit using right bundle branch and His bundle recordings. Circulation. 1978;58:295-304.
25. Lehmann MH, Tchou P, Mahmud R, Denker ST, Akhtar M. Electrophysiological determinants of antidromic reentry induced during atrial extrastimulation. Insights from a pacing model of Wolff-Parkinson-White syndrome. Circ Res. 1989;65:295-306.
26. Akhtar M, Sra. Preexcited Tachycardias: Differential Diagnosis, Mechanisms and Diagnostic Clues. In: Jasbir Sra, Masood Akhtar, Andrea Natale and David Wilber (Eds). Practical Electrophysiology; 2010. pp. 246-57.
27. Denker S, Lehmann M, Mahmud R, Gilbert C, Akhtar M. Effects of alternating cycle lengths on refractoriness of the His-Purkinje system. J Clin Invest. 1984;74:559-70.
28. Lehmann MH, Denker S, Mahmud R, Tchou P, Dongas J, Akhtar M. Electrophysiologic mechanisms of functional bundle branch block at onset of induced orthodromic tachycardia in the Wolff-Parkinson-White syndrome. Role of stimulation method. J Clin Invest. 1985;76:1566-74.
29. Niazi I, Jazayeri M, McKinnie J, Atassi K, Akhtar M. New insights into initiating mechanism of clinical ventricular tachycardia (abstr). Circulation. 1988;78(Suppl II):71.

30. Akhtar M, Jazayeri M, Sra J, Dhala A, et al. Role of Electrical Triggers in the Causation of Sudden Cardiac Death. In: Akhtar, Myerburg, Ruskin (Eds). Sudden Cardiac Death. Williams & Wilkins; 1994. pp. 385-93.
31. Lerman BB, Belardinelli L, West GA, Berne RM, DiMarco JP. Adenosine-sensitive ventricular tachycardia: evidence suggesting cyclic AMP-mediated triggered activity. Circulation. 1986;74:270-80.
32. Belhassen B, Rotmensch HH, Laniado S. Response of recurrent sustained ventricular tachycardia to verapamil. Br Heart J. 1981;46:679-82.
33. Svenson RH, Miller HC, Gallagher JJ, Wallace AG. Electrophysiological evaluation of the Wolff-Parkinson-White syndrome: problems in assessing antegrade and retrograde conduction over the accessory pathway. Circulation. 1975;52:552-62.
34. Tchou P, Lehmann MH, Jazayeri M, Akhtar M. Atriofascicular connection or a nodoventricular Mahaim fiber? Electrophysiologic elucidation of the pathway and associated reentrant circuit. Circulation. 1988;77:837-48.
35. Klein GJ, Guiraudon GM, Kerr CR, Sharma AD, Yee R, Szabo T, Wah JA. "Nodoventricular" accessory pathway: evidence for a distinct accessory atrioventricular pathway with atrioventricular node-like properties. J Am Coll Cardiol. 1988;11:1035-40.
36. Wellens HJJ. The preexcitation syndrome. In: Wellens HJJ, (Ed). Electrical Stimulation of the Heart in the Study and Treatment of Tachycardias. Baltimore, MD: University Park Press; 1971. pp. 97-109.
37. Akhtar M. Ventricular tachycardia. Card Electrophysiol Clin. 2010;2:245-65.
38. Mahaim I, Benatt A. Nouvelles recherches sur les connexions superieures de la branche gauche due faisceau de His-Tarawa avec cloison interventriculaire. Cardiologia. 1937;1: 61-73.
39. Jazayeri M, Akhtar M. Wide QRS Complex Tachycardia: Electrophysiology Mechanisms and electrocardiographic Features. In Cardiac Electrophysiology from Cell to Bedside, 2nd edn. pp. 977-989.
40. Akhtar M, Damato AN, Batsford WP, Ruskin JN, Ogunkelu JB. A comparative analysis of antegrade and retrograde conduction patterns in man. Circulation. 1975;52:766-78.
41. Panotopoulos P, Deshpande S, Akhtar M, Jazayeri MR. Wide QRS complex tachycardia in the presence of preexcitation: a diagnostic challenge. Pacing Clin Electrophysiol. 1997;20: 1716-20.
42. Jazayeri MR, Deshpande S, Dhala A, Blanck Z, Sra J, Akhtar M. Transcatheter mapping and radiofrequency ablation of cardiac arrhythmias. Curr Probl Cardiol. 1994;19:287-395.

EDITORS' SUMMARY

One of the great masters and founders of contemporary electrophysiology, Professor Masood Akhtar, has provided an incredibly insightful review of a commonly perceived as a difficult area in electrocardiography and clinical electrophysiology—wide QRS tachycardia. The readers will find an organized approach to the diagnostic consideration and specific arrhythmias that present as wide QRS tachycardia. In addition, an insightful analysis of the reasons and physiology behind the findings and the diagnostic criteria employed is provided. The student of electrophysiology will enjoy attempting to create a precis of this chapter and employ the main points in his or her practice both in the clinical consultative arena and in the invasive EP laboratory for approaching patients with wide QRS tachycardia.

CHAPTER 45

Venkata A Narla, Nitish Badhwar

Provocative Drug Testing in the Electrophysiology Lab

LIST OF ABBREVIATIONS

ARVC	Arrhythmogenic Right Ventricular Cardiomyopathy	ICD	Implantable Cardioverter-Defibrillator
AV	Atrioventricular	LQTS	Long QT Syndrome
CPVT	Catecholaminergic Polymorphic Ventricular Tachycardia	QTc	Corrected QT interval
ECG	Electrocardiogram	SCD	Sudden Cardiac Death
EP	Electrophysiology	WPW	Wolff-Parkinson-White

INTRODUCTION

Sudden cardiac death (SCD) accounts for approximately 400,000 deaths annually in the United States[1] and is responsible for approximately 50% of the mortality from cardiovascular disease in the US and other developed countries.[2] The majority of SCD is attributable to coronary artery disease and its sequelae, cardiomyopathies, congenital heart disease, and valvular heart disease. However, in 5 to 8% of sudden cardiac deaths, no structural abnormalities are evident.[3] Inherited channelopathies including long-QT syndrome (LQTS), Brugada syndrome, and catecholaminergic polymorphic ventricular tachycardia (CPVT) contribute to this incidence, and often elude detection by a standard 12-lead electrocardiogram (ECG). Individuals with these inherited channelopathies are often young and effective protection against sudden cardiac death can potentially be achieved with an implantable cardioverter-defibrillator (ICD). The typical type 1 ECG pattern of "coved-type" ST-segment elevation in the right precordial leads is often concealed in a significant proportion of patients with Brugada syndrome.[4] Every patient with CPVT has a normal resting ECG. Approximately 40% of patients with LQTS have a normal or borderline normal corrected QT interval (QTc). Provocative drug testing with sodium channel blockers and catecholaminergic agents are critical in unmasking Brugada syndrome, LQTS, and CPVT in a large portion of patients. This chapter will highlight the utility of provocative drug testing in the electrophysiology (EP) lab.

PROVOCATIVE DRUG TESTING IN BRUGADA SYNDROME

In a study of 179 patients with Brugada syndrome, who had undergone repetitive baseline ECGs, only 90 patients had the type 1 pattern on their baseline ECG.[5] Sodium channel blockers can effectively unmask or amplify ST-segment elevation in these patients who may have concealed Brugada syndrome. The sensitivity of provocative drug testing can

99% with a 12-month recurrence of 5%. Success was lowest for ablation of ventricular tachycardia (VT) at 78%; although the number of patients with VT in this study was quite small.[24]

The overall success rates with cryoablation in children are slightly lower than that of radiofrequency ablation. For example, the success rate for cryoablation for all accessory pathways is approximately 85%, though it is as high as 97% for left lateral accessory pathways.[25,26] The recurrence rate of cryoablation at 1 year is comparable with radiofrequency ablation and is around 10 to 12%. In most series, the acute success rate for cryoablation in AVNRT is slightly lower than with radiofrequency ablation (95% versus 98%) but in some reports, the success rate of cryoablation is as high as 97%.[27] As with accessory pathways, the recurrence rate for AVNRT with cryoablation and radiofrequency ablation is similar at around 5%.

COMPLICATIONS

Ablations can be performed in the pediatric population with a low incidence of complications. In addition, there have been no major negative long-term consequences as a result of performing ablations in children with over 20 years of follow-up. However, care must be taken due to the small size of the heart to avoid inadvertent damage to the valves, coronary arteries, or surrounding structures such as the phrenic nerve. The incidence of procedural complications during pediatric ablations is around 3%, with about half of these being hematoma at the catheter entry site. A list of the complications of catheter ablation in pediatric patients and their relative frequencies is listed in **Table 46.1**.

Catheter ablation of cardiac arrhythmias in very small children (≤ 15 kg) especially in infants (< 1 year of age) is controversial as they have been shown to have an increased risk for complications during radiofrequency ablation procedures.[28] However, the success rate of ablation in small children is not significantly different than the success rate in older children.[29] The risk of cryoablation in smaller patients also appears less than what has been reported with radiofrequency ablations.[30] The definitive indications of ablation in pediatric patients weighting over 15 kg are listed in **Table 46.2**.

Table 46.1: Complications of catheter ablation in pediatric patients

Complication	Frequency
Hematoma at catheter site	1.6%
Atrioventricular block	1.3%
Valvular regurgitation	0.6%
Perforation/effusion	0.3%
Embolism/thrombus	0.3%
Death	0.05%

Combined data from: Kugler et al. J Cardiovasc Electrophysiol. 2002;13:336-41 and Van Hare et al. J Cardiovasc Electrophysiol. 2004;15:759-70.

Atrioventricular Block

Outside of procedural mortality, complete AV block is one of the most serious complications that can result from an ablation procedure. As the junctional escape rate with surgical or catheter created AV block is unreliable and can result in long pauses resulting in sudden death, a pacemaker is required if AV block persists past 7 days of the procedure.[31] While studies in adult patients show the risk of complete AV block with radiofrequency ablation to be between 0.1 and 1%, the risk is 1–2% in children.[23] The highest risk for AV block exists during ablation of an accessory pathway in the para-Hisian region. The risk of AV block with radiofrequency ablation in adults in this region is around 2%.[32] In the pediatric registry, the risk is 3% in the midseptal region and 9% if the pathway is truly para-Hisian.[33] AV block has also been reported in other locations in the pediatric population with an incidence of 1% in the right posteroseptal region and 3% in the right anterior/anteroseptal region.[34] AV block has also been reported in right posterior, right lateral, left lateral and left paraseptal regions.[24] The risk of AV block with radiofrequency ablation of AVNRT is 1 to 2%. In pediatric radiofrequency ablation procedures, atrioventricular block

Table 46.2: Definitive indications for ablation in pediatric patients weighing over 15 kg

1. Supraventricular tachycardia that is
   a. Associated with ventricular dysfunction
   b. Recurrent and medications are
      i. Not effective or
      ii. Not tolerated or
      iii. Not desired
   c. Associated with hemodynamic compromise
   d. Prior to cardiac surgery or catheter intervention procedure when access to the arrhythmia substrate will be limited by issues with vascular access after surgery or procedure
2. Wolff-Parkinson-White syndrome
   a. After aborted sudden cardiac death
   b. With syncope and/or with high-risk factors for sudden death
3. Junctional Ectopic Tachycardia that is recurrent, not controlled with medications or associated with ventricular dysfunction
4. Ventricular tachycardia that is recurrent and not controlled with drugs or associated with ventricular dysfunction
5. Ventricular ectopy that is frequent and is associated with marked symptoms and/or ventricular dysfunction

Adapted from Philip SJ et al. PACES/HRS expert consensus statement on the use of catheter ablation in children and patients with congenital heart disease: Developed in partnership with the Pediatric and Congenital Electrophysiology Society (PACES) and the Heart Rhythm Society (HRS). Endorsed by the governing bodies of PACES, HRS, the American Academy of Pediatrics (AAP), the American Heart Association (AHA), and the Association for European Pediatric and Congenital Cardiology (AEPC). Heart Rhythm. 2016;13:e251-89.

has been seen from 5 seconds to 2 months (mean, 4.1 days; median, 15 seconds) after the onset of the energy application and may be permanent or transient lasting 1 hour to 1 month.[34]

The major advantage of using cryoablation in pediatric population is the decreased incidence of complete AV block. As most patients with supraventricular tachycardia have no other structural or functional limitations, the potential need for a pacemaker and subsequent follow-up as well as lead and generator replacement for multiple decades makes the additional safety of cryoablation desirable. To date, there has not been a reported case of permanent AV block using cryoablation if energy application is terminated immediately after an untoward effect on the AV node is seen. However, prolonged PR interval and bundle branch block have been reported in pediatric patients with cryoablation.[35]

Radiation Exposure

Despite the proven safety of catheter ablation in the pediatric population, fluoroscopy exposure during these procedures has been an emerging concern. Although, the amount of radiation from fluoroscopy is comparable to that in a computed tomography (CT) scan, there is still some concerns in developing children about exposure to ionizing radiation. The increased lifetime risk of fatal malignancy is around 0.02% per single radiofrequency ablation procedure.[36] Although this risk is low, it is advisable to limit the amount of radiation exposure as far as possible. The As Low As Reasonably Achievable (or ALARA) principle for radiation exposure is particularly important in the pediatric population. With newer 3-dimensional computer mapping systems, where anatomic model of heart chambers is created through magnetic or impedance-based measures from the mapping catheters, it is possible to perform ablation in pediatric patients with limited or negligible radiation exposure.[37] These systems have particular utility in the pediatric population and the success and complication rates are similar to fluoroscopic-based cases.

CONCLUSION

Ablations can be performed safely and effectively in the pediatric population with the potential for a permanent cure as in adults. There are special considerations that should be given due importance before and during these procedures in the pediatric patients with respect to the age and weight of the patient, mechanism of the arrhythmia, underlying structural heart disease, ablation techniques, equipment, and laboratory set-up in order to increase the success and prevent complications.

REFERENCES

1. Kugler JD, Danford DA, Houston K, Felix G. Radiofrequency catheter ablation for paroxysmal supraventricular tachycardia in children and adolescents without structural heart disease. Am J Cardiol. 1997;80:1438-43.
2. Schaffer MS, Gow RM, Moak JP, Saul JP. Mortality following radiofrequency catheter ablation (from the pediatric radiofrequency ablation registry). Am J Cardiol. 2000;86(6):639-43.
3. Garson A, Gillette PC. Electrophysiologic studies of supraventricular tachycardia in children. II. Prediction of specific mechanism by noninvasive features. Am Heart J. 1981;102: 383-8.
4. Roggen A, Pavlovic M, Pfammatter JP. Frequency of spontaneous ventricular tachycardia in a pediatric population. Am J Cardiol. 2008;101:852-4.
5. Benson DW, Smith WM, Dunnigan A, Sterba R, Gallagher JJ. Mechanism of regular, wide QRS tachycardia in infants and children. Am J Cardiol. 1982;49:1776-88.
6. Dicinson DF, Scott O. Ambulatory electrocardiographic monitoring in 100 healthy teenage boys. Br Heart J. 1984;51: 179-83.
7. Ko KJ, Deal BJ, Strasburger JF, Benson DW. Supraventricular tachycardia mechanisms and their age distribution in pediatric patients. Am J Cardiol. 1992;69:1028-32.
8. Porter MJ, Morton JB, Denman R, Lin AC, Tierney S, Santucci PA, Cai JJ, Madsen N, Wilber DJ. Influence of age and gender on the mechanism of supraventricular tachycardia. Heart Rhythm. 2004;4:393-6.
9. Benson DW, Dunnigan A, Benditt DG. Follow-up evaluation of infant paroxysmal atrial tachycardia: transesophageal study. Circulation. 1987;75:542-9.
10. Blaufox AD, Warsy I, D'Souza M, Kanter R. Transesophageal electrophysiology evaluation of children with a history of supraventricular tachycardia in infancy. Pediatr Cardiol. 2011;32:1110-4.
11. Bauersfeld U, Gow RM, Hamilton RM, Izukawa T. Treatment of atrial ectopic tachycardia in infants < 6 months old. Am Heart J. 1995;129:1145-8.
12. Kang KT, Etheridge SP, Kantoch MJ, Tisma-Dupanovic S, Bradley DJ, Balaji S, Hamilton RM, Singh AK, Cannon BC, Schaffer MS, Potts JE, Sanatani S. Current management of focal atrial tachycardia in children: A multicenter experience. Circ Arrhythm Electrophysiol. 2014;7:664-70.
13. Deal BJ, Keane JF, Gillette PC, Garson A Jr. Wolff-Parkinson-White syndrome and supraventricular tachycardia during infancy: management and follow-up. J Am Coll Cardiol. 1985;5:130-5.
14. Tortoriello TA, Snyder CS, Smith EO, Fenrich AL, Jr., Friedman RA, Kertesz NJ. Frequency of recurrence among infants with supraventricular tachycardia and comparison of recurrence rates among those with and without preexcitation and among those with and without response to digoxin and/or propranolol therapy. Am J Cardiol. 2003;92:1045-9.
15. Perry JC, Garson A. Supraventricular tachycardia due to Wolff-Parkinson-White syndrome in children: Early disappearance and late recurrence. J Am Cardiol. 1990;16:1215-20.
16. Erb TO, Hall JM, Ing RJ, Kanter RJ, Kern FH, Schulman SR, Gan TJ. Postoperative nausea and vomiting in children and adolescents undergoing radiofrequency catheter ablation: A randomized comparison of propofol- and isoflurane-based anesthetics. Anesth Analg. 2002;95:1577-81.
17. Triedman JK, Alexander ME, Love BA, Collins KK, Berul CI, Bevilacqua LM, Walsh EP. Influence of patient factors in ablative technologies on outcomes of radiofrequency ablation

of intra-atrial re-entrant tachycardia in patients with congenital heart disease. J Am Coll Cardiol. 2002;39:1827-35.
18. Miyake CY, Mah DY, Atallah J, Oikle HP, Melgar ML, Alexander ME, Berul CI, Cecchin F, Walsh EP, Triedman JK. Nonfluoroscopic imaging systems reduce radiation exposure in children undergoing ablation of supraventricular tachycardia. Heart Rhythm. 2011;8:519-25.
19. Papagiannis J, Avramidis D, Alexopoulos C, Kirvassilis G. Radiofrequency ablation of accessory pathways in children and congenital heart disease patients: Impact of nonfluoroscopic navigation system. Pacing Clin Electrophysiol. 2011;34:1288-96.
20. Moore JP, Patel PA, Shannon KM, Albers EL, Salerno JC, Stein MA, Stephenson EA, Mohan S, Shah MJ, Asakai H, et al. Predictors of myocardial recovery in pediatric tachycardia-induced cardiomyopathy. Heart Rhythm. 2014;11:1163-9.
21. Zimmerman FJ, Pahl E, Rocchini AP, et al. High incidence of incessant supraventricular tachycardia in pediatric patients referred for cardiac transplantation (Abstract). Pacing and Clin Electrophysiol. 1996;19:663.
22. Silva JN, Erickson CC, Carter CD, Greene EA, Kantoch M, Collins KK, Miyake CY, Carboni MP, Rhee EK, Papez A, Anand V, Bowman TM, Van Hare GF. Participating Members of Pediatric and Congenital Electrophysiology Society (PACES). Management of pediatric tachyarrhythmias on mechanical support. Circ Arrhythm Electrophysiol. 2014;7:658-63.
23. Van Hare GF, Javitz H, Carmelli D, Saul JP, Tanel RE, Fischbach PS, Kanter RJ, Schaffer M, Dunnigan A, Colan S, Serwer G. Prospective assessment after pediatric cardiac ablation: Demographics, medical profiles, and initial outcomes. J Cardiovasc Electrophysiol. 2004;15:759-70.
24. Van Hare GF, Javitz H, Carmelli D, Saul JP, Tanel RE, Fischbach PS, Kanter RJ, Schaffer M, Dunnigan A, Colan S, Serwer G. Prospective assessment after pediatric cardiac ablation: Recurrence at 1 year after initially successful ablation of supraventricular tachycardia. Heart Rhythm. 2004;1:188-96.
25. Gist KM, Bockoven JR, Lane J, Smith G, Clark JM. Acute success of cryoablation of left-sided accessory pathways: a single institution study. J Cardiovasc Electrophysiol. 2009;20:637-42.
26. Papez AL, Al-Ahdab M, Dick M II, Fischbach PS. Transcatheter cryotherapy for the treatment of supraventricular tachyarrhythmias in children: a single center experience. J Interv Card Electrophysiol. 2006;15:191-6.
27. Avari JN, Jay KS, Rhee EK. Experience and results during transition from radiofrequency ablation to cryoablation for treatment of pediatric atrioventricular nodal reentrant tachycardia. Pacing Clin Electrophysiol. 2008;31:454-60.
28. Aiyagari R, Saarel EV, Etheridge SP, Bradley DJ, Dick M, 2nd, Fischbach PS. Radiofrequency ablation for supraventricular tachycardia in children < or =15 kg is safe and effective. Pediatr Cardiol. 2005;26:622-6.
29. Blaufox AD, Felix GL, Saul JP, Pediatric Catheter Ablation R. Radiofrequency catheter ablation in infants </=18 months old: When is it done and how do they fare?: Short-term data from the pediatric ablation registry. Circulation. 2001;104:2803-8.
30. LaPage MJ, Reed JH, Collins KK, Law IH, Pilcher TA, Tanel RE, Anderson CC, Young ML, Emmel M, Paul T, Blaufox AD, Arora G, Saul JP. Safety and results of cryoablation in patients <5 years old and/or <15 kilograms. Am J Cardiol. 2011;108:565-71.
31. Epstein AE, Dimarco JP, Ellenbogen KA, Estes NA 3rd, Freedman RA, Gettes LS, Gillinov AM, Gregoratos G, Hammill SC, Hayes DL, Hlatky MA, Newby LK, Page L, Schoenfeld MH, Silka MJ, Stevenson LW, Sweeney MO; American College of Cardiology; American Heart Association Task Force on Practice Guidelines; American Association for Thoracic Surgery; Society of Thoracic Surgeons. ACC/AHA/HRS 2008 Guidelines for device-based therapy of cardiac rhythm abnormalities. Heart Rhythm. 2008;5:e1-62.
32. Brugada J, Puigfel M, Mont L, García-Bolao I, Figueiredo M, Matas M, Navarro-López F. Radiofrequency ablation of anteroseptal, para-Hisian, and mid-septal accessory pathways using a simplified femoral approach. Pacing Clin Electrophysiol. 1998;21:735-41.
33. Mandapati R, Berul CI, Triedman JK, Alexander ME, Walsh EP. Radiofrequency catheter ablation of septal accessory pathways in the pediatric age group. Am J Cardiol. 2003;92:947-50.
34. Schaffer MS, Silka MJ, Ross BA, Kugler JD. Inadvertent atrioventricular block during radiofrequency catheter ablation. Results of the Pediatric Radiofrequency Ablation Registry. Pediatric Electrophysiology Society. Circulation. 1996;94:3214-20.
35. Bar-Cohen Y, Cecchin F, Alexander ME, Berul CI, Triedman JK, Walsh EP. Cryoablation for accessory pathways located near normal conduction tissues or within the coronary venous system in children and young adults. Heart Rhythm. 2006;3:253-8.
36. Clay MA, Campbell RM, Strieper M, Frias PA, Stevens M, Mahle WT. Long-term risk of fatal malignancy following pediatric radiofrequency ablation. Am J Cardiol. 2008;102:913-5.
37. Von Bergen NH, Bansal S, Gingerich J, Law IH. Nonfluoroscopic and radiation-limited ablation of ventricular arrhythmias in children and young adults: a case series. Pediatr Cardiol. 2011;32:743-7.

EDITORS' SUMMARY

Drs Wackel and Cannon highlight the unique features of catheter ablation in children in this chapter. Rather than reiterating the clinical features and ablation approach for each of the various arrhythmias (which are covered elsewhere in this textbook), they outline the differences in our diagnostic approach, avoidance of complications, and maximizing success when ablating in children. The authors also summarize the specific value and need for cryoablation and minimizing radiation exposure in the pediatric population.

CHAPTER 47

Tahmeed Contractor, Roderick Tung,
Noel G Boyle, Kalyanam Shivkumar

Epicardial Ablation: Techniques and Applications

LIST OF ABBREVIATIONS

CS	Coronary Sinus	RV	Right Ventricle
LAA	Left Atrial Appendage	VT	Ventricular Tachycardia
LV	Left Ventricle		

INTRODUCTION

Cardiac arrhythmias, both atrial and ventricular, can often originate from subepicardial myocardial fibers.[1] Endocardial ablation in such cases may not be successful. Very limited aspects of the epicardial surface of the heart can be accessed through the coronary sinus and great cardiac veins.[2] In 1996, Sosa and colleagues described the method of percutaneous epicardial access into a dry pericardial space that provided extensive access to the epicardial surface for mapping and ablation.[3] Since then, this technique has been used worldwide for ablation of ventricular and even atrial tachyarrhythmias.[4]

The purpose of this chapter is to discuss the indications and techniques of epicardial access and ablation.

INDICATIONS FOR EPICARDIAL ACCESS AND ABLATION

Ventricular Arrhythmias

In patients presenting for ventricular tachycardia (VT) ablation, several clinical features, imaging studies, electrocardiographic characteristics and prior procedural findings can suggest the need for epicardial access and ablation. Patients with sustained VT due to nonischemic causes such as dilated cardiomyopathy[5] (excluding bundle branch reentry VT), arrhythmogenic right ventricular dysplasia/cardiomyopathy,[6] hypertrophic cardiomyopathy,[7] and Chagas disease[8] have a higher probability of requiring epicardial ablation due to the presence of subepicardial scar **(Figures 47.1A and B)**.[9] On the other hand, the scar of ischemic cardiomyopathy is predominantly subendocardial with variable epicardial sparing depending on the duration of coronary occlusion. Irrespective of etiology, subepicardial late gadolinium enhancement on cardiac MRI indicates an epicardial substrate and may necessitate epicardial ablation.[10]

There are several electrocardiographic features that suggest an epicardial exit of VT. These include a *pseudodelta* wave duration of more than 34 ms, QRS complex duration of more than 200 ms, delayed intrinsicoid deflection of more than 85 ms, and RS complex duration of more than 121 ms.[11] However, conduction delay due to cardiomyopathy or antiarrhythmic drugs and fusion of T-wave with the QRS complex can decrease the diagnostic specificity of these criteria.[12] Idiopathic VTs may also need epicardial access

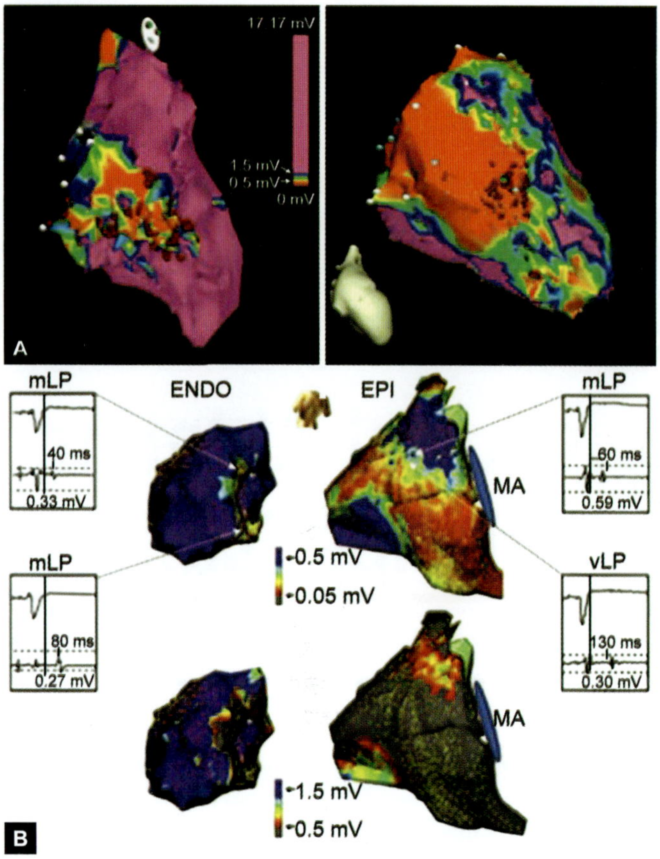

Figures 47.1A and B: (A) Electroanatomic map of a patient with arrhythmogenic right ventricular (RV) cardiomyopathy reveals more extensive epicardial scar (right anterior oblique caudal view). The *red circles* indicate ablation lesions and the termination of VT was achieved at the *green circle*; (B) Electroanatomic substrate mapping of a patient with nonischemic cardiomyopathy (NICM) reveals extensive epicardial scar in relation to endocardial scar. Multiple late potentials are seen within the low-voltage regions

Abbreviations: mLP, Moderate late potential; vLP, very late potential; ENDO, endocardial map; EPI, epicardial map; MA, mitral annulus

From: Nakahara S, Tung R, Ramirez RJ, et al. Characterization of the arrhythmogenic substrate in ischemic and nonischemic cardiomyopathy implications for catheter ablation of hemodynamically unstable ventricular tachycardia. J Am Coll Cardiol. 2010;55: 2355-65 with permission

when regular mapping of the outflow tracts, aortic cusps and the coronary sinus as well as its branches do not show any early local electrograms. Prior failed endocardial VT ablations with absence of early activation sites during VT or poor pace-mapped sites endocardially suggest an epicardial exit for VT. A proposed algorithm for selecting patients requiring epicardial ablation is depicted in **Figure 47.2.**[4]

Atrial Fibrillation

Since the initial description by Haissaguerre and colleagues,[13] endocardial pulmonary vein isolation has emerged as an effective strategy to decrease the burden of paroxysmal and persistent atrial fibrillation. However, in 20% of patients, epicardial connections between the pulmonary veins and left atrium can occur that may result in residual pulmonary vein-left atrial connection despite endocardial pulmonary vein isolation.[14] Epicardial access and ablation may be required in these patients. Additionally, epicardial access will lead to more effective ablation of left atrial ganglionated plexi which may play an important role in the pathogenesis of atrial fibrillation.[15] However, the value of epicardial ablation for atrial fibrillation needs to better defined in randomized studies.

Epicardial access also improves the safety of endocardial ablation by avoiding collateral damage to vital structures surrounding the left atrium. The esophagus lies in very close proximity to the posterior wall of the left atrium and pulmonary veins. We routinely visualize esophageal position (after barium is injected through the nasogastric tube) and not infrequently, the pulmonary veins lie in close proximity to the esophagus limiting adequate ablation. Additionally, the right phrenic nerve runs in close proximity to the right superior pulmonary vein and high output pacing can be used to localize its course. Proximity of the phrenic nerve to the antrum can also limit effective isolation of the right-sided pulmonary veins. In such situations at our institution, a Meditech balloon catheter (Meditech, Boston Scientific, Minneapolis, MN) has been inserted in the pericardial space to displace the esophagus or the phrenic nerve allowing safer endocardial ablation.[16,17]

Supraventricular Tachycardia

Ablation of supraventricular tachycardias rarely requires epicardial mapping and ablation. Accessory pathways are sometimes not effectively ablated endocardially; and epicardial ablation is required in such cases.[18] As mentioned previously, the right phrenic nerve courses near the anterolateral superior vena cava and right atrium. Rarely, patients with right atrial tachycardias emanating near the crista terminalis cannot be ablated due to phrenic nerve proximity.[19] Intrapericardial balloon protection of the phrenic nerve can then allow ablation to be safely performed in such situations.

Left Atrial Appendage Ligation

The left atrial appendage (LAA) has been implicated as the culprit for the origin of thrombus in nonvalvular atrial fibrillation.[20] In patients who cannot tolerate anticoagulants due to bleeding risk or noncompliance, LAA ligation/exclusion is an alternative option. One of the methods to achieve this is using the LARIAT LAA suture device (LARIAT®, SentreHEART, Redwood City, CA) which requires an anterior epicardial access.[21] The atrial appendage is then occluded by applying a knot ('lariat') around the base, in the epicardial space.

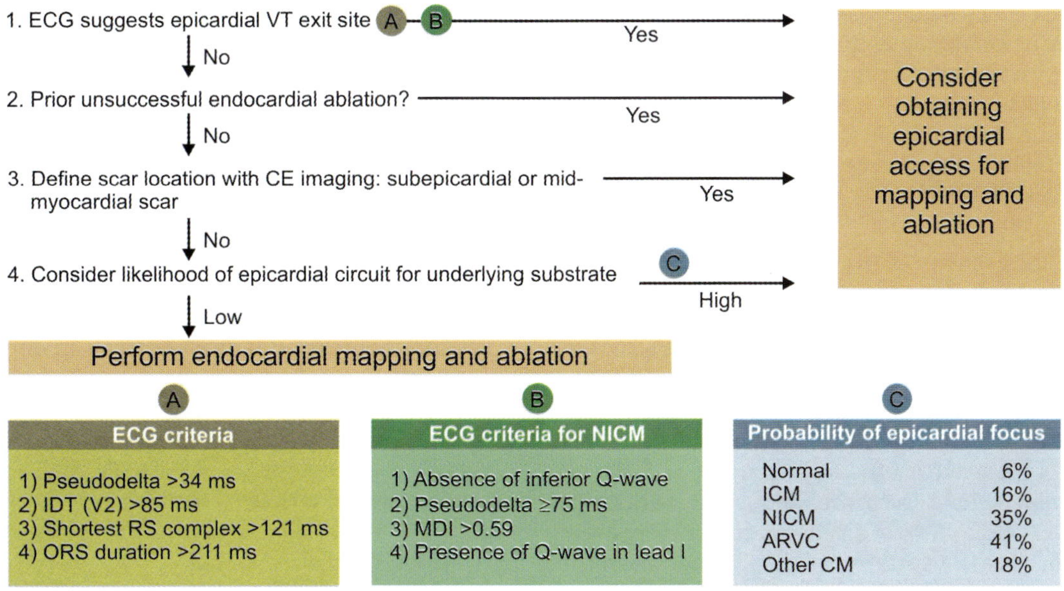

Figure 47.2: Proposed algorithm for selecting patients requiring epicardial access during ventricular tachycardia ablation
Abbreviations: ARVC, arrhythmogenic right ventricular cardiomyopathy; CE, contrast enhanced; CM, cardiomyopathy; ECG, electrocardiogram; ICM, ischemic cardiomyopathy; IDT, intrinsicoid deflection time; MDI, maximum deflection index; NICM, nonischemic cardiomyopathy; VT, ventricular tachycardia
From: Boyle N, Shivkumar K. Epicardial interventions in electrophysiology. Circulation. 2012;126:1752-69. With permission

TECHNIQUE OF EPICARDIAL ACCESS

Pericardial Anatomy

The pericardium is a self-enclosed sac that consists of two main layers—the serous and fibrous layers.[22] The serous layer consists of two sublayers—the serous visceral layer (on the epicardial side) and the serous parietal layer (on the fibrous pericardium side). Between these two layers is the pericardial space that contains ~50 mL of fluid. In a supine patient, this fluid accumulation occurs anteriorly and hence the 'best' potential space is anteriorly located. The goal of epicardial access is to enter this space without damage to the structures before (liver, colon or stomach) and beyond (right ventricle).

Preprocedural Planning

It is essential to review the patient's history and perform physical examination prior to the procedure. Occasionally, prior pericarditis or percutaneous epicardial access, and almost always prior cardiac surgery, will result in pericardial adhesions. It is critical to be aware of use of anticoagulants or antiplatelet agents. Abdominal examination and imaging studies may reveal musculoskeletal deformities (kyphoscoliosis, pectus) or abdominal organs in the trajectory of the epicardial access needle (anterior hiatal hernia, hepatomegaly, colonic dilation), and these are potential contraindications to this approach. These can result in inadvertent liver, colon or stomach damage prior to entering the pericardial space.

The presence of adhesions in the pericardium can make subxiphoid access extremely difficult. This can be sometimes revealed on MRI, but is mostly expected in patients with prior cardiac surgery. Basal adhesions are seen in patients with valve surgeries; adhesions are located in the anterior and midventricular regions after coronary artery bypass grafting. While the sheath can be used to break these adhesions during mapping and ablation, there is significant limitation to safe catheter manipulation in the pericardial space. In such patients, it is routine for us to collaborate with the cardiothoracic surgery team who can create a surgical pericardial window and later close the window at the end of ablation procedure. It should be ensured that anticoagulants and antiplatelet agents are stopped prior to epicardial access. We routinely obtain epicardial access prior to systemic heparinization that is required for left sided endocardial mapping and ablation.

Correlating the likely area of epicardial ablation with the coronary anatomy (from prior cardiac catheterizations, MRI or CT angiographic images) can help anticipate possible coronary damage during ablation. Angiography is usually done prior to ablation to ensure a safe distance from the coronary arteries (1 cm). Inadvertent ventricular perforation and pericardial bleeding are life-threatening complications and it is essential to have cardiac surgical team back-up available. Antibiotics (cefazolin or vancomycin) are administered prior to access to reduce the risk of bacterial pericarditis.

General anesthesia is usually preferred for epicardial access to reduce patient mobility and regulate respiration.

However, this has to be balanced against the disadvantage of noninducibility of automatic and triggered arrhythmias due to general anesthesia and needs to be individualized to the electrophysiological substrate.

The technique of epicardial ablation is relatively safe, especially in high volume centers, when performed by experienced operators.[23,24]

Epicardial Access and Ablation: Step-by-step

While this procedure can be done safely in different ways,[25,26] it is important for the operator to be mindful of the guiding principles that are outlined below in our step-by-step approach for epicardial access. Commonly, a 17-G curved tip Tuohy epidural needle is used to gain access as it directs the guidewire tangential to the myocardium once pericardial access is gained. Alternatively, a micropuncture needle set can be used for access, which is potentially safer given the fine tipped needle and the microguidewire. The feasibility of using a micropuncture needle has been tested in animals[27] and the safety of this technique has also been reported in humans.[28]

- *Landmarks:* Reviewing imaging studies prior to ablation helps the operator plan the location of needle entry in the skin and the trajectory of advancement to reach the pericardial space. The coronary sinus (CS) catheter and the right ventricular (RV) catheter (or the implantable cardioverter defibrillator lead in the RV) can be used as landmarks for the lateral border of the heart and the RV apex, respectively. Colonic and gastric dilation should be excluded on fluoroscopy. The subxiphoid area is explored for an area to introduce the needle and exclude hepatic enlargement. The puncture is performed one finger-breadth left of the subxiphoid process, allowing for access through the avascular Larrey's space (trigonum sternocostale).[29]
- *Skin preparation:* Lidocaine is infused for local anesthesia and a small incision is made on the skin to avoid skin resistance when introducing the Tuohy needle.
- *Advancing the needle:* The Tuohy needle is introduced through the incision with an initial shallow course towards the left shoulder (to avoid the liver). The trajectory of advancement depends on whether an anterior or posterior pericardial puncture is desired. In general, an anterior puncture has a lower likelihood of blood vessel injury. If an anterior puncture is desired, the needle is continued along a shallow course so that the needle tracks just posterior to the sternum on the steep lateral view. Conversely, if a posterior access is required, the needle should track more steeply (>45° angle to skin).
- *Just before access:* The needle is progressively and slowly advanced until the cardiac pulsations can be felt at the needle. Contrast injected at this point will reveal tenting of the fibrous pericardium **(Figures 47.3A and B)**.
- *Gaining access:* When the tip crosses the pericardial space, a popping sensation is felt; the needle must be carefully controlled at this point, and usually withdrawn slightly to avoid puncturing the right ventricle, while maintaining access to the pericardial space. Contrast can be injected to ensure the needle tip is in the pericardial space. A guidewire is then introduced through the needle and it should follow the left border of the heart in the left anterior oblique view, which confirms an intrapericardial location

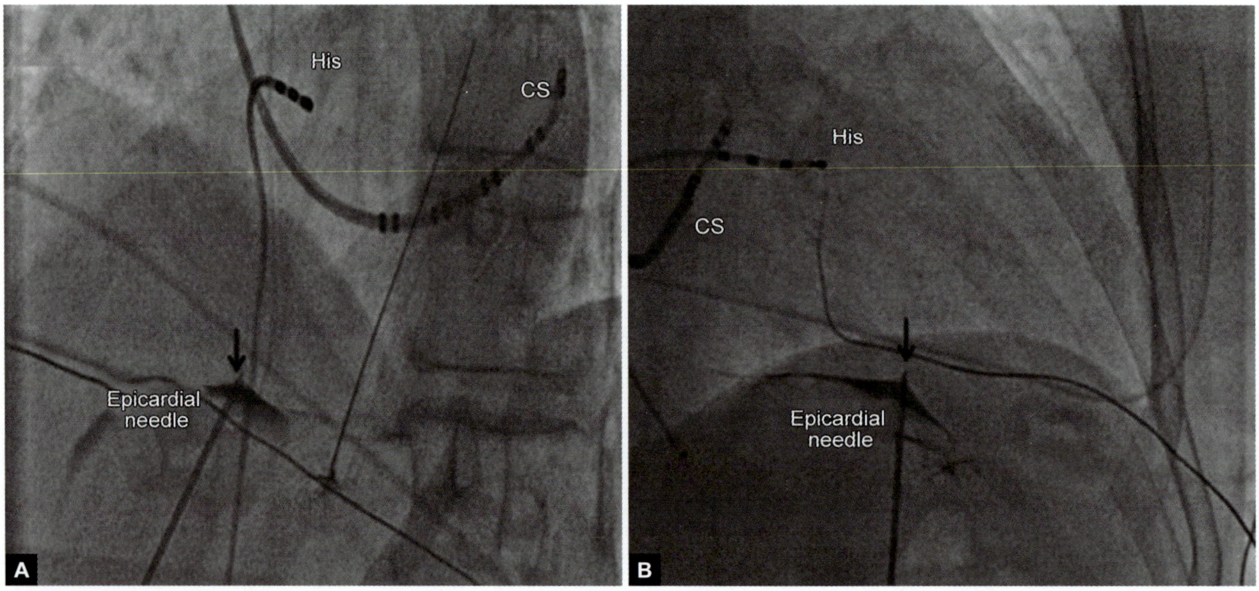

Figures 47.3A and B: Left anterior oblique (A) and right anterior oblique (B) views revealing tenting of pericardium just prior to access (arrows)
Abbreviation: CS, coronary sinus

(Figures 47.4A and B). Careful attention should be given to movement of the wire in the pericardial space. Lack of free movement could signify presence of wire in the RV, 'double puncture' of the RV with exit into the pericardial space, pericardial adhesions or presence of the wire in a pericardial sinus/recess. When in doubt, the wire should be withdrawn back to the needle, which is then adjusted. The wire can be then readvanced until the operator is comfortable about the location of the wire.

- *'Pericardiogram':* After confirming the presence of the wire in the pericardial space, a soft 5 Fr regular sheath is introduced and contrast in injected to confirm presence of the sheath in the pericardial space. The contrast will outline the pericardial space and the roots of the great vessel, and may show the location of adhesions **(Figures 47.5A and B)**. This sheath can be exchanged for longer or deflectable sheaths for better stability as well as increasing operator distance from fluoroscopy cameras. We also routinely double wire and retain an extrawire in the pericardial space in the event that access via the sheath is lost **(Figure 47.6)**.
- *Mapping and ablation:* The principles of epicardial mapping and ablation are similar to that in the endocardium, with a few notable exceptions. It is important to mark the atrioventricular and interventricular grooves during mapping where major vessels run. Ablation should be avoided in these grooves. We routinely use open irrigated catheters for epicardial ablation. Due to the lack of blood flow, there is less cooling as compared to that during endocardial ablation resulting in higher temperatures and larger lesion sizes.[30] The optimal power settings of epicardial ablation have not been well defined. We start with a power of 30 Watts and up-titrate to 50 Watts as required, carefully monitoring impedance and temperature changes; similar settings have been used in different series.[9,23,24] Aspiration every five minutes, or with any decrease in blood pressure, is recommended as the saline used for irrigation accumulates in the pericardial space resulting in ineffective ablation. If there is concern of being close to the coronary arteries or phrenic nerve, coronary angiography or high output pacing should be performed prior to ablation.
- *Exiting the pericardial space:* After epicardial mapping and ablation, the pericardial space is aspirated again to check for bleeding. We routinely inject steroids in the pericardial space (125–250 mg of methylprednisolone) postablation to prevent inflammatory pericarditis, which may result in significant pain as well as adhesion formation impeding future pericardial access. If there is bleeding, the catheter can be exchanged for a soft pigtail catheter, which is kept in place for 24 hours after which the system is finally removed if the bleeding has resolved.

COMPLICATIONS

RV Puncture

RV puncture can occur in up to 20% of cases.[9] The key to prevention of significant consequences from this is early recognition of the wire location, and to avoid advancing the sheath. After access, if it is discovered that the guidewire

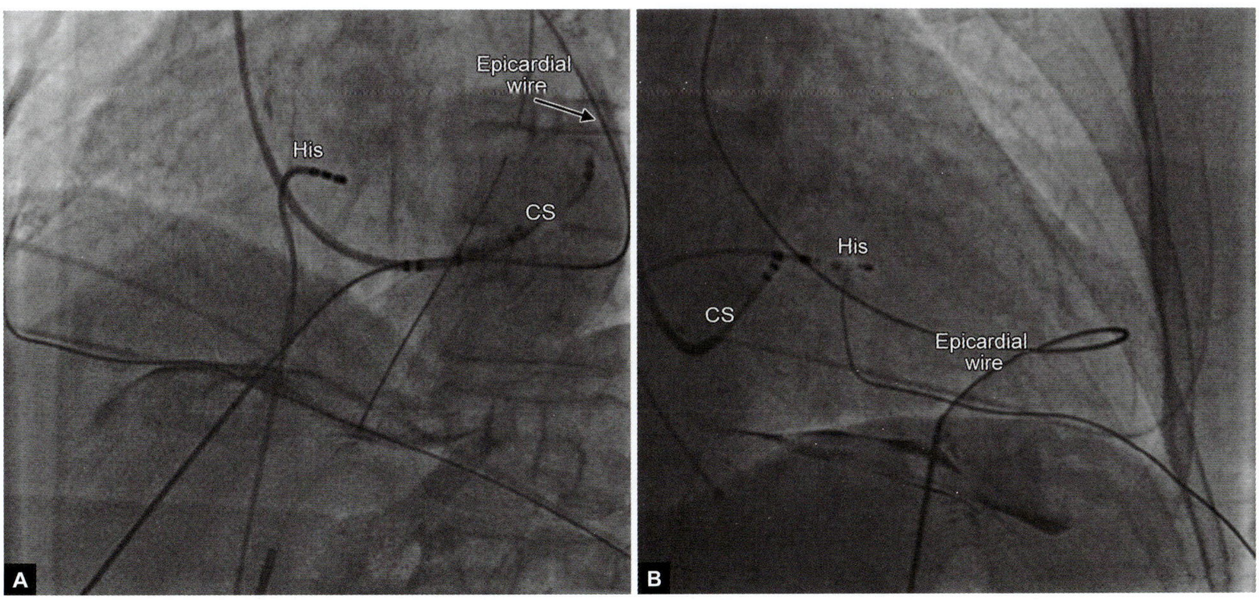

Figures 47.4A and B: Left anterior oblique (A) and right anterior oblique (B) views showing a wire in pericardial space traversing the lateral border of the heart in LAO view (arrow)
Abbreviation: CS, coronary sinus

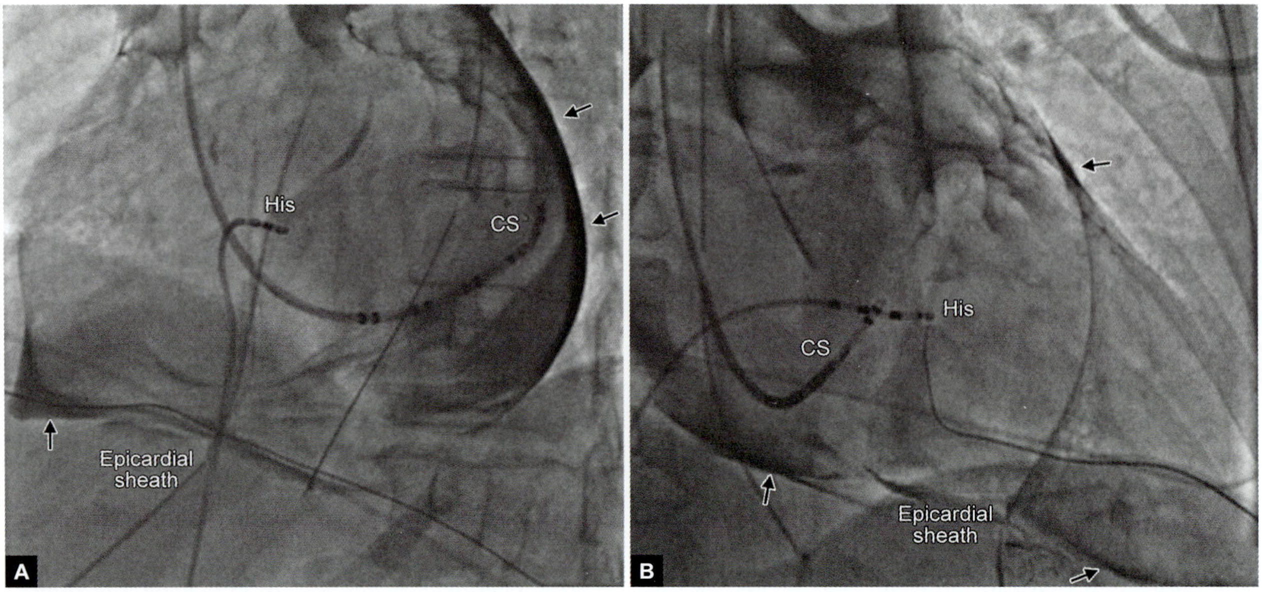

Figures 47.5A and B: Left anterior oblique (A) and right anterior oblique (B) views showing contrast in the pericardial space (arrows)
Abbreviation: CS, coronary sinus

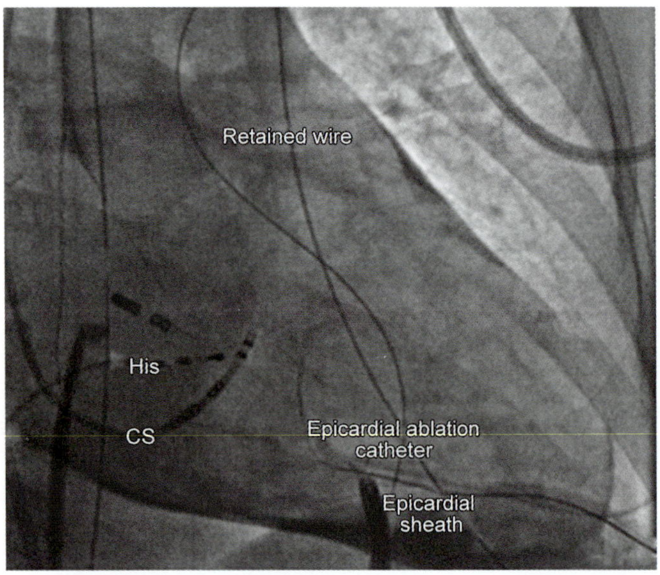

Figure 47.6: Right anterior oblique view showing ablation catheter and a retained wire in the pericardial space
Abbreviation: CS, coronary sinus

is in the RV, this can be pulled back until the pericardial space is reached and then readvanced. This may result in mild bleeding that generally stops with time. If the sheath is advanced into the RV, bleeding can be more profound after sheath removal, and surgical repair is usually required. Before removing the sheath from the RV, it is important to have another sheath in the pericardial space and to have the surgical team on stand-by if another sheath cannot be inserted.[26]

Pericardial Bleeding

A small amount of bleeding (<100 mL) is not uncommon with pericardial access and generally resolves in <30 minutes. Copious bleeding lasting for greater than one hour is very concerning and can be secondary to RV puncture or damage of an epicardial vessel.[26] In such circumstances, open heart surgery is generally required to repair the ventricle or artery. The operator should also be aware of the possibility of RV double puncture when there is no bleeding during mapping and ablation, but significant hemopericardium develops after the sheath is removed.[31] We routinely leave a wire in the pericardial space after removal of all the pericardial sheaths until all the other vascular sheaths are removed and the patient is almost ready to be transported out of the laboratory.

Other Complications

Collateral damage to surrounding structures can occur while gaining access and during mapping as well as ablation. In addition, a third of patients can experience symptoms of pericarditis. **Table 47.1** lists the possible complications and how these can be avoided. **Table 47.2** highlights important precautions that the operator must always remember during this procedure.

Table 47.1: Important complications of epicardial access and ablation

Possible complications	*Measures to avoid occurrence*	*Special comments*
Right ventricle puncture	Meticulous attention to detail and proper technique while gaining access; ensuring the guidewire tracks along the cardiac border in the LAO view; do NOT advance a sheath until certain of wire position	Insertion of sheath into the right ventricle can lead to significant bleeding after sheath removal-surgical team should be on standby if another sheath cannot be inserted into the pericardial space
Bleeding	Meticulous attention to detail and proper technique to avoid RV puncture and staying away from the atrioventricular/interventricular groove while gaining access	Copious bleeding (>100 mL) lasting for more than 1 hour is concerning for RV puncture or blood vessel damage requiring open heart surgery for repair
Liver, colon, stomach, epigastric artery or diaphragm damage while gaining access	Physical examination and review of imaging studies prior to puncture to identify hepatomegaly, anterior hiatal hernias and colonic dilation	Hypotension in the absence of pericardial bleeding should alert the operator for possibility of intra-abdominal hemorrhage
Coronary artery damage	Coronary angiogram prior to ablation (ensure ablation catheter distance of at least 1 cm from coronary artery)	Intracoronary cold saline during ablation resulted in lower intracoronary temperatures in animal models[32]
Phrenic nerve (left)	High output pacing prior to ablation on the LV free wall; Ensure the patient is not on paralytics/skeletal muscle relaxants prior to pacing	Epicardial balloon displacement of the phrenic nerve can be performed if ablation is required in an area of phrenic nerve capture
Pericarditis	Antibiotics prior to epicardial access; Intrapericardial steroids at the end of the procedure may be helpful	If patients have symptoms of pericarditis postprocedure, a short course of dual anti-inflammatory agents (colchicine and NSAIDs) can be used

Abbreviations: LAO, left anterior oblique; NSAID, non-steroidal anti-inflammatory drug; RV, right ventrilce

Table 47.2: Important precautions during epicardial access and ablation

During access
- Confirm free movement of wire in the pericardial space in the LAO view prior to insertion of sheath
- If a sheath is inadvertently placed in the right ventricle, insert another wire into the pericardium and have cardiac surgery on standby prior to removal of the sheath
- Maintain an additional guidewire in the pericardial space during the procedure in the event that access via the sheath is lost

During ablation
- Consider coronary angiography or high output pacing to ensure safe distance from coronary arteries and phrenic nerve respectively prior to ablation in areas of concern
- Aspiration every five minutes is required if open-irrigation ablation catheters are being used, or if blood pressure decreases
- Do not leave a 'bare' sheath in the pericardial space; insert a placeholder catheter through the sheath if the ablation catheter is removed (such as a Berman angiographic catheter)
- Unexplained hypotension during the procedure without hemopericardium should raise the concern for intra-abdominal hemorrhage

After ablation
- Beware of RV double puncture; hemopericardium may develop only after sheath removal
- Retain a guidewire in the pericardial space for 20 minutes after the pericardial sheaths are removed

Abbreviations: LAO, left anterior oblique; RV, right ventrilce

CONCLUSION

Epicardial access and ablation has emerged as an important tool in the treatment options for ventricular and occasionally supraventricular arrhythmias. There are several clinical, electrocardiographic and imaging tools that can suggest the need for epicardial ablation in patients with VT. While the technique is generally safe in high-volume centers, surgical back-up is strongly recommended in the event of inadvertent RV puncture and bleeding. The operator should be aware of the possibility of collateral damage to surrounding structures during epicardial ablation as well as techniques to prevent the same.

REFERENCES

1. Brugada J, Berruezo A, Cuesta A, Osca J, Chueca E, Fosch X, Wayar L, Mont L. Nonsurgical transthoracic epicardial radiofrequency ablation: an alternative in incessant ventricular tachycardia. J Am Coll Cardiol. 2003;41:2036-43.
2. Daniels DV, Lu Y-Y, Morton JB, Santucci PA, Akar JG, Green A, Wilber DJ. Idiopathic epicardial left ventricular tachycardia originating remote from the sinus of valsalva electrophysiological characteristics, catheter ablation, and identification from the 12-lead electrocardiogram. Circulation. 2006;113:1659-66.
3. Sosa E, Scanavacca M, d'Avila A, Pilleggi F. A new technique to perform epicardial mapping in the electrophysiology laboratory. J Cardiovasc Electrophysiol. 1996;7:531-6.
4. Boyle NG, Shivkumar K. Epicardial interventions in electrophysiology. Circulation. 2012;126:1752-69.
5. Cano O, Hutchinson M, Lin D, Garcia F, Zado E, Bala R, Riley M, Cooper J, Dixit S, Gerstenfeld E. Electroanatomic substrate and ablation outcome for suspected epicardial ventricular tachycardia in left ventricular nonischemic cardiomyopathy. J Am Coll Cardiol. 2009;54:799-808.
6. Garcia FC, Bazan V, Zado ES, Ren J-F, Marchlinski FE. Epicardial substrate and outcome with epicardial ablation of ventricular tachycardia in arrhythmogenic right ventricular cardiomyopathy/dysplasia. Circulation. 2009;120:366-75.
7. Santangeli P, Di Biase L, Lakkireddy D, Burkhardt JD, Pillarisetti J, Michowitz Y, Sanchez JE, Horton R, Mohanty P, Gallinghouse GJ. Radiofrequency catheter ablation of ventricular arrhythmias in patients with hypertrophic cardiomyopathy: safety and feasibility. Heart Rhythm. 2010;7:1036-42.
8. Sosa E, Scanavacca M, D'Avila A, Bellotti G, Pilleggi F. Radiofrequency catheter ablation of ventricular tachycardia guided by nonsurgical epicardial mapping in chronic Chagasic heart disease. Pacing Clin Electrophysiol. 1999;22:128-30.
9. Sacher F, Roberts-Thomson K, Maury P, Tedrow U, Nault I, Steven D, Hocini M, Koplan B, Leroux L, Derval N. Epicardial ventricular tachycardia ablation: a multicenter safety study. J Am Coll Cardiol. 2010;55:2366-72.
10. Assomull RG, Prasad SK, Lyne J, Smith G, Burman ED, Khan M, Sheppard MN, Poole-Wilson PA, Pennell DJ. Cardiovascular magnetic resonance, fibrosis, and prognosis in dilated cardiomyopathy. J Am Coll Cardiol. 2006;48:1977-85.
11. Berruezo A, Mont L, Nava S, Chueca E, Bartholomay E, Brugada J. Electrocardiographic recognition of the epicardial origin of ventricular tachycardias. Circulation. 2004;109:1842-7.
12. Martinek M, Stevenson WG, Inada K, Tokuda M, Tedrow UB. QRS characteristics fail to reliably identify ventricular tachycardias that require epicardial ablation in ischemic heart disease. J Cardiovasc Electrophysiol. 2012;23:188-93.
13. Haissaguerre M, Jais P, Shah DC, Takahashi A, Hocini M, Quiniou G, Garrigue S, Le Mouroux A, Le Metayer P, Clementy J. Spontaneous initiation of atrial fibrillation by ectopic beats originating in the pulmonary veins. N Engl J Med. 1998;339:659-66.
14. Perez-Castellano N, Villacastin J, Salinas J, Vega M, Moreno J, Doblado M, Ruiz E, Macaya C. Epicardial connections between the pulmonary veins and left atrium: relevance for atrial fibrillation ablation. J Cardiovasc Electrophysiol. 2011;22:149-59.
15. Po SS, Nakagawa H, Jackman WM. Localization of left atrial ganglionated plexi in patients with atrial fibrillation. J Cardiovasc Electrophysiol. 2009;20:1186-9.
16. Nakahara S, Ramirez RJ, Buch E, Michowitz Y, Vaseghi M, De Diego C, Boyle NG, Mahajan A, Shivkumar K. Intrapericardial balloon placement for prevention of collateral injury during catheter ablation of the left atrium in a porcine model. Heart Rhythm. 2010;7:81-7.
17. Buch E, Vaseghi M, Cesario DA, Shivkumar K. A novel method for preventing phrenic nerve injury during catheter ablation. Heart Rhythm. 2007;4:95-8.
18. Valderrábano M, Cesario DA, Ji S, Shannon K, Wiener I, Swerdlow CD, Oral H, Morady F, Shivkumar K. Percutaneous epicardial mapping during ablation of difficult accessory pathways as an alternative to cardiac surgery. Heart Rhythm. 2004;1:311-6.
19. Lee JC, Steven D, Roberts-Thomson KC, Raymond J-M, Stevenson WG, Tedrow UB. Atrial tachycardias adjacent to the phrenic nerve: recognition, potential problems, and solutions. Heart Rhythm. 2009;6:1186-91.
20. Al-Saady NM, Obel OA, Camm AJ. Left atrial appendage: structure, function, and role in thromboembolism. Heart. 1999;82:547-54.
21. Singh SM, Dukkipati SR, d'Avila A, Doshi SK, Reddy VY. Percutaneous left atrial appendage closure with an epicardial suture ligation approach: a prospective randomized preclinical feasibility study. Heart Rhythm. 2010;7:370-6.
22. Ernst S, Sanchez-Quintana D, Ho SY. Anatomy of the pericardial space and mediastinum: relevance to epicardial mapping and ablation. Card Electrophysiol Clin. 2010;2:1-8.
23. Della Bella P, Brugada J, Zeppenfeld K, Merino J, Neuzil P, Maury P, Maccabelli G, Vergara P, Baratto F, Berruezo A, Wijnmaalen AP. Epicardial ablation for ventricular tachycardia: An European multicenter study. Circ Arrhythm Electrophysiol. 2011;4:653-9.
24. Tung R, Michowitz Y, Yu R, Mathuria N, Vaseghi M, Buch E, Bradfield J, Fujimura O, Gima J, Discepolo W. Epicardial ablation of ventricular tachycardia: an institutional experience of safety and efficacy. Heart Rhythm. 2013;10:490-8.
25. Huang SKS, Wood MA. Catheter Ablation of Cardiac Arrhythmias: Expert Consult-Online: Elsevier Health Sciences; 2014.
26. Al-ahmad A, Callans DJ, Hsia HH, Natale A. Hands-On Ablation: The Experts' Approach: Cardiotext Publishing; 2013.
27. Sun F, Sánchez FM, Crisóstomo V, Luis L, Usón J, Maynar M. Subxiphoid access to normal pericardium with micropuncture set: technical feasibility study in pigs 1. Radiology. 2006;238:719-24.
28. Rasekh A, Kar S, Nagaraj H, Badhwar N, Massumi A, Lakkireddy D. Differences in experience with a new delivery device for LAA ligation among various US centers. J Am Coll Cardiol. 2015;65:404-5.
29. Baudoin Y-P, Hoch M, Protin X-M, Otton B-J, Ginon B, Voiglio E-J. The superior epigastric artery does not pass through Larrey's space (trigonum sternocostale). Surg Radiol Anat. 2003;25:259-62.
30. d'Avila A, Houghtaling C, Gutierrez P, Vragovic O, Ruskin JN, Josephson ME, Reddy VY. Catheter ablation of ventricular

epicardial tissue A comparison of standard and cooled-tip radiofrequency energy. Circulation. 2004;109:2363-9.

31. Koruth JS, d'Avila A. Management of hemopericardium related to percutaneous epicardial access, mapping, and ablation. Heart Rhythm. 2011;8:1652-7.

32. Thyer IA, Kovoor P, Barry MA, Pouliopoulos J, Ross DL, Thiagalingam A. Protection of the coronary arteries during epicardial radiofrequency ablation with intracoronary chilled saline irrigation: assessment in an in vitro model. J Cardiovasc Electrophysiol. 2006;17:544-9.

EDITORS' SUMMARY

Professor Shivkumar and colleagues have provided for this textbook an outstanding, thoroughly illustrated, and practical chapter on epicardial ablation. A highlight of this submission is a step-by-step approach for epicardial puncture and the all-important preprocedural planning to minimize complications and maximize success for what can be difficult ablation procedures. The extensive experience and pioneering ideas from this group are evident in how they simplify for the beginner the planning and execution of epicardial ablation. The reader would do well to thoroughly study this chapter and then refer to Table 47.2 as well as the paragraphs on "Epicardial Access and Ablation: Step-by-Step" whenever they are called to perform dry epicardial access for either ablation or appendage ligation.

Index

Page numbers followed by *f* refer to figure and *t* refer to table.

A

B

C

D

E

F

M

N

O

P

Q

R

U

V

W